Intervention and Reflection
BASIC ISSUES IN MEDICAL ETHICS
Fourth Edition

Ronald Munson
University of Missouri–St. Louis

Wadsworth Publishing Company, Belmont, California
A division of Wadsworth, Inc.

Philosophy Editor: Kenneth King
Editorial Assistant: Cynthia Campbell
Production: Cece Munson, The Cooper Company
Interior Designers: Katie Michels and John Edeen
Copy Editor: Micky Lawler
Cover Designer: Harry Voigt
Signing Representative: George Weiss
Print Buyer: Martha Branch
Compositor: Omegatype Typography

*This book is printed on acid-free paper that meets
Environmental Protection Agency standards
for recycled paper.*

1 2 3 4 5 6 7 8 9 10—96 95 94 93 92

Library of Congress Cataloging-in-Publication Data

Intervention and reflection : basic issues in medical ethics :
  [readings / selected by] Ronald Munson. — 4th ed.
     p.   cm.
  Includes bibliographical references and index.
  ISBN 0-534-16326-2
  1. Medical ethics. I. Munson, Ronald, 1939– .
  [DNLM: 1. Ethics, Medical—collected works. 2. Ethics, Medical—
problems. W 50 I618]
R724.I57   1991
174′.2—dc20
DNLM/DLC
for Library of Congress   91–10161
                                    CIP

To Miriam
"Giver of bright rings"

Ronald Munson is Professor of the Philosophy of Science and Medicine at the University of Missouri–St. Louis. He received his Ph.D. from Columbia University and was a Postdoctoral Fellow in Biology at Harvard University. He has been a Visiting Professor at the University of California, San Diego, and the Harvard Medical School.

His books include *Reasoning in Medicine* (with Daniel Albert and Michael Resnik), *The Way of Words*, and *The Elements of Reasoning* (with David Conway). He is also the author of the novel *Nothing Human*.

CONTENTS

PREFACE

In shaping the fourth edition of this book, I have tried to capture both the intellectual excitement and the great seriousness that surround the field of medical ethics. In particular, I've done my best to convey these aspects to students new to the field.

In the introductory materials and choice of topics, and by other means, I have attempted to familiarize readers with the issues and make them active participants in the enterprise. Whether someone is an undergraduate or graduate student, a nursing or medical student, with or without training in ethics, I think she or he will find this a useful and engaging book.

The Topics and Readings

The topics presented here are all fundamental ones in medical ethics. They reflect the range and variety of the problems we now confront and involve the basic moral and social issues that have excited the most concern. But more than this, the problems are morally serious ones that lead people to turn hopefully to philosophical consideration in search of satisfactory resolutions.

The reading selections present current thinking about the topics and show that such consideration can be worthwhile. All are readable and nontechnical, and several reveal medical ethics at its very best. Although philosophers are strongly represented in the readings, the authors also include jurists, scientists, social critics, and practicing physicians. The moral problems of medicine always have scientific, social, legal, and economic aspects; to deal with them sensibly, we need the knowledge and perceptions of people from a variety of disciplines.

I have also opted for diversity in another way: by trying to see to it that opposing viewpoints are given for major topics. Part of the intellectual excitement of medical ethics is generated by the searing controversies surrounding its issues, and to ignore these conflicts would be misleading. Even worse, it would deny students the opportunity of dealing directly with proposals and arguments incompatible with their own views.

The Introduction: Ethical Theories and Moral Principles

For some readers, the most important feature of the book may be the two-part general introduction. In the first part, I briefly sketch the basics of five major ethical theories and indicate how they might be used to answer particular moral questions in medicine. The main purpose is to give students without a background in ethics the information they need to understand and evaluate the arguments in the readings. In the second part, with this same end in view, I present and illustrate several major moral principles. The principles are ones endorsed by virtually all ethical theories, even though I don't try to demonstrate how the principles follow from particular theories.

The two parts of the general introduction complement each other, but they are self-contained and may be read separately. The aim of each (and of both) is to help prepare students for independent inquiry in medical ethics.

Case Presentations, Social Contexts, Chapter Introductions, and Decision Scenarios

Each chapter after the general introduction is like a sandwich with several layers. At the beginning are the Case Presentations and Social Contexts. Then comes the chapter Introduction, followed by the reading selections. At the end are the Decision Scenarios. A brief explanation of the components will give a sense of how they work together.

In the chapter Introductions, I discuss moral problems that occur in actual medical practice and research and present whatever factual information is needed to understand how they arise. I also suggest ways the five moral theories might be used to resolve some of the problems. These suggestions are offered only as starting points in the search for a satisfactory answer.

The Case Presentations are based upon (or closely parallel) actual events or situations. They are intended to provide a focus for discussion and to illustrate how genuine moral problems arise in ordinary life. Some of the cases (like Nancy Cruzan's) are well known, whereas others are obscure. I think they may also serve to remind us that, in dealing with medical ethics, we are not engaged in some purely intellectual abstract game.

The Social Contexts provide information relevant to understanding the current social, political, or biomedical situation in which issues are being debated. (They differ from Case Presentations in offering a broader view of a problem.) In my opinion, if we hope to raise the level of public discussion of an issue and genuinely inform the life of our society, it is essential to consider the social facts as well as the scientific and medical ones.

Several Decision Scenarios appear at the end of each chapter. These are brief, dramatic presentations of situations in which moral questions are crucial—in which ethical or social-policy decisions have to be made. The scenarios are followed by questions asking the reader to decide what the problems are and how they might be dealt with by a particular moral theory or by principles argued for in the readings. Thus, the Decision Scenarios are really exercises in medical ethics that can direct and structure class discussion.

After the final chapter, the Notes and References section lists sources for materials used in the Decision Scenarios, as well as in Cases, Contexts, and Introductions.

Finally, I have included at the end of the book a quite extensive bibliography arranged to correspond to the chapter divisions. Hence, anyone wanting to do further reading on a topic should have no trouble locating appropriate works.

Compensating for Limitations

An inherent limitation of a book of this sort is the impossibility of including selections dealing with all major issues in an area. I have tried to compensate for this by raising and discussing in the chapter Introductions more issues than are dealt with in the selections. I hope this will give readers a better sense of the scope and variety of issues in a complex area, even if little can be done to address them in a thorough way.

I also have tried to provide enough relevant medical, scientific, and social information to make it possible for both students and instructors to go beyond the scope of the text. No one need feel confined to the selections or to the problems specifically identified, and readers will be able to raise many serious issues that are not explicitly mentioned.

One way to touch on a larger number of issues is by using short excerpts for readings. With few exceptions, however, I chose to include entire articles, sections, or chapters. An excerpt summarizing a main argument may fairly represent a position, but the reader is deprived of participating in much of the dialectical process that is so crucial to arriving at a philosophically defensible conclusion.

The Current Edition

As times change, moral problems also change. The most notable addition to this edition is an entire chapter devoted to issues raised by AIDS. Since we are living in the midst of a major epidemic, the problems it presents demand our immediate attention.

Two other striking changes are also represented in this new edition. Recent Supreme Court decisions have altered the character and concerns of discussions about both abortion and euthanasia. Two new Social Context sections chart some of these changes, and selections from the Court's decisions in the *Webster* and *Cruzan* cases are included to represent the lines of argument that are themselves still hotly debated.

Other current issues with sharp moral edges have also been given a place in this revision. A few must stand for the rest: Should RU 486 ("the abortion pill") be allowed on the market? Does a pregnant woman have a duty to protect her fetus from damage caused by taking drugs? Should a Christian Scientist be required to act against his beliefs to provide his child with needed medical treatment? Is "gestational surrogacy" morally acceptable? Most important, is this country prepared to accept a comprehensive health-care plan to provide help to the more than 30 million Americans lacking insurance?

Chapter Introductions have been revised in dozens of ways to take into account changes in policies, statistics, and relevant scientific or medical information. Furthermore, a number of Cases, Contexts, and Decision Scenarios have been added or revised to bring them up to date. Finally, a large number of new items have been added to the Bibliography.

Teaching Possibilities

I've used this book to teach medical ethics, and I've also had many discussions and some correspondence with others who have chosen it as a text. Perhaps it would be appropriate to close my comments on this book by offering a few suggestions about its use in class.

Topic Organization

There is a logic in the organization of the book. Roughly, the first topics presented (abortion, euthanasia, etc.) involve individual moral decisions, while the later topics (genetic screening, distribution of resources, etc.) require decisions about social goals and policies. But of course virtually all the issues in medical ethics overlap and intertwine. (Abortion is a good example of this.)

For this reason, it seemed to me sensible to arrange the topics and write the introductions in a way that would make each chapter more or less independent of the others. Thus, the structure of the book does not have to be followed in teaching.

Particular moral problems, social-policy issues, or legal issues might all be used as organizing principle. For example, someone wanting to teach a policy-oriented course might start with the last two chapters (on health-care policies) and then go on to discuss regulating reproductive technology, protecting privacy in AIDS testing, and dealing with demands for euthanasia. It is possible to organize a course in this way without being faced with text or selections that presuppose familiarity with preceding chapters. Indeed, the chapters may be read in any order.

Chapter Organization

In each chapter, I've placed the Case Presentations before the Introduction, because I believe cases provide students with concrete examples that let them appreciate how particular moral issues arise. However, anyone who believes it is better to discuss cases after ethical issues and principles have been presented may want to ask students to read a Case Presentation after the introductory text or the philosophical materials.

The cases are written to stand alone, even when they are explicitly discussed in the selections. For example, it makes as much pedagogical sense to assign the Karen Quinlan Case Presentation after reading the Supreme Court decision as to reverse that order.

Social Contexts also appear before Introductions, and much of what I've said about Case Presentations also applies to them. Some may wish their students to have some basic information about the social and political aspects of an issue like organ transplants before dealing with philosophical claims about just distribution.

However, others may choose to focus exclusively on the philosophical issues and ignore the public aspects of the debate, on the grounds that students should make their own connections. The text is compatible with either approach.

I have provided more Cases and Contexts than some instructors may want to assign. This gives them the flexibility to decide which issues they want to emphasize within a particular chapter.

Using the Decision Scenarios

The Decision Scenarios naturally lend themselves to being considered after the reading selections, because then students can be expected to answer many of the questions. However, another strategy with something to recommend it is to ask students to read the scenarios before the selections. The cases and the questions about them can then serve as guides in reading—as flags marking notable issues.

Also, although time rarely permits it, if the scenarios are sometimes discussed both before and after the selections are read, students are given a chance to see the ways in which their own views change. They are also often in a better position to defend their initial views with relevant arguments.

Finally, the Decision Scenarios offer a rich source for written assignments. One or more questions can be selected and assigned, or an instructor may refer to the scenario but provide a new question.

I have tried to be helpful without being too intrusive. Anyone who teaches medical ethics wants enough flexibility to arrange a course in the way she or he sees fit. I have tried to offer that flexibility while at the same time supplying students with the kind of information and support they need.

This book, with its introductory materials and other appurtenances, is more ambitious than any similar work currently available. I've been pleased by responses from my colleagues to the earlier editions. Even their criticisms were tempered by a sympathetic understanding of the difficulty of producing a book of this scope that attempts to do so many things.

Thanks to the help of many people who took the trouble to write to me, I was able to correct errors in this edition that I missed in the last. (Will I *ever* get Kant right?) I am under no illusion that the book has achieved perfection, and I would still appreciate comments or suggestions from users on ways it can be improved.

I owe so many intellectual debts I must declare bankruptcy, and this means that those who invested their help in this project have to settle for an acknowledgment that is less than they are rightly owed. My greatest debt on behalf of this book is to those authors who allowed their work to be reprinted here. I hope they will find no grounds for objecting to the way I have dealt with them. I thank Michael Bayles, David B. Resnik, John T. Wilcox, and Lawrence Davis for criticism and advice.

I am also grateful to the following reviewers for their criticisms and recommendations:

John C. Modschiedler
College of DuPage

John Paris
Boston College

Harry Van der Linden
Butler University

Jane Sessions
University of California–Santa Barbara

William Werpehowski
Villanova University

Russell Wells
San Francisco State University

Ann Stankiewicz
Providence College

Michael Gillette
Randolph–Macon Woman's
 College

Donald Burt
Villanova University

Kenneth King, Wadsworth's philosophy editor, has shown a steady faith in this book from its conception. His interest in it has never flagged, and his help has been genuine. I particularly appreciate his willingness to stand aside and let the work get done without expecting a running account of progress.

Miriam Grove Munson has often pulled me from the slough of Despond, but I am likewise indebted to her sense of style and relevance and to her sharp critical judgment. Rebecca Grove Munson constantly reminded me in a forceful fashion that there is more to life than the making of books.

I have not always listened to those who have taken the trouble to warn and advise me, and this is reason enough for me to claim the errors here as my own.

Ronald Munson
University of Missouri–St. Louis, 1991

MORAL PRINCIPLES, ETHICAL THEORIES, AND MEDICAL DECISIONS: AN INTRODUCTION

"He's stopped breathing, Doctor," the nurse said. She sounded calm and not at all hysterical. By the time Dr. Sarah Cunningham had reached Mr. Sabatini's bedside, the nurse was already providing mouth-to-mouth resuscitation. But Mr. Sabatini still had the purplish-blue color of cyanosis, caused by a lack of oxygen in his blood.

Dr. Cunningham knew that, if he was to survive, Mr. Sabatini would have to be given oxygen fast and placed on a respirator. But should she order this done?

Mr. Sabatini was an old man, almost ninety. So far as anyone knew, he was alone in the world and would hardly be missed when he died. His health was poor. He had congestive heart disease and was dying slowly and painfully from intestinal cancer.

Wouldn't it be a kindness to Mr. Sabatini to allow him this quick and painless death? Why condemn him to lingering on for a few extra hours or weeks?

The decision that Sarah Cunningham faces is a moral one. She has to decide whether she should take the steps that might prolong Mr. Sabatini's life or not take them and accept the consequence that he will almost surely die within minutes. She knows the medical procedures that can be employed, but she has to decide whether she should employ them.

This kind of case rivets our attention because of its immediacy and drama. But there are many other situations that arise in the context of medical practice and research that present problems requiring moral decisions. Some are equal in drama to the problem facing Dr. Cunningham; others are not so dramatic but are of at least equal seriousness. There are far too many to catalogue, but consider this sample: Is it right for a woman to have an abortion for any reason? Should children with serious birth defects be put to death? Do people have a right to die? Does everyone have a right to medical care? Should physicians ever lie to their patients? Should people suffering from a genetic disease be allowed to have children? Can parents agree to allow their children to be used as experimental subjects?

Most of us have little tolerance for questions like these. They seem so cold and abstract. Our attitude changes, however, when we find ourselves in a position in which *we* are the decision makers. It changes, too, when we are in a position in which we must advise those who make the decisions. Or when we are on the receiving end of the decision.

But whether we view the problems abstractly or concretely, we are inclined to ask the same question: Are there any rules, standards, or principles that we can use as guides when we are faced with moral decisions? If there are, then Dr. Cunningham need not be wholly unprepared to decide whether she should order steps taken to save Mr. Sabatini. Nor need we be unprepared to decide issues like those in the questions above.

The branch of philosophy concerned with principles that allow us to make decisions about what is right and wrong is called *ethics* or *moral philosophy*. *Medical ethics* is specifically concerned with moral principles and decisions in the context of medical practice, policy, and research. Moral difficulties connected with medicine are so complex and important that they require special attention. Medical ethics gives them this attention, but it remains a part of the discipline of ethics. Thus, if we are to answer our question as to whether there are any rules or principles to use when making moral decisions in the medical context, we must turn to general ethical theories and to a consideration of moral principles that have been proposed to hold in all contexts of human action.

In the first major part of this chapter, we will discuss five major ethical theories that have been put forward by philosophers. Each of these theories represents an attempt to supply basic principles that we can rely on in making moral decisions. We'll consider these theories and examine how they might be applied to moral issues in the medical context. We will discuss the reasons that have been offered to persuade us to accept each theory, but we will also point out some of the difficulties that each theory presents.

In the second major part of the chapter, we will examine and illustrate several moral principles that are of special relevance to medical research and practice. These principles are frequently appealed to in discussions of practical ethical problems and are sufficiently uncontroversial as to be endorsed in a general way by any of the ethical theories mentioned in the first section.

The two sections are not dependent on each other, and it is possible to profit from either without reading the other. (The price for this independence is a small amount of repetition.) Nevertheless, reading both is recommended. The discussions and arguments presented in the selections that make up the majority of this book can most easily be followed by someone who has at least some familiarity with basic moral theories. At the same time, some points in discussions turn upon questions about the applicability of certain familiar moral principles. Being acquainted with those principles makes it easier to understand and evaluate such discussions.

PART I. BASIC ETHICAL THEORIES

Ethical theories attempt to articulate and justify principles that can be employed as guides for making moral decisions and as standards for the evaluation of actions and policies. In effect, such theories define what it means to act morally, and in doing so they stipulate in a general fashion the duties or obligations that fall upon us.

Ethical theories also offer a means to explain and justify actions. If our actions are guided by a particular theory, then we can explain them by demonstrating that the principles of the theory required us to act as we did. In such cases, the explanation also constitutes a justification. We justify our actions by showing that, according to the theory, we had an obligation to do what we did. (In some cases, we may justify our actions by showing that the theory *permitted* our actions—that is, didn't require them but didn't rule them out as wrong.)

Advocates of a particular ethical theory present what they consider to be good reasons and relevant evidence in its support. Their general aim is to show that the theory is one that any reasonable individual would find persuasive or would endorse as correct. Accordingly, appeals to religion, faith, or nonnatural factors are not considered to be either necessary or legitimate to justify the theory. Rational persuasion alone is regarded as the basis of justification.

In this section, we will briefly consider four general ethical theories and one theory of justice that has an essential ethical component. In each case, we will begin by examining the basic principles of the theory and the grounds offered for its acceptance. We will then explore some of the possibilities of applying the theory to problems that arise within the medical context. Finally, we will mention some of the practical consequences and conceptual difficulties that raise questions about the theory's adequacy or correctness.

UTILITARIANISM

The ethical theory known as utilitarianism was given its most influential formulation in the nineteenth century by the British philosophers Jeremy Bentham (1748–1832) and John Stuart Mill (1806–1873). Bentham and Mill did not produce identical theories, but both their versions have come to be spoken of as "classical utilitarianism." Subsequent elaborations and qualifications of utilitarianism are inevitably based on the formulations of Bentham and Mill, so their theories are worth careful examination.

The Principle of Utility

The foundation of utilitarianism is a single, apparently simple principle. Mill calls it the "principle of utility" and states it this way: *Actions are right in proportion as they tend to promote happiness, wrong as they tend to produce the reverse of happiness.*

The principle focuses attention on the *consequences* of actions, rather than on some feature of the actions themselves. The "utility" or "usefulness" of an action is determined by the extent to which it produces happiness. Thus, no action is *in itself* right or wrong. Nor is an action right or wrong by virtue of the actor's hopes, intentions, or past actions. Consequences alone are important. Breaking a promise, lying, causing pain, or even killing a person may, under certain circumstances, be the right action to take. Under other circumstances, the action might be wrong.

We need not think of the principle as applying to just one action that we are considering. It supplies the basis for a kind of cost-benefit analysis to employ in a situation in which several lines of action are possible. Using the principle, we are supposed to consider the possible results of each of the actions. Then we are to choose the one that produces the most benefit (happiness) at the least cost (unhappiness). The action we take may produce some unhappiness, but it is a balance of happiness over unhappiness that the principle tells us to seek.

Suppose, for example, that a woman in a large hospital is near death: she is in a coma, an EEG shows only minimal brain function, and a respirator is required to keep her breathing. Another patient has just been brought to the hospital from the scene of an automobile accident. His kidneys have been severely damaged, and he is in need of an immediate transplant. There is a good tissue match with the woman's kidneys. Is it right to hasten her death by removing a kidney?

The principle of utility would probably consider the removal justified. The woman is virtually dead, while the man has a good chance of surviving. It is true that the woman's life is threatened even more by the surgery. It may, in fact, kill her. But, on balance, the kidney transplant seems likely to produce more happiness than unhappiness. In fact, it seems better than the alternative of doing nothing. For in that case both patients are likely to die.

The principle of utility is also called the "greatest happiness principle" by Bentham and Mill. The reason for this name is clear when the principle is stated in this way: *Those actions are right that produce the greatest happiness for the greatest number of people.* This alternative formulation makes it obvious that in deciding how to act it is not just my happiness or the happiness of a particular person or group that must be considered. According to utilitarianism, every person is to count just as much as any other person. That is, when we are considering how we should act, everyone's interest must be considered. The right action, then, will be the one that produces the most happiness for the largest number of people.

Mill is particularly anxious that utilitarianism not be construed as no more than a sophisticated justification for crude self-interest. He stresses that in making a moral decision we must look at the situation in an objective way. We must, he says, be a "benevolent spectator" and then act in a way that will bring about the best results for all concerned. This view is summarized in a famous passage:

> The happiness which forms the utilitarian standard of what is right in conduct, is not the agent's own happiness, but that of all concerned. As between his own happiness and that of others, utilitarianism requires him to be as strictly impartial as a disinterested and benevolent spectator. In the golden rule of Jesus of Nazareth, we read the complete spirit of the ethics of utility. To do as you would be done by, and to love your neighbor as yourself, constitute the ideal perfection of utilitarian morality.

The key concept in both formulations of the principle of utility is "happiness." Bentham simply identifies happiness with pleasure—pleasure of any kind. The aim of ethics, then, is to increase the amount of pleasure in the world to the greatest possible extent. To facilitate this, Bentham recommends the use of a "calculus of pleasure and pain," in which characteristics of pleasure such as intensity, duration, and number of people affected are measured and assigned numerical values. To determine which of several possible actions is the right one, we need only determine which one receives the highest numerical score. Unfortunately, Bentham does not tell us what units to use or how to make the measurements.

Mill also identifies happiness with pleasure, but he differs from Bentham in a major respect. Unlike Bentham, he insists that some pleasures are "higher" than others. Thus, pleasures of the intellect are superior to, say, purely sensual pleasures. This difference in the concept of pleasure can become significant in a medical context. For example, in the choice of using limited resources to save the life of a lathe operator or of an art historian, Mill's view might assign more value to the life of the art historian. That person, Mill might say, is capable of "higher pleasures" than the lathe operator. (Of course other factors would be relevant here for Mill.)

Both Mill and Bentham regard happiness as an intrinsic good. That is, it is something good in itself or for its own sake. Actions, by contrast, are good only to the extent to which they tend to promote happiness. Therefore, they are only instrumentally good. Since utilitarianism determines the rightness of actions in terms of their tendency to promote the greatest happiness for the greatest number, it is considered to be a *teleological* ethical theory. ("Teleological" comes from the Greek word "telos," which means "end" or "goal.") A teleological ethical theory judges the rightness of an action in terms of an external goal or purpose —"general happiness" or utility for utilitarianism. However, utilitarianism is also a *consequentialist* theory, for the outcomes or consequences of actions are the only considerations relevant to determining their moral rightness. Not all teleological theories are consequentialist.

Some more recent formulations of utilitarianism have rejected the notion that happiness, no matter how defined, is the sole intrinsic good that actions or policies must promote. Critics of the classical view have argued that the list of things we recognize as valuable in themselves should be increased to include ones such as knowledge, beauty, love, friendship, liberty, and health. According to this *pluralistic* view, in applying the principle of utility we must consider the entire range of intrinsic goods that an action is likely to promote. Thus, the right action is the one that can be expected to produce the greatest sum of intrinsic goods. In most of the following discussion, we will speak of the greatest happiness or benefit, but it is easy enough to see how the same points can be made from a pluralistic perspective.

Act and Rule Utilitarianism

All utilitarians accept the principle of utility as the standard for determining the rightness of actions. But they divide into two groups over the matter of the application of the principle.

Act utilitarianism holds that the principle should be applied to particular acts in particular circumstances. *Rule utilitarianism* maintains that the principle should be used to test rules, which can in turn be used to decide the rightness of particular acts. Let's consider each of these views and see how it works in practice.

Act utilitarianism holds that an act is right if, and only if, no other act could have been performed that would produce a higher utility. Suppose that a child is born with severe impairments. The child has an open spine, severe brain damage, and dysfunctional kidneys. What should be done? (We will leave open the question of who should decide.)

The act utilitarian holds that we must attempt to determine the consequences of the various actions that are open to us. We should consider, for example, these possibilities: (1) give the child only the ordinary treatment that would be given to a normal child, (2) give the child special treatment for its problems, (3) give the child no treatment—allow it to die, (4) put the child to death in a painless way.

According to act utilitarianism, we must explore the potential results of each of these possibilities. We must realize, for example, that when such a child is given only ordinary treatment it will be worse off, if it survives, than if it had been given special treatment. Also, a child left alone and allowed to die is also likely to suffer more pain than one killed by a lethal injection. Furthermore, a child treated aggressively will have to undergo numerous surgical procedures of limited effectiveness. We must also consider the family of the child and judge the emotional and financial effects that each of the possible actions will have on them. Then, too, we must take into account such matters as the ''quality of life'' of a child with severe brain damage and multiple defects, the effect on physicians and nurses in killing the child or allowing it to die, and the financial costs to society in providing long-term care.

After these considerations, we should then choose the action that has the greatest utility. We should act in the way that will produce the most benefit for all concerned. Which of the possibilities we select will depend on the precise features of the situation: how impaired the child is, how good its chances are for living an acceptable life, the character and financial status of the family, and so on. The great strength of act utilitarianism is that it invites us to deal with each case as unique. When the circumstances of another case are different, we might, without being inconsistent, choose another of the possible actions.

Act utilitarianism shows a sensitivity to specific cases, but it is not free from difficulties. Some philosophers have pointed out that there is no way we can be certain that we have made the right choice of actions. We are sure to be ignorant of much relevant information. Besides, we can't know with much certainty what the results of our actions will really be. There is no way to be sure, for example, that even a severely impaired infant will not recover enough to live a better life than we predict.

The act utilitarian can reply that acting morally doesn't mean being omniscient. We need to make a reasonable effort to get relevant information, and we can usually predict the probable consequences of our actions. Acting morally doesn't require any more than this.

Another objection to act utilitarianism is more serious. According to the doctrine, we are obligated to keep a promise only if keeping it will produce more utility than some other action. If some other action will produce the same utility, then keeping the promise is permissible but not obligatory. Suppose that a surgeon promises a patient that only he will perform an operation, then allows a well-qualified resident to perform part of it. Suppose that all goes well and the patient never discovers that the promise was not kept. The outcome for the patient is exactly the same as if the surgeon had kept the promise. From the point of view of act utilitarianism, there is nothing wrong with the surgeon's failure to keep it. Yet critics charge that there is something wrong—that in making the promise the surgeon took on an obligation. Act utilitarianism is unable to account for obligations engendered by such actions as promising and pledging, critics say, for such actions involve something other than consequences.

A third objection to act utilitarianism arises in situations in which virtually everyone must follow the same rules in order to achieve a high level of utility, but even greater utility can be achieved if a few people do not follow the rules. Consider the relationship between physicians and the Medicaid program. The program pays physicians for services provided to those poor enough to qualify for the program. The program would collapse if nearly all physicians were not honest in billing Medicaid for their services. Not only would many poor people suffer, but physicians themselves would lose a source of income.

Suppose that a particular physician believes that the requirements to qualify for Medicaid are too restrictive and that many who urgently need medical care cannot afford it. As an act utilitarian, he reasons that it is right for him to get money to open a free clinic under the program. He intends to bill for services he does not provide, then use that money to treat those not covered by Medicaid. His claims will be small compared to the entire Medicaid budget, so it is unlikely that anyone who qualifies for Medicaid will go without treatment. Since he will tell no one what he is doing, others are not likely to be influenced by his example and make false claims for similar or less worthy purposes. The money he is paid will bring substantial benefit to those in need of health care. Thus, he concludes, by violating the rules of the program, his actions will produce greater utility than would be produced by following the rules.

The physician's action would be morally right, according to act utilitarianism. Yet, critics say, we expect an action that is morally right to be one that is right for everyone in similar circumstances. If every physician in the Medicaid program acted in this way, however, the program would be destroyed and thus pro-duce no utility at all. Furthermore, according to critics, the physician's action produces unfairness. While it is true that the patients he treats at his free clinic gain a benefit they would not otherwise have, similar patients must go without treatment. The Medicaid policy, whatever its flaws, is at least prima facie fair in providing benefits to all who meet its requirements. Once again, then, according to critics, more seems to be involved in judging the moral worth of an action than can be accounted for by act utilitarianism.

In connection with such objections, some critics have gone so far as to claim that it is impossible to see how a society in which everyone were an act utilitarian could function. We could not count on promises being kept nor take for granted that people were telling us the truth. Social policies would be no more than general guides to action, and we could never be sure that people would regard themselves as obligated to adhere to their provisions. Decisions made by individuals about each individual action would not obviously lead to the promotion of the highest degree of utility. Indeed, some critics say, such a society might collapse, for communication among individuals would be difficult (if not impossible), social cohesion would be weakened, and general policies and regulations would have very uncertain effects.

The critics are not necessarily right, of course, and defenders of act utilitarianism have made substantial efforts to answer the criticisms we have presented. Some have denied that the theory has those implications and have argued that some of our generally accepted moral perceptions should be changed. In connection with this last point, Carl Wellman provides an insight into the sort of conflict between moral feelings and rational judgment that the acceptance of act utilitarianism can produce. Concerning euthanasia, Wellman writes:

> Try as I may, I honestly cannot discover
> great hidden disutilities in the act of

killing an elderly person suffering greatly from an incurable illness, provided that certain safeguards like a written medical opinion by at least two doctors and a request by the patient are preserved. In this case I cannot find any way to reconcile my theory with my moral judgment. What I do in this case is to hold fast to act-utilitarianism and distrust my moral sense. I claim that my condemnation of such acts is an irrational disapproval, a condemnation that will change upon further reasoning about the act. . . . That I feel wrongness is clear, but I cannot state to myself any rational justification for my feeling. Hence, I discount this particular judgment as irrational.

Rule utilitarianism maintains that an action is right if it conforms to a rule of conduct that has been validated by the principle of utility as one that will produce at least as much utility as any other rule applicable to the situation. A rule like "Provide only ordinary care for severely brain-damaged newborns with multiple impairments," if it were established, would allow us to decide about the course of action to follow in situations like that of our earlier example.

The rule utilitarian is concerned with assessing the utility not of individual actions, but of particular rules. In practice, then, we do not have to go through the calculations involved in determining in each case whether a specific action will increase utility. All that we have to establish is that following a certain rule will, in general, result in a situation in which utility is maximized. Once rules are established, they can be relied on to determine whether a particular action is right.

The basic idea behind rule utilitarianism is that having a set of rules that are always observed produces the greatest social utility. Having everyone follow the same rule in each case of the same kind yields more utility for everybody in the long run. An act utilitarian can agree that having rules may produce more social utility than not having them. But the act utilitarian insists that the rules be regarded as no more than general guides to action, as "rules of thumb." Thus, for act utilitarianism it is perfectly legitimate to violate a rule if doing so will maximize utility in that instance. By contrast, the rule utilitarian holds that rules must generally be followed, even though following them may produce less net utility (more unhappiness than happiness) in a particular case.

Rule utilitarianism can endorse rules like "Keep your promises." Thus, unlike act utilitarianism, it can account for the general sense that in making promises we are placing ourselves under an obligation that cannot be set aside for the sake of increasing utility. If "Keep your promises" is accepted as a rule, then the surgeon who fails to perform all of an operation himself, when he has promised his patient he would do so, has not done the right thing, even if the patient never learns the truth.

Rule utilitarians recognize that circumstances can arise in which it would be disastrous to follow a general rule, even when it is true that in general greater happiness would result from following the rule all the time. Clearly we should not keep a promise to meet someone for lunch when we have to choose between keeping the promise and rushing a heart-attack victim to the hospital. It is consistent with the theory to formulate rules that include appropriate escape clauses. For example, "Keep your promises, unless breaking them is required to save a life" and "Keep your promises, unless keeping them would lead to a disastrous result unforeseen at the time the promise was made" are rules that a rule utilitarian might regard as more likely to lead to greater utility than "Always keep your promises, no matter what the consequences may be." What a rule utilitarian cannot endorse is a rule like "Keep your promises, except when breaking a promise would produce more utility." This would, in effect, transform the rule utilitarian into an act utilitarian.

Of course, rule utilitarians are not committed to endorsing general rules only. It is compatible with the view to offer quite specific rules, and in fact there is no constraint on just how specific a rule may be. A rule utilitarian might, for example, establish a rule like "If an infant is born with an open spine, severe brain damage, and dysfunctional kidneys, then the infant should receive no life-sustaining treatment."

The possibility of formulating a large number of rules and establishing them separately opens this basic version of rule utilitarianism to two objections. First, some rules are likely to conflict when they are applicable to the same case, and basic rule utilitarianism offers no way to resolve such conflicts. What should a physician do when faced both with a rule like that above and with another that directs him to "Provide life-sustaining care to all who require it"? Rules that, when considered individually, pass the test of promoting utility may, when taken together, express contradictory demands. A further objection to basic rule utilitarianism is that establishing rules to cover many different circumstances and situations results in such an abundance of rules that employing the rules to make moral decisions becomes virtually impossible in practice.

Partly because of such difficulties, rule utilitarians have taken the approach of establishing the utility of a *set* of rules or an entire moral code. The set can include rules for resolving possible conflicts, and an effort can be made to keep the rules few and simple to minimize the practical difficulty of employing them. Once again, as with individual actions or rules, the principle of utility is employed to determine which set of rules, out of the various sets considered, ought to be accepted.

In this more sophisticated form, rule utilitarianism can be characterized as the theory that an action is right when it conforms to a set of rules that has been determined to produce at least as much overall utility as any other set. It is possible to accept the present forms of social and economic institutions, such as private property and a market economy, as constraints, then argue for the set of rules that will

yield the most utility under those conditions. However, it is also possible to be more radical and argue for a particular set of rules that would lead to the greatest possible utility, quite apart from present social forms. Indeed, such a set of rules might be proposed and defended in an effort to bring about changes in present society that are needed to increase the overall level of utility. Utilitarianism, whether act or rule, is not restricted to being a theory about individual moral obligation. It is also a social and political theory.

We have already seen that rule utilitarianism, unlike act utilitarianism, makes possible the sort of obligation we associate with making a promise. But how might rule utilitarianism deal with the case of the physician who files false Medicaid claims to raise money to operate a free clinic? An obvious answer, although certainly not the only one possible, is that any set of rules likely to be adopted by a rule utilitarian will contain at least one rule making fraud morally wrong. Without a rule forbidding fraud, no social program that requires the cooperation of its participants is likely to achieve its aim. Such a rule protects the program from miscalculations of utility that individuals may make for self-serving reasons, keeps the program focused on its goal, and prevents it from becoming fragmented. Even if some few individuals commit fraud, the rule against it is crucial in discouraging as many as possible. Otherwise, as we pointed out earlier, such a program would collapse. By requiring that the program operate as it was designed, rule utilitarianism also preserves prima facie fairness, because only those who qualify receive benefits.

The most telling objection to rule utilitarianism, according to some philosophers, is that it is inconsistent. The justification of a set of moral rules is that the rules maximize utility. If rules are to maximize utility, then it seems obvious that they must require that an act produce more utility than any other possible act in a particular situation. Otherwise, the maximum amount of utility would not result. But if the rules satisfy this demand, then they will justify exactly the same actions as act utilitarianism. Thus, the rules will consider it right to break promises, make fraudulent claims, and so on. When rule utilitarianism moves to block these possibilities by requiring that rules produce only the most utility overall, it becomes inconsistent: the set of rules is said to maximize utility, but the rules will require actions that do not maximize utility. Thus, rule utilitarianism seems both to accept and to reject the principle of utility as the ultimate moral standard.

Preference Utilitarianism

Some philosophers have called into question the idea of using happiness or any other intrinsic value (knowledge or health, for example) as a criterion of the rightness of an action. The notion of an intrinsic value, they have argued, is too imprecise to be used as a practical guide. Furthermore, it is not at all clear that people share the same values; even if they do, they are not committed to them to the same degree. Someone may value knowledge more than health, while someone else may value physical pleasure over knowledge or health. As a result, there can be no clear-cut procedure for determining what action is likely to produce the best outcome for an individual or group.

The attempt to develop explicit techniques (such as those of decision theory) to help resolve questions about choosing the best action or policy has led some thinkers to replace considerations of intrinsic value with considerations of actual preferences. What someone wants, desires, or prefers can be determined, in principle, in an objective way by consulting the person directly. In addition, people are often able to do more than merely express a preference. Sometimes they can rank their preferences from that which is "most desired" to that which is "least desired."

Such a ranking is of special importance in situations involving risk, for people can be asked to decide how much risk they are will-ing to take to attempt to realize a given preference. A young woman with a hip injury who is otherwise in good health may be willing to accept the risk of surgery to increase her chances of being restored to many years of active life. By contrast, an elderly woman in frail health may prefer to avoid surgery and accept the limitations that the injury imposes on her physical activities. For the elderly woman, not only are the risks of surgery greater because of her poor health, but, even if the surgery is successful, she will have fewer years to benefit from it.

By contrast, the older woman may place such a premium on physical activity that she is willing to take the risk of surgery to improve her chances of securing even a few more years of it. Only she can say what is important to her and how willing she is to take the risk required to secure it.

These considerations about personal preferences can also be raised about social preferences. Statistical information about what people desire and what they are willing to forgo to see their desires satisfied becomes relevant to institutional and legislative deliberations about what policies to adopt. For example, a crucial question facing our own society is whether we are willing to provide everyone with at least a basic minimum of health care, even if this requires increasing taxes or reducing our support for other social goods, such as education and defense.

Employing the satisfaction of preferences as the criterion of the rightness of an action or policy makes it possible to measure some of the relevant factors in some situations. The life expectancy of infants with particular impairments at birth can be estimated by statistics; a given surgical procedure has a certain success rate and a certain mortality rate. Similarly, a particular social policy has a certain financial cost; if implemented, the policy is likely to mean the loss of other possible benefits and opportunities.

Ideally, information of this kind should allow a rational decision maker to calculate the best course of action for an individual or group. The best action will be the one that best combines the satisfaction of preferences with other conditions (financial costs and risks, for example) that are at least minimally acceptable. To use the jargon of the theorists, the best action is the one that maximizes the utilities of the person or group.

A utilitarianism that employs preferences has the advantage of suggesting more explicit methods of analysis and rules for decision making than the classical formulation. It also has the potential for being more sensitive to the expressed desires of individuals. However, preference utilitarianism is not free from special difficulties.

Most prominent is the problem posed by preferences that we would generally regard as unacceptable. What are we to say about those who prefer mass murder, child abuse, or the torture of animals? Obviously, subjective preferences cannot be treated equally, and we must have a way to distinguish acceptable from unacceptable ones. Whether this can be done by relying on the principle of utility alone is doubtful. In the view of some commentators, some other moral principle (or principles) is needed. (See the following discussion of justice.)

Difficulties

Classical utilitarianism is open to a variety of objections. We shall concentrate on only one, however, for it seems to reveal a fatal flaw in the structure of the entire theory. This most serious of all objections is that the principle of utility appears to justify the imposition of great suffering on a few people for the benefit of many people.

Certain kinds of human experimentation forcefully illustrate this possibility. Suppose that an investigator is concerned with acquiring a better understanding of brain functions. He could learn a great deal by systematically destroying the brain of one person and carefully noting the results. Such a study would offer many more opportunities for increasing our knowledge of the brain than those studies that use as subjects people who have damage to their brains in accidental ways. We may suppose that the experimenter chooses as his subject a person without education or training, without family or friends, who cannot be regarded as making much of a contribution to society. The subject will die from the experiment, but it is not unreasonable to suppose that the knowledge of the human brain gained from the experiment will improve the lives of countless numbers of people.

The principle of utility seems to make such experiments legitimate because the outcome is a greater amount of good than harm. One or a few have suffered immensely, but the many have profited to an extent that far outweighs that suffering.

Clearly what is missing from utilitarianism is the concept of *justice*. It cannot be right to increase the general happiness at the expense of one person or group. There must be some way of distributing happiness and unhappiness and avoiding exploitation.

Mill was aware that utilitarianism needs a principle of justice, but most contemporary philosophers do not believe that such a principle can be derived from the principle of utility. In their opinion, utilitarianism as an ethical theory suffers severely from this defect. Yet some philosophers, while acknowledging the defect, have still held that utilitarianism is the best substantive moral theory available.

KANT'S ETHICS

For utilitarianism, the rightness of an action depends upon its consequences. In stark contrast to this view is the ethical theory formulated by the German philosopher Immanuel Kant (1724–1804) in his book *Fundamental Principles of the Metaphysics of Morals*. For Kant, the consequences of an action are morally irrelevant. Rather, an action is right when it is in accordance with a rule that satisfies a principle he calls the "categorical imperative." Since this is the basic principle of Kant's ethics, we can begin our discussion with it.

The Categorical Imperative

If you decide to have an abortion and go through with it, it is possible to view your action as involving a rule. You can be thought of as endorsing a rule to the effect "Whenever I am in circumstances like these, then I shall have an abortion." Kant calls such a rule a "maxim." In his view, all reasoned and considered actions can be regarded as involving maxims.

The maxims in such cases are personal or subjective, but they can be thought of as being candidates for moral rules. If they pass the test imposed by the categorical imperative, then we can say that such actions are right. Furthermore, in passing the test, the maxims cease to be merely personal and subjective. They gain the status of objective rules of morality that hold for everyone.

Kant formulates the categorical imperative in this way: Act only on that maxim which you can will to be a universal law. Kant calls the principle "categorical" to distinguish it from "hypothetical" imperatives. These tell us what to do if we want to bring about certain consequences—such as happiness. A categorical imperative prescribes what we ought to do without reference to any consequences. The principle is an "imperative" because it is a command.

The test imposed on maxims by the categorical imperative is one of generalization or "universalizability." The central idea of the test is that a moral maxim is one that can be generalized to apply to all cases of the same kind. That is, you must be willing to see your rule adopted as a maxim by everyone who is in a situation similar to yours. You must be willing to see your maxim universalized, even though it may turn out on some other occasion to work to your disadvantage.

For a maxim to satisfy the categorical imperative, it is not necessary that we be agreeable in some psychological sense to see it made

into a universal law. Rather, the test is one that requires us to avoid inconsistency or conflict in what we will as a universal rule.

Suppose, for example, that I am a physician and I tell a patient that he has a serious illness, although I know that he doesn't. This may be to my immediate advantage, for the treatment and the supposed cure will increase my income and reputation. The maxim of my action might be phrased as "Whenever I have a healthy patient, I shall lie to him and say that he has an illness."

Now suppose that I try to generalize my maxim. In doing so, I will discover that I am willing the existence of a practice that has contradictory properties. If "Whenever any physician has a healthy patient, he shall lie to him and say he has an illness" is made a universal law, then every patient will be told that he has an illness. Trust in the diagnostic pronouncements of physicians will be destroyed, while my scheme depends on my patients' trusting me and accepting the truth of my lying diagnosis.

It is as if I were saying "Let there be a rule of truth telling such that people can assume that others are telling them the truth, but let there also be a rule that physicians may lie to their patients when it is in the interest of the physician to do so." In willing both rules, I am willing something contradictory. Thus, I can will my action in a particular case, but I can't will that my action be universal without generating a logical conflict.

Kant claims that such considerations show that it is always wrong to lie. Lying produces a contradiction in what we will. On one hand, we will that people believe what we say—that they accept our assurances and promises. On the other hand, we will that people be free to give false assurances and make false promises. Lying thus produces a self-defeating situation, for, when the maxim involved is generalized, the very framework required for lying collapses.

Similarly, consider the egoist who seeks only his self-interest and so makes "Never show love or compassion for others" the maxim of his actions. When universalized, this maxim results in the same kind of self-defeating situation that lying does. Since the egoist will sometimes find himself in need of love and compassion, if he wills the maxim of his action to be a universal law, then he will be depriving himself of something that is in his self-interest. Thus, in willing the abolition of love and compassion out of self-interest, he creates a logical contradiction in what he wills.

Another Formulation

According to Kant, there is only one categorical imperative, but it can be stated in three different ways. Each is intended to reveal a different aspect of the principle. The second formulation, the only other we shall consider, can be stated in this way: Always act so as to treat humanity, either yourself or others, always as an end and never as only a means.

This version illustrates Kant's notion that every rational creature has a worth in itself. This worth is not conferred by being born into a society with a certain political structure, or even by belonging to a certain biological species. The worth is inherent in the sheer possession of rationality. Rational creatures possess what Kant calls an "autonomous, self-legislating will." That is, they are able to consider the consequences of their actions, make rules for themselves, and direct their actions by those self-imposed rules. Thus, rationality confers upon everyone an intrinsic worth and dignity.

This formulation of the categorical imperative perhaps rules out some of the standards that are sometimes used to determine who is selected to receive certain medical resources (such as kidney machines) when the demand is greater than the supply. Standards that make a person's education, accomplishments, or social position relevant seem contrary to this version of the categorical imperative. They violate the basic notion that each person has an inherent worth equal to that of any other per-

son. Unlike dogs or horses, people cannot be judged on "show points."

For Kant, all of morality has its ultimate source in rationality. The categorical imperative, in any formulation, is an expression of rationality, and it is the principle that would be followed in practice by any purely rational being. Moral rules are not mere arbitrary conventions or subjective standards. They are objective truths that have their source in the rational nature of human beings.

Duty

Utilitarianism identifies the good with happiness or pleasure and makes the production of happiness the supreme principle of morality. But for Kant happiness is at best a conditional or qualified good. In his view, there is only one thing that can be said to be good in itself: a good will.

Will is what directs our actions and guides our conduct. But what makes a will a "good will"? Kant's answer is that a will becomes good when it acts purely for the sake of duty.

We act for the sake of duty (or from duty) when we act on maxims that satisfy the categorical imperative. This means, then, that it is the motive force behind our actions—the character of our will—that determines their moral character. Morality does not rest on results —such as the production of happiness—but neither does it rest on our feelings, impulses, or inclinations. An action is right, for Kant, only when it is done for the sake of duty.

Suppose that I decide to donate one of my kidneys for transplanting. If my hope is to gain approval or praise or even if I am moved by pity and a genuine wish to reduce suffering, and this is the only consideration behind my action, then, although I have done the morally right thing, my action has no inner moral worth. By contrast, if I make the donation because I perceive it is my duty to do so, then my action not only is right, but has moral worth. In the first case, I may have acted in accordance with duty (done the same thing as duty would have required), but I did not act from duty.

This view of duty and its connection with morality captures attitudes we frequently express. Consider a nurse who gives special care to a severely ill patient. Suppose you learned that the nurse was providing such extraordinary care only because he hoped that the patient or her family would reward him with a special bonus. Knowing this, you would be unlikely to say that the nurse was acting in a morally outstanding way. We might even think the nurse was being greedy or cynical, and we would say that he was doing the right thing for the wrong reasons.

Kant distinguishes between two types of duties: perfect and imperfect. (The distinction corresponds to the two ways in which maxims can be self-defeating when tested by the categorical imperative.) A perfect duty is one we must always observe, while an imperfect duty is one that we must observe only on some occasions. I have a perfect duty not to injure another person, but I have only an imperfect duty to show love and compassion. I must sometimes show it, but when I show it and which people I select to receive it are entirely up to me.

My duties determine what others can legitimately claim from me as a right. Some rights can be claimed as perfect rights, while others cannot. Everyone can demand of me that I do him or her no injury. But no one can tell me that I must make him or her the recipient of my love and compassion. In deciding how to discharge my imperfect duties, I am free to follow my emotions and inclinations.

For utilitarianism, an action is right when it produces something that is intrinsically valuable (happiness). Because actions are judged by their contributions to achieving a goal, utilitarianism is a teleological theory. By contrast, Kant's ethics holds that an action has features in itself that make it right or in accordance with duty. These features are distinct from the action's consequences. Such a theory is called

"deontological," a term derived from the Greek word for "duty" or "obligation."

Kant's Ethics in the Medical Context

Four features of Kant's ethics are of particular importance in dealing with issues in medical treatment and research:

1. No matter what the consequences may be, it is always wrong to lie.

2. We must always treat people (including ourselves) as ends and not as means only.

3. An action is right when it satisfies the categorical imperative.

4. Perfect and imperfect duties give a basis for claims that certain rights should be recognized.

We can present only two brief examples of how these features can be instrumental in resolving ethical issues, but these are suggestive of other possibilities.

Our first application of Kant's ethics bears on medical research. The task of medical investigators would be easier if they did not have to tell patients that they were going to be made part of a research program. Patients would then become subjects without even knowing it, and more often than not the risk to them would be negligible. Even though no overt lying would be involved, on Kantian principles this procedure would be wrong. It would require treating people as a means only and not as an end.

Likewise, it would never be right for an experimenter to deceive a potential experimental subject. If an experimenter told a patient "We would like to use this new drug on you because it might help you" and this were not really so, the experimenter would be performing a wrong action. Lying is always wrong.

Nor could the experimenter justify this deception by telling himself that the research is of such importance that it is legitimate to lie to the patient. On Kant's principles, good results never make an action morally right. Thus, a patient must give voluntary and informed consent to become a subject of medical experimentation. Otherwise, he or she is being deprived of autonomy and treated as a means only.

We may volunteer because we expect the research to bring direct benefits to us. But we may also volunteer even though no direct personal benefits can be expected. We may see participation in the research as an occasion for fulfilling an imperfect duty to improve human welfare.

But, just as Kant's principles place restrictions on the researcher, they place limits on us as potential subjects. We have a duty to treat ourselves as ends and act so as to preserve our dignity and worth as humans. Therefore, it would not be right for us to volunteer for an experiment that threatened our lives or threatened to destroy our ability to function as autonomous rational beings without first satisfying ourselves that the experiment was legitimate and necessary.

Our second application of Kant's ethics in a medical context bears on the relationship between people as patients and those who accept responsibility for caring for them. A physician, for example, has only an imperfect duty to accept me as a patient. He has a duty to make use of his skills and talents to treat the sick, but I cannot legitimately insist on being the beneficiary. How he discharges his duty is his decision.

If, however, I am accepted as a patient, then I can make some legitimate claims. I can demand that nothing be done to cause me pointless harm, because it is never right to injure a person. Furthermore, I can demand that I never be lied to or deceived. Suppose, for example, I am given a placebo (a harmless but inactive substance) and told that it is a powerful and effective medication. Or suppose that a biopsy shows that I have an inoperable form of cancer, but my physician tells me "There's

nothing seriously wrong with you." In both cases, the physician may suppose that he is deceiving me "for my own good": the placebo may be psychologically effective and make me feel better, and the lie about cancer may save me from useless worry. Yet, by being deceived, I am being denied the dignity inherent in my status as a rational being. Lying is wrong in general, and in such cases as these it also deprives me of my autonomy, of my power to make decisions and form my own opinions. As a result, such deception dehumanizes me.

As an autonomous rational being, a person is entitled to control over his or her own body. This means that medical procedures can be performed on me only with my permission. It would be wrong, for example, for my physician to have me held down and injected with a drug that I explicitly refused. It would be wrong even if the medication were needed for my "own good." I may voluntarily put myself under the care of a physician and submit to all that I am asked to, but the decision belongs to me alone.

In exercising control over my body, however, I also have a duty to myself. Suppose, for example, that I refuse to allow surgery to be performed on me, although I have been told it is necessary to preserve my life. Since I have a duty to preserve my life, as does every person, my refusal is morally unjustifiable. Even here, however, it is not legitimate for others to force me to "do my duty." In fact, in Kantian ethics it is impossible to force another to do his or her duty because it is not the action but the maxim involved that determines whether or not one's duty has been done.

It is obvious even from our sketchy examples that Kantian ethics is a fruitful source of principles and ideas for working out some of the specific moral difficulties of medical experimentation and practice. The absolute requirements imposed by the categorical imperative can be a source of strength and even of comfort. By contrast, utilitarianism requires us to weigh alternative courses of actions by anticipating their consequences and deciding whether what we are considering doing can be justified by those results. Kant's ethics saves us from this kind of doubt and indecision; we know we must never lie, no matter what good may come of it. Furthermore, the lack of a principle of justice that is the most severe defect of utilitarianism is met by Kant's categorical imperative. When every person is to be treated as an end and never as only a means, the possibility of legitimately exploiting some for the benefit of others is wholly eliminated.

Difficulties

Kant's ethical theory is complex and controversial. It has problems of a theoretical sort that manifest themselves in practice and lead us to doubt whether the absolute rules determined by the categorical imperative can always provide a straightforward solution to our moral difficulties. We will limit ourselves to discussing just three problems.

First, Kant's principles may produce resolutions to cases in which there is a conflict of duties that seems intuitively wrong. I have a duty to keep my promises, and I also have a duty to help those in need. Suppose, then, that I am a physician and I have promised a colleague to attend a staff conference. Right before the conference starts, I am talking with a patient who lapses into an insulin coma. If I get involved in treating the patient, I'll have to break my promise to attend the conference. What should I do?

The answer is obvious: I should treat the patient. Our moral intuition tells us this. But, for Kant, keeping promises is a perfect duty, while helping others is an imperfect one. This suggests, then, that according to Kantian principles I should abandon my patient and rush off to keep my appointment. Something is apparently wrong with a view that holds that a promise should never be broken—even when the promise concerns a relatively trivial matter and the consequences of keeping it are disastrous.

Another difficulty with the categorical imperative arises because we are free to choose how we formulate a maxim for testing. In all likelihood none of us would approve a maxim such as "Lie when it is convenient for you." But what about one like "Lie when telling the truth is likely to cause harm to another"? We would be more inclined to make this a universal law. Now consider the maxim "Whenever a physician has good reason to believe that a patient's life will be seriously threatened if he is told the truth about his condition, then the physician should lie." Virtually everyone would be willing to see this made into a universal law.

Yet these three maxims could apply to the same situation. Since Kant does not tell us how to formulate our maxims, it is clear that we can act virtually any way we choose if we are willing to describe the situation in detail. We might be willing to have everyone act just as we are inclined to act whenever they find themselves in *exactly* this kind of situation. The categorical imperative, then, does not seem to solve our moral problems quite so neatly as it first appears to.

A final problem arises from Kant's notion that we have duties to rational beings or persons. Ordinarily, we have little difficulty with this commitment to persons, yet there are circumstances, particularly in the medical context, in which serious problems arise. Consider, for example, a fetus developing in its mother's womb. Is the fetus to be considered a person? The way this question is answered makes all the difference in deciding about the rightness or wrongness of abortion.

A similar difficulty is present when we consider how we are to deal with an infant with serious birth defects. Is it our duty to care for this infant and do all we can to see that it lives? If the infant is not a person, then perhaps we do not owe it the sort of treatment it would be our duty to provide a similarly afflicted adult. It's clear from these two cases that the notion of a person as an autonomous rational being is both too restrictive and arbitrary. It begs important moral questions.

Another difficulty connected with Kant's concept of a rational person is the notion of an "autonomous self-regulating will." Under what conditions can we assume that an individual possesses such a will? Does a child, a mentally retarded person, or someone in prison? Without such a will, in Kant's view, such an individual cannot legitimately consent to be the subject of an experiment or even give permission for necessary medical treatment. This notion is very much in need of development before Kant's principles can be relied on to resolve ethical questions in medicine.

The difficulties that we have discussed require serious consideration. This does not mean, of course, that they cannot be resolved or that because of them Kant's theory is worthless. As with utilitarianism, there are some philosophers who believe the theory is the best available, despite its shortcomings. That it captures many of our intuitive beliefs about what is right (not to lie, to treat people with dignity, to act benevolently) and supplies us with a test for determining our duties (the categorical imperative) recommends it strongly as an ethical theory.

ROSS'S ETHICS

The English philosopher W. D. Ross (1877–1940) presented an ethical theory in his book *The Right and the Good* that can be seen as an attempt to incorporate aspects of utilitarianism and aspects of Kantianism. Ross rejected the utilitarian notion that an action is made right by its consequences alone, but he was also troubled by Kant's absolute rules. He saw not only that such rules fail to show sensitivity to the complexities of actual situations, but also that they sometimes conflict with one another. Like Kant, Ross is a deontologist, but with an important difference. Ross believes it is necessary to consider consequences in making a moral choice, even though it is not the results of an action taken alone that make it right.

Moral Properties and Rules

For Ross there is an unbridgeable distinction between moral and nonmoral properties. There are only two moral properties—rightness and goodness—and these cannot be replaced by, or explained in terms of, other properties. Thus, to say that an action is "right" is not at all the same as saying that it "causes pleasure" or "increases happiness," as utilitarianism claims.

At the same time, however, Ross does not deny that there is a connection between moral properties and nonmoral ones. What he denies is the possibility of establishing an identity between them. Thus, it may be right to relieve the suffering of someone, but right is not identical with relieving suffering. (More exactly put, the rightness of the action is not identical with the action's being a case of relieving suffering.)

Ross also makes clear that we must often know many nonmoral facts about a situation before we can legitimately make a moral judgment. If I see a physician injecting someone, I cannot say whether she is acting rightly without determining what she is injecting, why she is doing it, and so on. Thus, rightness is a property that depends partly on the nonmoral properties that characterize a situation. I cannot determine whether the physician is doing the right thing or the wrong thing until I determine what the nonmoral properties are.

Ross believes that there are cases in which we have no genuine doubt about whether the property of rightness or goodness is present. The world abounds with examples of cruelty, lying, and selfishness, and in these cases we are immediately aware of the absence of rightness or goodness. But the world also abounds with examples of compassion, reliability, and generosity in which rightness and goodness are clearly present. Ross claims that our experience with such cases puts us in a position to come to know rightness and goodness with the same degree of certainty as when we grasp the mathematical truth that a triangle has three angles.

Furthermore, according to Ross, our experience of many individual cases puts us in a position to recognize the validity of a general statement like "It is wrong to cause needless pain." We come to see such rules in much the same way that we come to recognize the letter "A" after having seen it written or printed in a variety of handwritings or typefaces.

Thus, our moral intuitions can supply us with moral rules of a general kind. But Ross refuses to acknowledge these rules as absolute. For him they can serve only as guides to assist us in deciding what we should do. Ultimately, in any particular case we must rely not only on the rules, but also on reason and our understanding of the situation.

Thus, even with rules, we may not recognize what the right thing to do is in a given situation. We recognize, he suggests, that there is always *some* right thing to do, but what it is may be far from obvious. In fact, doubt about what is the right way of acting may arise just because we have rules to guide us. We become aware of the fact that there are several possible courses of action, and all of them seem to be right.

Consider the problem of whether to lie to a terminally ill patient about her condition. Let us suppose that, if we lie to her, we can avoid causing her at least some useless anguish. But then aren't we violating her trust in us to act morally and to speak the truth?

In such cases, we seem to have a conflict in our duties. It is because of such familiar kinds of conflicts that Ross rejects the possibility of discovering absolute, invariant moral rules like "Always tell the truth" and "Always eliminate needless suffering." In cases like the one above, we cannot hold that both rules are absolute without contradicting ourselves. Ross says that we have to recognize that every rule has exceptions and must in some situations be overridden.

Actual Duties and Prima Facie Duties

If rules like "Always tell the truth" cannot be absolute, then what status can they have? When our rules come into conflict in particular situations, how are we to decide which rule applies? Ross answers this question by making use of a distinction between what is actually right and what is prima facie right. Since we have a duty to do what is right, this distinction can be expressed as one between *actual duty* and *prima facie duty*.

An actual duty is simply what my real duty is in a situation. It is the action that, out of the various possibilities, I ought to perform. More often than not, however, I may not know what my actual duty is. In fact, for Ross, the whole problem of ethics might be said to be the problem of knowing what my actual duty is in any given situation.

"Prima facie" literally means "at first sight," but Ross uses the phrase to mean something like "other things being equal." Accordingly, a prima facie duty is one that dictates what I should do when other relevant factors in a situation are not considered. If I promised to meet you for lunch, then I have a prima facie duty to meet you. But suppose I am a physician and, just as I am about to leave for our appointment, the patient I am with suffers cardiac arrest. In such circumstances, according to Ross's view, I should break my promise and render aid to the patient. My prima facie duty to keep my promise doesn't make that act obligatory. It constitutes a moral reason for meeting you, but there is also a moral reason for not meeting you. I also have a prima facie duty to aid my patient, and this is a reason that outweighs the first one. Thus, aiding the patient is both a prima facie duty and, in this situation, my actual duty.

The notion of a prima facie duty permits Ross to offer a set of moral rules stated in such a way that they are both universal and free from exceptions. For Ross, for example, lying is always wrong, but it is wrong prima facie. It may be that in a particular situation my actual duty requires that I lie. Even though what I have done is prima facie wrong, it is the morally right thing to do if some other prima facie duty that requires lying in the case is more stringent than the prima facie duty to tell the truth. (Perhaps only by lying am I able to prevent a terrorist from blowing up an airplane.) I must be able to explain and justify my failure to tell the truth, and it is of course possible that I may not be able to do so. It may be that I was confused and misunderstood the situation or failed to consider other alternatives. I may have been wrong to believe that my actual duty required me to lie. However, even if I was correct in my belief, that I lied is still prima facie wrong. It is this fact (and for Ross it is a fact) that requires me to explain and justify my action.

We have considered only a few simple examples of prima facie duties, but Ross is more thorough and systematic than our examples might suggest. He offers a list of duties that he considers binding on all moral agents. Here they are in summary form:

1. Duties of Fidelity: telling the truth, keeping actual and implicit promises, and not representing fiction as history.

2. Duties of Reparation: righting the wrongs we have done to others.

3. Duties of Gratitude: recognizing the services others have done for us.

4. Duties of Justice: preventing a distribution of pleasure or happiness that is not in keeping with the merit of the people involved.

5. Duties of Beneficence: helping to better the condition of other beings with respect to virtue, intelligence, or pleasure.

6. Duties of Self-Improvement: bettering ourselves with respect to virtue or intelligence.

7. Duties of Nonmaleficence: avoiding or preventing an injury to others.

Ross doesn't claim that this is a complete list of the prima facie duties that we recognize. However, he does believe that the duties on the list are all ones that we acknowledge and are willing to accept as legitimate and binding without argument. He believes that if we simply reflect on these prima facie duties we will see that they may be truly asserted. As he puts the matter:

I . . . am claiming that we *know* them to be true. To me it seems as self-evident as anything could be, that to make a promise, for instance, is to create a moral claim on us in someone else. Many readers will perhaps say that they do *not* know this to be true. If so I certainly cannot prove it to them. I can only ask them to reflect again, in the hope that they will ultimately agree that they also know it to be true.

Notice that Ross explicitly rejects the possibility of providing us with reasons or arguments to convince us to accept his list of prima facie duties. We are merely invited to reflect on certain kinds of cases (like keeping promises), and Ross is convinced that this reflection will bring us to accept his claim that these are true duties. Ross, like other intuitionists, tries to get us to agree with his moral perceptions in much the same way as we might try to get people to agree with us about our color perceptions. We might, for example, show a paint sample to a friend and say "Don't you think that looks blue? It does to me. Think about it for a minute."

We introduced the distinction between actual and prima facie duties to deal with those situations in which duties seem to conflict. The problem, as we can now state it, is this: What are we to do in a situation in which we recognize more than one prima facie duty and it is not possible for us to act in a way that will fulfill them all? We know, of course, that we should act in a way that satisfies our actual duty. But that is just our problem. What, after all, is our actual duty when our prima facie duties are in conflict?

Ross offers us two principles to deal with cases of conflicting duty. The first principle is designed to handle situations in which just two prima facie duties are in conflict: *That act is one's duty which is in accord with the more stringent prima facie obligation.*

The second principle is intended to deal with cases in which several prima facie duties are in conflict: *That act is one's duty which has the greatest balance of prima facie rightness over prima facie wrongness.*

Unfortunately, both these principles present problems in application. Ross does not tell us how we are to determine when an obligation is "more stringent" than another. Nor does he give us a rule for determining the "balance" of prima facie rightness over wrongness. Ultimately, according to Ross, we must simply rely on our perceptions of the situation. There is no automatic or mechanical procedure that can be followed. If we learn the facts in the case, consider the consequences of our possible actions, and reflect on our prima facie duties, we should be able to arrive at a conclusion as to the best course of action—in Ross's view something that we as moral agents must and can do.

To return to specific cases, perhaps there is no direct way to answer the abstract question, Is the duty not to lie to a patient "more stringent" than the duty not to cause needless suffering? So much depends on the character and condition of the individual patient that an abstract determination of our duty based on "balance" or "stringency" is useless. However, knowing the patient, we should be able to perceive what the right course of action is.

Ross further believes that there are situations in which there are no particular difficulties about resolving the conflict between prima facie duties. For example, most of us would agree that, if we can save someone from serious injury by lying, then we have more of an obligation to save someone from injury than we do to tell the truth.

Ross's Ethics in the Medical Context

Ross's moral rules are not absolute in the sense that Kant's are; consequently, as with utilitarianism, it is not possible to say what someone's duty would be in an actual concrete situation. We can discuss in general, however, the advantages that Ross's theory brings to medical-moral issues. We shall mention only two for illustration.

First and most important is Ross's list of prima facie duties. The list of duties can serve an important function in the moral education of physicians, researchers, and other medical personnel. The list encourages each person responsible for patient care to reflect on the prima facie obligations that he or she has toward those people and to set aside one of those obligations only when morally certain that another obligation takes precedence.

The specific duties imposed in a prima facie way are numerous and can be expressed in terms relevant to the medical context: do not injure patients; do not distribute scarce resources in a way that fails to recognize individual worth; do not lie to patients; show patients kindness and understanding; educate patients in ways useful to them; do not hold out false hopes to patients, and so on.

Second, like utilitarianism, Ross's ethics encourages us to show sensitivity to the unique features of situations before acting. Like Kant's ethics, however, Ross's also insists that we look at the world from a particular moral perspective. In arriving at decisions about what is right, we must learn the facts of the case and explore the possible consequences of our actions. Ultimately, however, we must guide our actions by what is right, rather than by what is useful, or by what will produce happiness, or anything of the kind.

Since for Ross actions are not always justified in terms of their results, we cannot say unequivocally "It's right to trick this person into becoming a research subject because the experiment may benefit thousands." Yet, we cannot say that it is always wrong for a researcher to trick a person into volunteering. An action is right or wrong regardless of what we think about it, but in a particular case circumstances might justify an experimenter's allowing some other duty to take precedence over the duty of fidelity.

Fundamentally, then, Ross's ethics offers us the possibility of gaining the advantages of utilitarianism without ignoring the fact that there seem to be duties with an undeniable moral force behind them that cannot be accounted for by utilitarianism. Ross's ethics accommodates not only our intuition that certain actions should be performed just because they are right but also our inclination to pay attention to the results of actions and not just the motives behind them.

Difficulties

The advantages Ross's ethics offers over both utilitarianism and Kantianism are offset by some serious difficulties. To begin with, it seems false that we all grasp the same principles. We are well aware that people's beliefs about what is right and about what their duties are result from the kind of education and experience that they have had. The ability to perceive what is good or right does not appear to be universally shared. Ross does say that the principles are the convictions of "the moral consciousness of the best people." In any ordinary sense of "best," there is reason to say that such people don't always agree on moral principles. If "best" means "morally best," then Ross is close to being circular: The best people are those who acknowledge the same prima facie obligations, and those who recognize the same prima facie obligations are the best people.

Some have objected that Ross's list of prima facie duties seems incomplete. For example, Ross does not explicitly say that we have a prima facie obligation not to steal, but most people would hold that if we have any prima facie duties at all, the duty not to steal

must surely be counted among them. Of course, it is possible to say that stealing is covered by some other obligation—the duty of fidelity, perhaps, since stealing may violate a trust. Nevertheless, from a theory based on intuition, the omission of such duties leaves Ross's list peculiarly incomplete.

Further, some critics have claimed that it is not clear that there is always even a prima facie obligation to do some of the things Ross lists. Suppose that I promise to lie about a friend's physical condition so that he can continue to collect insurance payments. Some would say that I have no obligation at all to keep such an unwise promise. In such a case, there would be no conflict of duties, because I don't have even a prima facie duty to keep such a promise.

Finally, Ross's theory, some have charged, seems to be false to the facts of moral disagreements. When we disagree with someone about an ethical matter, we consider reasons for and against some position. Sometimes the discussion results in agreement. But according to Ross's view this should not be possible. Although we may discuss circumstances and consequences and agree about the prima facie duties involved, ultimately I arrive at my judgment about the duty that is most stringent or has the greatest degree of prima facie rightness and you arrive at yours. At this point, it seems, there can be no further discussion, even though the two judgments are incompatible. Thus, a choice between the two judgments about what act should be performed becomes arbitrary.

Few contemporary philosophers would be willing to endorse Ross's ethical theory without serious qualifications. The need for a special kind of moral perception (or "intuition") marks the theory as unacceptable for most philosophers. Yet many would acknowledge that the theory has great value in illuminating such aspects of our moral experience as reaching decisions when we feel the pull of conflicting obligations. Furthermore, at least some would acknowledge Ross's prima facie duties as constituting an adequate set of moral principles.

RAWLS'S THEORY OF JUSTICE

In 1971 the Harvard philosopher John Rawls published a book called *A Theory of Justice*. The work continues to attract a considerable amount of attention and has been described by some as the most important book in moral and social philosophy of this century.

One commentator, R. P. Wolfe, points out that Rawls attempts to develop a theory that combines the strengths of utilitarianism with those of the deontological position of Kant and Ross, while avoiding the weaknesses of each view. Utilitarianism claims outright that happiness is fundamental and suggests a direct procedure for answering ethical-social questions. But it is flawed by its lack of a principle of justice. Kant and Ross make rightness a fundamental moral notion and stress the ultimate dignity of human beings. Yet neither provides a workable method for solving problems of social morality. Clearly, Rawls's theory promises much if it can succeed in uniting the two ethical traditions we have discussed.

The Original Position and the Principles of Justice

For Rawls the central task of government is to preserve and promote the liberty and welfare of individuals. Thus, principles of justice are needed to serve as standards for designing and evaluating social institutions and practices. They provide a way of resolving conflicts among the competing claims that individuals make and a means of protecting the legitimate interests of individuals. In a sense, the principles of justice constitute a blueprint for the development of a just society.

But how are we to formulate principles of justice? Rawls makes use of a hypothetical device he calls "the original position." Imagine a group of people like those who make up our society. These people display the ordinary range of intelligence, talents, ambitions, convictions, and social and economic advantages.

They include both sexes and members of various racial and ethnic groups.

Furthermore, suppose that this group is placed behind what Rawls calls "a veil of ignorance." Assume that each person is made ignorant of his or her sex, race, natural endowments, social position, economic condition, and so on. Furthermore, assume that these people are capable of cooperating with one another, that they follow the principles of rational decision making, and that they are capable of a sense of justice and will adhere to principles they agree to adopt. Finally, assume that they all desire what Rawls calls "primary goods": the rights, opportunities, powers, wealth, and such that both are worth possessing in themselves and are necessary to securing the more specific goods an individual may want.

Rawls argues that the principles of justice chosen by such a group will be just if the conditions under which they are selected and the procedures for agreeing on them are fair. The original position, with its veil of ignorance, characterizes a state in which alternative notions of justice can be discussed freely by all. Since the ignorance of the participants means that individuals cannot gain advantage for themselves by choosing principles that favor their own circumstances, the eventual choices of the participants will be fair. Since the participants are assumed to be rational, they will be persuaded by the same reasons and arguments. These features of the original position lead Rawls to characterize his view as "justice as fairness."

We might imagine at first that some people in the original position would gamble and argue for principles that would introduce gross inequalities in their society. For example, some might argue for slavery. If these people should turn out to be masters after the veil of ignorance is stripped away, they would gain immensely. But if they turn out to be slaves, then they would lose immensely. However, since the veil of ignorance keeps them from knowing their actual positions in society, it would not be rational for them to endorse a principle that might condemn them to the bottom of the social order.

Given the uncertainties of the original situation, there is a better strategy that these rational people would choose. In the economic discipline known as game theory, this strategy is called "maximin." When we choose in uncertain situations, this strategy directs us to select from the alternatives the one whose worst possible outcome is better than the worst possible outcome of the other alternatives. (If you don't know whether you're going to be a slave, you shouldn't approve a set of principles that permits slavery when you have other options.)

Acting in accordance with this strategy, Rawls argues that people in the original position would agree on the following two principles of justice:

1. Each person is to have an equal right to the most extensive total system of equal basic liberties compatible with a similar system of liberty for all.

2. Social and economic inequalities are to be arranged so that they are both: (a) to the greatest benefit of the least advantaged . . . , and (b) attached to offices and positions open to all under conditions of fair equality of opportunity.

For Rawls, these two principles are taken to govern the distribution of all social goods: liberty, property, wealth, and social privilege. The first principle has priority. It guarantees a system of equal liberty for all. Furthermore, because of its priority, it explicitly prohibits the bartering away of liberty for social or economic benefits. (For example, a society cannot withhold the right to vote from its members on the grounds that voting rights damage the economy.)

The second principle governs the distribution of social goods other than liberty. Although society could organize itself in a way that would eliminate differences in wealth and abolish the advantages that attach to different social positions, Rawls argues that those in the original position would not choose this form of egalitarianism. Instead, they would opt for the second principle of justice. This means that in a just society differences in wealth and social position can be tolerated only when they can be shown to benefit everyone and to benefit, in particular, those who have the fewest advantages. A just society is not one in which everyone is equal, but one in which inequalities must be demonstrated to be legitimate. Furthermore, there must be a genuine opportunity for acquiring membership in a group that enjoys special benefits. Those not qualified to enter medical schools because of past discrimination in education, for example, can claim a right for special preparation to qualify them. (Of course in a Rawlsian society there would be no discrimination to be compensated for.)

Rawls argues that these two principles are required to establish a just society. Furthermore, in distributing liberty and social goods, the principles guarantee the worth and self-respect of the individual. People are free to pursue their own conception of the good and fashion their own lives. Ultimately, the only constraints placed on them as members of society are those expressed in the principles of justice.

Yet Rawls also acknowledges that those in the original position would recognize that we have duties both to ourselves and to others. They would, for example, want to take measures to see that their interests are protected if they should meet with disabling accidents, become seriously mentally disturbed, and so on. Thus, Rawls approves a form of paternalism: Others should act for us when we are unable to act for ourselves. When our preferences are known to them, those acting for us should attempt to follow what we would wish. Otherwise, they should act for us as they would act for themselves if they were viewing our situation from the standpoint of the original position. Paternalism is thus a duty to ourselves that would be recognized by those in the original position.

Rawls is also aware of the need for principles that bind and guide individuals as moral decision makers. He claims that those in the original position would reach agreement on principles for such notions as fairness in our dealings with others, fidelity, respect for persons, and beneficence. From these principles we gain some of our obligations to one another.

But, Rawls claims, there are also "natural duties" that would be recognized by those in the original position. Among those Rawls mentions are (1) the duty of justice—supporting and complying with just institutions, (2) the duty of helping others in need or jeopardy, (3) the duty not to harm or injure another, and (4) the duty to keep our promises.

For the most part, these are duties that hold between or among people. They are only some of the duties that would be offered by those in the original position as unconditional duties. Thus, Rawls in effect endorses virtually the same duties as those that Ross presents as prima facie duties. Rawls realizes that the problem of conflicts of duty was left unsolved by Ross and so perceives the need for assigning priorities to duties—ranking them as higher and lower. Rawls believes that a full system of principles worked out from the original position would include rules for ranking duties. Rawls's primary concern, however, is with justice in social institutions, and he does not attempt to establish any rules for ranking.

Rawls's Theory of Justice in the Medical Context

Rawls's "natural duties" are virtually the same as Ross's prima facie duties. Consequently, most of what we said earlier about prima facie duties and moral decision making applies to Rawls.

Rawls endorses the legitimacy of paternalism, although he does not attempt to specify detailed principles to justify individual cases. He does tell us that we should consider the preferences of others when they are known to us and when we are in a situation in which we must act for them because they are unable to act for themselves. For example, suppose we know that a person approves of electroconvulsive therapy (shock treatments, or ECT) for the treatment of severe depression. If that person should become so depressed as to be unable to reach a decision about his own treatment, then we would be justified in seeing to it that he received ECT.

To take a similar case, suppose that you are a surgeon and have a patient who has expressed to you her wish to avoid numerous operations that may prolong her life six months or so but will be unable to restore her to health. If in operating you learned that she had a form of uterine cancer that had spread through her lower extremities and if in your best judgment nothing could be done to restore her to health, then it would be your duty to her to allow her to die as she chooses. Repeated operations would be contrary to her concept of her own good.

The most important question in exploring Rawls's theory is how the two principles of justice might apply to the social institutions and practices of medical care and research. Most obviously, Rawls's principles repair utilitarianism's flaw with respect to human experimentation. It would never be right, in Rawls's view, to exploit one group of people or even one person for the benefit of others. Thus, experiments in which people are forced to be subjects or are tricked into participating are ruled out. They involve a violation of basic liberties of individuals and of the absolute respect for persons that the principles of justice require.

A person has a right to decide what risks she is willing to take with her own life and health. Thus, voluntary consent is required before someone can legitimately become a research subject. However, society might decide to reward research volunteers with money, honors, or social privileges to encourage participation in research. Provided that the overall structure of society already conforms to the two principles of justice, this is a perfectly legitimate practice as long as it brings benefits (ideally) to everyone and the possibility of gaining the rewards of participation is open to all.

Regarding the allocation of social resources in the training of medical personnel (physicians, nurses, therapists, and so on), one may conclude that such investments are justified only if the withdrawal of the support would work to the disadvantage of those already most disadvantaged. Public money may be spent in the form of scholarships and institutional grants to educate personnel, who may then derive great social and economic benefits from their education. But for Rawls the inequality that is produced is not necessarily unjust. Society can invest its resources in this way if it brings benefits to those most in need of them.

The implication of this position seems to be that everyone is entitled to health care. First, it could be argued that health is among the "primary goods" that Rawls's principles are designed to protect and promote. After all, without health an individual is hardly in a position to pursue other more specific goods, and those in the original position might be imagined to be aware of this and to endorse only those principles of justice that would require providing at least basic health care to those in the society. Furthermore, it could be argued that the inequalities of the health-care system can be justified only if those in most need can benefit from them. Since this is not obviously the case with the present system, Rawls's principles seem to call for a reform that would provide health care to those who are unable to pay.

However, it is important to point out that it is not at all obvious that a demand to reform our health-care system follows from Rawls's position. For one thing, it is not clear that

Rawls's principles are intended to be directly applied to our society as it is. Our society includes among its members people with serious disabilities and ones with both acute and chronic diseases. If Rawls's principles are intended to apply only to people with normal physical and psychological abilities and needs, as he sometimes suggests, then it is not clear that those who are ill can be regarded as appropriate candidates. If they are considered appropriate, then the results may be unacceptable. The principles of justice may require that we devote vast amounts of social resources to making only marginal improvements in the lives of those who are ill.

Furthermore, Rawls does not explicitly mention the promotion of health as one of the primary goods. It may seem reasonable to include it among them, given the significance of health as a condition for additional pursuits, but this is a point that requires support. (Norman Daniels is one who has argued for considering health a primary good.) This seems the most promising position to take if Rawls's principles are to be used as a basis for evaluating our current health policies and practices.

It seems reasonable to hold that Rawls's principles, particularly the second, can be used to restrict access to certain kinds of health care. In general, individuals may spend their money in any way they wish to seek their notions of what is good. Thus, if someone wants cosmetic surgery to change the shape of his chin and has the money to pay a surgeon, then he may have it done. But if medical facilities or personnel should become overburdened and unable to provide needed care for the more seriously afflicted, then the society would be obligated to forbid cosmetic surgery. By doing this, it would then increase the net access to needed health care by all members of society. The rich who desired cosmetic surgery would not be permitted to exploit the poor who needed basic health care.

These are just a few of the possible implications that Rawls's theory has for medical research and practice. It seems likely that more and more applications of the theory will be worked out in detail in the future.

Difficulties

Rawls's theory is currently the subject of much discussion in philosophy. The debate is often highly technical, and a great number of objections have been raised. At present, however, there are no objections that would be acknowledged as legitimate by all critics. Rather than attempt to summarize the debate, we shall simply point to two aspects of Rawls's theory that have been acknowledged as difficulties.

One criticism concerns the original position and its veil of ignorance. Rawls does not permit those in the original position to know anything of their own purposes, plans, or interests—of their conception of the good. They do not know whether they prefer tennis to Tennyson, pleasures of mind over pleasures of the body. They are allowed to consider only those goods—self-respect, wealth, social position—that Rawls puts before them. Thus, critics have said, Rawls has excluded morally relevant knowledge. It is impossible to see how people could agree on principles to regulate their lives when they are so ignorant of their desires and purposes. Rawls seems to have biased the original position in his favor, and this calls into question his claim that the original position is a fair and reasonable way of arriving at principles of justice.

A second criticism focuses on whether Rawls's theory is really as different from utilitarianism as it appears to be. Rawls's theory may well permit inequalities of treatment under certain conditions in the same way that the principle of utility permits them. The principles of justice that were stated earlier apply, Rawls says, only when liberty can be effectively established and maintained. Rawls is very unclear about when a situation may be regarded as one of this kind. When it is not, his principles of justice are ones of a "general conception." Under this conception, liberties of individuals can be restricted, provided that the restrictions are for the benefit of all. It is possible to imagine, then, circumstances in which we might force individuals to become experimental subjects both for their own benefit and for that of others. We might, for example, require that all cigarette smokers participate in experiments intended to acquire knowledge about lung and heart damage. Since everyone would benefit, directly or indirectly, from such knowledge, forcing their participation would be legitimate. Thus, under the general conception of justice, the difference between Rawls's principles and the principle of utility may, in practice, become vanishingly small.

NATURAL LAW ETHICS AND MORAL THEOLOGY

The general view that the rightness of actions is something determined by nature itself, rather than by the laws and customs of societies or the preferences of individuals, is called "natural law theory." Moral principles are thus regarded as objective truths that can be discovered in the nature of things by reason and reflection. The basic idea of the theory was expressed succinctly by the Roman philosopher Cicero (106–43 B.C.): "Law is the highest reason, implanted in Nature, which commands what ought to be done and forbids the opposite. This reason, when firmly fixed and fully developed in the human mind, is Law."

The natural law theory originated in classical Greek and Roman philosophy and has immensely influenced the development of moral and political theories. Indeed, all the ethical theories we have discussed are indebted to the natural law tradition. The reliance upon reason as a means of settling upon or establishing ethical principles and the emphasis on the need to reckon with the natural abilities and inclinations of human nature are just two of the threads that are woven into the theories that we have discussed.

Purposes, Reason, and the Moral Law as Interpreted by Roman Catholicism

The natural law theory of Roman Catholicism was given its most influential formulation in the thirteenth century by St. Thomas Aquinas (1225–1274). Contemporary versions of the theory are mostly elaborations and interpretations of Aquinas's basic statement. Thus, an understanding of Aquinas's views is important for grasping the philosophical principles that underlie the Roman Catholic position on such issues as abortion.

Aquinas was writing at a time in which a great number of the texts of Aristotle (384–322 B.C.) were becoming available in the West, and Aquinas's philosophical theories incorporated many of Aristotle's principles. A fundamental notion borrowed by Aquinas is the view that the universe is organized in a teleological way. That is, the universe is structured in such a way that each thing in it has a goal or purpose. Thus, when conditions are right, a tadpole will develop into a frog. In its growth and change, the tadpole is following "the law of its nature." It is achieving its goal.

Humans have a material nature, just as a tadpole does, and in their own growth and development they too follow a law of their material nature. But Aquinas also stresses that humans possess a trait that no other creature does—reason. Thus, the full development of human potentialities—the fulfillment of human purpose—requires that we follow the direction of the law of reason, as well as being subjected to the laws of material human nature.

The development of reason is one of our ends as human beings, but we also rely upon reason to determine what our ends are and how we can achieve them. It is this function of reason that leads Aquinas to identify reason as the source of the moral law. Reason is practical in its operation, for it directs our actions so that we can bring about certain results. In giving us directions, reason imposes an obligation on us—the obligation to bring about the results that it specifies. But Aquinas says that reason cannot arbitrarily set goals for us. Reason directs us toward our good as the goal of our action, and what that good is, is discoverable within our nature. Thus, reason recognizes the basic principle "Good is to be done and evil avoided."

But this principle is purely formal, or empty of content. To make it a practical principle, we must consider what the human good is. According to Aquinas, the human good is that which is suitable or proper to human nature. It is what is "built into" human nature in the way that, in a sense, a frog is already "built into" a tadpole. Thus, the good is that to which we are directed by our natural inclinations as both physical and rational creatures.

Like other creatures, we have a natural inclination to preserve our lives; consequently, reason imposes on us an obligation to care for our health, not to kill ourselves, and not to put ourselves in positions in which we might be killed. We realize through reason that others have a rational nature like ours, and we see that we are bound to treat them with the same dignity and respect that we accord ourselves. Furthermore, when we see that humans require a society to make their full development possible, we realize that we have an obligation to support laws and practices that make society possible.

Thus, for example, as we have a natural inclination to propagate our species (viewed as a "natural" good), reason places on us an obligation not to thwart or pervert this inclination. As a consequence, to fulfill this obligation within society, reason supports the institution of marriage.

Reason also finds in our nature grounds for procedural principles. For example, because everyone has an inclination to preserve his life and well-being, no one should be forced to testify against himself. Similarly, because all individuals are self-interested, no one should be permitted to be a judge in his own case.

Physical inclinations, under the direction of reason, point us toward our natural good. But, according to Aquinas, reason itself can also be a source of inclinations. For example, Aquinas says that reason is the source of our natural inclination to seek the truth, particularly the truth about the existence and nature of God.

Just from the few examples we have considered, it should be clear how Aquinas believed it was possible to discover in human nature natural goods. Relying upon these as goals or purposes to be achieved, reason would then work out the practical way of achieving them. Thus, through the subtle application of reason, it should be possible to establish a body of moral principles and rules. These are the doctrines of natural law.

Because natural law is founded on human nature, which is regarded as unchangeable, Aquinas regards natural law itself as unchangeable. Moreover, it is seen as the same for all people, at all times, and in all societies. Even those without knowledge of God can, through the operation of reason, recognize their natural obligations.

For Aquinas and for Roman Catholicism, this view of natural law is just one aspect of a broader theological framework. The teleological organization of the universe is attributed to the planning of a creator—goals or purposes are ordained by God. Furthermore, although natural law is discoverable in the universe, its ultimate source is divine wisdom and God's eternal law. Everyone who is rational is capable of grasping natural law. But because passions and irrational inclinations may corrupt human nature and because some people lack the abilities or time to work out the demands of natural law, God also chose to reveal our duties to us in explicit ways. The major source of revelation, of course, is taken to be the Biblical scriptures.

Natural law, scriptural revelation, the interpretation of the scriptures by the Church, Church tradition, and the teachings of the Church are regarded in Roman Catholicism as the sources of moral ideals and principles. By guiding one's life by them, one can develop the rational and moral part of one's nature and move toward the goal of achieving the sort of perfection that is suitable for humans.

This general moral-theological point of view is the source for particular Roman Catholic doctrines that have special relevance to medicine. We shall consider just two of the most important principles.

The Principle of Double Effect. A particular kind of moral conflict arises when the performance of an action will produce both good and bad effects. On the basis of the good effect, it seems it is our duty to perform the action; but on the basis of the bad effect, it seems our duty not to perform it.

Let's assume that the death of a fetus is in itself a bad effect and consider a case like the following: A woman who is three months pregnant is found to have a cancerous uterus. If the woman's life is to be saved, the uterus must be removed at once. But if the uterus is removed, then the life of the unborn child will be lost. Should the operation be performed?

The principle of double effect is intended to help in the resolution of these kinds of conflicts. The principle holds that such an action should be performed only if the intention is to bring about the good effect and the bad effect will be an unintended or indirect consequence. More specifically, four conditions must be satisfied:

1. The action itself must be morally indifferent or morally good.

2. The bad effect must not be the means by which the good effect is achieved.

3. The motive must be the achievement of the good effect only.

4. The good effect must be at least equivalent in importance to the bad effect.

Are these conditions satisfied in the case that we mentioned? The operation itself, if this is considered to be the action, is at least morally indifferent. That is, in itself it is neither good nor bad. That takes care of the first condition. If the mother's life is to be saved, it will not be *by means of* killing the fetus. It will be by means of removing the cancerous uterus. Thus, the second condition is met. The motive of the surgeon, we may suppose, is not the death of the fetus but saving the life of the woman. If so, then the third condition is satisfied. Finally, since two lives are at stake, the good effect (saving the life of the woman) is at least equal to the bad effect (the death of the fetus). The fourth condition is thus met. Under ordinary conditions, then, these conditions would be considered satisfied and such an operation would be morally justified.

The principle of double effect is most often mentioned in a medical context in cases of abortion. But, in fact, it has a much wider range of application in medical ethics. It bears on cases of contraception, sterilization, organ transplants, and the use of extraordinary measures to maintain life.

The Principle of Totality.   The principle of totality can be expressed in this way: An individual has a right to dispose of his organs or to destroy their capacity to function only to the extent that the general well-being of the whole body demands it. Thus, it is clear that we have a natural obligation to preserve our lives, but, by the Roman Catholic view, we also have a duty to preserve the integrity of our bodies. This duty is based on the belief that each of our organs was designed by God to play a role in maintaining the functional integrity of our bodies, that each has a place in the divine plan. As we are the custodians of our bodies, not their owners, it is our duty to care for them as a trust.

The principle of totality has implications for a great number of medical procedures. Strictly speaking, even cosmetic surgery is morally right only when it is required to main-tain or assure the normal functioning of the rest of the body. More important, procedures that are typically employed for contraceptive purposes—vasectomies and tubal ligations—are ruled out. After all, such procedures involve "mutilation" and the destruction of the capacity of the organs of reproduction to function properly. The principle of totality thus also forbids the sterilization of the mentally retarded.

As an ethical theory, natural law theory is sometimes described as teleological. In endorsing the principle "Good is to be done and evil avoided," the theory identifies a goal with respect to which the rightness of an action is to be judged. As the principle of double effect illustrates, the intention of the individual who acts is crucial to determining whether the goal is sought. In a sense, the intention of the action, what the individual wills, defines the action. Thus, "performing an abortion" and "saving a woman's life" are not necessarily the same action, even in those instances in which their external features are the same. Unlike utilitarianism, which is also a teleological theory, natural law theory is not consequentialist: the outcome of an action is not the sole feature to consider in determining the moral character of the action.

Applications of Roman Catholic Moral-Theological Viewpoints in the Medical Context

Roman Catholic ethicists and moral theologians have written on numerous aspects of medical ethics and developed a body of widely accepted doctrine. We shall consider only four topics.

First, the application of the principle of double effect and the principle of totality has definite consequences in the area of medical experimentation. Since we hold our bodies in trust, we are responsible for assessing the degree of risk present in an experiment in which we are asked to be a subject. Thus, we need to be fully informed of the nature of the experiment and the risks that it holds for us. If after obtaining this knowledge we decide to give our consent, it must be given freely and not as the result of deception or coercion.

Because human experimentation carries with it the possibility of injury and death, the principle of double effect and its four strictures apply. If scientific evidence indicates that a sick person may benefit from participating in an experiment, then the experiment is morally justifiable. If, however, the evidence indicates that the chances of helping that person are slight and he or she may die or be gravely injured, then the experiment is not justified. In general, the likelihood of a person's benefiting from the experiment must exceed the danger of that person's suffering greater losses.

A person who is incurably ill may volunteer to be an experimental subject, even though she or he cannot reasonably expect personal gain in the form of improved health. The good that is hoped for is good for others, in the form of increased medical knowledge. Even here, however, there are constraints imposed by the principle of double effect. There must be no likelihood that the experiment will seriously injure, and the probable value of the knowledge expected to result must balance the risk run by the patient. Not even the incurably ill can be made subjects of trivial experiments.

The good sought by healthy volunteers is also the good of others. The same restrictions mentioned in connection with the incurably ill apply to experimenting on healthy people. Additionally, the principle of totality places constraints on what a person may volunteer to do with his or her body. No healthy person may submit to an experiment that involves the probability of serious injury, impaired health, mutilation, or death.

A second medical topic addressed by Roman Catholic theologians is whether "ordinary" or "extraordinary" measures are to be taken in the preservation of human life.

While it is believed that natural law and divine law impose on us a moral obligation to preserve our lives, Catholic moralists have interpreted this obligation as requiring that we rely upon only ordinary means. In the medical profession, the phrase "ordinary means" is used to refer to medical procedures that are standard or orthodox, in contrast to those that are untried or experimental. But from the viewpoint of Catholic ethics, "ordinary" used in the medical context applies to "all medicines, treatments, and operations which offer a reasonable hope of benefit for the patient and which can be obtained and used without excessive expense, pain, or other inconvenience." Thus, by contrast, extraordinary means are those that offer the patient no reasonable hope or whose use causes serious hardship for the patient or others.

Medical measures that would save the life of a patient but subject her to years of pain or would produce in her severe physical or mental incapacities are considered extraordinary. A patient or her family is under no obligation to choose them, and physicians are under a positive obligation not to encourage their choice.

The third medical topic for consideration is euthanasia. In the Roman Catholic ethical view, euthanasia in any form is considered immoral. It is presumed to be a direct violation of God's dominion over creation and the human obligation to preserve life. The Ethical Directives for Catholic Hospitals is explicit on the matter of taking a life:

> The direct killing of any innocent person, even at his own request, is always morally wrong. Any procedure whose sole immediate effect is the death of a human being is a direct killing. . . . Euthanasia ("mercy killing") in all its forms is forbidden. . . . The failure to supply the ordinary means of preserving life is equivalent to euthanasia.

According to this view, it is wrong to allow babies suffering from serious birth defects to die. If they can be saved by ordinary means, there is an obligation to do so. It is also wrong to act to terminate the lives of those hopelessly ill, either by taking steps to bring about their deaths or by failing to take steps to maintain their lives by ordinary means.

It is never permissible to hasten the death of a person as a direct intention. It is, however, permissible to administer drugs that alleviate pain. The principle of double effect suggests that giving such drugs is a morally justifiable action even though the drugs may indirectly hasten the death of a person.

Last, we may inquire how Roman Catholicism views abortion. According to the Roman Catholic view, from the moment of conception the conceptus (later, the fetus) is considered to be a person with all the rights of a person. For this reason, direct abortion at any stage of pregnancy is regarded as morally wrong. Abortion is "direct" when it results from a procedure "whose sole immediate effect is the termination of pregnancy." This means that what is generally referred to as therapeutic abortion, in which an abortion is performed to safeguard the life or health of the woman, is considered wrong. For example, a woman with serious heart disease who becomes pregnant cannot morally justify an abortion on the grounds that the pregnancy is a serious threat to her life. Even when the ultimate aim is to save the life of the woman, direct abortion is wrong.

We have already seen, however, that the principle of double effect permits the performance of an action that may result in the death of an unborn child if the action satisfies the four criteria for applying the principle. Thus, *indirect* abortion is considered to be morally permissible. That is, the abortion must be the outcome of some action (for example, removal of a cancerous uterus) that is performed for the direct and total purpose of treating a pathological condition affecting the woman. The end sought in direct abortion is the destruction of life, but the end sought in indirect abortion is the preservation of life.

Difficulties

Our discussion has centered on the natural law theory of ethics as it has been interpreted in Roman Catholic theology. Thus, there are two possible types of difficulties: those associated with natural law ethics in its own right and those associated with its incorporation into theology. The theological difficulties go beyond the scope of our aims and interests. We shall restrict ourselves to considering the basic difficulty that faces natural law theory as formulated by Aquinas. Since it is this formulation that has been used in Roman Catholic moral theology, we shall be raising a problem for it in an indirect way.

The fundamental difficulty with Aquinas's argument for natural law is caused by the assumption, borrowed from Aristotle, that the universe is organized in a teleological fashion. (This is the assumption that every kind of thing has a goal or purpose.) This assumption is essential to Aquinas's ethical theory, for he identifies the good of a thing with its natural mode of operation. Without the assumption, we are faced with the great diversity and moral indifference of nature. Inclinations, even when shared by all humans, are no more than inclinations. There are no grounds for considering them "goods," and they have no moral status. The universe is bereft of natural values.

Yet, there are many reasons to consider this assumption false. Physics surrendered the notion of a teleological organization in the world as long ago as the seventeenth century—the rejection of Aristotle's physics also entailed the rejection of Aristotle's teleological view of the world. This left biology as the major source of arguments in favor of teleology. But contemporary evolutionary theory shows that the apparent purposive character of evolutionary change can be accounted for by the operation of natural selection on random mutations. Also, the development and growth of organisms can be explained by the presence of genetic information that controls the processes. The tadpole develops into a frog because evolution has produced a genetic program that directs the sequence of complicated chemical changes. Thus, there seem to be no adequate grounds for asserting that the teleological organization of nature is anything more than apparent.

Science and "reason alone" do not support teleology. It can be endorsed only if one is willing to assume that any apparent teleological organization is the product of a divine plan. Yet, because all apparent teleology can be explained in nonteleological ways, this assumption seems neither necessary nor legitimate.

Without its foundation of teleology, Aquinas's theory of natural law ethics seems to collapse. This is not to say, of course, that some other natural law theory, one not requiring the assumption of teleology, might not be persuasively defended.

PART II. MAJOR MORAL PRINCIPLES

Making moral decisions is always a difficult and stressful task. Abstract discussions of issues never quite capture the feelings of uncertainty and self-doubt we characteristically experience when called upon to decide what ought to be done or to judge whether someone did the right thing. There are no mechanical processes or algorithms we can apply in a situation of moral doubt. There are no computer programs to supply us with the proper decision when given the relevant data.

In a very real sense, we are on our own when it comes to making ethical decisions. This does not mean that we are without resources and must decide blindly or even naively. When we have the luxury of time, when the need to make a decision is not pressing, then we may attempt to work out an answer to a moral question by relying upon a general ethical theory like those discussed earlier. However, in ordinary life we rarely have the opportunity or time to engage in an elaborate process of reasoning and analysis.

A more practical approach is to employ moral principles that have been derived from and justified by a moral theory. A principle such as "Avoid causing needless harm" can serve as a more direct guide to action and decision making than, say, Kant's categorical imperative. With such a principle in mind, we realize that, if we are acting as a physician, then we have a duty to use our knowledge and skills to protect our patients from injury. For example, we should not expose a patient to the needless risk of a diagnostic test that does not promise to yield useful information.

In this section, we will present and illustrate five moral principles. All are ones of special relevance to the ethical issues presented by decisions concerning medical care. The principles have their limitations. For one thing, they are in no sense complete. Moral issues arise, even in the context of medicine, for which they can supply no direct guidance. In other situations, the principles themselves may come into conflict and point toward incompatible solutions. (How can we both avoid causing harm and allow a terminally ill patient to die?) The principles themselves indicate no way such conflicts can be resolved, for, even taken together, they do not constitute a coherent moral theory. To resolve conflicts, it may be necessary to employ the more basic principles of such a theory.

It is fair to say that each of the five basic moral theories we have discussed endorses the legitimacy of these principles. Not all would formulate them in the same way, and not all would give them the same moral weight. Nevertheless, each theory would accept them as expressing appropriate guidelines for moral decision making.

Indeed, the best way to think about the principles is as guidelines. They are in no way rules that can be applied automatically. Rather, they express standards to be consulted in attempting to arrive at a justified decision. As such, they provide a basis for evaluating actions or policies as well as for making individual moral decisions. They help guarantee that our decisions are made in accordance with principles and not according to our whims or prejudices. By following them, we are more likely to reach decisions that are reasoned, consistent, and applicable to similar cases.

THE PRINCIPLE OF NONMALEFICENCE

"Above all, do no harm" is perhaps the most famous and most quoted of all moral maxims in medicine. It captures in a succinct way what is universally considered to be an overriding duty of anyone who undertakes the care of a patient. We believe that in treating a patient a physician should not by carelessness, malice, inadvertence, or avoidable ignorance do anything that will cause injury to the patient.

The maxim is one expression of what is sometimes called in ethics the principle of nonmaleficence. The principle can be formulated in various ways, but here is one relatively noncontroversial way of stating it: *We ought to act in ways that do not cause needless harm or injury to others.* Stated in a positive fashion, the principle tells us that we have a duty to avoid maleficence—that is, to avoid harming or injuring other people.

In the most obvious case, we violate the principle of nonmaleficence when we intentionally do something we know will cause someone harm. For example, suppose that a surgeon during the course of an operation deliberately severs a muscle, knowing that by doing so he will cripple the patient. The surgeon is guilty of maleficence and is morally (as well as legally) blameworthy for his action.

The principle may also be violated when no malice or intention to do harm is involved. A nurse who carelessly gives a patient the wrong medication and causes the patient to suffer irreversible brain damage may have had no intention of causing the patient any injury. However, the nurse was negligent in his actions and failed to exercise due care in dis-

charging his responsibilities. His actions resulted in an avoidable injury to his patient. Hence, he failed to meet his obligation of nonmaleficence.

The duty imposed by the principle of nonmaleficence is not a demand to accomplish the impossible. We realize that we cannot reasonably expect perfection in the practice of medicine. We know that the results of treatments are often uncertain and may cause more harm than good. We know that the knowledge we have of diseases is only partial and that decisions about diagnosis and therapy typically involve the exercise of judgment, with no guarantee of correctness. We know there is an uncertainty built into the very nature of things and that our power to control the outcome of natural processes is limited. Consequently, we realize that we cannot hold physicians and other health professionals accountable for every instance of death and injury involving patients under their care.

Nevertheless, we can demand that physicians and others live up to reasonable standards of performance. In the conduct of their professions, we can expect them to be cautious and diligent, patient and thoughtful. We can expect them to pay attention to what they are doing and to deliberate about whether a particular procedure should be done. In addition, we can expect them to possess the knowledge and skills relevant to the proper discharge of their duties.

These features and others like them make up the standards of performance that define what we have a right to expect from physicians and other health professionals. In the language of the law, these are the standards of "due care," and it is by reference to them that we evaluate the medical care given to patients. Failure to meet the standards opens practitioners (physicians, nurses, dentists, therapists) to the charge of moral or legal maleficence.

In our society, we have attempted to guarantee that at least some of the due-care standards are met by relying upon such measures as degree programs, licensing laws, certifying boards, and hospital credentials committees. Such an approach offers a way of seeing to it that physicians and others have acquired at least a minimum level of knowledge, skill, and experience before undertaking the responsibilities attached to their roles. The approach also encourages such values as diligence, prudence, and caution, but there is of course no way of guaranteeing that in a particular case a physician will exhibit those virtues. Haste, carelessness, and inattention are always possible, and the potential that a patient will suffer an injury from them is always present.

The standards of due care are connected in some respects with such factual matters as the current state of medical knowledge and training and the immediate circumstances in which a physician provides care. For example, in the 1920s and 1930s, it was not at all unusual for a general practitioner to perform relatively complicated surgery. This was particularly true of someone practicing in a rural area. In performing surgery, he would be acting in a reasonable and expected fashion and could not be legitimately charged with violating the principle of nonmaleficence.

However, the change in medicine from that earlier time to the present has also altered our beliefs about what is reasonable and expected. Today a general practitioner who has had no special training and is not board certified and yet performs surgery on his patients may be legitimately criticized for maleficence. The standards of due care in surgery are now higher and more exacting than they once were, and the general practitioner who undertakes to perform most forms of surgery causes his patients to undergo an unusual and unnecessary risk literally at his hands. Their interest would be better served if their surgery were performed by a trained and qualified surgeon.

Such a case also illustrates that no actual harm or injury must occur for someone to be acting in violation of the principle of nonmaleficence. The general practitioner performing surgery may not cause any injury to his patients, but he puts them in a position in which the possibility of harm to them is greater than it needs to be. It is in this respect that he is not exercising due care in his treatment and so can be charged with maleficence. He has subjected his patients to *unnecessary* risk—risk greater than they would be subject to in the hands of a trained surgeon.

It is important to stress that the principle of nonmaleficence does not require that a physician subject a patient to no risks at all. Virtually every form of diagnostic testing and medical treatment involves some degree of risk to the patient; to provide medical care at all, a physician must often act in ways that involve a possible injury to the patient. For example, a physician who takes a thorough medical history and performs a physical examination, then treats a patient with an antibiotic for bacterial infection, cannot be held morally responsible if the patient suffers a severe drug reaction. That such a thing might happen is a possibility that cannot be foreseen in an individual case.

Similarly, a serious medical problem may justify subjecting the patient to a serious risk. (Gaining the consent of the patient is an obvious consideration, however.) A life-threatening condition, such as an occluded right coronary artery, may warrant coronary-bypass surgery, with all its attendant dangers.

In effect, the principle of nonmaleficence tells us to avoid needless risk and, when risk is an inevitable aspect of an appropriate diagnostic test or treatment, to minimize the risk as much as is reasonably possible. A physician who orders a lumbar puncture for a patient who complains of occasional headaches is acting inappropriately, given the nature of the complaint, and is subjecting his patient to needless risk. By contrast, a physician who orders such a test after examining a patient who has severe and recurring headaches, a fever, pain and stiffness in the neck, and additional key clinical signs is acting appropriately. The risk to the patient from the lumbar puncture is the same in both cases, but the risk is warranted in the second case and not in the first. A failure to act with due care violates the principle of nonmaleficence, even if no harm results, whereas acting with due care does not violate the principle, even if harm does result.

THE PRINCIPLE OF BENEFICENCE

"As to diseases, make a habit of two things—to help or at least to do no harm." This directive from the Hippocratic writings stresses that the physician has two duties. The second of them ("at least to do no harm") we discussed in connection with the principle of nonmaleficence. The first of them ("to help") we will consider here in connection with the principle of beneficence.

Like the previous principle, the principle of beneficence can be stated in various and different ways. Here is one formulation: *We should act in ways that promote the welfare of other people.* That is, we should help other people when we are able to do so.

Some philosophers have expressed doubt that we have an actual duty to help others. We certainly have a duty not to harm other people, but it has seemed to some that there are no grounds for saying that we have a duty to promote their welfare. We would deserve praise if we did, but we would not deserve blame if we did not. From this point of view, being beneficent is beyond the scope of duty.

We need not consider whether this view is correct in general. For our purposes, it is enough to realize that the nature of the relationship between a physician and a patient does impose the duty of acting in the patient's welfare. That is, the duty of beneficence is inherent in the role of physician. A physician who was not acting for the sake of the patient's good would, in a very real sense, not be acting as a physician.

That we recognize this as a duty appropriate to the physician's role is seen most clearly in cases in which the physician is also a researcher and the patient is also an experimental subject. In such instances, there is a possibility of a role conflict, for the researcher's aim of acquiring knowledge is not always compatible with the physician's aim of helping the patient. (See Chapter 5 for a discussion of this problem.)

The duty required by the principle of beneficence is inherent in the role not only of physicians but of all health professionals. Nurses, therapists, clinical psychologists, social workers, and others accept the duty of promoting the welfare of their patients or clients as an appropriate part of their responsibilities. We expect nurses and others to do good for us, and it is this expectation that leads us to designate them as belonging to what are often called "the helping professions."

The extent to which beneficence is required as a duty for physicians and others is not a matter easily resolved. In practice, we recognize that there are limits to what can be expected from even those who have chosen to make a career of helping others. We do not expect physicians to sacrifice completely their self-interest and welfare on behalf of their patients. We do not think their duty demands that they be totally selfless. If some are, we may praise them as secular saints or moral heroes, but that is because they go beyond the demands of duty. At the same time, we would have little good to say of a physician who always put her interest above that of her patients, who never made a personal sacrifice to serve their interests.

Just as there are standards of due care that explicitly and implicitly define what we consider to be right conduct in protecting patients from harm, so there seem to be implicit standards of beneficence. We obviously expect physicians to help patients by providing them with appropriate treatment. More than this, we expect physicians to be prepared to make *reasonable* sacrifices for the sake of their patients. Even in the age of "health-care teams," a single physician assumes responsibility for a particular patient when the patient is hospitalized or treated for a serious illness. It is this physician who is expected to make the crucial medical decisions, and we expect him or her to realize that discharging that responsibility may involve an interruption of private plans and activities. A surgeon who is informed that her postoperative patient has started to bleed can be expected to cancel her plan to attend a concert. Doing so is a reasonable duty imposed by the principle of beneficence. If she failed to discharge the duty, in the absence of mitigating circumstances, she would become the object of disapproval by her patient and by her medical colleagues.

It would be very difficult to spell out exactly what duties are required by the principle of beneficence. Even if we limited ourselves to the medical context, there are so many ways of promoting someone's welfare and so many different circumstances to consider that it would be virtually impossible to provide anything like a catalogue of appropriate actions. However, such a catalogue is hardly necessary. Most people most often have a sense of what is reasonable and what is not, and it is this sense that we rely on in making judgments about whether physicians and others are fulfilling the duty of beneficence in their actions.

The principles of nonmaleficence and beneficence impose social duties also. In the most general terms, we look to society to take measures to promote the health and safety of its citizens. The great advances made in public health during the nineteenth century were made because the society recognized a responsibility to attempt to prevent the spread of disease. Water-treatment plants, immunization programs, and quarantine restrictions were all in recognition of society's duty of nonmaleficence.

These and similar programs have been continued and augmented, and our society has also recognized a duty of beneficence in connection with health care. The Medicaid program for the poor and Medicare for the elderly are major efforts to see to at least some of the health needs of a large segment of the population. Prenatal programs for expectant mothers and public clinics are among the other social responses we have made to promote the health of citizens.

Less obvious than programs that provide direct medical care are ones that support medical research and basic science. Directly or indirectly, such programs contribute to meeting the health needs of our society. Much basic research is relevant to acquiring an understanding of the processes involved in both health and disease, and much medical research is specifically aimed at the development of effective diagnostic and therapeutic measures.

In principle, social beneficence has no limits, but, in practice, it must. Social resources like tax revenues are in restricted supply, and the society must decide how they are to be spent. Housing and food for the poor, education, defense, the arts, and the humanities are just some of the areas demanding support in the name of social beneficence. Medical care is just one among many claimants, and we must decide as a society what proportion of our social resources we want to commit to medical care. Are we prepared to guarantee to all whatever medical care they need? Are we willing to endorse only a basic level of care? Do we want to say that what is available to some (the rich or well-insured) must be available to all (the poor and uninsured)? Just how beneficent we wish to be—and can afford to be—is a matter still under discussion (see Chapter 10).

THE PRINCIPLE OF UTILITY

The principle of utility can be formulated in this way: *We should act in such a way as to bring about the greatest benefit and the least harm.* As we discussed earlier, the principle is the very foundation of the moral theory of utilitarianism. However, the principle need not be regarded as unique to utilitarianism. It can be thought of as one moral principle among others that presents us with a prima facie duty, and as such it need not be regarded as always taking precedence over others. In particular, we would never think it was justified to deprive someone of a right, even if by doing so we could bring benefit to many others.

We need not repeat the discussion of the principle of utility presented earlier, but it may be useful to consider here how the principle relates to the principles of nonmaleficence and beneficence. When we consider the problem of distributing social resources, it becomes clear that acting in accordance with the principles of nonmaleficence and beneficence usually involves tradeoffs. To use our earlier example, as a society we are concerned with providing for the health-care needs of our citizens. To accomplish this end, we support various programs —Medicare, Medicaid, hospital-building programs, medical research, and so on.

However, there are limits to what we can do. Medical care is not the only concern of our society. We are interested in protecting people from harm and in promoting their interests, but there are many forms of harm and many kinds of interest to be promoted. With finite resources at our disposal, the more money we spend on health care, the less we can spend on education, the arts, the humanities, and so on.

Even if we decided to spend more money on health care than we are currently spending, there would come a point at which we would receive only a marginal return for our money. General health would eventually reach such a level that it would be difficult to raise it still higher. To save even one additional life, we would have to spend a vast sum of money. By contrast, at the start of a health-care program, relatively little money can make a relatively big difference. Furthermore, money spent for marginal improvements would be directed away from other needs that had become even more crucial because of underfunding. Thus, we could not spend all our resources on health care without ignoring other social needs.

The aim of social planning is to balance the competing needs of the society. Taken alone, the principles of nonmaleficence and beneficence are of no help in resolving the conflicts among social needs. The principle of utility must come into play to establish and rank

needs and to serve as a guide for determining to what extent it is possible to satisfy one social need in comparison with others. In effect, the principle imposes a social duty on us all to use our resources to do as much good as possible. That is, we must do the most good *overall*, even when this means we are not able to meet all needs in a particular area.

The application of the principle of utility is not limited to large-scale social issues, such as how to divide our resources among medical care, defense, education, and so on. We may also rely on the principle when we are deliberating about the choice of alternative means of accomplishing an aim. For example, we might decide to institute a mandatory screening program to detect infants with phenylketonuria (PKU) but decide against a program to detect those with Tay-Sachs. PKU can often be treated successfully if discovered early enough, whereas early detection of Tay-Sachs makes little or no difference in the outcome of the disease. Furthermore, PKU is distributed in the general population, whereas Tay-Sachs occurs mostly in a special segment of the population. In general, then, the additional money spent on screening for Tay-Sachs would not be justified by the results. The money could do more good, producing more benefits, were it spent some other way.

The principle of utility is also relevant to making decisions about the diagnosis and treatment of individuals. For example, as we mentioned earlier, no diagnostic test can be justified if it causes the patient more risk than the information likely to be gained is worth. Invasive procedures are associated with a certain rate of injury and death (morbidity and mortality). It would make no sense to subject a patient to a kidney biopsy if the findings were not likely to affect the course of treatment or if the risk from the biopsy were greater than the risk of the suspected disease itself.

Attempts are well underway in medicine to employ the formal theories of decision analysis to assist physicians in determining whether a particular mode of diagnosis, therapy, or surgery can be justified in individual cases. Underlying the details of formal analysis is the principle of utility, which directs us to act in a way that will bring about the greatest benefit and the least harm.

PRINCIPLES OF DISTRIBUTIVE JUSTICE

We expect (and can demand) to be treated justly in our dealings with other people and with institutions. If our insurance policy covers up to thirty days of hospitalization, then we expect a claim against the policy for that amount of time to be honored. If we arrive in an emergency room with a broken arm before the arrival of someone else with a broken arm, we expect to be attended to before that person.

We do not always expect that being treated justly will work to our direct advantage. Although we would prefer to keep all the money we earn, we realize that we must pay our share of taxes. If a profusely bleeding person arrives in the emergency room after we do, we recognize that he is in need of immediate treatment and should be attended to before we are.

Justice has at least two major aspects. Seeing to it that people receive that to which they are entitled, that their rights are recognized and protected, falls under the general heading of *noncomparative justice*. By contrast, *comparative justice* is concerned with the application of laws and rules and with the distribution of burdens and benefits.

The concern of comparative justice that is most significant to the medical context is *distributive justice*. As the name suggests, distributive justice concerns the distribution of such social benefits and burdens as medical services, welfare payments, public offices, taxes, and military service. In general, the distribution of income has been the focus of recent discussions of distributive justice. In medical ethics, the focus has been the distribution of health care. Is everyone in the society entitled to receive health-care benefits, whether or not she or he can pay for them? If so, then is

everyone entitled to the same amount of health care? (See Chapter 10 for a discussion of this issue.)

Philosophical theories of justice attempt to resolve questions of distributive justice by providing a detailed account of the features of individuals and society that will justify our making distinctions in the ways we distribute benefits and burdens. If some people are to be rich and others poor, if some are to rule and others serve, then there must be some rational and moral basis for such distinctions. We look to theories of justice to provide us with such a basis. (See the earlier discussion of John Rawls's theory for an outstanding recent example.)

Theories of justice differ significantly, but at the core of all theories is the basic principle that "Similar cases ought to be treated in similar ways." The principle expresses the notion that justice involves fairness of treatment. For example, it is manifestly unfair to award two different grades to two people who score the same on a multiple-choice exam. If two cases are the same, then it is arbitrary or irrational to treat them differently. To justify different treatment, we would have to show that in some relevant respect the cases are also dissimilar.

This fairness principle is known as the *formal* principle of justice. It is called "formal" because, like a sentence with blanks, it must be filled in with information. Specifically, we must be told what factors or features are to be considered *relevant* in deciding whether or not two cases are similar. If two cases differ in *relevant* respects, we may be justified in treating them differently. We may do so without being either irrational or arbitrary.

Theories of distributive justice present us with *substantive* (or *material*) principles of justice. The theories present us with arguments to show why certain features or factors should be considered relevant in deciding whether cases are similar. The substantive principles can then be referred to in determining whether particular laws, practices, or public policies can be considered just. Further, the substantive principles can be employed as guidelines for framing laws and policies and for developing a just society.

Arguments in favor of particular theories of justice are too lengthy to present here. However, it is useful to consider briefly four substantive principles that have been offered by various theorists as ones worthy of acceptance. To a considerable extent, differences among these principles help explain present disagreements in our society about the ways in which such social "goods" as income, education, and health care should be distributed. Although the principles themselves direct the distribution of burdens (taxation, public service, and so on) as well as benefits, we will focus on benefits. The basic question answered by each principle is "Who is entitled to what proportion of society's goods?"

The Principle of Equality

According to the principle of equality, all benefits and burdens are to be distributed equally. Everyone is entitled to the same size slice of the pie, and everyone must bear an equal part of the social load. The principle, strictly interpreted, requires a radical egalitarianism—everyone is to be treated the same in all respects.

The principle is most plausible for a society above the margin of production. When there is enough to go around but not much more, then it is manifestly unfair for some to have more than they need and for others to have less than they need. When a society is more affluent, the principle may lose some of its persuasiveness. When greater efforts by a few produce more goods than the efforts of the ordinary person, it may be unfair not to recognize the accomplishments of a few with greater rewards. Rawls's theory remains an egalitarian one while providing a way to resolve this apparent conflict. According to Rawls, any departure from equality is arbitrary, unless it can be shown that the inequality will work out to everyone's advantage.

The Principle of Need

The principle of need is an extension of the egalitarian principle of equal distribution. If goods are parceled out according to individual need, those who have greater needs will receive a greater share. However, the outcome will be one of equality. Since the basic needs of everyone will be met, everyone will end up at the same level. The treatment of individuals will be equal, in this respect, even though the proportion of goods they receive will not be.

What is to count as a need is a significant question that cannot be answered by a principle of distribution alone. Obviously, basic biological needs (food, clothing, shelter) must be included, but what about psychological or intellectual needs? The difficulty of resolving the question of needs is seen in the fact that—even in our affluent society, the richest in the history of the world—we are still debating the question of whether health care should be available to all.

The Principle of Contribution

According to the principle of contribution, everyone should get back that proportion of social goods that is the result of his or her productive labor. If two people work to grow potatoes and the first works twice as long or twice as hard as the second, then the first should be entitled to twice as large a share of the harvest.

The difficulty with this principle in an industrialized, capitalistic society is that contributions to production can take forms other than time and labor. Some people risk their money in investments needed to make production possible, and others contribute crucial ideas or inventions. How are comparisons to be made? Furthermore, in highly industrialized societies it is the functioning of the entire system, rather than the work of any particular individual, that creates the goods to be distributed. A single individual's claim on the outcome of the whole system may be very small.

Nonetheless, it is individuals who make the system work, so it does seem just that individuals should benefit from their contributions. If it is true that it is the system of social organization itself that is most responsible for creating the goods, then this is an argument for supporting the system through taxation and other means. If individual contributions count for relatively little (although for something), there may be no real grounds for attempting to distinguish among them in distributing social benefits.

The Principle of Effort

According to the principle of effort, the degree of effort made by the individual should determine the proportion of goods received by the individual. Thus, the file clerk who works just as hard as the president of a company should receive the same proportion of social goods as the president. Those who are lazy and refuse to exert themselves will receive proportionally less than those who work hard.

The advantage of the principle is that it captures our sense of what is fair—that those who do their best should be similarly rewarded, while those who do less than their best should be less well rewarded. The principle assumes that people have equal opportunities to do their best and that if they do not it is their own fault. One difficulty with this assumption is that, even if the society presents equal opportunities, nature does not. Some people are born with handicaps or meet with accidents, and their misfortunes may make it difficult for them to want to do their best, even when they are given the opportunity.

Each principle has its shortcomings, but this does not mean that adjustments cannot be made to correct their weaknesses. A complete theory of justice need not be limited in the number of principles that it accepts, and it is doubtful that any theory can be shown to be both fair and plausible if it restricts itself to only one principle. Although all theories require

adjustment, theories fall into types in accordance with the principles they emphasize. For example, Marxist theories select need as basic, while libertarian theories stress personal contribution as the grounds for distribution. Utilitarian theories employ that combination of principles that promises to maximize both private and public interests.

Joel Feinberg, to whom the preceding discussion is indebted, may be mentioned as an example of a careful theorist who recommends the adoption of a combination of principles. Feinberg sees the principle of equality based on needs as the basic determination of distributive justice. After basic needs have been satisfied, the principles of contribution and effort should be given the most weight.

According to Feinberg, when there is an economic abundance, then the claim to "minimally decent conditions" can reasonably be made for every person in the society. To have one's basic needs satisfied under such conditions amounts to a fundamental right. However, when everyone's basic needs are taken care of and society produces a surplus of goods, then considerations of contribution and effort become relevant. Those who contribute most to the increase of goods or those who work hardest to produce it (or some combination) can legitimately lay claim to a greater share.

The principles of justice we have discussed may seem at first to be intolerably abstract and thus irrelevant to the practical business of society. However, it is important to keep in mind that it is by referring to such principles that we criticize our society and its laws and practices. The claim that society is failing to meet some basic need of all of its citizens and that this is unfair or unjust is a powerful charge. It can be a call to action in the service of justice. If the claim can be demonstrated, it has more than rhetorical power. It imposes upon us all an obligation to eliminate the source of the injustice.

Similarly, in framing laws and formulating policies, we expect those who occupy the offices of power and influence to make their decisions in accordance with principles. Prominent among these must be principles of justice. It may be impossible in the conduct of daily business to apply any principle directly or exclusively, for we can hardly remake our society overnight. Yet if we are committed to a just society, then the principles of justice can at least serve as guidelines when policy decisions are made. They remind us that it is not always fair for the race to go to the swift.

THE PRINCIPLE OF AUTONOMY

The principle of autonomy can be stated this way: *Rational individuals should be permitted to be self-determining.* According to this formulation, we act autonomously when our actions are the result of our own choices and decisions. Thus, autonomy and self-determination are equivalent.

Autonomy is associated with the status we ascribe to rational beings as persons in the morally relevant sense. We are committed to the notion that persons are by their very nature uniquely qualified to decide what is in their own best interest. This is because, to use Kant's terms, they are ends in themselves, not means to some other end. As such, they have an inherent worth, and it is the duty of others to respect that worth and avoid treating them as though they were just ordinary parts of the world to be manipulated according to the will of someone else. A recognition of autonomy is a recognition of that inherent worth, and a violation of autonomy is a violation of our concept of what it is to be a person. To deny someone autonomy is to treat her or him as something less than a person.

This view of the nature of autonomy and its connection with our recognition of what is involved in being a person is shared by several significant moral theories. At the core of each theory is the concept of the rational individual as a moral agent who, along with other moral agents, possesses an unconditional worth. Moral responsibility itself is based on the as-sumption that such agents are free to determine their own actions and pursue their own aims.

Autonomy is significant not only because it is a condition for moral responsibility, but because it is through the exercise of autonomy that individuals shape their lives. We might not approve of what people do with their lives. It is sad to see talent wasted and opportunities for personal development rejected. Nevertheless, as we sometimes say, "It's *his* life." We recognize that people are entitled to attempt to make their lives what they want them to be and that it would be wrong for us to take control of their lives and dictate their actions, even if we could. We recognize that a person must walk to heaven or hell by his own freely chosen path.

Simply put, to act autonomously is to decide for oneself what to do. Of course, decisions are never made outside of a context, and the world and the people in it exert influence, impose constraints, and restrict opportunities. It is useful to call attention to three interrelated aspects of autonomy in order to get a better understanding of the ways in which autonomy can be exercised, denied, and restricted. We will look at autonomy in the contexts of actions, options, and decision making.

Autonomy and Actions

Consider the following situations:

A police officer shoves a demonstrator off the sidewalk during an abortion protest.

An attendant in a psychiatric ward warns a patient to stay in bed or be strapped down.

A corrections officer warns a prison inmate that if he does not donate blood he will not be allowed out of his cell to eat dinner.

A state law requires that anyone admitted to a hospital be screened for the AIDS antibody.

In each of these situations, either actual force, the threat of force, or potential penalties are employed to direct the actions of an individual toward some end. All involve some form of coercion, and the coercion is used to restrict the freedom of individuals to act as they might choose.

Under such circumstances, the individual ceases to be the agent who initiates the action as a result of his or her choice. The individual's initiative is set aside, wholly or partially, in favor of someone else's.

Autonomy is violated in such cases even if the individual intends to act in the way that is imposed or demanded. Perhaps the prison inmate would have donated blood anyway, and surely some people would have wanted to be screened for AIDS. However, the use of coercion makes the wishes or intentions of the individual partly or totally irrelevant to whether the act is performed.

Autonomy as the initiation of action through one's own intention and choice can clearly be restricted to a greater or lesser degree. Someone who is physically forced to become a subject in a medical experiment, as in a Nazi concentration camp, is totally deprived of autonomy. The same is true of someone tricked into becoming a subject without knowing it. In the infamous Tuskegee syphilis studies, some participants were led to believe that they were receiving appropriate medical treatment, when in fact they were part of a control group in the experiment. The situation is somewhat different for someone who agrees to become a subject in order to receive needed medical care. Such a person is acting under strong coercion, but the loss of autonomy is not complete. It is at least possible to refuse to participate, even if the cost of doing so may be extremely high.

In situations more typical than those above, autonomy may be compromised rather than denied. For example, someone who is by nature nonassertive or someone who is poor and uneducated may find it very difficult to preserve his power of self-determination when he becomes a patient in a hospital. Medical authority, represented by physicians and the hospital staff, may be so intimidating to such a person that he does not feel free to exercise his autonomy. In such a case, although no one may be deliberately attempting to infringe on the patient's autonomy, social and psychological factors may constitute a force so coercive that the patient feels he has no choice but to do what he is told.

Autonomy and Options

Autonomy involves more than freedom from duress in making decisions. There must be genuine possibilities to decide among. A forced option is no option at all, and anyone who is in the position of having to take what she can get can hardly be regarded as self-determining or as exercising free choice.

In our society, economic and social conditions frequently limit the options available in medical care. As a rule, the poor simply do not have the same choices available to them as the rich. Someone properly insured or financially well off who might be helped by a heart transplant can decide whether or not to undergo the risk of having one. That is an option not generally available to someone who is uninsured and poor.

Similarly, a woman who depends on Medicaid and lives in a state in which Medicaid funds cannot be used to pay for abortions may not have the option of having an abortion. Her choice is not a genuine one, for she lacks the means to implement it. The situation is quite different for a middle-class woman faced with the same question. She may decide against having an abortion, but, whatever she decides, the choice is real. She is autonomous in a way that the poor woman is not.

Those who believe that one of the goals of our society is to promote and protect the autonomy of individuals have frequently argued that we must do more to offer all individuals the same range of health-care options. If we do not, they have suggested, then our society cannot be one in which everyone has an equal degree of autonomy. In a very real sense, those who are rich will have greater freedom of action than those who are poor.

Autonomy and Decision Making

More is involved in decision making than merely saying yes or no. In particular, relevant information is an essential condition for genuine decision making. We are exercising our autonomy in the fullest sense only when we are making *informed* decisions.

It is pointless to have options if we are not aware of them, and we can hardly be said to be directing the course of our lives if our decisions must be made in ignorance of information that is available and relevant to our choices. These are the reasons that lying and other forms of deception are so destructive of autonomy. If someone with a progressive and ordinarily fatal disease is not told about it by her physician, then she is in no position to decide how to shape what remains of her life. The lack of a crucial piece of information—that she is dying—is likely to lead her to make decisions different from the ones she would make were she in possession of the information.

Information is the key to protecting and preserving autonomy in most medical situations. A patient who is not informed of alternative forms of treatment and their associated risks is denied the opportunity to make his own wishes and values count for something in his own life. For example, someone with coronary artery disease who is not told of the relative merits of medical treatment with drugs but is told only that he is a candidate for coronary-artery bypass surgery, is in no position to decide what risks he wishes to take and what ordeals he is prepared to undergo. A physician who does not supply the patient with the information the patient needs is restricting the patient's autonomy. The principle of autonomy requires *informed* consent, for consent alone does not involve genuine self-determination.

Making decisions for "the good" of others (paternalism), without consulting their wishes, deprives them of their status as autonomous agents. For example, some people at the final stages of a terminal illness might prefer to be allowed to die without heroic intervention, while others might prefer to prolong their lives as long as medical skills and technological powers make possible. If a physician or family undertakes to make a decision in this matter on behalf of the patient, then, no matter what their motive, they are denying to the patient the power of self-determination.

Because autonomy is so bound up with informed consent and decision making, special problems arise in the case of those unable to give consent and make decisions. Patients who are comatose, severely brain-damaged, psychotic, or seriously mentally impaired are not capable of making decisions on their own behalf. The nature of their condition has already deprived them of their autonomy. Of course this does not mean that they have no status as moral persons or that they have no interests. It falls to others to see that their interests are served.

The situation is similar for those, such as infants and young children, who are incapable of understanding. Any consent that is given must be given by others. But what are the limits of consent that can be legitimately given for some other person? Consenting to needed medical care seems legitimate, but what about rejecting needed medical care? What about consenting to becoming a subject in a research program? These questions are as crucial as they are difficult to resolve.

Restrictions on Autonomy

Autonomy is not an absolute or unconditional value. We would regard it as absurd for someone to claim that he was justified in committing a murder because he was only exercising his power of self-determination. Such a defense would be morally ludicrous.

However, we do value autonomy and recognize a general duty to respect it and even to promote its exercise. We demand compelling reasons to justify restricting the power of individuals to make their own choices and direct their own lives.

We will briefly examine four principles that are frequently appealed to in justifying restrictions on autonomy. The principles have been discussed most in the context of social and legal theory, for it is through laws and penalties that a society most directly regulates the conduct of its citizens. However, the principles can also be appealed to to justify policies and practices of institutions (such as hospitals) and the actions of individuals that affect other people.

Appealing to a principle can provide, at best, only a prima facie justification. Even if a principle can be shown to apply to a particular case in which freedom of action is restricted, we may value the lost freedom more than what is gained by restricting it. Reasons suggested by the principle may not be adequately persuasive. Furthermore, the principles themselves are frequently the subjects of controversy, and, with the exception of the harm principle, it is doubtful that any of the principles would be universally endorsed by philosophers and legal theorists.

The Harm Principle. According to the harm principle, we may restrict the freedom of people to act if the restriction is necessary to prevent harm to others. In the most obvious case, we may take action to prevent violence like rape, robbery, killing, or assault. We may act to protect someone who is in apparent risk of harm from the action of someone else. The risk of harm need not be the result of the intention to harm. Thus, we might take steps to see that a surgeon whose skills and judgment have been impaired through drug use is not permitted to operate. The risk that he poses to his patients warrants the effort to keep him from acting as he wishes.

The harm principle may also be used to justify laws that exert coercive force and so restrict freedom of action. Laws against homicide and assault are clear examples, but the principle extends also to the regulation of institutions and practices. People may be robbed at the point of a pen, as well as at the point of a knife, and the harm produced by fraud may be as great as that produced by outright theft. Careless or deceptive medical practitioners may cause direct harm to their patients, and laws that regulate the standards of medical practice restrict the freedom of practitioners for the protection of patients.

The Principle of Paternalism. In its weak version, the principle of paternalism is no more than the harm principle applied to the individual himself. According to the principle, we are justified in restricting someone's freedom to act if doing so is necessary to prevent him from harming himself. Thus, we might force an alcoholic into a treatment program and justify our action by claiming that we did so to prevent him from continuing to harm himself by his drinking.

In its strong version, the principle of paternalism justifies restricting someone's autonomy if by doing so we can benefit her. In such a case, our concern is not only with preventing the person from harming herself, but also with promoting her good in a positive way. The principle might be appealed to even in cases in which our actions go against the other's known wishes. For example, a physician might decide to treat a patient with a placebo (an inactive drug), even if she has asked to be told the truth about her medical condition and her therapy. He might attempt to justify his action by claiming that if the patient knew she was receiving a placebo, then the placebo would be less likely to be effective. Since taking the placebo while believing that it is an active drug makes her feel better, the physician may claim that by deceiving her he is doing something to help her.

Paternalism may be expressed in laws and public policies, as well as in private actions. Some have pointed to the drug laws as a prime example of governmental paternalism. By making certain drugs illegal and inaccessible and by placing other drugs under the control of physicians, the laws aim to protect people from themselves. Self-medication is virtually eliminated, and the so-called recreational use of drugs is prohibited. The price for such laws is a restriction on individual autonomy. Some have argued that the price is too high and that the most the government should do is warn and educate the individual about the consequences of using certain drugs.

The Principle of Legal Moralism. The principle of legal moralism holds that a legitimate function of the law is to enforce morality by turning the immoral into the illegal. Hence, the restrictions placed on actions by the law are justified by the presumed fact that the actions are immoral and so ought not to be performed.

To a considerable extent, laws express the values of a society and the society's judgments about what is morally right. In our society, homicide and theft are recognized as crimes, and those who commit them are guilty of legal, as well as moral, wrongdoing. Society attempts to prevent such crimes and to punish offenders.

The degree to which the law should embody moral judgments is a hard question. It is particularly difficult to answer in a pluralistic society like ours, in which there may be sharp differences of opinion about the moral legitimacy of some actions. Until quite recently, for example, materials considered obscene could not be freely purchased, birth-control literature could not be freely distributed nor contraceptives legally prescribed in some states, and the conditions of divorce were generally stringent and punitive. Even now many states outlaw homosexual solicitation and acts, and prostitution is generally illegal. The foundation for such laws is the belief by many that the practices proscribed are morally wrong.

The current heated debate over abortion reflects, in some of its aspects, the conflict between those who favor strong legal moralism and those who oppose it. Many who consider abortion morally wrong would also like to see it made illegal once more. Others, even though they may oppose abortion, believe that it is a private moral matter and that the attempt to regulate it by law is an unwarranted intrusion of state power.

The Welfare Principle. The welfare principle holds that it is justifiable to restrict individual autonomy if doing so will result in providing benefits to others. Those who endorse this principle are not inclined to think that it demands a serious self-sacrifice for the welfare of others. Rather, in their view, an ideal application of the principle would be the case in which we give up just a little autonomy to bring about a great deal of benefit to others.

For example, transplant organs are in short supply at the moment because their availability depends mostly on their being freely donated. The situation could be dramatically changed by a law requiring that organs from the recently dead be salvaged and made available for use as transplants.

Such a law would end the present system of voluntary donation, and by doing so it would restrict our freedom to decide what is to be done with our bodies after death. However, it would be easy to argue that the tremendous value that others might gain from such a law easily outweighs the slight restriction on autonomy that it would involve.

These four principles are not the only ones that offer grounds for abridging the autonomy of individuals, but they are the most relevant to decision making and policy planning in medicine. It is important to keep in mind that merely appealing to a principle is not enough to warrant a limit on autonomy. A principle points in the direction of an argument, but it is no substitute for one. The high value we place on autonomy gives its preservation a high priority, and compelling considerations are required to justify compromising it. In the view of some philosophers, who endorse the position taken by Mill, only the harm principle can serve as grounds for legitimately restricting autonomy. Other theorists find persuasive reasons to do so in other principles.

PART III.   RETROSPECT

The two major tasks of this chapter have been to provide information about several important ethical theories and to formulate and illustrate several generally accepted moral principles. One aim in performing these tasks was to make it easier to follow the arguments and discussions in the selections that make up the major part of this book.

Another, and ultimately more serious, aim has been to call attention to ethical theories and principles you may wish to consider adopting. From this standpoint, the problems and issues presented in the selections can be considered test cases for the theories and principles. You may find that some of the theories that we have discussed are inadequate to deal with certain moral issues in the medical context, although they may seem satisfactory in more common or simpler cases. Or you may discover that certain commonly accepted moral principles lead to contradictory results or to conclusions that you find difficult to accept. Other theories or principles may appear to give definite and persuasive answers to medical-moral problems, but you may find that they rest on assumptions that it does not appear reasonable to accept. Such a dialectical process of claims

and criticism is slow and frustrating. Yet it offers the best hope of settling on theories and principles that we can accept with confidence and employ without misgivings.

During the last ten years, a great amount of effort has been expended addressing the moral problems of medical practice and research. Without question, progress has been made in developing a better understanding of a number of issues and securing agreement about how they are to be dealt with. Nevertheless, a large number of moral issues in medicine remain unsettled or even unexplored. Even in the absence of moral consensus on these issues, the demands of practical decision making generate a force that presses us for immediate solutions.

In such a situation, we cannot afford to try to settle all doubts about moral principles in an abstract way and only then apply them to problems in medicine. The dialectical process must be made practical. Formulating and testing theories and principles must go on at the same time as we are actually making moral decisions. We must do our best to discover the principles of aerodynamics while staying aloft.

To a considerable extent, that is what this book is about. Positions are taken and defended by the authors. But they, too, are aware that they are participating in a search for a satisfactory resolution to the problems they discuss, and few, if any, would regard their solutions as beyond criticism. Medical ethics is still an area in which there are more legitimate questions than there are satisfactory answers, but the answers that we do have are better supported and better reasoned than those available even ten years ago.

PART I

TERMINATION

CHAPTER 1

ABORTION

SOCIAL CONTEXT: THE *WEBSTER* DECISION AND THE CONTINUING ABORTION BATTLE

The Background: *Roe* v. *Wade*

Norma McCorvey of Dallas was unmarried, poor, and pregnant. She wished to have an abortion, but under Texas law abortion was a criminal offense, except when required to save the woman's life. California law was less restrictive and McCorvey believed she could get an abortion there; however, she lacked money for travel and expenses. Unwillingly, she bowed to legal and economic necessity and carried the fetus to term. She then gave up the newborn child for adoption.

When McCorvey was later approached by a public-interest attorney and asked if she would agree to be the plaintiff in a class-action suit against Henry Wade, the District Attorney of Dallas County, challenging the constitutionality of the Texas abortion law, she readily consented. Federal courts ruled that the Texas statute was void, but Wade appealed to the Supreme Court.

McCorvey wished her identity to be protected by a pseudonym, so the 1973 Supreme Court decision in the case was titled *Roe* v. *Wade*. In a 7-to-2 decision, written by Justice Harry A. Blackmun, the Court found the Texas

law unconstitutional. In doing so, the Court effectively decriminalized abortion, for abortion laws in most other states differed little from the Texas statute.

The *Roe* decision did not require that abortion be unregulated, but it placed limits on the restrictions states could impose. According to the ruling, during the first twelve weeks (the first trimester) of pregnancy, states cannot restrict a woman's decision about abortion. During the second trimester, states may restrict abortion to protect the health of the woman. In the final trimester, because the fetus may be considered viable, states may limit abortions to those necessary to preserve the health of the woman.

After the *Roe* decision, abortions became easily obtainable by most women who wanted them. Yet the decision also triggered a firestorm of controversy between proponents of relatively unregulated choice ("prochoice" advocates) and opponents of so-called abortion on demand ("prolife" or "right-to-life" advocates) that shows no sign of dying down. While those who favored making abortion a matter of individual decision were pleased by the *Roe* decision, those morally opposed to abortion were not.

Many, if not most, who believe abortion is morally wrong also think it should be illegal, except in very special cases. Within the limits of regulation imposed by the *Roe* decision, opponents of abortion took various legal measures to attempt to slow or halt its practice. Opponents of abortion became politically active, and requirements that abortions be performed in hospitals, that women considering abortions be given counseling or information, and that a waiting period be instituted between a patient's decision and the procedure were some of the legal methods proposed to make it difficult to secure abortions. When opponents of abortion were successful in getting such restrictions written into laws in states like Pennsylvania, the Supreme Court struck down the laws as unconstitutional.

Webster v. Reproductive Health Services

The Missouri law in the *Webster* case is similar to those the Supreme Court had previously held to be void. However, because of new appointees during the Reagan administration, the political character of the Court had changed. Also, the law had been carefully crafted to avoid the specific difficulties that had led the Court to reject earlier arguments. To a considerable extent, the law was the result of the efforts of Missouri right-to-life activists Lee and Andrew Puzder.

Lee was arrested in 1979 for trespassing in connection with sit-ins at abortion clinics, and Andrew, an attorney, managed to keep him out of jail until 1983. At that time, he was sentenced to 314 days for violating an injunction to stay clear of abortion facilities. Lee was assigned to a work-release program, and during the day he began going to a law library to study the past Supreme Court decisions on abortion. He and Andrew then wrote a draft of a bill restricting abortion that they believed would be accepted by the majority of the Court.

Prolife advocates in the Missouri legislature approved of the bill and in 1986 succeeded in getting it passed into law. Reproductive Health Services, a private organization, challenged the constitutionality of the law in Federal District Court, but the ruling upheld the

law, finding in favor of Missouri Attorney General William Webster. The Eighth Circuit Court of Appeals agreed with the lower court's decision, and the case was then appealed to the Supreme Court.

The character of the law is indicated by its preamble, asserting that "life begins at conception," but at issue in the Court dispute were three provisions of the law restricting abortion:

1. Public employees, including physicians, nurses, technicians, or other health-care providers, are forbidden to perform or assist in performing an abortion, except when necessary to save a woman's life.

2. Public hospitals, clinics, or other tax-supported facilities cannot be used to perform abortions not necessary to save a woman's life, even if no public funds are involved.

3. Physicians are required to perform tests to determine the viability of a fetus, if they have reason to believe the woman has been pregnant for at least twenty weeks.

On July 3, 1989, the Supreme Court, in a 5-to-4 decision, upheld the constitutionality of the Missouri law. Chief Justice William Rehnquist, writing the majority opinion, held that the Court did not have to rule against the claim in the law's preamble that life begins at conception, for such language is an expression of a permissible value judgment not limited to abortion. Furthermore, he argued, "Nothing in the Constitution requires States to enter or remain in the business of performing abortions. Nor . . . do private physicians and their patients have some kind of constitutional right of access to public facilities for the performance of abortions."

So far as viability is concerned, Rehnquist saw a problem, not with the Missouri law but with *Roe* v. *Wade*'s "rigid trimester analysis of the course of a pregnancy." That is, the Missouri law he found more sensitive to the issue of viability than the trimester rule, which holds that the state can regulate abortion after the point of viability. Furthermore, "the key elements" of *Roe* v. *Wade* are "not found in the text of the Constitution or in any place else one would expect to find a constitutional principle."

Justice Harry A. Blackmun, the author of the majority opinion in *Roe* v. *Wade,* wrote the dissenting opinion in *Webster.* He made clear that he regarded the Court's decision as an outright attack on *Roe.* "The plurality [of this Court] repudiates every principle for which *Roe* stands. . . . I fear for the future. I fear for the liberty and equality of the millions of women who have lived and come of age in the sixteen years since *Roe* was decided. I fear for the integrity of, and public esteem for, this Court."

Rehnquist, he argued, failed to consider the case for viability an appropriate grounds —namely, the right to privacy, on which *Roe* and its successors were decided. Instead, he misread the Missouri law in a way that seemed to conflict with the trimester structure established in *Roe* to balance the state's interest in maternal health and potential life against the right to privacy.

In the end, Blackmun claims, the decision is "deceptive" and "filled with winks and nods at those who would do away with *Roe* explicitly." The decision is an example of "because we say so" reasoning.

Blackmun sees the decision as heralding bleak times. It "casts into darkness the hopes and visions of every woman in the country who had come to believe that the Constitution guaranteed her the right to exercise some control over her unique ability to bear children."

Consequences

The hope of abortion opponents was that the Supreme Court would use the *Webster* case to overturn *Roe* v. *Wade.* The Court stopped short of doing this, but the *Webster* decision made it clear that the Court is willing to accept state and local restrictions on abortion of a sort that it held to be unconstitutional during the previous sixteen years. Consequently, both abortion opponents and rights advocates expect debate over the next few years to move to the area of state and local politics.

Abortion opponents are pleased with the trend toward more regulation. In their view, the fewer abortions, the more fetal lives saved. By contrast, prochoice advocates see additional regulations as portending disaster. The regulations will explicitly restrict the rights of women to control their reproductive power and will put much of the decision-making power in the hands of others.

Furthermore, prochoice advocates hold, many women will be kept from having abortions for practical reasons. Even private institutions typically receive some tax money, so a law like Missouri's would severely restrict the number of places an abortion could be performed. In big cities this might not be much of a problem. In smaller towns and rural areas, however, if local physicians refused to perform abortions in their offices, then a woman seeking an abortion would have to travel elsewhere.

This would also be true if, as is expected, some states pass laws requiring that abortions be performed only in highly equipped clinics. Such requirements as these will increase the cost of abortion, and this too will make abortion available to fewer women.

The Missouri law further requires that, if physicians suspect a fetus is at least twenty weeks old, they perform tests to determine its viability. Other states are expected to pass similar laws. However, tests of the type mandated are hardly reliable for the purpose intended and add costs and hazards to an abortion.

Sonography can reveal a great deal about fetal development, but it cannot be counted on to determine viability. Similarly, amniocentesis is supposed to reveal the presence of surfactant, indicating that the lungs are sufficiently developed for viability, but in the opinion of many experts amniocentesis cannot provide useful information about lung maturity until around the twenty-eighth week.

Sonography costs about $200, and amniocentesis about $450. Sonography is relatively free of risks, but amniocentesis can cause hemorrhage and infection. Also, the requirement that a test be performed may delay an abortion for a week or more and so significantly increase its cost. Again, this is particularly true for women who are not in urban areas and so are not likely to have easy access either to sonography or to amniocentesis.

Such restrictions are viewed by both prolife and prochoice advocates as roadblocks to abortion. The difference is that one group considers the roadblocks justifiable in terms of the end served (preserving fetal life), while the other considers them unwarranted interference with the exercise of individual autonomy.

The Continuing Trend

On June 25, 1990, the Supreme Court ruled in two other cases concerning abortion: *Hodgson* v. *Minnesota* and *Ohio* v. *Akron Center for Reproductive Health*. In the *Minnesota* case, the Court held in a 5-to-4 decision that a state can require a pregnant teenager to notify both her parents before having an abortion, on the condition that the law provide the alternative of a judicial hearing. In the *Akron* case, the Court upheld by 6-to-3 a law requiring the notification of one parent, as long as a judicial hearing is provided as an alternative.

The Court's decisions in these two cases confirmed the expectation that it would continue to follow the course it had set in *Webster* and let stand laws restricting access to abortion. Most observers believe that over the next few years the Court will agree to consider more such cases to make clear how much of the doctrine of *Roe* v. *Wade* it is willing to accept.

The outcome of battles at the state level will determine the nature of the cases that reach the Supreme Court. Already states like Idaho and Louisiana have attempted to pass highly restrictive abortion legislation, only to have it vetoed by the respective governors. For many abortion opponents, this means that the abortion issue should be made even more political and a candidate's position on abortion should be the central issue in political contests.

Prochoice advocates also see the issues as political in much the same way. In addition, some also advocate the passage of a "reproductive rights" amendment to the Constitution. Only in this way, they believe, can women be sure of protecting the rights that were acknowledged in the *Roe* v. *Wade* decision.

CASE PRESENTATION
The Ordeal of Alice Wilson

Late in the afternoon on a September day, twelve-year-old Alice Wilson (as we will call her) was walking the eight blocks home from the public school she attended. She liked the walk, for the south St. Louis neighborhood she lived in was a generally pleasant place. Large, turn-of-the-century brick houses predominated, and the streets were lined with leafy sycamore trees.

But, like many urban areas, the neighborhood showed signs of decay. Several houses were abandoned, their windows boarded up with unpainted plywood. The streets were littered, and once well-tended front lawns were often hardly more than scraggly patches of weeds.

At the corner of Grand and Hervy, Alice left the well-traveled sidewalk through the business district and crossed the street to Shaw Park. By walking through the park, rather than around it, she could cut the distance to her house almost by half. She wouldn't dare go through the park after dark, but on that bright afternoon the park seemed beautiful and safe. She had walked through the park dozens of times, both alone and with her friends, and had never had any trouble.

That day was different. Alice stayed on the main asphalt path leading across the park and passed by the first picnic area. Then, just beyond that area, she was attacked by three teenage males. They were older and larger than Alice, and she had never seen them before. One grabbed her from behind and put his hand over her mouth so she couldn't scream. Another said they would kill her if she didn't keep quiet. They dragged her off the path and into a place surrounded by bushes. Then all three of them raped her.

Afterward the boys ran from the park, leaving Alice crying on the ground. She eventually recovered enough to dress herself and walk the rest of the way home. When her mother came home from work, Alice told her what had happened. Because Alice seemed to be basically unhurt, except for being frightened and distraught, Mrs. Wilson decided that Alice didn't need medical attention. Alice's father was dead, so Mrs. Wilson was responsible for making decisions about her welfare.

Alice went back to school and resumed her normal life. But not long thereafter she developed a high fever and vaginal pains and discharges. Mrs. Wilson was sufficiently alarmed to take her daughter to the clinic of nearby South General Hospital.

After a physical examination and laboratory tests, Dr. Charles Kranski, a resident at South General working at the clinic, first talked with Alice, then presented the results to Mrs. Wilson. He explained that Alice was in generally good health, but the chances were quite high that she had been infected with gonorrhea as a result of the sexual assault. It would be necessary to wait for a culture to grow to be certain; meanwhile, Alice would be treated with a course of penicillin.

The most troubling news, however, was that Alice was pregnant from the rape. That would be an unfortunate thing to happen for any rape victim, but in Alice's case it was particularly terrible. Dr. Kranski explained that, although Alice was old enough to conceive a child, she was not really old enough to have one. She was simply not sufficiently developed physiologically to undergo pregnancy. She might well have a spontaneous abortion (a miscarriage), but, if she did not, the chances were very good that attempting to have the child might kill her.

Dr. Kranski told Mrs. Wilson that he had discussed Alice's case with two obstetricians and that they both agreed with him that the only reasonable course of action was for Alice to have an abortion as soon as possible. In fact, Dr. Kranski said, as soon as the venereal disease was controlled, he would like to schedule Alice for an abortion for therapeutic reasons. He had already explained the situation to Alice, he said, and she agreed to the abortion. But because she was still a minor, it was necessary to have Mrs. Wilson's consent before the operation could be performed.

To Dr. Kranski's surprise, Mrs. Wilson told him that she would not give her consent. "I belong to the Church of the Spiritual Life," she said. "We follow the commandment 'Thou shall not kill.' "

Thinking that she had not understood the implications of Alice's pregnancy, Dr. Kranski again explained that Alice would probably die unless she had an abortion. Because of Alice's youth and small size, he said, the developing fetus would severely compress her internal organs and perhaps rupture them. If that happened, she would probably bleed to death. Even if that did not happen, she might suffer irreversible liver or kidney damage.

Mrs. Wilson remained totally unmoved. "God will save my daughter's life, if He wants it saved," she said. "And God will abort the child she's carrying, if He wants it aborted."

Dr. Kranski gave up his attempt to secure Mrs. Wilson's approval for the abortion. Later, he explained the situation to the director of the clinic, Dr. Saul Mendlovitz. Dr. Mendlovitz took up the matter with the legal staff of South General Hospital, and it was decided to seek a court order permitting the abortion.

The appropriate legal steps were taken, and after a court hearing at which Mrs. Wilson was represented by a state-appointed attorney, South General Hospital was granted permission to take necessary medical steps to save the life of Alice Wilson. No appeal was filed.

Despite her mother's continued personal opposition, Alice Wilson underwent an abortion.

CASE RETROSPECTIVE

When Abortion Was Illegal: Mrs. Sherri Finkbine and the Thalidomide Tragedy

Background Note: The following case concerns an event that took place before the U.S. Supreme Court decision in Roe v. Wade *was handed down in 1973. That decision had the effect of legalizing abortion in the United States. Before the decision, most state laws permitted abortion only for the purpose of saving the life of the mother. The case presented here illustrates the kinds of problems faced by many women who sought an abortion for other reasons.*

In 1962 Mrs. Sherri Finkbine was the mother of four normal children and was pregnant. Her health was good, but she was having some trouble sleeping. Rather than talking with her doctor, she simply took some of the tranquilizers that her husband had brought back from a trip to Europe. The tranquilizers were widely used there, and, like aspirin, they could simply be bought over the counter.

Subsequently, Mrs. Finkbine read an article that told of the great increase in the number of deformed children being born in Europe. Some of the children's arms and legs failed to develop or developed only in malformed ways; other children were blind and deaf or had seriously defective internal organs. The birth defects had been traced to the use in pregnancy of a supposedly harmless and widely used tranquilizer. Its active ingredient was thalidomide.

Mrs. Finkbine was worried enough to ask her doctor to find out if the pills she had been taking contained thalidomide. They did. When he learned this, her doctor told her "The odds are so against you that I am recommending termination of pregnancy." He explained that getting approval for an abortion should not be difficult. She had good medical reasons, and all she had to do was explain them to the three-member medical board of Phoenix.

Mrs. Finkbine agreed with her doctor's advice. But then she began to think that maybe it was her duty to inform other women who may have been taking thalidomide about its disastrous consequences. She called a local newspaper and told her story to the editor. He agreed not to use her name, but on a front page, bordered in black, he used the headline "BABY-DEFORMING DRUG MAY COST WOMAN HER CHILD HERE."

The story was picked up by the wire services, and it was not long before Mrs. Finkbine's identity became known. The medical board had already approved her request for an abortion, but because of the great publicity her case received they canceled their approval. The State of Arizona abortion statute legally sanctioned abortion only when it was required to save the life of the mother. The board was afraid that their decision might be challenged in court and that the decision could not stand up to the challenge.

Mrs. Finkbine became the object of a great outpouring of antiabortion feelings. *Il Osservatore Romano,* the official Vatican newspaper, condemned Mrs. Finkbine and her husband as murderers. Although she received some letters of support, others were abusive. One writer said: "I hope someone takes the other four children and strangles them, because it is all the same thing." Another wrote from the perspective of the fetus: "Mommy, please dear Mommy, let me live. Please, please, I want to live. Let me love you, let me see the light of day, let me smell a rose, let me sing a song, let me look into your face, let me say Mommy."

Although Mrs. Finkbine tried to obtain a legal abortion outside her own state, she was unable to do so. Eventually, she went to Sweden. After a rigorous investigation by a medical board, Mrs. Finkbine was given an abortion in a Swedish hospital.

Mrs. Finkbine saw her own problem as solved at last. But she continued to have sympathy with those thousands of potential parents of thalidomide children who lacked the money to follow the course of action she had been forced to take by abortion laws she considered to be restrictive and inhumane.

SOCIAL CONTEXT: THE NEW CHALLENGE—RU 486, "THE ABORTION PILL"

Sandra Crane, as we'll call her, decided she had missed her period. She was thirty-one years old, and ordinarily her menstrual cycle was as regular as the calendar. Since she was now two weeks overdue, she felt sure she was pregnant.

The feeling was familiar. She had two children already, six-year-old Jennifer and two-year-old Thomas. She and her husband had decided they weren't going to have more. They had discussed the matter, and she resolved that if she became pregnant she would seek medical help to end her pregnancy.

The next morning Sandra Crane consulted her gynecologist, and a day later she received a phone call informing her that she was indeed pregnant. She explained that she wanted the pregnancy ended as soon as possible, and she was told to return to the clinic to pick up a 600-milligram dose of the drug RU 486.

She took the drug that evening, and two days later she was back in the clinic. She was given an injection of prostaglandin and asked to lie down on an examining table. Later she began to experience cramping and bleeding, but soon the uterine lining was expelled. She felt some discomfort, but the process differed little from an unusually heavy menstrual period.

Her husband met her at the clinic and escorted her home. After a day of rest, she felt almost her usual self again.

RU 486 was developed by the French endocrinologist Etienne-Émile Baulieu. The drug works by blocking the action of progesterone, the hormone that prepares the uterine wall for the implantation of the fertilized egg. The injection of prostaglandin induces uterine contractions that expel the sloughed-off lining, including the zygote. To be effective, the drug must be taken during the first five weeks of pregnancy, although physicians urge that it be taken as early as possible.

In initial testing, 100 women volunteers less than a month pregnant were given RU 486. Of these, 85% aborted within four days, without reporting the pain or psychological difficulties that can accompany surgical abortion. The later use of prostaglandin in conjunction with the drug increased the speed of the process. Additional clinical trials in France and the use of the drug by more than 50,000 women have shown it to be safe and 90–95% effective. Some women bleed excessively, and a proportion do not abort as expected and require surgical intervention. For these reasons the drug is intended for use only under close medical supervision. All in all, however, the evidence suggests that the use of the drug is safer and cheaper than surgical abortion.

The drug was developed in 1980 by the pharmaceutical company Roussel Uclaf and approved for use in France in September 1988. A month later, in response to a boycott of the company's products by abortion opponents, Roussel took the drug off the market.

This provoked public protests. Health Minister Claude Evin notified the company that if it did not release the drug the government, which owned 36.25% of the company, would permanently transfer the patent to another company. "From the moment the governmental approval of the drug was granted, RU 486 became the moral property of women, not just the property of the drug company," Evin said. Two days later the company resumed marketing the drug.

Roussel licensed the drug for use in China and announced that it was considering marketing the drug in Great Britain, the Netherlands, and the Scandinavian countries. Initial plans to market the drug in the United States have been delayed, if not abandoned, because of opposition from right-to-life groups.

Since opponents of abortion generally consider RU 486 as no more than a biochemical means for producing an abortion, they oppose its use. According to the president of the National Right to Life Coalition, RU 486 represents "chemical warfare against an entire class of innocent humans."

In accord with this view, National Right to Life (NRL) and other groups opposed to abortion have informed drug companies that they will boycott all the company's products if the company tries to market an abortion-inducing drug. "Our basic position is that death drugs designed to kill unborn babies have no place in America," the NRL education director said.

Baulieu, the drug's developer, charges that fears of such reprisals have kept RU 486 from being distributed worldwide. Indeed, the fear of boycotts of Roussel and Hoechst, the German pharmaceutical company that is its majority stockholder, has led the company to decide against applying for approval so that the drug could be sold in the United States. No U.S. drug company has applied to the FDA for approval out of fear of the response of the prolife movement.

Baulieu also charges that Roussel should not have put approval of the drug for international use in the hands of the World Health Organization (WHO). WHO has delayed its approval because it is so financially dependent on the United States that a reprisal in the form of a withdrawal of U.S. funds would severely cripple its operations.

"I believe the key to the future of RU 486 lies in the United States," Baulieu stated during a news conference. He said that, because of the drug's simplicity, it could dramatically reduce the number of illegal abortions and related maternal deaths throughout the world.

"How can we ignore that 500 women a day die as a result of badly executed abortions?" he said. "At present, things are so bad in the Third World that anything that improves the situation is welcome. I think it is our moral duty to act."

Along the same lines, Louise B. Tyrer of Planned Parenthood characterized the lack of availability of the drug as "discriminatory to women" and "a threat to their safety and health." In her view and in the opinion of prochoice advocates, "Women should have a choice between medical and surgical abortion."

In June 1990 the policy-making House of Delegates of the American Medical Association endorsed the testing of RU 486. Yet no experimental investigations of the drug have been initiated, and clinical trials seem a long way off.

INTRODUCTION

Less than two decades ago, most Americans considered abortion a crime so disgusting that it was rarely mentioned in public. Back-alley abortionists with dirty hands and unclean instruments were real enough, but they were also the villains of cautionary tales to warn women against being tempted into the crime. Abortion was the dramatic stuff of novels and movies portraying "girls in trouble" or women pushed to the brink. To choose to have an abortion was to choose to be degraded.

The Supreme Court decision in *Roe* v. *Wade* changed all that in 1973. The decision had the effect of legalizing abortion, and since then abortion has gained acceptance from a majority of the population. Yet controversy over the legitimacy of abortion continues to flare. Indeed, no other topic in medical ethics has attracted more attention or so polarized public opinion. The reason is understandable. In the abortion question, major moral, legal, and social issues are intertwined to form a problem of great subtlety and complexity.

Before focusing on some of the specific issues raised by abortion, we would do well to have in hand some of the relevant factual information about human developmental biology and the techniques of abortion.

Human Development and Abortion

Fertilization occurs when an ovum is penetrated by a sperm cell and the nuclei of the two unite to form a single cell containing forty-six chromosomes. This normally occurs in the Fallopian tube (or oviduct), a narrow tube leading from the ovary into the uterus (womb). The fertilized ovum—zygote, or conceptus—continues its passage down the Fallopian tube, and during its two- to three-day passage it undergoes a number of cell divisions that increase its size. (Rarely, the zygote does not descend but continues to develop in the Fallopian tube. Because the tube is so small, the pregnancy usually has to be terminated surgically.) After reaching the uterus, a pear-shaped organ, the zygote floats free in the intrauterine fluid. Here it develops into a blastocyst, a ball of cells surrounding a fluid-filled cavity.

By the end of the second week, the blastocyst becomes embedded in the wall of the uterus. At this point and until the end of the eighth week, it is known as an embryo. During the fourth and fifth weeks, organ systems begin to develop, and the external features take on a definitely human shape.

During the eighth week, brain activity usually becomes detectable. At this time, the embryo comes to be known as a fetus.

Birth generally occurs about nine months after fertilization. It is customary to divide this time into three three-month periods, or trimesters. At present, pregnancy cannot be diagnosed with certainty by ordinary methods until ten to fourteen days after a woman has missed her menstrual period.

Abortion is the termination of pregnancy. It can occur because of internal biochemical factors or as a result of physical injury to the woman. Terminations from such causes are usually referred to as "spontaneous abortions," but they are also commonly called miscarriages.

Abortion can also be a deliberate process resulting from human intervention. The methods used in contemporary medicine depend to a great extent on the stage of the pregnancy. The earliest intervention involves the use of drugs (like RU 486) to prevent the embedding of the blastocyst in the uterine wall. Subsequent intervention during the first trimester (up to about twelve weeks) commonly employs one of two techniques. The first of the two is uterine or vacuum aspiration. The cervix, the narrow outer opening of the uterus, is dilated (widened) by instruments. Then a small tube is inserted into the uterus, and its contents are emptied by suction. The second commonly used procedure is dilation and curettage. The cervix is dilated and its contents

are gently scraped out by the use of a curette, a spoon-shaped surgical instrument.

After sixteen weeks, when the fetus is too large to make the other methods practical, the most common abortion technique is saline injection. The fluid in the membrane sac (amnion) surrounding the fetus is withdrawn through a hollow needle and replaced by a solution of salt and water. This induces a miscarriage.

Another second method, hysterotomy, is a surgical procedure in which the fetus is removed from the uterus through an incision. The procedure is the same as that known as Caesarean section and is rarely performed for the purpose of abortion.

These facts about pregnancy and abortion put us in a position to discuss some of the moral problems connected with them. We shall not be able to untangle the skein of issues wrapped around the abortion question. We shall only attempt to state a few of the more serious ones and to indicate the lines of argument that have been offered to support positions taken with respect to them. Afterward we will sketch out some possible responses that might be offered on the basis of the ethical theories we considered in the introductory chapter. Finally, we will present summary statements of the views taken by the authors of the selections that make up the bulk of this chapter.

The Status of the Fetus

It is absolutely crucial for the application of the principles of any moral theory that we have a settled opinion about the objects and subjects of morality. Although principles are generally stated with respect to rational individuals, every theory recognizes that there are people who in fact cannot be considered rational agents. For example, mental and physical incapacities may diminish or destroy rationality. But ethical theories generally recognize that we still have duties to people who are so incapacitated.

The basic problem that this raises is: Who or what is to be considered a person? Are there characteristics that we can point to and say that it is by virtue of possessing these characteristics that an individual must be considered a person and thus accorded moral treatment?

The abortion issue raises this question most particularly with regard to the fetus. (We will use the term "fetus," for the moment, to refer to the developing organism at any stage.) Just what is the status of the fetus in the world? We must find a satisfactory answer to this question, some writers have suggested, before we can resolve the general moral problem of abortion.

Let's consider the possible consequences of answering this question one way or the other. First, if a fetus is a person, then it has a serious claim to life. We must assert the claim on its behalf, for, like an unconscious person, the fetus is unable to do so. The claim of the fetus as a person must be given weight and respect in deliberating about any action that would terminate its life. Perhaps only circumstances as extreme as a threat to the life of the mother would justify abortion.

Assuming that the fetus is a person, then an abortion would be a case of killing and not something to be undertaken without reasons sufficient to override the fetus's claim to life. In effect, only conditions of the same sort as would justify our killing an adult person (for example, self-defense) would justify our killing a fetus. Thus, the moral burden in every case would be to demonstrate that abortion is not a case of wrongful killing.

By contrast, if a fetus is not a person in a morally relevant sense, then abortion need not be considered a case of killing equivalent to the killing of an adult. In one view, it might be said that an abortion is not essentially different from an appendectomy. According to this way of thinking, a fetus is no more than a complicated clump of organic material, and its removal involves no serious moral difficulty.

In another view, it could be argued that, even though the fetus is not a person, it is a *potential* person, and thus is a significant and morally relevant property. The fetus's very potentiality makes it unique and distinguishes it from a diseased appendix or a cyst or any other kind of organic material. Thus, because the fetus can become a person, abortion does present a moral problem. A fetus can be destroyed only for serious reasons. Thus, preventing a person from coming into existence must be justified to an extent comparable to the justification required for killing a person. (Some have suggested that the justification does not have to be identical because the fetus is only a potential person. The justifications we might present for killing a person would thus serve only as a guide for those that might justify abortion.)

So far we have used the word "fetus," and this usage tends to obscure the fact that human development is a process with many stages. Perhaps it is only in the later stages of development that the entity becomes a person. But exactly when might this happen?

The differences between a fertilized ovum and a fully developed baby just a few minutes before birth are considerable. The ovum and the blastocyst seem just so much tissue. But the embryo and the fetus present more serious claims to being persons. Should abortion be allowed until the fetus becomes visibly human, or until the fetus shows heartbeat and brain waves, or until the fetus can live outside the uterus (becomes viable)?

The process of development is continuous, and so far it has proved impossible to find differences between stages that can be generally accepted as morally relevant. Some writers on abortion have suggested that it is useless to look for such differences, because any place where the line is drawn will be arbitrary. Others have claimed that it is possible to draw the line by relying on criteria that can be rationally defended. A few have even argued that a reasonable set of criteria for determining who shall be considered a person might even deny the status to infants.

Pregnancy, Abortion, and the Rights of Women

Pregnancy and fetal development are normal biological processes, and most women who choose to have a child carry it to term without unusual difficulties. However, it is important to keep in mind that even a normal pregnancy involves changes and stresses that are uniquely burdensome. Once the process of fetal growth is initiated, a woman's entire physiology is altered by the new demands placed on it and by the biochemical changes taking place within her body. For example, metabolic rate increases, the thyroid gland grows larger, the heart pumps more blood to meet fetal needs, and a great variety of hormonal changes take place. The growing fetus physically displaces the woman's internal organs and alters the size and shape of her body.

As a result of such changes, the pregnant woman may suffer a variety of ailments. More common ones include severe nausea and vomiting ("morning sickness"), muscle cramps, abdominal pain, anemia, tiredness, and headaches. For many women such complaints are relatively mild or infrequent, while for others they are severe or constant. Nausea and vomiting can lead to dehydration and malnutrition so serious as to be life-threatening. Women who suffer from diseases like diabetes are apt to face special health problems as a result of pregnancy.

Partly because of hormonal changes, women are also more likely to experience psychological difficulties when pregnant, such as emotional lability (mood swings), severe depression, and acute anxiety. Such conditions are often accompanied by quite realistic concerns about the loss of freedom associated with becoming a parent, compromised job status, loss of sexual attractiveness due to the change in body shape, and the pains and risks of childbirth.

The woman who intends to carry a child to term is also likely to have to alter her behavior in many ways. She may have to curtail the time she spends working, take a leave of absence, or even quit her job. Any career plans she has are likely to suffer. She may be unable to participate in social activities to the extent she previously did, and give up some entirely. In addition, if she recognizes an obligation to the developing fetus and is well informed, she may have to alter her diet, stop smoking, and strictly limit the amount of alcohol she consumes.

In summary, the physical and emotional price paid by a woman for a full-term pregnancy is high. Even a normal pregnancy, one that proceeds without any special difficulties, exacts a toll of discomfort, stress, restricted activity, and worry.

Women who wish to have a child are generally willing to undergo the rigors of pregnancy to satisfy this desire. But is it a woman's duty to nurture and carry to term an unwanted child? Pregnancies resulting from rape and incest are the kinds of dramatic cases frequently mentioned to emphasize the seriousness of the burden imposed on women. But the question is also important when the conditions surrounding the pregnancy are more ordinary.

Suppose that a woman becomes pregnant unintentionally and decides that having a child will be harmful to her career or her way of life. Or suppose that she simply does not wish to subject herself to the pains of pregnancy. Does a woman have a moral duty to see to it that the developing child comes to be born?

A number of writers have taken the position that women have an exclusive right to control their own reproductive function. In their view, such a right is based upon the generally recognized right to control what is done to our bodies. Since pregnancy is something that involves a woman's body, the woman concerned may legitimately decide whether to continue the pregnancy or terminate it. The decision is hers alone, and social or legal policies that restrict the free exercise of her right are unjustifiable.

Essentially the same point is sometimes phrased by saying that women own their bodies. Because their bodies are their own "property," women alone have the right to decide whether to become pregnant and, if pregnant unintentionally, whether to have an abortion.

Critics have pointed out that this general line of argument, taken alone, does not support the strong conclusion that women should be free from all constraints in making abortion decisions. Even granting that women's bodies are their own property, we nevertheless recognize restrictions on exercising property rights. We have no right to shoot trespassers, and we cannot endanger our neighbors by burning down our house. Similarly, if any legitimate moral claims can be made on behalf of the fetus, then the right of women to decide whether to have an abortion may not be unrestricted.

Some philosophers (Judith J. Thomson, for example) have taken the view that, although women are entitled to control their bodies and make abortion decisions, the decision to have an abortion must be supported by weighty reasons. They have suggested that, even if we grant that a fetus is a person, its claim to life cannot be given unconditional precedence over the woman's claim to control her own life. She is entitled to autonomy and the right to arrange her life in accordance with her own concept of the good. It would be wrong for her to destroy the fetus for a trivial reason, but legitimate and adequate reasons for taking the life of the fetus might be offered.

Others, by contrast, have argued that when a woman becomes pregnant she assumes an obligation for the life of the fetus. It is, after all, completely dependent on her for its continued existence. She has no more right to take its life in order to seek her own best interest than she has to murder someone whose death may bring benefits to her.

Therapeutic Abortion

Abortion is sometimes required in order to save the life of the mother or in order to provide her with medical treatment that may correct some life-threatening condition. Abortion performed for such a purpose is ordinarily regarded as a case of self-defense. For this reason, it is almost universally considered to be morally unobjectionable. (Strictly speaking, the Roman Catholic view condemns abortion in all of its forms. It does approve of providing medical treatment for the mother, even if this results in the death of the fetus, but the death of the fetus must never be intended.)

If the principle of preserving the life and health of the mother justifies abortion, then what conditions fall under that principle? If a woman has cancer of the uterus and her life can be saved only by an operation that will result in the death of the fetus, then this clearly falls under the principle. But what about psychological conditions? Is a woman's mental health relevant to deciding whether an abortion is justified? What if a psychiatrist believes that a woman cannot face the physical rigors of pregnancy or bear the psychological stresses that go with it without developing severe psychiatric symptoms? Would such a judgment justify an abortion? Or is the matter of psychological health irrelevant to the abortion issue?

Consider, too, the welfare of the fetus. Suppose that prenatal tests or other reliable means indicate that the developing child suffers from serious abnormalities. (This was the case of the "thalidomide babies.") Is abortion for the purpose of preventing the birth of such children justifiable?

It might be argued that it is not, that an impaired fetus has as much right to its life as an impaired person. We do not, after all, consider it legitimate to kill people who become seriously injured or suffer from diseases that render them helpless. Rather, we care for them and work to improve their lives—at least we ought to.

Someone might argue, however, that abortion in such cases is not only justifiable, but a duty. (See, for example, the article by H. T. Engelhardt in Chapter 2.) It is our duty to kill the fetus to spare the person that it will become a life of unhappiness and suffering. We might even be said to be acknowledging the dignity of the fetus by doing what it might do for itself if it could—what any rational creature would do. Destroying such a fetus would spare future pain to the individual and his or her family and save society from an enormous expense. Thus, we have not only the justification to kill such a fetus, but also the positive obligation to do so.

In this chapter, we will not deal explicitly with the issues that are raised by attempting to decide whether it is justifiable to terminate the life of an impaired fetus. Because such issues are directly connected with prenatal genetic diagnosis and treatment, we will discuss them more fully in Chapter 7. Nonetheless, in considering the general question of the legitimacy of abortion, it is important to keep such special considerations in mind.

Abortion and the Law

Abortion in our society has been a legal issue as well as a moral issue. Until the Supreme Court decision in *Roe* v. *Wade,* nontherapeutic abortion was illegal in virtually all states. The *Webster* decision (see the earlier Social Context) is a recent indication that the Court is willing to accept more state restrictions than previously, but even so abortions are far from being illegal. Yet there are groups lobbying strongly for a constitutional amendment that would protect a fetus's "right to life" and prohibit elective abortion.

The rightness or wrongness of abortion is a moral matter, one whose issues can be resolved only by appealing to a moral theory. Different theories may yield incompatible answers, and even individuals who accept the same theory may arrive at different conclusions.

Such a state of affairs raises the question of whether the moral convictions or conclusions of some people should be embodied in laws that govern the lives of all people in the society. The question can be put succinctly: Should the moral beliefs of some people serve as the basis for laws that will impose those beliefs on everyone?

There is no straightforward way of answering this general question. To some extent, which moral beliefs are at issue is a relevant consideration. So too are the political principles that we are willing to accept as basic to our society. Every ethical theory recognizes that there is a scope of action that must be left to individuals as moral agents acting freely on the basis of their own understanding and perceptions. Laws requiring the expression of benevolence or gratitude, for example, seem peculiarly inappropriate.

Yet, one of the major aims of a government is to protect the rights of its citizens. Consequently, a society must have just laws that recognize and enforce those rights. In a very real way, then, the moral theory that we hold and the conclusions arrived at on the basis of it will determine whether we believe that certain types of laws are justified. They are justified when they protect the rights recognized in our moral theories—when political rights reflect moral rights. (See the Introduction to Chapter 10 for a fuller discussion of moral rights and their relation to political rights.)

An ethical theory that accords the status of a person to a fetus is likely to claim also that the laws of the society should recognize the rights of the fetus. A theory that does not grant the fetus this position is not likely to regard laws forbidding abortion as justifiable.

Ethical Theories and Abortion

Theories like those of Mill, Kant, Ross, and Rawls attribute to individuals autonomy or self-direction. An individual is entitled to control his or her own life, and it seems reasonable to extend this principle to apply to one's own body. If so, then a woman should have the right to determine whether or not she wishes to have a child. If she is pregnant with an unwanted child, then, no matter how she came to be pregnant, she might legitimately decide on an abortion. Utilitarianism also suggests this answer on consequential grounds. In the absence of other considerations, if it seems likely that having a child will produce more unhappiness than an abortion would, then an abortion would be justifiable.

If the fetus is considered to be a person, however, the situation is different for some theories. The Roman Catholic view holds that the fetus is an innocent person and that direct abortion is never justifiable. Even if the pregnancy is due to rape, the fetus cannot be held at fault and made to suffer through its death. Even though she may not wish to have the child, the mother has a duty to preserve the life of the fetus.

For deontological theories like those of Kant and Ross, the situation becomes more complicated. If the fetus is a person, then it has an inherent dignity and worth. It is an innocent life which cannot be destroyed except for the weightiest moral reasons. Those reasons may include the interests and wishes of the woman, but deontological theories provide no clear answer as to how those are to be weighed.

For utilitarianism, by contrast, even if the fetus is considered a person, the principle of utility may still justify an abortion. Killing a person is not, for utilitarianism, inherently wrong. (Yet it is compatible with rule utilitarianism to argue that permitting elective abortion as a matter of policy would produce more unhappiness than forbidding abortion altogether. Thus, utilitarianism does not offer a definite answer to the abortion issue.)

As we have already seen, both utilitarianism and deontological theories can be used to justify therapeutic abortion. When the mother's life or health is at stake, then the situation may be construed as one of self-defense. Both Kant and Ross recognize that we each have a right to protect ourselves, even if it means taking the life of another person. For utilitarianism, preserving one's life is justifiable, for being alive is a necessary condition for all forms of happiness.

We have also indicated that abortion "for the sake of the fetus" can be justified by both utilitarianism and deontological theories. If by killing the fetus we can spare it a life of suffering, minimize the sufferings of its family, and preserve the resources of the society, then abortion is legitimate on utilitarian grounds. In the terms of Kant and Ross, destroying the fetus might be a way of recognizing its dignity. If we assume that it is a person, then by sparing it a life of indignity and pain we are treating it in the way that a rational being would want to be treated.

The legitimacy of laws forbidding abortion is an issue that utilitarianism would resolve by considering their effects. If such laws promote the general happiness of the society, then they are justifiable. Otherwise, they are not. In general, Kant, Ross, Rawls, and natural law theory recognize intrinsic human worth and regard as legitimate laws protecting that worth, even if those holding this view are only a minority of the society. Thus, laws discriminating against blacks and women, for example, would be considered unjust on the basis of these theories. Laws enforcing equality, by contrast, would be considered just.

But what about fetuses? The Roman Catholic interpretation of natural law would regard the case as exactly the same. As full human persons, they are entitled to have their rights protected by law. Those who fail to recognize this are guilty of moral failure, and laws permitting abortion are the moral equivalent of laws permitting murder.

For Kant and other deontologists, the matter is less clear. As long as there is substantial doubt about the status of the fetus, it is not certain that it is legitimate to demand that the rights of fetuses be recognized and protected by law. It is clear that the issue of whether or not the fetus is considered a person is most often taken as the crucial one in the abortion controversy.

Abortion Statistics

The social problems of abortion show no signs of being resolved. At present, about 1.5 million abortions are performed every year in the United States. About 30% of all pregnancies end in abortion, and the abortion rate for sixteen- to nineteen-year-olds is twice the national average. More than 60% of women who have abortions are under twenty-five. A similar proportion live in families with incomes under $11,000 a year. About one-quarter of all abortions are paid for with tax money in the form of Medicaid payments. (See also Abortion Profile Box.)

In 1977 the Supreme Court ruled that states are under no obligation to fund elective abortions for the poor under the Medicaid program, and in 1980 the Court held that the federal government is not required to fund abortions of any kind. Medicaid is presently both a state and federally funded program. Some fourteen states, accounting for 75% of the women eligible for Medicaid, chose to continue to finance elective abortions with state funds. In those states, nearly 98% of the women seeking an abortion obtained one. In states providing no funding, about 20% of women wanting abortions were forced to continue their pregnancies. Those securing abortions either obtained money from private sources to pay for legal abortions or (in 4% of the cases) had illegal ones.

Opponents of abortion have generally approved the Supreme Court decisions regarding abortion payments. By contrast, those who support elective abortion point out that the result of the decisions is to deny to some women an opportunity open to others. Women with financial means will have no difficulty obtaining abortions, whereas those without money will have either to bear children they don't want or to take their chances with back-alley abortionists whose services they can afford.

Yet, should those who consider abortion a form of murder have to pay through taxes for an operation that commits it? This is just one of the moral dilemmas that must be worked out before the issue of the place of abortion in society can be resolved.

United States Supreme Court Decision in *Roe* v. *Wade*

In *Roe* v. *Wade* the U.S. Supreme Court declared unconstitutional a Texas statute that restricted legal abortions to cases in which the life of the mother was threatened. The decision implied that all such state laws regulating abortion were unconstitutional. In effect, then, the decision made abortion legal in the United States.

The decision rested, in part, on the reasoning that a woman has a right to act for her own health and well-being as part of a more general right of privacy. The Court also considered the question of the legitimate limits of state interference to protect a woman's health and to protect the life of a fetus. The Court refused to recognize the fetus as a "person in the full sense" or to grant the right of the state to act on its behalf until the time (around the twenty-eighth week) that it can live outside the mother's body.

The ruling laid down three guidelines for regulating abortion: (1) until the end of the first trimester, the abortion decision is a medical one that must be left to the woman and her physician; (2) after the end of the first trimester, the state may

Abortion Profile

Number per year: 1.5 million (about 30% of all pregnancies)

Age*

15–17	32.2
18–19	62.4
20–24	54.6
25–29	30.0
30–34	17.9
35–39	9.8
40–40 +	3.4

Race*

White	23.0
Nonwhite	52.6

Family Income*

Under $11,000	62.2
$11,000–$24,999	32.5
$25,000 and over	16.5

*Estimated rate per 1,000 women; figures based on 1987 data.

Length of Pregnancy (in weeks)

8 or less	50.3%
9–10	26.9%
11–12	13.3%
13–15	5.3%
16–20	3.4%
21 and over	0.8%
(above 24	0.02%)

Source: Alan Guttmacher Institute; 1985 data.

Who Has Abortions?

More than 25% are teenagers.
More than 60% are under 25.
More than 80% are unmarried.
More than 75% said they could not afford a child or were not ready for motherhood.
About 20% of women above the age of 15 have had an abortion.
Hispanic women are 60% more likely to have an abortion than non-Hispanics but are less likely than black women.
Roman Catholic women are more likely to have an abortion than either Protestant or Jewish women.
One of every six women who have abortions describes herself as an evangelical Christian.
The abortion rate for 18- and 19-year-olds is twice the national average.

Source: Alan Guttmacher Institute.

Laws and Beliefs

Do you favor or oppose passing laws making it more difficult for women to have abortions?

FAVOR: 47%   OPPOSE: 48%   NOT SURE: 5%

Do you personally believe that having an abortion is wrong?

YES: 50%   NO: 43%   NOT SURE: 7%

Source: Time–Yankelovich Telephone Poll; published May 1, 1989.

regulate the abortion procedure in ways reasonably related to maternal health; (3) after the fetus is viable, the state may regulate or even prohibit abortion, except where it is necessary to preserve the life or health of the mother.

Background Note: A pregnant single woman, Roe, brought a class-action suit against Wade, the District Attorney of Dallas County. Roe challenged the constitutionality of the Texas criminal abortion laws, which pro-hibited procuring or performing an abortion except on medical advice for the purpose of saving the mother's life. A three-judge District Court ruled that the abortion stat-utes were void, and Wade appealed directly to the Supreme

Court. By 7 to 2 the Court ruled in favor of Roe, and Justice Blackmun delivered the majority opinion. That opinion is abridged here and citations to other cases omitted. The decision was handed down on January 22, 1973.

Three reasons have been advanced to explain historically the enactment of criminal abortion laws in the 19th century and to justify their continued existence.

It has been argued occasionally that these laws were the product of a Victorian social concern to discourage illicit sexual conduct. Texas, however, does not advance this justification in the present case, and it appears that no court or commentator has taken the argument seriously. The appellants and *amici* contend, moreover, that this is not a proper state purpose at all and suggest that, if it were, the Texas statutes are overbroad in protecting it since the law fails to distinguish between married and unwed mothers.

A second reason is concerned with abortion as a medical procedure. When most criminal abortion laws were first enacted, the procedure was a hazardous one for the woman. This was particularly true prior to the development of antisepsis. Antiseptic techniques, of course, were based on discoveries by Lister, Pasteur, and others first announced in 1867, but were not generally accepted and employed until about the turn of the century. Abortion mortality was high. Even after 1900, and perhaps until as late as the development of antibiotics in the 1940's, standard modern techniques such as dilation and curettage were not nearly so safe as they are today. Thus it has been argued that a State's real concern in enacting a criminal abortion law was to protect the pregnant woman, that is, to restrain her from submitting to a procedure that placed her life in serious jeopardy.

Modern medical techniques have altered this situation. Appellants and various *amici* refer to medical data indicating that abortion in early pregnancy, that is, prior to the end of first trimester, although not without its risk, is now relatively safe. Mortality rates for women undergoing early abortions, where the procedure is legal, appear to be as low as or lower than the rates for normal childbirth. Consequently, any interest of the State in protecting the woman from an inherently hazardous procedure, except when it would be equally dangerous for her

to forego it, has largely disappeared. Of course, important state interests in the area of health and medical standards do remain. The state has a legitimate interest in seeing to it that abortion, like any other medical procedure, is performed under circumstances that insure maximum safety for the patient. This interest obviously extends at least to the performing physician and his staff, to the facilities involved, to the availability of after-care, and to adequate provision for any complication or emergency that might arise. The prevalence of high mortality rates at illegal "abortion mills" strengthens, rather than weakens, the State's interest in regulating the conditions under which abortions are performed. Moreover, the risk to the woman increases as her pregnancy continues. Thus the State retains a definite interest in protecting the woman's own health and safety when an abortion is proposed at a late stage of pregnancy.

The third reason is the State's interest—some phrase it in terms of duty—in protecting prenatal life. Some of the argument for this justification rests on the theory that a new human life is present from the moment of conception. The State's interest and general obligation to protect life then extends, it is argued, to prenatal life. Only when the life of the pregnant mother herself is at stake, balanced against the life she carries within her, should the interest of the embryo or fetus not prevail. Logically, of course, a legitimate state interest in this area need not stand or fall on acceptance of the belief that life begins at conception or at some other point prior to live birth. In assessing the State's interest, recognition may be given to the less rigid claim that as long as at least *potential* life is involved, the State may assert interests beyond the protection of the pregnant woman alone.

Parties challenging state abortion laws have sharply disputed in some courts the contention that a purpose of these laws, when enacted, was to protect prenatal life. Pointing to the absence of legislative history to support the contention, they claim that most state laws were designed solely to protect the woman. Because medical advances have lessened this concern, at least with respect to abortion in early pregnancy, they argue that with respect to such abortions the laws can no longer be justified by any state interest. There is some scholarly support for this view of original purpose. The few state

United States Supreme Court, 410 U.S. 113, 93 S. Ct. 705. January 22, 1973.

courts called upon to interpret their laws in the late 19th and early 20th centuries did focus on the State's interest in protecting the woman's health rather than in preserving the embryo and fetus. Proponents of this view point out that in many States, including Texas, by statute or judicial interpretation, the pregnant woman herself could not be prosecuted for self-abortion or for cooperating in an abortion performed upon her by another. They claim that adoption of the "quickening" distinction through received common law and state statutes tacitly recognizes the greater health hazards inherent in late abortion and impliedly repudiates the theory that life begins at conception.

It is with these interests, and the weight to be attached to them, that this case is concerned.

The Constitution does not explicity mention any right of privacy. In a line of decisions, however, going back perhaps as far as *Union Pacific R. Co.* v. *Botsford*, 141 U.S. 250, 251 (1891), the Court has recognized that a right of personal privacy, or a guarantee of certain areas or zones of privacy, does exist under the Constitution. In varying contexts the Court or individual Justices have indeed found at least the roots of that right in the First Amendment, in the Fourth and Fifth Amendments, in the penumbras of the Bill of Rights, in the Ninth Amendment, or in the concept of liberty guaranteed by the first section of the Fourteenth Amendment. These decisions make it clear that only personal rights that can be deemed "fundamental" or "implicit in the concept of ordered liberty" are included in this guarantee of personal privacy. They also make it clear that the right has some extension to activities relating to marriage, procreation, contraception, family relationships, and child rearing and education.

This right of privacy, whether it be founded in the Fourteenth Amendment's concept of personal liberty and restrictions upon state action, as we feel it is, or, as the District Court determined, in the Ninth Amendment's reservation of rights to the people, is broad enough to encompass a woman's decision whether or not to terminate her pregnancy. The detriment that the State would impose upon the pregnant woman by denying this choice altogether is apparent. Specific and direct harm medically diagnosable even in early pregnancy may be involved. Maternity, or additional offspring, may force upon the woman a distressful life and future. Psychological harm may be imminent. Mental and physical health may be taxed by child care. There is also the distress, for all concerned, associated with the unwanted child, and there is the problem of bringing a child into a family already unable, psychologically and otherwise, to care for it. In other cases, as in this one, the additional difficulties and continuing stigma of unwed motherhood may be involved. All these are factors the woman and her responsible physician necessarily will consider in consultation.

On the basis of elements such as these, appellants and some *amici* argue that the woman's right is absolute and that she is entitled to terminate her pregnancy at whatever time, in whatever way, and for whatever reason she alone chooses. With these we do not agree. Appellants' arguments that Texas either has no valid interest at all in regulating the abortion decision, or no interest strong enough to support any limitation upon the woman's sole determination, is unpersuasive. The Court's decisions recognizing a right of privacy also acknowledge that some state regulation in areas protected by that right is appropriate. As noted above, a state may properly assert important interests in safeguarding health, in maintaining medical standards, and in protecting potential life. At some point in pregnancy, these respective interests become sufficiently compelling to sustain regulation of the factors that govern the abortion decision. The privacy right involved, therefore, cannot be said to be absolute. In fact, it is not clear to us that the claim asserted by some *amici* that one has an unlimited right to do with one's body as one pleases bears a close relationship to the right of privacy previously articulated in the Court's decisions. The Court has refused to recognize an unlimited right of this kind in the past.

We therefore conclude that the right of personal privacy includes the abortion decision, but that this right is not unqualified and must be considered against important state interests in regulation.

We note that those federal and state courts that have recently considered abortion law challenges have reached the same conclusion. A majority, in addition to the District Court in the present case, have held state laws unconstitutional, at least in part, because of vagueness or because of overbreadth and abridgement of rights.

Although the results are divided, most of these courts have agreed that the right of privacy, however based, is broad enough to cover the abortion decision; that the right, nonetheless, is not absolute and is subject to some limitations; and that at some point the state interests as to protection of health, medical standards, and prenatal life, become dominant. We agree with this approach.

Where certain "fundamental rights" are involved, the Court has held that regulation limiting these rights may be justified only by a "compelling state interest" . . . and that legislative enactments must be narrowly drawn to express only the legitimate state interests at stake.

In the recent abortion cases courts have recognized these principles. Those striking down state laws have generally scrutinized the State's interest in protecting health and potential life and have concluded that neither interest justified broad limitations on the reasons for which a physician and his pregnant patient might decide that she should have an abortion in the early stages of pregnancy. Courts sustaining state laws have held that the State's determinations to protect health or prenatal life are dominant and constitutionally justifiable.

The District Court held that the appellee failed to meet his burden of demonstrating that the Texas statute's infringement upon Roe's rights was necessary to support a compelling state interest, and that, although the defendant presented "several compelling justifications for state presence in the area of abortions," the statutes outstripped these justifications and swept "far beyond any areas of compelling state interest." Appellant and appellee both contest that holding. Appellant, as has been indicated, claims an absolute right that bars any state imposition of criminal penalties in the area. Appellee argues that the State's determination to recognize and protect prenatal life from and after conception constitutes a compelling state interest. As noted above, we do not agree fully with either formulation.

A. The appellee and certain *amici* argue that the fetus is a "person" within the language and meaning of the Fourteenth Amendment. In support of this they outline at length and in detail the well-known facts of fetal development. If this suggestion of personhood is established, the appellant's case, of course, collapses, for the fetus' right to life is then guaranteed specifically by the Amendment. The appellant conceded as much on reargument. On the other hand, the appellee conceded on reargument that no case could be cited that holds that a fetus is a person within the meaning of the Fourteenth Amendment.

The Constitution does not define "person" in so many words. Section I of the Fourteenth Amendment contains three references to "person." . . . But in nearly all these instances, the use of the word is such that it has application only postnatally. None indicates, with any assurance, that it has any possible prenatal application.

All this, together with our observation, *supra,* that throughout the major portion of the 19th century prevailing legal abortion practices were far freer than they are today, persuades us that the word "person," as used in the Fourteenth Amendment, does not include the unborn. . . .

B. The pregnant woman cannot be isolated in her privacy. She carries an embryo and, later, a fetus, if one accepts the medical definitions of the developing young in the human uterus. See Dorland's Illustrated Medical Dictionary, 478–479, 547 (24th ed. 1965). The situation therefore is inherently different from marital intimacy, or bedroom possession of obscene material, or marriage, or procreation, or education, with which *Eisenstadt, Giswold, Stanley, Loving, Skinner, Pierce,* and *Meyer* were respectively concerned. As we have intimated above, it is reasonable and appropriate for a State to decide that at some point in time another interest, that of health of the mother or that of potential human life, becomes significantly involved. The woman's privacy is no longer sole and any right of privacy she possesses must be measured accordingly.

Texas urges that, apart from the Fourteenth Amendment, life begins at conception and is present throughout pregnancy, and that, therefore, the State has a compelling interest in protecting that life from and after conception. We need not resolve the difficult question of when life begins. When those trained in the respective disciplines of medicine, philosophy, and theology are unable to arrive at any consensus, the judiciary, at this point in the development of man's knowledge, is not in a position to speculate as to the answer.

It should be sufficient to note briefly the wide divergence of thinking on this most sensitive and difficult question. There has always been strong support for the view that life does not begin until live birth. This was the belief of the Stoics. It appears to be the predominant, though not the unanimous, attitude of the Jewish faith. It may be taken to represent also the position of a large segment of the Protestant community, insofar as that can be ascertained; organized groups that have taken a formal position on the abortion issue have generally regarded abortion as a matter for the conscience of the individual and her family. As we have noted, the common law found greater significance in quickening. Physicians and their scientific colleagues have regarded that event with less interest and have tended to focus either upon conception or upon live birth or upon the interim point at which the fetus becomes "viable," that is, potentially able to live outside the mother's womb, albeit with artificial aid. Viability is usually placed at about seven months (28 weeks) but may occur earlier, even at 24 weeks. The Aristotelian theory of "mediate animation," that held sway throughout the Middle Ages and the Renaissance in Europe, continued to be official Roman Catholic dogma until the 19th century, despite opposition to this "ensoulment" theory from those in the Church who would recognize the existence of life from the moment of conception. The latter is now, of course, the official belief of the Catholic Church. As one of the briefs *amicus* discloses, this is a view strongly held by many non-Catholics as well, and by many physicians. Substantial problems for precise definition of this view are posed, however, by new embryological data that purport to indicate that conception is a "process" over time, rather than an event, and by new medical techniques such as menstrual extraction, the "morning-after" pill, implantation of embryos, artificial insemination, and even artificial wombs.

In areas other than criminal abortion the law has been reluctant to endorse any theory that life, as we recognize it, begins before live birth or to accord legal rights to the unborn except in narrowly defined situations and except when the rights are contingent upon live birth. For example, the traditional rule of tort law had denied recovery for prenatal injuries even though the child was born alive. That rule has been changed in almost every jurisdiction. In most States recovery is said to be permitted only if the fetus was viable, or at least quick, when the injuries were sustained, though few courts have squarely so held. In a recent development, generally opposed by the commentators, some States permit the parents of a stillborn child to maintain an action for wrongful death because of prenatal injuries. Such an action, however, would appear to be one to vindicate the parents' interest and is thus

consistent with the view that the fetus, at most, represents only the potentiality of life. Similarly, unborn children have been recognized as acquiring rights or interests by way of inheritance or other devolution of property, and have been represented by guardians *ad litem*. Perfection of the interests involved, again, has generally been contingent upon live birth. In short, the unborn have never been recognized in the law as persons in the whole sense.

In view of all this, we do not agree that, by adopting one theory of life, Texas may override the rights of the pregnant woman that are at stake. We repeat, however, that the State does have an important and legitimate interest in preserving and protecting the health of the pregnant woman, whether she be a resident of the State or a nonresident who seeks medical consultation and treatment there, and that it has still *another* important and legitimate interest in protecting the potentiality of human life. These interests are separate and distinct. Each grows in substantiality as the woman approaches term and, at a point during pregnancy, each becomes "compelling."

With respect to the State's important and legitimate interest in the health of the mother, the "compelling" point, in the light of present medical knowledge, is at approximately the end of the first trimester. This is so because of the now established medical fact . . . that until the end of the first trimester mortality in abortion is less than mortality in normal childbirth. It follows that, from and after this point, a State may regulate the abortion procedure to the extent that the regulation reasonably relates to the preservation and protection of maternal health. Examples of permissible state regulation in this area are requirements as to the qualifications of the person who is to perform the abortion; as to the licensure of that person; as to the facility in which the procedure is to be performed, that is, whether it must be a hospital or may be a clinic or some other place of less-than-hospital status; as to the licensing of the facility; and the like.

This means, on the other hand, that, for the period of pregnancy prior to this "compelling" point, the attending physician, in consultation with his patient, is free to determine, without regulation by the State, that in his medical judgment the patient's pregnancy should be terminated. If that decision is reached, the judgment may be effectuated by an abortion free of interference by the State.

With respect to the State's important and legitimate interest in potential life, the "compelling" point is at viability. This is so because the fetus then presumably has the capability of meaningful life outside the mother's womb. State regulation protective of fetal life after viability thus has both logical and biological justifications. If the State is interested in protecting fetal life after viability, it may go so far as to proscribe abortion during that period except when it is necessary to preserve the life or health of the mother.

Measured against these standards, Art. 1196 of the Texas Penal Code, in restricting legal abortions to those "procured or attempted by medical advice for the purpose of saving the life of the mother," sweeps too broadly. The statute makes no distinction between abortions performed early in pregnancy and those performed later, and it limits to a single reason, "saving" the mother's life, the legal justification for the procedure. The statute, therefore, cannot survive the constitutional attack made upon it here. . . .

To summarize and to repeat:

1. A state criminal abortion statute of the current Texas type, that excepts from criminality only a *life saving* procedure on behalf of the mother, without regard to pregnancy stage and without recognition of the other interests involved, is violative of the Due Process Clause of the Fourteenth Amendment.

   a. For the stage prior to approximately the end of the first trimester, the abortion decision and its effectuation must be left to the medical judgment of the pregnant woman's attending physician.

   b. For the stage subsequent to approximately the end of the first trimester, the State, in promoting its interest in the health of the mother, may, if it chooses, regulate the abortion procedure in ways that are reasonably related to maternal health.

   c. For the stage subsequent to viability the State, in promoting its interest in the potentiality of human life, may, if it chooses, regulate, and even proscribe, abortion except where it is necessary, in appropriate medical judgment, for the preservation of the life or health of the mother.

2. The State may define the term "physician" . . . to mean only a physician currently licensed by the State, and may proscribe any abortion by a person who is not a physician as so defined. . . .

This holding, we feel, is consistent with the relative weights of the respective interests involved, with the lessons and example of medical and legal history, with the lenity of the common law, and with the demands of the profound problems of the present day. The decision leaves the State free to place increasing restrictions on abortion as the period of pregnancy lengthens, so long as those restrictions are tailored to the recognized state interests. The decision vindicates the right of the physician to administer medical treatment according to his professional judgment up to the points where important state interests provide compelling justifications for intervention. Up to those points the abortion decision in all its aspects is inherently, and primarily, a medical decision, and basic responsibility for it must rest with the physician. If an individual practitioner abuses the privilege of exercising proper medical judgment, the usual remedies, judicial and intra-professional, are available. . . .

An Almost Absolute Value in History

John T. Noonan, Jr.

John T. Noonan makes the moment of fertilization the stage at which the developing organism becomes a person. Noonan reviews the distinctions used by abortion proponents (viability, experience, quickening, attitudes of adults toward the fetus, social viability) and concludes that they are all illegitimate. By contrast, he argues that conception is the decisive moment of humanization—for it is then that the new being receives the genetic code of its parents.

The basic principle that should govern our attitude toward the fetus, Noonan claims, is a theological and humanistic one: Do not injure your fellow man without a reason. Thus, once the humanity of the fetus is perceived, abortion is never right except in "self-defense." With the exception of saving the mother's life, then, abortion is immoral because it "violates the rational humanist tenet of the quality of human lives."

The most fundamental question involved in the long history of thought on abortion is: How do you determine the humanity of a being? To phrase the question that way is to put in comprehensive humanistic terms what the theologians either dealt with as an explicitly theological question under the heading of "ensoulment" or dealt with implicitly in their treatment of abortion. The Christian position as it originated did not depend on a narrow theological or philosophical concept. It had no relation to theories of infant baptism.[1] It appealed to no special theory of instantaneous ensoulment. It took the world's view on ensoulment as that view changed from Aristotle to Zacchia. There was, indeed, theological influence affecting the theory of ensoulment finally adopted, and, of course, ensoulment itself was a theological concept, so that the position was always explained in theological terms. But the theological notion of ensoulment could easily be translated into humanistic language by substituting "human" for "rational soul"; the problem of knowing when a man is a man is common to theology and humanism.

If one steps outside the specific categories used by the theologians, the answer they gave can be analyzed as a refusal to discriminate among human beings on the basis of their varying potentialities. Once conceived, the being was recognized as man because he had man's potential. The criterion for humanity, thus, was simple and all-embracing: if you are conceived by human parents, you are human.

The strength of this position may be tested by a review of some of the other distinctions offered in the contemporary controversy over legalizing abortion. Perhaps the most popular distinction is in terms of viability. Before an age of so many months, the fetus is not viable, that is, it cannot be removed from the mother's womb and live apart from her. To that extent, the life of the fetus is absolutely dependent on the life of the mother. This dependence is made the basis of denying recognition to its humanity.

There are difficulties with this distinction. One is that the perfection of artificial incubation may make the fetus viable at any time: it may be removed and artificially sustained. Experiments with animals already show that such a procedure is possible. This hypothetical extreme case relates to an actual difficulty: there is considerable elasticity to the idea of viability. Mere length of life is not an exact measure. The viability of the fetus depends on the extent of its anatomical and functional development. The weight and length of the fetus are better guides to the state of its development than age, but weight and length vary. Moreover, different racial groups have different ages at which their fetuses are viable. Some evidence, for example, suggests that Negro fetuses mature more quickly than white fetuses. If viability is the norm, the standard would vary with race and with many individual circumstances.

The most important objection to this approach is that dependence is not ended by viability. The fetus is still absolutely dependent on someone's care in order to continue existence; indeed a child of one or three or even five years of age is absolutely dependent on another's care for existence; uncared for, the older fetus or the younger child will die as surely as the early fetus detached from the mother. The unsubstantial lessening in dependence at viability does not seem to signify any special acquisition of humanity.

Reprinted by permission from John T. Noonan, Jr., editor, The Morality of Abortion: Legal and Historical Perspectives, *pp. 51–59. Cambridge, Mass.: Harvard University Press. Copyright © 1970 by the President and Fellows of Harvard College.*

A second distinction has been attempted in terms of experience. A being who has had experience, has lived and suffered, who possesses memories, is more human than one who has not. Humanity depends on formation by experience. The fetus is thus "unformed" in the most basic human sense.

This distinction is not serviceable for the embryo which is already experiencing and reacting. The embryo is responsive to touch after eight weeks and at least at that point is experiencing. At an earlier stage the zygote is certainly alive and responding to its environment. The distinction may also be challenged by the rare case where aphasia has erased adult memory: has it erased humanity? More fundamentally, this distinction leaves even the older fetus or the younger child to be treated as an unformed inhuman thing. Finally, it is not clear why experience as such confers humanity. It could be argued that certain central experiences such as loving or learning are necessary to make a man human. But then human beings who have failed to love or to learn might be excluded from the class called man.

A third distinction is made by appeal to the sentiments of adults. If a fetus dies, the grief of the parents is not the grief they would have for a living child. The fetus is an unnamed "it" till birth, and is not perceived as personality until at least the fourth month of existence when movements in the womb manifest a vigorous presence demanding joyful recognition by the parents.

Yet feeling is notoriously an unsure guide to the humanity of others. Many groups of humans have had difficulty in feeling that persons of another tongue, color, religion, sex, are as human as they. Apart from reactions to alien groups, we mourn the loss of a ten-year-old boy more than the loss of his one-day-old brother or his 90-year-old grandfather. The difference felt and the grief expressed vary with the potentialities extinguished, or the experience wiped out; they do not seem to point to any substantial difference in the humanity of baby, boy, or grandfather.

Distinctions are also made in terms of sensation by the parents. The embryo is felt within the womb only after about the fourth month. The embryo is seen only at birth. What can be neither seen nor felt is different from what is tangible. If the fetus cannot be seen or touched at all, it cannot be perceived as man.

Yet experience shows that sight is even more untrustworthy than feeling in determining humanity. By sight, color became an appropriate index for saying who was a man, and the evil of racial discrimination was given foundation. Nor can touch provide the test; a being confined by sickness, "out of touch" with others, does not thereby seem to lose his humanity. To the extent that touch still has appeal as a criterion, it appears to be a survival of the old English idea of "quickening"—a possible mistranslation of the Latin *animatus* used in the canon law. To that extent touch as a criterion seems to be dependent on the Aristotelian notion of ensoulment, and to fall when this notion is discarded.

Finally, a distinction is sought in social visibility. The fetus is not socially perceived as human. It cannot communicate with others. Thus, both subjectively and objectively, it is not a member of society. As moral rules are rules for the behavior of members of society to each other, they cannot be made for behavior toward what is not yet a member. Excluded from the society of men, the fetus is excluded from the humanity of men.[2]

By force of the argument from the consequences, this distinction is to be rejected. It is more subtle than that founded on an appeal to physical sensation, but it is equally dangerous in its implications. If humanity depends on social recognition, individuals or whole groups may be dehumanized by being denied any status in their society. Such a fate is fictionally portrayed in *1984* and has actually been the lot of many men in many societies. In the Roman empire, for example, condemnation to slavery meant the practical denial of most human rights; in the Chinese Communist world, landlords have been classified as enemies of the people and so treated as nonpersons by the state. Humanity does not depend on social recognition, though often the failure of society to recognize the prisoner, the alien, the heterodox as human has led to the destruction of human beings. Anyone conceived by a man and a woman is human. Recognition of this condition by society follows a real event in the objective order, however imperfect and halting the recognition. Any attempt to limit humanity to exclude some group runs the risk of furnishing authority and precedent for excluding other groups in the name of the consciousness or perception of the controlling group in the society.

A philosopher may reject the appeal to the humanity of the fetus because he views "humanity" as a secular view of the soul and because he doubts the existence of anything real and objective which can be identified as humanity. One answer to such a philosopher is to ask how he reasons about moral questions without supposing that there is a sense in which he and the others of whom he speaks are human. Whatever group is taken as the society which determines who may be killed is thereby taken as human. A second answer is to ask if he does not believe that there is a right and wrong way of deciding moral questions. If there is such a difference, experience may be appealed to: to decide who is human on the basis of the sentiment of a given society has led to consequences which rational men would characterize as monstrous.

The rejection of the attempted distinctions based on viability and visibility, experience and feeling, may be buttressed by the following considerations: Moral judgments often rest on distinctions, but if the distinctions are not to appear arbitrary *fiat*, they should relate to some real difference in probabilities. There is a kind of continuity in all life, but the earlier stages of the elements of human life possess tiny probabilities of development. Consider for example, the spermatozoa in any normal ejaculate: There are about 200,000,000 in any single ejaculate, of which one has a chance of developing into a zygote. Consider the oocytes which may become ova: there are 100,000 to 1,000,000 oocytes in a female infant, of which a maximum of 390 are ovulated. But once spermatozoon and ovum meet and the conceptus is formed, such studies as have been made show that roughly in only 20 percent of the cases will spontaneous abortion occur. In other words, the chances are about 4 out of 5 that this new being will develop. At this stage in the life of the being there is a sharp shift in probabilities, an immense jump in potentialities. To make a distinction between the rights of spermatozoa and the rights of the fertilized ovum is to respond to an enormous shift in possibilities. For about twenty days after conception the egg may split to form twins or combine with another egg to form a chimera, but the probability of either event happening is very small.

It may be asked, What does a change in biological probabilities have to do with establishing humanity? The argument from probabilities is not aimed at establishing humanity but at establishing an objective discontinuity which may be taken into account in moral discourse. As life itself is a matter of probabilities, as most moral reasoning is an estimate of probabilities, so it seems in accord with the structure of reality and the nature of moral thought to found a moral judgment on the change in probabilities at conception. The appeal to probabilities is the most commonsensical of arguments, to a greater or smaller degree all of us base our actions on probabilities, and in morals, as in law, prudence and negligence are often measured by the account one has taken of the probabilities. If the chance is 200,000,000 to 1 that the movement in the bushes into which you shoot is a man's, I doubt if many persons would hold you careless in shooting; but if the chances are 4 out of 5 that the movement is a human being's, few would acquit you of blame. Would the argument be different if only one out of ten children conceived came to term? Of course this argument would be different. This argument is an appeal to probabilities that actually exist, not to any and all state of affairs which may be imagined.

The probabilities as they do exist do not show the humanity of the embryo in the sense of a demonstration in logic any more than the probabilities of the movement in the bush being a man demonstrate beyond all doubt that the being is a man. The appeal is a "buttressing" consideration, showing the plausibility of the standard adopted. The argument focuses on the decisional factor in any moral judgment and assumes that part of the business of a moralist is drawing lines. One evidence of the nonarbitrary character of the line drawn is the difference of probabilities on either side of it. If a spermatozoon is destroyed, one destroys a being which had a chance of far less than 1 in 200 million of developing into a reasoning being, possessed of the genetic code, a heart and other organs, and capable of pain. If a fetus is destroyed, one destroys a being already possessed of the genetic code, organs, and sensitivity to pain, and one which had an 80 percent chance of developing further into a baby outside the womb who, in time, would reason.

The positive argument for conception as the decisive moment of humanization is that at conception the new being receives the genetic code. It is this genetic information which determines his characteristics, which is the biological carrier of the possibility of human wisdom, which makes him a self-evolving being. A being with a human genetic code is man.

This review of current controversy over the humanity of the fetus emphasizes what a fundamental question the theologians resolved in asserting the inviolability of the fetus. To regard the fetus as possessed of equal rights with other humans was not, however, to decide every case where abortion might be employed. It did decide the case where the argument was that the fetus should be aborted for its own good. To say a being was human was to say it had a destiny to decide for itself which could not be taken from it by another man's decision. But human beings with equal rights often come in conflict with each other, and some decision must be made as whose claims are to prevail. Cases of conflict involving the fetus are different only in two respects: the total inability of the fetus to speak for itself and the fact that the right of the fetus regularly at stake is the right to life itself.

The approach taken by the theologians to these conflicts was articulated in terms of "direct" and "indirect." Again, to look at what they were doing from outside their categories, they may be said to have been drawing lines or "balancing values." "Direct" and "indirect" are spatial metaphors; "line-drawing" is another. "To weigh" or "to balance" values is a metaphor of a more complicated mathematical sort hinting at the process which goes on in moral judgments. All the metaphors suggest that, in the moral judgments made, comparisons were necessary, that no value completely controlled. The principle of double effect was no doctrine fallen from heaven, but a method of analysis appropriate where two relative values were being compared. In Catholic moral theology, as it developed, life even of the innocent was not taken as an absolute. Judgments of acts affecting life issued from a process of weighing. In the weighing, the fetus was always given a value greater than zero, always a value separate and independent from its parents. This valuation was crucial and fundamental in all Christian thought on the subject and marked it off from any approach which considered that only the parents' interests needed to be considered.

Even with the fetus weighed as human, one interest could be weighed as equal or superior: that of the mother in her own life. The casuists between 1450 and 1895 were willing to weigh this interest as superior. Since 1895, that interest was given decisive weight only in the two special cases of the cancerous uterus and the ectopic pregnancy. In both of these cases the fetus itself had little chance of survival even if the abortion were not performed.

As the balance was once struck in favor of the mother whenever her life was endangered, it could be so struck again. The balance reached between 1895 and 1930 attempted prudentially and pastorally to forestall a multitude of exceptions for interests less than life.

The perception of the humanity of the fetus and the weighing of fetal rights against other human rights constituted the work of the moral analysts. But what spirit animated their abstract judgments? For the Christian community it was the injunction of Scripture to love your neighbor as yourself. The fetus as human was a neighbor; his life had parity with one's own. The commandment gave life to what otherwise would have been only rational calculation.

The commandment could be put in humanistic as well as theological terms: Do not injure your fellow man without reason. In these terms, once the humanity of the fetus is perceived, abortion is never right except in self-defense. When life must be taken to save life, reason alone cannot say that a mother must prefer a child's life to her own. With this exception, now of great rarity, abortion violates the rational humanist tenet of the equality of human lives.

For Christians the commandment to love had received a special imprint in that the exemplar proposed of love was the love of the Lord for his disciples. In the light given by this example, self-sacrifice carried to the point of death seemed in the extreme situations not without meaning. In the less extreme cases, preference for one's own interests to the life of another seemed to express cruelty or selfishness irreconcilable with the demands of love.

Notes

1. According to Granville Williams (*The Sanctity of Human Life*, p. 193), "The historical reason for the Catholic objection to abortion is the same as for the Christian Church's historical opposition to infanticide: the horror of bringing about the death of an unbaptized child." This statement is made without any citation of evidence. [As previously argued], desire to administer baptism could, in the Middle Ages, even be urged as a reason for procuring an abortion. It is highly regrettable that the American Law Institute was apparently misled by Williams' account and repeated after him the same baseless statement. See American Law Institute, *Model Penal Code: Tentative Draft No. 9* (1959), p. 148, n. 12.

2.   Thomas Aquinas gave an analogous reason against
     baptizing a fetus in the womb: "As long as it exists
     in the womb of the mother, it cannot be subject to

the operation of the ministers of the Church as it is
not known to men" (*In sententias Petri Lombardi* 4.6
1.1.2).

A Defense of Abortion[1]

Judith Jarvis Thomson

Judith Jarvis Thomson, in this very influential article, avoids the problem of determining when the fetus becomes a person. For the sake of argument only, she grants the conservative view that the fetus is a person from the moment of conception. She points out, however, that the conservative argument using this claim as a premise actually involves an additional unstated premise. The argument typically runs: The fetus is an innocent person; therefore, killing a fetus is always wrong. The argument requires that we assume that killing an innocent person is always wrong. But, Thomson claims, killing an innocent person is sometimes allowable. This is most clearly so when self-defense requires it.

Using several moral analogies, Thomson attempts to show that a fetus's right to life does not consist in the right not to be killed, but in the right not to be killed unjustly. The fetus's claim to life is not an absolute one which must always be granted unconditional precedence over the interests of its mother. Thus, abortion is not always permissible, but neither is it always impermissible. When the reasons for having an abortion are trivial, then abortion is not legitimate. When the reasons are serious and involve the health or welfare of the woman, then abortion is justifiable.

Most opposition to abortion relies on the premise that the fetus is a human being, a person, from the moment of conception. The premise is argued for, but, as I think, not well. Take, for example, the most common argument. We are asked to notice that the development of a human being from conception through birth into childhood is continuous; then it is said that to draw a line, to choose a point in this development and say "before this point the thing is not a person, after this point it is a person" is to make an arbitrary choice, a choice for which in the nature of things no good reason can be given. It is concluded that the fetus is, or anyway that we had better say it is, a person from the moment of conception. But this conclusion does not follow. Similar things might be said about the development of an acorn into an oak tree, and it does not follow that

acorns are oak trees, or that we had better say they are. Arguments of this form are sometimes called "slippery slope arguments"—the phrase is perhaps self-explanatory—and it is dismaying that opponents of abortion rely on them so heavily and uncritically.

I am inclined to agree, however, that the prospects for "drawing a line" in the development of the fetus look dim. I am inclined to think also that we shall probably have to agree that the fetus has already become a human person well before birth. Indeed, it comes as a surprise when one first learns how early in its life it begins to acquire human characteristics. By the tenth week, for example, it already has a face, arms and legs, fingers and toes; it has internal organs, and brain activity is detectable.[2] On the other hand, I think that the premise is false, that the fetus is not a person from the moment of conception. A newly fertilized ovum, a newly implanted clump of cells, is no more a person than an acorn is an oak tree. But I shall not discuss any of this. For it seems to me to be of great interest to ask what happens if, for the sake of argument, we allow the premise. How, precisely, are we supposed to get from there to the conclusion that abortion is morally impermissible? Opponents of abortion commonly spend most of their time establishing that the fetus is a person, and hardly any time explaining the step from there to the impermissibility of abortion. Perhaps they think the step too simple and obvious to require much comment. Or perhaps instead they are simply being economical in argument. Many of those who defend abortion rely on the premise that the fetus is not a person, but only a bit of tissue that will become a person at birth; and why pay out more arguments than you have to? Whatever the explanation, I suggest that the step they take is neither easy nor obvious, that it calls for closer examination than it is commonly given, and that when we do give it this closer examination we shall feel inclined to reject it.

I propose, then, that we grant that the fetus is a person from the moment of conception. How does the argument go from here? Something like this, I take it. Every person has a right to life. So the fetus has a right to life. No doubt the mother has a right to decide what shall happen in and to her body; everyone would grant that. But surely a person's right to life is stronger and more stringent than the mother's right to decide what happens in and to her body, and so outweighs it. So the fetus may not be killed; an abortion may not be performed.

It sounds plausible. But now let me ask you to imagine this. You wake up in the morning and find yourself back to back in bed with an unconscious violinist. A famous unconscious violinist. He has been found to have a fatal kidney ailment, and the Society of Music Lovers has canvassed all the available medical records and found that you alone have the right blood type to help. They have therefore kidnapped you, and last night the violinist's circulatory system was plugged into yours, so that your kidneys can be used to extract poisons from his blood as well as your own. The director of the hospital now tells you, "Look, we're sorry the Society of Music Lovers did this to you—we would never have permitted it if we had known. But still, they did it, and the violinist now is plugged into you. To unplug you would be to kill him. But never mind, it's only for nine months. By then he will have recovered from his ailment, and can safely be unplugged from you." Is it morally incumbent on you to accede to this situation? No doubt it would be very nice of you if you did, a great kindness. But do you *have* to accede to it? What if it were not nine months, but nine years? Or longer still? What if the director of the hospital says, "Tough luck, I agree, but you've now got to stay in bed, with the violinist plugged into you, for the rest of your life. Because remember this. All persons have a right to life, and violinists are persons. Granted you have a right to decide what happens in and to your body, but a person's right to life outweighs your right to decide what happens in and to your body. So you cannot ever be unplugged from him." I imagine you would regard this as outrageous, which suggests that something really is wrong with that plausible-sounding argument I mentioned a moment ago.

In this case, of course, you were kidnapped; you didn't volunteer for the operation that plugged the violinist into your kidneys. Can those who oppose abortion on the ground I mentioned make an exception for a pregnancy due to rape? Certainly. They can say that persons have a right to life only if they didn't come into existence because of rape; or they can say that all persons have a right to life, but that some have less of a right to life than others, in particular, that those who came into existence because of rape have less. But these statements have a rather unpleasant sound. Surely the question of whether you have a right to life at all, or how much of it you have, shouldn't turn on the question of whether or not you are a product of a rape. And in fact the people who oppose abortion on the ground I mentioned do not make this distinction, and hence do not make an exception in case of rape.

Nor do they make an exception for a case in which the mother has to spend the nine months of her pregnancy in bed. They would agree that would be a great pity, and hard on the mother; but all the same, all persons have a right to life, the fetus is a person, and so on. I suspect, in fact, that they would not make an exception for a case in which, miraculously enough, the pregnancy went on for nine years, or even the rest of the mother's life.

Some won't even make an exception for a case in which continuation of the pregnancy is likely to shorten the mother's life; they regard abortion as impermissible even to save the mother's life. Such cases are nowadays very rare, and many opponents of abortion do not accept this extreme view. All the same, it is a good place to begin: a number of points of interest come out in respect to it.

1.

Let us call the view that abortion is impermissible even to save the mother's life "the extreme view." I want to suggest first that it does not issue from the argument I mentioned earlier without the addition of some fairly powerful premises. Suppose a woman has become pregnant, and now learns that she has a cardiac condition such that she will die if she carries the baby to term. What may be done for her? The fetus, being a person, has a right to life, but as the mother is a person too, so has she a right to life. Presumably they have an equal right to life. How is it supposed to come out that an abortion may not be performed? If mother and child have an equal right to life, shouldn't we perhaps flip a coin? Or should we add to the mother's right to life her right to decide what happens in and to her body, which everybody seems to be ready to grant—the sum of her rights now outweighing the fetus's right to life?

The most familiar argument here is the following. We are told that performing the abortion would be directly killing[3] the child, whereas doing nothing would not be killing the mother, but only letting her die. Moreover, in killing the child, one would be killing an innocent person, for the child has committed no crime, and is not aiming at his mother's death. And then there are a variety of ways in which this might be continued. (1) But as directly killing an innocent person is always and absolutely impermissible, an abortion may not be performed. Or, (2) as directly killing an innocent person is murder, and murder is always and absolutely impermissible, an abortion may not be performed.[4] Or, (3) as one's duty to refrain from directly killing an innocent person is more stringent than one's duty to keep a person from dying, an abortion may not be performed. Or, (4) if one's only options are directly killing an innocent person or letting a person die, one must prefer letting the person die, and thus an abortion may not be performed.[5]

Some people seem to have thought that these are not further premises which must be added if the conclusion is to be reached, but that they follow from the very fact that an innocent person has a right

to life.[6] But this seems to me to be a mistake, and perhaps the simplest way to show this is to bring out that while we must certainly grant that innocent persons have a right to life, the theses in (1) through (4) are all false. Take (2), for example. If directly killing an innocent person is murder, and thus is impermissible, then the mother's directly killing the innocent person inside her is murder, and thus is impermissible. But it cannot seriously be thought to be murder if the mother performs an abortion on herself to save her life. It cannot seriously be said that she *must* refrain, that she *must* sit passively by and wait for her death. Let us look again at the case of you and the violinist. There you are, in bed with the violinist, and the director of the hospital says to you, "It's all most distressing, and I deeply sympathize, but you see this is putting an additional strain on your kidneys, and you'll be dead within the month. But you *have* to stay where you are all the same. Because unplugging you would be directly killing an innocent violinist, and that's murder, and that's impermissible." If anything in the world is true, it is that you do not commit murder, you do not do what is impermissible, if you reach around to your back and unplug yourself from that violinist to save your life.

The main focus of attention in writings on abortion has been on what a third party may or may not do in answer to a request from a woman for an abortion. This is in a way understandable. Things being as they are, there isn't much a woman can safely do to abort herself. So the question asked is what a third party may do, and what the mother may do, if it is mentioned at all, is deduced, almost as an afterthought, from what it is concluded that third parties may do. But it seems to me that to treat the matter in this way is to refuse to grant to the mother that very status of person which is so firmly insisted on for the fetus. For we cannot simply read off what a person may do from what a third party may do. Suppose you find yourself trapped in a tiny house with a growing child. I mean a very tiny house, and a rapidly growing child—you are already up against the wall of the house and in a few minutes you'll be crushed to death. The child on the other hand won't be crushed to death; if nothing is done to stop him from growing he'll be hurt, but in the end he'll simply burst open the house and walk out a free man. Now I could well understand it if a bystander were to say, "There's nothing we can do for you. We cannot choose between your life and his, we cannot be the ones to decide who is to live, we cannot intervene." But it cannot be concluded that you too can do nothing, that you cannot attack it to save your life. However innocent the child may be, you do not have to wait passively while it crushes you to death. Perhaps a pregnant woman is vaguely felt to have the status of house, to which we don't allow the right of self-defense. But if the woman houses the child, it should be remembered that she is a person who houses it.

I should perhaps stop to say explicitly that I am not claiming that people have a right to do anything whatever to save their lives. I think, rather, that there are drastic limits to the right of self-defense. If someone threatens you with death unless you torture someone else to death, I think you have not the right, even to save your life, to do so. But the case under consideration here is very different. In our case there are only two people involved, one whose life is threatened, and one who threatens it. Both are innocent: the one who is threatened is not threatened because of any fault, the one who threatens does not threaten because of any fault. For this reason we may feel that we bystanders cannot intervene. But the person threatened can.

In sum, a woman surely can defend her life against the threat to it posed by the unborn child, even if doing so involves its death. And this shows not merely that the theses in (1) through (4) are false; it shows also that the extreme view of abortion is false, and so we need not canvass any other possible ways of arriving at it from the argument I mentioned at the outset.

2.

The extreme view could of course be weakened to say that while abortion is permissible to save the mother's life, it may not be performed by a third party, but only by the mother herself. But this cannot be right either. For what we have to keep in mind is that the mother and the unborn child are not like two tenants in a small house which has, by an unfortunate mistake, been rented to both: the mother *owns* the house. The fact that she does adds to the offensiveness of deducing that the mother can do nothing from the supposition that third parties can do nothing. But it does more than this: it casts a bright light on the supposition that third parties can do nothing. Certainly it lets us see that a third party who says "I cannot choose between you" is fooling

himself if he thinks this is impartiality. If Jones has found and fastened on a certain coat, which he needs to keep him from freezing, but which Smith also needs to keep him from freezing, then it is not impartiality that says "I cannot choose between you" when Smith owns the coat. Women have said again and again "This body is *my* body!" and they have reason to feel angry, reason to feel that it has been like shouting into the wind. Smith, after all, is hardly likely to bless us if we say to him, "Of course it's your coat, anybody would grant that it is. But no one may choose between you and Jones who is to have it."

We should really ask what it is that says "no one may choose" in the face of the fact that the body that houses the child is the mother's body. It may be simply a failure to appreciate this fact. But it may be something more interesting, namely the sense that one has a right to refuse to lay hands on people, even where it would be just and fair to do so, even where justice seems to require that somebody do so. Thus justice might call for somebody to get Smith's coat back from Jones, and yet you have a right to refuse to be the one to lay hands on Jones, a right to refuse to do physical violence to him. This, I think, must be granted. But then what should be said is not "no one may choose," but only "I cannot choose," and indeed not even this, but "*I* will not *act*," leaving it open that somebody else can or should, and in particular that anyone in a position of authority, with the job of securing people's rights, both can and should. So this is no difficulty. I have not been arguing that any given third party must accede to the mother's request that he perform an abortion to save her life, but only that he may.

I suppose that in some views of human life the mother's body is only on loan to her, the loan not being one which gives her any prior claim to it. One who held this view might well think it impartiality to say "I cannot choose." But I shall simply ignore this possibility. My own view is that if a human being has any just, prior claim to anything at all, he has a just, prior claim to his own body. And perhaps this needn't be argued for here anyway, since, as I mentioned, the arguments against abortion we are looking at do grant that the woman has a right to decide what happens in and to her body.

But although they do grant it, I have tried to show that they do not take seriously what is done in granting it. I suggest the same thing will reappear even more clearly when we turn away from cases in which the mother's life is at stake, and attend, as I propose we now do, to the vastly more common cases in which a woman wants an abortion for some less weighty reason than preserving her own life.

3.

Where the mother's life is not at stake, the argument I mentioned at the outset seems to have a much stronger pull. "Everyone has a right to life, so the unborn person has a right to life." And isn't the child's right to life weightier than anything other than the mother's own right to life, which she might put forward as ground for an abortion?

This argument treats the right to life as if it were unproblematic. It is not, and this seems to me to be precisely the source of the mistake.

For we should now, at long last, ask what it comes to, to have a right to life. In some views having a right to life includes having a right to be given at least the bare minimum one needs for continued life. But suppose that what in fact *is* the bare minimum a man needs for continued life is something he has no right at all to be given? If I am sick unto death, and the only thing that will save my life is the touch of Henry Fonda's cool hand on my fevered brow, then all the same, I have no right to be given the touch of Henry Fonda's cool hand on my fevered brow. It would be frightfully nice of him to fly in from the West Coast to provide it. It would be less nice, though no doubt well meant, if my friends flew out to the West Coast and carried Henry Fonda back with them. But I have no right at all against anybody that he should do this for me. Or again, to return to the story I told earlier, the fact that for continued life that violinist needs the continued use of your kidneys does not establish that he has a right to be given the continued use of your kidneys. He certainly has no right against you that *you* should give him continued use of your kidneys. For nobody has any right to use your kidneys unless you give him this right—if you do allow him to go on using your kidneys, this is a kindness on your part, and not something he can claim from you as his due. Nor has he any right against anybody else that *they* should give him continued use of your kidneys. Certainly he had no right against the Society of Music Lovers that they should plug him into you in the first place. And if you now start to unplug yourself, having learned that you will otherwise have to spend nine years in bed with him, there is

nobody in the world who must try to prevent you, in order to see to it that he is given something he has a right to be given.

Some people are rather stricter about the right to life. In their view, it does not include the right to be given anything, but amounts to, and only to, the right not to be killed by anybody. But here a related difficulty arises. If everybody is to refrain from killing that violinist, then everybody must refrain from doing a great many different sorts of things. Everybody must refrain from slitting his throat, everybody must refrain from shooting him—and everybody must refrain from unplugging you from him. But does he have a right against everybody that they shall refrain from unplugging you from him? To refrain from doing this is to allow him to continue to use your kidneys. It could be argued that he has a right against us that *we* should allow him to continue to use your kidneys. That is, while he had no right against us that we should give him the use of your kidneys, it might be argued that he anyway has a right against us that we shall not now intervene and deprive him of the use of your kidneys. I shall come back to third-party interventions later. But certainly the violinist has no right against you that *you* shall allow him to continue to use your kidneys. As I said, if you do allow him to use them, it is a kindness on your part, and not something you owe him.

The difficulty I point to here is not peculiar to the right of life. It reappears in connection with all the other natural rights, and it is something which an adequate account of rights must deal with. For present purposes it is enough just to draw attention to it. But I would stress that I am not arguing that people do not have a right to life—quite to the contrary, it seems to me that the primary control we must place on the acceptability of an account of rights is that it should turn out in that account to be a truth that all persons have a right to life. I am arguing only that having a right to life does not guarantee having either a right to be given the use of or a right to be allowed continued use of another person's body—even if one needs it for life itself. So the right to life will not serve the opponents of abortion in the very simple and clear way in which they seem to have thought it would.

4.

There is another way to bring out the difficulty. In the most ordinary sort of case, to deprive someone of what he has a right to is to treat him unjustly. Suppose a boy and his small brother are jointly given a box of chocolates for Christmas. If the older boy takes the box and refuses to give his brother any of the chocolates, he is unjust to him, for the brother has been given a right to half of them. But suppose that, having learned that otherwise it means nine years in bed with that violinist, you unplug yourself from him. You surely are not being unjust to him, for you gave him no right to use your kidneys, and no one else can have given him any such right. But we have to notice that in unplugging yourself, you are killing him; and violinists, like everybody else, have a right to life, and thus in the view we were considering just now, the right not to be killed. So here you do what he supposedly has a right you shall not do, but you do not act unjustly to him in doing it.

The emendation which may be made at this point is this: the right to life consists not in the right not to be killed, but rather in the right not to be killed unjustly. This runs a risk of circularity, but never mind: it would enable us to square the fact that the violinist has a right to life with the fact that you do not act unjustly toward him in unplugging yourself, thereby killing him. For if you do not kill him unjustly, you do not violate his right to life, and so it is no wonder you do him no injustice.

But if this emendation is accepted, the gap in the argument against abortion stares us plainly in the face: it is by no means enough to show that the fetus is a person, and to remind us that all persons have a right to life—we need to be shown also that killing the fetus violates its right to life, i.e., that abortion is unjust killing. And is it?

I suppose we may take it as a datum that in a case of pregnancy due to rape the mother has not given the unborn person a right to the use of her body for food and shelter. Indeed, in what pregnancy could it be supposed that the mother has given the unborn person such a right? It is not as if there were unborn persons drifting about the world, to whom a woman who wants a child says "I invite you in."

But it might be argued that there are other ways one can have acquired a right to the use of another person's body than by having been invited to use it by that person. Suppose a woman voluntarily indulges in intercourse, knowing of the chance it will issue in pregnancy, and then she does become pregnant; is she not in part responsible for the presence, in fact the very existence, of the unborn person inside? No doubt she did not invite it in. But doesn't her partial responsibility for its being there itself give it a right to the use of her body?[7] If so, then her aborting it would be more like the boys taking away the chocolates, and less like your unplugging yourself from the violinist—doing so would be depriving it of what it does have a right to, and thus would be doing it an injustice.

And then, too, it might be asked whether or not she can kill it even to save her own life: If she voluntarily called it into existence, how can she now kill it, even in self-defense?

The first thing to be said about this is that it is something new. Opponents of abortion have been so concerned to make out the independence of the fetus, in order to establish that it has a right to life, just as its mother does, that they have tended to overlook the possible support they might gain from making out that the fetus is *dependent* on the mother, in order to establish that she has a special kind of responsibility for it, a responsibility that gives it rights against her which are not possessed by any independent person—such as an ailing violinist who is a stranger to her.

On the other hand, this argument would give the unborn person a right to its mother's body only if her pregnancy resulted from a voluntary act, undertaken in full knowledge of the chance a pregnancy might result from it. It would leave out entirely the unborn person whose existence is due to rape. Pending the availability of some further argument, then, we would be left with the conclusion that unborn persons whose existence is due to rape have no right to the use of their mothers' bodies, and thus that aborting them is not depriving them of anything they have a right to and hence is not unjust killing.

And we should also notice that it is not at all plain that this argument really does go even as far as it purports to. For there are cases and cases, and the details make a difference. If the room is stuffy, and I therefore open a window to air it, and a burglar climbs in, it would be absurd to say, "Ah, now he can stay, she's given him a right to the use of her house—for she is partially responsible for his presence there, having voluntarily done what enabled him to get in, in full knowledge that there are such things as burglars, and that burglars burgle." It would be still more absurd to say this if I had had bars installed outside my windows, precisely to prevent burglars from getting in, and a burglar got in only because of a defect in the bars. It remains equally absurd if we imagine it is not a burglar who climbs in, but an innocent person who blunders or falls in. Again, suppose it were like this: people-seeds drift about in the air like pollen, and if you open your windows, one may drift in and take root in your carpets or upholstery. You don't want children, so you fix up your windows with fine mesh screens, the very best you can buy. As can happen, however, and on very, very rare occasions does happen, one of the screens is defective, and a seed drifts in and takes root. Does the person-plant who now develops have a right to the use of your house? Surely not—despite the fact that you voluntarily opened your windows, you knowingly kept carpets and upholstered furniture, and you knew that screens were sometimes defective. Someone may argue that you are responsible for its rooting, that it does have a right to your house, because after all you could have lived out your life with bare floors and furniture, or with sealed windows and doors. But this won't do —for by the same token anyone can avoid a pregnancy due to rape by having a hysterectomy, or anyway by never leaving home without a (reliable!) army.

It seems to me that the argument we are looking at can establish at most that there are *some* cases in which the unborn person has a right to the use of its mother's body, and therefore *some* cases in which abortion is unjust killing. There is room for much discussion and argument as to precisely which, if any. But I think we should sidestep this issue and leave it open, for at any rate the argument certainly does not establish that all abortion is unjust killing.

5.

There is room for yet another argument here, however. We surely must all grant that there may be cases in which it would be morally indecent to detach a person from your body at the cost of his life. Suppose you learn that what the violinist needs is not nine years of your life, but only one hour: all you need do to save his life is to spend one hour in that bed with him. Suppose also that letting him use your kidneys for that one hour would not affect your health in the slightest. Admittedly you were kidnapped. Admittedly you did not give anyone per-

mission to plug him into you. Nevertheless it seems to me plain you *ought* to allow him to use your kidneys for that hour—it would be indecent to refuse.

Again, suppose pregnancy lasted only an hour, and constituted no threat to life or health. And suppose that a woman becomes pregnant as a result of rape. Admittedly she did not voluntarily do anything to bring about the existence of a child. Admittedly she did nothing at all which would give the unborn person a right to the use of her body. All the same it might well be said, as in the newly amended violinist story, that she *ought* to allow it to remain for that hour—that it would be indecent of her to refuse.

Now some people are inclined to use the term "right" in such a way that it follows from the fact that you ought to allow a person to use your body for the hour he needs, that he has a right to use your body for the hour he needs, even though he has not been given that right by any person or act. They may say that it follows also that if you refuse, you act unjustly toward him. This use of the term is perhaps so common that it cannot be called wrong; nevertheless it seems to me to be an unfortunate loosening of what we would do better to keep a tight rein on. Suppose that box of chocolates I mentioned earlier had not been given to both boys jointly, but was given only to the older boy. There he sits, stolidly eating his way through the box, his small brother watching enviously. Here we are likely to say, "You ought not to be so mean. You ought to give your brother some of those chocolates." My own view is that it just does not follow from the truth of this that the brother has any right to any of the chocolates. If the boy refuses to give his brother any, he is greedy, stingy, callous—but not unjust. I suppose that the people I have in mind will say it does follow that the brother has a right to some of the chocolates, and thus that the boy does act unjustly if he refuses to give his brother any. But the effect of saying this is to obscure what we should keep distinct, namely the difference between the boy's refusal in this case and the boy's refusal in the earlier case, in which the box was given to both boys jointly, and in which the small brother thus had what was from any point of view clear title to half.

A further objection to so using the term "right" that from the fact that A ought to do a thing for B, it follows that B has a right against A that A do it for him, is that it is going to make the question of whether or not a man has a right to a thing turn on how easy it is to provide him with it; and this seems not merely unfortunate, but morally unacceptable. Take the case of Henry Fonda again. I said earlier that I had no right to the touch of his cool hand on my fevered brow, even though I needed it to save my life. I said it would be frightfully nice of him to fly in from the West Coast to provide me with it, but that I had no right against him that he should do so. But suppose he isn't on the West Coast. Suppose he has only to walk across the room, place a hand briefly on my brow—and lo, my life is saved. Then surely he ought to do it, it would be indecent to refuse. Is it to be said, "Ah, well, it follows that in this case she has a right to the touch of his hand on her brow, and so it would be an injustice in him to refuse"? So that I have a right to it when it is easy for him to provide it, though no right when it's hard? It's rather a shocking idea that anyone's rights should fade away and disappear as it gets harder and harder to accord them to him.

So my own view is that even though you ought to let the violinist use your kidneys for the one hour he needs, we should not conclude that he has a right to do so—we should say that if you refuse, you are, like the boy who owns all the chocolates and will give none away, self-centered and callous, indecent in fact, but not unjust. And similarly, that even supposing a case in which a woman pregnant due to rape ought to allow the unborn person to use her body for the hour he needs, we should not conclude that he has a right to do so; we should conclude that she is self-centered, callous, indecent, but not unjust, if she refuses. The complaints are no less grave; they are just different. However, there is no need to insist on this point. If anyone does wish to deduce "he has a right" from "you ought," then all the same he must surely grant that there are cases in which it is not morally required of you that you allow that violinist to use your kidneys, and in which he does not have a right to use them, and in which you do not do him an injustice if you refuse. And so also for mother and unborn child. Except in such cases as the unborn person has a right to demand it—and we were leaving open the possibility that there may be such cases—nobody is morally *required* to make large sacrifices, of health, of all other interests and concerns, of all other duties and commitments, for nine years, or even for nine months, in order to keep another person alive.

6.

We have in fact to distinguish between two kinds of Samaritan: the Good Samaritan and what we might call the Minimally Decent Samaritan. The story of the Good Samaritan, you will remember, goes like this:

> A certain man went down from Jerusalem to Jericho, and fell among thieves, which stripped him of his raiment, and wounded him, and departed, leaving him half dead.
>
> And by chance there came down a certain priest that way: and when he saw him, he passed by on the other side.
>
> And likewise a Levite, when he was at the place, came and looked on him, and passed by on the other side.
>
> But a certain Samaritan, as he journeyed, came where he was; and when he saw him he had compassion on him.
>
> And went to him, and bound up his wounds, pouring in oil and wine, and set him on his own beast, and brought him to an inn, and took care of him.
>
> And on the morrow, when he departed, he took out two pence, and gave them to the host, and said unto him, "Take care of him; and whatsoever thou spendest more, when I come again, I will repay thee." (Luke 10:30–35)

The Good Samaritan went out of his way, at some cost to himself, to help one in need of it. We are not told what the options were, that is, whether or not the priest and the Levite could have helped by doing less than the Good Samaritan did, but assuming they could have, then the fact they did nothing at all shows they were not even Minimally Decent Samaritans, not because they were not Samaritans, but because they were not even minimally decent.

These things are a matter of degree, of course, but there is a difference, and it comes out perhaps most clearly in the story of Kitty Genovese, who, as you will remember, was murdered while thirty-eight people watched or listened, and did nothing at all to help her. A Good Samaritan would have rushed out to give direct assistance against the murderer. Or perhaps we had better allow that it would have been a Splendid Samaritan who did this, on the ground that it would have involved a risk of death for himself. But the thirty-eight not only did not do this, they did not even trouble to pick up a phone to call the police. Minimally Decent Samaritanism would call for doing at least that, and their not having done it was monstrous.

After telling the story of the Good Samaritan, Jesus said, "Go, and do thou likewise." Perhaps he meant that we are morally required to act as the Good Samaritan did. Perhaps he was urging people to do more than is morally required of them. At all events it seems plain that it was not morally required of any of the thirty-eight that he rush out to give direct assistance at the risk of his own life, and that it is not morally required of anyone that he give long stretches of his life—nine years or nine months—to sustaining the life of a person who has no special right (we were leaving open the possibility of this) to demand it.

Indeed, with one rather striking class of exceptions, no one in any country in the world is *legally* required to do anywhere near as much as this for anyone else. The class of exceptions is obvious. My main concern here is not the state of the law in respect to abortion, but it is worth drawing attention to the fact that in no state in this country is any man compelled by law to be even a Minimally Decent Samaritan to any person; there is no law under which charges could be brought against the thirty-eight who stood by while Kitty Genovese died. By contrast, in most states in this country women are compelled by law to be not merely Minimally Decent Samaritans, but Good Samaritans to un-born persons inside them. This doesn't by itself settle anything one way or the other, because it may well be argued that there should be laws in this country—as there are in many European countries—compelling at least Minimally Decent Sa-maritanism.[8] But it does show that there is a gross injustice in the existing state of the law. And it shows also that the groups currently working against liberalization of abortion laws, in fact work-ing toward having it declared unconstitutional for a state to permit abortion, had better start working for the adoption of Good Samaritan laws generally, or earn the charge that they are acting in bad faith.

I should think, myself, that Minimally Decent Samaritan laws would be one thing, Good Samari-tan laws quite another, and in fact highly improper. But we are not here concerned with the law. What we should ask is not whether anybody should be compelled by law to be a Good Samaritan, but whether we must accede to a situation in which somebody is being compelled—by nature, per-haps—to be a Good Samaritan. We have, in other words, to look now at third-party interventions. I have been arguing that no person is morally re-quired to make large sacrifices to sustain the life of another who has no right to demand them, and this even where the sacrifices do not include life itself; we are not morally required to be Good Samaritans or anyway Very Good Samaritans to one another. But what if a man cannot extricate himself from such a situation? What if he appeals to us to extricate him? It seems to me plain that there are cases in which we can, cases in which a good Samaritan would extri-cate him. There you are, you were kidnapped, and nine years in bed with that violinist lie ahead of you. You have your own life to lead. You are sorry, but you simply cannot see giving up so much of your life to the sustaining of his. You cannot extricate yourself, and ask us to do so. I should have thought that—in light of his having no right to the use of your body—it was obvious that we do not have to accede to your being forced to give up so much. We can do what you ask. There is no injustice to the violinist in our doing so.

7.

Following the lead of the opponents of abor-tion, I have throughout been speaking of the fetus merely as a person, and what I have been asking is whether or not the argument we began with, which proceeds only from the fetus's being a person, really does establish its conclusion. I have argued that it does not.

But of course there are arguments and argu-ments, and it may be said that I have simply fas-tened on the wrong one. It may be said that what is important is not merely the fact that the fetus is a person, but that it is a person for whom the woman has a special kind of responsibility issuing from the fact that she is its mother. And it might be argued that all my analogies are therefore irrelevant—for you do not have that special kind of responsibility for that violinist, Henry Fonda does not have that special kind of responsibility for me. And our atten-tion might be drawn to the fact that men and women both *are* compelled by law to provide support for their children.

I have in effect dealt (briefly) with this argu-ment in section 4 above; but a (still briefer) recapit-ulation now may be in order. Surely we do not have any such "special responsibility" for a person unless we have assumed it, explicitly or implicitly. If a set of parents do not try to prevent pregnancy, do not obtain an abortion, but rather take it home with them, then they have assumed responsibility for it, they have given it rights, and they cannot *now* withdraw support from it at the cost of its life because they now find it difficult to go on providing for it. But if they have taken all reasonable precautions against having a child, they do not simply by virtue of their biological relationship to the child who comes into existence have a special responsibility for it. They may wish to assume responsibility for it, or they may not wish to. And I am suggesting that if assuming responsibility for it would require large sacrifices, then they may refuse. A Good Samaritan would not refuse—or anyway, a Splendid Samaritan, if the sacrifices that had to be made were enormous. But then so would a Good Samaritan assume responsibility for that violinist; so would Henry Fonda, if he is a Good Samaritan, fly in from the West Coast and assume responsibility for me.

8.

My argument will be found unsatisfactory on two counts by many of those who want to regard abortion as morally permissible. First, while I do argue that abortion is not impermissible, I do not argue that it is always permissible. There may well be cases in which carrying the child to term requires only Minimally Decent Samaritanism of the mother, and this is a standard we must not fall below. I am inclined to think it a merit of my account precisely that it does *not* give a general yes or a general no. It allows for and supports our sense that, for example, a sick and desperately frightened fourteen-year-old schoolgirl, pregnant due to rape, may *of course* choose abortion, and that any law which rules this out is an insane law. And it also allows for and supports our sense that in other cases resort to abortion is even positively indecent. It would be indecent in the woman to request an abortion, and indecent in a doctor to perform it, if she is in her seventh month, and wants the abortion just to avoid the nuisance of postponing a trip abroad. The very fact that the arguments I have been drawing attention to treat all cases of abortion, or even all cases of abortion in which the mother's life is not at stake, as morally on a par ought to have made them suspect at the outset.

Second, while I am arguing for the permissibility of abortion in some cases, I am not arguing for the right to secure the death of the unborn child. It is easy to confuse these two things in that up to a certain point in the life of the fetus it is not able to survive outside the mother's body; hence removing it from her body guarantees its death. But they are importantly different. I have argued that you are not morally required to spend nine months in bed, sustaining the life of that violinist; but to say this is by no means to say that if, when you unplug yourself, there is a miracle and he survives, you then have a right to turn round and slit his throat. You may detach yourself even if this costs him his life; you have no right to be guaranteed his death, by some other means, if unplugging yourself does not kill him. There are some people who will feel dissatisfied by this feature of my argument. A woman may be utterly devastated by the thought of a child, a bit of herself, put out for adoption and never seen or heard of again. She may therefore want not merely that the child be detached from her, but more, that it die. Some opponents of abortion are inclined to regard this as beneath contempt—thereby showing insensitivity to what is surely a powerful source of despair. All the same, I agree that the desire for the child's death is not one which anybody may gratify, should it turn out to be possible to detach the child alive.

At this place, however, it should be remembered that we have only been pretending throughout that the fetus is a human being from the moment of conception. A very early abortion is surely not the killing of a person, and so is not dealt with by anything I have said here.

Notes

1. I am very much indebted to James Thomson for discussion, criticism, and many helpful suggestions.

2. Daniel Callahan, *Abortion: Law, Choice and Morality* (New York, 1970), p. 373. This book gives a fascinating survey of the available information on abortion. The Jewish tradition is surveyed in David M. Feldman, *Birth Control in Jewish Law* (New York, 1968). Part 5, the Catholic tradition in John T. Noonan, Jr., "An Almost Absolute Value in History," in *The Morality of Abortion*, ed. John T. Noonan, Jr. (Cambridge, Mass., 1970).

3. The term "direct" in the arguments I refer to is a technical one. Roughly, what is meant by "direct killing" is either killing as an end in itself, or killing as a means to some end, for example, the end of saving someone else's life. See note 6, below, for an example of its use.

4. Cf. *Encyclical Letter of Pope Pius XI on Christian Marriage*, St. Paul Editions (Boston, n.d.), p. 32:

"However much we may pity the mother whose health and even life is gravely imperiled in the performance of the duty allotted to her by nature, nevertheless what could ever be a sufficient reason for excusing in any way the direct murder of the innocent? This is precisely what we are dealing with here." Noonan (*The Morality of Abortion*, p. 43) reads this as follows: "What cause can ever avail to excuse in any way the direct killing of the innocent? For it is a question of that."

5.   The thesis in (4) is in an interesting way weaker than those in (1), (2), and (3): they rule out abortion even in cases in which both mother *and* child will die if the abortion is not performed. By contrast, one who held the view expressed in (4) could consistently say that one needn't prefer letting two persons die to killing one.

6.   Cf. the following passage from Pius XII, *Address to the Italian Catholic Society of Midwives*: "The baby in the maternal breast has the right to life immediately

from God.—Hence there is no man, no human authority, no science, no medical, eugenic, social, economic or moral 'indication' which can establish or grant a valid juridical ground for a direct deliberate disposition of an innocent human life, that is a disposition which looks to its destruction either as an end or as a means to another end perhaps in itself not illicit.—The baby, still not born, is a man in the same degree and for the same reason as the mother" (quoted in Noonan, *The Morality of Abortion*, p. 45).

7.   The need for a discussion of this argument was brought home to me by members of the Society for Ethical and Legal Philosophy, to whom this paper was originally presented.

8.   For a discussion of the difficulties involved, and a survey of the European experience with such laws, see *The Good Samaritan and the Law*, ed. James M. Ratcliffe (New York, 1966).

On the Moral and Legal Status of Abortion

Mary Anne Warren

Mary Anne Warren takes an even stronger position than Thomson (see preceding article), arguing that a woman's right to have an abortion is unrestricted. She attempts to show that there is no adequate basis for holding that the fetus has "a significant right to life" and that, whatever right can be appropriately granted to the fetus, it can never override a woman's right to protect her own interest and well-being. Accordingly, laws that restrict access to abortion are an unjustified violation of a woman's rights.

Warren is critical of both Noonan (see earlier article) and Thomson. Noonan, she claims, fails to demonstrate that whatever is genetically human (the fetus) is also morally human (a person). Thomson, Warren argues, is mistaken in believing that it is possible both to grant that the fetus is a person and to produce a satisfactory defense of the right to obtain an abortion. Contrary to Thomson's aim, her central argument supports the right to abortion only in cases in which the woman is in no way responsible for her pregnancy.

Like Noonan, Warren conceives the basic issue in abortion to be the question of what properties something must possess to be a person in the moral sense. She offers five traits she believes anyone would accept as central and argues that the fetus, at all stages of development, possesses none of them. Since the fetus is not a person, it is not entitled to the full range of moral rights. That the fetus has the potential to become a person may give it a prima facie right to life, but the rights of an actual person always outweigh those of a potential person.

We will be concerned with both the moral status of abortion, which for our purposes we may define as the act which a woman performs in voluntarily terminating, or allowing another person to terminate, her pregnancy, and the legal status which is appropriate for this act. I will argue that, while it is not possible to produce a satisfactory defense of a woman's right to obtain an abortion without showing that a fetus is not a human being, in the morally relevant sense of that term, we ought not to conclude that the difficulties involved in determining whether or not a fetus is human make it impossible to produce any satisfactory solution to the problem of the moral status of abortion. For it is possible to show that, on the basis of intuitions which we may expect even the opponents of abortion to share, a fetus is not a person, and hence not the sort of entity to which it is proper to ascribe full moral rights.

Of course, while some philosophers would deny the possibility of any such proof,[1] others will deny that there is any need for it, since the moral permissibility of abortion appears to them to be too obvious to require proof. But the inadequacy of this attitude should be evident from the fact that both the friends and the foes of abortion consider their position to be morally self-evident. Because proabortionists have never adequately come to grips with the conceptual issues surrounding abortion, most if not all, of the arguments which they advance in opposition to laws restricting access to abortion fail to refute or even weaken the traditional antiabortion argument, i.e., that a fetus is a human being, and therefore abortion is murder.

These arguments are typically of one of two sorts. Either they point to the terrible side effects of the restrictive laws, e.g., the deaths due to illegal abortions, and the fact that it is poor women who suffer the most as a result of these laws, or else they state that to deny a woman access to abortion is to deprive her of her right to control her own body. Unfortunately, however, the fact that restricting access to abortion has tragic side effects does not, in itself, show that the restrictions are unjustified, since murder is wrong regardless of the consequences of prohibiting it; and the appeal to the right to control one's body, which is generally construed as a property right, is at best a rather feeble argument for the permissibility of abortion. Mere ownership does not give me the right to kill innocent people whom I find on my property, and indeed I am apt to be held responsible if such people injure themselves while on my property. It is equally unclear that I have any moral right to expel an innocent person from my property when I know that doing so will result in his death.

Furthermore, it is probably inappropriate to describe a woman's body as her property, since it seems natural to hold that a person is something distinct from her property, but not from her body. Even those who would object to the identification of a person with his body, or with the conjunction of his body and his mind, must admit that it would be very odd to describe, say, breaking a leg, as damaging one's property, and much more appropriate to describe it as injuring one*self*. Thus it is probably a mistake to argue that the right to obtain an abortion is in any way derived from the right to own and regulate property.

But however we wish to construe the right to abortion, we cannot hope to convince those who consider abortion a form of murder of the existence of any such right unless we are able to produce a clear and convincing refutation of the traditional antiabortion argument, and this has not, to my knowledge, been done. With respect to the two most vital issues which that argument involves, i.e., the humanity of the fetus and its implication for the moral status of abortion, confusion has prevailed on both sides of the dispute.

Thus, both proabortionists and antiabortionists have tended to abstract the question of whether abortion is wrong to that of whether it is wrong to destroy a fetus, just as though the rights of another person were not necessarily involved. This mistaken abstraction has led to the almost universal assumption that if a fetus is a human being, with a right to life, then it follows immediately that abortion is wrong (except perhaps when necessary to save the woman's life), and that it ought to be prohibited. It has also been generally assumed that unless the question about the status of the fetus is answered, the moral status of abortion cannot possibly be determined.

Reprinted from The Monist, *LaSalle, Illinois 61301, Vol. 57, no. 1, with permission. "Postscript on Infanticide" reprinted from* The Problem of Abortion, *Second Edition, edited by Joel Fienberg (Belmont, Calif.: Wadsworth, 1984).*

Two recent papers, one by B. A. Brody,[2] and one by Judith Thomson,[3] have attempted to settle the question of whether abortion ought to be prohibited apart from the question of whether or not the fetus is human. Brody examines the possibility that the following two statements are compatible: (1) that abortion is the taking of innocent human life, and therefore wrong; and (2) that nevertheless it ought not to be prohibited by law, at least under the present circumstances.[4] Not surprisingly, Brody finds it impossible to reconcile these two statements, since, as he rightly argues, none of the unfortunate side effects of the prohibition of abortion is bad enough to justify legalizing the *wrongful* taking of human life. He is mistaken, however, in concluding that the incompatibility of (1) and (2), in itself, shows that "the legal problem about abortion cannot be resolved independently of the status of the fetus problem" (p. 369).

What Brody fails to realize is that (1) embodies the questionable assumption that if a fetus is a human being, then of course abortion is morally wrong, and that an attack on *this* assumption is more promising, as a way of reconciling the humanity of the fetus with the claim that laws prohibiting abortion are unjustified, than is an attack on the assumption that if abortion is the wrongful killing of innocent human beings then it ought to be prohibited. He thus overlooks the possibility that a fetus may have a right to life and abortion still be morally permissible, in that the right of a woman to terminate an unwanted pregnancy might override the right of the fetus to be kept alive. This immorality of abortion is no more demonstrated by the humanity of the fetus, in itself, than the immorality of killing in self-defense is demonstrated by the fact that the assailant is a human being. Neither is it demonstrated by the *innocence* of the fetus, since there may be situations in which the killing of innocent human beings is justified.

It is perhaps not surprising that Brody fails to spot this assumption, since it has been accepted with little or no argument by nearly everyone who has written on the morality of abortion. John Noonan is correct in saying that "the fundamental question in the long history of abortion is, How do you determine the humanity of a being?"[5] He summarizes his own antiabortion argument, which is a version of the official position of the Catholic Church, as follows:

. . . it is wrong to kill humans, however poor, weak, defenseless, and lacking in opportunity to develop their potential they may be. It is therefore morally wrong to kill Biafrans. Similarly, it is morally wrong to kill embryos.[6]

Noonan bases his claim that fetuses are human upon what he calls the theologians' criterion of humanity: that whoever is conceived of human beings is human. But although he argues at length for the appropriateness of this criterion, he never questions the assumption that if a fetus is human then abortion is wrong for exactly the same reason that murder is wrong.

Judith Thomson is, in fact, the only writer I am aware of who has seriously questioned this assumption; she has argued that, even if we grant the antiabortionist his claim that a fetus is a human being, with the same right to life as any other human being, we can still demonstrate that, in at least some and perhaps most cases, a woman is under no moral obligation to complete an unwanted pregnancy.[7] Her argument is worth examining, since if it holds up it may enable us to establish the moral permissibility of abortion without becoming involved in problems about what entitles an entity to be considered human, and accorded full moral rights. To be able to do this would be a great gain in the power and simplicity of the proabortion position, since, although I will argue that these problems can be solved at least as decisively as can any other moral problem, we should certainly be pleased to be able to avoid having to solve them as part of the justification of abortion.

On the other hand, even if Thomson's argument does not hold up, her insight, i.e., that it requires argument to show that if fetuses are human then abortion is properly classified as murder, is an extremely valuable one. The assumption she attacks is particularly invidious, for it amounts to the decision that it is appropriate, in deciding the moral status of abortion, to leave the rights of the pregnant woman out of consideration entirely, except possibly when her life is threatened. Obviously, this will not do; determining what moral rights, if any, a fetus possesses is only the first step in determining the moral status of abortion. Step two, which is at least equally essential, is finding a just solution to the conflict between whatever rights the fetus may have, and the rights of the woman who is unwillingly pregnant. While the historical error has been to pay far too little attention to the second step, Ms. Thomson's suggestion is that if we look at the second step first we may find that a woman has a right to obtain an abortion *regardless* of what rights the fetus has.

Our own inquiry will also have two stages. In Section I, we will consider whether or not it is possible to establish that abortion is morally permissible even on the assumption that a fetus is an entity with a full-fledged right to life. I will argue that in fact this cannot be established, at least not with the conclusiveness which is essential to our hopes of convincing those who are skeptical about the morality of abortion, and that we therefore cannot avoid dealing with the question of whether or not a fetus really does have the same right to life as a (more fully developed) human being.

In Section II, I will propose an answer to this question, namely, that a fetus cannot be considered a member of the moral community, the set of beings with full and equal moral rights, for the simple reason that it is not a person, and that it is personhood, and not genetic humanity, i.e., humanity as defined by Noonan, which is the basis for membership in this community. I will argue that a fetus, whatever its stage of development, satisfies none of the basic criteria of personhood, and is not even enough *like* a person to be accorded even some of the same rights on the basis of this resemblance. Nor, as we will see, is a fetus's *potential* personhood a threat to the morality of abortion, since, whatever the rights of potential people may be, they are invariably overridden in any conflict with the moral rights of actual people.

I

We turn now to Professor Thomson's case for the claim that even if a fetus has full moral rights, abortion is still morally permissible, at least sometimes, and for some reasons other than to save the woman's life. Her argument is based upon a clever, but I think faulty, analogy. She asked us to picture ourselves waking up one day, in bed with a famous violinist. Imagine that you have been kidnapped, and your bloodstream hooked up to that of the violinist, who happens to have an ailment which will certainly kill him unless he is permitted to share your kidneys for a period of nine months. No one else can save him, since you alone have the right

type of blood. He will be unconscious all that time, and you will have to stay in bed with him, but after the nine months are over he may be unplugged, completely cured, that is provided that you have cooperated.

Now then, she continues, what are your obligations in this situation? The antiabortionist, if he is consistent, will have to say that you are obligated to stay in bed with the violinist: for all people have a right to life, and violinists are people, and therefore it would be murder for you to disconnect yourself from him and let him die (p. 49). But this is outrageous, and so there must be something wrong with the same argument when it is applied to abortion. It would certainly be commendable of you to agree to save the violinist, but it is absurd to suggest that your refusal to do so would be murder. His right to life does not obligate you to do whatever is required to keep him alive; nor does it justify anyone else in forcing you to do so. A law which required you to stay in bed with the violinist would clearly be an unjust law, since it is no proper function of the law to force unwilling people to make huge sacrifices for the sake of other people toward whom they have no such prior obligation.

Thomson concludes that, if this analogy is an apt one, then we can grant the antiabortionist his claim that a fetus is a human being, and still hold that it is at least sometimes the case that a pregnant woman has the right to refuse to be a Good Samaritan towards the fetus, i.e., to obtain an abortion. For there is a great gap between the claim that x has a right to life, and the claim that y is obligated to do whatever is necessary to keep x alive, let alone that he ought to be forced to do so. It is y's duty to keep x alive only if he has somehow contracted a *special* obligation to do so; and a woman who is unwillingly pregnant, e.g., who was raped, has done nothing which obligates her to make the enormous sacrifice which is necessary to preserve the conceptus.

This argument is initially quite plausible, and in the extreme case of pregnancy due to rape it is probably conclusive. Difficulties arise, however, when we try to specify more exactly the range of cases in which abortion is clearly justifiable even on the assumption that the fetus is human. Professor Thomson considers it a virtue of her argument that it does not enable us to conclude that abortion is *always* permissible. It would, she says, be "indecent" for a woman in her seventh month to obtain an abortion just to avoid having to postpone a trip to Europe. On the other hand, her argument enables us to see that "a sick and desperately frightened schoolgirl pregnant due to rape may *of course* choose abortion, and that any law which rules this out is an insane law" (p. 65). So far, so good; but what are we to say about the woman who becomes pregnant not through rape but as a result of her own carelessness, or because of contraceptive failure, or who gets pregnant intentionally and then changes her mind about wanting a child? With respect to such cases, the violinist analogy is of much less use to the defender of the woman's right to obtain an abortion.

Indeed, the choice of a pregnancy due to rape, as an example of a case in which abortion is permissible even if a fetus is considered a human being, is extremely significant; for it is only in the case of pregnancy due to rape that the woman's situation is adequately analogous to the violinist case for our intuitions about the latter to transfer convincingly. The crucial difference between a pregnancy due to rape and the normal case of an unwanted pregnancy is that in the normal case we cannot claim that the woman is in no way responsible for her predicament; she could have remained chaste, or taken her pills more faithfully, or abstained on dangerous days, and so on. If on the other hand, you are kidnapped by strangers, and hooked up to a strange violinist, then you are free of any shred of responsibility for the situation, on the basis of which it would be argued that you are obligated to keep the violinist alive. Only when her pregnancy is due to rape is a woman clearly just as nonresponsible.[8]

Consequently, there is room for the antiabortionist to argue that in the normal case of unwanted pregnancy a woman has, by her own actions, assumed responsibility for the fetus. For if x behaves in a way which he could have avoided, and which he knows involves, let us say, a 1 percent chance of bringing into existence a human being, with a right to life, and does so knowing that if this should happen then that human being will perish unless x does certain things to keep him alive, then it is by no means clear that when it does happen x is free of any obligation to what he knew in advance would be required to keep that human being alive.

The plausibility of such an argument is enough to show that the Thomson analogy can provide a clear and persuasive defense of a woman's right to obtain an abortion only with respect to those cases in which the woman is in no way responsible for her pregnancy, e.g., where it is due to rape. In all other cases, we would almost certainly conclude that it was necessary to look carefully at the particular circumstances in order to determine the extent of the woman's responsibility, and hence the extent of her obligation. This is an extremely unsatisfactory outcome, from the viewpoint of the opponents of restrictive abortion laws, most of whom are convinced that a woman has a right to obtain an abortion regardless of how and why she got pregnant.

Of course a supporter of the violinist analogy might point out that it is absurd to suggest that forgetting her pill one day might be sufficient to obligate a woman to complete an unwanted pregnancy. And indeed it *is* absurd to suggest this. As we will see, the moral right to obtain an abortion is not in the least dependent upon the extent to which the woman is responsible for her pregnancy. But unfortunately, once we allow the assumption that a fetus has full moral rights, we cannot avoid taking this absurd suggestion seriously. Perhaps we can make this point more clear by altering the violinist story just enough to make it more analogous to a normal unwanted pregnancy and less to a pregnancy due to rape, and then seeing whether it is still obvious that you are not obligated to stay in bed with the fellow.

Suppose, then, that violinists are peculiarly prone to the sort of illness the only cure for which is the use of someone else's bloodstream for nine months, and that because of this there has been formed a society of music lovers who agree that whenever a violinist is stricken they will draw lots and the loser will, by some means, be made the one and only person capable of saving him. Now then, would you be obligated to cooperate in curing the violinist if you had voluntarily joined this society, knowing the possible consequences, and then your name had been drawn and you had been kidnapped? Admittedly, you did not promise ahead of time that you would, but you did deliberately place yourself in a position in which it might happen that a human life would be lost if you did not. Surely this is at least a prima facie reason for supposing that you have an obligation to stay in bed with the violinist. Suppose that you had gotten your name drawn deliberately; surely *that* would be quite a strong reason for thinking that you had such an obligation.

It might be suggested that there is one important disanalogy between the modified violinist case and the case of an unwanted pregnancy, which makes the woman's responsibility significantly less, namely, the fact that the fetus *comes into existence* as the result of the result of the woman's actions. This fact might give her a right to refuse to keep it alive, whereas she would not have had this right had it existed previously, independently, and then as a result of her actions become dependent upon her for its survival.

My own intuition, however, is that x has no more right to bring into existence, either deliberately or as a foreseeable result of actions he could have avoided, a being with full moral rights (y), and then refuse to do what he knew beforehand would be required to keep that being alive, than he has to enter into an agreement with an existing person, whereby he may be called upon to save that person's life, and then refuse to do so when so called upon. Thus x's responsibility for y's existence does not seem to lessen his obligation to keep y alive, if he is also responsible for y's being in a situation in which only he can save him.

Whether or not this intuition is entirely correct, it brings us back once again to the conclusion that once we allow the assumption that a fetus has full moral rights it becomes an extremely complex and difficult question whether and when abortion is justifiable. Thus the Thomson analogy cannot help us produce a clear and persuasive proof of the moral permissibility of abortion. Nor will the opponents of the restrictive laws thank us for anything less; for their conviction (for the most part) is that abortion is obviously *not* a morally serious and extremely unfortunate, even though sometimes justified act, comparable to killing in self-defense or to letting the violinist die, but rather is closer to being a morally neutral act, like cutting one's hair.

The basis of this conviction, I believe, is the realization that a fetus is not a person, and thus does not have a full-fledged right to life. Perhaps the reason why this claim has been so inadequately defended is that it seems self-evident to those who accept it. And so it is, insofar as it follows from what I take to be perfectly obvious claims about the nature of personhood, and about the proper grounds for ascribing moral rights, claims which ought, indeed, to be obvious to both the friends and foes of abortion. Nevertheless, it is worth examining these claims, and showing how they demonstrate the moral innocuousness of abortion, since this apparently has not been adequately done before.

II

The question which we must answer in order to produce a satisfactory solution to the problem of the moral status of abortion is this: How are we to define the moral community, the set of beings with full and equal moral rights, such that we can decide whether a human fetus is a member of this community or not? What sort of entity, exactly, has the inalienable rights to life, liberty, and the pursuit of happiness? Jefferson attributed these rights to all *men*, and it may or may not be fair to suggest that he intended to attribute them *only* to men. Perhaps he ought have attributed them to all human beings. If so, then we arrive, first, at Noonan's problem of defining what makes a being human, and, second, at the equally vital question which Noonan does not consider, namely, What reason is there for identifying the moral community with the set of all human beings, in whatever way we have chosen to define that term?

1. On the Definition of "Human"

One reason why this vital second question is so frequently overlooked in the debate over the moral status of abortion is that the term "human" has two distinct, but not often distinguished, senses. This fact results in a slide of meaning, which serves to conceal the fallaciousness of the traditional argument that since (1) it is wrong to kill innocent human beings, and (2) fetuses are innocent human beings, then (3) it is wrong to kill fetuses. For if "human" is used in the same sense in both (1) and (2) then, whichever of the two senses is meant, one of these premises is question-begging. And if it is used in two different senses then of course the conclusion doesn't follow.

Thus, (1) is a self-evident moral truth,[9] and avoids begging the question about abortion, only if "human being" is used to mean something like "a full-fledged member of the moral community." (It may or may not also be meant to refer exclusively to members of the species *Homo sapiens*.) We may call this the *moral* sense of "human." It is not to be confused with what we will call the *genetic* sense; i.e., the sense in which *any* member of the species is a human being, and no member of any other species could be. If (1) is acceptable only if the moral sense is intended, (2) is non-question-begging only if what is intended is the genetic sense.

In "Deciding Who is Human," Noonan argues for the classification of fetuses with human beings by pointing to the presence of the full genetic code, and the potential capacity for rational thought (p. 135). It is clear that what he needs to show, for his version of the traditional argument to be valid, is that fetuses are human in the moral sense, the sense in which it is analytically true that all human beings have full moral rights. But, in the absence of any argument showing that whatever is genetically human is also morally human, and he gives none, nothing more than genetic humanity can be demonstrated by the presence of the human genetic code. And, as we will see, the *potential* capacity for rational thought can at most show that an entity has the potential for *becoming* human in the moral sense.

2. Defining the Moral Community

Can it be established that genetic humanity is sufficient for moral humanity? I think that there are very good reasons for not defining the moral community in this way. I would like to suggest an alternative way of defining the moral community, which I will argue for only to the extent of explaining why it is, or should be, self-evident. The suggestion is simply that the moral community consists of all and *only* people, rather than all and only human beings;[10] and probably the best way of demonstrating its self-evidence is by considering the concept of personhood, to see what sorts of entity are and are not persons, and what the decision that a being is or is not a person implies about its moral rights.

What characteristics entitle an entity to be considered a person? This is obviously not the place to attempt a complete analysis of the concept of personhood, but we do not need such a fully adequate analysis just to determine whether and why a fetus is or isn't a person. All we need is a rough and approximate list of the most basic criteria of personhood, and some idea of which, or how many, of these an entity must satisfy in order to properly be considered a person.

In searching for such criteria, it is useful to look beyond the set of people with whom we are acquainted, and ask how we would decide whether a totally alien being was a person or not. (For we have no right to assume that genetic humanity is necessary for personhood.) Imagine a space traveler who lands on an unknown planet and encounters a race of beings utterly unlike any he has ever seen or heard of. If he wants to be sure of behaving morally toward these beings, he has to somehow decide whether they are people, and hence have full moral

rights, or whether they are the sort of thing which he need not feel guilty about treating as, for example, a source of food.

How should he go about making this decision? If he has some anthropological background, he might look for such things as religion, art, and the manufacturing of tools, weapons, or shelters, since these factors have been used to distinguish our human from our prehuman ancestors, in what seems to be closer to the moral than the genetic sense of "human." And no doubt he would be right to consider the presence of such factors as good evidence that the alien beings were people, and morally human. It would, however, be overly anthropocentric of him to take the absence of these things as adequate evidence that they were not, since we can imagine people who have progressed beyond, or evolved without ever developing, these cultural characteristics.

I suggest that the traits which are most central to the concept of personhood, or humanity in the moral sense, are, very roughly, the following:

1. consciousness (of objects and events external and/or internal to the being), and in particular the capacity to feel pain;

2. reasoning (the *developed* capacity to solve new and relatively complex problems);

3. self-motivated activity (activity which is relatively independent of either genetic or direct external control);

4. the capacity to communicate, by whatever means, messages of an indefinite variety of types, that is, not just with an indefinite number of possible contents, but on indefinitely many possible topics;

5. the presence of self-concepts, and self-awareness, either individual or racial, or both.

Admittedly, there are apt to be a great many problems involved in formulating precise definitions of these criteria, let alone in developing universally valid behavioral criteria for deciding when they apply. But I will assume that both we and our explorer know approximately what (1)–(5) mean, and that he is also able to determine whether or not they apply. How, then, should he use his findings to decide whether or not the alien beings are people? We needn't suppose that an entity must have *all* of these attributes to be properly considered a person; (1) and (2) alone may well be sufficient for personhood, and quite probably (1)–(3) are sufficient. Neither do we need to insist that any one of these criteria is necessary for personhood, although once again (1) and (2) look like fairly good candidates for necessary conditions, as does (3), if "activity" is construed so as to include the activity of reasoning.

All we need to claim, to demonstrate that a fetus is not a person, is that any being which satisfies *none* of (1)–(5) is certainly not a person. I consider this claim to be so obvious that I think anyone who denied it, and claimed that a being which satisfied none of (1)–(5) was a person all the same, would thereby demonstrate that he had no notion at all of what a person is—perhaps because he had confused the concept of a person with that of genetic humanity. If the opponents of abortion were to deny the appropriateness of these five criteria, I do not know what further arguments would convince them. We would probably have to admit that our conceptual schemes were indeed irreconcilably different, and that our dispute could not be settled objectively.

I do not expect this to happen, however, since I think that the concept of a person is one which is very nearly universal (to people), and that it is common to both proabortionists and antiabortionists, even though neither group has fully realized the relevance of this concept to the resolution of their dispute. Furthermore, I think that on reflection even the antiabortionists ought to agree not only that (1)–(5) are central to the concept of personhood, but also that it is a part of this concept that all and only people have full moral rights. The concept of a person is in part a moral concept; once we have admitted that x is a person we have recognized, even if we have not agreed to respect, x's right to be treated as a member of the moral community. It is true that the claim that x is a *human being* is more commonly voiced as part of an appeal to treat x decently than is the claim that x is a person, but this is either because "human being" is here used in the sense which implies personhood, or because the genetic and moral senses of "human" have been confused.

Now if (1)–(5) are indeed the primary criteria of personhood, then it is clear that genetic humanity is neither necessary nor sufficient for establishing that an entity is a person. Some human beings are not people, and there may well be people who are not human beings. A man or woman whose consciousness has been permanently obliterated but who remains alive is a human being which is no longer a person; defective human beings, with no appreciable mental capacity, are not and presumably never will be people; and a fetus is a human being which is not yet a person, and which therefore cannot coherently be said to have full moral rights. Citizens of the next century should be prepared to recognize highly advanced, self-aware robots or computers, should such be developed, and intelligent inhabitants of other worlds, should such be found, as people in the fullest sense, and to respect their moral rights. But to ascribe full moral rights to an entity which is not a person is as absurd as to ascribe moral obligations and responsibilities to such an entity.

3. Fetal Development and the Right to Life

Two problems arise in the application of these suggestions for the definition of the moral community to the determination of the precise moral status of a human fetus. Given that the paradigm example of a person is a normal adult being, then (1) How like this paradigm, in particular how far advanced since conception, does a human being need to be before it begins to have a right to life by virtue, not of being fully a person as of yet, but of being *like* a person? and (2) To what extent, if any, does the fact that a fetus has the *potential* for becoming a person endow it with some of the same rights? Each of these questions requires some comment.

In answering the first question, we need not attempt a detailed consideration of the moral rights of organisms which are not developed enough, aware enough, intelligent enough, etc., to be considered people, but which resemble people in some respects. It does seem reasonable to suggest that the more like a person, in the relevant respects, a being is, the stronger is the case for regarding it as having a right to life, and indeed the stronger its right to life is. Thus we ought to take seriously the suggestion that, insofar as "the human individual develops biologically in a continuous fashion . . . the rights of a human person might develop in the same way."[11] But we must keep in mind that the attributes which are relevant in determining whether or not an entity is enough like a person to be regarded as having some of the same moral rights are no different from those which are relevant to determining whether or not it is fully a person—i.e., are no different from (1)–(5)—and that being genetically human, or having recognizably human facial and other physical features, or detectable brain activity, or the capacity to survive outside the uterus, are simply not among these relevant attributes.

Thus it is clear that even though a seven- or eight-month fetus has features which make it apt to arouse in us almost the same powerful protective instinct as is commonly aroused by a small infant, nevertheless it is not significantly more personlike than is a very small embryo. It is *somewhat* more personlike; it can apparently feel and respond to pain, and it may even have a rudimentary form of consciousness, insofar as its brain is quite active. Nevertheless, it seems safe to say that it is not fully conscious, in the way that an infant of a few months is, and that it cannot reason, or communicate messages of indefinitely many sorts, does not engage in self-motivated activity, and has no self-awareness. Thus, in the *relevant* respects, a fetus, even a fully developed one, is considerably less personlike than is the average mature mammal, indeed the average fish. And I think that a rational person must conclude that if the right to life of a fetus is to be based upon its resemblance to a person, then it cannot be said to have any more right to life than, let us say, a newborn guppy (which also seems to be capable of feeling pain), and that a right of that magnitude could never override a woman's right to obtain an abortion, at any stage of her pregnancy.

There may, of course, be other arguments in favor of placing legal limits upon the stage of pregnancy in which an abortion may be performed. Given the relative safety of the new techniques of artificially inducing labor during the third trimester, the danger to the woman's life or health is no longer such an argument. Neither is the fact that people tend to respond to the thought of abortion in the later stages of pregnancy with emotional repulsion, since mere emotional responses cannot take the place of moral reasoning in determining what ought to be permitted. Nor, finally, is the frequently heard argument that legalizing abortion, especially late in the pregnancy, may erode the level of respect for human life, leading, perhaps, to an increase in unjustified euthanasia and other crimes. For this threat, if it is a threat, can be better met by educating people to the kinds of moral distinctions which we are making here than by limiting access to abortion (which limitation may, in its disregard for the rights of women, be just as damaging to the level of respect for human rights).

Thus, since the fact that even a fully developed fetus is not personlike enough to have any significant right to life on the basis of its personlikeness shows that no legal restrictions upon the stage of pregnancy in which an abortion may be performed can be justified on the grounds that we should protect the rights of the older fetus; and since there is no other apparent justification for such restrictions, we may conclude that they are entirely unjustified. Whether or not it would be *indecent* (whatever that means) for a woman in her seventh month to obtain an abortion just to avoid having to postpone a trip to Europe, it would not, in itself, be *immoral*, and therefore it ought to be permitted.

4. Potential Personhood and the Right to Life

We have seen that a fetus does not resemble a person in any way which can support the claim that it has even some of the same rights. But what about its *potential*, the fact that if nurtured and allowed to develop naturally it will very probably become a person? Doesn't that alone give it at least some right to life? It is hard to deny that the fact that an entity is a potential person is a strong prima facie reason for not destroying it; but we need not conclude from this that a potential person has a right to life, by virtue of that potential. It may be that our feeling that it is better, other things being equal, not to destroy a potential person is better explained by the fact that potential people are still (felt to be) an invaluable resource, not to be lightly squandered. Surely, if every speck of dust were a potential person, we would be much less apt to conclude that every potential person has a right to become actual.

Still, we do not need to insist that a potential person has no right to life whatever. There may well be something immoral, and not just imprudent, about wantonly destroying potential people, when doing so isn't necessary to protect anyone's rights. But even if a potential person does have some prima facie right to life, such a right could not possibly outweigh the right of a woman to obtain an abortion, since the rights of any actual person invariably outweigh those of any potential person, whenever the two conflict. Since this may not be immediately obvious in the case of a human fetus, let us look at another case.

Suppose that our space explorer falls into the hands of an alien culture, whose scientists decide to create a few hundred thousand or more human beings, by breaking his body into its component cells, and using these to create fully developed human beings, with, of course, his genetic code. We may imagine that each of these newly created men will have all of the original man's abilities, skills, knowledge, and so on, and also have an individual self-concept, in short that each of them will be a bona fide (though hardly unique) person. Imagine that the whole project will take only seconds, and that its chances of success are extremely high, and that our explorer knows all of this, and also knows that these people will be treated fairly. I maintain that in such a situation he would have every right to escape if he could, and thus to deprive all of these potential people of their potential lives; for his right to life outweighs all of theirs together, in spite of the fact that they are all genetically human, all innocent, and all have a very high probability of becoming people very soon, if only he refrains from acting.

Indeed, I think he would have a right to escape even if it were not his life which the alien scientists planned to take, but only a year of his freedom, or, indeed, only a day. Nor would he be obligated to stay if he had gotten captured (thus bringing all these people-potentials into existence) because of his own carelessness, or even if he had done so deliberately, knowing the consequences. Regardless of how he got captured, he is not morally obligated to remain in captivity for *any* period of time for the sake of permitting any number of potential people to come into actuality, so great is the margin by which one actual person's right to liberty outweighs whatever right to life even a hundred thousand potential people have. And it seems reasonable to conclude that the rights of a woman will outweigh by a similar margin whatever right to life a fetus may have by virtue of its potential personhood.

Thus, neither a fetus's resemblance to a person, nor its potential for becoming a person provides any basis whatever for the claim that it has any significant right to life. Consequently, a woman's right to protect her health, happiness, freedom, and even her life,[12] by terminating an unwanted pregnancy, will always override whatever right to life it may be appropriate to ascribe to a fetus, even a fully developed one. And thus, in the absence of any overwhelming social need for every possible child, the laws which restrict the right to obtain an abortion, or limit the period of pregnancy during which an

abortion may be performed, are a wholly unjustified violation of a woman's most basic moral and constitutional rights.[13]

Notes

1. For example, Roger Wertheimer, who in "Understanding the Abortion Argument" (*Philosophy and Public Affairs*, 1, No. I [Fall, 1971], 67–95), argues that the problem of the moral status of abortion is insoluble, in that the dispute over the status of the fetus is not a question of fact at all, but only a question of how one responds to the facts.

2. B. A. Brody, "Abortion and the Law," *The Journal of Philosophy*, 68, No. 12 (June 17, 1971), 357–69.

3. Judith Thomson, "A Defense of Abortion," *Philosophy and Public Affairs*, 1, No. 1 (Fall, 1971), 47–66.

4. I have abbreviated these statements somewhat, but not in a way which affects the argument.

5. John Noonan, "Abortion and the Catholic Church: A Summary History," *Natural Law Forum*, 12 (1967), 125.

6. John Noonan, "Deciding Who Is Human," *Natural Law Forum*, 13 (1968), 134.

7. "A Defense of Abortion."

8. We may safely ignore the fact that she might have avoided getting raped, e.g., by carrying a gun, since by similar means you might likewise have avoided getting kidnapped, and in neither case does the victim's failure to take all possible precautions against a highly unlikely event (as opposed to reasonable precautions against a rather likely event) mean that he is morally responsible for what happens.

9. Of course, the principle that it is (always) wrong to kill innocent human beings is in need of many other modifications, e.g., that it may be permissible to do so to save a greater number of other innocent human beings, but we may safely ignore these complications here.

10. From here on, we will use "human" to mean genetically human, since the moral sense seems closely connected to, and perhaps derived from, the assumption that genetic humanity is sufficient for membership in the moral community.

11. Thomas L. Hayes, "A Biological View," *Commonweal*, 85 (March 17, 1967), 677–78; quoted by Daniel Callahan, in *Abortion, Law, Choice, and Morality* (London: Macmillan & Co., 1970).

12. That is, insofar as the death rate, for the woman, is higher for childbirth than for early abortion.

13. My thanks to the following people, who were kind enough to read and criticize an earlier version of this paper: Herbert Gold, Gene Glass, Anne Lauterbach, Judith Thomson, Mary Mothersill, and Timothy Binkley.

United States Supreme Court Decision in the *Webster* Case _____

Chief Justice William Rehnquist is author of the Court's opinion in a challenge (on the grounds that it violates the principles of *Roe* v. *Wade*) to a Missouri law regulating abortion. He holds, first, that the Court need not rule against the claim in the preamble of the Missouri law that life begins at conception, because the claim is not stated as applying only to abortion and expresses an allowable value judgment. He argues, second, that there is no constitutional basis for requiring states to support abortion by supplying medical personnel and facilities and, third, that there is no constitutional right of physicians or patients to use public facilities to perform abortions. In addition, he claims that the trimester test of justification for regulating abortion used in *Roe* is less sensitive to the matter of viability than the Missouri law at issue. Furthermore, "the key elements" of *Roe* are "not found in the text of the Constitution or in any place else one would expect to find a constitutional principle."

Justice Harry A. Blackmun, in a dissenting opinion, sees the Court decision as an attack on *Roe* that will have harmful consequences for millions of women. Rehnquist, he argues, fails to consider the case for viability on appropriate grounds—namely, the right to privacy, on which *Roe* and its successors were decided. Instead, he misreads the legislation being considered in a way that seems to conflict with the trimester structure established in *Roe* to balance the state's interest in maternal health and potential life against the right to privacy.

William Rehnquist: Court Opinion

This appeal concerns the constitutionality of a Missouri statute regulating the performance of abortions. The United States Court of Appeals for the Eighth Circuit struck down several provisions of the statute on the ground that they violated this Court's decision in Roe v. Wade, 410 U.S. 113 (1973), and cases following it. We noted probable jurisdiction, and now reverse. . . .

Decision of this case requires us to address four sections of the Missouri Act: (a) the preamble; (b) the prohibition on the use of public facilities or employees to perform abortions; (c) the prohibition on public funding of abortion counseling; and (d) the requirements that physicians conduct viability tests prior to performing abortions. We address these *seriatim*.

The Act's preamble . . . sets forth "findings" by the Missouri legislature that "[t]he life of each

human being begins at conception," and that "[u]nborn children have protectable interests in life, health, and well-being." The Act then mandates that state laws be interpreted to provided unborn children with "all the rights, privileges and immunities available to other persons, citizens and residents of this state," subject to the Constitution and this Court's precedents. In invalidating the preamble, the Court of Appeals relied on this Court's dictum that "a state may not adopt one theory of when life begins to justify its regulation of abortions." . . . It rejected Missouri's claim that the preamble was "abortion-neutral," and "merely determine[d] when life begins in a nonabortion context, a traditional state prerogative." . . .

We think the extent to which the preamble's language might be used to interpret other state stat-

United States Supreme Court, U.S. 109, S. Ct. 3040. July 3, 1989.

utes or regulations is something that only the courts of Missouri can definitively decide. . . . It will be time enough for Federal courts to address the meaning of the preamble should it be applied to restrict the activities of appellees in some concrete way. . . .

Section 188.210 provides that "[i]t shall be unlawful for any public employee within the scope of his employment to perform or assist an abortion, not necessary to save the life of the mother," while Section 188.215 makes it "unlawful for any public facility to be used for the purpose of performing or assisting an abortion not necessary to save the life of the mother." The Court of Appeals held that these provisions contravened this Court's abortion decisions. We take the contrary view. . . .

As we said earlier this term in DeShaney v. Winnebago County Dept. of Social Services, "our cases have recognized that the due process clauses generally confer no affirmative right to governmental aid, even where such aid may be necessary to secure life, liberty or property interests of which the government itself may not deprive the individual."

In Maher v. Roe (1977), the Court upheld a Connecticut welfare regulation under which Medicaid recipients received payments for medical services related to childbirth, but not for nontherapeutic abortions. The Court rejected the claim that this unequal subsidization of childbirth and abortion was impermissible under Roe v. Wade. . . .

Just as Congress' refusal to fund abortions in McRae left "an indigent woman with at least the same range of choice in deciding whether to obtain a medically necessary abortion as she would have had if Congress had chosen to subsidize no health care costs all," Missouri's refusal to allow public employees to perform abortions in public hospitals leaves a pregnant woman with the same choices as if the State had chosen not to operate any public hospitals at all.

The challenged provisions only restrict a woman's ability to obtain an abortion to the extent that she chooses to use a physician affiliated with a public hospital. This circumstance is more easily remedied, and thus considerably less burdensome, than indigency, which "may make it difficult—and in some cases, perhaps, impossible—for some women to have abortions" without public funding.

Having held that the State's refusal to fund abortions does not violate Roe v. Wade, it strains

logic to reach a contrary result for the use of public facilities and employees. If the State may "make a value judgment favoring childbirth over abortion and . . . implement that judgment by the allocation of public funds," surely it may do so through the allocation of other public resources such as hospitals and medical staff. . . . Section 188.029 of the Missouri Act provides:

"Before a physician performs an abortion on a woman he has reason to believe is carrying an unborn child of 20 or more weeks gestational age, the physician shall first determine if the unborn child is viable by using and exercising that degree of care, skill and proficiency commonly exercised by the ordinarily skillful, careful and prudent physician engaged in similar practice under the same or similar conditions. In making this determination of viability, the physician shall perform or cause to be performed such medical examinations and tests as are necessary to make a finding of the gestational age, weight and lung maturity of the unborn child and shall enter such findings and determination of viability in the medical record of the mother." . . .

The Court of Appeals read Section 188.029 as requiring that after 20 weeks "doctors *must* perform tests to find gestational age, fetal weight and lung maturity." The court indicated that the tests needed to determine fetal weight at 20 weeks are "unreliable and inaccurate" and would add $125 to $250 to the cost of an abortion.

It also stated that "amniocentesis, the only method available to determine lung maturity, is contrary to accepted medical practice until 28–30 weeks of gestation, expensive, and imposes significant health risks for both the pregnant woman and the fetus." . . .

The viability-testing provision of the Missouri Act is concerned with promoting the State's interest in potential human life rather than in maternal health. Section 188.029 creates what is essentially a presumption of viability at 20 weeks, which the physician must rebut with tests indicating that the fetus is not viable prior to performing an abortion. It also directs the physician's determination as to viability by specifying consideration, if feasible, of gestational age, fetal weight and lung capacity. . . .

The District Court found that "the medical evidence is uncontradicted that a 20-week fetus is *not* viable," and that $23\frac{1}{2}$ to 24 weeks gestation is the earliest point in pregnancy where a reasonable possibility of viability exists." But it also found that there may be a 4-week error in estimating gestational age, which supports testing at 20 weeks.

In Roe v. Wade, the Court recognized that the State has "important and legitimate" interests in protecting maternal health and in the potentiality of human life. During the second trimester, the State "may, if it chooses, regulate the abortion procedure in ways that are reasonably related to maternal health." After viability, when the State's interest in potential human life was held to become compelling, the State "may, if it chooses, regulate, and even proscribe, abortion except where it is necessary, in appropriate medical judgment, for the preservation of the life or health of the mother."

In Colautti v. Franklin (1979), upon which appellees rely, the Court held that a Pennsylvania statute regulating the standard of care to be used by a physician performing an abortion of a possibly viable fetus was void for vagueness. But in the course of reaching that conclusion, the Court reaffirmed its earlier statement in Planned Parenthood of Central Missouri v. Danforth, that "the determination of whether a particular fetus is viable is, and must be, a matter for the judgment of the responsible attending physician."

To the extent that Section 188.029 regulates the method for determining viability, it undoubtedly does superimpose state regulation on the medical determination of whether a particular fetus is viable. The Court of Appeals and the District Court thought it unconstitutional for this reason. . . .

We think that the doubt cast upon the Missouri statute by these cases is not so much a flaw in the statute as it is a reflection of the fact that the rigid trimester analysis of the course of a pregnancy enunciated in Roe has resulted in subsequent cases like Colautti and Akron making constitutional law in this area a virtual Procrustean bed. . . .

In the first place, the rigid Roe framework is hardly consistent with the notion of a Constitution case in general terms, as ours is, and usually speaking in general principles, as ours does. The key elements of the Roe framework—trimester and viability—are not found in the text of the Constitution or in any place else one would expect to find a constitutional principle. Since the bounds of the inquiry are essentially indeterminate, the result has been a web of legal rules that have become increasingly intricate, resembling a code of regulations rather than a body of constitutional doctrine. . . .

In the second place, we do not see why the state's interest in protecting potential human life should come into existence only at the point of viability, and that there should therefore be a rigid line allowing state regulation after viability but prohibiting it before viability. . . .

The tests that Section 188.029 requires the physician to perform are designed to determine viability. The State here has chosen viability as the point at which its interest in potential human life must be safeguarded. . . . It is true that the tests in question increase the expense of abortion and regulate the discretion of the physician in determining the viability of the fetus. Since the tests will undoubtedly show in many cases that the fetus is not viable, the tests will have been performed for what were in fact second-trimester abortions. But we are satisfied that the requirement of these tests permissibly furthers the State's interest in protecting potential human life, and we therefore believe Section 188.029 to be constitutional. . . .

Both appellants and the United States as *Amicus Curiae* have urged that we overrule our decision Roe v. Wade. . . . The facts of the present case, however, differ from those at issue in Roe. Here, Missouri has determined that viability is the point at which its interest in potential human life must be safeguarded. In Roe, on the other hand, the Texas statute criminalized the performance of all abortions, except when the mother's life was at stake. . . . This case therefore affords us no occasion to revisit the holding of Roe, which was that the Texas statute unconstitutionally infringed the right to an abortion derived from the Due Process Clause. . . . and we leave it undisturbed. To the extent indicated in our opinion, we would modify and narrow Roe and succeeding cases.

Harry A. Blackmun: Dissenting Opinion

Today, Roe v. Wade, and the fundamental constitutional right of women to decide whether to terminate a pregnancy, survive but are not secure. Although the Court extricates itself from this case without making a single, even incremental, change in the law of abortion, the plurality and Justice Scalia would overrule Roe (the first silently, the other explicitly) and would return to the states virtually unfettered authority to control the quintessentially intimate, personal and life-directing decision whether to carry a fetus to term.

Although today, no less than yesterday, the Constitution and the decisions of this Court prohibit a state from enacting laws that inhibit women from the meaningful exercise of that right, a plurality of this Court implicitly invites every state legislature to enact more and more restrictive abortion regulations in order to provoke more and more test cases, in the hope that sometime down the line the Court will return the law of procreative freedom to the severe limitations that generally prevailed in this country before January 22, 1973. Never in my memory has a plurality announced a judgment of this Court that so foments disregard for the law and for our standing decisions. . . .

In the plurality's view, the viability-testing provision imposes a burden on second-trimester abortions as a way of furthering the State's interest in protecting the potential life of the fetus. Since under the Roe framework, the State may not fully regulate abortion in the interest of potential life (as opposed to maternal health) until the third trimester, the plurality finds it necessary, in order to save the Missouri testing provision, to throw out Roe's trimester framework.

In flat contradiction to Roe, the plurality concludes that the State's interest in potential life is compelling before viability, and upholds the testing provision because it "permissibly furthers" that state interest. . . .

Had the plurality read the statute as written, it would have had no cause to reconsider the Roe framework. As properly construed, the viability-testing provision does not pass constitutional muster under even a rational-basis standard, the least restrictive level of review applied by this Court.

By mandating tests to determine fetal weight and lung maturity for every fetus thought to be more than 20 weeks of gestational age, the statute requires physicians to undertake procedures, such as amniocentesis, that, in the situation presented, have no medical justification, impose significant additional health risks on both the pregnant woman and the fetus, and bear no rational relation to the State's interest in protecting fetal life.

As written, Section 188.029 is an arbitrary imposition of discomfort, risk and expense, furthering no discernible interest except to make the procurement of an abortion as arduous and difficult as possible. Thus, were it not for the plurality's tortured effort to avoid the plain import of Section 188.029, it could have struck down the testing provision as patently irrational irrespective of the Roe framework. . . .

The plurality opinion is far more remarkable for the arguments that it does not advance than for those that it does. The plurality does not even mention, much less join, the true jurisprudential debate underlying this case; whether the Constitution includes an "unenumerated" general right to privacy as recognized in many of our decisions, most notably Griswold v. Connecticut (1965) and Roe, and, more specifically, whether and to what extent such a right of privacy extends to matters of childbearing and family life, including abortion. . . .

But rather than arguing that the text of the Constitution makes no mention of the right to privacy, the plurality complains that the critical elements of the Roe framework—trimesters and viability—do not appear in the Constitution and are, therefore, somehow inconsistent with a Constitution cast in general terms. Were this a true concern, we would have to abandon most of our constitutional jurisprudence. . . .

With respect to the Roe framework, the general constitutional principle—indeed, the fundamental constitutional right—for which it was developed is the right to privacy. See, e.g., Griswold v. Connecticut (1965), a species of "liberty" protected by the due process clause, which under our past decisions safeguards the right of women to exercise some control over their own role in procreation.

As we recently reaffirmed in Thornburg v. American College of Obstetricians and Gynecologists, 476 U.S. 747 (1986), few decisions are "more basic to individual dignity and autonomy" or more appropriate to that "certain private sphere of individual liberty" that the Constitution reserves from the intrusive reach of government than the right to make the uniquely personal, intimate and self-defining decision whether to end a pregnancy. It is this general principle, the "moral fact that a person belongs to himself and not others nor to society as a whole," that is found in the Constitution.

The trimester framework simply defines and limits that right to privacy in the abortion context to accommodate, not destroy, a state's legitimate interest in protecting the health of pregnant women and in preserving potential human life. Fashioning such accommodations between individual rights and the legitimate interests of government, establishing benchmarks and standards with which to evaluate the competing claims of individuals and government, lies at the very heart of constitutional adjudication.

To the extent that the trimester framework is useful in this enterprise, it is not only consistent with constitutional interpretation, but necessary to the wise and just exercise of this Court's paramount authority to define the scope of constitutional rights.

The plurality next alleges that the result of the trimester framework has "been a web of legal rules that have become increasingly intricate, resembling a code of regulations rather than a body of constitutional doctrine." Again, if this were a true and genuine concern, we would have to abandon vast areas of our constitutional jurisprudence.

Finally, the plurality asserts that the trimester framework cannot stand because the State's interest in potential life is compelling throughout pregnancy, not merely after viability. The opinion contains not one word of rationale for its view of the State's interest. This "it-is-so-because-we-say-so" jurisprudence constitutes nothing other than an attempted exercise of brute force; reason, much less persuasion, has no place. . . .

For my own part, I remain convinced, as six other members of this Court 16 years ago were convinced, that the Roe framework, and the viability standard in particular, fairly, sensibly and effectively functions to safeguard the constitutional liberties of pregnant women while recognizing and accommodating the State's interest in potential human life.

The viability line reflects the biological facts and truths of fetal development; it marks that threshold moment prior to which a fetus cannot survive separate from the woman and cannot reasonably and objectively be regarded as a subject of rights or interests distinct from, or paramount to, those of the pregnant woman.

At the same time, the viability standard takes account of the undeniable fact that as the fetus evolves into its postnatal form, and as it loses its dependence on the uterine environment, the State's interest in the fetus's potential human life, and in fostering a regard for human life in general, becomes compelling. . . .

Having contrived an opportunity to reconsider the Roe framework, and then having discarded that framework, the plurality finds the testing provision unobjectionable because it "permissibly furthers the State's interest in protecting potential human life." This newly minted standard is circular and totally meaningless. Whether a challenged abortion regulation "permissibly furthers" a legitimate state interest is the *question* that courts must answer in abortion cases, not the standard for courts to apply.

In keeping with the rest of its opinion, the plurality makes no attempt to explain or to justify its new standard, either in the abstract or as applied in this case. Nor could it. The "permissibly furthers" standard has no independent meaning, and consists of nothing other that what a majority of this Court may believe at any given moment in any given case.

The plurality's novel test appears to be nothing more than a dressed-up version of rational-basis review, this Court's most lenient level of scrutiny. One thing is clear, however: were the plurality's "permissibly furthers" standard adopted by the Court, for all practical purposes, Roe would be overruled. . . .

Thus, "not with a bang, but a whimper," the plurality discards a landmark case of the last generation and casts into darkness the hopes and visions of every woman in this country who had come to believe that the Constitution guaranteed her the right to exercise some control over her unique ability to bear children.

The plurality does so either oblivious or insensitive to the fact that millions of women and their families have ordered their lives around the right to reproductive choice, and that this right has become vital to the full participation of women in the economic and political walks of American life.

The plurality would clear the way once again for government to force upon women the physical labor and specific and direct medical and psychological harms that may accompany carrying a fetus to term. The plurality would clear the way again for the State to conscript a woman's body and to force upon her a "distressful life and future."

The result, as we know from experience, would be that every year hundreds of thousands of women, in desperation, would defy the law and place their health and safety in the unclean and unsympathetic hands of back-alley abortionists, or they would attempt to perform abortions upon themselves, with disastrous results. Every year many women, especially poor and minority women, would die or suffer debilitating physical trauma, all in the name of enforced morality or religious dictates or lack of compassion, as it may be.

Of the aspirations and settled understandings of American women, of the inevitable and brutal consequences of what it is doing, the tough-approach plurality utters not a word. This silence is callous. It is also profoundly destructive of this Court as an institution.

To overturn a constitutional decision is a rare and grave undertaking. To overturn a constitutional decision that secured a fundamental personal liberty to millions of persons would be unprecedented in our 200 years of constitutional history. . . .

For today, at least, the law of abortion stands undisturbed. For today, the women of this Nation still retain the liberty to control their destinies. But the signs are evident and very ominous, and a chill wind blows.

I dissent.

Decision Scenario 1 . . . .

Ruth Perkins is twenty-four years old, and her husband, Carl Freedon, is four years older. Both are employed, Ruth as an executive for Laporte Gas Transmission and Carl as a systems analyst at a St. Louis bank. Their combined income is over $140,000 a year.

Perkins and Freedon live up to their income. They have an eleven-room house with a tennis court in a high-priced suburb, they both dress well, and Carl is a modest collector of sports cars (three MG-TDs). Both like to travel, and they try to get out of the country at least twice a year—Europe for a month in the summer and Mexico or the Caribbean for a couple of weeks during the winter.

Perkins and Freedon have no children. They agreed when they were married that children would not be a part of their plan for life together. They were distressed when Ruth became pregnant and at first refused to face the problem. They worried about it for several months, considering arguments for and against abortion. At last they decided that Ruth should have an abortion.

"I don't see why I have to go through with this interview," Ruth said to the woman at the Morton Hospital Counseling Center.

"It's required of all who request an abortion," the counselor explained. "We think it's better for a person to be sure what she is doing so she won't regret it later."

"My husband and I are certain," Ruth said. "A child doesn't fit in at all with our life-style. We go out a lot, and we like to do things. A child would just get in the way."

"A child can offer many pleasures," the woman said.

"I don't doubt it. If some want them, that's fine with me. We don't. Besides, we both have careers that we're devoted to. I'm not about to quit my job to take care of a child, and the same is true of my husband."

"How long have you been pregnant?"

Ruth looked embarrassed. "Almost six months," she said. "Carl and I weren't sure what we wanted to do at first. It took a while for us to get used to the idea."

"You don't think you waited too long?"

"That's stupid," Ruth said. She could hardly keep her voice under control. "I didn't mean that personally. But Carl and I have a right to live our lives the way we want. So far as we are concerned a six-month fetus is not a person. If we want to get rid of it, that's our business."

"Would you feel the same if it were a child already born?"

"I might," Ruth said. "I mean, a baby doesn't have much personality or anything, does it?"

"I take it you're certain you want the abortion."

"Absolutely. My husband and I think it's the right thing for us. If others think we're wrong . . . well, it's their right to think what they please."

1. *How might Warren's arguments be used to support Perkins's position?*

2. *Could someone who accepts Thomson's arguments consider abortion justified in this case?*

3. *Do you believe Perkins is right about a six-month fetus's not being a person? If not, why not?*

4. *If a person believes abortion is a kind of murder, can she legitimately endorse the tolerant position taken by Perkins?*

5. *Under Missouri law, Ruth and Carl will have to have viability tests to determine whether an abortion can be*

obtained. On what grounds does Justice Rehnquist support this requirement? What individual right does

Justice Blackmun see as infringed by the requirement?

Decision Scenario 2 . . . .

It happened after a concert. Sixteen-year-old Mary Pluski had gone with three of her friends to hear Bruce Springsteen at Chicago's Blanton Auditorium. After the concert, in a crowd estimated at 11,000, Mary became separated from the other three girls. She decided that the best thing to do was to meet them at the car.

But when she got to the eight-story parking building, Mary realized she wasn't sure what level they had parked on. She thought it might be somewhere in the middle so she started looking on the fourth floor. While she was walking down the aisles of cars, two men in their early twenties, one white and the other black, stopped her and asked if she was having some kind of trouble.

Mary explained the situation to them, and one of the men suggested that they get his car and drive around inside the parking building. Mary hesitated, but both seemed so polite and genuinely concerned to help that she decided to go with them.

Once they were in the car, however, the situation changed. They drove out of the building and toward the South Side. Mary pleaded with them to let her out of the car, but they refused. They threatened her with violence if she called for help or tried to escape from the car. Then, some seven miles from the auditorium, the driver stopped the car in a dark area behind a vacant building. Mary was then raped by both men.

Mary was treated at Allenworth Hospital and released into the custody of her parents. She filed a complaint with the police, but her troubles were not yet over. Two weeks after she missed her menstrual period, tests showed that Mary was pregnant.

"How do you feel about having this child?" asked Sarah Ruben, the Pluski family physician.

"I hate the idea," Mary said. "I feel guilty about it, though. I mean, it's not the child's fault."

"Let me ask a delicate question," said Dr. Ruben. "I know from what you've told me before that you and your boyfriend have been having sex. Can you be sure this pregnancy is not really the result of that?"

Mary shook her head. "Not really. I use my diaphragm, but I know it doesn't give a hundred percent guarantee."

"That's right. Now, does it make any difference to you who the father might be, so far as a decision about terminating the pregnancy is concerned?"

"If I were sure that it was Bob, I guess the problem would be even harder," Mary said.

"There are some tests we can use to give us that information," Dr. Ruben said. "But that would mean waiting for the embryo to develop into a fetus. It would be easier and safer to terminate the pregnancy now."

Mary started crying. "I don't want a child," she said. "I don't want any child. I don't care who's the father. It was forced on me, and I want to get rid of it."

"I'll make the arrangements," said Dr. Ruben.

1. *Would Thomson's position recognize abortion here as a form of self-defense?*

2. *Would Noonan consider abortion immoral in this case?*

3. *Suppose the fetus is a person; would the maxim in this case satisfy the categorical imperative?*

4. *Does Mary's uncertainty about the father add any special moral difficulties?*

5. *Would Warren consider an abortion justifiable?*

Decision Scenario 3 . . . .

"I don't want no more children," Mrs. Hinson said. "I've already got five, and I can't look after them the way they should be looked after. My husband's been gone three years. I don't know where he is, but I know he ain't coming back."

After two years as a psychiatric social worker, David Rossum found Mrs. Hinson's situation familiar. He looked around the small living room. It was clean but crowded with broken second-hand furniture. Cheap dime-store metal frames lined the top of the television set. Children smiled in the blurry color snapshots.

"You're sure you're pregnant?" Rossum asked.

"The doctor at the clinic told me so," Mrs. Hinson said. "He gave me a paper to prove it. But I'm already on the welfare and the ADC. I can't do right by my children if I have another one to take care of."

"And you can't count on the father of this child to help you?"

"I can't count on him for nothing," said Mrs. Hinson. "I don't even see him anymore."

"So what do you want to do?" Rossum asked. He knew the answer, but the main part of his job was just listening.

"I want an abortion. That's what I want. But the people at the clinic, they told me I'd have to talk to you people first. If you won't say it's okay they won't do it, because there won't be nobody to pay for it."

"That's right," Rossum said. "You've got to have an authorization from our agency for any kind of special medical procedure of a nonemergency kind."

1. *Suppose that you are David Rossum. On what grounds would you authorize (or refuse to authorize) Mrs. Hinson's request? If you were opposed to all abortions on moral grounds, ought you to allow this to influence your decision?*

2. *Does the reasoning in* Roe v. Wade *apply in this case?*

3. *Do Rawls's principles of justice suggest a legitimate social policy to cover such cases?*

4. *Does the principle of utility suggest a policy?*

5. *If the fetus is a person, are there sufficient reasons for considering abortion here a case of justified killing?*

6. *If Mrs. Hinson is visiting a public clinic in Missouri, she will not be able to get an abortion at the clinic. How does Justice Rehnquist argue in support of this ban? How might one argue against it?*

Decision Scenario 4 . . . .

Clare Macwurter was twenty-two years old chronologically, but mentally she remained a child. As a result of her mother's prolonged and difficult labor, Clare had been deprived of an adequate blood-oxygen supply during her birth. The consequence was that she suffered irreversible brain damage.

Clare enjoyed life and was generally a happy person. She couldn't read, but she liked listening to music and watching television, although she could rarely understand the stories. She was physically attractive and, with the help of her parents, she could care for herself.

Clare was also interested in sex. When she was seventeen, she and a fellow student at the special school they attended had been caught having intercourse. Clare's parents had been told about the incident, but after Clare left the school the following year, they took no special precautions to ensure that Clare would not become sexually involved with anyone. After all, she stayed at home with her mother every day, and, besides, it was a matter they didn't much like to think about.

The Macwurters were both surprised and upset when Clare became pregnant. At first they couldn't imagine how it could have happened. Then they recalled that on several occasions Clare had been sent to stay at the house of Mr. Macwurter's brother and his wife while Mrs. Macwurter went shopping.

John Macwurter at first denied that he had had anything to do with Clare's pregnancy. But during the course of a long and painful conversation with his brother, he admitted that he had had sexual relations with Clare.

"I wasn't wholly to blame," John Macwurter said. "I mean, I know I shouldn't have done it. But still, she was interested in it too. I didn't really rape her. Nothing like that."

The Macwurters were at a loss about what they should do. The physician they consulted told them that Clare would probably have a perfectly normal baby. But of course Clare couldn't really take care of herself, much less a baby. She was simply unfit to be a mother. Mrs. Macwurter, for her part, was not eager to assume the additional responsibilities of caring for another child. Mr. Macwurter would be eligible to retire in four more years, and the couple had been looking forward to selling their house and moving back to the small town in Oklahoma where they had first met and then married. The money they had managed to save, plus insurance and a sale of their property, would permit them to place Clare in a long-term care facility after their deaths. Being responsible for another child would both ruin their plans and jeopardize Clare's future well-being.

"I never thought I would say such a thing," Mrs. Macwurter told her husband, "but I think we should arrange for Clare to have an abortion."

"That's killing," Mr. Macwurter said.

"I'm not so sure it is. I don't really know. But even if it is, I think it's the best thing to do."

Mrs. Macwurter made the arrangements with Clare's physician for an abortion to be performed. When Mr. Macwurter asked his brother to pay for the operation, John Macwurter refused. He explained that he was opposed to abortion and so it would not be right for him to provide money to be used in that way.

1. *Can the reasoning in* Roe v. Wade *be applied in this case? After all, the person involved is not mentally competent and cannot be expected to exercise any right of privacy.*

2. *Could Thomson's defense of abortion be employed here to show that the proposed abortion is permissible?*

3. *Why would Noonan oppose abortion here? What alternatives might he recommend? What if it were likely that the baby would be defective? Would this alter the situation for Noonan?*

4. *Do the traits Warren lists as central to the concept of personhood require that we think of Clare Macwurter as not being a person in a morally relevant sense?*

Decision Scenario 5 . . . .

Daniel Bocker was worried. The message his secretary had taken merely said "Go to see Dr. Tai at 3:30 today." He hadn't been asked if 3:30 was convenient for him, and he hadn't been given a reason for coming in.

Mr. Bocker knew it would have to do with his wife, Mary. She had been suffering a lot of pain during her pregnancy, and the preceding week she had been examined by a specialist that Dr. Tai, her gynecologist, had sent her to see. The specialist had performed a thorough examination and taken blood, tissue, and urine samples, but he had told Mary nothing.

"Thank you for coming in," Dr. Tai said. "I want to talk to you before I talk to your wife, because I need your help."

"The tests showed something bad, didn't they?" Mr. Bocker said. "Something is wrong with the baby."

"The baby is fine, but there is something wrong with your wife, something very seriously wrong. She has what we call uterine neoplasia."

"Is that cancer?"

"Yes it is," said Dr. Tai. "But I don't want either of you to panic about it. It's not at a very advanced stage, and at the moment it's localized. If an operation is performed very soon, then she has a good chance to make a full recovery. The standard figures show about 80% success."

"But what about the baby?"

"The pregnancy will have to be terminated," Dr. Tai said. "And I should tell you that your wife will not be able to have children after the operation."

Mr. Bocker sat quietly for a moment. He had always wanted children; for him a family without children was not a family at all. He and Mary had talked about having at least three, and the one she was pregnant with now was the first.

"Is it possible to save the baby?" he asked Dr. Tai.

"Mrs. Bocker is only in her fourth month; there is no chance the child could survive outside her body."

"But what if she didn't have the operation? Would the baby be normal?"

"Probably so, but the longer we wait to perform the operation, the worse your wife's chances become. I don't want to seem to tell you what to do, but my advice is for your wife to have an abortion and to undergo the operation as soon as it is reasonably possible."

"But she might recover, even if she had the child and then had the operation, mightn't she?"

"It's possible, but her chances of recovery are much less. I don't know what the exact figures would be, but she would be running a terrible risk."

Mr. Bocker understood what Dr. Tai was saying, but he also understood what he wanted.

"I'm not going to encourage Mary to have an abortion," he said. "I want her to have a child, and I think she wants that, too."

"What if she wants to have a better chance to live? I think the decision is really hers. After all, it's her life that is at stake."

"But it's not just her decision," Mr. Bocker said. "It's a family decision, hers and mine. I'm not going to agree to an abortion, even if she does want one. I'm going to try to get her to take the extra risk and have the child before she has the operation."

"I think that's the cruelest, most immoral thing I've ever heard," Dr. Tai said.

1. *Would the doctrine of double effect justify taking steps to treat Mrs. Bocker's illness, even at the cost of terminating her pregnancy?*

2. *Would both Noonan and Thomson see the situation as one in which considerations of self-defense are relevant?*

3. *It is sometimes said that the father of a child also has a right to decide whether an abortion is to be performed. Would Daniel Bocker be justified in urging his wife to take the risk of having the child?*

4. *Does the categorical imperative have any relevance in determining whether an abortion is morally right in this case?*

Decision Scenario 6 ·

Mrs. Lois Bishop (as we will call her) learned that she was carrying twins at the same time that she learned one of the twins had Down's syndrome.

"There's no question in my mind," she said. "I want to have an abortion. I had the tests done in the first place to do what I could to guarantee that I would have a normal, healthy child. I knew from the first that there was a possibility that I would have to have an abortion, so I'm prepared for it."

Her obstetrician, Dr. George Savano, nodded. "I understand that," he said. "You are certainly within your rights to ask for an abortion, and I can arrange for you to have one. But there is another possibility, an experimental one, that you might want to consider as an option."

The possibility consisted of the destruction of the abnormally developing fetus. In the end, it was the possibility that Mrs. Bishop chose. A long, thin needle was inserted through Mrs. Bishop's abdomen and guided into the heart of the fetus. A solution was then injected directly into the fetal heart.

Although there was a risk that Mrs. Bishop would have a miscarriage, she did not. The surviv-

ing twin continued to develop normally, and Mrs. Bishop had an uneventful delivery. The child, a boy, is now over five years old.

Dr. Savano was criticized by some physicians as "misusing medicine," but he rejects such charges. Mrs. Bishop also has no regrets, for if the procedure had not been performed, she would have been forced to abort both twins.

1. *What sort of utilitarian argument might be offered to justify Dr. Savano's experimental procedure in this case?*

2. *Can the doctrine of double effect justify the procedure that terminates the life of the Down's syndrome twin? After all, Mrs. Bishop is concerned with preserving the life of the twin that is developing normally. She chooses the experimental procedure in order to avoid an abortion.*

3. *The procedure leads to the death of a developing fetus, so one might say that it is morally equivalent to abortion. Are there any morally relevant features that distinguish this case from more ordinary cases involving abortion?*

Decision Scenario 7 ·

Helen and John Kent waited nervously in the small consulting room while Laurie Stent, their Genetic Counselor, went to tell Dr. Charles Blatz that they had arrived to talk to him.

"I regret that I have some bad news for you," Dr. Blatz told them. "The karyotyping that we do after the amniocentesis shows a chromosomal abnormality."

He looked at them, and Helen felt she could hardly breathe. "What is it?" she asked.

"It's a condition known as Trisomy-21, and it produces a birth defect we call Down's syndrome. You may have heard of it under the old name of mongolism."

"Oh, God," John said. "How bad is it?"

"Such children are always mentally retarded," Dr. Blatz said. "Some are severely retarded and others just twenty or so points below average. They have some minor physical deformities, and they sometimes have heart damage. They typically don't live beyond their thirties, but by and large they seem happy and have good dispositions."

Helen and John looked at each other with great sadness. "What do you think we should do?" Helen asked. "Should I have an abortion, and then we could try again?"

"I don't know," John said. "I really don't know. You've had a hard time being pregnant these last five months, and you'd have to go through that again. Besides, there's no guarantee this wouldn't happen again."

"But this won't be the normal baby we wanted," Helen said. "Maybe in the long run we'll be even unhappier than we are now."

1. *According to the doctrine in* Roe *v.* Wade, *who is to decide whether Helen Kent has an abortion? Are there any restrictions on the decision?*

2. *Explain the nature of the conflict between the positions taken by Noonan and Warren that arises in this case.*

3. *If one accepts Thomson's view, what factors are relevant to deciding whether an abortion is justifiable in this instance?*

CHAPTER 2

TREATING OR TERMINATING:
THE PROBLEM OF IMPAIRED INFANTS

CASE PRESENTATION
Baby Owens: Down's Syndrome and Duodenal Atresia

On a chilly December evening in 1976, Dr. Joan Owens pushed through the plateglass doors of Midwestern Medical Center and walked over to the admitting desk. Dr. Owens was a physician in private practice and regularly visited Midwestern to attend to her patients.

But this night was different. Dr. Owens was coming to the hospital to be admitted as a patient. She was pregnant, and shortly after 9:00 she began having periodic uterine contractions. Dr. Owens recognized them as the beginnings of labor pains. She was sure of this not only because of her medical knowledge but also because the pains followed the same pattern they had before her other three children were born.

While her husband, Phillip, parked the car, Dr. Owens went through the formalities of admission. She was not particularly worried, for the birth of her other children had been quite normal and uneventful. But the pains were coming more frequently now, and she was relieved when she completed the admission process and was taken to her room. Phillip came with her, bringing her small blue suitcase of personal belongings.

At 11:30 that evening, Dr. Owens gave birth to a 4½-pound baby girl. The plastic bracelet fastened around her wrist identified her as Baby Owens and listed her patient number as 23-764-2509.

Dr. Owens was groggy from exhaustion and from the medication she had received. But when the baby was shown to her, she saw at once that it was not normal. The baby's head was misshapen and the skin around her eyes strangely formed. Dr. Owens recognized that her daughter had Down's syndrome.

"Clarence," she called to her obstetrician. "Is the baby mongoloid?"

"We'll talk about it after your recovery," Dr. Clarence Ziner said.

"Tell me now," said Dr. Owens. "Examine it!"

Dr. Ziner made a hasty examination of the child. He had already seen that Dr. Owens was right and was doing no more than making doubly certain. A more careful examination would have to be made later.

When Dr. Ziner confirmed Joan Owens's suspicion, she did not hesitate to say what she was thinking. "Get rid of it," she told Dr. Ziner. "I don't want a mongoloid child."

Dr. Ziner tried to be soothing. "Just sleep for a while now," he told her. "We'll talk about it later."

Four hours later, a little after 5:00 in the morning and before it was fully light, Joan Owens woke up. Phillip was with her, and he had more bad news to tell. A more detailed examination had shown that the child's small intestine had failed to develop properly and was closed off in one place—the condition known as duodenal atresia. It could be corrected by a relatively simple surgical procedure, but until surgery was performed the child could not be fed. Phillip had refused to consent to the operation until he had talked to his wife.

Joan Owens had not changed her mind: she did not want the child. "It wouldn't be fair to the other children to raise them with a mongoloid," she told Phillip. "It would take all of our time, and we wouldn't be able to give David, Sean, and Melinda the love and attention they need."

"I'm willing to do whatever you think best," Phillip said. "But what can we do?"

"Let the child die," Joan said. "If we don't consent to the surgery, the baby will die soon. And that's what we have to let happen."

Phillip put in a call for Dr. Ziner, and, when he arrived in Joan's room, they told him of their decision. He was not pleased with it.

"The surgery has very low risk," he said. "The baby's life can almost certainly be saved. We can't tell how retarded she'll be, but most DS children get along quite well with help from their families. The whole family will grow to love her."

"I know," Joan said. "And I don't want that to happen. I don't want us to center our lives around a defective child. Phillip and I and our other children will be forced to lose out on many of life's pleasures and possibilities."

"We've made up our minds," Phillip said. "We don't want the surgery."

"I'm not sure the matter is as simple as that," Dr. Ziner said. "I'm not sure we can legally just let the baby die. I'll have to talk to the Director and the hospital attorney."

At 6:00 in the morning, Dr. Ziner called Dr. Felix Entraglo, the Director of Midwestern Medical Center, and Isaac Putnam, the head of the center's legal staff. They agreed to meet at 9:00 to talk over the problem presented to them by the Owenses.

They met for two hours. It was Putnam's opinion that the hospital would not be legally liable if Baby Owens were allowed to die because her parents refused to give consent for necessary surgery.

"What about getting a court order requiring surgery?" Dr. Entraglo asked. "That's the sort of thing we do when an infant requires a blood transfusion or immunization and his parents' religious beliefs make them refuse consent."

"This case is not exactly parallel," said Mr. Putnam. "Here we're talking about getting a court to force parents to allow surgery to save the life of a defective infant. The infant will still be defective after the surgery, and I think a court would be reluctant to make a family undergo significant emotional and financial hardships when the parents have seriously deliberated about the matter and decided against surgery."

"But doesn't the child have some claim in this situation?" Dr. Ziner asked.

"That's not clear," said Mr. Putnam. "In general we assume that parents will act for the sake of their child's welfare, and when they are reluctant to do so we look to the courts to act for the child's welfare. But in a situation like this . . . who can say? Is the Owens baby really a person in any legal or moral sense?"

"I think I can understand why a court would hesitate to order surgery," said Dr. Entraglo. "What sort of life would it be for a family when they had been pressured into accepting a child they didn't want? It would turn a family into a cauldron of guilt and resentment mixed in with love and concern. In this case, the lives of five normal people would be profoundly altered for the worse."

"So we just stand by and let the baby die?" asked Dr. Ziner.

"I'm afraid so," Dr. Entraglo said.

It took twelve days for Baby Owens to die. Her lips and throat were moistened with water to lessen her suffering, and in a small disused room set apart from the rooms of patients, she was allowed to starve to death.

Many nurses and physicians thought it was wrong that Baby Owens was forced to die such a lingering death. Some thought it was wrong for her to have to die at all, but such a protracted death seemed needlessly cruel. Yet they were cautioned by Dr. Entraglo that anything done to shorten the baby's life would probably constitute a criminal action. Thus, fear of being charged with a crime kept the staff from administering any medication to Baby Owens.

The burden of caring for the dying baby fell on the nurses in the obstetrics ward. The physicians avoided the child entirely, and it was the nurses who had to see to it that she received her water and was turned in her bed. This was the source of much resentment among the nursing staff, and a few nurses refused to have anything to do with the dying child. Most kept their ministrations to an absolute minimum.

But one nurse, Sara Ann Moberly, was determined to make Baby Owens's last days as comfortable as possible. She held the baby, rocked her, and talked soothingly to her when she cried. Doing all for the baby that she could do soothed Sara Ann as well.

But even Sara Ann was glad when Baby Owens died. "It was a relief to me," she said. "I almost couldn't bear the frustration of just sitting there day after day and doing nothing that could really help her."

SOCIAL CONTEXT: THE BABY DOE CASES

In Bloomington, Indiana, in 1982, a child was born with Down's syndrome and esophageal atresia. The parents and the physicians of the infant, who became known as Baby Doe, decided against the surgery that was needed to open the esophagus and allow the baby to be fed. The decision was upheld by the courts, and six days after birth Baby Doe died of starvation and dehydration.

A month later, in May of 1982, the Secretary of Health and Human Services (HHS) notified hospitals that any institution receiving federal funds could not lawfully "withhold from a handicapped infant nutritional sustenance or medical or surgical treatment required to correct a life-threatening condition if (1) the withholding is based on the fact that the infant is handicapped and (2) the handicap does not render treatment or nutritional sustenance contraindicated."

Ten months later, acting under instructions from President Reagan, an additional and more detailed regulation was issued. Hospitals were required to display a poster in neonatal intensive-care units and pediatric wards indicating that "discrimination" against handicapped infants was a violation of federal law. The poster also listed a toll-free, twenty-four-hour "hotline" number for reporting suspected violations. In addition, the regulations authorized representatives of HHS to take "immediate remedial action" to protect infants. Further, hospitals were required to permit HHS investigators access to the hospital and to relevant patient records.

A group of associations, including the American Academy of Pediatrics, brought suit against HHS in an attempt to stop the regulations from becoming legally effective. Judge Gerhard Gesell of the U.S. District Court ruled, in April 1983, that HHS had not followed the proper procedures in putting the regulations into effect and so they were invalid. In particular, the regulations were issued without notifying and consulting with those affected by them, a procedure that is legally required to avoid arbitrary bureaucratic actions. The judge held that, while HHS had considered relevant factors in identifying a problem, it had failed to consider the effects of the use of the hotline number. An "anonymous tipster" could cause "the sudden descent of Baby Doe squads" on hospitals, and "monopolizing physician and nurse time, and making hospital charts and records unavailable during treatment, can hardly be presumed to produce quality care for the infant."

Furthermore, Judge Gesell held, the main purpose of the regulations was apparently to "require physicians treating newborns to take into account wholly medical risk-benefit considerations and to prevent parents from having any influence upon decisions as to whether further medical treatment is desirable." The regulations explored no other ways to prevent "discriminatory medical care." In his conclusion, Judge Gesell held that federal regulations dealing with imperiled newborns should "reflect caution and sensitivity" and that "wide public comment prior to rule-making is essential."

The Department of Health and Human Services responded to the court decision by drafting another regulation (July 5, 1983) that attempted to resolve the procedural objection that invalidated the first. Sixty days was allowed for the filing of written comments. Since the substance of the regulation was virtually the same, the proposal was widely contested, and on January 12, 1984, another set of regulations was published. Although changing some of the more controversial requirements of the original regulations and providing for infant-care advisory committees, the regulations were still the object of controversy and criticism.

Meanwhile, a second Baby Doe case had become the focus of public attention and legal action. On October 11, 1983, an infant who became known as Baby Jane Doe was born in Port Jefferson (Long Island), New York. Baby

Jane Doe suffered from meningomyelocele, anencephaly, and hydrocephaly. (See the introduction to this chapter for an explanation of these conditions.) Her parents were told that without surgery the child might be expected to live from two weeks to two years, while with surgery she might survive twenty years. However, she would be severely retarded, epileptic, paralyzed, and likely to have constant urinary and bladder infections.

The parents consulted with neurologists, a Roman Catholic priest, nurses, and social workers. In the end they decided that surgery was not in the best interest of the child and opted, instead, for the use of antibiotics to prevent infection of the exposed spinal nerves. "We love her very much," her mother said, "and that's why we made the decision we did."

Lawrence Washburn, Jr., a lawyer who for a number of years had initiated lawsuits on behalf of the unborn and handicapped, somehow learned that Baby Jane Doe was being denied life-prolonging surgery and entered a petition on her behalf before the New York State Supreme Court. Because Mr. Washburn was not related to the infant and had no personal knowledge of her condition or of her parents' decision, his legal standing in the case was questionable, and the court appointed William E. Weber to represent the interest of Baby Jane Doe. After a hearing, the judge ruled that the infant was in need of surgery to preserve her life and authorized Mr. Weber to consent.

This decision was reversed on appeal. The court held that the parents' decision was in the best interest of the infant. Hence, the state had no basis to intervene. The ruling was then appealed to the New York Court of Appeals and upheld. The court held that the parents' right to privacy was invaded when a person totally unrelated and with no knowledge of the infant's condition and treatment entered into litigation in an attempt to challenge the discharge of parental responsibility. However, the main grounds for allowing the ruling to stand were procedural, for the suit had not followed New York law requiring that the state intervene in the treatment of children only through the family court.

In the cases of both Baby Doe and Baby Jane Doe, the federal government went to court to demand the medical records of the infants. In both cases, the government charged that decisions against treatment represented discrimination against the handicapped. However, the courts consistently rejected the government's demands. In June of 1985, the Supreme Court agreed to hear arguments to decide whether the federal laws that protect the handicapped against discrimination also apply to the treatment of imperiled newborns who are denied life-prolonging treatment.

On May 15, 1985, the third anniversary of the death of Baby Doe, the Department of Health and Human Services' final "Baby Doe" regulation went into effect. The regulation was an implementation of an amendment to the Child Abuse Prevention and Treatment Act that was passed into law in October 1985. The amendment was the result of negotiations among some nineteen groups representing right-to-life advocates, the disabled, the medical professions, and members of Congress.

The regulation extended the term "medical neglect" to cover cases of "withholding of medically indicated treatment from a disabled infant with a life-threatening condition." Such treatment was defined as

> the failure to respond to the infant's life-threatening conditions by providing treatment (including appropriate nutrition, hydration, and medication) which, in the treating physician's (or physicians') reasonable medical judgment, will be most likely to be effective in ameliorating or correcting all such conditions . . . .

Withholding treatment, but not food and water, was not "medical neglect" in three kinds of cases:

1. The infant is chronically and irreversibly comatose.

2. The provision of such treatment would merely prolong dying, not be effective in ameliorating or correcting all of the infant's life-threatening conditions, or otherwise be futile in terms of the survival of the infant.

3. The provision of such treatment would be virtually futile in terms of the survival of the infant, and the treatment itself under such circumstances would be inhumane.

The regulation defined "reasonable medical judgment" as "a medical judgment that would be made by a reasonably prudent physician knowledgeable about the case and the treatment possibilities with respect to the medical conditions involved." State child-protection service agencies were designated as the proper organizations to see to it that infants were not suffering "medical neglect," and, in order to receive any federal funds, such agencies were required to develop a set of procedures to carry out this function.

On June 9, 1986, the Supreme Court, in a 5-to-3 ruling with one abstention, struck down the Baby Doe regulations. The Court held that there was no evidence that hospitals had discriminated against impaired infants or had refused treatments sought by parents. Accordingly, there was no basis for federal intervention.

Justice John Paul Stevens, in the majority opinion, stressed the absence of any law that might serve as a basis for federal intervention. According to Justice Stevens, no federal law requires hospitals to treat impaired infants without parental consent. Nor does the government have the right "to give unsolicited advice either to parents, to hospitals, or to state officials who are faced with difficult treatment decisions concerning handicapped children." Furthermore, state child-protection agencies "may not be conscripted against their will as the foot soldiers in a Federal crusade."

Representatives of hospitals and those directly involved in neonatal care were generally relieved by the Supreme Court decision. In their arguments before the Court, they had claimed that federal "Baby Doe squads arriving within hours after birth" had second-guessed the agonizing decisions made by parents and physicians and that this had "a devastating impact on the parents."

The Court decision once again places the major responsibility for making decisions about withholding life-sustaining treatment from imperiled newborns on families and physicians acting in consultation.

One recommendation made in the Baby Doe regulations may continue to have influence. The regulations encouraged hospitals to establish Infant Care Review Committees, and similar recommendations have been made by the President's Commission for the Study of Ethical Problems in Medicine and by the American Academy of Pediatrics. Exactly how such committees might operate, how they would be composed, and what powers they should have continues to be a matter of discussion and disagreement.

The proper role of government, the power of committees, and the responsibilities of parents are merely some of the problems that form the complex of moral issues associated with imperiled and impaired infants.

INTRODUCTION

If we could speak of nature in human terms, we would often say that it is cruel and pitiless. Nowhere does it seem more heartless than in the case of babies born into the world with severe physical impairments and deformities. The birth of such a child transforms an occasion of expected joy into one of immense sadness. It forces the child's parents to make a momentous decision at a time they are least prepared to reason clearly: Shall they insist that everything be done to save the child's life? Or shall they request that the child be allowed an easeful death?

Nor can physicians and nurses escape the burden that the birth of such a child delivers. Committed to saving lives, can they condone the death of that child? What shall the physician say to the parents when they turn to him or her for advice? No one involved in the situation can escape the moral agonies that it brings.

To see more clearly what the precise moral issues are in such cases, we need to consider some of the factual details that may be involved in them. We need also to mention other kinds of moral considerations that may be relevant to deciding how an impaired newborn child is to be dealt with by those who have the responsibility to decide.

GENETIC AND CONGENITAL IMPAIRMENTS

The development of a child to the point of birth is an unimaginably complicated process, and there are many ways in which it can go wrong. Two kinds of errors are most frequently responsible for producing impaired children: genetic errors and congenital errors.

1. *Genetic errors.* The program of information that is coded into DNA (the genetic material) may be in some way abnormal because of the occurrence of a mutation. Consequently, when the DNA blueprint is "read" and its instructions followed, the child that develops will be impaired. The defective gene may have been inherited, or it may be due to a new mutation.

2. *Congenital errors.* "Congenital" means only "present at birth," and, since genetic defects have results that are present at birth, the term is misleading. Ordinarily, however, the phrase is used to designate errors that result during the developmental process. The impairment, then, is not in the original blueprint (genes) but results either from genetic damage or from the reading of

the blueprint. The manufacture and assembly of the materials that constitute the child's development are affected.

We know that many factors can influence fetal development. Radiation (such as X rays), drugs (such as thalidomide), chemicals (such as mercury), and nutritional deficiencies can all cause changes in an otherwise normal process. Also, biological disease agents, such as certain viruses or spirochetes, may intervene in development. They may alter the machinery of the cells, interfere with the formation of tissues, and defeat the carefully programmed process that leads to a normal child.

Genetic impairments are inherited; they are the outcome of the genetic endowment of the child. A carrier of defective genes who has children can pass on the genes. Congenital impairments are not inherited and cannot be passed on. This point is of great theoretical and practical importance. With proper genetic counseling, individuals belonging to families in which certain diseases "run" can assess the risk that their children might be impaired. Also, some genetic diseases can be diagnosed before birth. A blood test for the presence of the substance alphafetoprotein can indicate the likelihood of neural tube defects characteristic of spina bifida. Ultrasound can be used to confirm or detect these or other developmental anomalies. In a procedure known as amniocentesis, fluid is drawn from the uterus, and cells from the developing embryo are examined for genetic abnormalities. (The newer procedure of chorion sampling takes the cells directly from the fetal membrane.) If abnormalities are present, the woman may decide to have an abortion rather than give birth to an impaired child. A recognition of some kinds of developmental errors can lead to efforts to eliminate the impairments by controlling the factors responsible for them. (For additional information on genetic errors, screening, and attempts to correct their results, see the introduction to Chapter 7.)

Once the impaired child is born, the medical and moral problems are immediate. Let us consider now some of the defects commonly found in newborn children. Our focus will be on what they are rather than on what caused them, for, as far as the moral issue is concerned in a particular case, how the child came to be impaired is of no importance.

Down's Syndrome

This is a genetic disease first identified in 1866 by the English physician J. L. H. Down. Normally, humans have twenty-three pairs of chromosomes, but Down's syndrome results from the presence of an extra chromosome. The condition is called Trisomy-21, for, instead of a twenty-first pair of chromosomes, the affected person has a twenty-first *triple*. (Less often, the syndrome is produced when the string of chromosomes gets twisted and chromosome pair number 21 sticks to number 15.)

In ways not wholly understood, the normal process of development is altered by this extra chromosome. The child is born with retardation and various physical abnormalities. Typically, these are relatively minor and include such features as a broad skull, a large tongue, and an upward slant of the eyelids. It is this last feature that led to the name "mongolism" for the condition.

Down's syndrome occurs in about one of every 1,000 births. It occurs most frequently in women over the age of thirty-five, although it is not known why this should be so. In 1984 researchers discovered that certain chromosomes sometimes contain an extra copy of a segment known as the "nucleolar organizing region." This abnormality seems linked to Down's syndrome, and families in which either parent has the abnormality are twenty times more likely to have an afflicted child. Researchers hope to use this information to develop a reliable screening test.

There is no cure for Down's syndrome—no way to compensate for the abnormality of the development process. Those with the defect generally have an 1Q of about 50–80 and usually require the care and help of others. They can be taught easy tasks, and despite their impairment, those with Down's syndrome usually seem to be quite happy people.

Spina Bifida

Spina bifida is a general name for birth defects that involve an opening in the spine. In development, the spine of the child fails to fuse properly, and often the open vertebrae permit the membrane covering the spinal cord to protrude to the outside. The membrane sometimes forms a bulging, thin sac that contains spinal fluid and nerve tissue. When nerve tissue is present, the condition is called myelomeningocele. This form of spina bifida is a very severe one.

Complications arising from spina bifida must often be treated surgically. The initial condition, the opening in the spine, must be closed up. In severe cases, the sac is removed and the nerve tissue inside is placed within the spinal canal. Normal skin is then grafted over the area. The danger of an infection of the meninges (meningitis) is great; thus, treatment with antibiotic drugs is also necessary.

Furthermore, a child with spina bifida is also likely to require orthopedic operations to attempt to correct the deformities of the legs and feet that occur because of muscle weakness and lack of muscular control due to nerve damage. The bones of such children are thin and brittle, and fractures are frequent.

A child born with spina bifida is virtually always paralyzed to some extent. Generally the paralysis is below the waist. Because of the nerve damage, the child will have limited sensation in the lower part of the body. This means that he will have no control over his bladder or bowels. The lack of bladder control may result in infection of the bladder, urinary tract, and kidneys, because the undischarged urine may serve as a breeding place for micro-organisms. Surgery may help with the problem of lack of control of the bladder and bowels.

Spina bifida occurs in between one and ten per 1,000 births. For reasons not understood, the rate in white families of low socioeconomic status is three times higher than that in families of higher socioeconomic status. The rate in the black population is less than half of that in the white population. A recent study also shows that women who took multivitamins during pregnancy ran less than half the risk of having an affected child than those who did not, but the significance of this result remains uncertain.

Spina bifida is almost always accompanied by hydrocephaly.

Hydrocephaly

This term literally means "water on the brain." When, for whatever reasons, the flow of fluid through the spinal canal is blocked, the cerebrospinal fluid produced within the brain cannot escape. Pressure buildup from the fluid can cause brain damage, and if it is not released the child will die. Although hydrocephaly is frequently the result of spina bifida, it can have several causes and can develop late in a child's life.

Treatment requires surgically inserting a thin tube, or shunt, to drain the fluid from the skull to the heart or abdomen where it can be absorbed. The operation can save the baby's life, but physical and mental damage is frequent. Placing the shunt and getting it to work properly are difficult tasks that may require many operations. If hydrocephaly accompanies spina bifida (and it almost always does), it is treated first.

Anencephaly

This term means literally "without brain." In this condition, the brain is partially or al-most totally absent. The defect is related to spina bifida, for in some forms the bones of the skull are not completely formed and leave an opening through which brain material bulges to the outside.

In some cases, death is a virtual certainty. Other cases can be dealt with in much the same way as is spina bifida. Ordinarily, the individual is so severely retarded that he has minimum control over bodily movements and functions. There is never hope for improvement by any known means.

Esophageal Atresia

In medical terms, an atresia is the closing of a normal opening or canal. The esophagus is the muscular tube that extends from the back of the throat to the stomach. Sometimes the tube forms without an opening, or it does not completely develop so that it does not extend to the stomach. The condition must be corrected by surgery in order for the child to get food into its stomach. The chances of success in such surgery are very high.

Duodenal Atresia

The duodenum is the upper part of the small intestine. Food from the stomach empties into it. When the duodenum is closed off, food cannot pass through and be digested. Surgery can repair this condition and is successful in most cases.

An estimated 6% of all live births, some 200,000 infants a year, require intensive neonatal care. The afflictions that we have singled out for special mention are those that are most often the source of major moral problems. Those correctable by standard surgical procedures present no special moral difficulties. But even they are often involved with other impairments, such as Down's syndrome, that make them important factors in moral deliberations.

ETHICAL THEORIES AND THE PROBLEM OF BIRTH IMPAIRMENTS

A great number of serious moral issues are raised by impaired newborns. Should they be given only ordinary care, or should special efforts be made to save their lives? Should they be given no care and allowed to die? Should they be killed in a merciful manner? Who should decide what is in the interest of the child? Might acting in the interest of the child require not acting to save the child's life?

A more basic question that cuts even deeper than these concerns the status of the newborn. It is virtually the same as the question raised in Chapter 1 about the fetus. Namely, are severely impaired newborns persons? It might be argued that some infants are so severely impaired that they should not be considered persons in a relevant moral sense. Not only do they lack the capacity to function, but they lack even the potentiality for ordinary psychological and social development. In this respect, they are worse off than most maturing fetuses.

If this view is accepted, then the principles of our moral theories do not require that we act to preserve the lives of impaired newborns. We might, considering their origin, be disposed to show them some consideration and treat them benevolently—perhaps in the same way we might deal with animals that are in a similarly hopeless condition. We might kill them or allow them to die as a demonstration of our compassion.

One major difficulty with this view is that it is not at all clear which impaired infants could legitimately be considered nonpersons. Birth defects vary widely in severity, and, unless one is prepared to endorse infanticide generally, it is necessary to have defensible criteria for distinguishing among newborns. Also, one must defend a general concept of a person that would make it reasonable to regard human offspring as occupying a different status.

By contrast, it might be claimed that the fact that a newborn is a human progeny is sufficient to consider it a person. Assuming that this is so, the question becomes "How ought we to treat a severely impaired infant person?" Just because they are infants, impaired newborns cannot express wishes, make claims, or enter into deliberations. All that is done concerning them must be done by others.

A utilitarian might decide that the social and personal cost (the suffering of the infant, the anguish of the parents and family, the monetary cost to society) of saving the life of such an infant is greater than the social and personal benefits that can be expected. Accordingly, such a child should not be allowed to live, and it should be killed as painlessly as possible to minimize its suffering. Yet a rule utilitarian might claim, on the contrary, that the rule "Save every child where possible" would, in the long run, produce more utility than disutility.

The natural law position of Roman Catholicism is that even the most defective newborn is a human person. Yet this view does not require that extraordinary means be used to save the life of such a child. The suffering of the family, great expense, and the need for multiple operations would be reasons for providing only ordinary care. Ordinary care does not mean that every standard medical procedure that might help should be followed. It means only that the defective newborn should receive care of the same type provided for a normal infant. It would be immoral to kill the child or to cause its death by withholding all care.

If the infant is a person, then Kant would regard it as possessing an inherent dignity and value. But the infant in its condition lacks the capacity to reason and to express its will. How, then, should we, acting as its agents, treat it? Kant's principles provide no clear-cut answer. The infant does not threaten our own existence, and we have no grounds for killing it. But, it could be argued, we should allow the child to die. We can imaginatively put ourselves in the place of the infant. Although it would be morally wrong to will our own death (which, Kant claimed, would involve a self-defeating maxim), we might express our autonomy and rationality by choosing to refuse treatment that would prolong a painful and hopeless life. If this is so, then we might act in this way on behalf of the defective child. We might allow the child to die. Indeed, it may be our duty to do so. A similar line of argument from Ross's viewpoint might lead us to decide that, although we have a prima facie duty to preserve the child's life, our actual duty is to allow it to die.

Another basic question remains: Who is to make the decision about how an impaired newborn is to be treated? Traditionally, the assumption has been that this is a decision best left to the infant's parents and physicians. Because they can be assumed to have the highest concern for his welfare and the most knowledge about his condition and prospects, they are the ones who should have the primary responsibility for deciding his fate. If there is reason to believe that they are not acting in a responsible manner, then it becomes the responsibility of the courts to guarantee that the interests of the infant are served.

Hardly any responsible person advocates heroic efforts to save the lives of infants who are most severely impaired, and hardly anyone advocates not treating infants with relatively simple and correctable impairments. The difficult cases are those that fall somewhere along the continuum. Advances in medical management and technology can now save the lives of many infants who earlier would have died relatively quickly, and yet we still lack the power to provide those infants with a life that we might judge to be worthwhile. Yet a failure to treat such infants does not invariably result in their deaths, and a failure to provide them with early treatment may mean that they are even more impaired than they would be otherwise.

No one believes that we currently have a satisfactory solution to this dilemma. It is important to keep in mind that it is not a purely intellectual problem. The context in which particular decisions are made is one of doubt and confusion and genuine anguish.

Examination of Arguments in Favor of Withholding Ordinary Medical Care from Defective Infants _____

John A. Robertson

John A. Robertson defends a conservative natural law position in criticizing two arguments in favor of withholding "necessary but ordinary" medical care from impaired infants. He rejects the claim made by Michael Tooley that infants are not persons and argues that, on the contrary, there is no nonarbitrary consideration that requires us to protect the past realization of conceptual capability but not its potential realization.

The second argument that Robertson considers is one to the effect that we have no obligation to treat defective newborns when the cost of doing so greatly outweighs the benefits (a utilitarian argument). In criticism, Robertson claims that we have no way of judging this. Life itself may be of sufficient worth to an impaired person to offset his or her suffering, and the suffering and cost to society are not sufficient to justify withholding care.

This [selection] considers two arguments in favor of with-holding necessary but ordinary medical care from defective infants, and concludes that neither is persuasive. . . .

1. Defective Infants Are Not Persons

Children born with congenital malformations may lack human form and the possibility of ordinary, psychosocial development. In many cases mental retardation is or will be so profound, and physical incapacity so great, that the term "persons" or "humanly alive" have odd or questionable meaning when applied to them. In these cases the infant's physical and mental defects are so severe that they will never know anything but a vegetative existence, with no discernible personality, sense of self, or capacity to interact with others. Withholding ordinary medical care in such cases, one may argue, is justified on the ground that these infants are not persons or human beings in the ordinary or legal sense of the term, and therefore do not possess the right of care that persons possess.

Central to this argument is the idea that living products of the human uterus can be classified into offspring that are persons, and those that are not. Conception and birth by human parents does not automatically endow one with personhood and its accompanying rights. Some other characteristic or feature must be present in the organism for personhood to vest, and this the defective infant arguably lacks. Lacking that property, an organism is not a person or deserving to be treated as such.

Before considering what "morally significant features" might distinguish persons from nonpersons, and examining the relevance of such features to the case of the defective infant, we must face an initial objection to this line of inquiry. The objection questions the need for any distinction among human offspring because of

the monumental misuse of the concept of "humanity" in so many practices of discrimination and atrocity throughout history. Slavery, witchhunts and wars have all been justified by their perpetrators on the grounds that they held their victims to be less than fully human. The insane and the criminal have for long periods

been deprived of the most basic necessities for similar reasons, and been excluded from society. . . .

. . . Even when entered upon with the best of intentions, and in the most guarded manner, the enterprise of basing the protection of human life upon such criteria and definitions is dangerous. To question someone's humanity or personhood is a first step to mistreatment and killing.

Hence, according to this view, human parentage is a necessary and sufficient condition for personhood, whatever the characteristics of the offspring, because qualifying criteria inevitably lead to abuse and untold suffering to beings who are unquestionably human. Moreover, the human species is sufficiently different from other sentient species that assigning its members greater rights on birth alone is not arbitrary.

This objection is indeed powerful. The treatment accorded slaves in the United States, the Nazi denial of personal status to non-Aryans, and countless other incidents, testify that man's inhumanity to man is indeed greatest when a putative nonperson is involved. Arguably, however, a distinction based on gross physical form, profound mental incapacity, and the very existence of personality or selfhood, besides having an empirical basis in the monstrosities and mutations known to have been born to women is a basic and fundamental one. Rather than distinguishing among the particular characteristics that persons might attain through the contingencies of race, culture, and class, it merely separates out those who lack the potential for assuming any personal characteristics beyond breathing and consciousness.

This reply narrows the issue: should such creatures be cared for, protected, or regarded as "ordinary" humans? If such treatment is not warranted, they may be treated as nonpersons. The arguments supporting care in all circumstances are based on the view that all living creatures are sacred, contain a spark of the divine, and should be so regarded. Moreover, identifying those human offspring unworthy of care is a difficult task and will inevitably take a toll on those whose humanity cannot seriously be questioned. At this point the argument becomes metaphysical or religious and

Reprinted by permission of the publisher from "Involuntary Euthanasia of Defective Newborns: A Legal Analysis," Stanford Law Review 27 (1975): 246–261. *Copyright 1975 by the Board of Trustees of the Leland Stanford Junior University. Editor's Note: The footnotes in this essay are too lengthy to be included here.*

immune to resolution by empirical evidence, not unlike the controversy over whether a fetus is a person. It should be noted, however, that recognizing all human offspring as persons, like recognizing the fetus to be a person, does not conclude the treatment issue.

Although this debate can be resolved only by reference to religious or moral beliefs, a procedural solution may reasonably be considered. Since reasonable people can agree that we ordinarily regard human offspring as persons, and further, that defining categories of exclusion is likely to pose special dangers of abuse, a reasonable solution is to presume that all living human offspring are persons. This rule would be subject to exception only if it can be shown beyond a reasonable doubt that certain offspring will never possess the minimal properties that reasonable persons ordinarily associate with human personality. If this burden cannot be satisfied, then the presumption of personhood obtains.

For this purpose I will address only one of the many properties proposed as a necessary condition of personhood—the capacity for having a sense of self—and consider whether its advocates present a cogent account of the nonhuman. Since other accounts may be more convincingly articulated, this discussion will neither exhaust nor conclude the issue. But it will illuminate the strengths and weaknesses of the personhood argument and enable us to evaluate its application to defective infants.

Michael Tooley has recently argued that a human offspring lacking the capacity for a sense of self lacks the rights to life or equal treatment possessed by other persons. In considering the morality of abortion and infanticide, Tooley considers "what properties a thing must possess in order to have a serious right to life," and he concludes that:

> [h]aving a right to life presupposes that one is capable of desiring to continue existing as a subject of experiences and other mental states. This in turn presupposes both that one has the concept of such a continuing entity and that one believes that one is oneself such an entity. So an entity that lacks such a consciousness of itself as a continuing subject of mental states does not have a right to life.

However, this account is at first glance too narrow, for it appears to exclude all those who do not presently have a desire "to continue existing as a subject of experiences and other mental states." The sleeping or unconscious individual, the deranged, the conditioned, and the suicidal do not have such desires, though they might have had them or could have them in the future. Accordingly, Tooley emphasizes the capability of entertaining such desires, rather than their actual existence. But it is difficult to distinguish the capability for such desires in an unconscious, conditioned, or emotionally disturbed person from the capability existing in a fetus or infant. In all cases the capability is a future one; it will arise only if certain events occur, such as normal growth and development in the case of the infant, and removal of the disability in the other cases. The infant, in fact, might realize its capability long before disabled adults recover emotional balance or consciousness.

To meet this objection, Tooley argues that the significance of the capability in question is not solely its future realization (for fetuses and infants will ordinarily realize it), but also its previous existence and exercise. He seems to say that once the conceptual capability has been realized, one's right to desire continued existence permanently vests, even though the present capability for desiring does not exist, and may be lost for substantial periods or permanently. Yet, what nonarbitrary reasons require that we protect the past realization of conceptual capability but not its potential realization in the future? As a reward for its past realization? To mark our reverence and honor for someone who has realized that state? Tooley is silent on this point.

Another difficulty is Tooley's ambiguity concerning the permanently deranged, comatose, or conditioned. Often he phrases his argument in terms of a temporary suspension of the capability of conceptual thought. One wonders what he would say of someone permanently deranged, or with massive brain damage, or in a prolonged coma. If he seriously means that the past existence of a desire for life vests these cases with the right to life, then it is indeed difficult to distinguish the comatose or deranged from the infant profoundly retarded at birth. Neither will ever possess the conceptual capability to desire to be a continuing subject of experiences. A distinction based on reward or desert seems arbitrary, and protection of life applies equally well in both cases. Would Tooley avoid this problem by holding that the permanently comatose and deranged lose their rights after a certain point because conceptual capacity will never be regained? This would permit killing (or at least withholding of care) from the insane and comatose—doubtless an unappealing prospect. Moreover, we do not ordinarily think of the insane, and possibly the comatose, as losing personhood before their death. Although their personality or identity may be said to change, presumably for the worse, or become fragmented or minimal, we still regard them as specific persons. If a "self" in some minimal sense exists here then the profoundly retarded, who at least is conscious, also may be considered a self, albeit a minimal one. Thus, one may argue that Tooley fails to provide a convincing account of criteria distinguishing persons and nonpersons. He both excludes beings we ordinarily think of as persons—infants, deranged, conditioned, possibly the comatose—and fails to articulate criteria that convincingly distinguish the nonhuman. But, even if we were to accept Tooley's distinction that beings lacking the potential for desire and a sense of self are not persons who are owed the duty to be treated by ordinary medical means, this would not appear to be very helpful in deciding whether to treat the newborn with physical or mental defects. Few infants, it would seem, would fall into this class. First, those suffering from malformations, however gross, that do not affect mental capabilities would not fit the class of nonpersons. Second, frequently even the most severe cases of mental retardation cannot be reliably determined until a much later period; care thus could not justifiably be withheld in the neonatal period, although this principle would permit nontreatment at the time when nonpersonality is clearly established. Finally, the only group of defective newborns who would clearly qualify as nonpersons is anencephalics, who altogether lack a brain or those so severely brain-damaged that it is immediately clear that a sense of self or personality can never develop. Mongols, myelomeningoceles, and other defective infants from whom ordinary care is now routinely withheld would not qualify as nonpersons. Thus, even the most coherent and cogent criteria of humanity are only marginally helpful in the situation of the defective infant. We must therefore consider whether treatment can be withheld on grounds other than the claim that such infants are not persons.

2. No Obligation to Treat Exists When the Costs of Maintaining Life Greatly Outweigh the Benefits

If we reject the argument that defective newborns are not persons, the question remains whether circumstances exist in which the consequences of treatment as compared with nontreatment are so undesirable that the omission of care is justified. As we have seen, the doctrine of necessity permits one to violate the criminal law when essential to prevent the occurrence of a greater evil. The circumstances, however, when the death of a nonconsenting person is a lesser evil than his continuing life are narrowly circumscribed, and do not include withholding care from defective infants. Yet many parents and physicians deeply committed to the loving care of the newborn think that treating severely defective infants causes more harm than good, thereby justifying the withholding of ordinary care. In their view the suffering and diminished quality of the child's life do not justify the social and economic costs of treatment. This claim has a growing commonsense appeal, but it assumes that the utility or quality of one's life can be measured and compared with other lives, and that health resources may legitimately be allocated to produce the greatest personal utility. This argument will now be analyzed from the perspective of the defective patient and others affected by his care.

a. The Quality of the Defective Infant's Life

Comparisons of relative worth among persons, or between persons and other interests, raise moral and methodological issues that make any argument that relies on such comparisons extremely vulnerable. Thus the strongest claim for not treating the defective newborn is that treatment seriously harms the infant's own interests, whatever may be the effects on others. When maintaining his life involves great physical and psychosocial suffering for the patient, a reasonable person might conclude that such a life is not worth living. Presumably the patient, if fully informed and able to communicate, would agree. One then would be morally justified in withholding lifesaving treatment if such action served to advance the best interests of the patient.

Congenital malformations impair development in several ways that lead to the judgment that deformed retarded infants are "a burden to themselves." One is the severe physical pain, much of it resulting from repeated surgery that defective infants will suffer. Defective children also are likely to develop other pathological features, leading to repeated fractures, dislocations, surgery, malfunctions, and other sources of pain. The shunt, for example, inserted to relieve hydrocephalus, a common problem in defective children, often becomes clogged, necessitating frequent surgical interventions.

Pain, however, may be intermittent and manageable with analgesics. Since many infants and adults experience great pain, and many defective infants do not, pain alone, if not totally unmanageable, does not sufficiently show that a life is so worthless that death is preferable. More important are the psychosocial deficits resulting from the child's handicaps. Many defective children never can walk even with prosthesis, never interact with normal children, never appreciate growth, adolescence, or the fulfillment of education and employment, and seldom are even able to care for themselves. In cases of severe retardation, they may be left with a vegetative existence in a crib, incapable of choice or the most minimal response to stimuli. Parents or others may reject them, and much of their time will be spent in hospitals, in surgery, or fighting the many illnesses that beset them. Can it be said that such a life is worth living?

There are two possible responses to the quality-of-life argument. One is to accept its premises but to question the degree of suffering in particular cases, and thus restrict the justification for death to the most extreme cases. The absence of opportunities for schooling, career, and interaction may be the fault of social attitudes and the failings of healthy persons, rather than a necessary result of congenital malformations. Psychosocial suffering occurs because healthy, normal persons reject or refuse to relate to the defective, or hurry them to poorly funded institutions. Most nonambulatory, mentally retarded persons can be trained for satisfying roles. One cannot assume that a nonproductive existence is necessarily unhappy; even social rejection and nonacceptance can be mitigated. Moreover, the psychosocial ills of the handicapped often do not differ in kind from those experienced by many persons. With training and care, growth, development, and a full range of experiences are possible for most people with physical and mental handicaps. Thus, the claim that death is a far better fate than life cannot in most cases be sustained.

This response, however, avoids meeting the quality-of-life argument on its strongest grounds. Even if many defective infants can experience growth, interaction, and most human satisfactions if nurtured, treated, and trained, some infants are so severely retarded or grossly deformed that their response to love and care, in fact their capacity to be conscious, is always minimal. Although mongoloid and nonambulatory spina bifida children may experience an existence we would hesitate to adjudge worse than death, the profoundly retarded, nonambulatory, blind, deaf infant who will spend his few years in the back-ward cribs of a state institution is clearly a different matter.

To repudiate the quality-of-life argument, therefore, requires a defense of treatment in even these extreme cases. Such a defense would question the validity of any surrogate or proxy judgments of the worth or quality of life when the wishes of the person in question cannot be ascertained. The essence of the quality-of-life argument is a proxy's judgment that no reasonable person can prefer the pain, suffering, and loneliness of, for example, life in a crib at an IQ level of 20, to an immediate, painless death.

But in what sense can the proxy validly conclude that a person with different wants, needs, and interests, if able to speak, would agree that such a life were worse than death? At the start one must be skeptical of the proxy's claim to objective disinterestedness. If the proxy is also the parent or physician, as has been the case in pediatric euthanasia, the impact of treatment on the proxy's interests, rather than solely on those of the child, may influence his assessment. But even if the proxy were truly neutral and committed only to caring for the child, the problem of egocentricity and knowing another's mind remains. Compared with the situation and life prospects of a "reasonable man," the child's potential quality of life indeed appears dim. Yet a standard based on healthy, ordinary development may be entirely inappropriate to this situation. One who has never known the pleasures of mental operation, ambulation, and social interaction surely does not suffer from their loss as much as one who has. While one who has known these capacities may prefer death to a life without them, we have no assurance that the handicapped person, with no point of comparison, would agree. Life, and life alone, whatever its limitations, might be of sufficient worth to him.

One should also be hesitant to accept proxy assessments of quality-of-life because the margin of error in such predictions may be very great. For instance, while one expert argues that by a purely clinical assessment he can accurately forecast the minimum degree of future handicap an individual will experience, such forecasting is not infallible, and risks denying care to infants whose disability might otherwise permit a reasonably acceptable quality-of-life. Thus given the problems in ascertaining another's wishes, the proxy's bias to personal or culturally relative interests, and the unreliability of predictive criteria, the quality-of-life argument is open to serious question. Its strongest appeal arises in the case of a grossly deformed, retarded, institutionalized child, or one with incessant unmanageable pain, where continued life is itself torture. But these cases are few, and cast doubt on the utility of any such judgment. Even if the judgment occasionally may be defensible, the potential danger of quality-of-life assessments may be a compelling reason for rejecting this rationale for withholding treatment.

b. The Suffering of Others

In addition to the infant's own suffering, one who argues that the harm of treatment justifies violation of the defective infant's right to life usually relies on the psychological, social, and economic costs of maintaining his existence to family and society. In their view the minimal benefit of treatment to persons incapable of full social and physical development does not justify the burdens that care of the defective infant imposes on parents, siblings, health professionals, and other patients. Matson, a noted pediatric neurosurgeon, states:

> [I]t is the doctor's and the community's responsibility to provide [custodial] care and to minimize suffering, but, at the same time, it is also their responsibility not to prolong such individual, familial, and community suffering unnecessarily, and not to carry out multiple procedures and prolonged, expensive, acute hospitalization in an infant whose chance for acceptable growth and development is negligible.

Such a frankly utilitarian argument raises problems. It assumes that because of the greatly curtailed

orbit of his existence, the costs or suffering of others [are] greater than the benefit of life to the child. This judgment, however, requires a coherent way of measuring and comparing interpersonal utilities, a logical-practical problem that utilitarianism has never surmounted. But even if such comparisons could reliably show a net loss from treatment, the fact remains that the child must sacrifice his life to benefit others. If the life of one individual, however useless, may be sacrificed for the benefit of any person, however useful, or for the benefit of any number of persons, then we have acknowledged the principle that rational utility may justify any outcome. As many philosophers have demonstrated, utilitarianism can always permit the sacrifice of one life for other interests, given the appropriate arrangement of utilities on the balance sheet. In the absence of principled grounds for such a decision, the social equation involved in mandating direct, involuntary euthanasia becomes a difference of degree, not kind, and we reach the point where protection of life depends solely on social judgments of utility.

These objections may well be determinative. But if we temporarily bracket them and examine the extent to which care of the defective infant subjects others to suffering, the claim that inordinate suffering outweighs the infant's interest in life is rarely plausible. In this regard we must examine the impact of caring for defective infants on the family, health professions, and society-at-large.

The Family. The psychological impact and crisis created by birth of a defective infant is devastating. Not only is the mother denied the normal tension release from the stresses of pregnancy, but both parents feel a crushing blow to their dignity, self-esteem and self-confidence. In a very short time, they feel grief for the loss of the normal expected child, anger at fate, numbness, disgust, waves of helplessness, and disbelief. Most feel personal blame for the defect, or blame their spouse. Adding to the shock is fear that social position and mobility are permanently endangered. The transformation of a "joyously awaited experience into one of catastrophe and profound psychological threat" often will reactivate unresolved maturational conflicts. The chances for social pathology— divorce, somatic complaints, nervous and mental disorders—increase and hard-won adjustment patterns may be permanently damaged.

The initial reactions of guilt, grief, anger, and loss, however, cannot be the true measure of family suffering caused by care of a defective infant, because these costs are present whether or not the parents choose treatment. Rather, the question is to what degree treatment imposes psychic and other costs greater than would occur if the child were not treated. The claim that care is more costly rests largely on the view that parents and family suffer inordinately from nurturing such a child.

Indeed, if the child is treated and accepted at home, difficult and demanding adjustments must be made. Parents must learn how to care for a disabled child, confront financial and psychological uncertainty, meet the needs of other siblings, and work through their own conflicting feelings. Mothering demands are greater than with a normal child, particularly if medical care and hospitalization are frequently required. Counseling or professional support may be nonexistent or difficult to obtain. Younger siblings may react with hostility and guilt, older with shame and anger. Often the normal feedback of child growth that renders the turmoil of childrearing worthwhile develops more slowly or not at all. Family resources can be depleted (especially if medical care is needed), consumption patterns altered, or standards of living modified. Housing may have to be found closer to a hospital, and plans for further children changed. Finally, the anxieties, guilt, and grief present at birth may threaten to recur or become chronic.

Yet, although we must recognize the burdens and frustrations of raising a defective infant, it does not necessarily follow that these costs require non-treatment, or even institutionalization. Individual and group counseling can substantially alleviate anxiety, guilt, and frustration, and enable parents to cope with underlying conflicts triggered by the birth and the adaptations required. Counseling also can reduce psychological pressures on siblings, who can be taught to recognize and accept their own possibly hostile feelings and the difficult position of their parents. They may even be taught to help their parents care for the child.

The impact of increased financial costs also may vary. In families with high income or adequate health insurance, the financial costs are manageable. In others, state assistance may be available. If severe financial problems arise or pathological adjustments are likely, institutionalization, although undesirable for the child, remains an option. Finally, in many cases, the experience of living through a crisis is a deepening and enriching one, accelerating personality maturation, and giving one a new sensitivity to the needs of spouse, siblings, and others. As one parent of a defective child states: "In the last months I have come closer to people and can understand them more. I have met them more deeply. I did not know there were so many people with troubles in the world."

Thus, while social attitudes regard the handicapped child as an unmitigated disaster, in reality the problem may not be insurmountable, and often may not differ from life's other vicissitudes. Suffering there is, but seldom is it so overwhelming or so imminent that the only alternative is death of the child.

Health Professionals. Physicians and nurses also suffer when parents give birth to a defective child, although, of course, not to the degree of the parents. To the obstetrician or general practitioner the defective birth may be a blow to his professional identity. He has the difficult task of informing the parents of the defects, explaining their causes, and dealing with the parents' resulting emotional shock. Often he feels guilty for failing to produce a normal baby. In addition, the parents may project anger or hostility on the physician, questioning his professional competence or seeking the services of other doctors. The physician also may feel that his expertise and training are misused when employed to maintain the life of an infant whose chances for a productive existence are so diminished. By neglecting other patients, he may feel that he is prolonging rather than alleviating suffering.

Nurses, too, suffer role strain from care of the defective newborn. Intensive-care-unit nurses may work with only one or two babies at a time. They face the daily ordeals of care—the progress and relapses—and often must deal with anxious parents who are themselves grieving or ambivalent toward the child. The situation may trigger a nurse's own ambivalence about death and mothering, in a context in which she is actively working to keep alive a child whose life prospects seem minimal.

Thus, the effects of care on physicians and nurses are not trivial, and must be intelligently confronted in medical education or in management of a pediatric unit. Yet to state them is to make clear that they can but weigh lightly in the decision of whether to treat a defective newborn. Compared with the situation of the parents, these burdens seem insignificant, are short term, and most likely do not evoke such profound emotions. In any case, these difficulties are hazards of the profession—caring for the sick and dying will always produce strain. Hence, on these grounds alone it is difficult to argue that a defective person may be denied the right to life.

Society. Care of the defective newborn also imposes societal costs, the utility of which is questioned when the infant's expected quality-of-life is so poor. Medical resources that can be used by infants with a better prognosis, or throughout the health-care system generally, are consumed in providing expensive surgical and intensive-care services to infants who may be severely retarded, never lead active lives, and die in a few months or years. Institutionalization imposes costs on taxpayers and reduces the resources available for those who might better benefit from it, while reducing further the quality of life experienced by the institutionalized defective.

One answer to these concerns is to question the impact of the costs of caring for defective newborns. Precise data showing the costs to taxpayers or the trade-offs with health and other expenditures do not exist. Nor would ceasing to care for the defective necessarily lead to a reallocation within the health budget that would produce net savings in suffering or life; in fact, the released resources might not be reallocated for health at all. In any case, the trade-offs within the health budget may well be small. With advances in prenatal diagnosis of genetic disorders, many deformed infants who would formerly require care will be aborted beforehand. Then, too, it is not clear that the most technical and expensive procedures always constitute the best treatment for certain malformations. When compared with the almost seven percent of the GNP now spent on health, the money in the defense budget, or tax revenues generally, the public resources required to keep defective newborns alive seem marginal, and arguably worth the commitment to life that such expenditures reinforce. Moreover, as the Supreme Court recently recognized, conservation of the taxpayer's purse does not justify serious infringement of fundamental rights. Given legal and ethical norms against sacrificing the lives of nonconsenting others, and the imprecisions in diagnosis and prediction concerning the eventual outcomes of medical care, the social-cost argument does not compel nontreatment of defective newborns.

Ethical Issues in Aiding the Death of Young Children

H. Tristram Engelhardt, Jr.

H. T. Engelhardt contends that children are not persons in the full sense. They must exist in and through their families. Thus, parents, in conference with a physician who provides information, are the appropriate ones to decide whether to treat an impaired newborn when (1) there is not only little likelihood of a full human life, but also the likelihood of suffering if the life is prolonged, or (2) the cost of prolonging the life is very great.

Engelhardt further argues that it is reasonable to speak of a *duty* not to treat an impaired infant when this will only prolong a painful life or would only lead to a painful death. He bases his claim on the legal notion of a "wrongful life." This notion suggests that there are cases in which nonexistence would be better than existence under the conditions in which a person must live. Life can thus be seen as an injury, rather than as a gift.

Euthanasia in the pediatric age group involves a constellation of issues that are materially different from those of adult euthanasia.[1] The difference lies in the somewhat obvious fact that infants and young children are not able to decide about their own futures and thus are not persons in the same sense that normal adults are. While adults usually decide their own fate, others decide on behalf of young children. Although one can argue that euthanasia is or should be a personal right, the sense of such an argument is obscure with respect to children. Young children do not have any personal rights, at least none that they can exercise on their own behalf with regard to the manner of their life and death. As a result, euthanasia of young children raises special questions concerning the standing of the rights of children, the status of parental rights, the obligations of adults to prevent the suffering of children, and the possible effects on society of allowing or expediting the death of seriously defective infants.

What I will refer to as the euthanasia of infants and young children might be termed by others infanticide, while some cases might be termed the withholding of extraordinary life-prolonging treatment.[2] One needs a term that will encompass both death that results from active intervention and death that ensues when one simply ceases further therapy.[3] In using such a term, one must recognize that death is often not directly but only obliquely intended. That is, one often intends only to treat no further, not actually to have death follow, even though one knows death will follow.[4]

Finally, one must realize that deaths as the result of withholding treatment constitute a significant proportion of neonatal deaths. For example, as high as 14 percent of children in one hospital have been identified as dying after a decision was made not to treat further, the presumption being that the children would have lived longer had treatment been offered.[5]

Even popular magazines have presented accounts of parental decisions not to pursue treatment.[6] These decisions often involve a choice between expensive treatment with little chance of achieving a full, normal life for the child and "letting nature take its course," with the child dying as a result of its defects. As this suggests, many of these problems are products of medical progress. Such

children in the past would have died. The quandaries are in a sense an embarrassment of riches; now that one *can* treat such defective children, *must* one treat them? And, if one need not treat such defective children, may one expedite their death?

I will here briefly examine some of these issues. First, I will review differences that contrast the euthanasia of adults to euthanasia of children. Second, I will review the issue of the rights of parents and the status of children. Third, I will suggest a new notion, the concept of the "injury of continued existence," and draw out some of its implications with respect to a duty to prevent suffering. Finally, I will outline some important questions that remain unanswered even if the foregoing issues can be settled. In all, I hope more to display the issues involved in a difficult question than to advance a particular set of answers to particular dilemmas.

For the purpose of this paper, I will presume that adult euthanasia can be justified by an appeal to freedom. In the face of imminent death, one is usually choosing between a more painful and more protracted dying and a less painful or less protracted dying, in circumstances where either choice makes little difference with regard to the discharge of social duties and responsibilities. In the case of suicide, we might argue that, in general, social duties (for example, the duty to support one's family) restrain one from taking one's own life. But in the face of imminent death and in the presence of the pain and deterioration of a fatal disease, such duties are usually impossible to discharge and are thus rendered moot. One can, for example, picture an extreme case of an adult with a widely disseminated carcinoma, including metastases to the brain, who because of severe pain and debilitation is no longer capable of discharging any social duties. In these and similar circumstances, euthanasia becomes the issue of the right to control one's own body, even to the point of seeking assistance in suicide. Euthanasia is, as such, the issue of assisted suicide, the universalization of a maxim that all persons should be free, *in extremis*, to decide with regard to the circumstances of their death.

Further, the choice of positive euthanasia could be defended as the more rational choice: the choice of a less painful death and the affirmation of the value of a rational life. In so choosing, one would be

This article first appeared in the book Beneficient Euthanasia, *edited by Marvin Kohl, published by Prometheus Books, Buffalo, N.Y., 1975, and is reprinted by permission.*

acting to set limits to one's life in order not to live when pain and physical and mental deterioration make further rational life impossible. The choice to end one's life can be understood as a noncontradictory willing of a smaller set of states of existence for oneself, a set that would not include a painful death. As such, it would not involve a desire to destroy oneself. That is, adult euthanasia can be construed as an affirmation of the rationality and autonomy of the self.[7]

The remarks above focus on the active or positive euthanasia of adults. But they hold as well concerning what is often called passive or negative euthanasia, the refusal of life-prolonging therapy. In such cases, the patient's refusal of life-prolonging therapy is seen to be a right that derives from personal freedom, or at least from a zone of privacy into which there are no good grounds for social intervention.[8]

Again, none of these considerations apply directly to the euthanasia of young children, because they cannot participate in such decisions. Whatever else pediatric, in particular neonatal, euthanasia involves, it surely involves issues different from those of adult euthanasia. Since infants and small children cannot commit suicide, their right to assisted suicide is difficult to pose. The difference between the euthanasia of young children and that of adults resides in the difference between children and adults. The difference, in fact, raises the troublesome question of whether young children are persons, or at least whether they are persons in the sense in which adults are. Answering that question will resolve in part at least the right of others to decide whether a young child should live or die and whether he should receive life-prolonging treatment.

The Status of Children

Adults belong to themselves in the sense that they are rational and free and therefore responsible for their actions. Adults are *sui juris*. Young children, though, are neither self-possessed nor responsible. While adults exist in and for themselves, as self-directive and self-conscious beings, young children, especially newborn infants, exist for their families and those who love them. They are not, nor can they in any sense be, responsible for themselves. If being a person is to be a responsible agent, a bearer of rights and duties, children are not persons in a strict sense. They are, rather, persons in a

social sense: others must act on their behalf and bear responsibility for them. They are, as it were, entities defined by their place in social roles (for example, mother-child, family-child) rather than beings that define themselves as persons, that is, in and through themselves. Young children live as persons in and through the care of those who are responsible for them, and those responsible for them exercise the children's rights on their behalf. In this sense children belong to families in ways that most adults do not. They exist in and through their family and society.

Treating young children with respect has, then, a sense different from treating adults with respect. One can respect neither a newborn infant's or very young child's wishes nor its freedom. In fact, a newborn infant or young child is more an entity that is valued highly because it will grow to be a person and because it plays a social role as if it were a person.[9] That is, a small child is treated as if it were a person in social roles such as mother-child and family-child relationships, though strictly speaking the child is in no way capable of claiming or being responsible for the rights imputed to it. All the rights and duties of the child are exercised and "held in trust" by others for a future time and for a person yet to develop.

Medical decisions to treat or not to treat a neonate or small child often turn on the probability and cost of achieving that future status—a developed personal life. The usual practice of letting anencephalic children (who congenitally lack all or most of the brain) die can be understood as a decision based on the absence of the possibility of achieving a personal life. The practice of refusing treatment to at least some children born with meningomyelocele can be justified through a similar, but more utilitarian, calculus. In the case of anencephalic children one might argue that care for them as persons is futile since they will never be persons. In the case of a child with meningomyelocele, one might argue that when the cost of cure would likely be very high and the probable lifestyle open to attainment very truncated, there is not a positive duty to make a large investment of money and suffering. One should note that the cost here must include not only financial costs but also the anxiety and suffering that prolonged and uncertain treatment of the child would cause the parents.

This further raises the issue of the scope of positive duties not only when there is no person present in a strict sense, but when the likelihood of a full human life is also very uncertain. Clinical and parental judgment may and should be guided by the expected lifestyle and the cost (in parental and societal pain and money) of its attainment. The decision about treatment, however, belongs properly to the parents because the child belongs to them in a sense that it does not belong to anyone else, even to itself. The care and raising of the child falls to the parents, and when considerable cost and little prospect of reasonable success are present, the parents may properly decide against life-prolonging treatment.

The physician's role is to present sufficient information in a usable form to the parents to aid them in making a decision. The accent is on the absence of a positive duty to treat in the presence of severe inconvenience (costs) to the parents; treatment that is very costly is not obligatory. What is suggested here is a general notion that there is never a duty to engage in extraordinary treatment and that "extraordinary" can be defined in terms of costs. This argument concerns children (1) whose future quality of life is likely to be seriously compromised and (2) whose present treatment would be very costly. The issue is that of the circumstances under which parents would not be obliged to take on severe burdens on behalf of their children or those circumstances under which society would not be so obliged. The argument should hold as well for those cases where the expected future life would surely be of normal quality, though its attainment would be extremely costly. The fact of little likelihood of success in attaining a normal life for the child makes decisions to do without treatment more plausible because the hope of success is even more remote and therefore the burden borne by parents or society becomes in that sense more extraordinary. But very high costs themselves could be a sufficient criterion, though in actual cases judgments in that regard would be very difficult when a normal life could be expected.[10]

The decisions in these matters correctly lie in the hands of the parents, because it is primarily in terms of the family that children exist and develop—until children become persons strictly, they are persons in virtue of their social roles. As long as parents do not unjustifiably neglect the humans in those roles so that the value and purpose of that role (that is, child) stands to be eroded (thus endangering other children), society need not intervene. In short,

parents may decide for or against the treatment of their severely deformed children.

However, society has a right to intervene and protect children for whom parents refuse care (including treatment) when such care does not constitute a severe burden and when it is likely that the child could be brought to a good quality of life. Obviously, "severe burden" and "good quality of life" will be difficult to define and their meanings will vary, just as it is always difficult to say when grains of sand dropped on a table constitute a heap. At most, though, society need only intervene when the grains clearly do not constitute a heap, that is, when it is clear that the burden is light and the chance of a good quality of life for the child is high. A small child's dependence on his parents is so essential that society need intervene only when the absence of intervention would lead to the role "child" being undermined. Society must value mother-child and family-child relationships and should intervene only in cases where (1) neglect is unreasonable and therefore would undermine respect and care for children, or (2) where societal intervention would prevent children from suffering unnecessary pain.[11]

The Injury of Continued Existence

But there is another viewpoint that must be considered: that of the child or even the person that the child might become. It might be argued that the child has a right not to have its life prolonged. The idea that forcing existence on a child could be wrong is a difficult notion, which, if true, would serve to amplify the foregoing argument. Such an argument would allow the construal of the issue in terms of the perspective of the child, that is, in terms of a duty not to treat in circumstances where treatment would only prolong suffering. In particular, it would at least give a framework for a decision to stop treatment in cases where, though the costs of treatment are not high, the child's existence would be characterized by severe pain and deprivation.

A basis for speaking of continuing existence as an injury to the child is suggested by the proposed legal concept of "wrongful life." A number of suits have been initiated in the United States and in other countries on the grounds that life or existence itself is, under certain circumstances, a tort or injury to the living person.[12] Although thus far all such suits have ultimately failed, some have succeeded in their initial stages. Two examples may be instructive. In each case the ability to receive recompense for the injury (the tort) presupposed the existence of the individual, whose existence was itself the injury. In one case a suit was initiated on behalf of a child against his father alleging that his father's siring him out of wedlock was an injury to the child.[13] In another case a suit on behalf of a child born of an inmate of a state mental hospital impregnated by rape in that institution was brought against the state of New York.[14] The suit was brought on the grounds that being born with such historical antecedents was itself an injury for which recovery was due. Both cases presupposed that nonexistence would have been preferable to the conditions under which the person born was forced to live.

The suits for tort for wrongful life raise the issue not only of when it would be preferable not to have been born but also of when it would be *wrong* to cause a person to be born. This implies that someone should have judged that it would have been preferable for the child never to have had existence, never to have been in the position to judge that the particular circumstances of life were intolerable.[15] Further, it implies that the person's existence under those circumstances should have been prevented and that, not having been prevented, life was not a gift but an injury. The concept of tort for wrongful life raises an issue concerning the responsibility for giving another person existence, namely the notion that giving life is not always necessarily a good and justifiable action. Instead, in certain circumstances, so it has been argued, one may have a duty *not* to give existence to another person. This concept involves the claim that certain qualities of life have a negative value, making life an injury, not a gift; it involves, in short, a concept of human accountability and responsibility for human life. It contrasts with the notion that life is a gift of God and thus similar to other "acts of God" (that is, events for which no man is accountable). The concept thus signals the fact that humans can now control reproduction and that where rational control is possible humans are accountable. That is, the expansion of human capabilities has resulted in an expansion of human responsibilities such that one must now decide when and under what circumstances persons will come into existence.

The concept of tort for wrongful life is transferable in part to the painfully compromised existence

of children who can only have their life prolonged for a short, painful, and marginal existence. The concept suggests that allowing life to be prolonged under such circumstances would itself be an injury of the person whose painful and severely compromised existence would be made to continue. In fact, it suggests that there is a duty not to prolong life if it can be determined to have a substantial negative value for the person involved.[16] Such issues are moot in the case of adults, who can and should decide for themselves. But small children cannot make such a choice. For them it is an issue of justifying prolonging life under circumstances of painful and compromised existence. Or, put differently, such cases indicate the need to develop social canons to allow a decent death for children for whom the only possibility is protracted, painful suffering.

I do not mean to imply that one should develop a new basis for civil damages. In the field of medicine, the need is to recognize an ethical category, a concept of wrongful continuance of existence, not a new legal right. The concept of injury for continuance of existence, the proposed analogue of the concept of tort for wrongful life, presupposes that life can be of a negative value such that the medical maxim *primum non nocere* ("first do no harm") would require not sustaining life.[17]

The idea of responsibility for acts that sustain or prolong life is cardinal to the notion that one should not under certain circumstances further prolong the life of a child. Unlike adults, children cannot decide with regard to euthanasia (positive or negative), and if more than a utilitarian justification is sought, it must be sought in a duty not to inflict life on another person in circumstances where that life would be painful and futile. This position must rest on the facts that (1) medicine now can cause the prolongation of the life of seriously deformed children who in the past would have died young and that (2) it is not clear that life so prolonged is a good for the child. Further, the choice is made not on the basis of costs to the parents or to society but on the basis of the child's suffering and compromised existence.

The difficulty lies in determining what makes life not worth living for a child. Answers could never be clear. It seems reasonable, however, that the life of children with diseases that involve pain and no hope of survival should not be prolonged. In the case of Tay-Sachs disease (a disease marked by a progressive increase in spasticity and dementia usually leading to death at age three or four), one can hardly imagine that the terminal stages of spastic reaction to stimuli and great difficulty in swallowing are at all pleasant to the child (even insofar as it can only minimally perceive its circumstances). If such a child develops aspiration pneumonia and is treated, it can reasonably be said that to prolong its life is to inflict suffering. Other diseases give fairly clear portraits of lives not worth living: for example, Lesch-Nyhan disease, which is marked by mental retardation and compulsive self-mutilation.

The issue is more difficult in the case of children with diseases for whom the prospects for normal intelligence and a fair lifestyle do exist, but where these chances are remote and their realization expensive. Children born with meningomyelocele present this dilemma. Imagine, for example, a child that falls within Lorber's fifth category (an IQ of sixty or less, sometimes blind, subject to fits, and always incontinent). Such a child has little prospect of anything approaching a normal life, and there is a good chance of its dying even with treatment.[18] But such judgments are statistical. And if one does not treat such children, some will still survive and, as John Freeman indicates, be worse off if not treated.[19] In such cases one is in a dilemma. If one always treats, one must justify extending the life of those who will ultimately die anyway and in the process subjecting them to the morbidity of multiple surgical procedures. How remote does the prospect of a good life have to be in order not to be worth great pain and expense?[20] It is probably best to decide, in the absence of a positive duty to treat, on the basis of the cost and suffering to parents and society. But, as Freeman argues, the prospect of prolonged or even increased suffering raises the issue of active euthanasia.[21]

If the child is not a person strictly, and if death is inevitable and expediting it would diminish the child's pain prior to death, then it would seem to follow that, all else being equal, a decision for active euthanasia would be permissible, even obligatory.[22] The difficulty lies with "all else being equal," for it is doubtful that active euthanasia could be established as a practice without eroding and endangering children generally, since, as John Lorber has pointed out, children cannot speak in their own behalf.[23] Thus although there is no argument in principle against the active euthanasia of small children, there could be an argument against such practices based on questions of prudence. To put it

another way, even though one might have a duty to hasten the death of a particular child, one's duty to protect children in general could override that first duty. The issue of active euthanasia turns in the end on whether it would have social consequences that refraining would not, on whether (1) it is possible to establish procedural safeguards for limited active euthanasia and (2) whether such practices would have a significant adverse effect on the treatment of small children in general. But since these are procedural issues dependent on sociological facts, they are not open to an answer within the confines of this article. In any event, the concept of the injury of continued existence provides a basis for the justification of the passive euthanasia of small children—a practice already widespread and somewhat established in our society—beyond the mere absence of a positive duty to treat.[24]

Conclusion

Though the lack of certainty concerning questions such as the prognosis of particular patients and the social consequence of active euthanasia of children prevents a clear answer to all the issues raised by the euthanasia of infants, it would seem that this much can be maintained: (1) Since children are not persons strictly but exist in and through their families, parents are the appropriate ones to decide whether or not to treat a deformed child when (a) there is not only little likelihood of full human life but also great likelihood of suffering if the life is prolonged, or (b) when the cost of prolonging life is very great. Such decisions must be made in consort with a physician who can accurately give estimates of cost and prognosis and who will be able to help the parents with the consequences of their decision. (2) It is reasonable to speak of a duty not to treat a small child when such treatment will only prolong a painful life or would in any event lead to a painful death. Though this does not by any means answer all the questions, it does point out an important fact—that medicine's duty is not always to prolong life doggedly but sometimes is quite the contrary.

Notes

1. I am grateful to Laurence B. McCullough and James P. Morris for their critical discussion of this paper. They may be responsible for its virtues, but not for its shortcomings.

2. The concept of extraordinary treatment as it has been developed in Catholic moral theology is useful: treatment is extraordinary and therefore not obligatory if it involves great costs, pain, or inconvenience, and is a grave burden to oneself or others without a reasonable expectation that such treatment would be successful. See Gerald Kelly, S. J., *Medico-Moral Problems* (St. Louis: The Catholic Hospital Association Press, 1958), pp. 128–141. Difficulties are hidden in terms such as "great costs" and "reasonable expectation," as well as in terms such as "successful." Such ambiguity reflects the fact that precise operational definitions are not available. That is, the precise meaning of "great," "reasonable," and "successful" are inextricably bound to particular circumstances, especially particular societies.

3. I will use the term euthanasia in a broad sense to indicate a deliberately chosen course of action or inaction that is known at the time of decision to be such as will expedite death. This use of euthanasia will encompass not only positive or active euthanasia (acting in order to expedite death) and negative or passive euthanasia (refraining from action in order to expedite death), but acting and refraining in the absence of a direct intention that death occur more quickly (that is, those cases that fall under the concept of double effect). See note 4.

4. But both active and passive euthanasia can be appreciated in terms of the Catholic moral notion of double effect. When the doctrine of double effect is invoked, one is strictly not intending euthanasia, but rather one intends something else. That concept allows actions or omissions that lead to death (1) because it is licit not to prolong life *in extemis* (allowing death is not an intrinsic evil), (2) if death is not actually willed or actively sought (that is, the evil is not directly willed), (3) if that which is willed is a major good (for example, avoiding useless major expenditure of resources or serious pain), and (4) if the good is not achieved by means of the evil (for example, one does not will to save resources or diminish pain *by* the death). With regard to euthanasia the doctrine of double effect means that one need not expend major resources in an endeavor that will not bring health but only prolong dying and that one may use drugs that decrease pain but hasten death. See Richard McCormick, *Ambiguity in Moral Choice* (Milwaukee: Marquette University Press, 1973). I exclude the issue of double effect from my discussion because I am interested in those cases in which the good may follow directly from the evil—the death of the child. In part, though, the second section of this paper is concerned with the concept of proportionate good.

5. Raymond S. Duff and A. G. M. Campbell, "Moral and Ethical Dilemmas in the Special-Care Nursery," *The New England Journal of Medicine*, 289 (Oct. 25, 1973), pp. 890–894.

6. Roger Pell, "The Agonizing Decision of Joanne and Roger Pell," *Good Housekeeping* (January 1972), pp. 76–77, 131–135.

7. This somewhat Kantian argument is obviously made in opposition to Kant's position that suicide involves a default of one's duty to oneself ". . . to preserve his life simply because he is a person and must therefore recognize a duty to himself (and a strict one at that)," as well as a contradictory volition: "that man ought to have the authorization to withdraw himself from all obligation, that is, to be free to act as if no authorization at all were required for this withdrawal, involves a contradiction. To destroy the subject of morality in his own person is tantamount to obliterating from the world . . ." Immanuel Kant, *The Metaphysical Principles of Virtue: Part II of the Metaphysics of Morals*, trans. James Ellington (Indianapolis: Bobbs-Merrill, 1964), p. 83; Akademie Edition, VI, 422–423.

8. Norman L. Cantor, "A Patient's Decision to Decline Life-Saving Medical Treatment: Bodily Integrity Versus the Preservation of Life," *Rutgers Law Review*, 26 (Winter 1972), p, 239.

9. By "young child" I mean either an infant or child so young as not yet to be able to participate, in any sense, in a decision. A precise operational definition of "young child" would clearly be difficult to develop. It is also not clear how one would bring older children into such decisions. See, for example, Milton Viederman, "Saying 'No' to Hemodialysis: Exploring Adaptation," and Daniel Burke, "Saying 'No' to Hemodialysis: An Acceptable Decision," both in *The Hastings Center Report*, 4 (September 1974), pp. 8–10, and John E. Schowalter, Julian B. Ferholt, and Nancy M. Mann, "The Adolescent Patient's Decision To Die," *Pediatrics*, 51 (January 1973), pp. 97–103.

10. An appeal to high costs alone is probably hidden in judgments based on statistics: even though there is a chance for a normal life for certain children with apparently severe cases of meningomyelocele, one is not obliged to treat since that chance is small, and the pursuit of that chance is very expensive. Cases of the costs being low but the expected suffering of the child being high will be discussed under the concept of the injury of continued existence. It should be noted that none of the arguments in this paper bear on cases where neither the cost nor the suffering of the child is considerable. Cases in this last category probably

include, for example, children born with mongolism complicated only by duodenal atresia.

11. I have in mind here the issue of physicians, hospital administrators, or others being morally compelled to seek an injunction to force treatment of the child in the absence of parental consent. In these circumstances, the physician, who is usually best acquainted with the facts of the case, is the natural advocate of the child.

12. G. Tedeschi, "On Tort Liability for 'Wrongful Life,' " Israel Law Review, 1 (1966), p. 513.

13. Zepeda v. Zepeda: 41 Ill. App. 2d 240, 190 N.E. 2d 849 (1963).

14. Williams v. State of New York: 46 Misc. 2d 824, 260 N.Y.S. 2d 953 (Ct. Cl., 1965).

15. Torts: "Illegitimate Child Denied Recovery Against Father for 'Wrongful Life,' "Iowa Law Review, 49 (1969), p. 1009.

16. It is one thing to have a conceptual definition of the injury of continued existence (for example, causing a person to continue to live under circumstances of severe pain and deprivation when there are no alternatives but death) and another to have an operational definition of that concept (that is, deciding what counts as such severe pain and deprivation). This article has focused on the first, not the second, issue.

17. H. Tristram Engelhardt, Jr., "Euthanasia and Children: The Injury of Continued Existence," The Journal of Pediatrics, 83 (July 1973), pp. 170–171.

18. John Lorber, "Results of Treatment of Myelomeningocele," Developmental Medicine and Child Neurology, 13 (1971), p. 286.

19. John M. Freeman, "The Shortsighted Treatment of Myelomeningocele: A Long-Term Case Report," Pediatrics, 53 (March 1974), pp. 311–313.

20. John M. Freeman, "To Treat or Not To Treat," Practical Management of Meningomyelocele, ed. John Freeman (Baltimore: University Park Press, 1974), p. 21.

21. John Lorber, "Selective Treatment of Myelomeningocele: To Treat or Not To Treat," Pediatrics, 53 (March 1974), pp. 307–308.

22. I am presupposing that no intrinsic moral distinctions exist in cases such as these, between acting and refraining, between omitting care in the hope that death will ensue (that is, rather than the child living to be even more defective) and acting to ensure that death will ensue rather than having the child live under painful and seriously compromised circumstances. For a good discussion of the distinction between acting and refraining, see Jonathan Bennett, "Whatever the Consequences," Analysis, 26 (January 1966), pp. 83–102; P. J. Fitzgerald, "Acting and Refraining," Analysis, 27 (March 1967), pp. 133–139; Daniel Dinello, "On Killing and Letting Die," Analysis, 31 (April 1971), pp. 83–86.

23. Lorber, "Selective Treatment of Myelomeningocele," p. 308.

24. Positive duties involve a greater constraint than negative duties. Hence it is often easier to establish a duty not to do something (not to treat further) than a duty to do something (to actively hasten death). Even allowing a new practice to be permitted (for example, active euthanasia) requires a greater attention to consequences than does establishing the absence of a positive duty. For example, at common law there is no basis for action against a person who watches another drown without giving aid; this reflects the difficulty of establishing a positive duty.

Toward an Ethic of Ambiguity

John D. Arras

John Arras raises the question of whether there are differences between normal and gravely impaired infants that justify withholding life-sustaining treatment from the impaired. The "best-interest" of the child standard seems to point to morally relevant distinctions. It is clearly in the best-interest of the normal child to live, but is this always the case with the impaired child? The standard has the advantage of focusing on the child's interest, rather than (as with utilitarianism) on the interest of the parents or society. However, Arras points to a number of serious problems in interpreting and applying the standard in individual cases.

Furthermore, Arras claims, in the final analysis the best-interest standard makes the absence of pain the only real moral consideration.

Arras argues that this is an unacceptable result and that other features, such as the ability to communicate and to give and receive love, are also morally relevant. Without acknowledging their relevance, we cannot even attribute any human interests to the child. Thus, according to Arras, we need a supplementary standard that is "geared to the presence or absence of distinctly human capacities." Such a "relational potential standard" rests on the ethical principle that biological human life is only a relative good. This means that in applying the standard we must face up to the difficult task of assessing the factors that make human life valuable to its possessors. In effect, we must attempt to determine a "threshold of meaningful human life."

The Best Interests of the Child

How are we to show equal concern and respect for gravely impaired newborns? Are there any differences between otherwise normal children and certain gravely impaired babies that might justify allowing the latter to die through the intentional withholding of medical treatments?

One important and plausible candidate for a morally relevant distinction between normal and certain anomalous newborns resides in the notion of their respective "best interests."[1] Continued life is obviously in the interests of the normal child, but what of the child impaired by profound brain damage, whose days will be measured by operations and whose pain will be unrelieved by the communication of human sympathy? Would it not be in this child's best interests to die, rather than endure a life of meaningless suffering? And if so, would that not provide us with a morally relevant distinction?

The case for allowing the deaths of anomalous newborns on the ground of their "best interests" is by far the most compelling argument for infant euthanasia. By focusing on *the child's* interests, this standard avoids morally dubious utilitarian justifications based on the well-being of other interested parties, such as parents, siblings, or even of society at large. And by giving *full weight* to the child's interests, this approach can justify nontreatment in certain cases without having to make the (usually pernicious) assumption that the child is a nonperson with no standing in the human community.

Despite these advantages, however, the best-interest standard presents staggering problems of interpretation and application.

A Preliminary Objection

Before coming to these problems, we must confront a direct challenge to the legitimacy of the best-interest standard itself. Certain theologians and jurists who oppose any resort to "quality-of-life" judgments on behalf of voiceless patients have argued that the best-interest standard forces us to make an impossible comparison. Although we can and should compare better life against worse life, they argue, we cannot compare the advantages of life, even with severe disabilities, against the state of nonbeing initiated by death. Since all our everyday evaluations take place against the backdrop of the assumed value of life, it is said, we cannot make the comparison of life against nonlife demanded by the best-interest standard without foundering on conceptual incoherence.[2]

While this is not the occasion to launch a lengthy metaphysical explanation of how a state of nonexistence might be "preferable" to certain states of existence—how can someone be better off dead?—two points can be made in response to those who claim that death can never be in the best interests of a nondying child. First, we can concede that a belief in the desirability of life grounds our everyday judgments of "better" and "worse," while still maintaining that the moral choices posed by the

Reproduced by permission. © The Hastings Center. Hastings Center Report, 14 (April 1984): 25–33.
Editor's Note: This is a shortened version of the original article, and the footnotes have been renumbered.

plight of the impaired newborn are anything but ordinary. Although we usually profess an implicit faith in the conceptual connection between our notions of "life" and "good," the profoundly anomalous and severely brain-damaged child shatters this everyday faith and severs the assumed connection.

In such cases, it is not at all obvious that mere life remains a good to the afflicted person; rather, it seems as though the child's illness has eclipsed the possibility of enjoying those normal human goods that ordinarily predispose us to say that life is good.[3] Moreover, while the existence of severe disabilities threatens to sever our everyday connection between "life" and "good," another item of everyday faith remains unshaken: We continue to believe that pain and suffering are evil, and that beneficence largely consists in abolishing, or at least ameliorating, these twin scourges of humankind. If an act of mercy killing were to deliver a child from a life of unmitigated pain—if only to a state of nonexistence rather than beatitude—it would take a profoundly dogmatic temperament to deny that death was in the child's best interest. Opponents of infant euthanasia could perhaps find other reasons to oppose such an act—for example, the belief that humans have no right to dispose of their own or anyone else's life—but merely on the grounds of individual well-being, there is no denying that death would be better than a life of intense and constant pain.

Second, if it were impossible for us to detach ourselves from our everyday grounding in the belief that life is good, if we could not wish someone else dead for his or her own sake, then the same difficulty would attach to first-person judgments as well. If it were in principle impossible to say that death would serve the best interests of any child, then it would be equally impossible for any rational adult to conclude that, given a bleak prognosis and the prospect of burdensome treatments, he or she would be better off dead. I doubt that the more thoughtful opponents of euthanasia would wish to embrace such a result. Even conservative theologians such as Paul Ramsey restrict their rejection of quality-of-life reasoning—and hence their rejection of "excessive burdensomeness" as a test of extraordinary means—to the class of voiceless patients who have not developed a value system that would allow them to assess the quality of future life for themselves.[4]

Ramsey explicitly grants to the competent adult the right to refuse treatments that would render continued life a burden. In order to assume this stance, he must admit the possibility that death would be in the best interest of certain persons, but this admission pulls the rug out from under the claim that, in principle, we cannot judge death to be in a child's best interest. The most that can be said is that no one has the right to make such judgments, or that allowing adults to make them for children will result in mistaken choices or downright abuse. We cannot say that, in principle, life (even with crushing impairments and constant pain) cannot even be compared with death. At best, such a denial is an unfortunate overstatement; at worst, it could be placed in the service of an overbearing medical paternalism. Indeed, what better way to thwart the choices of mature adults than to deny them the very capacity rationally to choose between an earlier death without treatment and a life of suffering with treatment?

In sum, we can say that death is not always and everywhere the greatest evil that could befall a person. Afflictions of the body and mind might conspire to render continued life a burden for certain individuals, for whom death might be viewed as a benefit—or at least as the lesser of two evils. As the President's Commission recently concluded, the best interests of the child—rather than a spurious nondiscrimination principle—should be our guide. Normally, of course, treatment will clearly be in a child's best interest. But the Commission granted the possibility that some permanent handicaps might be "so severe that continued existence would not be a net benefit to the infant."[5] Our next problem, then, is to determine with more precision how a best-interest standard might be applied and to discuss some weighty problems of interpretation.

Prognostic Uncertainty

One problem will plague efforts to implement any proposed criterion of nontreatment: medical and prognostic uncertainty.[6] Decisions must often be made regarding life or death in the absence of reliable data regarding a particular child's future life prospects. No matter where we draw the line separating "meaningful" from "excessively burdensome" life, we will often have to decide under conditions of great uncertainty. The spectrum of neonatal disabilities is very wide, as is the spectrum of disability *within* particular disease categories. The mere presence of Down's syndrome or of spina bifida does not by itself indicate how disabled a child will be. Some Down's children are profoundly retarded, while others turn out to be sufficiently intelligent to live at home with their families or in group homes and eventually to work productively in a sheltered setting. The problem is that, except for a few classes of disease, physicians cannot accurately predict the degree of a child's eventual impairment. This problem is compounded by our ability to diminish a child's eventual degree of disability by some means of vigorous medical and educational interventions. In the absence of reliable prognostic indicators of future quality of life, the rationality of nontreatment decisions for defective neonates is bound to be diminished. Any medical ethic that places a great value on human life must look with suspicion upon nontreatment decisions taken in the absence of reliable medical information.

While medical uncertainty threatens to undermine the application of *any* set of criteria for nontreatment based on quality of life, the best-interest standard is subject to further difficulties of interpretation. It may well turn out that, all things considered, death may serve the best interests of a severely afflicted infant; but before we can reach this conclusion, two important questions must be resolved. First, we must know what burdens to the child are admissible in our moral calculations of benefit and burden. Do any and all burdens to the child count, or only certain kinds? Second, we must have a clearer idea of the point of view from which these burdens will be assessed. Shall it be the viewpoint of the gravely impaired child or of the normal adult?

Which Burdens Shall Count?

So far, we have listed physical ailments that might befall a child and render excessively burdensome a prolongation of his or her life. Now we must consider whether burdens attributable to the child's socioeconomic status can be counted alongside strictly medical burdens as contributing to an excessively burdensome life and, if so, whether such burdens morally *ought* to be so counted.

In addition to suffering from the retardation associated with Down's syndrome, the repeated surgeries associated with spina bifida, or the iatrogenic toll of respirator therapy for premature infants, a child may suffer from a host of nonmedical problems. She may, if allowed to live, suffer from parental rejection. Plagued by frustration, guilt, and disappointment, parents can and do neglect their impaired children—or, worse yet, abuse them. Or

the parents may love and wish to care for their child, yet be too ill-equipped to care for her at home and too poor to place her in an acceptable institution. Such parents face the dilemma of keeping their child at home, where the demands of caring for her disabilities are likely to drain their economic and emotional resources, or handing her over to an institution that is likely to be underfinanced and understaffed. At such an institution, the severely impaired child is likely to be relegated to some back ward where she will suffer from lack of love, human contact, and even basic care.[7]

"Clearly," it might be argued, "subjecting the anomalous child to this sort of institutionalized deprivation amounts to a harm of considerable proportion. In the absence of better alternatives to institutionalization, such as it is today in many economically deprived areas, these children should be relieved of potentially crushing burdens by means of an early, merciful death."

This is a plausible argument. Unquestionably the abuse and neglect attributable to a family's inability to cope or to pay for humane care can amount to substantial burdens for the child. And so long as burdensomeness to the child remains the crucial criterion involved in the best-interest standard, why shouldn't social as well as purely medical burdens count in our overall calculations? Indeed, if socially induced burdens can make continued life excessively burdensome for a severely retarded child relegated to some back ward, logic would seem to compel us to weigh them as heavily as any other kind of burden. The important thing, it might be said, is not the source of the burden, but its effect on the child. If parental neglect, social ostracism, and degrading conditions can make life unbearable, why shouldn't they be a part of our moral deliberations?

In spite of its initial plausibility, this line of reasoning runs afoul of the nondiscrimination principle. If it would be in a wealthy child's best interest to receive life-sustaining therapies, justice demands that a poor child with a similar medical condition and prognosis also receive the same treatment. Like cases should be treated alike. (The same can be said on behalf of children born to parents rich and poor alike who are unable or unwilling to nurture them. The parents' inadequacies are not the fault of their children.)

True, in our previous discussion of medically induced burdens we suggested that certain disabilities could be so severe as to render an anomalous child significantly different from a normal child for purposes of moral analysis. We said then that such disabilities could prompt us to deny the premise that the severely impaired child was still "like" the normal child in all relevant respects, and thus to deny the conclusion that such children must receive "like" treatment. We argued, finally, that the severely impaired child was unlike the normal child precisely in the sense that her best interests would not be served by further treatment or continued existence. Why not repeat the same argument here with regard, this time, to socially related burdens?

The answer to this eminently sensible question is that, whereas an extremely poor medical prognosis and quality of life can make for a significant moral difference between two babies, the same cannot be said of differences in wealth. Degree of wealth is never a morally significant difference between two potential recipients of basic health care. If a certain medical procedure is deemed to be truly beneficial and offered to a wealthy child with severe disabilities, it must also be offered to the similarly situated poor child. The latter is not responsible for the lack of concern of her parents, or for their inability to afford dignified and humane follow-up care. To say that the wealthy child should live (because her anomalies are not so severe as to make life too burdensome) but that the poor child with similar prognosis should die (because of further burdens imposed by her poverty) is to indulge in the rankest kind of discrimination. For purposes of moral analysis, these two patients are identical, and they should therefore receive similar treatment. That is the demand of simple justice—unless we hold that being rich in itself makes the wealthy impaired child more deserving of health care than the poor child, an unlikely concession for us to make.

A policy that allowed us to consider socially induced burdens would not only be profoundly unjust; it would also most likely impede efforts to improve the plight of the institutionalized, poor, imperiled child. Historically, one of the most potent arguments in favor of social reform has rested on the existence of human suffering and deprivation. Could we expect vigorous efforts to reform public institutions housing severely impaired children once the suffering and neglect that characterize such institutions have become publicly recognized as good reasons for killing these newborns? My sympathies lie entirely with Paul Ramsey's response to the suggestion that a child's poverty ought to count in her constellation of publicly recognized burdens. "That's one way," says Ramsey, "to remove every evening the human debris that has accumulated since morning." For the great majority of these handicapped infants, radical social reform—not "beneficent" euthanasia—is the answer.

The procedural implication of this argument about justice is that we should attempt to distinguish clearly between "treatment decisions" and decisions regarding the child's ultimate placement.[8] In other words, worries about the child's future life with a potentially abusive parent or in a hopelessly inadequate state institution should not be allowed to influence treatment decisions. Even though socially induced burdens can join forces with strictly physical disabilities to make a life excessively burdensome to its bearer, we must base our treatment decisions solely on the extent of medical disabilities. To take social factors into account is to act unjustly toward the child.

At this point in the argument, we have clearly entered a "moral blind alley"—that is, a situation so structured that whatever course we take, we end up doing something morally unacceptable.[9] Ordinarily this structure takes the form of a conflict between two disparate moral concerns—namely, doing good and doing justice. Morality, through the principle of beneficence, requires us to increase people's happiness and mitigate their unhappiness. But another moral principle enjoins us to respect persons' rights and to do justice. When these conflicting demands meet head-on in a concrete situation, the stage is set for an ethical dilemma. How can they be reconciled?

As Ronald Dworkin has contended, a concern for rights and justice can function as a "trump card" in moral and political argument with regard to competing utilitarian considerations.[10] When there is a conflict between the demands of utility and the requirements of justice, we usually say that the former must simply yield to the latter. Pointing to the good or bad consequences said to flow from the performance or omission of an act is usually said to be an insufficient (or even irrelevant) justification if that act or omission happens to be unjust. For example, we say that a citizen's right to speak freely must be respected, even though rather serious consequences (such as public disturbances) may ensue from the exercise of that right. In this sort of case, the right course is clear—we should let the individual speak—and there is no serious moral dilemma. One moral concern has simply eclipsed another.

Sometimes circumstances may be so extreme and the consequences so dreadful that the priority of justice can no longer be maintained. When this happens, an agent enters a moral blind alley. He must choose, but all of his alternatives are morally unacceptable. If he does the "right" thing, the act required by strict justice, then catastrophic results will follow: if he violates the demands of justice, he avoids terrible consequences at the cost of doing a deed that should never be done. In such cases, one may prudently decide to violate rights and justice in order to avoid catastrophe, but this does not always count as a complete justification. "Moral traces" of the demands of justice remain, even when circumstances make it plain that justice must be violated. Simply put, it does not become *all right:* we are left with dirty hands.[11]

Winston Churchill faced such a moral dilemma in World War II—should he launch rocket attacks on German civilian populations, thereby killing hundreds of innocent persons, or risk losing the war? I suspect that we face a similar dilemma in the case of the impoverished impaired newborn. If we take the child's socially caused burdens into account—such as the likelihood of being neglected in a state institution—we may rightly decide that death would be better than such a fate. Allowing such a child to die would be a merciful act, averting an unbearable life for the child; but it would also be unjust. As we have seen, it is profoundly unjust to afford differential treatment to impaired newborns on the basis of socioeconomic factors. However, if we avert our eyes from the child's subsequent fate in a barren state institution, we act justly but possibly consign the child to a miserable life in a warehouse for discarded humans—a catastrophic result, to be sure.

It would appear, then, that we are confronted by a genuine moral dilemma occasioned by social conditions of poverty and inequity. Here, as elsewhere in the field of biomedical ethics, straightforward appeals to notions of right and justice —abstracted from a social context of profound injustice—can lead to morally disastrous results.[12] So long as these unjust social conditions persist, so long as the rich gravely impaired child enjoys a bearable quality of life denied to a poor counterpart, the door of the neonatal nursery will continue to open onto a moral blind alley. Rather than serve as an invitation to resignation, however, this conclusion underscores the necessity of increased social (governmental) support of the handicapped. Surely, any society that insists upon a controversial strict standard of justice concerning nontreatment decisions—a standard that will weigh heaviest upon those parents most in need of psychological and financial support—surely, such a society thereby incurs a corresponding duty to support those who must bear the burden it imposes.

What Standard Will Measure the Burden?

There are essentially two possibilities: we can adopt either the point of view of the rational adult or that of the anomalous child. According to some philosophers, we ought to adopt the viewpoint of the mature adult or the so-called "reasonable person."[13] "Since incompetent creatures are incompetent," writes Joseph Margolis, "we judge as rational adults of normal sensibilities would. It is in this sense that the decision to bring to an end the lives of selected fetuses and infants . . . is *conceptually parasitic* on the decision of the competent to end their own lives. . . ."

Although this approach is flawed, it has a certain appealing modesty. It does not require us to plumb the depths of the incompetent person's psyche to discern there what the incompetent patient "really wants." Such modesty is becoming when the patient for whom we are to decide has not left us any evidence of how he or she would decide: it is especially becoming when the patient lacks the very capacity to develop a value system in the first place. Although courts have recently ascribed to themselves or to guardians the right to make so-called "substituted judgments" for voiceless patients, and although the proxy decision makers have been legally charged with the (impossible?) task of deciding as the patient would decide, were he or she miraculously to become competent for an instant, I suspect that they end up attempting to judge as any rational adult of normal sensibilities would. And for good reason.

In the absence of explicit or implicit value judgments from the incompetent patient, what else do we have to go on? How do we know whether or not the permanently incompetent patient would judge life under present circumstances to be worth the candle? Far from being endowed with the Herculean powers of discernment required by such a task, we can only ask what the "vast majority" of adults would want, should such a fate befall them. This sort of judgment might still be very difficult to render, but at least we would be familiar with the grounds of our decision. Presumably, we all have some rough idea of when life would no longer be meaningful or worth living *for us*.

Despite its commonsensical appeal, two different objections have been lodged against invoking a "reasonable person" standard in the case of impaired newborns. The first merely points to the probability of abuse: a reasonable-person standard, based on what the vast majority of people would want, leaves the child unprotected against the whims and vagaries of normal adults. This prospect leads some critics to reject out of hand any consideration of quality of life in the treatment of newborns.

This objection is itself somewhat ambiguous. It could be taken to mean that a reasonable-person standard is theoretically acceptable, but would tend to be too easily abused in practice. This objection may or may not be sound. Empirical studies would have to be adduced showing that the likelihood of abuse is so great that any and all quality-of-life judgments based on adult sensibilities should be banished. In the absence of such evidence, an abrupt dismissal of a best-interest standard would appear to be unsupported.

Another objection goes to the heart of the matter. According to this version, put forth by John Robertson and others, the problem lies in the reasonable-person standard itself, not in our penchant for misusing it. Any standard of judgment based on the sensibilities of normal adults, it is claimed, will necessarily be prejudicial to the best interests of impaired children. In contrast to the point about the inevitability of abuse, this objection assumes the appropriateness of a best-interest standard but insists that any criterion based on the values of normal adults is bound systematically to distort our judgments of what is truly in a child's best interests. This version of the objection thus poses a direct challenge to Margolis's assumption that decisions on behalf of incompetent children must be conceptually parasitic on the standards appealed to by normal adults in deciding to end their own lives.

Come to think of it, why should the sentiments of normal adults be used as the touchstone of meaningful life for imperiled newborns? Although most normal adults are no doubt wellmeaning and genu-inely concerned not to abuse their standard of judgment, they are undoubtedly biased in favor of normalcy. Being normal themselves, competent adults have naturally pitched their value systems on the solid ground of normalcy. But it is precisely through the mediation of these values that adults are supposed to evaluate the disabilities of the child and assess their implications for the value of continued life. It is only natural to expect that, were the question put to them, many normal adults, having grown accustomed to the social and intellectual satisfactions that normalcy makes possible, would rather die than live without these basic human capacities. But as John Robertson pointed out in a classic article:

> Yet a standard based on healthy, ordinary development may be entirely inappropriate to this situation. One who has never known the pleasures of mental operation, ambulation, and social interaction surely does not suffer from their loss as much as one who has. While one who has known these capacities may prefer death to a life without them, we have no assurance that the handicapped person, with no point of comparison, would agree. Life, and life alone, whatever its limitations, might be of sufficient worth to him.[14]

Echoing Robertson's point, the President's Commission recently warned against adopting the viewpoint of normal adults in assessing the best interests of anomalous children. While conceding that responsible parties must try to ground their judgments on considerations that would move a competent decision maker to forego treatment—thereby barring the consideration of idiosyncratic value judgments—the President's Commission strongly recommended that benefits and burdens be weighed from the incompetent infant's own perspective. We must ask not whether a normal adult would rather die than suffer from severe mental and physical impairments, but rather whether this child, who has never known the satisfactions and aspirations of the normal world, would prefer nothing to what he or she has.

If the best interests of the child is to be our standard of judgment, the viewpoint of the child is clearly the most appropriate measure of benefits and burdens. The standard of the reasonable adult, based as it is on the capacities and expectations of normalcy, would introduce a systematic bias into our considerations. Everywhere, it would have us see dashed hopes and frustration, rather than op-portunities for growth and strategies of meaningful accommodation. Adopting the child's viewpoint would be difficult in practice, but it would conform more closely to the spirit of the best-interest stan-dard. The issue, after all, is the welfare of this child, not the hopes and fears of adults that might be projected onto the child.

As the Commission rightly points out, this in-terpretation of the best-interest standard yields a very strict policy. For one thing, it stresses the child's well-being, to the exclusion of any and all considerations of the child's negative impact on others. Nontreatment of a nondying impaired child could not be justified on the ground that ongoing care would drain the family (or the state) of its financial resources or deprive siblings of the love and attention that they deserve.[15] In addition, this gloss of the best-interest standard would clearly have mandated life-saving treatments in most of the cases that have generated public controversy in re-cent years. While normal adults might prefer, for themselves, death to mental retardation, it cannot plausibly be argued that the average Down's syn-drome child would see death as being in his or her best interest. To the contrary, persons with Down's syndrome derive great satisfaction from their lives. From their point of view, life is good and worth living, no matter how limited others might think their lives to be. The main difference separating them from us lies not in our capacity for enjoying life and for sharing love, but rather, it has been plausibly suggested, in their "congenital inability to hate."[16]

The Limits of the Best-Interest Standard

This standard, interpreted from the impaired child's viewpoint, is indeed strict—and rightly so. When human lives are at stake, we do not want to substitute, no matter how unconsciously, the fears of normal adults for the genuine best interests of impaired children. It has not been generally appre-ciated, however—not even by the President's Com-mission—just how strict this child-relative standard can become when pushed to the extreme limits of human disability.

The first hint of a problem with the application of this standard can be found in Robertson's initial article championing the viewpoint of the impaired child. Immediately following his convincing ref-utation of the claim that death would be a better fate than life for most "mongoloid" and nonambulatory spina bifida children, Robertson reached the same conclusion in the "worse case"—that is, "the profoundly retarded, nonambulatory, blind, deaf infant who will spend his few years in the back-ward cribs of a state institution . . . "[17] Even in such an extreme case, where the Commission would no doubt be most likely to concede that "continued existence would not be a net benefit to the infant," Robertson refuses to sanction nontreatment and death. How do we know, he asks, that such a child with wants, needs, and interests so different from our own would prefer the abyss to his back-ward existence? How can we be sure that, for such a child, life and life alone would not be of sufficient worth?

Assuming that the infant is not in pain and has no conscious experience of suffering, Robertson's doubts appear to be well founded. Of course, if this child were also suffering inordinately from the side effects of invasive therapies or from the underlying condition itself—in addition to other multiple hand-icaps—that would be a different story. As we have already seen, unremitting and unrelievable pain can transform a person's continued existence from an unquestioned benefit into a harsh burden. But sup-pose the child suffers no pain. He lies there in his crib, blind, deaf, and uncomprehending. Never having experienced the satisfactions of normalcy, the infant is neither horrified by his plight, nor depressed by his neglect in the state institution or by the thought of his impending doom. He just lies there. Can we say with moral certitude that it is in the child's best interest to die?

I think not. We can say that, for such a severely impaired child, life cannot have much significance or value. Indeed, it is difficult to understand in what sense such a child can have any interests to which a best-interest standard might apply. Nevertheless, strictly from this infant's point of view, it is far from clear that death would be preferable to such a life. As Robertson implies, the mere act of subsisting on the back ward—vegetating, if you will—might well be deemed "worth the candle" by this child if, mi-raculously, he could survey his situation with the clarity of a competent person. "It's certainly not much," he might ruefully admit to himself, "but it's better than nothing. They feed me, change me, occasionally cuddle me. And I'm not in any pain to speak of. So why not just play out the meager hand that I've been dealt?''

This eerie soliloquy, spoken by a child who will never speak, will play to mixed reviews. For some, it will furnish convincing evidence that the best-interest standard, interpreted from the child's point of view, mandates treatment even in the worst cases (provided that the child is not in pain). Others, while (correctly) agreeing with this conclusion, will see in it evidence, not that such children should be kept alive, but rather that, in such extreme cases, the best-interest standard has been pushed beyond the pale of its capabilities. They will contend, rightly I think, that when pushed this far the best-interest standard generates results that conflict with moral common sense.

Consider, for example, the plight of the child born with Trisomy 13, a chromosomal disorder associated with severe mental retardation and severe physical impairments. The child's brain is so malformed that she will never possess the capacity to think or to communicate with others. And, as if these deficits were not sufficient, she is doomed to an early death. If treated aggressively and vigilantly, however, she might well live for months, or perhaps even for a year. Although she is probably not properly classified as a ''dying patient'' according to Surgeon General Koop's taxonomy,[18] this child will soon die never having had an intelligible thought, never having given or acknowledged love, never having experienced anything beyond simply ''being there.''

The fact that the child-based best-interest standard would mandate treatment even in the face of a prognosis bereft of any distinctly human potentiality reveals a feature of that standard that has so far gone unnoticed. In such extreme cases, the best-interest standard tends to view the absence of pain as the only morally relevant consideration. No matter that the infant is doomed to a life of very short duration, and lacks the capacity for any distinctively human development or activity; so long as the child does not experience any severe burdens, interpreted from her point of view, the fact that she can anticipate no distinctly human benefits is of no moral consequence.

But this seems wrong. The presence or absence of such characteristics as the ability to think, to communicate, to give and receive love, seems to be highly relevant from a moral point of view. Indeed, in the absence of these capacities, how can we attribute any human interests to the child on which a best-interest standard might operate? By narrowing the range of meaningful data to the presence or absence of unrelievable pain, the best-interest standard consigns itself in extreme cases to operating in a moral vacuum. The result is an indiscriminate mandate to treat, to keep alive, that flies in the face of common sense. When confronted with such cases, one wants to ask, not whether treatment will further the infant's best interests, but rather whether the child's impoverished level of existence is worth sustaining.

Beyond the Best-Interest Standard

Far from advancing the conclusion that even the worst case ought to receive life-sustaining treatments, our hypothetical soliloquy reveals the limits of the best-interest standard; in so doing, it underscores our need for a supplementary standard geared to the presence or absence of distinctly human capacities.[19] The ethical principle that justifies this standard is the proposition that biological human life is only a relative good. In the absence of certain distinctly human capacities—for self-consciousness and relating to other people—the usual connection between biological life and our notion of the good is effectively severed. Just as the presence of unrelievable pain can preclude the attainment of those basic human goods that make life worth living, so the absence of fundamental human capacities can render a life valueless, both to its possessor and to others. (This is not to deny that families can derive great satisfactions from caring for such severely impaired children and may well desire to keep them alive. But this particular reason for sustaining their lives has nothing to do with the child's best interests.) Without these qualities, no distinctly human good can be achieved. When this point is reached, the duty to sustain life loses its hold on caregivers.

Since such grievously afflicted children have no distinctly human capacities, and thus no human interests, the activity of keeping them alive is pointless from the moral point of view. Indeed, in these worst cases, it is a mistake to inquire about the best interests of such children or to insist that decisions to terminate treatment be made solely in terms of the child's good. As the previous discussion of the best-interest standard revealed, the only interest that can intelligibly be attributed to children lacking self-consciousness or relational potential is an interest in avoiding pain and suffering. Since, for them, continued existence does not offer the prospect of achieving any human good, we cannot sensibly attribute to such children an interest in sustaining their lives. Consequently, those who bear the responsibility for them are under no ethical obligation to prolong their lives by means of medical treatments.

In contrast to the misapplied best-interest standard, which sought to fasten onto the subjective preferences of the severely impaired child, this "relational potential standard" must issue from a social, intersubjective inquiry into the conditions of a valuable human life. Although any attempt to define the parameters of "meaningful human life" will doubtless meet with suspicion—or even with extreme hostility—this sort of inquiry makes a great deal more sense than the convoluted speculations required by a best-interest standard pushed beyond its limits. The search for a threshold of meaningful human life might well be difficult and fraught with the danger of abuse—how many pogroms and genocidal campaigns have been justified by their victims' alleged lack of "basic humanity"?—but the search for the secret preferences of patients lacking the capacity for self-knowledge and human relations is, I would argue, an essentially misguided venture.

The futility of this search is illustrated by the paradoxical subjective tests the courts have applied in extreme cases. In the famous *Saikewicz* case, for example, the judge bids us to reach a decision that "would be made by the incompetent person, if that person were competent, but taking into account the present and future incompetency of the individual as one of the factors which would necessarily enter into the decision-making process of the competent person."[20] Although the language of the President's Commission avoids the transparent absurdity of the *Saikewicz* formula, its recommendation amounts to the same thing: we are to base our judgments on grounds that "would lead a competent decision-maker . . . to forego treatment" while, at the same time, "adopting the viewpoint of the *incompetent* patient" (emphasis added). Given the impossibility of this charge in the case of children lacking any relational potential or capacity for choosing a system of values, we are faced with two alternatives. We can either attempt to sustain the lives of such pa-

tients in spite of their empty prognoses, or we can engage in the risky business of designating a threshold of meaningful human life. The latter alternative might well be dangerous, but the former is pointless and burdensome to parents and society.

The Beginning of Wisdom

Two distinctions between normal infants and certain severely anomalous children are morally relevant. Just as a child might be excessively burdened by his treatments or underlying disease, so a child may lack certain basic human capacities. Such pain and lack of capacities mark significant moral differences between these anomalous children and their normal counterparts. Just as we ought to extend similar treatment to similar cases, we should also be prepared to extend dissimilar treatment to dissimilar cases. Since the nondiscrimination principle forbids differential treatment only in the absence of morally relevant distinctions between people, and since excessive burdens or the lack of relational potential constitute relevant distinctions, the nondiscrimination principle does not forbid nontreatment in the sorts of cases we have been discussing.

We are confronted here with an enormously difficult and complex moral issue. Contrary to the opinion of those who would simplify this problem beyond all recognition—either by mandating treatment for all children, or by allowing parents or health professionals unbridled discretion—I have tried, following Kierkegaard's example, ". . . to create [or at least acknowledge] difficulties everywhere. . . ."[21]

Ethical ambiguity pervades the issue. Most seriously impaired children should be treated, some should be allowed to die. Substantive principles are available, but their application is fraught with difficulty and danger. Although this pervasive ambiguity is difficult to live with, we can be sure that attempts to ignore it, to reduce the problem to a simple formula, will lead to an illusory and counterproductive quest for moral certainty.

Notes

1. President's Commission, *Deciding to Forego Life-Sustaining Treatments,* pp. 134–36, 217–23.
2. Versions of this argument appear in Paul Ramsey, *Ethics at the Edges of Life* (New Haven: Yale University Press, 1978), pp. 206–07, 240 n. 11; and in Paul Camenisch, "Abortion for the Sake of the Fetus." *Hastings Center Report* 6 (April 1976), 38–41.

See also *Gleitman* v. *Cosgrove*, 49 N.J. 22, 227 A.2d 689 (1967): "It is basic to the human condition to seek life and hold on to it however heavily burdened."

3. Philippa Foot, "Euthanasia." *Philosophy and Public Affairs* 6 (1977), 94–96.

4. Ramsey, *Ethics at the Edges of Life*, pp. 154–59, 225.

5. President's Commission, *Deciding to Forego Life-Sustaining Treatment*, p. 218. On closer inspection, this particular gloss of the best-interest standard turns out to be dangerously overinclusive. Continued existence is not a "net benefit" for many people who would nevertheless opt for life over death. Here we should be talking about handicaps so severe that continued existence would be marked by constant pain and suffering. This lapse in the Commission report was called to my attention by Alan Fleischman.

6. See, e.g., Norman Fost, "How Decisions Are Made: A Physician's View," in C. A. Swinyard, ed., *Decision Making and the Defective Newborn* (Springfield, Ill.: Charles C Thomas, 1978), pp. 220–30.

7. For a vivid description of how bad the conditions can get in such institutions, see *New York State Association of Retarded Children* v. *Rockefeller* 357 Fed. Supp. 752 (Eisterii Division, N.Y. 1973).

8. Ramsey, *Ethics at the Edges of Life*, pp. 202–03.

9. Thomas Nagel, "War and Massacre," in Marshall Cohen, et al., eds., *War and Moral Responsibility* (Princeton, N.J.: Princeton University Press, 1974), p. 23.

10. Dworkin, *Taking Rights Seriously*, pp. xi, 171–72.

11. Nagel, "War and Massacre," 16–17. See also Robert Nozick. "Moral Complications and Moral Structures," *Natural Law Forum* 13 (1968), 1–50.

12. This theme is developed at length in my essay, "The Right to Die on the Slippery Slope," *Social Theory and Practice* 8 (Fall 1982), 285–328. See also Nancy Rhoden, "The Limits of Liberty: Deinstitutionalization, Homelessness, and Libertarian Theory," *Emory Law Journal* 32 (Spring 1982), 375–440.

13. See Robert Veatch, *Death, Dying, and the Biological Revolution* (New Haven: Yale University Press, 1976), pp. 124–36; and Joseph Margolis, "Human Life: Its Worth and Bringing It to an End," in Marvin Kohl, ed., *Infanticide and the Value of Life* (Buffalo, N.Y.: Prometheus, 1978), pp. 180–91.

14. John Robertson, "Involuntary Euthanasia of Defective Newborns," *Stanford Law Review* 27 (1975), 254.

15. For an opposing view, see Carson Strong, "Defective Infants and Their Impact on Families: Ethical and Legal Considerations," *Law, Medicine and Health Care* (September 1983), pp. 168–81.

16. Louis Lasagna, "Murder Most Foul," *The Sciences* 22 (August–September 1982). Dr. Lasagna is the father of a twenty-year-old with Down's syndrome.

17. Robertson, "Involuntary Euthanasia of Defective Newborns," p. 254.

18. According to Dr. Koop, "For such [dying] infants, neither medicine nor law can be of any help. And neither medicine nor law should prolong these infants' process of dying." Statement before Hearing on Handicapped Newborns, Subcommittee on Select Education Committee on Education and Labor, U.S. House of Representatives (September 16, 1982). Quoted in President's Commission, *Deciding to Forego Life-Sustaining Treatment*, pp. 219–20, n. 81.

19. Such a standard is worked out by Richard McCormick, S. J., in "To Save or Let Die: The Dilemma of Modern Medicine," *Journal of the American Medical Association* 229, No. 2 (July 8, 1974), 172–76.

20. *Superintendent of Belchertown State School* v. *Saikewicz*, 370 NE 2d 417 (1977).

21. Robert Bretall, ed., *A Kierkegaard Anthology* (New York: Modern Library, 1936), p. 194.

Decision Scenario 1 . . . .

I had been working as a bioethics advisor at University Hospital for three months before I was called in to consult on a pediatrics case. Dr. Savano, the attending obstetrician, asked me to meet with him and Dr. Hinds, one of the staff surgeons, to talk with the father of a newborn girl.

I went to the consulting room with Dr. Savano, and he introduced me and Dr. Hinds to Joel Blake. From what Dr. Savano had already told me, I knew that Mr. Blake was in his early twenties and worked as a clerk at a discount store called the Bargain Barn. The baby's mother was Hilda Godgeburn, and she and Mr. Blake were not married.

Mr. Blake was very nervous. He knew that the baby had been born just three hours or so before and that Ms. Godgeburn was in very good condition. But Dr. Savano had not told him anything about the baby.

"I'm sorry to have to tell you this," Dr. Savano said. "But the baby was born with severe defects."

"My God," Blake said. "What's the matter?"

"It's a condition called spina bifida," Dr. Savano said. "There's a hole in the baby's back just below the shoulder blades, and some of the nerves from the spine are protruding through it. The baby will have little or no control over her legs, and she won't be able to control her bladder or bowels." Dr. Savano paused to see if Mr. Blake was understanding him. "The legs and feet are also deformed to some extent because of the defective spinal nerves."

Mr. Blake was shaking his head, paying close attention but hardly able to accept what he was being told.

"There's one more thing," Dr. Savano said. "The spinal defect is making the head fill up with liquid from the spinal canal. That's putting pressure on the brain. We can be sure that the brain is already damaged, but if the pressure continues the child will die."

"Is there anything that can be done?" Blake asked. "Anything at all?"

Dr. Savano nodded to Dr. Hinds. "We can do a lot," Dr. Hinds said. "We can drain the fluid from the head, repair the opening in the spine, and later we can operate on the feet and legs."

"Then why aren't you doing it?" Mr. Blake asked. "Do I have to agree to it? If I do, then I agree. Please go ahead."

"It's not that simple," Dr. Hinds said. "You see, we can perform surgery, but that won't turn your baby into a normal child. She will always be paralyzed and mentally retarded. To what extent, we can't say now. Her bodily wastes will have to be drained to the outside by means of artificial devices that we'll have to connect surgically. There will have to be several operations, probably, to get the drain from her head to work properly. A number of operations on her feet will be necessary."

"Oh, God," Mr. Blake said. "Hilda and I can't take it. We don't have enough money for the oper-ations. And even if we did, we would have to spend the rest of our lives taking care of the child."

"The child could be put into a state institution," Dr. Hinds said.

"That's even worse," Mr. Blake said. "Just handing our problem to somebody else. And what kind of life would she have? A pitiful, miserable life."

None of the rest of us said anything. "You said she would die without the operation to drain her head," Mr. Blake said. "How long would that take?"

"A few hours, perhaps," Dr. Savano said. "But we can't be sure. It may take several days, and conceivably she might not die at all."

"Oh, God," Mr. Blake said again. "I don't want her to suffer. Can she just be put to sleep pain-lessly?"

Dr. Savano didn't answer the question. He seemed not even to hear it. "We'll have to talk to Ms. Godgeburn also," he said. "And before you make up your mind for good, I want you to talk with the bioethics advisor. You two discuss the matter, and the advisor will perhaps bring out some things you haven't thought about. Dr. Hinds will leave you both together now. Let me know when you've reached your final decision and we'll talk again."

1. *Assume that you are the bioethics advisor in this case. Would you attempt to persuade Mr. Blake that attempts should be made to save the child's life?*

2. *Do you think he is right in asking that the child be painlessly killed? If such killing is not legally permissible, is this relevant to deciding whether the child should be saved if possible? What considerations for and against such an attempt might you mention to help Mr. Blake to reach a decision?*

3. *Are there any arguments in what you have read that seem to you entirely persuasive in such a case?*

4. *What factual considerations (if any) do you consider relevant to resolving the moral issues here?*

Decision Scenario 2 • • • • • • • • • • • • • • • •

Brookhaven, as we will call it, is a long-term health-care institution in the Washington metropolitan area. Most of Brookhaven's patients are in residence there for only a few months; either they succumb to their ailments and die, or they recover sufficiently to return to their homes.

But for some patients death has no immediate likelihood, nor is recovery a possibility. They linger on at Brookhaven, day after day and year after year. Juli Meyers is such a patient, although that is not really her name.

Juli is seventeen and has been in Brookhaven for six years. But before Brookhaven there were other institutions. In fact, Juli has spent most of her life in hospitals and special-care facilities. But Juli does not seem to be aware of any of this.

At Brookhaven she spends her days lying in a bed surrounded with barred metal panels. The bars have been padded with foam rubber. Although most of the time Juli is curled tightly in a fetal position, she sometimes flails around wildly and makes guttural sounds. The padding keeps her from injuring herself.

Juli's body is thin and underdeveloped, with sticklike arms and legs. She is blind and deaf and has no control over her bowels and bladder. She is totally dependent on others to clean her and care for her. She can swallow the food put into her mouth, but she cannot feed herself. She makes no response to the people or events around her.

There is no hope that Juli will walk or talk, laugh or cry, or even show the slightest sign of intelligence or awareness. She is the victim of one of the forms of Schilder's disease. The nerve fibers that make up her central nervous system have mostly degenerated. The cause of the degeneration is not fully known, nor is it known how to halt the process. The condition is irreversible, and Juli will never be better than she is.

At birth Juli seemed perfectly normal and healthy, but at three months she began to lose her sight and hearing. She made the gurgling noises typical of babies less and less frequently. By the end of her first year, she made no sounds at all and was completely blind and deaf. Also, she was losing control of her muscles, and her head lolled on her shoulders, like a doll with a broken neck.

She became highly subject to infections, and more than once she had pneumonia. Once when she was on the critical list, a specialist suggested to her mother that it would be pointless to continue treating her. Even if she recovered from the pneumonia, she would remain hopelessly impaired. Mrs. Meyers angrily rejected the suggestion and insisted that everything possible be done to save Juli's life.

Although not wealthy, the family bore the high cost of hospitalization and treatments. Mrs. Meyers devoted herself almost totally to caring for Juli at home, and the other four children in the family received little of her attention. Eventually, Mrs. Meyers began to suffer from severe depression, and when Juli was eight and a half her parents decided she would have to be placed in an institution. Since then, Juli has changed little. No one expects her to change. Her mother visits her three times a month and brings Juli freshly laundered and ironed clothes.

1. Would Robertson's arguments support Mrs. Meyers's decision not to allow Juli to die? How might a utilitarian criticize the decision?

2. Would treatment for pneumonia in Juli's case be considered "normal medical measures" on the Roman Catholic view?

3. Are there any grounds for supposing that Juli is being made to suffer what Engelhardt calls "the injury of continued existence"?

4. Would your decision have been the same as Mrs. Meyers's?

5. Is it possible to justify using society's limited medical resources to keep Juli alive?

6. Evaluate the following argument: Opponents of abortion oppose spending public funds for abortion on the grounds that they (the opponents) are being forced to support murder, which is a serious moral evil. Keeping Juli alive is a serious moral evil. Therefore, no public funds should be used for this purpose.

Decision Scenario 3 . . . .

Susan Roth was looking forward to being a mother. She had quit her secretarial job three months before her baby was due so she could spend the time getting everything ready. Her husband, David, was equally enthusiastic, and they spent many hours happily speculating about the way things would be when their baby came. It was their first child.

"I hope they don't mix her up with some other baby," Mrs. Roth said to her husband after delivery.

She didn't know yet that there was little chance of confusion. The Roth infant was seriously deformed. Her arms and legs had failed to develop, her skull was misshapen, and her face deformed. Her large intestine emptied through her vagina, and she had no muscular control over her bladder.

When she was told, Mrs. Roth said "We cannot let it live, for her sake and ours." On the day she left the hospital with the child, Mrs. Roth mixed a lethal dose of a tranquilizing drug with the baby's formula and fed it to her. The child died that evening.

Mrs. Roth and her husband were charged with infanticide. During the court proceedings, Mrs. Roth admitted to the killing but said she was satisfied she had done the right thing. "I know I could not let my baby live like that," she said. "If only she had been mentally abnormal, she would not have known her fate. But she had a normal brain. She would have known. Placing her in an institution

might have helped me, but it wouldn't have helped her."

The jury, after deliberating for two hours, found Mrs. Roth and her husband guilty of the charge.

1. *Are laws against infanticide unjust?*

2. *Does the fact that the intelligence of the child is normal support the mother's claim that killing was justifiable? Might normal intelligence make the "injury of continued existence" even greater than subnormal intelligence?*

3. *Why might Robertson consider the mother's action morally wrong?*

4. *Would the "best-interest" of the infant standard, as presented by Arras, offer any support for the mother's action?*

Decision Scenario 4 ·

I can't believe God has done this to me, Mike Chovo said to himself. Tears came to his eyes, and his nose started running.

His wife, Carol, handed him a tissue from the box by her bed. "It's all right, Mikey," she said. "We'll make it all right."

Mike wiped his eyes and blew his nose. The yellow tissue struck him as being absurdly cheerful. Given the circumstances, it seemed totally out of place in the hospital room.

"I know," he said. "But it's going to be so hard, so very hard. And it's going to be terrible for Chris and Jan."

"They'll adjust," Carol said. "In some ways it will be good for them to have a brother like Terry. They'll learn somebody doesn't have to be perfect for you to love them."

"Oh, Jesus," Mike said. "Maybe we should have told them not to do anything. He's in such bad shape. The doctors told me they're not sure he has enough of a brain even to learn who we are. I mean, it may be like he's unconscious all of his life."

Mike pulled another tissue out of the box and held it over his eyes. He pressed hard with his fingertips. He wanted Terry to die, but he couldn't tell Carol that. He could barely allow himself to think it. He wished he hadn't given permission for

the operation to drain the fluid from Terry's head. But he couldn't oppose Carol at a time like this.

"But we'll love him anyway," Carol said. "We'll take care of him until God calls him away."

"I wonder if we're doing him a favor. I wonder if he's really fit for this world."

"We couldn't just stand by and let him die," Carol said.

"No, I guess we couldn't." Mike hesitated, then went on. "You know, this one operation won't be the end of them. Dr. Flanners told me that it's not unusual to have to operate ten or twelve times in cases like this."

"It's going to be expensive."

"That's right, and I don't know where we're going to get the money."

"We can probably borrow some from my parents. And if we have to, I guess we can get a second mortgage on the house."

"I guess so," Mike admitted.

Carol looked at Mike and smiled at him. After a moment, he smiled back.

1. *Would the line of reasoning taken by Robertson tend to support the decision made by Carol Chovo?*

2. *Might the considerations mentioned by Engelhardt be used to argue that it would have been better for the Chovos to allow their son to die?*

3. *Does the natural law view require treatment in such a case?*

4. *On what grounds might Kantian principles be appealed to in order to justify a decision not to treat Terry Chovo?*

5. *In what ways, if any, are such considerations as the financial status of the Chovos and the likely influence on the other two children of having a wholly dependent and impaired brother relevant to the decision that faced the parents?*

6. *Would the "best-interest" standard discussed by Arras provide grounds for justifing a decision to withhold medical treatment?*

Decision Scenario 5 •

Irene Towers had been a nurse for almost twelve years; for the last three of those years she had worked in the Neonatal Unit of Halifax County Hospital. It was a job she loved. Even when the infants were ill or required special medical or surgical treatment, she found the job of caring for them immensely rewarding. She knew that without her efforts many of the babies would simply die.

Irene Towers was on duty the night that Siamese twins were born to Corrine Couchers and brought at once to the Neonatal Unit. Even Irene, with all her experience, was distressed to see them. The twin boys were joined at their midsections in a way that made it impossible to separate them surgically. Because of the position of the single liver and the kidneys, not even one twin could be saved at the expense of the life of the other. Moreover, both children were severely deformed, with incompletely developed arms and legs and misshapen heads. As best as the neurologist could determine, both suffered severe brain damage.

The father of the children was Dr. Harold Couchers. Dr. Couchers, a slightly built man in his early thirties, was a specialist in internal medicine with a private practice.

Irene felt sorry for him the night the children were born. When he went into the room with the obstetrician to examine his sons, he had already been told what to expect. He showed no signs of grief as he stood over the slat-sided crib, but the corners of his mouth were drawn tight, and his face was almost unnaturally empty of expression. Most strange for a physician, Irene thought, he merely looked at the children and did not touch them. She was sure that in some obscure way he must be blaming himself for what had happened to them.

Later that evening, Irene saw Dr. Couchers sitting in the small conference room at the end of the hall with Dr. Cara Rosen, Corrine Couchers's obstetrician. They were talking earnestly and quietly when Irene passed the open door. Then, while she was looking over the assignment sheet at the nursing station, the two of them walked up. Dr. Rosen took a chart from the rack behind the desk and made a notation. After returning the chart, she shook hands with Dr. Couchers, and he left.

It was not until the end of her shift that Irene read the chart; Dr. Rosen's note said that the twin boys were to be given neither food nor water. At first Irene couldn't believe the order. But when she asked her supervisor, she was told that the supervisor had telephoned Dr. Rosen and that the obstetrician had confirmed the order.

Irene said nothing to the supervisor or to anyone else, but she made her own decision. She believed it was wrong to let the children die, particularly in such a horrible way. They deserved every chance to fight for their lives, and she was going to help them the way she had helped hundreds of other babies in the unit.

For the next week and a half, Irene saw to it that the children were given water and fed the standard infant formula. She did it all herself, on her own initiative. Although some of the other nurses on the floor saw what she was doing, none of them said anything to her. One even smiled and nodded to her when she saw Irene feeding the children.

Apparently someone else also disapproved of the order to let the twins die. Thirteen days after their birth, an investigator from the state Family Welfare Agency appeared in the neonatal ward. The rumor was that his visit had been prompted by an anonymous telephone call.

Late in the afternoon of the day of that visit, the deformed twins were made temporary wards of the Agency, and the orders on the chart were changed—the twins were now to be given food and water. On the next day, the county prosecutor's office announced publicly that it would conduct an investigation of the situation and decide whether criminal charges should be brought against Dr. Couchers or members of the hospital staff.

Irene was sure that she had done the right thing. Nevertheless, she was glad to be relieved of the responsibility.

1. *Might a utilitarian argument be offered in defense of Dr. Couchers's decision to allow the twins to die?*

2. *What criticism of such an argument might Robertson offer?*

3. *Is there a morally relevant distinction between not treating (and allowing to die) and not providing such minimal needs as food and water (and allowing to die)?*

4. *Does Engelhardt's line of reasoning support the action taken by Irene Towers?*

5. *Did Irene Towers exceed the limits of her responsibility, or did she act in a morally heroic way?*

6. *Proposed federal regulations require that impaired infants be given food and water, even if medical treatment can justifiably be withheld. Are there any moral grounds for making the distinction between treatment and nutritional support?*

Decision Scenario 6 •

Dr. Daniel McKay and his wife, Carol, had only a few moments of joy at the birth of their son. They learned almost immediately that the child was severely impaired. Half an hour later, the infant was dead—Dr. McKay, a veterinarian, had slammed him onto the floor of the delivery room.

Mrs. McKay had had problems during pregnancy. An ultrasound test indicated excessive fluid in the uterus, a sign that something might be wrong. Dr. Joaquin Ramos assured the McKays that everything was all right and that the pregnancy should continue. On June 27, 1983, he ordered Mrs. McKay admitted to the Markham, Illinois, hospital so that labor could be induced.

"Don't do any heroic measures," Dr. McKay told Dr. Ramos when Dr. McKay learned that the infant was impaired. Dr. Ramos explained that that was not his choice, for hospital policy required that everything possible be done for babies, even ones like the McKay baby that might not live more than a few months. The child had webbed fingers, heart and lung malfunctions, and missing testicles. It was suspected that the child also had a genetic disorder that might mean kidney malfunctions, mental retardation, and death within months.

Dr. McKay smashed the infant's head against the floor several times, splattering the wall and floor with brain tissue and blood. "Dan, what have you done?" a nurse shouted. Dr. McKay later said that while holding the child he asked himself "Can I accept and love this child, or would it be better off dead?" He had just talked to his wife. "I said to Dan,

'Is it a boy or a girl?' He said it was a little boy. I said, 'Oh, Dan, we got our boy!' Dan really wasn't saying anything. He had tears in his eyes." She then realized that the baby was not crying and asked her husband to go see what was wrong.

Dr. McKay was charged with murder. Two defense psychiatrists testified that he had been temporarily insane. Two others said that he had succumbed to stress. A prosecution psychiatrist said that he was legally sane but that "he made a decision that he had a moral imperative to do what he did." The jury could not agree whether Dr. McKay was guilty, not guilty, guilty but not mentally ill, or not guilty by reason of insanity. A mistrial was declared, but another trial was scheduled.

1. *How might the hospital policy of "doing everything possible" for all impaired infants be criticized in terms of the two standards presented by Arras?*

2. *Would any of the authors here endorse such a policy? If so, on what grounds?*

3. *Would Arras's relational potential standard justify withholding medical care from the McKay infant?*

4. *Might one argue that Dr. McKay's action was morally right, whether or not it was legally justifiable?*

5. *Under what conditions, if any, ought the parents of an impaired infant be allowed to decide how the child is to be treated?*

CHAPTER 3

EUTHANASIA

SOCIAL CONTEXT: THE CRUZAN CASE: THE SUPREME COURT UPHOLDS A RIGHT TO DIE

In the early morning of January 11, 1983, twenty-five-year-old Nancy Cruzan was driving on a deserted county road in Missouri. The road was icy and the car skidded, then flipped over and crashed. Nancy Cruzan was thrown from the driver's seat and landed face down in a ditch by the side of the road.

An ambulance arrived quickly, but not quickly enough to save her from suffering irreversible brain damage. Nancy Cruzan never regained consciousness, and her physicians eventually concluded that she had entered into what is known medically as a persistent vegetative state, awake but unaware. The higher brain functions responsible for recognition, memory, comprehension, anticipation, and other cognitive functions had all been lost.

Her arms and legs were drawn into a fetal position, her knees against her chest, and her body stiff and contracted. Only loud sounds and painful stimuli evoked responses, but even those were no more than neurological reflexes.

"We've literally cried over Nancy's body, and we've never seen anything," her father, Joe Cruzan, said. "She has no awareness of herself."

Nancy Cruzan was incapable of eating, but her body was sustained by a feeding tube surgically implanted in her stomach. She was a patient at the Missouri Rehabilitation Center, but no one expected her to be rehabilitated. She could only be kept alive.

"If only the ambulance had arrived five minutes earlier—or five minutes later," her father lamented.

The cost of Nancy Cruzan's care was $130,000 a year. The bill was paid by the state. Because she was a legal adult when her accident occurred, her family was not responsible for her medical care. Had she been under twenty-one, the Cruzans would have been responsible for her medical bills, as long as they had any financial resources to pay them.

In 1991 Nancy Cruzan was thirty-two years old. Her physicians estimated that she might live another thirty years. She was like some 10,000 other Americans at any given time. They are lost in a dark, dimensionless limbo that lies between living and dying. Those who love them can think of them only with sadness and despair. Given a choice between lingering in this twilight world and dying, most people find it difficult to imagine that some might choose not to die.

Hope eventually faded for Nancy Cruzan's parents. They faced the fact that she would never recover her awareness, and the time came when they wanted their daughter to die, rather than be kept alive in her hopeless condition. They asked that the feeding tube used to keep Nancy alive be withdrawn. Officials at the Missouri Rehabilitation Center refused, and Joe and Louise Cruzan were forced to go to court.

During the court hearings, the family testified that Nancy would not have wanted to be kept alive in her present condition. Her sister Christy said Nancy had told her that she never wanted to be kept alive "just as a vegetable." A friend also testified that Nancy had said that if she were injured or sick she wouldn't want to continue her life, unless she could live "halfway normally." Family and friends spoke in general terms of Nancy's vigor and her sense of independence.

In July 1988, Charles E. Teel of the Jasper County Circuit Court ruled that artificially prolonging the life of Nancy Cruzan violated her constitutional right. As he wrote, "There is a fundamental right expressed in our Constitution as 'the right to liberty,' which permits an individual to refuse or direct the withholding or withdrawal of artificial death-prolonging procedures when the person has no cognitive brain function."

Missouri Attorney General William Webster said that Judge Teel's interpretation of the Missouri living-will law was much broader than the legislature intended. Acting on behalf of the state, Webster appealed the ruling to the state supreme court.

In November 1988, the Missouri Supreme Court in a 4-to-3 decision overruled the decision of the lower court—Nancy Cruzan's parents would not be allowed to disconnect the feeding tube.

The court focused on the state's living-will statute. The law permits the withdrawing of artificial life-support systems in cases in which individuals are hopelessly ill or injured and there is "clear and convincing evidence" that this is what they would want done. The act specifically forbids the withholding of food and water. Judge Teel's reasoning in the lower court decision was that the surgically implanted tube was an invasive medical treatment that the Missouri law permitted her parents, as guardians, to order withdrawn.

The Missouri Supreme Court held that the evidence as to what Nancy Cruzan would have wanted did not meet the "clear and convincing" standard required by the law. In addition, the evidence did not show that the implanted feeding tube was "heroically invasive" or "burdensome." In the circumstance, then, the state's interest in preserving life should override other considerations.

In the words of the decision, the court found "no principled legal basis" to permit the Cruzans "to choose the death of their ward." In the absence of such a basis, "and in the face of the state's strongly stated policy in favor of life, we choose to err on the side of life, respecting the right of incompetent persons who may wish to live despite a severely diminished quality of life."

The Cruzans' attorney, William Colby, appealed the ruling to the United States Supreme Court. For the first time the Court agreed to hear a case involving "right to die" issues. On June 25, 1990, the Court issued what is considered a landmark ruling. In a 5-to-4 decision, the Court rejected Colby's argument that the Court should reject as unconstitutional the State of Missouri's stringent standard requiring "clear and convincing evidence" as to a comatose patient's wishes. This meant that Nancy Cruzan's parents had lost their case.

Despite the cruel disappointment of the Cruzans, the Court acknowledged for the first time a strong constitutional basis for living wills and for the designation of another person to act as a surrogate in making medical decisions on behalf of another. Unlike the decisions in *Roe* v. *Wade* and *Quinlan*, which found a right of privacy in the Constitution, the Court decision in *Cruzan* appealed to a Fourteenth Amendment "liberty interest." The interest involves being free to reject unwanted medical treatment. The Court found grounds for this interest in the common-law tradition, according to which, if one person even touches another without consent or legal justification, then battery is committed.

The Court regarded this as the basis for requiring that a patient give informed consent to medical treatment. The "logical corollary" of informed consent, the Court held, is that the patient also possesses the right to withhold consent. A difficulty arises, though, when a patient is in no condition to give consent. The problem becomes one of knowing what the patient's wishes would be.

Rehnquist, in the majority opinion, held that the Constitution permits states to decide on the standard that must be met in determining the wishes of a comatose patient. Hence, Missouri's rigorous standard that requires "clear and convincing proof" of the wishes of the patient was allowed to stand. The Court held that it was legitimate for the state to err on the side of caution, "because an erroneous decision not to terminate treatment results in the maintenance of the status quo," while an erroneous decision to end treatment "is not susceptible of correction."

Justice William Brennan dissented strongly from this line of reasoning. He pointed out that making a mistake about a comatose patient's wishes and continuing treatment also has a serious consequence. Maintaining the status quo "robs a patient of the very qualities protected by the right to avoid unwanted medical treatment."

Justice Stevens, in another dissenting opinion, argued that the Court's focus on how much weight to give previous statements by the patient missed the point. The Court should have focused on the issue of the best interest of the patient. Otherwise, the only people who are eligible to exercise their constitutional right to be free of unwanted medical treatment are those "who had the foresight to make an unambiguous statement of their wishes while competent."

One of the more significant aspects of the decision was that the Court made no distinction between providing nutrition and hydration and other forms of medical treatment. One argument on behalf of the state was that providing food and water was not medical treatment. However, briefs filed by medical associations made it clear that determining the formula required by a person in Nancy Cruzan's condition and regulating her feeding are medically complex procedures. The situation is more comparable to determining the contents of an intravenous drip than to giving someone food and water.

The Missouri living-will statute explicitly forbids the withdrawal of food and water.

However, the law was not directly at issue in the Cruzan case, because Nancy Cruzan's accident occurred before the law was passed. The Court's treatment of nutrition and hydration as just another form of medical treatment is expected to serve as a basis for challenging the constitutionality of the Missouri law, as well as laws in several other states containing a similar provision.

The Court decision placed much emphasis on the wishes of the individual in accepting or rejecting medical treatment. In doing so, it underscored the importance of the living will as a way of indicating our wishes, if something should happen to render us incapable of making them known directly. In some states, though, living wills have legal force only when the individual has a terminal illness (Nancy Cruzan did not) or when the individual has been quite specific about what treatments are unwanted. (As noted above, in some states a directive rejecting nourishment and hydration is not legally enforceable.) Because of such limitations, some legal observers recommend that individuals sign a durable power of attorney designating someone to make medical decisions for them if they become legally incompetent.

The Court decision left undecided the question of the constitutionality of what is sometimes called assisted suicide. Some state courts have held that, although individuals have a right to die, they do not have a right to the assistance of others in killing themselves. (See the Elizabeth Bouvia Case Presentation.) Some AIDS advocates have been particularly concerned with making it legal for the medical profession to provide people with AIDS who wish it a means of dying quickly at a certain time, rather than lingering and suffering until the end.

What of Nancy Cruzan? The State of Missouri withdrew from the case, and both the family's attorney and the state-appointed guardian filed separate briefs with the Jasper County Circuit Court asking that the implanted feeding tube be removed. A hearing was held to consider both her medical condition and evidence from family and friends about what Nancy Cruzan would wish to be done. On December 14, 1990, Judge Charles Teel ruled that there was evidence to show that her intent, "if mentally able, would be to terminate her nutrition and hydration," and he authorized the request to remove the feeding tube.

Even after the tube was removed, controversy did not end. About twenty-five protesters tried to force their way into Nancy Cruzan's hospital room to reconnect the feeding tube. "The best we can do is not cooperate with anyone trying to starve an innocent person to death," one of the protest leaders said.

Twelve days after the tube was removed, on December 26, 1990, Nancy Cruzan died. Her parents, sisters, and grandparents were at her bedside. Almost eight years had passed since the accident that destroyed her brain and made the remainder of her life a matter of debate.

"We all feel good that Nancy is free at last," her father said at her graveside.

William Webster, Missouri's Attorney General, urged the state legislature to pass a bill that would alter the existing living-will statute. The new bill would provide a remedy in a case in which a patient has been in a "persistent oblivious state" for thirty-six months, three physicians have agreed there is no hope of recovery, and family members agree that extraordinary measures should be ended.

The bill would also weaken the current standard of proof concerning a patient's wishes from "clear and convincing evidence" to "a preponderance of evidence." According to its usual legal interpretation, this standard requires more evidence for a particular claim than against it.

The *Cruzan* decision, by acknowledging a "right to die" and by finding a basis for it in the Constitution, provides states with new opportunities to resolve the issues surrounding the thousands of cases as sad and tragic as Nancy Cruzan's.

CASE PRESENTATION
Karen Quinlan

At two in the morning on Tuesday, April 14, 1975, Mrs. Julie Quinlan was awakened by a telephone call. When she hung up she was crying. "Karen is very sick," Mrs. Quinlan said to her husband, Joseph. "She's unconscious, and we have to go to Newton Hospital right away."

The Quinlans thought that their twenty-one-year-old adopted daughter might have been in an automobile accident. But the doctor in the intensive care unit told them that wasn't so. Karen was in a critical comatose state of unknown cause and was being given oxygen through a mask taped over her nose and mouth. She had been brought to the hospital by two friends who had been with her at a birthday party. After a few drinks, she had started to pass out, and her friends decided she must be drunk and put her to bed. Then a girl checked on her later in the evening and found that Karen wasn't

breathing. Her friends gave her mouth-to-mouth resuscitation and took her to the nearest hospital.

Blood and urine tests showed that Karen had not consumed a dangerous amount of alcohol. They also showed the presence of .6 milligram percent of aspirin and the tranquilizer Valium. Two milligrams would have been toxic, and five lethal. Why Karen stopped breathing was mysterious. But it was during that time that part of her brain died from oxygen depletion.

After Karen had been unconscious for about a week, she was moved to St. Clare's Hospital in nearby Denville, where testing and life-support facilities were better. Dr. Robert J. Morse, a neurologist, and Dr. Arshad Javed, a pulmonary internist, became her physicians. Additional tests were made. Extensive brain damage was confirmed, and several possible causes of the coma were ruled out.

During the early days, the Quinlans were hopeful. Karen's eyes opened and closed, and her mother and her nineteen-year-old sister, Mary Ellen, thought that they detected signs that she recognized them. But Karen's condition began to deteriorate. Her weight gradually dropped from 120 pounds to seventy. Her body began to contract into a rigid fetal position, until her five-foot-two-inch frame was bent into a shape hardly longer than three feet. She was now breathing mechanically, by means of an MA-1 respirator that pumped air through a tube in her throat.

By early July, Karen's physicians and her mother, sister, and brother had come to believe it was hopeless to expect her ever to regain consciousness. Only her father continued to believe it might be possible. But when he told Dr. Morse about some encouraging sign he had noticed, Dr. Morse said to him "Even if God did perform a miracle so that Karen would live, her damage is so extensive she would spend the rest of her life in an institution." Mr. Quinlan then realized that Karen would never again be as he remembered her. He now agreed with Karen's sister: "Karen would never want to be kept alive on machines like this. She would hate this."

The Quinlan's parish priest, Father Thomas Trapasso, had also assured them that the moral doctrines of the Roman Catholic Church did not require the continuation of extraordinary measures to support a hopeless life. Before making his decision, Mr. Quinlan asked the priest "Am I playing God?" Father Thomas said "God has made the decision that Karen is going to die. You're just agreeing with God's decision, that's all."

On July 31, after Karen had been unconscious for three and a half months, the Quinlans gave Drs. Morse and Jared their permission to take Karen off the respirator. The Quinlans signed a letter authorizing the discontinuance of extraordinary procedures and absolving the hospital from all legal liability. "I think you have come to the right decision," Dr. Morse said to Mr. Quinlan.

But the next morning Dr. Morse called Mr. Quinlan. "I have a moral problem about what we agreed on last night," he said. "I feel I have to consult somebody else and see how he feels about it." The next day, Dr. Morse called again. "I find I will not do it," he said. "And I've informed the administrator at the hospital that I will not do it."

The Quinlans were upset and bewildered by the change in Dr. Morse. Later they talked with the hospital attorney and were told by him that, because Karen was over twenty-one, they were no longer her legal guardians. The Quinlans would have to go to court and be appointed to guardianship. After that, the hospital might or might not remove Karen from the respirator.

Mr. Quinlan consulted attorney Paul Armstrong. Because Karen was an adult without income, Mr. Quinlan explained, Medicare was paying the $450 a day it cost to keep her alive. The Quinlans thus had no financial motive in asking that the respirator be taken away. Mr. Quinlan said that his belief that Karen should be allowed to die rested on his conviction that it was God's will, and it was for this reason that he wanted to be appointed Karen's guardian.

Mr. Armstrong filed a plea with Judge Robert Muir of the New Jersey Superior Court on September 12, 1975. He explicitly requested that Mr. Quinlan be appointed Karen's guardian so that he would have "the express power of authorizing the discontinuance of all extraordinary means of sustaining her life." Later, on October 20, Mr. Armstrong argued the case on three constitutional grounds. First, he claimed that there is an implicit right to privacy guaranteed by the Constitution and that this right permits individuals or others acting for them to terminate the use of extraordinary medical measures, even when death may result. This right holds, Armstrong said, unless there are compelling state interests that set it aside.

Second, Armstrong argued that the First Amendment guarantee of religious freedom extended to the Quinlan case. If the court did not allow them to act in accordance with the doctrines of their church, their religious liberty would be infringed. Finally, Armstrong appealed to the "cruel and unusual punishment" clause of the Eighth Amendment. He claimed that "for the state to require that Karen Quinlan be kept alive, against her will and the will of her family, after the dignity, beauty, promise and meaning of earthly life have vanished, is cruel and unusual punishment."

Karen's mother, sister, and a friend testified that Karen had often talked about not wanting to be kept alive by machines. An expert witness, a neurologist, testified that Karen was in a "chronic vegetative state" and that it was unlikely that she would ever regain consciousness. Doctors testifying for St. Clare's Hospital and Karen's physicians agreed with this. But, they argued, her brain still showed patterns of electrical activity, and she still had a discernible pulse. Thus, she could not be considered dead by legal or medical criteria.

On November 10, Judge Muir ruled against Joseph Quinlan. He praised Mr. Quinlan's character and concern, but he decided that Mr. Quinlan's anguish over his daughter might cloud his judgment about her welfare so he should not be made her guardian. Furthermore, Judge Muir said, because Karen is still medically and legally alive, "the Court should not authorize termination of the respirator. To do so would be homicide and an act of euthanasia."

Mr. Armstrong appealed the decision to the New Jersey Supreme Court. On January 26, 1976, the court convened to hear arguments, and Mr. Armstrong argued substantially as before. But this time the court's ruling was favorable. The court agreed that Mr. Quinlan could assert a right of privacy on Karen's behalf and that whatever he decided for her should be accepted by society. It also set aside any criminal liability for removing the respirator, claiming that if death resulted it would not be homicide and that, even if it were homicide, it would not be unlawful. Finally, the court stated that, if Karen's physicians believed that she would never emerge from her coma, they should consult an ethics committee to be established by St. Clare's Hospital. If the committee accepted their prognosis, then the respirator could be removed. If Karen's

present physicians were then unwilling to take her off the respirator, Mr. Quinlan was free to find a physician who would.

Six weeks after the court decision, the respirator still had not been turned off. In fact, another machine, one for controlling body temperature, had been added. Mr. Quinlan met with Morse and Jared and demanded that they remove the respirator. They agreed to "wean" Karen from the machine, and soon she was breathing without mechanical assistance. Dr. Morse and St. Clare's Hospital were determined that Karen would not die while under their care. Although she was moved to a private room, it was next door to the intensive-care unit. They intended to put her back on the respirator at the first sign of breathing difficulty.

Because Karen was still alive, the Quinlans began a long search for a chronic-care hospital. Twenty or more institutions turned them away, and physicians expressed great reluctance to become involved in the case. Finally, Dr. Joseph Fennelly volunteered to treat Karen, and on June 9 she was moved from St. Clare's to the Morris View Nursing Home.

Karen Quinlan continued to breathe. She received high-nutrient feedings and regular doses of antibiotics to ward off infections. During some periods she was more active than at others, making reflexive responses to touch and sound.

On June 11, 1985, at 7:01 in the evening, ten years after she lapsed into a coma, Karen Quinlan finally died. She was thirty-one years old.

CASE PRESENTATION
Elizabeth Bouvia's Demand to Starve

On September 3, 1983, Elizabeth Bouvia was admitted, at her own request, to Riverside General Hospital in Riverside, California. She sought admission on the grounds that she was suicidal. She was twenty-six years old, a victim of cerebral palsy, and almost totally paralyzed. She had the partial use of one arm, could speak, and could chew her food if someone fed it to her. In addition to her paralysis, she suffered almost constant pain from arthritis.

Despite the severity of her handicap, Mrs. Bouvia had earned a degree in social work, been married, and lived independently with the assistance of relatives and others. Then matters became particularly difficult for her. She had not been successful in an attempt to have a child, her husband left her, and she lost the state grant that paid for her special transportation needs.

After her admission, Mrs. Bouvia announced to the hospital staff that she wished to starve herself to death. She asked to be provided with hygienic care and pain-killing medicines but no food. She explained that she wanted the hospital to be a place where she would "just be left alone and not bothered by friends or family or anyone else" so that she could "ultimately starve to death" and be free from her "useless body."

Mrs. Bouvia refused to eat the solid food offered to her, and her attending physician declared that, if she did not eat, he would have her declared mentally ill and a danger to herself. She could then be force-fed. She responded by calling local newspapers and asking for legal assistance. The American Civil Liberties Union agreed to provide her an attorney, and Richard Stanley Scott became her legal representative.

Mr. Scott convinced her to allow herself to be fed while he made efforts to secure a court order restraining the hospital from either discharging her or force-feeding her. At the court hearing, Mrs. Bouvia testified as to her reasons for refusing nourishment:

> I hate to have someone care for every personal need . . . it's humiliating. It's disgusting, and I choose to no longer do that, no longer to be dependent on someone to take care of me in that manner. . . . I am choosing this course of action due to my physical limitation and disability.

Dr. Donald E. Fisher, head of psychiatry at the hospital, testified that he would force-feed Mrs. Bouvia, even if the court ordered him not to.

On behalf of his client, Mr. Scott argued that her decision to refuse nourishment was "exactly medically and morally analogous to the patient deciding to forgo further kidney dialysis," knowingly accepting death as the consequence.

Judge John H. Hews refused to grant the restraining order. He expressed the view that Mrs. Bouvia was a competent, rational, and sincere person whose decision was based on her physical condition and not upon her recent misfortunes. Nevertheless, allowing her to starve herself to death in the hospital would "have a profound effect" on the staff, other patients, and other handicapped people. Mrs. Bouvia, Judge Hews held, was "not terminal" and might expect to live another fifteen to twenty years. Accordingly, he held that "the established ethics of the medical profession clearly outweigh and overcome her own rights of self-determination," and "forced feeding, however invasive, would be administered for the purpose of saving the life of an otherwise nonterminal patient and should be permitted. There is no other reasonable option." In effect, in Judge Hews's view, Mrs. Bouvia had a right to commit suicide, but she did not have the right to have others assist her.

Mrs. Bouvia later refused to eat, and Judge Hews authorized the hospital to feed her against her will. Her attorney argued that this was an unlawful invasion of her privacy and appealed to the California Supreme Court. The court unanimously refused to grant a hearing on the appeal, thus allowing the lower court ruling to stand.

In February 1986, Mrs. Bouvia was back in court. Through her attorney, she sought an injunction to stop High Desert Hospital of Lancaster, California, where she had become a patient, from using a nasogastric tube to feed her against her wishes. In a public statement, she asserted that she had no intention to attempt to starve herself to death but wished only to receive a liquid diet. The hospital's physicians and lawyers maintained that a liquid diet would be a form of starvation and that the law precluded them from agreeing to her demand. The eventual court decision was again in favor of Mrs. Bouvia, and in April the feeding tube was removed.

However, Mrs. Bouvia eventually decided she would begin to eat voluntarily. The hospital resumed feeding her, and, when her health was considered stable once more, she was released. She announced at that time that she had changed her mind about dying, but in 1987 she again reversed herself. She tried starving herself to death but gave up the effort when she was told it might take several weeks. She felt she could not endure such side effects as the constant vomiting caused by taking pain-killing medications without food. "Starving myself would take too long," she said. "I wish there were a quicker way."

She moved to Los Angeles and for the past several years has lived in a small cell-like room at the Los Angeles County–USC Medical Center. The cost of the room, more than $800 a day, is paid for by MediCal.

Her father and two sisters visit her from out of state a couple of times a year, and various friends visit about once a week. Mostly, though, she just lies in her bed and watches TV. "The thought of being here another ten years, I just can't fathom," she says. "I would rather be dead than lie here."

CASE PRESENTATION
The Death of J. K. Collums

On November 16, 1981, sixty-nine-year-old Woodrow Collums went into the Oak Hills Care Center in the small town of Poteet, Texas, to visit his seventy-two-year-old brother, J. K. Collums. J. K. was a victim of Alzheimer's disease, a poorly understood illness in which the brain undergoes progressive degeneration. J. K. had already reached the point of being unable to care for any of his bodily needs, and he could no longer speak or respond to others. A nasogastric tube fed him the nutrients needed to keep him alive.

"I just stood there and looked at him a few minutes," Woody Collums said about his brother. "He was beyond saying anything to me. So I left and went back to the car, thinking I'd just go on and let the Lord take care of it. But I got to the car, and this gun was in the car."

Mr. Collums decided to shoot his brother and he took the gun back into the room. But once there, he changed his mind. "So I started to leave, and I looked back at him, and I just couldn't go off and leave him like that. I turned around and shot him five times, just as fast as I could shoot him. He never moved. He was the most peaceful-looking guy you've ever seen."

Mr. Collums then checked his brother's pulse to be sure that he was dead. He put the pistol down on a bedside tray and waited for someone to call the police. While waiting, he said to a staff member "I've killed horses, cows, and dogs that were suffering. He's suffered long enough."

Mr. Collums freely admitted shooting his brother, but he refused to acknowledge that he had murdered him. "I feel like he's been dead since he's been in this condition," he said.

A Bexar County, Texas, grand jury indicted Mr. Collums for the shooting of his brother. But even the county prosecutors regarded the action as a clear case of mercy killing. The two brothers had been very close all their lives, and, although J. K. Collums had not signed an actual "living will," which is legal in Texas, he had written a letter to his physician in which he expressed his views about being kept alive by extraordinary means. According to J. K. Collums's wife, Helen, he said that "if they couldn't do something to help his brain, to please put him to sleep forever." The letter was written before the disease had progressed to the point that he was no longer able to reason and communicate.

When asked if she blamed her brother-in-law for his actions, Helen Collums said "Oh, no! God, no, no!" She went on to say "I thank God Jim's out of his misery. I hate to think it had to be done the way it was done, but I understand it. I couldn't ever have shot him. I could have asked for the life supports to be taken away, because I don't believe in life supports. I just think it's cruelty for someone who's terminally ill, to stuff a tube down his nose from May to November. That's agony and cruelty. People don't know about these things. I just hope it helps somebody else, so they don't have to go through what he went through."

Helen Collums now believes she should not have allowed the stomach tube to be put into place. But, once it had been, other members of the family refused to allow it to be removed. They thought removing it would constitute murder. Besides, it was not clear that the nursing home would agree to its removal. Court decisions allow the removal of support systems that are "extraordinary means" of prolonging life when the patient has "clearly and convincingly" rejected the use of such means beforehand. But is a feeding tube "extraordinary"?

Woodrow Collums received much public sympathy, but not everyone approved of his action. Theresa Brock, the administrator of the Oak Hills Care Center, expressed the opposition view. "None of us knows," she said, "and nobody here can tell you, nobody on this earth can tell you, what Jim was able to feel, or perceive, or think or know, and it's not up to any of us to end somebody's life for them."

Everyone agreed that J. K. Collums could still recognize his wife and could still pucker his lips as if to kiss her. He did just that on the day that he died.

In February of 1982, Woodrow Collums pleaded guilty to a charge of murder. He waived a jury trial, and at a punishment hearing he told Judge Tom Rickhoff about what he had done. Mr. Collums said of his brother "He looked like he was just begging me to get him out of his misery. I regret having to do what I did, but I don't regret doing it. I felt he would have done it himself if he could have."

Mr. Collums's lawyer, Roy Barrera, expressed the hope that the hearing would help people understand the need for euthanasia. "If we can do mercy killings for animals to relieve pain and suffering," he said, "I just can't see where under the proper conditions a human being would be given any less than what we give animals."

Judge Rickhoff was faced with the decision of whether to send Mr. Collums to jail or to put him on probation. On March 4, Judge Rickhoff ruled that Mr. Collums was to be placed on probation for a period of ten years. During that time, he would be required to spend ten hours each week working at homes for the elderly.

INTRODUCTION

Death comes to us all. We hope that when it comes it will be swift and allow us to depart without prolonged suffering, our dignity intact. We also hope that it will not force burdens on our family and friends, making them pay both financially and emotionally by our lingering and hopeless condition.

Such considerations give euthanasia a strong appeal. Should we not be able to snip the thread of life when the weight of suffering and hopelessness grows too heavy to bear? The answer to this question is not so easy as it may seem, for hidden within it are a number of complicated moral issues.

Just what is euthanasia? The word comes from the Greek for "good death," and in English it has come to have the meaning "easy death." But this does very little to help us understand the concept. For consider this: If we give ourselves an easy death, are we committing suicide? If we assist someone else to an easy death (with or without that person's permission), are we committing murder? Anyone who opposed killing (either of oneself or of others) on moral grounds might also consider it necessary to object to euthanasia.

It may be, however, that the answer to both of these questions is no. But if it is, then it is necessary to specify the conditions that distinguish euthanasia from both suicide and murder. Only then would it be possible to argue, without contradiction, that euthanasia is morally acceptable but the other two forms of killing are not. (Someone believing that suicide is morally legitimate would not object to euthanasia carried out by the person herself, but he would still have to deal with the problem posed by the euthanasia/murder issue.)

ACTIVE AND PASSIVE EUTHANASIA

We have talked of euthanasia as though it involved directly taking the life of a person, either one's own life or the life of another. However, some philosophers distinguish between "active euthanasia" and "passive euthanasia," which in turn rests on a distinction between *killing* and *letting die*. To kill someone (including oneself) is to take a definite action to end his or her life (administering a lethal injection, for example). To allow someone to die, by contrast, is to take no steps to prolong a person's life when those steps seem called for (failing to give an injection of antibiotics, for example). Active euthanasia, then, is direct killing and is an act of commission. Passive euthanasia is an act of omission.

This distinction is used in most contemporary codes of medical ethics (that of the American Medical Association, for example) and is also recognized in the Anglo-American tradition of law. Except in special circumstances, it is illegal to deliberately cause the death of another person. It is not, however, illegal (except in special circumstances) to allow a person to die. Clearly, one might consider active euthanasia morally wrong while recognizing passive euthanasia as morally legitimate.

Some philosophers, however, have argued that the active-passive distinction is morally irrelevant with respect to euthanasia. Both are cases of causing death, and it is the circumstances in which death is caused, not the manner of causing it, that is of moral importance. (This is the claim defended by James Rachels in his essay "Active and Passive Euthanasia," included in this chapter.) Furthermore, the active-passive distinction is not always clear-cut. If a person dies after special life-sustaining equipment has been withdrawn, is this a case of active or passive euthanasia? Or is it a case of euthanasia at all?

VOLUNTARY AND NONVOLUNTARY EUTHANASIA

Philosophers and other writers on euthanasia have often thought it important to distinguish between *voluntary* and *nonvoluntary* euthanasia. Voluntary euthanasia includes cases in which a person takes his or her own life, either directly or by refusing treatment. But it also includes cases in which a person deputizes another to act in accordance with his wishes. Thus, a person might instruct her family not to permit the use of artificial support systems should she become unconscious, suffer from brain damage, and be unable to speak for herself. Or a person might request that he be given a lethal injection, after suffering third-degree burns over most of his body and being told that he has virtually no hope of recovery. That the individual explicitly consents to death is a necessary feature of voluntary euthanasia.

Nonvoluntary (or involuntary) euthanasia includes those cases in which the decision about death is not made by the person who is to die. Here the person gives no specific consent or instructions, and the decision is made by family, friends, or physician. The distinction between voluntary and nonvoluntary euthanasia is not always a clear one. Physicians sometimes assume that people are "asking" to die, even when no explicit request has been made. Also, the wishes and attitudes that people express when they are *not* in extreme life-threatening medical situations may be too vague for us to be certain that they would choose death when they are in such a situa-

tion. Is "I never want to be hooked up to one of those machines" an adequate indication that the person who says this does not want to be put on a respirator should he meet with an accident and fall into a comatose state?

If the distinctions we have made are considered legitimate and relevant, it is clear that there are six cases in which euthanasia becomes a moral decision:

1. Self-administered euthanasia
   a. active
   b. passive

2. Other-administered euthanasia
   a. active and voluntary
   b. active and nonvoluntary
   c. passive and voluntary
   d. passive and nonvoluntary

Even these possibilities do not exhaust the cases that euthanasia presents us with. For example, notice that the voluntary/nonvoluntary distinction does not appear in connection with self-administered euthanasia in our scheme. It might be argued that it should, for a person's decision to end his life (actively or passively) may well not be a wholly voluntary or free decision. People who are severely depressed by their illness and decide to end their lives, for example, might not be thought of as having made a voluntary choice. Hence, one might approve of self-administered voluntary euthanasia yet think that the nonvoluntary form should not be permitted. It should not be allowed not because it is necessarily morally wrong, but because it would not be a genuine decision by the person. The person might be thought of as suffering from a psychiatric disability.

ETHICAL THEORIES AND EUTHANASIA

Roman Catholicism explicitly rejects all forms of euthanasia as being against the natural law duty to preserve life. It considers euthanasia as morally identical with either suicide or murder. This position is not so rigid as it may seem, however. As we have already seen in the introductory chapter and in the last chapter, the principle of double effect makes it morally acceptable to give medication for the relief of pain—even if the indirect result of the medication will be to shorten the life of the recipient. The intended result is not the death of the person but the relief of suffering. The difference in intention is thus considered to be a morally significant one. Those not accepting the principle of double effect would be likely to classify the administration of a substance that would relieve pain but would also cause death as a case of euthanasia.

Furthermore, on the Catholic view there is no moral obligation to continue treatment when a person is medically hopeless. It is legitimate to allow people to die as a result of their illness or injury, even though their lives might be lengthened by the use of extraordinary means. Additionally, we may legitimately make the same decisions about ourselves that we make about others who are in no condition to decide. Thus, without intending to kill ourselves, we may choose measures for the relief of pain that may secondarily hasten our end. Or we may refuse extraordinary treatment and let "nature" take its course, let "God's will" determine the outcome. (See the introductory chapter for a fuller discussion of the Roman Catholic position on euthanasia and extraordinary means of sustaining life.)

At first sight, utilitarianism would seem to endorse euthanasia in all of its forms. Whenever suffering is great and the condition of the person is one without legitimate medical hope, then the principle of utility might be invoked to approve putting the person to death. After all, in such a case we seem to be acting to end suffering and to bring about a state of affairs in which happiness exceeds unhappiness. Thus, whether the person concerned is ourself or another, euthanasia would seem to be a morally right action.

A utilitarian might argue in this way, but this is not the only way in which the principle of utility might be applied. It could be argued, for example, that, since life is a necessary condition for happiness, it is wrong to destroy that condition because, by doing so, the possibility of all future happiness is lost. Furthermore, a rule utilitarian might well argue that a rule like "The taking of a human life is permissible when suffering is intense and the condition of the person permits no legitimate hope" would be open to abuse. Consequently, in the long run the rule would actually work to increase the amount of unhappiness in the world. Obviously, it is not possible to say there is such a thing as "the utilitarian view of euthanasia." The principle of utility supplies a guide for an answer, but it is not itself an answer.

Euthanasia presents a considerable difficulty for Kant's ethics. For Kant, an autonomous rational being has a duty to preserve his or her life. Thus, one cannot rightly refuse needed medical care or commit suicide. Yet our status as autonomous rational beings also endows us with an inherent dignity. If that status is destroyed or severely compromised, as it is when people become comatose and unknowing because of illness or injury, then it is not certain that we have a duty to maintain our lives under such conditions. It may be more in keeping with our freedom and dignity for us to instruct others either to put us to death or to take no steps to keep us alive should we ever be in such a state. Voluntary euthanasia may be compatible with (if not required by) Kant's ethics.

By a similar line of reasoning, it may be that nonvoluntary euthanasia might be seen as a duty that we have to others. We might argue that by putting to death a comatose and hopeless person we are recognizing the dignity that person possessed in his or her previous state. Also, as we mentioned in the last chapter, it might also be argued that a human being in a vegetative state is not a person in the relevant moral sense. Thus, our ordinary duty to preserve life does not hold.

According to Ross, we have a strong prima facie obligation not to kill a person except in justifiable self-defense—unless we have an even stronger prima facie moral obligation to do something that cannot be done without killing. Since active euthanasia typically requires taking the life of an innocent person, there is a moral presumption against it. However, another of Ross's prima facie obligations is that we keep promises made to others. Accordingly, if someone who is now in an irreversible coma with no hope of recovery has left instructions that in case of such an event's happening she wishes her life to be ended, then we are under a prima facie obligation to follow her instructions. Thus, in such a case, we may be justified in overriding the presumption against taking an innocent life.

What if there are no such instructions? It could be argued that our prima facie obligation of acting beneficently toward others requires us to attempt to determine what someone's wishes would be from what we know about him as a person. We would then treat him the way that we believe that he would want us to. In the absence of any relevant information, we might make the decision on the basis of how a rational person would want to be treated in similar circumstances. Of course, if anyone has left instructions that his life is to be maintained, if possible, under any circumstances, then we have a prima facie obligation to respect this preference also.

THE DUTCH EXPERIENCE

The Dutch criminal code provides as much as twelve years in prison for anyone who "takes the life of another at his or her explicit and serious request." However, in a 1972 case concerning a physician who put her mother to death at the mother's request, a court refused to impose the penalty. Since that time, and with the reinforcement of a major court decision in 1984, the extralegal practice of voluntary, active, physician-administered euthanasia has become established in the Netherlands. The de facto practice requires that a conscious and competent patient make the request of a physi-

cian and then discuss the decision with family and advisors. Relatives cannot make a request on behalf of a patient and patients in a coma or suffering from dementia are not considered candidates. The patient must have no reasonable hope of recovery and suffer unbearable pain not relievable by medication. The patient must also sign a witnessed explicit authorization for the act to be carried out. Typically, the physician then injects a barbiturate to induce sleep, combined with curare to produce death.

Attempts to make the procedure a legal one have failed in recent years. Nevertheless, opinion polls show that over 60% of the Dutch favor this limited form of active euthanasia. About 50% of those who are Roman Catholics favor it.

The influence of the Dutch practice can be seen in an effort made in California to place a voluntary-euthanasia proposal on the November 1988 ballot. The "Humane and Dignified Death Act" would have allowed terminally ill patients to execute a directive authorizing a physician to assist them in dying "by any medical procedure that will terminate the life . . . swiftly, painlessly, and humanely." The act was sponsored by Americans Against Human Suffering and the Hemlock Society, organizations favoring making voluntary euthanasia an individual option. The act was opposed by the California Nurses Association and the California Medical Association. The proposal failed to get enough signatures to get on the ballot.

Despite this failure, the Dutch practice is often mentioned in the United States as an example of what a reasonable euthanasia policy might include. In particular the practice is offered as a model for providing an option to continuing treatment of individuals suffering from a lingering terminal illness. People with AIDS, for example, have often expressed a wish for a social and legal policy that would permit active, voluntary euthanasia or assisted suicide. These are just the sort of people the Dutch practice has evolved to deal with.

However, the Dutch practice is not relevant to the types of cases that have caused much concern and controversy in this country. Until recently, the proper treatment of individuals in irreversible comas, as in the *Quinlan* and *Cruzan* cases, has been the focus of dispute. Since the practice in Holland requires that individuals be conscious and intellectually competent, it embodies no principles that could be appealed to for resolving the troublesome issues involved in dealing with patients in persistent vegetative states.

LIVING WILLS

Like so many issues in medical ethics, euthanasia has traditionally been discussed only in the back rooms of medicine. Often decisions about whether to allow a patient to die are made by physicians acting on their own authority. Such decisions do not represent so much an arrogant claim to godlike wisdom as an acknowledgment of the physician's obligation to do what is best for the patient. Most physicians admit that allowing or helping a patient to die is sometimes the best assistance that can be given. Decisions made in this fashion depend on the beliefs and judgment of particular physicians. Because these may differ from those of the patient concerned, it is quite possible that the physician's decision may not reflect the wishes of the patient.

But covert decisions made by a physician acting alone are becoming practices of the past as euthanasia is discussed more widely and openly. (The overwhelmingly negative response that met "It's Over, Debbie," an anonymous account of a physician deciding, without consulting anyone, to administer a lethal injection to a comatose patient, is an indication of how far traditional attitudes have altered.) Court cases, such as *Quinlan* and now *Cruzan*, have both widened the scope of legally permissible actions and reinforced the notion that an individual has a right to refuse or discontinue life-sustaining medical treatment. Such cases have also made it clear that there are limits to the benefits that can be derived from medicine—that, under some conditions,

individuals may be better off if everything that technologically can be done is not done. Increasingly, people want to be sure that they have some say in what happens to them should they fall victim to hopeless injury or illness.

One indication of this interest is that the number of states permitting individuals to sign "living wills" has now increased to more than forty, and it is reasonable to believe that before long every state will have some living-will procedure. The first living-will legislation was the "Natural Death Act," passed by the California legislature on August 30, 1977. The act is generally representative of all such legislation. It permits a competent adult to sign a directive that will authorize physicians to withhold or discontinue "mechanical" or "artificial" life-support equipment if the person is judged to be "terminal" and if "death is imminent."

The strength of living wills is that they allow a person to express in an explicit manner how he or she wishes to be treated before treatment is needed. In this way, the autonomy of the individual is recognized. Even though unconscious or comatose, a person can continue to exert control over his or her life. This, in turn, means that physicians need not and should not be the decisive voice in determining the continuation or use of special medical equipment.

Critics of living-will legislation have claimed that it does not go far enough in protecting autonomy and making death easier (where this is what is wanted). They point out that the directive specified in the California bill and most others would have made no difference in the case of Karen Quinlan. She had not been diagnosed as having a "terminal condition" at least two weeks prior to being put on a respirator, yet this is one of the requirements of the act. Consequently, the directive would have been irrelevant to her condition.

Nor, for that matter, would those people be allowed to die who wish to, if their disease or injury does not involve treatment by "artificial" or "mechanical" means. Thus, a person suffering from throat cancer would simply have to bear the pain and wait for a "natural" death. Finally, at the moment, some states explicitly exclude nutrition and hydration as medical treatments that can be discontinued. The Supreme Court in the *Cruzan* case accepted the notion that the nutrition received by Nancy Cruzan through a feeding tube implanted in her stomach was a form of medical treatment that could be withdrawn. However, the Court did not rule on the Missouri law that forbids withdrawal. Until this law or some other like it is successfully challenged in court, a living will does not necessarily guarantee that such treatment will be discontinued, even when requested.

Limitations of such kinds on living wills have led some writers to recommend that individuals sign a legal instrument known as a durable power of attorney. In such a document, an individual can name someone to act on his behalf should he become legally incompetent to act. Hence, unlike the living will, a durable power of attorney allows a surrogate to exercise control over novel and unanticipated situations. For example, the surrogate may order the discontinuation of artificial feeding, something that a living will might not permit.

The widespread wish to have some control over the end of one's life is reflected in a new federal law that took effect in 1991. The Self-Determination Act is sometimes referred to as a "medical Miranda warning." It requires that hospitals, nursing homes, and other healthcare facilities receiving federal funding provide patients at the time of admission with written information about relevant state laws and the rights of citizens under those laws to refuse or discontinue treatment. Patients must also be told about the practices and policies at that particular institution so they can choose a facility willing to abide by their decisions. The institutions must also record whether a patient has provided a written "advance directive" (e.g., a living will or power of attorney for health care) that will take effect should the patient become incapacitated.

Should a Physician Help Someone Die?

If a person has a disease that will ultimately destroy the person's mind, and the person wants to take his or her own life, should a doctor be allowed to assist the person in taking his or her own life?

Yes: 53%
No: 42%
Don't know/No answer: 6%

Source: New York Times/CBS News Poll (June 9, 1990).

Removing a Feeding Tube

Suppose a patient is in a coma, doctors say brain activity has stopped, and the patient is getting food and water through a feeding tube. Should a close family member have the right to tell the doctor to take away the feeding tube and let the person die?

Yes: 81%
No: 13%
Don't know: 6%

Suppose you were in a coma with no brain activity and were being kept alive by a feeding tube. Would you want your doctor to remove the feeding tube and let you die?

Yes: 85%
No: 11%
Don't know: 4%

Source: New York Times/CBS News Poll (June 26, 1990).

Another sign of change is the recent concern with the medical circumstances in which people die. The medical ideal of a "hospital death," one in which the patient's temperature, pulse rate, and respiration are brought within normal limits by medication and machinery, is being severely challenged. This is reflected in the policy reaffirmed in 1988 by the

AMA that holds that it may be morally appropriate to withhold "all means of life prolonging medical treatment," including artificial feeding, from patients in irreversible comas.

A new ideal of natural death also seems to be emerging. In this view, the kind of support a dying patient needs is psychological counseling and contact with family and friends, rather than heroic medical efforts. An acceptance of death as a normal end of life and the development of new means of caring for the dying may ease the problem of euthanasia. If those who are hopeless and near death are offered an alternative to either euthanasia or an all-out medical effort to preserve their lives, they may choose that alternative. "Death with dignity" need not always mean choosing a lethal injection.

The Wrongfulness of Euthanasia

J. Gay-Williams

J. Gay-Williams defines "euthanasia" as intentionally taking the life of a person who is believed to be suffering from some illness or injury from which recovery cannot reasonably be expected. Gay-Williams rejects passive euthanasia as a *name* for actions that are usually designated by the phrase but seems to approve of the actions themselves. He argues that euthanasia as intentional killing goes against natural law because it violates the natural inclination to preserve life. Furthermore, both self-interest and possible practical consequences of euthanasia provide reasons for rejecting it.

My impression is that euthanasia—the idea, if not the practice—is slowly gaining acceptance within our society. Cynics might attribute this to an increasing tendency to devalue human life, but I do not believe this is the major factor. The acceptance is much more likely to be the result of unthinking sympathy and benevolence. Well-publicized, tragic stories like that of Karen Quinlan elicit from us deep feelings of compassion. We think to ourselves, "She and her family would be better off if she were dead." It is an easy step from this very human response to the view that if someone (and others) would be better off dead, then it must be all right to kill that person.[1] Although I respect the compassion that leads to this conclusion, I believe the conclusion is wrong. I want to show that euthanasia is wrong. It is inherently wrong, but it is also wrong judged from the standpoints of self-interest and of practical effects.

Before presenting my arguments to support this claim, it would be well to define "euthanasia." An essential aspect of euthanasia is that it involves taking a human life, either one's own or that of another. Also, the person whose life is taken must be someone who is believed to be suffering from some disease or injury from which recovery cannot reasonably be expected. Finally, the action must be deliberate and intentional. Thus, euthanasia is intentionally taking the life of a presumably hopeless person. Whether the life is one's own or that of another, the taking of it is still euthanasia.

It is important to be clear about the deliberate and intentional aspect of the killing. If a hopeless person is given an injection of the wrong drug by mistake and this causes his death, this is wrongful killing but not euthanasia. The killing cannot be the result of accident. Furthermore, if the person is given an injection of a drug that is believed to be necessary to treat his disease or better his condition and the person dies as a result, then this is neither wrongful killing nor euthanasia. The intention was to make the patient well, not kill him. Similarly, when a patient's condition is such that it is not reasonable to hope that any medical procedures or treatments will save his life, a failure to implement the procedures or treatments is not euthanasia. If the person dies, this will be as a result of his injuries or disease and not because of his failure to receive treatment.

The failure to continue treatment after it has been realized that the patient has little chance of benefiting from it has been characterized by some as "passive euthanasia." This phrase is misleading and mistaken.[2] In such cases, the person involved is not killed (the first essential aspect of euthanasia), nor is the death of the person intended by the withholding of additional treatment (the third essential aspect of euthanasia). The aim may be to spare the person additional and unjustifiable pain, to save him from the indignities of hopeless manipulations, and to avoid increasing the financial and emotional burden on his family. When I buy a pencil it is so that I can use it to write, not to contribute to an increase in the gross national product. This may be the unintended consequence of my action, but it is not the aim of my action. So it is with failing to continue the treatment of a dying person. I intend his death no more than I intend to reduce the GNP by not using medical supplies. His is an unintended dying, and so-called "passive euthanasia" is not euthanasia at all.

1. The Argument from Nature

Every human being has a natural inclination to continue living. Our reflexes and responses fit us to fight attackers, flee wild animals, and dodge out of the way of trucks. In our daily lives we exercise the caution and care necessary to protect ourselves. Our bodies are similarly structured for survival right down to the molecular level. When we are cut, our capillaries seal shut, our blood clots, and fibrogen is produced to start the process of healing the wound. When we are invaded by bacteria, antibodies are produced to fight against the alien organisms, and their remains are swept out of the body by special cells designed for clean-up work.

Euthanasia does violence to this natural goal of survival. It is literally acting against nature because

all the processes of nature are bent towards the end of bodily survival. Euthanasia defeats these subtle mechanisms in a way that, in a particular case, disease and injury might not.

It is possible, but not necessary, to make an appeal to revealed religion in this connection.[3] Man as trustee of his body acts against God, its rightful possessor, when he takes his own life. He also violates the commandment to hold life sacred and never to take it without just and compelling cause. But since this appeal will persuade only those who are prepared to accept that religion has access to revealed truths, I shall not employ this line of argument.

It is enough, I believe, to recognize that the organization of the human body and our patterns of behavioral responses make the continuation of life a natural goal. By reason alone, then, we can recognize that euthanasia sets us against our own nature.[4] Furthermore, in doing so, euthanasia does violence to our dignity. Our dignity comes from seeking our ends. When one of our goals is survival, and actions are taken that eliminate that goal, then our natural dignity suffers. Unlike animals, we are conscious through reason of our nature and our ends. Euthanasia involves acting as if this dual nature—inclination towards survival and awareness of this as an end—did not exist. Thus, euthanasia denies our basic human character and requires that we regard ourselves or others as something less than fully human.

2. The Argument from Self-Interest

The above arguments are, I believe, sufficient to show that euthanasia is inherently wrong. But there are reasons for considering it wrong when judged by standards other than reason. Because death is final and irreversible, euthanasia contains within it the possibility that we will work against our own interest if we practice it or allow it to be practiced on us.

Contemporary medicine has high standards of excellence and a proven record of accomplishment, but it does not possess perfect and complete knowledge. A mistaken diagnosis is possible, and so is a mistaken prognosis. Consequently, we may believe that we are dying of a disease when, as a matter of fact, we may not be. We may think that we have no hope of recovery when, as a matter of fact, our chances are quite good. In such circumstances, if euthanasia were permitted, we would die needlessly. Death is final and the chance of error too great to approve the practice of euthanasia.

Also, there is always the possibility that an experimental procedure or a hitherto untried technique will pull us through. We should at least keep this option open, but euthanasia closes it off. Furthermore, spontaneous remission does occur in many cases. For no apparent reason, a patient simply recovers when those all around him, including his physicians, expected him to die. Euthanasia would just guarantee their expectations and leave no room for the "miraculous" recoveries that frequently occur.

Finally, knowing that we can take our life at any time (or ask another to take it) might well incline us to give up too easily. The will to live is strong in all of us, but it can be weakened by pain and suffering and feelings of hopelessness. If during a bad time we allow ourselves to be killed, we never have a chance to reconsider. Recovery from a serious illness requires that we fight for it, and anything that weakens our determination by suggesting that there is an easy way out is ultimately against our own interest. Also, we may be inclined towards euthanasia because of our concern for others. If we see our sickness and suffering as an emotional and financial burden on our family, we may feel that to leave our life is to make their lives easier.[5] The very presence of the possibility of euthanasia may keep us from surviving when we might.

3. The Argument from Practical Effects

Doctors and nurses are, for the most part, totally committed to saving lives. A life lost is, for them, almost a personal failure, an insult to their skills and knowledge. Euthanasia as a practice might well alter this. It could have a corrupting influence so that in any case that is severe doctors and nurses might not try hard enough to save the patient. They might decide that the patient would simply be "better off dead" and take the steps necessary to make that come about. This attitude could then carry over to their dealings with patients less seriously ill. The result would be an overall decline in the quality of medical care.

Finally, euthanasia as a policy is a slippery slope. A person apparently hopelessly ill may be allowed to take his own life. Then he may be permitted to deputize others to do it for him should he no longer be able to act. The judgment of others then becomes the ruling factor. Already at this point euthanasia is not personal and voluntary, for others are acting "on behalf of" the patient as they see fit. This may well incline them to act on behalf of other patients who have not authorized them to exercise their judgment. It is only a short step, then, from voluntary euthanasia (self-inflicted or authorized), to directed euthanasia administered to a patient who has given no authorization, to involuntary euthanasia conducted as part of a social policy.[6] Recently many psychiatrists and sociologists have argued that we define as "mental illness" those forms of behavior that we disapprove of.[7] This gives us license then to lock up those who display the behavior. The category of the "hopelessly ill" provides the possibility of even worse abuse. Embedded in a social policy, it would give society or its representatives the authority to eliminate all those who might be considered too "ill" to function normally any longer. The dangers of euthanasia are too great to all to run the risk of approving it in any form. The first slippery step may well lead to a serious and harmful fall.

I hope that I have succeeded in showing why the benevolence that inclines us to give approval of euthanasia is misplaced. Euthanasia is inherently wrong because it violates the nature and dignity of human beings. But even those who are not convinced by this must be persuaded that the potential personal and social dangers inherent in euthanasia are sufficient to forbid our approving it either as a personal practice or as a public policy.

Suffering is surely a terrible thing, and we have a clear duty to comfort those in need and to ease their suffering when we can. But suffering is also a natural part of life with values for the individual and for others that we should not overlook. We may legitimately seek for others and for ourselves an easeful death, as Arthur Dyck has pointed out.[8] Euthanasia, however, is not just an easeful death. It is a wrongful death. Euthanasia is not just dying. It is killing.

Notes

1. For a sophisticated defense of this position see Philippa Foot, "Euthanasia," *Philosophy and Public Affairs,* vol. 6 (1977), pp. 85–112. Foot does not endorse the radical conclusion that euthanasia, voluntary and involuntary, is always right.

2. James Rachels rejects the distinction between active and passive euthanasia as morally irrelevant in his "Active and Passive Euthanasia," *New England Journal of Medicine*, vol. 292, pp. 78–80. But see the criticism by Foot, pp. 100–103.

3. For a defense of this view see J. V. Sullivan, "The Immorality of Euthanasia," in *Beneficent Euthanasia*, ed. Marvin Kohl (Buffalo, N.Y.: Prometheus Books, 1975), pp. 34–44.

4. This point is made by Ray V. McIntyre in "Voluntary Euthanasia: The Ultimate Perversion," *Medical Counterpoint*, vol. 2, pp. 26–29.

5. See McIntyre, p. 28.

6. See Sullivan, "Immorality of Euthanasia," pp. 34–44, for a fuller argument in support of this view.

7. See, for example, Thomas S. Szasz, *The Myth of Mental Illness*, rev. ed. (New York: Harper & Row, 1974).

8. Arthur Dyck, "Beneficent Euthanasia and Benemortasia," Kohl, op. cit., pp. 117–129.

Justifying Voluntary Euthanasia

Peter Singer

Peter Singer is concerned exclusively with voluntary euthanasia. Nonvoluntary euthanasia, as characterized by Singer, involves the killing of a "merely conscious being," whereas voluntary euthanasia involves "the killing of a person, a rational and self-conscious being." Hence, according to Singer, it is a more serious matter.

The presumption against killing a person is supported by the classical utilitarian claim that to kill someone puts others in fear of their lives and the preference utilitarian claim that the desire of a person to live is a reason not to kill her. Further, the presumption is supported by the notion that having a right to life means being able to desire one's continued existence and by the respect we have for the decisions of autonomous agents to maintain their lives.

Singer argues that these four grounds for holding that it is usually wrong to kill a person do not prohibit killing in cases in which a competent person is suffering from a painful and incurable disease. Indeed, these same considerations show that voluntary euthanasia is fully justified. In Singer's view, the objections are basically technical ones that can be met by employing certain procedural safeguards. Hence, Singer supports the general thesis that active voluntary euthanasia is morally permissible, even in those cases in which it is fundamentally the same as assisted suicide.

Most of the groups currently campaigning for changes in the law to allow euthanasia are campaigning for voluntary euthanasia—that is, euthanasia carried out at the request of the person killed.

Sometimes voluntary euthanasia is scarcely distinguishable from assisted suicide. In *Jean's Way*, Derek Humphry has told how his wife Jean, when dying of cancer, asked him to provide her with the means to end her life swiftly and without pain. They had seen the situation coming and discussed it beforehand. Derek obtained some tablets and gave them to Jean, who took them and died soon afterwards.

In other cases, people wanting to die may be unable to kill themselves. In 1973 George Zygmaniak was injured in a motorcycle accident near his home in New Jersey. He was taken to hospital, where he was found to be totally paralyzed from the neck down. He was also in considerable pain. He told his doctor and his brother, Lester, that he did not want to live in this condition. He begged them both to kill him. Lester questioned the doctor and hospital staff about George's prospects of recovery: he was told that they were nil. He then smuggled a gun into the hospital, and said to his brother: 'I am here to end your pain, George. Is it all right with you?' George, who was now unable to speak because of an operation to assist his breathing, nodded affirmatively. Lester shot him through the temple.

The Zygmaniak case appears to be a clear instance of voluntary euthanasia, although without some of the procedural safeguards that advocates of the legalization of voluntary euthanasia propose. For instance, medical opinions about the patient's prospects of recovery were obtained only in an informal manner. Nor was there a careful attempt to establish, before independent witnesses, that George's desire for death was of a fixed and rational kind, based on the best available information about his situation. The killing was not carried out by a doctor. An injection would have been less distressing to others than shooting. But these choices were not open to Lester Zygmaniak, for the law in New Jersey, as in most other places, regards mercy killing as murder, and if he had made his plans known, he would not have been able to carry them out.

Euthanasia can be voluntary even if a person is not able, as Jean Humphry and George Zygmaniak were able, to indicate the wish to die right up to the moment the tablets are swallowed or the trigger pulled. A person may, while in good health, make a written request for euthanasia if, through accident or illness, she should come to be incapable of making or expressing a decision to die, in pain, or without the use of her mental faculties, and there is no reasonable hope of recovery. In killing a person who has made such a request, has reaffirmed it from time to time, and is now in one of the states described, one could truly claim to be acting with her consent. . . .

. . . Under existing laws people suffering unrelievable pain or distress from an incurable illness who ask their doctors to end their lives are asking their doctors to become murderers. Although juries are extremely reluctant to convict in cases of this kind the law is clear that neither the request, nor the degree of suffering, nor the incurable condition of the person killed, is a defence to a charge of murder.

Advocates of voluntary euthanasia propose that this law be changed so that a doctor could legally act on a patient's desire to die without further suffering.

The case for voluntary euthanasia has some common ground with the case for nonvoluntary euthanasia, in that the reason for killing is to end suffering. The two kinds of euthanasia differ, however, in that voluntary euthanasia involves the killing of a person, a rational and self-conscious being and not a merely conscious being. (To be strictly accurate it must be said that this is not always so, because although only rational and self-conscious beings can consent to their own deaths, they may not be rational and self-conscious at the time euthanasia is contemplated—the doctor may, for instance, be acting on a prior written request for euthanasia if, through accident or illness, one's rational faculties should be irretrievably lost. For simplicity we shall, henceforth, disregard this complication.)

We have seen [in an earlier section] that it is possible to justify nonvoluntary euthanasia, when the being killed lacks the capacity to consent. We must now ask in what way the ethical issues are different when the being is capable of consenting, and does in fact consent.

Let us return to the general principles about killing proposed in Chapter 4 [of *Practical Ethics*]. I argued there that the wrongness of killing a conscious being which is not self-conscious, rational or autonomous, depends on utilitarian considerations. It is on this basis that I have defended nonvoluntary euthanasia. On the other hand it is, as we saw, plausible to hold that killing a self-conscious being is a more serious matter than killing a merely conscious being. We found four distinct grounds on which this could be argued:

i.   The classical utilitarian claim that since self-conscious beings are capable of fearing their own death, killing them has worse effects on others.

ii. The preference utilitarian calculation which counts the thwarting of the victim's desire to go on living as an important reason against killing.

iii. A theory of rights according to which to have a right one must have the ability to desire that to which one has a right, so that to have a right to life one must be able to desire one's own continued existence.

iv. Respect for the autonomous decisions of rational agents.

Now suppose we have a situation in which a person suffering from a painful and incurable disease wishes to die. If the individual were not a person—not rational or self-conscious—euthanasia would, as I have said, be justifiable. Do any of the four grounds for holding that it is normally worse to kill a person provide reasons against killing when the individual is a person?

The classical utilitarian objection does not apply to killing that takes place only with the genuine consent of the person killed. That people are killed under these conditions would have no tendency to spread fear or insecurity, since we have no cause to be fearful of being killed with our own genuine consent. If we do not wish to be killed, we simply do not consent. In fact, the argument from fear points in favour of voluntary euthanasia, for if voluntary euthanasia is not permitted we may, with good cause, be fearful that our deaths will be unnecessarily drawn-out and distressing.

Preference utilitarianism also points in favour of, not against, voluntary euthanasia. Just as preference utilitarianism must count a desire to go on living as a reason against killing, so it must count a desire to die as a reason for killing.

Next, according to the theory of rights we have considered, it is an essential feature of a right that one can waive one's rights if one so chooses. I may have a right to privacy; but I can, if I wish, film every detail of my daily life and invite the neighbours to my home movies. Neighbours sufficiently intrigued to accept my invitation could do so without violating my right to privacy, since the right has on this occasion been waived. Similarly, to say that I have a right to life is not to say that it would be wrong for my doctor to end my life, if she does so at my request. In making this request I waive my right to life.

Lastly, the principle of respect for autonomy tells us to allow rational agents to live their own lives according to their own autonomous decisions, free from coercion or interference; but if rational agents should autonomously choose to die, then respect for autonomy will lead us to assist them to do as they choose.

So, although there are reasons for thinking that killing a self-conscious being is normally worse than killing any other kind of being, in the special case of voluntary euthanasia most of these reasons count for euthanasia rather than against. Surprising as this result might at first seem, it really does no more than reflect the fact that what is special about self-conscious beings is that they can know that they exist over time and will, unless they die, continue to exist. Normally this continued existence is fervently desired; when the foreseeable continued existence is dreaded rather than desired however, the desire to die may take the place of the normal desire to live, reversing the reasons against killing based on the desire to live. Thus the case for voluntary euthanasia is arguably much stronger than the case for nonvoluntary euthanasia.

Some opponents of the legalization of voluntary euthanasia might concede that all this follows, if we have a genuinely free and rational decision to die: but, they add, we can never be sure that a request to be killed is the result of a free and rational decision. Will not the sick and elderly be pressured by their relatives to end their lives quickly? Will it not be possible to commit outright murder by pretending that a person has requested euthanasia? And even if there is no pressure or falsification, can anyone who is ill, suffering pain, and very probably in a drugged and confused state of mind, make a rational decision about whether to live or die?

These questions raise technical difficulties for the legalization of voluntary euthanasia, rather than objections to the underlying ethical principles; but they are serious difficulties nonetheless. Voluntary euthanasia societies in Britain and elsewhere have sought to meet them by proposing that euthanasia should be legal only for a person who:

i. is diagnosed by two doctors as suffering from an incurable illness expected to cause severe distress or the loss of rational faculties;

and

ii. has, at least 30 days before the proposed act of euthanasia, and in the presence of two independent witnesses, made a written request for euthanasia in the event of the situation described in (i) occurring.

Only a doctor could administer euthanasia, and if the patient was at the time still capable of consenting, the doctor would have to make sure that the patient still wished the declaration to be acted upon. A declaration could be revoked at any time.

These provisions, though in some respects cumbersome, appear to meet most of the technical objections to legalization. Murder in the guise of euthanasia would be far-fetched. Two independent witnesses to the declaration, the 30-day waiting period, and—in the case of a mentally competent person—the doctor's final investigation of the patient's wishes would together do a great deal to reduce the danger of doctors acting on requests which did not reflect the free and rational decisions of their patients.

It is often said, in debates about euthanasia, that doctors can be mistaken. Certainly some patients diagnosed by competent doctors as suffering from an incurable condition have survived. Possibly the legalization of voluntary euthanasia would, over the years, mean the deaths of one or two people who would otherwise have recovered. This is not, however, the knockdown argument against euthanasia that some imagine it to be. Against a very small number of unnecessary deaths that might occur if euthanasia is legalized we must place the very large amount of pain and distress that will be suffered by patients who really are terminally ill if euthanasia is not legalized. Longer life is not such a supreme good that it outweighs all other considerations. (If it were, there would be many more effective ways of saving life—such as a ban on smoking, or on cars that can drive faster than 10 m.p.h.—than prohibiting voluntary euthanasia.) The possibility that two doctors may make a mistake means that the person who opts for euthanasia is deciding on the balance of probabilities, and giving up a very slight chance of survival in order to avoid suffering that will almost certainly end in death. This may be a perfectly rational choice. Probability is, as Bishop Butler said, the guide of life, and we must follow its guidance right to the end. Against this, some will reply that improved care for the terminally ill has eliminated pain and made voluntary euthanasia unnecessary. Elisabeth Kübler-Ross, whose *On Death and Dying* is perhaps the best-known book on care for the dying, has claimed that none of her patients request euthanasia. Given personal attention and the right medication, she says, people come to accept their deaths and die peacefully without pain.

Kübler-Ross may be right. It may be possible, now, to eliminate pain. It may even be possible to do it in a way which leaves patients in possession of their rational faculties and free from vomiting, nausea, or other distressing side-effects. Unfortunately only a minority of dying patients now receive this kind of care. Nor is physical pain the only problem. There can also be other distressing conditions, like bones so fragile they fracture at sudden movements, slow starvation due to a cancerous growth, inability to control one's bowels or bladder, difficulty in breathing and so on.

Take the case of Jean Humphry, as described in *Jean's Way*. This is not a case from the period before effective painkillers: Jean Humphry died in 1975. Nor is it the case of someone unable to get good medical care: she was treated at an Oxford hospital and if there were anything else that could have been done for her, her husband, a well-connected Fleet Street journalist, would have been better placed than most to obtain it. Yet Derek Humphry writes:

> when the request for help in dying meant relief from relentless suffering and pain and I had seen the extent of this agony, the option simply could not be denied . . . and certainly Jean deserved the dignity of selecting her own ending. She must die soon—as we both now realized—but together we would decide when this would be.

Perhaps one day it will be possible to treat all terminally ill patients in such a way that no one requests euthanasia and the subject becomes a nonissue; but this still distant prospect is no reason to deny euthanasia to those who die in less comfortable conditions. It is, in any case, highly paternalistic to tell dying patients that they are now so well looked after they need not be offered the option of euthanasia. It would be more in keeping with respect for individual freedom and autonomy to legalize euthanasia and let patients decide whether their situation is bearable—let them, as Derek Humphry puts it, have the dignity of selecting their own endings. Better that voluntary euthanasia be an unexercised legal right than a prohibited act which, for all we know, some might desperately desire.

Finally, do these arguments for voluntary euthanasia perhaps give too much weight to individual freedom and autonomy? After all, we do not allow people free choices on matters like, for instance, the taking of heroin. This is a restriction of freedom but, in the view of many, one that can be justified on paternalistic grounds. If preventing people becoming heroin addicts is justifiable paternalism, why isn't preventing people having themselves killed?

The question is a reasonable one, because respect for individual freedom can be carried too far. John Stuart Mill thought that the state should never interfere with the individual except to prevent harm to others. The individual's own good, Mill thought, is not a proper reason for state intervention. But Mill may have had too high an opinion of the rationality of a human being. It may occasionally be right to prevent people making choices which are obviously not rationally based and which we can be sure they will later regret. The prohibition of voluntary euthanasia cannot be justified on paternalistic grounds, however, for voluntary euthanasia is, by definition, an act for which good reasons exist. Voluntary euthanasia occurs only when, to the best of medical knowledge, a person is suffering from an incurable and painful or distressing condition. In these circumstances one cannot say that to choose to die quickly is obviously irrational. The strength of the case for voluntary euthanasia lies in this combination of respect for the preferences, or autonomy, of those who decide for euthanasia; and the clear rational basis of the decision itself.

Active and Passive Euthanasia

James Rachels

James Rachels challenges both the use and the moral significance of the distinction between active and passive euthanasia. Since both forms of euthanasia result in the death of a person, Rachels argues that active euthanasia ought to be preferred to passive. It is more humane because it allows suffering to be brought to a speedy end. Furthermore, Rachels claims, the distinction itself can be shown to be morally irrelevant. Is there, he asks, any genuine moral difference between drowning a child and merely watching a child drown and doing nothing to save it?

Finally, Rachels attempts to show that the bare fact that there is a difference between killing and letting die doesn't make active euthanasia wrong. Killing of any kind is right or wrong depending on the intentions and circumstances in which it takes place; if the intentions and circumstances are of a certain kind, then active euthanasia can be morally right.

For these reasons, Rachels suggests that the approval given to the active-passive euthanasia distinction in the Code of Ethics of the American Medical Association is unwise. He encourages physicians to rely upon the distinction only to the extent that they are forced to do so by law but not to give it any significant moral weight. In particular, they should not make use of it when writing new policies or guidelines.

The distinction between active and passive euthanasia is thought to be crucial for medical ethics. The idea is that it is permissible, at least in some cases, to withhold treatment and allow a patient to die, but it is never permissible to take any direct action designed to kill the patient. This doctrine seems to be accepted by most doctors, and it is endorsed in a statement adopted by the House of Delegates of the American Medical Association on December 4, 1973:

The intentional termination of the life of one human being by another—mercy killing—is contrary to that for which the medical profession stands and is contrary to the policy of the American Medical Association.

The cessation of the employment of extraordinary means to prolong the life of the body when there is irrefutable evidence that biological death is imminent is the decision of the patient and/or his immediate family. The advice

Reprinted by permission from the New England Journal of Medicine 292, *no. 2 (January 9, 1975): 78–80.*

and judgment of the physician should be freely available to the patient and/or his immediate family.

However, a strong case can be made against this doctrine. In what follows I will set out some of the relevant arguments, and urge doctors to reconsider their views on this matter.

To begin with a familiar type of situation, a patient who is dying of incurable cancer of the throat is in terrible pain, which can no longer be satisfactorily alleviated. He is certain to die within a few days, even if present treatment is continued, but he does not want to go on living for those days since the pain is unbearable. So he asks the doctor for an end to it, and his family joins in the request.

Suppose the doctor agrees to withhold treatment, as the conventional doctrine says he may. The justification for his doing so is that the patient is in terrible agony, and since he is going to die anyway, it would be wrong to prolong his suffering needlessly. But now notice this. If one simply withholds treatment, it may take the patient longer to die, and so he may suffer more than he would if more direct action were taken and a lethal injection given. This fact provides strong reason for thinking that, once the initial decision not to prolong his agony has been made, active euthanasia is actually preferable to passive euthanasia, rather than the reverse. To say otherwise is to endorse the option that leads to more suffering rather than less, and is contrary to the humanitarian impulse that prompts the decision not to prolong his life in the first place.

Part of my point is that the process of being "allowed to die" can be relatively slow and painful, whereas being given a lethal injection is relatively quick and painless. Let me give a different sort of example. In the United States about one in 600 babies is born with Down's syndrome. Most of these babies are otherwise healthy—that is, with only the usual pediatric care, they will proceed to an otherwise normal infancy. Some, however, are born with congenital defects such as intestinal obstructions that require operations if they are to live. Sometimes, the parents and the doctor will decide not to operate, and let the infant die. Anthony Shaw describes what happens then:

. . . When surgery is denied [the doctor] must try to keep the infant from suffering while natural forces sap the baby's life away. As a surgeon whose natural inclination is to use the scalpel to fight off death, standing by and watching a salvageable baby die is the most emotionally exhausting experience I know. It is easy at a conference, in a theoretical discussion, to decide that such infants should be allowed to die. It is altogether different to stand by in the nursery and watch as dehydration and infection wither a tiny being over hours and days. This is a terrible ordeal for me and the hospital staff—much more so than for the parents who never set foot in the nursery.[1]

I can understand why some people are opposed to all euthanasia, and insist that such infants must be allowed to live. I think I can also understand why other people favor destroying these babies quickly and painlessly. But why should anyone favor letting "dehydration and infection wither a tiny being over hours and days"? The doctrine that says that a baby may be allowed to dehydrate and wither, but may not be given an injection that would end its life without suffering, seems so patently cruel as to require no further refutation. The strong language is not intended to offend, but only to put the point in the clearest possible way.

My second argument is that the conventional doctrine leads to decisions concerning life and death made on irrelevant grounds.

Consider again the case of the infants with Down's syndrome who need operations for congenital defects unrelated to the syndrome to live. Sometimes, there is no operation, and the baby dies, but when there is no such defect, the baby lives on. Now, an operation such as that to remove an intestinal obstruction is not prohibitively difficult. The reason why such operations are not performed in these cases is, clearly, that the child has Down's syndrome and the parents and doctor judge that because of that fact it is better for the child to die.

But notice that this situation is absurd, no matter what view one takes of the lives and potentials of such babies. If the life of such an infant is worth preserving, what does it matter if it needs a simple operation? Or, if one thinks it better that such a baby should not live on, what difference does it make that it happens to have an unobstructed intestinal tract? In either case, the matter of life and death is being decided on irrelevant grounds. It is the Down's syndrome, and not the intestines, that is the issue. The matter should be decided, if at all, on that basis, and not be allowed to depend on the essentially irrelevant question of whether the intestinal tract is blocked.

What makes this situation possible, of course, is the idea that when there is an intestinal blockage, one can "let the baby die," but when there is no such defect there is nothing that can be done, for one must not "kill" it. The fact that this idea leads to such results as deciding life or death on irrelevant grounds is another good reason why the doctrine should be rejected.

One reason why so many people think that there is an important moral difference between active and passive euthanasia is that they think killing someone is morally worse than letting someone die. But is it? Is killing, in itself, worse than letting die? To investigate this issue, two cases may be considered that are exactly alike except that one involves killing whereas the other involves letting someone die. Then, it can be asked whether this difference makes any difference to the moral assessments. It is important that the cases be exactly alike, except for this one difference, since otherwise one cannot be confident that it is this difference and not some other that accounts for any variation in the assessments of the two cases. So, let us consider this pair of cases:

In the first, Smith stands to gain a large inheritance if anything should happen to his six-year-old cousin. One evening while the child is taking his bath, Smith sneaks into the bathroom and drowns the child, and then arranges things so that it will look like an accident.

In the second, Jones also stands to gain if anything should happen to his six-year-old cousin. Like Smith, Jones sneaks in planning to drown the child in his bath. However, just as he enters the bathroom Jones sees the child slip and hit his head, and fall face down in the water. Jones is delighted; he stands by, ready to push the child's head back under if it is necessary, but it is not necessary. With only a little thrashing about, the child drowns all by himself, "accidentally," as Jones watches and does nothing.

Now Smith killed the child, whereas Jones "merely" let the child die. That is the only difference between them. Did either man behave better, from a moral point of view? If the difference between killing and letting die were in itself a morally important matter, one should say that Jones's behavior was less reprehensible than Smith's. But does one really want to say that? I think not. In the first place, both men acted from the same motive, personal gain, and both had exactly the same end in view when they acted. It may be inferred from Smith's conduct that he is a bad man, although that judg-ment may be withdrawn or modified if certain further facts are learned about him—for example, that he is mentally deranged. But would not the very same thing be inferred about Jones from his conduct? And would not the same further considerations also be relevant to any modification of this judgment? Moreover, suppose Jones pleaded, in his own defense, "After all, I didn't do anything except just stand there and watch the child drown. I didn't kill him; I only let him die." Again, if letting die were in itself less bad than killing, this defense should have at least some weight. But it does not. Such a "defense" can only be regarded as a grotesque per-version of moral reasoning. Morally speaking, it is no defense at all.

Now, it may be pointed out, quite properly, that the cases of euthanasia with which doctors are concerned are not like this at all. They do not involve personal gain or the destruction of normal healthy children. Doctors are concerned only with cases in which the patient's life is of no further use to him, or in which the patient's life has become or will soon become a terrible burden. However, the point is the same in these cases: the bare difference between killing and letting die does not, in itself, make a moral difference. If a doctor lets a patient die, for humane reasons, he is in the same moral position as if he had given the patient a lethal injection for humane reasons. If his decision was wrong—if, for example, the patient's illness was in fact curable—the decision would be equally regrettable no matter which method was used to carry it out. And if the doctor's decision was the right one, the method used is not in itself important.

The AMA policy statement isolates the crucial issue very well; the crucial issue is "the intentional termination of the life of one human being by an-other." But after identifying this issue, and forbid-ding "mercy killing," the statement goes on to deny that the cessation of treatment is the intentional termination of a life. This is where the mistake comes in, for what is the cessation of treatment, in these circumstances, if it is not "the intentional ter-mination of the life of one human being by another"? Of course it is exactly that, and if it were not, there would be no point to it.

Many people will find this judgment hard to accept. One reason, I think, is that it is very easy to conflate the question of whether killing is, in itself, worse than letting die, with the very different ques-tion of whether most actual cases of killing are more reprehensible than most actual cases of letting die. Most actual cases of killing are clearly terrible (think, for example, of all the murders reported in the newspapers), and one hears of such cases every day. On the other hand, one hardly ever hears of a case of letting die, except for the actions of doctors who are motivated by humanitarian reasons. So one learns to think of killing in a much worse light than of letting die. But this does not mean that there is something about killing that makes it in itself worse than letting die, for it is not the bare difference between killing and letting die that makes the difference in these cases. Rather, the other factors—the murderer's motive of personal gain, for example, contrasted with the doctor's humanitarian motivation—account for different reactions to the different cases.

I have argued that killing is not in itself any worse than letting die; if my contention is right, it follows that active euthanasia is not any worse than passive euthanasia. What arguments can be given on the other side? The most common, I believe, is the following:

"The important difference between active and passive euthanasia is that, in passive euthanasia, the doctor does not do anything to bring about the patient's death. The doctor does nothing, and the patient dies of whatever ills already afflict him. In active euthanasia, however, the doctor does something to bring about the patient's death: he kills him. The doctor who gives the patient with cancer a lethal injection has himself caused his patient's death; whereas if he merely ceases treatment, the cancer is the cause of the death."

A number of points need to be made here. The first is that it is not exactly correct to say that in passive euthanasia the doctor does nothing, for he does do one thing that is very important: he lets the patient die. "Letting someone die" is certainly different, in some respects, from other types of action—mainly in that it is a kind of action that one may perform by way of not performing certain other actions. For example, one may let a patient die by way of not giving medication, just as one may insult someone by way of not shaking his hand. But for any purpose of moral assessment, it is a type of action nonetheless. The decision to let a patient die is subject to moral appraisal in the same way that a decision to kill him would be subject to moral appraisal: it may be assessed as wise or unwise, compassionate or sadistic, right or wrong. If a doctor

deliberately let a patient die who was suffering from a routinely curable illness, the doctor would certainly be to blame for what he had done, just as he would be to blame if he had needlessly killed the patient. Charges against him would then be appropriate. If so, it would be no defense at all for him to insist that he didn't "do anything." He would have done something very serious indeed, for he let his patient die.

Fixing the cause of death may be very important from a legal point of view, for it may determine whether criminal charges are brought against the doctor. But I do not think that this notion can be used to show a moral difference between active and passive euthanasia. The reason why it is considered bad to be the cause of someone's death is that death is regarded as a great evil—and so it is. However, if it has been decided that euthanasia—even passive euthanasia—is desirable in a given case, it has also been decided that in this instance death is no greater an evil than the patient's continued existence. And if this is true, the usual reason for not wanting to be the cause of someone's death simply does not apply.

Finally, doctors may think that all of this is only of academic interest—the sort of thing that philosophers may worry about but that has no practical bearing on their own work. After all, doctors must be concerned about the legal consequences of what they do, and active euthanasia is clearly forbidden by the law. But even so, doctors should also be concerned with the fact that the law is forcing upon them a moral doctrine that may well be indefensible, and has a considerable effect on their practices. Of course, most doctors are not now in the position of being coerced in this matter, for they do not regard themselves as merely going along with what the law requires. Rather, in statements such as the AMA policy statement that I have quoted, they are endorsing this doctrine as a central point of medical ethics. In that statement, active euthanasia is condemned not merely as illegal but as "contrary to that for which the medical profession stands," whereas passive euthanasia is approved. However, the preceding considerations suggest that there is really no moral difference between the two, considered in themselves (there may be important moral differences in some cases in their *consequences*, but, as I pointed out, these differences may make active euthanasia, and not passive euthanasia, the morally preferable option). So, whereas doctors may have

to discriminate between active and passive euthanasia to satisfy the law, they should not do any more
than that. In particular, they should not give the
distinction any added authority and weight by writing it into official statements of medical ethics.

Note

1. A. Shaw, "Doctor, Do We Have a Choice?" *The
    New York Times Magazine,* January 30, 1972, p. 54.

"It's Over, Debbie" and Two Commentaries

An anonymous medical resident tells of being called in the middle of the night to
attend to a twenty-year-old woman dying of ovarian cancer. The woman is in
distress and says to him "Let's get this over with." The resident injects her with
morphine, and she dies.

This is the first account of an apparent act of active euthanasia to appear in a
medical journal (*JAMA, Journal of the American Medical Association*). By the next
issue, *JAMA* had received more than 150 letters. By 4-to-1 writers condemned the
resident's act, and by 3-to-1 they held that *JAMA* should not have published the
piece. The story was carried by the national media and elicited a similar outpouring
of responses.

The authors of "Doctors Must Not Kill" condemn the action as immoral and
illegal and recommend that *JAMA* turn over all information to legal authorities. It
is not possible, they say, to have a value-free discussion about an act that violates
procedural safeguards protecting consent. The author of "Debbie's Dying" also
condemns the action but argues that in a restricted range of cases there is a place
for voluntary euthanasia.

The Chicago prosecutor's office requested the name of the author, but George
Lundberg, the editor of *JAMA*, refused to release it. A judge ruled that the journal
and its editor were protected by the First Amendment and the Illinois Reporters'
Act.

"It's Over, Debbie"

Anonymous

The call came in the middle of the night. As a gynecology resident rotating through a large, private
hospital, I had come to detest telephone calls, because invariably I would be up for several hours and
would not feel good the next day. However, duty
called, so I answered the phone. A nurse informed
me that a patient was having difficulty getting rest,
could I please see her. She was on 3 North. That was
the gynecologic oncology unit, not my usual duty
station. As I trudged along, bumping sleepily
against walls and corners and not believing I was up
again, I tried to imagine what I might find at the end
of my walk. Maybe an elderly woman with an anxiety reaction, or perhaps something particularly
horrible.

I grabbed the chart from the nurses station on
my way to the patient's room, and the nurse gave
me some hurried details: A 20-year-old girl named

Debbie was dying of ovarian cancer. She was having unrelenting vomiting, apparently as the result of an alcohol drip administered for sedation. Hmmm, I thought. Very sad. As I approached the room I could hear loud, labored breathing. I entered and saw an emaciated, dark-haired woman who appeared much older than 20. She was receiving nasal oxygen, had an IV, and was sitting in bed suffering from what was obviously severe air hunger. The chart noted her weight at 80 pounds. A second woman, also dark-haired but of middle age stood at her right, holding her hand. Both looked up as I entered. The room seemed filled with the patient's desperate effort to survive. Her eyes were hollow, and she had suprasternal and intercostal retractions with her rapid inspirations. She had not eaten or slept in two days. She had not responded to chemotherapy and was being given supportive care only. It was a gallows scene, a cruel mockery of her youth and unfulfilled potential. Her only words to me were, "Let's get this over with."

I retreated with my thoughts to the nurses station. The patient was tired and needed rest. I could not give her health, but I could give her rest. I asked the nurse to draw 20 mg of morphine sulfate into a syringe. Enough, I thought, to do the job. I took the syringe into the room and told the two women I was going to give Debbie something that would let her rest and to say good-bye. Debbie looked at the syringe, then laid her head on the pillow with her eyes open, watching what was left of the world. I injected the morphine intravenously and watched to see if my calculations on its effects would be correct. Within seconds her breathing slowed to a normal rate, her eyes closed, and her features softened as she seemed restful at last. The older woman stroked the hair of the now-sleeping patient. I waited for the inevitable next effect of depressing the respiratory drive. With clocklike certainty, within four minutes the breathing rate slowed even more, then became irregular, then ceased. The dark-haired woman stood erect and seemed relieved.

It's over, Debbie.

Name Withheld by Request

Commentary: "Doctors Must Not Kill" _____

Willard Gaylin, Leon R. Kass, Edmund D. Pellegrino, and Mark Siegler

In the middle of the night, a sleepy gynecology resident is called to attend a young woman, dying of cancer, whom he has never seen before. Horrified by her severe distress, and proceeding alone without consultation with anyone, he gives her a lethal injection of morphine, clearly intending the death that promptly ensues. The resident submits a first-person account of his killing to the *Journal of the American Medical Association*. Without any editorial comment, *JAMA* publishes the account, withholding the author's name at his request. What in the world is going on?

Before the sophisticated obscure our vision with clouds of arguments and subtle qualifications, we must fix our gaze on the brute facts.

First, on his own admission, the resident appears to have committed a felony: premeditated murder. Direct intentional homicide is a felony in all American jurisdictions, for which the plea of merciful motive is no excuse. That the homicide was clearly intentional is confirmed by the resident's act of unrepentant publication.

Second, law aside, the physician behaved altogether in a scandalously unprofessional and unethical manner. He did not know the patient: he had never seen her before, he did not study her chart, he did not converse with her or her family. He never spoke to *her* physician. He took as an unambiguous command her only words to him, "Let's get this over with": he did not bother finding out what precisely she meant or whether she meant it wholeheartedly. He did not consider alternative ways of bringing her relief or comfort; instead of comfort, he gave her death. This is no humane and thoughtful

Reprinted by permission. JAMA: Journal of the American Medical Association, *Apr. 8, 1988, Vol. 259, No. 14, pp. 2139–2140. Copyright 1988, American Medical Association.*

physician succumbing with fear and trembling to the pressures and well-considered wishes of a patient well known to him, for whom there was truly no other recourse. This is, by his own account, an impulsive yet cold technician, arrogantly masquerading as a knight of compassion and humanity. (Indeed, so cavalier is the report and so cold-blooded the behavior, it strains our credulity to think that the story is true.)

Third, law and professional manner both aside, the resident violated one of the first and most hallowed canons of the medical ethic: doctors must not kill. Generations of physicians and commentators on medical ethics have underscored and held fast to the distinction between ceasing useless treatments (or allowing to die) and active, willful taking of life; at least since the Oath of Hippocrates, Western medicine has regarded the killing of patients, even on request, as a profound violation of the deepest meaning of the medical vocation. As recently as 1986, the Judicial Council of the American Medical Association, in an opinion regarding treatment of dying patients, affirmed the principle that a physician "should not intentionally cause death." Neither legal tolerance nor the best bedside manner can ever make medical killing medically ethical.

The conduct of the physician is inexcusable. But the conduct of the editor of *JAMA* is incomprehensible. By publishing this report, he knowingly publicizes a felony and shields the felon. He deliberately publicizes the grossest medical malfeasance and shields the malefactor from professional scrutiny and judgment, presumably allowing him to continue his practices without possibility of rebuke and remonstrance, not even from the physician whose private patient he privately dispatched. Why? For what possible purpose central to *JAMA*'s professional mission?

According to newspaper reports, the editor of *JAMA* published the article "to promote discussion" of a timely and controversial topic. But is this a responsible way for the prestigious voice of our venerable profession to address the subject of medical killing? Is it morally responsible to promulgate challenges to our most fundamental moral principles without editorial rebuke or comment, "for the sake of discussion"? Decent folk do not deliberately stir discussion of outrageous practices, like slavery, incest, or killing those in our care.

What is to be done? Regarding the case at hand, the proper course is clear. *JAMA* should voluntarily turn all the information it has regarding the case over to the legal authorities in the pertinent jurisdictions. The physician's name should also be reported to his hospital directors and to his state and county medical societies for their scrutiny and action. The Council on Ethical and Judicial Affairs of the American Medical Association should examine the case, as well as the decision to publish it. Justice requires nothing less.

But much more is at stake than punishing an offender. The very soul of medicine is on trial. For this is not one of those peripheral issues about which pluralism and relativism can be tolerated, about which a value-free stand on the substance can be hedged around with procedural safeguards to ensure informed consent or "sound decision-making." Nor is this an issue, like advertising, fee-splitting, or cooperation with chiropractors, that touches medicine only as a trade. This issue touches medicine at its very moral center; if this moral center collapses, if physicians become killers or are even merely licensed to kill, the profession—and, therewith, each physician—will never again be worthy of trust and respect as healer and comforter and protector of life in all its frailty. For if medicine's power over life may be used equally to heal or to kill, the doctor is no more a moral professional but rather a morally neutered technician.

These are perilous times for our profession. The Hemlock Society and others are in the courts and legislatures trying to legalize killing by physicians at patient request. Such a proposal is almost certainly going to be on the ballot in California next November. High costs of care for the old and incurable already tempt some physicians to regard as "dispensable" some patients who never express the wish to die. In the Netherlands, where the barriers to physician killing are gone, there are now many well-documented cases of such cryptic and "uninvited" killing by doctors.[1]

Now is not the time for promoting neutral discussion. Rather, now is the time for the medical profession to rally in defense of its fundamental moral principles, to repudiate any and all acts of direct and intentional killing by physicians and their agents. We call on the profession and its leadership to obtain the best advice, regarding both theory and practice, about how to defend the profession's moral center and to resist growing pressures both from without and from within. We call on fellow physicians to say that we will not deliberately kill. We must say also to each of our fellow physicians that we will not tolerate killing of patients and that we shall take disciplinary action against doctors who kill. And we must say to the broader community that if it insists on tolerating or legalizing active euthanasia, it will have to find nonphysicians to do its killing.

Note

1.   Fenigsen R: *Euthanasie: Een Weldaad (Charitable Euthanasia)*. Deventer, the Netherlands: Van Loghum Slaterus, 1987.

Commentary: Debbie's Dying: Mercy Killing and the Good Death

Kenneth L. Vaux

Most of the condemnatory response to "It's Over, Debbie"[1] has rightly claimed that what (apparently) transpired that night was unconscionable. One does not stumble angrily into the night and decide profound matters of life and death for another human being. This strange narrative does not tell us whether Debbie wanted simply to be relieved of pain or released from intolerable suffering; whether the family consented or what the nurses or chaplains on call advised; or whether the attending or primary physician, if one existed, authorized the action. The whole process, from beginning to end, was morally unacceptable.

A deeper question, however, lies behind the widespread interest in this one reprehensible action—the question that troubles us all. As I lie dying, will I be offered humane care, will I be done in too soon by some expediency, or will I be subjected to terminal torture?

Euthanasia does not refer to Nazi-like elimination of the sick, old, or unproductive, and, because it lacks any account of patient consent, "It's Over, Debbie" is in no way an accurate representation of any form of euthanasia. Traditionally, euthanasia means the search for a good death, an easier death for one who is dying, a death released in some measure from intractable suffering. It assumes and requires the patient's unequivocal request and the consent of the family. Our best medical and religious traditions accept euthanasia when it assists the person who is imminently dying toward a less devastating and more peaceful demise. Passive euthanasia *often*, double-effect euthanasia *sometimes*, and active euthanasia *rarely* have become established as a morally acceptable continuum of action in our ethical tradition.

One reading of this ambiguous and melodramatic diary suggests that Debbie's case may be one of *double-effect* euthanasia: the patient died as a result of medication given in an attempt to relieve pain and with the knowledge that it would hasten death. Morphine is not normally a poison but an analgesic drug, and 20 mg is scarcely a murderous dose. The physician could not possibly have known with the brash confidence that his narrative displays that his injection would kill. More likely, he sought to provide relief and rest to this dying young woman, knowing that it would speed her death. In the pursuit of a legitimate, indeed obligatory, purpose of relieving suffering, he shortened the remaining hours of her life. If this is a true rendition of Debbie's case, it represents an instance of morally acceptable double-effect euthanasia (or what is technically called *agathanasia*, a better death). The side effect is unfortunate, indeed grievous, but it is not unethical.

The President's Commission report on *Decisions to Forego Life-Sustaining Treatment*[2] and many cancer care texts hold that it is permissible to use analgesic treatment for end-stage cancer pain and respiratory distress even if it hastens death. As the President's Commission report states,

> No death is more agonizing for the aware patient . . . than one from respiratory insufficiency. Untreated, the patient will struggle for air until exhausted, when carbon dioxide narco-

Reprinted by permission. JAMA: Journal of the American Medical Association, *Apr. 8, 1988, Vol. 259, No. 14, pp. 2140–2141. Copyright 1988, American Medical Association.*

sis and progressive hypoxia finally bring death fairly quickly. With the consent of the family morphine may be given. . . . If the patient is already quite exhausted, the slowed respirations will induce hypercapnia, which will perpetuate the sedation and the patient will die in the ensuing sleep.

What about intentional mercy killing—active and direct euthanasia? Is such action ever medically or ethically acceptable? Even if it is proscribed, can it be excused from legal prosecution or professional censure? Down through the ages, when the patient and physician have established a clear understanding and the physician's desire has been to relieve the patient's incurable pain, most cases of mercy killing have been excused by virtue of the spirit rather than the letter of the law. In all noble jurisprudence and even more in the ethics of caring for the dying, absolutist principles must always be chastened by mercy.

I argue that while positive euthanasia must be proscribed in principle, in exceptional cases it may be abided in deed. There has always been a place, albeit carefully restricted to a limited range of cases, for voluntary euthanasia. From classical times throughout the Christian centuries and into modern secular society, this allowance has always existed alongside the dominant ethic of prolonging and sustaining life. There are numerous cases today in the medical and legal case files in which active euthanasia has been reluctantly allowed and the physicians involved have not been prosecuted. In his classic of medical ethics, *The Patient as Person*,[3] Paul Ramsey, PhD, a spokesman for traditional ethics, makes unrelenting cancer pain an exception to the dominant ethic of "doing nothing to place the dying more quickly beyond our love and care." Here, "one can hardly be held morally blameworthy if in these instances dying is directly accomplished or hastened."

Philosophical ethics aside, the most moving evidence I have witnessed for this viewpoint in my 25 years as a consultant in medical ethics is the testimony of highly ethical and humane physicians. Although impeded by law and custom from giving a lethal dose to their patient, these physicians would, in fact, do so even at risk of prosecution for their wife or father or child if the patient was suffering in such end-of-life agony as Debbie.

That physicians and nurses would request euthanasia of their colleagues or would assist their own loved ones to have a more merciful death but would deny it to their patients says something about the moral nature of the act. Such loving acts illustrate a kind of "exception" ethic that has a place in the tradition of alleviating suffering.

The position of "exceptional-case" active euthanasia is grounded in classical clinical wisdom. In the Hippocratic tradition, the physician was discouraged from therapeutically or technologically invading the atrium of death. Attempts to cure had to yield to attempts to comfort. An ethical principle that later transformed Western medicine held that the living ought never to be treated as if they were dying, nor the dying as if they were living. To know the difference entailed discerning the *signum Hippocraticum* (the signs of mortality).

In recent years the qualities that morally distinguished the living from the dying have been blurred. With our life-prolonging techniques and medications, we have transformed death; we have taken it out of the acute, natural, and non-interventional mode and made it more into a chronic, contrived, and manipulated phenomenon. Deaths as inevitable as Debbie's have been protracted by a range of interventions, including chemotherapy (disrupting the cellular-pathogenic process), analgesia (altering the release of natural body endorphins and narcotics), the administration of intravenous fluids and nutrients, and hospitalization itself. Logically and emotionally, we cannot intervene at one phase and then be inactive at another, more painful phase. We cannot modify nature and then plead that nature must be allowed to run its unhindered course.

Medicine is a pastoral art, especially when a good physician, like a good shepherd, accompanies a patient "into the valley of the shadow." Here the dying one must indeed "fear no evil," either the evil of weary dispatch or of principled withdrawal.

Where does this leave us? The outrage of Debbie's case reminds us that we must never abandon the cardinal purpose of medical care—to save and sustain life and never intentionally to harm or kill. The other lesson of this case is that we must not destroy the virtue of that commitment by using medical art to prolong dying and puritanically refuse to relieve suffering. This distortion is very possible today, when technological prowess is joined to low rates of bed occupancy and economic distress in hospitals and when our society tends to deny the inevitability of death. If biomedical acts of life extension become acts of death prolongation, we may force some patients to outlive their deaths, and we may ultimately repudiate the primary life-saving and merciful ethic itself.

Notes

1. It's over Debbie, A PIECE OF MY MIND. *JAMA* 1988; 259:272.

2. Supportive care for dying patients, in *Decisions to Forego Life-Sustaining Treatment*. President's Commission for the Study of Ethical Problems in Medicine and Biomedical and Behavioral Research, 1983, pp. 294–295.

3. Ramsey, P., *The Patient as Person*. New Haven, Conn.: Yale University Press, 1983, p. 163.

In the Matter of Karen Quinlan, an Alleged Incompetent

The Supreme Court of New Jersey

The 1976 decision of the New Jersey Supreme Court in the case of Karen Quinlan was significant in establishing that a legally based right of privacy permits a patient to decide to refuse medical treatment. The court also held that this right can be exercised by a parent or guardian when the patient herself is in no position to do so. Thus, in the opinion of the court, removal of life-sustaining equipment would not be a case of homicide (or any other kind of wrongful killing), even if the patient should die as a result.

The ruling in the *Quinlan* case has had an enormous impact on decisions about discontinuing extraordinary medical measures. However, the ruling has been generally construed rather narrowly so as to apply only to mentally incompetent patients who are brain-dead, comatose, or in an irreversible coma.

Background Note. The decision of the court was issued on March 31, 1976. It was delivered by Chief Justice Hughes. The following abridgment omits references and case citations.

Constitutional and Legal Issues

I. The Free Exercise of Religion

Simply stated, the right to religious beliefs is absolute but conduct in pursuance thereof is not wholly immune from governmental restraint. So it is that, for the sake of life, courts sometimes (but not always) order blood transfusions for Jehovah's Witnesses (whose religious beliefs abhor such procedure), forbid exposure to death from handling virulent snakes or ingesting poison (interfering with deeply held religious sentiments in such regard), and protect the public health as in the case of com-

pulsory vaccination (over the strongest of religious objections). . . . The Public interest is thus considered paramount, without essential dissolution of respect for religious beliefs.

We think, without further examples, that, ranged against the State's interest in the preservation of life, the impingement of religious belief, much less religious "neutrality" as here, does not reflect a constitutional question, in the circumstances at least of the case presently before the Court. Moreover, like the trial court, we do not recognize an independent parental right of religious freedom to support the relief requested.

II. Cruel and Unusual Punishment

Similarly inapplicable to the case before us is the Constitution's Eighth Amendment protection

From In the Matter of Karen Quinlan, an Alleged Incompetent. *Supreme Court of New Jersey, 70 N.J. 10, 355 A. 2d 647.*

against cruel and unusual punishment which, as held by the trial court, is not relevant to situations other than the imposition of penal sanctions. Historic in nature, it stemmed from punitive excesses in the infliction of criminal penalties. We find no precedent in law which would justify its extension to the correction of social injustice or hardship, such as, for instance, in the case of poverty. The latter often condemns the poor and deprived to horrendous living conditions which could certainly be described in the abstract as "cruel and unusual punishment." Yet the constitutional base of protection from "cruel and unusual punishment" is plainly irrelevant to such societal ills which must be remedied, if at all, under other concepts of constitutional and civil right.

So it is in the case of the unfortunate Karen Quinlan. Neither the State, nor the law, but the accident of fate and nature, has inflicted upon her conditions which though in essence cruel and most unusual, yet do not amount to "punishment" in any constitutional sense.

Neither the judgment of the court below, nor the medical decision which confronted it, nor the law and equity perceptions which impelled its action, nor the whole factual base upon which it was predicated, inflicted "cruel and unusual punishment" in the constitutional sense.

III. The Right of Privacy

It is the issue of the constitutional right of privacy that has given us most concern, in the exceptional circumstances of this case. Here a loving parent, *qua* parent and raising the rights of his incompetent and profoundly damaged daughter, probably irreversibly doomed to no more than a biologically vegetative remnant of life, is before the court. He seeks authorization to abandon specialized technological procedures which can only maintain for a time a body having no potential for resumption or continuance of other than a "vegetative" existence.

We have no doubt, in these unhappy circumstances, that if Karen were herself miraculously lucid for an interval (not altering the existing prognosis of the condition to which she would soon return) and perceptive of her irreversible condition, she could effectively decide upon discontinuance of the life-support apparatus, even if it meant the prospect of natural death. To this extent we may distinguish [a case] which concerned a severely injured young woman (Delores Heston), whose life depended on surgery and blood transfusion; and who was in such extreme shock that she was unable to express an informed choice (although the Court apparently considered the case as if the patient's own religious decision to resist transfusion were at stake), but most importantly a patient apparently salvable to long life and vibrant health;—a situation not at all like the present case.

We have no hesitancy in deciding, in the instant diametrically opposite case, that no external compelling interest of the State could compel Karen to endure the unendurable, only to vegetate a few measurable months with no realistic possibility of returning to any semblance of cognitive or sapient life. We perceive no thread of logic distinguishing between such a choice on Karen's part and a similar choice which, under the evidence in this case, could be made by a competent patient terminally ill, riddled by cancer and suffering great pain; such a patient would not be resuscitated or put on a respirator in the example described by Dr. Korein, and *a fortiori* would not be kept *against his will* on a respirator.

Although the Constitution does not explicitly mention a right of privacy, Supreme Court decisions have recognized that a right of personal privacy exists and that certain areas of privacy are guaranteed under the Constitution. The Court has interdicted judicial intrusion into many aspects of personal decision, sometimes basing this restraint upon the conception of a limitation of judicial interest and responsibility, such as with regard to contraception and its relationship to family life and decision.

The Court in *Griswold* found the unwritten constitutional right of privacy to exist in the penumbra of specific guarantees of the Bill of Rights "formed by emanations from those guarantees that help give them life and substance." Presumably this right is broad enough to encompass a patient's decision to decline medical treatment under certain circumstances, in much the same way as it is broad enough to encompass a woman's decision to terminate pregnancy under certain conditions.

The claimed interests of the State in this case are essentially the preservation and sanctity of human life and defense to the right of the physician to administer medical treatment according to his best judgment. In this case the doctors say that removing Karen from the respirator will conflict with their professional judgment. The plaintiff answers that Karen's present treatment serves only a maintenance function; that the respirator cannot cure or improve her condition but at best can only prolong her inevitable slow deterioration and death; and that the interests of the patient, as seen by her surrogate, the guardian, must be evaluated by the court as predominant, even in the face of an option *contra* by the present attending physicians. Plaintiff's distinction is significant. The nature of Karen's care and the realistic chances of her recovery are quite unlike those of the patients discussed in many of the cases where treatments were ordered. In many of those cases the medical procedure required (usually a transfusion) constituted a minimal bodily invasion and the chances of recovery and return to functioning life were very good. We think that the State's interest *contra* weakens and the individual's right to privacy grows as the degree of bodily invasion increases and the prognosis dims. Ultimately there comes a point at which the individual's rights overcome the State interest. It is for that reason that we believe Karen's choice, if she were competent to make it, would be vindicated by the law. Her prognosis is extremely poor,—she will never resume cognitive life. And the bodily invasion is very great,—she requires 24-hour intensive nursing care, antibiotics, and the assistance of a respirator, a catheter and feeding tube.

Our affirmance of Karen's independent right of choice, however, would ordinarily be based upon her competency to assert it. The sad truth, however, is that she is grossly incompetent and we cannot discern her supposed choice based on the testimony of her previous conversation with friends, where such testimony is without sufficient probative weight. Nevertheless we have concluded that Karen's right of privacy may be asserted on her behalf by her guardian under the peculiar circumstances here present.

If a putative decision by Karen to permit this non-cognitive, vegetative existence to terminate by natural forces is regarded as a valuable incident of her right of privacy, as we believe it to be, then it should not be discarded solely on the basis that her condition prevents her conscious exercise of the choice. The only practical way to prevent destruction of the right is to permit the guardian and family of Karen to render their best judgment, subject to

the qualifications hereinafter stated, as to whether she would exercise it in these circumstances. If their conclusion is in the affirmative this decision should be accepted by a society the overwhelming majority of whose members would, we think, in similar circumstances, exercise such a choice in the same way for themselves or for those closest to them. It is for this reason that we determine that Karen's right of privacy may be asserted in her behalf, in this respect, by her guardian and family under the particular circumstances presented by this record. [Sections IV (Medical Factors), V (Alleged Criminal Liability), and VI (Guardianship of the Person) omitted.]

Declaratory Relief

We thus arrive at the formulation of the declaratory relief which we have concluded is appropriate to this case. Some time has passed since Karen's physical and mental condition was described to the Court. At that time her continuing deterioration was plainly projected. Since the record has not been expanded we assume that she is now even more fragile and nearer to death than she was then. Since her present treating physicians may give reconsideration to her present posture in the light of this opinion, and since we are transferring to the plaintiff as guardian the choice of the attending physician and therefore other physicians may be in charge of the case who may take a different view from that of the present attending physicians, we herewith declare the following affirmative relief on behalf of the plaintiff. Upon the concurrence of the guardian and family of Karen, should the responsible attending physicians conclude that there is no reasonable possibility of Karen's ever emerging from her present comatose condition to a cognitive, sapient state and that the life-support apparatus now being administered to Karen should be discontinued, they shall consult with the hospital "Ethics Committee" or like body of the institution in which Karen is then hospitalized. If that consultative body agrees that there is no reasonable possibility of Karen's ever emerging from her present comatose condition to a cognitive, sapient state, the present life-support system may be withdrawn and said action shall be without any civil or criminal liability therefor on the part of any participant, whether guardian, physician, hospital or others. We herewith specifically so hold.

United States Supreme Court Decision in the
Cruzan Case

This is the first decision by the Supreme Court addressing the "right to die" issue. By 5-to-4, the Court rejected the petition of the parents of Nancy Cruzan, a comatose patient, that Missouri's standard for determining the wishes of a mentally incompetent patient be ruled unconstitutional. (For discussion and background details, see earlier *Social Context: The Cruzan Case*.)

Chief Justice William Rehnquist, author of the majority opinion, finds a basis in the common law and in the Fourteenth Amendment for an individual's refusing medical treatment. Where a comatose person is concerned, wishes can be ascertained only indirectly, and Rehnquist and the rest of the majority hold that it is not unconstitutional for states to determine what standard of evidence must be met. In pursuing the legitimate state interest of protecting life, Missouri errs on the side of caution. This is acceptable for it preserves the status quo, whereas an error in the other direction cannot be remedied.

Justice William J. Brennan, in a dissenting opinion, argues that there can be no state interest in keeping Nancy Cruzan alive. Further, maintaining the status quo may produce definite harm. It may force patients to receive medical treatment they would reject, were they able.

Justice John Paul Stevens, in another dissenting opinion, argues that the Court's abstract interest acknowledging the legitimate interest of the state in protecting life ignores the best interest of Nancy Cruzan. This is where the focus should have been, not on her past statements about her wishes. By not making this the issue, the Court is limiting the constitutional right to be free of medical treatment to those who have the foresight to express their wishes while competent.

William Rehnquist: Court Opinion

Petitioner Nancy Beth Cruzan was rendered incompetent as a result of severe injuries sustained during an automobile accident. Co-petitioners Lester and Joyce Cruzan, Nancy's parents and co-guardians, sought a court order directing the withdrawal of their daughter's artificial feeding and hydration equipment after it became apparent that she had virtually no chance of recovering her cognitive faculties. The Supreme Court of Missouri held that because there was no clear and convincing evidence of Nancy's desire to have life-sustaining treatment withdrawn under such circumstances, her parents lacked authority to effectuate such a request. . . .

After it had become apparent that Nancy Cruzan had virtually no chance of regaining her mental faculties her parents asked hospital employees to terminate the artificial nutrition and hydration procedures. All agree that such a removal would cause her death. The employees refused to honor the request without court approval. The parents then sought and received authorization from

United States Supreme Court, Cruzan v. Director, Missouri Dept. of Health, *U.S. 580 SLW 4916.*
June 25, 1990.

the state trial court for termination. The court found that a person in Nancy's condition had a fundamental right under the State and Federal Constitutions to refuse or direct the withdrawal of "death prolonging procedures." The court also found that Nancy's "expressed thoughts at age 25 in somewhat serious conversation with a housemate friend that if sick or injured she would not wish to continue her life unless she could live at least halfway normally" suggests that given her present condition she would not wish to continue on with her nutrition and hydration.

Missouri Court's Decision

The Supreme Court of Missouri reversed by a divided vote. The court recognized a right to refuse treatment embodied in the common-law doctrine of informed consent, but expressed skepticism about the application of that doctrine in the circumstances of this case. . . . The court also declined to read a broad right of privacy into the State Constitution which would "support the right of a person to refuse medical treatment in every circumstance," and expressed doubt as to whether such a right existed under the United States Constitution. It then decided that the Missouri Living Will statute embodied a state policy strongly favoring the preservation of life. The court found that Cruzan's statements to her roommate regarding her desire to live or die under certain conditions were "unreliable for the purpose of determining her intent," "and thus insufficient to support the co-guardians' claim to exercise substituted judgment on Nancy's behalf." . . .

We granted *certiorari* to consider the question of whether Cruzan has a right under the United States Constitution which would require the hospital to withdraw life-sustaining treatment from her under these circumstances.

At common law, even the touching of one person by another without consent and without legal justification was a battery.

The logical corollary of the doctrine of informed consent is that the patient generally possesses the right not to consent, that is, to refuse treatment. Until about 15 years ago and the seminal decision in *In re Quinlan*, 70 N.J. 10, the number of right-to-refuse-treatment decisions were relatively few. . . .

More recently, however, with the advance of medical technology capable of sustaining life well past the point where natural forces would have brought certain death in earlier times, cases involving the right to refuse life-sustaining treatment have burgeoned. . . .

Doctrine of Informed Consent

As these cases demonstrate, the common-law doctrine of informed consent is viewed as generally encompassing the right of a competent individual to refuse medical treatment. Beyond that, these decisions demonstrate both similarity and diversity in their approach to decision of what all agree is a perplexing question with unusually strong moral and ethical overtones. State courts have available to them for decision a number of sources—state constitutions, statutes, and common law—which are not available to us.

In this Court, the question is simply and starkly whether the United States Constitution prohibits Missouri from choosing the rule of decision which it did. This is the first case in which we have been squarely presented with the issue of whether the United States Constitution grants what is in common parlance referred to as a "right to die."

The 14th Amendment provides that no state shall "deprive any person of life, liberty, or property, without due process of law." The principle that a competent person has a constitutionally protected liberty interest in refusing unwanted medical treatment may be inferred from our prior decisions. . . .

Just this term, in the course of holding that a state's procedures for administering antipsychotic medication to prisoners were sufficient to satisfy due process concerns, we recognized that prisoners possess "a significant liberty interest in avoiding the unwanted administration of antipsychotic drugs under the Due Process Clause of the 14th Amendment." *Washington* v. *Harper*, (1990) . . .

But determining that a person has a "liberty interest" under the Due Process Clause* does not end the inquiry; "whether respondent's constitutional rights have been violated must be determined by balancing his liberty interests against the relevant state interests."

*Although many state courts have held that a right to refuse treatment is encompassed by a generalized constitutional right of privacy, we have never so held. We believe this issue is more properly analyzed in terms of a 14th Amendment liberty interest.

Forced Medical Treatment

Petitioners insist that under the general holdings of our cases, the forced administration of life-sustaining medical treatment, and even of artificially delivered food and water essential to life, would implicate a competent person's liberty interest. Although we think the logic of the cases discussed above would embrace such a liberty interest, the dramatic consequences involved in refusal of such treatment would inform the inquiry as to whether the deprivation of that interest is constitutionally permissible. But for purposes of this case, we assume that the United States Constitution would grant a competent person a constitutionally protected right to refuse life-saving hydration and nutrition.

Petitioners go on to assert that an incompetent person should possess the same right in this respect as is possessed by a competent person. . . .

The difficulty with petitioners' claim is that in a sense it begs the question: an incompetent person is not able to make an informed and voluntary choice to exercise a hypothetical right to refuse treatment or any other right. Such a "right" must be exercised for her, if at all, by some sort of surrogate. Here, Missouri has in effect recognized that under certain circumstances a surrogate may act for the patient in electing to have hydration and nutrition withdrawn in such a way as to cause death, but it has established a procedural safeguard to assure that the action of the surrogate conforms as best it may to the wishes expressed by the patient while competent.

Missouri requires that evidence of the incompetent's wishes as to the withdrawal of treatment be proved by clear and convincing evidence. The question, then, is whether the United States Constitution forbids the establishment of this procedural requirement by the state. We hold that it does not.

Whether or not Missouri's clear and convincing evidence requirement comports with the United States Constitution depends in part on what interests the state may properly seek to protect in this situation. Missouri relies on its interest in the protection and preservation of human life, and there can be no gainsaying this interest. As a general matter, the states—indeed, all civilized nations—demonstrate their commitment to life by treating homicide as serious crime. Moreover, the majority of states in this country have laws imposing criminal penalties on one who assists another to commit suicide. We do not think a state is required to remain neutral in the face of an informed and voluntary decision by a physically able adult to starve to death.

Heightened Evidentiary Requirements

But in the context presented here, a state has more particular interests at stake. The choice between life and death is a deeply personal decision of obvious and overwhelming finality. We believe Missouri may legitimately seek to safeguard the personal element of this choice through the imposition of heightened evidentiary requirements. It cannot be disputed that the Due Process Clause protects an interest in life as well as an interest in refusing life-sustaining medical treatment. Not all incompetent patients will have loved ones available to serve as surrogate decision makers. . . .

In our view, Missouri has permissibly sought to advance these interests through the adoption of a "clear and convincing" standard of proof to govern such proceedings. . . .

In sum, we conclude that a state may apply a clear and convincing evidence standard in proceedings where a guardian seeks to discontinue nutrition and hydration of a person diagnosed to be in a persistent vegetative state. . . .

The Supreme Court of Missouri held that in this case the testimony adduced at trial did not amount to clear and convincing proof of the patient's desire to have hydration and nutrition withdrawn. . . .

No doubt is engendered by anything in this record but that Nancy Cruzan's mother and father are loving and caring parents. If the state were required by the United States Constitution to repose a right of "substituted judgment" with anyone, the Cruzans would surely qualify. But we do not think the Due Process Clause requires the state to repose judgment on these matters with anyone but the patient herself. Close family members may have a strong feeling—a feeling not at all ignoble or unworthy, but not entirely disinterested, either—that they do not wish to witness the continuation of the life of a loved one which they regard as hopeless, meaningless and even degrading. But there is no automatic assurance that the view of close family members will necessarily be the same as the patient's would have been had she been confronted with the prospect of her situation while competent. All of the reasons previously discussed for allowing Missouri to require clear and convincing evidence of the patient's wishes lead us to conclude that the state may choose to defer only to those wishes, rather than confide the decision to close family members.

William Brennan: Dissenting Opinion

The question before this Court is a relatively narrow one: whether the Due Process Clause allows Missouri to require a now-incompetent patient in an irreversible persistent vegetative state to remain on life-support absent rigorously clear and convincing evidence that avoiding the treatment represents the patient's prior, express choice. If a fundamental right is at issue, Missouri's rule of decision must be scrutinized under the standards this Court has always applied in such circumstances. . . .

There are also affirmative reasons why someone like Nancy might choose to forgo artificial nutrition and hydration under these circumstances. Dying is personal. And it is profound. For many, the thought of an ignoble end, steeped in decay, is abhorrent. A quiet, proud death, bodily integrity intact, is a matter of extreme consequence. . . .

Although the right to be free of unwanted medical intervention, like other constitutionally protected interests, may not be absolute, no state interest could outweigh the rights of an individual in Nancy Cruzan's position. Whatever a state's possible interests in mandating life-support treatment under other circumstances, there is no good to be obtained here by Missouri's insistence that Nancy Cruzan remain on life-support systems if it is indeed her wish not to do so. Missouri does not claim, nor could it, that society as a whole will be benefited by Nancy's receiving medical treatment. No third party's situation will be improved and no harm to others will be averted.

The only state interest asserted here is a general interest in the preservation of life. But the state has no legitimate general interest in someone's life, completely abstracted from the interest of the person living that life, that could outweigh the person's choice to avoid medical treatment. . . . Thus, the state's general interest in life must accede to Nancy Cruzan's particularized and intense interest in self-determination in her choice of medical treatment. There is simply nothing legitimately within the state's purview to be gained by superseding her decision.

John Paul Stevens: Dissenting Opinion

Our Constitution is born of the proposition that all legitimate governments must secure the equal right of every person to "life, liberty, and the pursuit of happiness." In the ordinary case we quite naturally assume that these three ends are compatible, mutually enhancing and perhaps even coincident.

The Court would make an exception here. It permits the state's abstract, undifferentiated interest in the preservation of life to overwhelm the best interests of Nancy Beth Cruzan, interests which would, according to an undisputed finding, be served by allowing her guardians to exercise her constitutional right to discontinue medical treatment.

Ironically, the Court reaches this conclusion despite endorsing three significant propositions which should save it from any such dilemma. First, a competent individual's decision to refuse life-sustaining medical procedures is an aspect of liberty protected by the Due Process Clause of the 14th Amendment. Second, upon a proper evidentiary showing, a qualified guardian may make that decision on behalf of an incompetent ward. Third, in answering the important question presented by this tragic case, it is wise "not to attempt by any general statement, to cover every possible phase of the subject." Together, these considerations suggest that Nancy Cruzan's liberty to be free from medical treatment must be understood in light of the facts and circumstances particular to her.

I would so hold: in my view, the Constitution requires the state to care for Nancy Cruzan's life in a way that gives appropriate respect to her own best interests.

This case is the first in which we consider whether, and how, the Constitution protects the liberty of seriously ill patients to be free from life-sustaining medical treatment. So put, the question is both general and profound. We need not, however, resolve the question in the abstract. Our responsibility as judges both enables and compels us to treat the problem as it is illuminated by the facts of the controversy before us. . . .

Best Interest of the Patient

The portion of this Court's opinion that considers the merits of this case is similarly unsatisfactory. It, too, fails to respect the best interest of the patient. It, too, relies on what is tantamount to a waiver rationale: the dying patient's best interests are put to one side and the entire inquiry is focused on her prior expressions of intent.

An innocent person's constitutional right to be free from unwanted medical treatment is thereby categorically limited to those patients who had the foresight to make an unambiguous statement of their wishes while competent. The Court's decision affords no protection to children, to young people who are victims of unexpected accidents or illnesses, or to the countless thousands of elderly persons who either fail to decide, or fail to explain, how they want to be treated if they should experience a similar fate.

Because Nancy Beth Cruzan did not have the foresight to preserve her constitutional right in a living will, or some comparable "clear and convincing" alternative, her right is gone forever and her fate is in the hands of the state Legislature instead of in those of her family, her independent neutral guardian ad litem, and an impartial judge— all of whom agree on the course of action that is in her best interests. The Court's willingness to find a waiver of this constitutional right reveals a distressing misunderstanding of the importance of individual liberty. . . .

Only because Missouri has arrogated to itself the power to define life, and only because the Court permits this usurpation, are Nancy Cruzan's life and liberty put into disquieting conflict. If Nancy Cruzan's life were defined by reference to her own interests, so that her life expired when her biological existence ceased serving any of her own interests, then her constitutionally protected interest in freedom from unwanted treatment would not come into conflict with her constitutionally protected interest in life.

Conversely, if there were any evidence that Nancy Cruzan herself defined life to encompass every form of biological persistence by a human being, so that the continuation of treatment would serve Nancy's own liberty, then once again there would be no conflict between life and liberty. The opposition of life and liberty in this case are thus not the result of Nancy Cruzan's tragic accident, but are instead the artificial consequence of Missouri's effort, and this Court's willingness, to abstract Nancy Cruzan's life from Nancy Cruzan's person. . . .

The Right to Death ———————————————

Ronald Dworkin

Commentators about the Supreme Court's decision in *Cruzan* say the Court recognized a "right to die," but Ronald Dworkin questions this. Rehnquist stressed that the right was assumed only hypothetically and that the question of whether the state's duty to protect life could be set aside by even a competent person's decision was an open one. Dworkin focuses on Rehnquist's two arguments supporting the ruling opinion that states can require "clear and convincing evidence" that a person would prefer death to being maintained in a chronic vegetative condition.

In the argument that the state has a duty to protect individuals, Dworkin finds the question begging. It invokes the "implausible assumption" that continuing life is an advantage under any conditions, but this ignores the fact that people also care about dignity, the perceptions of others, and the burdens and costs imposed on friends, family, and society.

The second argument holds that the state may impose requirements concerning medical treatment, even though they go against the interest of some individuals, because of the state's interest in protecting life. Dworkin claims Rehnquist goes far beyond the usual notion that the state must protect its citizens from harm. States recognize that competent people may refuse treatment, so Rehnquist must justify forcing patients to accept medical treatment when they or their guardians think they would be better off dead. The support of this view offered by Scalia is based on the legal tradition that suicide is wrong. Dworkin finds the grounds for the traditional view questionable and the notion that suicide is involved in *Cruzan* "bizarre."

To support his position, Rehnquist must hold that life is of intrinsic value. The religious view that life is from God and we cannot choose to end it cannot be appealed to in resolving a constitutional question, and Dworkin reviews two secular arguments supporting the idea. He concludes that neither offers grounds for keeping a comatose patient alive. He predicts, however, that future discussions of the issue will focus on the intrinsic-value question.

1.

The tragedy of Nancy Cruzan's life is now part of American constitutional law. Before her automobile accident in 1983, she was an energetic twenty-four-year-old recently married woman. Her injuries deprived her brain of oxygen for fourteen minutes, and left her in what doctors describe as a permanent vegetative state. Only the lower part of her brain stem continued to function. She was unconscious and oblivious to the environment, though she had reflexive responses to sound and perhaps to painful stimuli. She was fed and hydrated through tubes implanted in her stomach, and other machines performed her other bodily functions. She was washed and turned regularly, but all of her limbs were contracted and her fingernails cut into her wrists.

For months after the accident her parents and her then husband pressed doctors to do everything possible to restore her to some kind of life. But when it became plain that she would remain in a vegetative state until she died, which might mean for thirty more years, her parents, who had become her legal guardians, asked the state hospital to remove the tubes and allow her to die at once. Since the hospital refused to do so without a court order, the parents petitioned a Missouri court, which appointed a guardian *ad litem* (a special guardian appointed to represent her in these proceedings) to offer arguments why it should not grant that order. After a hearing the court granted the order on the ground that it was in Cruzan's best interests to be permitted to die with some dignity now rather than to live on in an unconscious state.

The guardian *ad litem* felt it his duty to appeal the order to the Missouri supreme court, although he told that court that he did not disagree with the decision. But the supreme court reversed the lower court's decision: it held that Cruzan's legal guardians had no power to order feeding stopped without "clear and convincing" evidence that she herself had decided, when competent, not to be fed in her present circumstances. Though a friend had testified that Cruzan had said, in a conversation soon

*From Ronald Dworkin, The Right to Death, The New York Review of Books, January 31, 1991
(Vol. 35, No. 3), pp. 14–17. Reprinted with permission from The New York Review of Books.
Copyright © 1991 Nyrev, Inc.*

after the death of her grandmother, that she would not want to be kept alive if she could not really live, the supreme court held that this testimony was not adequate evidence of the necessary decision.

Cruzan's parents appealed to the United States Supreme Court: their lawyers argued that the Missouri decision violated her right not be subjected to unwanted medical treatment. The Court had not previously ruled on the question [of] how far states must respect that right. Last June 25, by a five-to-four vote, the Court refused to reverse the Missouri decision: it denied that Cruzan had a constitutional right that could be exercised by her parents in these circumstances.

The main opinion was written by Chief Justice Rehnquist, and was joined by Justices Kennedy and White. Many newspaper reports and comments on the case declared that, although the Court had refused the Cruzan family's request, it had nevertheless endorsed a general constitutional right of competent people to decide that they should not be kept alive through medical technology. *The New York Times*, for example, said that the Court had decided that "the Constitution protects a person's liberty to reject life-sustaining technology," and congratulated the Court for a "monumental examples of law adjusting to life." *The Washington Post* headline read, "Court Rules Patient's Wishes Must Control 'Right to Die.' "

It is important to notice, however, that Rehnquist took care to say that he and the two justices who joined his opinion were not actually deciding that people have a right to die. He said they were assuming such a right only *hypothetically*, "for purposes of this case," and he emphasized that he thought it still an open question whether even a competent person's freedom to die with dignity could be overridden by a state's own constitutional right to keep people alive.[1] Although the logic of past cases would embrace a "liberty interest" of a competent person to refuse artificially delivered food and water, he said, "the dramatic consequences involved in refusal of such treatment would inform the inquiry as to whether the deprivation of that interest is constitutional."

Even if we do assume that people have a constitutional right to refuse to be kept alive if they become permanently vegetative, Rehnquist said, Missouri did not infringe that right. It only insisted that people must exercise the right for themselves, while still competent, and do so in a formal and unmistakable way, by executing a "living will," for example. The United States Constitution does not prohibit states from adopting strict evidentiary requirements of that sort, he said. The Constitution does not require Missouri to recognize what most people would think was very strong evidence of Cruzan's convictions, that is, her serious and apparently well-considered statement to a close friend soon after a relative's death.

Justices O'Connor and Scalia, though they agreed to uphold the Missouri supreme court's decision, filed separate concurring opinions. O'Connor made an important practical point: that instead of drafting a living will describing precisely what should not be done to keep them alive, many people would prefer to designate someone else—a relative or close friend—to make those decisions for them when the need arises.[2] She stated her own view that the Constitution gave people that right, and emphasized that the Court's decision against Cruzan's parents was not to the contrary, since Cruzan had made no formal designation.

Scalia's concurring opinion was of a very different character. He repeated his extraordinarily narrow view of constitutional rights: that the Constitution, properly interpreted, allows the states to do anything that it does not expressly forbid. Since, he said, the Constitution "says nothing" about people's rights to control their own deaths, there is no question of any constitutional right of that sort, and state legislatures are free to make any decision they wish about what can be done to people to keep them technically alive. Scalia left little doubt about his own views of what a sensible state legislature would decide; he said that no reasonable person would wish to inhabit a body that was only technically alive. But, he said, the Constitution does not require state legislatures to be either reasonable or humane.

Justice Brennan dissented in an opinion joined by Justices Marshall and Blackmun. Brennan's opinion, one of the last he delivered before his retirement, was a valedictory address that made even plainer how much his humanity and intelligence will be missed. He pointed out the main fallacy in Rehnquist's opinion: it is inconsistent to assume that people have a constitutional right not to be given medical care contrary to their wishes, but yet for the state to be allowed to impose evidentiary rules that make it unlikely that an incompetent person's past wishes will actually be discovered.

"Even someone with a resolute determination to avoid life-support under circumstances such as Nancy's," he said, "would still need to know that such things as living wills exist and how to execute one. . . . For many, the thought of an ignoble end, steeped in decay, is abhorrent. A quiet, proud death, bodily integrity intact, is matter of extreme consequence."

Justice Stevens dissented separately. He criticized the majority for not having enough regard for Cruzan's best interests, and stressed the religious basis of Missouri's case. "[N]ot much may be said with confidence about death," he wrote, "unless it is said from faith, and that alone is reason enough to protect the freedom to conform choices about death to individual conscience."

Last August Cruzan's parents petitioned the lower court that had initially decided in their favor with what they called new evidence: three more friends of Cruzan had come forward prepared to testify that she had told them, too, that she would not want to live as a vegetable. Though this evidence was of the same character as that which the Missouri Supreme Court had earlier said was not sufficiently "clear and convincing," the state attorney general decided this time not to oppose the parents' petition. On December 14, the lower court granted the parents' petition. Within a few days feeding and hydration were stopped, and Cruzan was given medication to prevent pain. She died on December 26.

2.

When competent people refuse medical treatment that is necessary to save their lives, doctors and legal officials may face a dilemma. They have an ethical and legal obligation both to act in the patient's best interests and to respect his autonomy, his right to decide for himself what will be done with or to his body. These obligations may be in conflict, because a patient may refuse treatment the doctors think essential. Rehnquist introduced a third consideration into the constitutional issue. He contrasted the patient's autonomy not just with his or her own best interests but also with the *state's* interest in "protecting and preserving life." In most cases when a competent person refuses life-saving aid— for example, when he refuses an essential blood transfusion on religious grounds—there is no difference between what most people would regard as his best interests and the state's interest in keeping him alive, because it is assumed that it is in his best interests to live. But in some cases—when the patient is in great pain, for example, and cannot live very long even with treatment—then the state's supposed interest in keeping him alive may conflict with his own best interests, not only as he but as most people would judge these.

If we accept that some state policy might be served by prolonging life even in such cases, then two constitutional issues are presented. Does a state have the constitutional power to impose life-saving medical treatment on a person against his will, that is, in defiance of his autonomy, when it believes that treatment is in his own best interest? Does it have the constitutional power to impose such treatment for its own purposes, even when it concedes that this is *against* his best interests, that is, in defiance of the normal rule that patients should not be given medical treatment that is bad for them?

The law of most American states seems settled that the autonomy of a competent patient will be decisive in all such cases, and that doctors may not treat him against his will either for his sake or for the sake of some social interest in keeping him alive. The Supreme Court had never explicitly decided that the Constitution compels states to take that position, though in the present case, as I said, Rehnquist assumed hypothetically that it does.

In the case of people who are unconscious or otherwise incompetent, however, and who did not exercise their right of self-determination when they were able to do so, the distinction between their own best interests and the alleged interest of the state in keeping them alive is of great importance, as Rehnquist's opinion, carefully examined, makes clear. He offered two different, though not clearly distinct, arguments why Missouri has a right to tip the scales in favor of keeping comatose people alive by demanding "clear and convincing" evidence that they had decided they would rather die. His first argument appealed to the best interests of incompetent people. He said that a rule requiring evidence of a formal declaration of a past decision to die, before life support can be terminated, benefits people who have become comatose because it protects them against guardians who abuse their trust, and because a decision not to terminate is always reversible if documented evidence of a formal past decision emerges later. His second argument is very different: it appeals not the interests of comatose patients but to Missouri's supposed independent interests in keeping such patients alive. He said that a state has its own legitimate reasons for protecting and preserving life, which "no one can gainsay," and that Missouri is therefore entitled for its own sake to tip the evidentiary scales against termination.

He treats these as cumulative arguments: he thinks that taken together they justify Missouri's evidentiary rule. I shall consider them separately, however, because they raise very different issues, and because, though Rehnquist mentions the second only obliquely and in passing, it has important implications for other constitutional issues, including the abortion controversy, and so deserves separate study.

Rehnquist devotes most of his opinion to the first argument: that the Missouri rule is in the best interests of most of the thousands of people who live in a permanent vegetative state and did not sign living wills when they could. That seems implausible. Many people who are now in that position talked and acted in ways that make it very likely that they would have signed a living will had they anticipated their own accidents, as Nancy Cruzan did in conversations with her friends. The Missouri rule flouts rather than honors their autonomy. Many others, at least in the opinions of their family and others who know them best, almost certainly would have decided that way if they had ever considered the matter. The Missouri rule denies them what they probably would have chosen. Why is so indiscriminate a rule necessary? Why would it not be better to allow lower courts to decide each case on the balance of probabilities, so that a court might decide that on the best evidence Nancy Cruzan would have chosen to die, as the initial Missouri court in fact did decide?

While Rehnquist concedes that Missouri's rigid rule may sometimes lead to a "mistake," he says that the Constitution does not require states to adopt procedures that work perfectly. But his arguments that the Missouri rule would even in general work to the benefit of incompetent people are question-begging: they reflect a presumption that it is normally in the best interests of permanently comatose people to live, so that they should be kept alive unless there is decisive evidence that they have actually decided to the contrary. It is true that in some situations a presumption of that kind is sensible. A state need not accept the judgment of devout

Jehovah's Witnesses, for example, that it would be in the best interests of an unconscious relative not to have a blood transfusion that would bring him back to conscious life, even if the state would accept his own decision not to be treated were he conscious. But we think the presumption sensible in that case because we believe that life and health are fundamentally so important that no one should be allowed to reject them on behalf of someone else.

No such assumption is plausible when the life in question is only the insensate life of the permanently vegetative. That kind of life is not valuable to anyone. Some people, no doubt, would want to be kept alive indefinitely in such a state out of religious convictions: they might think that failing to prolong life as long as possible is insulting to God, for example. But even they do not think that it is in *their* interests to live on; most such people would hope, I think, for an early death in that situation, though one in which everything had been done to prolong life. They would regard an early death as an instance of God's mercy.

But Rehnquist is so far in the grip of the presumption that life is of great importance even to people in a vegetative state that he argues, at times, as if the Cruzan family's petition was a proceeding *against* their daughter. He says that the state is entitled to act as a "shield" for the incompetent, and he cites cases in which the Supreme Court required that government have "clear and convincing" evidence of fault before deporting someone, or depriving him of citizenship, or terminating his parental rights. In such cases constitutional law properly tips the scales against punitive action, because, as in an ordinary criminal trial, a mistake on one side, against the defendant, is much more serious than a mistake on the other. Cruzan's case is not a adversary proceeding, however. Her own parents are seeking relief on her *behalf*, and fairness argues for only one thing: the most accurate possible identification of what Nancy Cruzan's wishes were and where her interests now lie.

Some of Rehnquist's arguments depend not on the assumption that it is normally in the interests of a permanently comatose person to continue living, but on the equally implausible assumption that continued life in those circumstances is never against such a person's interests. This is the premise of his argument, for example, that it is better to keep a comatose patient alive than to allow her to die, even if the chances of recovery are infinitesimal, because the latter decision is irreversible. He assumes that someone in Nancy Cruzan's position suffers no disadvantage in continuing to live, so that if there is only the barest conceivable possibility of some extraordinary medical discovery in the future, however remote that may seem now, it must be on balance in their interests to continue living as long as possible.

If the only things people worried about, or wanted to avoid, were pain and other unpleasant physical experiences, then of course they would be indifferent about whether, if they became permanently comatose, their bodies continued to live or not. But people care about many other things as well. They worry about their dignity and integrity, and about the view other people have of them, how they are conceived and remembered. Many of them are anxious that their relatives and friends not have to bear the burdens, whether emotional or financial, of keeping them alive. Many are appalled by the thought of resources being wasted on them that might be used for the benefit of other people, who have genuine, conscious lives to lead.

These various concerns explain the horror so many people feel at the idea of existing pointlessly for years as a vegetable. They think that a bare biological existence, with no intelligence or sensibility or sensation, is not a matter of indifference, but something bad for them, something that damages their lives considered as a whole. This was the view Nancy Cruzan expressed to her friend after her grandmother's death. Rehnquist seems depressingly insensitive to all these concerns. In any case his assumption—that people lose nothing when permission to terminate their lives is refused—ignores them. A great many people, at least, believe the contrary: that a decision to keep them alive would cheat them forever of a chance to die with both dignity and consideration for others, and that to be deprived of that chance would be a great and irreversible loss.

Of course, given the devastating importance of the decision to terminate life support, a state may impose strenuous procedural constraints on any doctor's or guardian's decision to do so. The state may require them to show, for example, in an appropriate hearing before a judge or hospital committee or some other suitable body, and with appropriate medical support, that there is no genuine hope that the victim will ever become competent again. It may require guardians to show, moreover,

that there is no persuasive reason to think the patient would have preferred to have life support continued. It may also adopt suitable precautions to insure that the decision is made by people solely concerned with the patient's wishes and interests; it may specify, for example, that the decision not be made by guardians who would gain financially by the patient's early death. Though these and other procedural constraints may somewhat increase the chance that a patient who would have wished to die is kept alive, they can plausibly be described as in the best interests of patients overall, or in the interests of protecting their autonomy.

The Cruzan family satisfied all such requirements, however. There is no evidence that Nancy Cruzan had any religious beliefs that would have led her to prefer mere biological life to death. On the contrary, the evidence of her serious conversations strongly suggested—to put it at its weakest—that she would vigorously oppose being kept alive. Since Missouri itself paid the full cost of her treatment, the family had no financial incentive to allow her to die. So the state's evidentiary procedures cannot reasonably be said to have been in Cruzan's best interests, or in the best interests of vegetative patients generally. If Missouri's rule is constitutional, it must be for some other reason.

3.

We must therefore turn to Rehnquist's second, much less developed, argument: that Missouri can impose evidentiary requirements, even if that is against Cruzan's interests and those of other permanently incompetent people, in order to protect its own interests in preserving life. He said that "societal" and "institutional" issues are at stake, as well as individual ones, that no one can "gainsay" Missouri's "interest in the protection and preservation of human life."

No doubt Missouri pressed this agreement, and perhaps Rehnquist adopted it, with an eye to the abortion controversy. In 1989's abortion case, *Webster* v. *Missouri Reproductive Services*, Missouri cited its own sovereign interest in preserving all human life as justification for refusing to allow abortions to be performed in state financed medical facilities. Even *Roe* v. *Wade*, the 1973 decision that established a woman's limited right to an abortion, acknowledged that a state has a legitimate concern with protecting the life of a fetus. Though Justice

Blackmun said, in that case, that a state's right to protect a fetus is outweighed by a woman's right of privacy during the first two trimesters of pregnancy, he held that the state's right was sufficiently strong thereafter to allow a state to make most third-trimester abortions illegal. In the *Webster* decision, several justices said that the state's legitimate interest in protecting human life is more powerful than Blackmun recognized, and justifies more sweeping regulation of abortion than he allowed.

Nevertheless, in spite of the crucial part that the idea of a legitimate state interest in preserving all human life now plays in constitutional law, there has been remarkably little attention, either in Supreme Court opinions or in the legal literature, to the question of what that supposed interest is or why it is legitimate for a state to pursue it. It is particularly unclear how the supposed state interest bears on the questions that were at stake in the *Cruzan* case. Of course government is properly concerned with the welfare and well-being of its citizens, and it has the right, for that reason, to try to prevent them from being killed or put at risk of death from disease or accident. But the state's obvious and general concern with its citizens' well-being does not give it a reason to preserve someone's life when his or her welfare would be better served by being permitted to die in dignity. So the state interest that Rehnquist has in mind, as justifying Missouri's otherwise unreasonable evidentiary rule, must be a different, less familiar one: it must supply a reason for forcing people to accept medical treatment when they or their guardians plausibly think they would be better off dead.

Scalia, in his concurring opinion, said that we must assume that states are constitutionally entitled to preserve people's lives, even against their own interests, because otherwise familiar laws making either suicide or aiding suicide a crime, which no one doubts are valid, would be unconstitutional. As I said, he disagreed with Rehnquist's hypothetical assumption that, at least, competent people have a constitutional right to refuse life-saving medical treatment. But Scalia's argument is doubly suspect.

First, his assumption that states have the constitutional power to prevent suicide in all circumstances is too broad and it is premature. It is true that both suicide and assisting suicide were crimes according to common law, and Scalia relies heavily on the views of William Blackstone, the famous and influential eighteenth-century legal commentator,

who declared that it was a crime even for someone suffering a terminal illness and in terrible pain to take his own life. But there are many examples in constitutional history of constraints on liberty that were unquestioned for long periods of history but were then reexamined and found unconstitutional because lawyers and the public as a whole had developed a more sophisticated understanding of the underlying ethical and moral issues.[3] That is particularly likely when the historical support for the constraint has been mainly religious. It was long unquestioned that states have the power to outlaw contraception, for example, before the Supreme Court held otherwise in 1965 in *Griswold* v. *Connecticut*.

Longstanding practice is an even worse guide to constitutional law when technological change has created entirely new problems or exacerbated old ones. Doctors can now keep people alive in terminal illness for long periods that would have seemed incredible in the recent past, and their new abilities have made the position of people who would rather die than continue living in pain both more tragic and more common. So when the Supreme Court is next asked to rule on whether states can constitutionally forbid someone in that position from taking his own life, or can make it criminal for a doctor to assist him, even if the doctor takes every precaution to be sure that the person has freely decided to do so, the Court will face a very different situation from that in which the common law principles about suicide developed. It seems premature for Scalia simply to declare that the power of states to forbid suicide has no exceptions at all. Government is entitled to try to prevent people from killing themselves in many circumstances—in periods of severe but transient depression, for example. But it does not follow that it has the power to prolong the suffering of someone in terrible and pointless pain.

In any case, it is bizarre to classify as suicide someone's decision to reject treatment that would keep him alive but at a cost he and many other people think too great. Many people whose lives could be lengthened through severe amputations or incapacitating operations decide to die instead, and they are not thought to have taken their own lives for that reason. It seems plain that states have no constitutional power to direct doctors to perform such operations without the consent and against the wishes of the patient. People imagining themselves as permanently comatose are in the same position:

their biological lives could then be prolonged only through medical treatment they would think degrading, and only in a form they would think worse than death. So it is a mistake, for that reason, to describe someone who signs a living will as committing hypothetical suicide. It seems a mistake for another reason as well. Even if Scalia were right, that a conscious and competent patient who refuses an amputation that would prolong his life should be treated as a suicide, it would still not follow that someone who decides to die if he were to become a permanent vegetable is in fact taking his own life, because it is at least a reasonable view that a permanently comatose person is, for all that matters, dead already.

4.

Scalia's argument is therefore a red herring, and in spite of Rehnquist's confident remark that no one can "gainsay" Missouri's interest in protecting and preserving life, we still lack an explanation of what that interest is and why it is proper for Missouri to pursue it. It might be said that keeping people alive, even when they would be better off dead, helps to protect the community's sense of the importance of life. I agree that society is better and more secure when its members share a sense that human life is sacred, and that no effort should be spared to save lives. People who lack that sense may themselves be more ready to kill, and will be less anxious to make sacrifices to protect the lives of others. That seems to me the most powerful available argument why states should be permitted to outlaw elective abortion of very late-stage fetuses, for example.[4] But it is extremely implausible that allowing a permanently comatose patient to die, after a solemn proceeding devoted only to her wishes and interests, will in any way erode a community's sense of the importance of life.

So a state cannot justify keeping comatose people alive on the instrumental ground that this is necessary to prevent murder or to encourage people to vote for famine relief. If Rehnquist is right that a state has a legitimate interest in preserving all human life, then this must be in virtue not of any instrumental argument but of the *intrinsic* value of such life, its importance for its own sake. Most people do believe that human life has intrinsic importance, and perhaps Rehnquist thinks it unnecessary either to clarify or to justify that idea.[5] It is

unclear, however, that they accept the idea on any ground, or in any sense, that supports his case. For some people, for example, life has intrinsic value because it is a gift of God; they believe, as I said, that it is wrong not to struggle to prolong life, because this is an insult to Him, who alone should decide when life ends. But the Constitution does not allow states to justify policy on grounds of religious doctrine; some more secular account of the intrinsic value of life would be needed to support Rehnquist's second argument.

It will be helpful to distinguish two forms that a more secular version of the claim might take. The first supposes that a human life, in any form or circumstance, is a unique and valuable addition to the universe, so that the stock of value is needlessly diminished when any life is shorter than it might be. That does not seem a convincing view. Even if we think that a conscious, reflective, engaged human life is inherently valuable, we might well doubt that an insensate, vegetative life has any value at all.

The view that all forms of life are inherently valuable is also disqualified for a different reason. On that view we would have as much reason to bring new lives into being, increasing the population, as for prolonging lives already in progress. After all, people who think that great art is inherently valuable have the same reason for encouraging the production of more masterpieces as for preserving art that now exists. But most people who think life has intrinsic significance do not think that they therefore have any general duty to procreate or to encourage procreation. In any case, the Supreme Court's decision in *Griswold*, which is now accepted by almost everyone, holds that the states have no power to prohibit contraception.

People who think that life has intrinsic value or importance, but do not think that this fact offers any reason for increasing the population, understand life's value in a second and more conditional way. They mean, I think, that once a human life has begun it is terribly important that it go well, that it be a good rather than a bad life, a successful rather than a wasted one. Most people accept that human life has inherent importance in that sense. That explains why they try not just to make their lives pleasant but to give them worth and also why it seems a tragedy when people decide, late in life, that they can take neither pride nor satisfaction in the way they have lived.[6] Of course nothing in the idea that life has intrinsic importance in this second sense can justify a policy of keeping permanently comatose people alive. The worth of their lives—the character of the lives they have led—cannot be improved just by keeping the bodies they used to inhabit technically alive. On the contrary, that makes their lives worse, because it is a bad thing, for all the reasons I described earlier, to have one's body medicated, fed, and groomed, as an object of pointless and degrading solicitude, after one's mind is dead. Rehnquist's second argument is therefore a dramatic failure: Missouri's policy is not supported but condemned by the idea that human life is importance for its own sake, on the only understanding of that idea that is available in our constitutional system.

5.

It is a relatively new question how the medical technology that now allows doctors to keep wholly incompetent people alive for decades should be used. Of course the Constitution leaves considerable latitude to the state legislatures in fixing detailed schemes for regulating how and what doctors and guardians decide. But the Constitution does limit a state's power in certain ways, as it must in order to protect the autonomy and the most fundamental interests of the patient.

In the *Cruzan* case the Supreme Court recognized, even if only hypothetically, an important part of that constitutional protection: that in principle a state has no right to keep a comatose patient alive against his previously expressed wish that he be allowed to die in the circumstances he has now reached. But the Court undercut the full value of that principle by allowing Missouri to impose an evidentiary rule that substantially decreases the chance a patient will receive only the treatment he or she would have wanted. Even worse, the justification the Chief Justice offered for the Court's decision put forward two principles that, unless they are soon rejected, will damage the rest of the law as it develops. It is therefore worth summarizing the argument I have made against these principles.

Rehnquist assumed that it is in the best interests of at least most people who become permanent vegetables to remain alive in that condition. But there is no way in which continued life can be good for such people, and several ways in which it might well be thought bad. He also assumed that a state can have its own legitimate reasons for keeping such

people alive even when it concedes that this is against their best interests. But that judgment rests on a dangerous misunderstanding of the irresistible idea that human life has intrinsic moral significance. We do not honor that idea—on the contrary we insult it—when we waste resources in prolonging a bare, technical, insensate form of life.

More than just the right to die, or even the right to abortion, is at stake in these issues. In the next decades the question of why and how human life has intrinsic value is likely to be debated, by philosophers, lawyers, and the public, not just with respect to those issues but others as well, including genetic engineering, for example. Constitutional law will both encourage and reflect the debate, and though it is far too early to anticipate what form that law will take, Rehnquist's unreasoned opinion was a poor beginning.

Notes

1. In fact five justices—Justice O'Connor and the four dissenters—did declare that people have that right. But one of the dissenters, Justice Brennan, has retired, and it is not known whether Justice Souter, who took his place, agrees.

2. On July 1, 1990, the New York state legislature enacted a law, the "health care proxy bill," that provides for such delegation. Governor Cuomo said that the *Cruzan* decision helped to break a logjam on the bill. See *The New York Times*, July 2, 1990.

3. The recent, well-publicized case of Janet Adkins, who killed herself using Dr. Jack Kevorkian's suicide machine in the back of his Volkswagen van, suggests the moral complexity of suicide provoked by illness, and the degree to which Americans are divided about the issues raised by such suicide. Adkins was fifty-three and in the relatively early stages of Alzheimer's disease. Her mental capacity had begun to diminish—she found tennis scoring and the foreign languages she used to speak too difficult, for example, though she had lost little physical capacity, and had recently beaten her thirty-three-year-old son at tennis. She was still alert and intelligent, and had retained her sense of humor. But she wanted to die before the irreversible disease worsened; the life she would soon lead, she said, "is not the way I wanted it at all. . . ." She telephoned Kevorkian, whom she had seen on television discussing his device. They met in Michigan, chosen because assisting suicide is not a crime there, in a motel room where he taped a forty-minute conversation which recorded her competence and her wish to die. Two days

later he inserted a needle into her vein as she lay in the back of his van, and told her which button to push for a lethal injection. Michigan prosecutors charged Kevorkian with murder, but the judge acquitted him after listening to the tape.

The case raises serious moral issues that the Cruzan case does not. Janet Adkins apparently had several years of meaningful life left, and Kevorkian's examination may not have been long or substantial enough to rule out the possibility that she was in a temporary depression from which she might recover while still competent. It is of interest that about half of the 250 doctors who wrote in response to a critical article in a medical journal approved of what Kevorkian did, while the rest disapproved.

4. See my article "The Great Abortion Case," in *The New York Review*, June 29, 1989.

5. I do not mean to deny that animal life might have intrinsic importance, too.

6. I do not mean that many people often reflect on their lives as a whole, or live according to some overall theory about what makes their lives good or bad. Most people define living well in much more concrete terms: living well means having a good job, a successful family life, warm friendships, and time and money for recreation or travel, for example. But I believe that people take pride as well as pleasure in these concrete achievements and experiences, and have a sense of failure as well as displeasure when a job goes wrong or a friendship sours. Very few of them, perhaps, except those for whom religion is important, self-consciously think of their lives as an opportunity that they may either waste or make into something worthwhile. But most people's

attitudes toward successes and failures do seem to presuppose that view of life's importance. Most of us think it is important that the lives of other people, as well as our own, be worthwhile: we think it is a central role of government to encourage people to make something of their lives rather than just survive, and to provide some of the institutions, including the schools, necessary for them to do so. These assumptions are premises of liberal education, and also of the limited paternalism involved in stopping people from using drugs or wasting their lives in other ways, and in trying to prevent or discourage people who are depressed or despondent from killing themselves when they could in fact lead lives worth living.

That human life has intrinsic value in this sense—that it is important that a life go well once it has begun—obviously has important though complex implications for the abortion issue. In a recent Holmes Lecture at Harvard Law School I explored these implications. I argued that the idea that life has intrinsic value in the sense I described does explain many of our attitudes about abortion, including the opinion many people have that abortion even in an early stage poses moral problems. It does not follow that abortion is always wrong; indeed it sometimes follows that abortion is morally recommended or required. I argued, moreover, that understanding our moral notions about abortion as flowing from respect for the inherent value of life reinforces the Supreme Court decision in *Roe* v. *Wade* that the state has no business coercing pregnant women to take a particular view about what the principle of respect for the inherent value of life requires.

Must Patients Always Be Given Food and Water? _____

Joanne Lynn and James F. Childress

Lynn and Childress consider whether it is ever permissible to withhold or withdraw food or nutrition from a patient. After rejecting the notion that such an action would be intrinsically wrong, they describe how providing nutrition as a medical treatment differs from ordinary feeding. They then mention three circumstances in which such treatment is not obligatory: when it would be futile, when it could bring no benefit to the patient, and when any benefit brought is outweighed by the burden imposed on the patient. They reject four arguments that hold that nutrition and hydration must be provided: because it is a part of ordinary care, because treatment begun must be continued, because we should not cause death, and because such treatment is symbolically significant.

Many people die from the lack of food or water. For some, this lack is the result of poverty or famine, but for others it is the result of disease or deliberate decision. In the past, malnutrition and dehydration must have accompanied nearly every death that followed an illness of more than a few days. Most dying patients do not eat much on their own, and nothing could be done for them until the first flexible tubing for instilling food or other liquid into the stomach was developed about a hundred years ago. Even then, the procedure was so scarce, so costly in physician and nursing time, and so poorly tolerated that it was used only for patients who clearly could benefit. With the advent of more reliable and efficient procedures in the past few decades, these conditions can be corrected or ameliorated in nearly every patient who would otherwise be malnourished or dehydrated. In fact, intravenous lines and nasogastric tubes have become common images of hospital care.

Providing adequate nutrition and fluids is a high priority for most patients, both because they suffer directly from inadequacies and because these deficiencies hinder their ability to overcome other diseases. But are there some patients who need not receive these treatments? This question has become a prominent public policy issue in a number of recent cases. In May 1981, in Danville, Illinois, the parents and the physician of newborn conjoined twins with shared abdominal organs decided not to feed these children. Feeding and other treatments were given after court intervention, though a grand jury refused to indict the parents.[1] Later that year, two physicians in Los Angeles discontinued intravenous nutrition to a patient who had severe brain damage after an episode involving loss of oxygen following routine surgery. Murder charges were brought, but the hearing judge dismissed the charges at a preliminary hearing. On appeal, the charges were reinstated and remanded for trial.[2]

In April 1982, a Bloomington, Indiana, infant who had tracheoesophageal fistula and Down Syndrome was not treated or fed, and he died after two courts ruled that the decision was proper but before all appeals could be heard.[3] When the federal government then moved to ensure that such infants would be fed in the future,[4] the Surgeon General, Dr. C. Everett Koop, initially stated that there is never adequate reason to deny nutrition and fluids to a newborn infant.

While these cases were before the public, the nephew of Claire Conroy, an elderly incompetent woman with several serious medical problems, petitioned a New Jersey court for authority to discontinue her nasogastric tube feedings. Although the intermediate appeals court has reversed the ruling,[5] the trial court held that he had this authority since the evidence indicated that the patient would not have wanted such treatment and that its value to her was doubtful.

In all these dramatic cases and in many more that go unnoticed, the decision is made to deliberately withhold food or fluid known to be necessary for the life of the patient. Such decisions are unsettling. There is now widespread consensus that sometimes a patient is best served by not undertaking or continuing certain treatments that would sustain life, especially if these entail substantial suffering.[6] But food and water are so central to an array of human emotions that it is almost impossible to consider them with the same emotional detachment that one might feel toward a respirator or a dialysis machine.

Nevertheless, the question remains: Should it ever be permissible to withhold or withdraw food and nutrition? The answer in any real case should acknowledge the psychological contiguity between feeding and loving and between nutritional satisfaction and emotional satisfaction. Yet this acknowledgment does not resolve the core question.

Some have held that it is intrinsically wrong not to feed another. The philosopher G. E. M. Anscombe contends: ''For wilful starvation there can be no excuse. The same can't be said quite without qualification about failing to operate or to adopt

Reprinted by permission of the authors and The Hastings Center from Hastings Center Report 13 *(October 1983), pp. 17–21.*

some courses of treatment."[7] But the moral issues are more complex than Anscombe's comment suggests. Does correcting nutritional deficiencies always improve patients' well-being? What should be our reflective moral response to withholding or withdrawing nutrition? What moral principles are relevant to our reflections? What medical facts about ways of providing nutrition are relevant? And what policies should be adopted by the society, hospitals, and medical and other health care professionals?

In our effort to find answers to these questions, we will concentrate upon the care of patients who are incompetent to make choices for themselves. Patients who are competent to determine the course of their therapy may refuse any and all interventions proposed by others, as long as their refusals do not seriously harm or impose unfair burdens upon others.[8] A competent patient's decision regarding whether or not to accept the provision of food and water by medical means such as tube feeding or intravenous alimentation is unlikely to raise questions of harm or burden to others.

What then should guide those who must decide about nutrition for a patient who cannot decide? As a start, consider the standard by which other medical decisions are made: one should decide as the incompetent person would have if he or she were competent, when that is possible to determine, and advance that person's interests in a more generalized sense when individual preferences cannot be known.

The Medical Procedures

There is no reason to apply a different standard to feeding and hydration. Surely, when one inserts a feeding tube, or creates a gastrostomy opening, or inserts a needle into a vein, one intends to benefit the patient. Ideally, one should provide what the patient believes to be of benefit, but at least the effect should be beneficial in the opinions of surrogates and caregivers.

Thus, the question becomes, is it ever in the patient's interest to become malnourished and dehydrated, rather than to receive treatment? Posing the question so starkly points to our need to know what is entailed in treating these conditions and what benefits the treatments offer.

The medical interventions that provide food and fluids are of two basic types. First, liquids can be delivered by a tube that is inserted into a functioning gastrointestinal tract, most commonly through the nose and esophagus into the stomach or through a surgical incision in the abdominal wall and directly into the stomach. The liquids used can be specially prepared solutions of nutrients or a blenderized version of an ordinary diet. The nasogastric tube is cheap; it may lead to pneumonia and often annoys the patient and family, sometimes even requiring that the patient be restrained to prevent its removal.

Creating a gastrostomy is usually a simple surgical procedure, and, once the wound is healed, care is very simple. Since it is out of sight, it is aesthetically more acceptable and restraints are needed less often. Also, the gastrostomy creates no additional risk of pneumonia. However, while elimination of a nasogastric tube requires only removing the tube, a gastrostomy is fairly permanent, and can be closed only by surgery.

The second type of medical intervention is intravenous feeding and hydration, which also has two major forms. The ordinary hospital or peripheral IV, in which fluid is delivered directly to the bloodstream through a small needle, is useful only for temporary efforts to improve hydration and electrolyte concentrations. One cannot provide a balanced diet through the veins in the limbs: to do that requires a central line, or a special catheter placed into one of the major veins in the chest. The latter procedure is much more risky and vulnerable to infections and technical errors, and it is much more costly than any of the other procedures. Both forms of intravenous nutrition and hydration commonly require restraining the patient, cause minor infections and other ill effects, and are costly, especially since they ordinarily require the patient to be in a hospital.

None of these procedures, then, is ideal; each entails some distress, some medical limitations, and some costs. When may a procedure be forgone that might improve nutrition and hydration for a given patient? Only when the procedure and the resulting improvement in nutrition and hydration do not offer the patient a net benefit over what he or she would otherwise have faced.

Are there such circumstances? We believe that there are; but they are few and limited to the following three kinds of situations: (1) the procedures that would be required are so unlikely to achieve improved nutritional and fluid levels that they could be correctly considered futile; (2) the improvement in nutritional and fluid balance, through achievable, could be of no benefit to the patient; (3) the burdens of receiving the treatment may outweigh the benefit.

When Food and Water May Be Withheld

Futile Treatment.   Sometimes even providing "food and water" to a patient becomes a monumental task. Consider a patient with a severe clotting deficiency and a nearly total body burn. Gaining access to the central veins is likely to cause hemorrhage or infection, nasogastric tube placement may be quite painful, and there may be no skin to which to suture the stomach for a gastrostomy tube. Or consider a patient with severe congestive heart failure who develops cancer of the stomach with a fistula that delivers food from the stomach to the colon without passing through the intestine and being absorbed. Feeding the patient may be possible, but little is absorbed. Intravenous feeding cannot be tolerated because the fluid would be too much for the weakened heart. Or consider the infant with infarction of all but a short segment of bowel. Again, the infant can be fed, but little if anything is absorbed. Intravenous methods can be used, but only for a short time (weeks or months) until their complications, including thrombosis, hemorrhage, infections, and malnutrition, cause death.

In these circumstances, the patient is going to die soon, no matter what is done. The ineffective efforts to provide nutrition and hydration may directly cause suffering that offers no counterbalancing benefit for the patient. Although the procedures might be tried, especially if the competent patient wanted them or the incompetent patient's surrogate had reason to believe that this incompetent patient would have wanted them, they cannot be considered obligatory. To hold that a patient must be subjected to this predictably futile sort of intervention just because protein balance is negative or the blood serum is concentrated is to lose sight of the moral warrant for medical care and to reduce the patient to an array of measurable variables.

No Possibility of Benefit.   Some patients can be reliably diagnosed to have permanently lost con-

sciousness. This unusual group of patients includes those with anencephaly, persistent vegetative state, and some preterminal comas. In these cases, it is very difficult to discern how any medical intervention can benefit or harm the patient. These patients cannot and never will be able to experience any of the events occurring in the world or in their bodies. When the diagnosis is exceedingly clear, we sustain their lives vigorously mainly for their loved ones and the community at large.

While these considerations probably indicate that continued artificial feeding is best in most cases, there may be some cases in which the family and the caregivers are convinced that artificial feeding is offensive and unreasonable. In such cases, there seems to be more adequate reason to claim that withholding food and water violates any obligations that these parties or the general society have with regard to permanently unconscious patients. Thus, if the parents of an anencephalic infant or of a patient like Karen Quinlan in a persistent vegetative state feel strongly that no medical procedures should be applied to provide nutrition and hydration, and the caregivers are willing to comply, there should be no barrier in law or public policy to thwart the plan.[9]

Disproportionate Burden.   The most difficult cases are those in which normal nutritional status or fluid balance could be restored, but only with a severe burden for the patient. In these cases, the treatment is futile in a broader sense—the patient will not actually benefit from the improved nutrition and hydration. A patient who is competent can decide the relative merits of the treatment being provided, knowing the probable consequences, and weighing the merits of life under various sets of constrained circumstances. But a surrogate decision maker for a patient who is incompetent to decide will have a difficult task. When the situation is irremediably ambiguous, erring on the side of continued life and improved nutrition and hydration seems the less grievous error. But are there situations that would warrant a determination that this patient, whose nutrition and hydration could surely be improved, is not thereby well served?

Though they are rare, we believe there are such cases. The treatments entailed are not benign. Their effects are far short of ideal. Furthermore, many of the patients most likely to have inadequate food and fluid intake are also likely to suffer the most serious side effects of these therapies.

Patients who are allowed to die without artificial hydration and nutrition may well die more comfortably than patients who receive conventional amounts of intravenous hydration.[10] Terminal pulmonary edema, nausea, and mental confusion are more likely when patients have been treated to maintain fluid and nutrition until close to the time of death.

Thus, those patients whose "need" for artificial nutrition and hydration arises only near the time of death may be harmed by its provision. It is not at all clear that they receive any benefit in having a slightly prolonged life, and it does seem reasonable to allow a surrogate to decide that, for this patient at this time, slight prolongation of life is not warranted if it involves measures that will probably increase the patient's suffering as he or she dies.

Even patients who might live much longer might not be well served by artificial means to provide fluid and food. Such patients might include those with fairly severe dementia for whom the restraints required could be a constant source of fear, discomfort, and struggle. For such a patient, sedation to tolerate the feeding mechanisms might preclude any of the pleasant experiences that might otherwise have been available. Thus, a decision not to intervene, except perhaps briefly to ascertain that there are no treatable causes, might allow such a patient to live out a shorter life with fair freedom of movement and freedom from fear, while a decision to maintain artificial nutrition and hydration might consign the patient to end his or her life in unremitting anguish. If this were the case a surrogate decision-maker would seem to be well justified in refusing the treatment.

Inappropriate Moral Constraints

Four considerations are frequently proposed as moral constraints on forgoing medical feeding and hydration. We find none of these to dictate that artificial nutrition and hydration must always be provided.

The Obligation to Provide "Ordinary" Care. Debates about appropriate medical treatment are often couched in terms of "ordinary" and "extraordinary" means of treatment. Historically, this distinction emerged in the Roman Catholic tradition to differentiate optional treatment from treatment that was obligatory for medical professionals to offer and for patients to accept.[11] These terms also appear in many secular contexts, such as court decisions and medical codes. The recent debates about ordinary and extraordinary means of treatment have been interminable and often unfruitful, in part because of a lack of clarity about what the terms mean. Do they represent the premises of an argument or the conclusion, and what features of a situation are relevant to the categorization as "ordinary" or "extraordinary"?[12]

Several criteria have been implicit in debates about ordinary and extraordinary means of treatment; some of them may be relevant to determining whether and which treatments are obligatory and which are optional. Treatments have been distinguished according to their simplicity (simple/complex), their naturalness (natural/artificial), their customariness (usual/unusual), their invasiveness (noninvasive/invasive), their chance of success (reasonable chance/futile), their balance of benefits and burdens (proportionate/disproportionate), and their expense (inexpensive/costly). Each set of paired terms or phrases in the parentheses suggests a continuum: as the treatment moves from the first of the paired terms to the second, it is said to become less obligatory and more optional.

However, when these various criteria, widely used in discussions about medical treatment, are carefully examined, most of them are not morally relevant in distinguishing optional from obligatory medical treatments. For example, if a rare, complex, artificial, and invasive treatment offers a patient a reasonable chance of nearly painless cure, then one would have to offer a substantial justification not to provide that treatment to an incompetent patient.

What matters, then, in determining whether to provide a treatment to an incompetent patient is not a prior determination that this treatment is "ordinary" per se, but rather a determination that this treatment is likely to provide this patient benefits that are sufficient to make it worthwhile to endure the burdens that accompany the treatment. To this end, some of the considerations listed above are relevant: whether a treatment is likely to succeed is an obvious example. But such considerations taken in isolation are not conclusive. Rather, the surrogate decision-maker is obliged to assess the desirability to this patient of each of the options presented, including nontreatment. For most people at most times, this assessment would lead to a clear obligation to provide food and fluids.

But sometimes, as we have indicated, providing food and fluids through medical interventions may fail to benefit and may even harm some patients. Then the treatment cannot be said to be obligatory, no matter how usual and simple its provision may be. If "ordinary" and "extraordinary" are used to convey the conclusion about the obligation to treat, providing nutrition and fluids would have become, in these cases, "extraordinary." Since this phrasing is misleading, it is probably better to use "proportionate" and "disproportionate," as the Vatican now suggests,[13] or "obligatory" and "optional."

Obviously, providing nutrition and hydration may sometimes be necessary to keep patients comfortable while they are dying even though it may temporarily prolong their dying. In such cases, food and fluids constitute warranted palliative care. But in other cases, such as a patient in a deep and irreversible coma, nutrition and hydration do not appear to be needed or helpful, except perhaps to comfort the staff and family.[14] And sometimes the interventions needed for nutrition and hydration are so burdensome that they are harmful and best not utilized.

The Obligation to Continue Treatments Once Started. Once having started a mode of treatment, many caregivers find it very difficult to discontinue it. While this strongly felt difference between the ease of withholding a treatment and the difficulty of withdrawing it provides a psychological explanation of certain actions, it does not justify them. It sometimes even leads to a thoroughly irrational decision process. For example, in caring for a dying, comatose patient, many physicians apparently find it harder to stop a functioning peripheral IV than not to restart one that has infiltrated (that is, has broken through the blood vessel and is leaking fluid into surrounding tissue), especially if the only way to reestablish an IV would be to insert a central line into the heart or to do a cutdown (make an incision to gain access to the deep large blood vessels).[15]

What factors might make withdrawing medical treatment morally worse than withholding it? Withdrawing a treatment seems to be an action, which,

when it is likely to end in death, initially seems more serious than an omission that ends in death. However, this view is fraught with errors. Withdrawing is not always an act: failing to put the next infusion into a tube could be correctly described as an omission, for example. Even when withdrawing is an act, it may well be morally correct and even morally obligatory. Discontinuing intravenous lines in a patient now permanently unconscious in accord with that patient's well-informed advance directive would certainly be such a case. Furthermore, the caregiver's obligation to serve the patient's interests through both acts and omissions rules out the exculpation that accompanies omissions in the usual course of social life. An omission that is not warranted by the patient's interests is culpable.

Sometimes initiating a treatment creates expectations in the minds of caregivers, patients, and family that the treatment will be continued indefinitely or until the patient is cured. Such expectations may provide a reason to continue the treatment as a way to keep a promise. However, as with all promises, caregivers could be very careful when initiating a treatment to explain the indications for its discontinuation, and they could modify preconceptions with continuing reevaluation and education during treatment. Though all patients are entitled to expect the continuation of care in the patient's best interests, they are not and should not be entitled to the continuation of a particular mode of care.

Accepting the distinction between withholding and withdrawing medical treatment as morally significant also has a very unfortunate implication: caregivers may become unduly reluctant to begin some treatments precisely because they fear that they will be locked into continuing treatments that are no longer of value to the patient. For example, the physician who had been unwilling to stop the respirator while the infant Andrew Stinson died over several months is reportedly "less eager to attach babies to respirators now."[16] But if it were easier to ignore malnutrition and dehydration and to withhold treatments for these problems than to discontinue the same treatments when they have become especially burdensome and insufficiently beneficial for the patient, then the incentives would be perverse. Once a treatment has been tried, it is often much clearer whether it is of value to the patient, and the decision to stop it can be made more reliably.

The same considerations should apply to starting as to stopping a treatment, and whatever assessment warrants withholding should also warrant withdrawing.

The Obligation to Avoid Being the Unambiguous Cause of Death.   Many physicians will agree with all that we have said and still refuse to allow a choice to forgo food and fluid because such a course seems to be a "death sentence." In this view death seems to be more certain from malnutrition and dehydration than from forgoing other forms of medical therapy. This implies that it is acceptable to act in ways that are likely to cause death, as in not operating on a gangrenous leg, only if there remains a chance that the patient will survive. This is a comforting formulation for caregivers, to be sure, since they can thereby avoid feeling the full weight of the responsibility for the time and manner of a patient's death. However, it is not a persuasive moral argument.

First, in appropriate cases discontinuing certain medical treatments is generally accepted despite the the fact that death is as certain as with nonfeeding. Dialysis in a patient without kidney function or transfusions in a patient with severe aplastic anemia are obvious examples. The dying that awaits such patients often is not greatly different from dying of dehydration and malnutrition.

Second, the certainty of a generally undesirable outcome such as death is always relevant to a decision, but it does not foreclose the possibility that this course is better than others available to this patient.[17] Ambiguity and uncertainty are so common in medical decision-making that caregivers are tempted to use them in distancing themselves from direct responsibility. However, caregivers are in fact responsible for the time and manner of death for many patients. Their distaste for this fact should not constrain otherwise morally justified decisions.

The Obligation to Provide Symbolically Significant Treatment.   One of the most common arguments for always providing nutrition and hydration is that it symbolizes, expresses, or conveys the essence of care and compassion. Some actions not only aim at goals, they also express values. Such expressive actions should not simply be viewed as means to ends; they should also be viewed in light of what they communicate. From this perspective food and water are not only goods that preserve life and provide comfort; they are also symbols of care and compassion. To withhold or withdraw them—to "starve" a patient—can never express or convey care.

Why is providing food and water a central symbol of care and compassion? Feeding is the first response of the community to the needs of newborns and remains a central mode of nurture and comfort. Eating is associated with social interchange and community, and providing food for someone else is a way to create and maintain bonds of sharing and expressing concern. Furthermore, even the relatively low levels of hunger and thirst that most people have experienced are decidedly uncomfortable, and the common image of severe malnutrition or dehydration is one of unremitting agony. Thus, people are rightly eager to provide food and water. Such provision is essential to minimally tolerable existence and a powerful symbol of our concern for each other.

However, *medical* nutrition and hydration, we have argued, may not always provide net benefits to patients. Medical procedures to provide nutrition and hydration are more similar to other medical procedures than to typical human ways of providing nutrition and hydration, for example, a sip of water. It should be possible to evaluate their benefits and burdens, as we evaluate any other medical procedure. Of course, if family, friends, and caregivers feel that such procedures affirm important values even when they do not benefit the patient, their feelings should not be ignored. We do not contend that there is an obligation to withhold or to withdraw such procedures (unless consideration of the patient's advance directives or current best interest unambiguously dictates that conclusion); we only contend that nutrition and hydration may be forgone in some cases.

The symbolic connection between care and nutrition or hydration adds useful caution to decision making. If decision makers worry over withholding or withdrawing medical nutrition and hydration, they may inquire more seriously into the circumstances that putatively justify their decisions. This is generally salutary for health care decision making. The critical inquiry may well yield the sad but justified conclusion that the patient will be served best by not using medical procedures to provide food and fluids.

A Limited Conclusion

Our conclusion—that patients or their surrogates, in close collaboration with their physicians and other caregivers and with careful assessment of the relevant information, can correctly decide to forgo the provision of medical treatments intended to correct malnutrition and dehydration in some circumstances—is quite limited. Concentrating on incompetent patients, we have argued that in most cases such patients will be best served by providing nutrition and fluids. Thus, there should be a presumption in favor of providing nutrition and fluids as part of the broader presumption to provide means that prolong life. But this presumption may be rebutted in particular cases.

We do not have enough information to be able to determine with clarity and conviction whether withholding or withdrawing nutrition and hydration was justified in the cases that have occasioned public concern, though it seems likely that the Danville and Bloomington babies should have been fed and that Claire Conroy should not.

It is never sufficient to rule out "starvation" categorically. The question is whether the obligation to act in the patient's best interests was discharged by withholding or withdrawing particular medical treatments. All we have claimed is that nutrition and hydration by medical means need not always be provided. Sometimes they may not be in accord with the patient's wishes or interests. Medical nutrition and hydration do not appear to be distinguishable in any morally relevant way from other life-sustaining medical treatments that may on occasion be withheld or withdrawn.

Notes

1. John A. Robertson, " Dilemma in Danville," *Hastings Cent. Rep.* 11: 5–8 (October 1981).

2. T. Rohrlich, "2 Doctors Face Murder Charges in Patient's Death." *L.A. Times*, August 19, 1982. A-1; Jonathan Kirsch, "A Death at Kaiser Hospital." *Calif. Mag.* (1982), 79ff; Magistrate's findings. California v. Barber and Nejdl, No. A 925586, Los Angeles Man. Ct. Cal. (March 9, 1983); Superior Court of California, County of Los Angeles,

California v. Barber and Nejdl, No. A0 25586k tentative decision May 5, 1983.

3. *In re* Infant Doe, No. GU 8204-00 (Cir. Ct. Monroe County, Ind., April 12, 1982), *writ of mandamus dismissed sub nom.* State ex rel. Infant Doe v. Baker, No. 482 S140 (Indiana Supreme Ct., May 27, 1982).

4. Office of the Secretary, Department of Health and Human Services, "Nondiscrimination on the Basis of Handicap," *Federal Register* 48 (1983), 9630-32. (Interim final rule modifying 45 C.F.R. #84.61.) See Judge Gerhard Gesell's decision, American Academy of Pediatrics v. Heckler, No. 83-0774, U.S. District Court, D.C., April 24, 1983; and also George J. Annas, "Disconnecting the Baby Doe Hotline," *Hastings Cent. Rep.* 13: 14–16 (June 1983).

5. *In re* Conroy, 190 N.J. Super. 453, 464 A.2d 303 (App. Div. 1983).

6. President's Commission for the Study of Ethical Problems in Medicine and Biomedical and Behavioral Research. *Deciding to Forego Life-Sustaining Treatment.* Washington, D.C.: U.S. Government Printing Office (1982).

7. G. E. M. Anscombe, "Ethical Problems in the Management of Some Severely Handicapped Children: Commentary 2," *J. Med. Ethics* 7: 117–124 (1981).

8. See, e.g., President's Commission for the Study of Ethical Problems in Medicine and Biomedical and Behavioral Research, *Making Health Care Decisions*, Washington, D.C.: U.S. Government Printing Office (1982).

9. President's Commission, *Deciding to Forego*, at 171–196.

10. Joyce V. Zerwekh, "The Dehydration Question," *Nursing 83*, 47–51 (1983) with comments by Judith R. Brown and Marion B. Dolan. See also chapter 3.

11. James J. McCartney, "The Development of the Doctrine of Ordinary and Extraordinary Means of Preserving Life in Catholic Moral Theology before the Karen Quinlan Case," *Linacre Q.* 47: 215 (1980).

12. President's Commission. *Deciding to Forego*, at 82–90. For an argument that fluids and electrolytes can be "extraordinary," see Carson Strong, "Can Fluids and Electrolytes be 'Extraordinary' Treatment?" *J. Med. Ethics* 7: 83–85 (1981).

13. The Sacred Congregation for the Doctrine of the Faith, Declaration on Euthanasia, Vatican City, May 5, 1980.

14. Paul Ramsey, *The Patient as Person*, New Haven: Yale University Press (1970), 128–129; Paul Ramsey, *Ethics at the Edges of Life: Medical and Legal Intersections*, New Haven: Yale University press (1978), 275;

Bernard Towers, "Irreversible Coma and Withdrawal of Life Support: Is It Murder If the IV Line Is Disconnected?" *J. Med. Ethics* 8: 205 (1982).

15.   See Kenneth C. Micetich, Patricia H. Steinecker, and David C. Thomasma, "Are Intravenous Fluids Morally Required for a Dying Patient?" *Arch. Intern. Med.* 143: 975–978 (1983), also chapter 4.

16.   Robert and Peggy Stinson, *The Long Dying of Baby Andrew*, Boston: Little, Brown and Co. (1983), 355.

17.   See chapter 4 [in original volume].

Natural Death Act

The State of California

The people of the State of California do enact as follows:

CHAPTER 3.9. NATURAL DEATH ACT

7188. Any adult person may execute a directive directing the withholding or withdrawal of life-sustaining procedures in a terminal condition. The directive shall be signed by the declarant in the presence of two witnesses not related to the declarant by blood or marriage and who would not be entitled to any portion of the estate of the declarant upon his decease under any will of the declarant or codicil thereto then existing or, at the time of the directive, by operation of law then existing. In addition, a witness to a directive shall not be the attending physician, an employee of the attending physician or a health facility in which the declarant is a patient, or any person who has a claim against any portion of the estate of the declarant upon his decease at the time of the execution of the directive. The directive shall be in the following form:

DIRECTIVE TO PHYSICIANS

Directive made this _____ day of _____ _____ (month, year).

I _____ , being of sound mind, willfully, and voluntarily make known my desire that my life shall not be artificially prolonged under the circumstances set forth below, do hereby declare:

1. If at any time I should have an incurable injury, disease, or illness certified to be a terminal condition by two physicians, and where the application of life-sustaining procedures would serve only to artificially prolong the moment of my death and where my physician determines that my death is imminent whether or not life-sustaining procedures are utilized, I direct that such procedures be withheld or withdrawn, and that I be permitted to die naturally.

2. In the absence of my ability to give directions regarding the use of such life-sustaining procedures, it is my intention that this directive shall be honored by my family and physician(s) as the final expression of my legal right to refuse medical or surgical treatment and accept the consequences from such refusal.

3. If I have been diagnosed as pregnant and that diagnosis is known to my physician, this directive shall have no force or effect during the course of my pregnancy.

4. I have been diagnosed and notified at least 14 days ago as having a terminal condition by _____ M.D., whose address is _____ , and whose telephone number is _____ . I understand that if I have not filled in the physician's name and address, it shall be presumed that I did not have a terminal condition when I made out this directive.

5. This directive shall have no force or effect five years from the date filled in above.

6. I understand the full import of this directive and I am emotionally and mentally competent to make this directive.

Signed _____

City, County and State of Residence _____

The declarant has been personally known to me and I believe him or her to be of sound mind.

Witness _____

Witness _____

From California Health and Safety Code, *Part I, Division 7, Chapter 3.9, Section 7188. Approved by the Governor on the 30th of September, 1976.*

The California Medical Association's Durable Power of Attorney for Health Care Form

California Medical Association

TERMS OF DURABLE POWER OF ATTORNEY FOR HEALTH CARE

1. CREATION OF DURABLE POWER OF ATTORNEY FOR HEALTH CARE

By this document I intend to create a durable power of attorney by appointing the person designated below to make health care decisions for me as allowed by Sections 2410 to 2443, inclusive, of the California Civil Code. This power of attorney shall not be affected by my subsequent incapacity.

2. DESIGNATION OF HEALTH CARE AGENT

(Insert the name and address of the person you wish to designate as your agent to make health care decisions for you. None of the following may be designated as your agent: (1) your treating health care provider, (2) a nonrelative employee of your treating health care provider, (3) an operator of a community care facility or residential care facility for the elderly, or (4) a nonrelative employee of an operator of a community care facility or residential care facility for the elderly).

I, _____
(insert your name)

do hereby designate and appoint: _____
(name)

as my attorney-in-fact (agent) to make health care decisions for me as authorized in this document.

Address: _____

Telephone Number: _____

3. GENERAL STATEMENT OF AUTHORITY GRANTED

If I become incapable of giving informed consent to health care decisions, I hereby grant to my agent full power and authority to make health care decisions for me including the right to consent, refuse consent, or withdraw consent to any care, treatment, service, or procedure to maintain, diagnose or treat a physical or mental condition, and to receive and to consent to the release of medical information, subject to the statement of desires, special provisions and limitations set out in paragraph 4.

4. STATEMENT OF DESIRES CONCERNING MEDICAL TREATMENT

(Your agent must make health care decisions that are consistent with your known desires. You can, but are not required to, state your desires in the space provided below. You should consider whether you want to include a statement of your desires concerning decisions to withhold or remove life-sustaining treatment. For your convenience, some general statements concerning the withholding and removal of life-sustaining treatment are set out below. If you agree with one of these statements, you may INITIAL that statement. READ ALL OF THESE STATEMENTS CAREFULLY BEFORE YOU SELECT ONE TO INITIAL. You can also write your own statement concerning life-sustaining and/or other matters relating to your health care. BY LAW, YOUR AGENT IS NOT PERMITTED TO CONSENT ON YOUR BEHALF TO ANY OF THE FOLLOWING: COMMITMENT TO OR PLACEMENT IN A MENTAL HEALTH TREATMENT FACILITY, CONVULSIVE TREATMENT, PSY-CHOSURGERY, STERILIZATION OR ABORTION. In every other respect, your agent may make health care decisions for you to the same extent you could make them for yourself if you were capable of doing so. If you want to limit in any other way the authority given your agent by this document, you should state the limits in the space below. If you do not initial one of the printed statements or write your own statement, your agent will have the broad powers to make health care decisions on your behalf which are set forth in Paragraph 3, except to the extent that there are limits provided by law.)

1

I do **not** want my life to be prolonged and I do **not** want life-sustaining treatment to be provided or continued: (1) if I am in an irreversible coma or persistent vegetative state; or (2) if I am terminally ill and the application of life sustaining procedures would serve only to artificially delay the moment of my death; or (3) under any other circumstances where the burdens of the treatment outweigh the expected benefits. I want my agent to consider the relief of suffering and the quality as well as the extent of the possible extension of my life in making decisions concerning life-sustaining treatment.

If this statement reflects your desires initial here: _____

I want my life to be prolonged and I want life sustaining treatment to be provided **unless I am in a coma or vegetative state** which my doctor reasonably believes to be irreversible. Once my doctor has reasonably concluded that I will remain unconscious for the rest of my life, I do **not** want life-sustaining treatment to be provided or continued.

If this statement reflects your desires initial here: _____

I want my life to be prolonged to the greatest extent possible without regard to my condition, the chances I have for recovery or the cost of the procedures.

If this statement reflects your desires initial here: _____

Other or additional statements of desires, special provisions, or limitations:

_____

_____

_____

_____

_____

_____

(You may attach additional pages if you need more space to complete your statement. If you attach additional pages, you must DATE and SIGN EACH PAGE.)

DATE AND SIGNATURE OF PRINCIPAL

(YOU MUST DATE AND SIGN THIS POWER OF ATTORNEY)

I sign my name to this Durable Power of Attorney for Health Care on _____ at

(Date)

_____ , _____

(City)   *(State)*

_____

(Signature of Principal)

(THIS POWER OF ATTORNEY WILL NOT BE VALID FOR MAKING HEALTH CARE DECISIONS UNLESS IT IS EITHER: (1) SIGNED BY TWO QUALIFIED ADULT WITNESSES WHO ARE PERSONALLY KNOWN TO YOU AND WHO ARE PRESENT WHEN YOU SIGN OR ACKNOWLEDGE YOUR SIGNATURE OR (2) ACKNOWLEDGED BEFORE A NOTARY PUBLIC IN CALIFORNIA.)

Decision Scenario 1 •

"Apparently he was inside the tank with an oxygen hose to provide ventilation," Dr. Mangel said. "There was some oil residue on the walls. When Mr. Golenga struck an arc to weld the seam, there was a flash fire."

Mrs. Golenga gripped the hand of her nineteen-year-old son, Cervando. Both had been crying, but now listening was so important that they forced back their tears.

"How badly hurt is he?" Mrs. Golenga asked.

"Very badly," Dr. Mangel said. "Most of his body is covered with severe burns, and his lungs are damaged from breathing in the fire and smoke."

"Will he live?" Cervando asked.

"I have to be honest with you and say that I don't think he will," Dr. Mangel said. "We are giving him plasma and saline solutions to rehydrate him and antibiotics to try to stop infections. But he hasn't got much of a chance."

"The pain, what about the pain?" asked Mrs. Golenga.

"There's only so much we can do."

"There's really no hope?" Cervando asked.

"I wouldn't say that," Dr. Mangel said. "There is always hope. But in this case it is very limited. He might die in a few hours, or he might die tomorrow or the next day."

"Please," Mrs. Golenga said. "Can you help him die? I know he doesn't want to suffer if he has no real hope. He told me often 'If something happens to me, don't let them stick me full of needles and keep me alive. Tell them to put me out of my misery.' Can you do that, Doctor?"

"Are you sure that's what he would want?" Dr. Mangel asked.

"My mother is right," Cervando said. "I've heard my father say that many times. He said he never wanted to just lie around and suffer, being a burden to himself and everyone. We want to do as he wanted us to."

"We could stop treating him," Dr. Mangel said. "Then let nature take its course."

"That sounds terrible," Mrs. Golenga said. "To make a man fight for his life when he has no hope and no help. It is cold and cruel."

"I'm sorry," said Dr. Mangel. "It is all that the law permits me to do."

1. Would Rachels regard this as the kind of case in which active euthanasia would be more humane than passive?

2. According to the conservative view of Gay-Williams, is there anything that might be done to put an end to Mr. Golenga's life that would also be morally acceptable?

3. Would the line of reasoning taken by Chief Justice Hughes in the Quinlan case make Mrs. Golenga and Cervando the appropriate people to decide whether Mr. Golenga receives additional treatment, is allowed to die, or is killed?

4. Would the Court's reasoning in Cruzan be likely to lead to the same opinion? How might Dworkin respond?

5. According to the considerations advanced by Lynn and Childress, would it be morally acceptable for Mr. Golenga's physicians to stop the procedure to rehydrate him?

Decision Scenario 2 •

Mr. Jeffry Box was eighty-one years old when he was brought to Doctor's Hospital. His right side was paralyzed, he spoke in a garbled way, and he had trouble understanding even the simplest matters. His only known relative was a sister four years younger, and she lived half a continent away. When a hospital social worker called to tell her about her brother's condition, she was quite uninterested. "I haven't seen him in fifteen years," she said. "I thought he might already be dead. Just do whatever you think best for him. I'm too old to worry about him."

Neurological tests and X-ray studies showed Mr. Box was suffering from a brain hemorrhage caused by a ruptured blood vessel.

"Can you fix it?" asked Dr. Hollins. She was the resident responsible for Mr. Box's primary care. The man she addressed was Dr. Carl Oceana, the staff's only neurosurgeon.

"Sure," said Dr. Oceana. "I can repair the vessel and clean out the mess. But it won't do much good, you know."

"You mean he'll still be paralyzed?"

"That's right. And he'll still be mentally incoherent. After the operation he'll have to be put in a nursing home or some other chronic-care place, because he won't be able to see to his own needs."

"And if you don't operate?" Dr. Hollins asked.

Dr. Oceana shrugged. "He'll be dead by tomorrow. Maybe sooner, depending on how long it takes for the pressure in his skull to build up."

"What would you do?"

"I know what I would want done to me if I were the patient," said Dr. Oceana. "I'd want people to keep their knives out of my head and let me die a nice, peaceful death."

"But we don't know what he would want," Dr. Hollins said. "He's never been our patient before, and the social worker hasn't been able to find any friends who might tell us what he'd want done."

"Let's just put ourselves in his place," said Dr. Oceana. "Let's do unto others what we would want done unto us."

"That means letting Mr. Box die."

"Exactly."

1. *On what grounds might Gay-Williams object to Dr. Oceana's view?*

2. *Would Rachels's principles justify active euthanasia?*

3. *Would the natural law view make the operation discussed a moral mandate?*

4. *How might Gaylin et al. assess Dr. Oceana's reasoning?*

5. *Could Justice Stevens's arguments against the majority opinion in* Cruzan *be used to support Oceana's position? What might Dworkin say about the issue?*

Decision Scenario 3 . . . .

On April 8, 1984, Mr. William Bartling was admitted to the Glendale Adventist Medical Center in Los Angeles. He was seventy years old and suffered from five ordinarily fatal diseases: emphysema, diffuse arteriosclerosis, coronary arteriosclerosis, an abdominal aneurysm, and inoperable lung cancer. During the performance of a biopsy to diagnose the lung cancer, Mr. Bartling's left lung collapsed. He was placed in the ICU, and a chest tube and mechanical respirator were used to assist his breathing.

Mr. Bartling complained about the pain the respirator caused him, and he repeatedly asked to have it removed. When his physician refused, he pulled out the chest tube himself. This happened so often that eventually Mr. Bartling's hands were tied to the bed to keep him from doing it. He had signed a living will in an attempt to avoid just such a situation.

Although after discussions with Richard S. Scott, Mr. Bartling's attorney, Mr. Bartling's physician and the hospital administration agreed to disconnect the respirator, the hospital's attorney refused to permit it. He argued that, since Mr. Bartling was not terminally ill, brain-dead, or in a persistent vegetative state, the hospital might be open to legal action.

Mr. Scott took the case to Los Angeles Superior Court. He argued that Mr. Bartling was legally competent to make a decision about his welfare and that, although he did not want to die, he understood that disconnecting the respirator might lead to his death. The hospital's attorney took the position that Mr. Bartling was ambivalent on the question of his death. His statements "I don't want to die" and "I don't want to live on the respirator" were taken as inconsistent and so as evidence of ambivalence. Removing the respirator, the attorney argued, would be tantamount to aiding suicide or even committing homicide.

The court refused either to allow the respirator to be removed or to order that Mr. Bartling's hands be freed. To do so, the court ruled, would be to take a positive step to end treatment, and the only precedents for doing so were in cases in which the patients were comatose, brain-dead, or in a chronic vegetative state.

The case was then taken to the California Court of Appeal, which ruled: "If the right of a patient to self-determination as to his own medical treatment is to have any meaning at all, it must be paramount to the interests of the patient's hospitals and doctors. The right of a competent adult patient to refuse medical treatment is a constitutionally guaranteed right which must not be abridged."

The rule came too late for Mr. Bartling. He died twenty-three hours before the court heard his appeal.

1. *Is there any merit to the hospital's position that to remove Mr. Bartling's respirator or to free his hands would be equivalent to assisting suicide? How might Singer's arguments apply to this position?*

2. *On the natural law view, would the request to remove the respirator be, in effect, a request for assistance in committing suicide?*

3. *How can the reasoning in the* Quinlan *case be extended to Mr. Bartling's case?*

4. *Can the arguments offered by Gay-Williams be used to support the view that it would be morally wrong even to untie Mr. Bartling's hands?*

5. *If Mr. Bartling had an implanted feeding tube, would it be morally right to disconnect it at his request? Would the* Cruzan *decision permit it? Would the criteria offered by Lynn and Childress?*

Decision Scenario 4 . . . .

When two plainclothes detectives arrived at Virginia Crawford's suburban apartment at 6:30 on a Sunday morning to arrest her for murder, she was not terribly surprised to see them.

She cried when they insisted on putting her in handcuffs before transporting her to the jail in the county court building. Yet she had more or less expected to be arrested eventually.

For almost a month, a police investigation had been conducted at Mercy Hospital, where Ms. Crawford worked as a nurse in the intensive-care unit. The entire hospital staff knew about the investigation, and Ms. Crawford herself had been questioned on three occasions by officers conducting the inquiry. At the time, her answers had seemed to be satisfactory to the police, and there was no hint that she was under suspicion. Still, she always believed that eventually they would catch up with her.

The investigation centered on the deaths of four elderly patients during the period February 1979 to March 1980. All of the patients were in the intensive-care unit at the times of their deaths. Each had been diagnosed as suffering from a terminal illness, and the chart notation on each case indicated that they had all suffered irreversible brain damage and were totally without higher brain functions.

The three women and one man were all unmarried and had no immediate family to take an interest in their welfare. All of them were being kept alive by respirators, and their deaths were caused directly by their respirators being turned off. In each instance of death, Ms. Crawford had been the person in charge of the ICU.

After securing the services of an attorney, Ms. Crawford was released on bail, and a time was set for her appearance in court. Through her attorney, Marvin Washington, she made a statement to the media.

"My client has asked me to announce that she fully and freely admits that she was the one who turned off the respirators of the four patients in question at Mercy Hospital. She acted alone and without the knowledge of any other individual. She is prepared to take full responsibility for her actions."

Mr. Washington went on to say that he would request a jury trial for his client. "I am sure," he said, "that no jury will convict Ms. Crawford of murder merely for turning off the life-support systems of people who were already dead."

When asked what he meant by that, Mr. Washington explained. "These patients were no longer people," he said. "Sometime during the course of the treatment, their brains simply stopped functioning in a way that we associate with human life."

Ms. Crawford was present during the reading of her statement, and after a whispered conversation with her attorney, she spoke once for herself. "I consider what I did an act of compassion and humanity," she said. "I consider it altogether moral, and I feel no guilt about it. I did for four people what they would have wanted done, if they had only been in a condition to know."

1. *Does the natural law view offer grounds for removing life-support systems for people who are beyond a reasonable hope of recovery? If so, what are they?*

2. *Why would Gay-Williams's arguments lead us to condemn the actions of Ms. Crawford?*

3. Can Singer's arguments favoring voluntary active euthanasia be extended to justify Ms. Crawford's actions?

4. Are Ms. Crawford's actions consistent with the position taken by Vaux in the "Debbie" debate?

5. Is this the sort of case Dworkin would view as involving the issue of the "intrinsic value of life"? What does he consider wrong about the two "secular" arguments he examines?

Decision Scenario 5 . . . .

Consider the following four cases.

1. Harvey Shick of Tyler, Texas, on June 1, 1983, shot his wife in the head twice with a .22-caliber pistol. Mrs. Marie Shick had suffered from severe arteriosclerosis since the late 1970s and, according to her physician, suffered extreme pain in her lower legs. The couple had been happily married for forty-five years. Although Mr. Shick was charged with murder, the charges were dismissed by the state district court judge. "I found nothing would be gained in this case by further punishing this man," Judge Donald Carroll said. "This was an act motivated by love," Mr. Shick's attorney said. "He was distressed at the sickness, and additional treatment would have brought only a precarious and burdensome prolonging of life." Mrs. Shick's family supported the action.

2. On September 14, 1984, Mr. Thomas P. Engel, a registered nurse, removed the respirator from Joseph Dohr, a seventy-eight-year-old stroke victim at St. Michael Hospital in Milwaukee. Mr. Engel said that Mr. Dohr's family asked that treatment be stopped. Mr. Dohr's physician said that he had refused the request because he believed that death was imminent.

Mr. Engel described the bedside scene with Mr. Dohr's daughter that had led him to act:

> She was standing there by her father's bed, stroking his arm and cheek and crying and talking to him. He was in a coma, in a steady decline. The only thing keeping him alive was the ventilator breathing for him. "This isn't right," she said. Then she looked across the bed at me, right in my eyes, and she said "If I could do this thing, I would." Now, what would you do?

Mr. Engel was charged with practicing medicine without a license. He pleaded guilty and received a twenty-month suspended sentence. His nursing license was revoked for one year by the state nursing board.

3. On August 8, 1985, seventy-nine-year-old Abel Montigny walked into the intensive-care unit of Worcester Memorial Hospital in Worcester, Massachusetts, and shot his wife in the head. He then shot himself. Both died from the injuries. Mrs. Leona Montigny, seventy-six, had been in the hospital for several months. She suffered from serious stomach and blood disorders and was recovering from surgery. Her illnesses were considered treatable, and she was in no immediate danger of death from them.

4. Roswell Gilbert, a seventy-five-year-old retired engineer, was convicted in Ft. Lauderdale, Florida, on May 9, 1985, for killing his incurably ill seventy-three-year-old wife. The couple had been married fifty-one years. Emily Gilbert had a debilitating bone disease and Alzheimer's disease; as a consequence, she suffered both severe pain and mental disorientation. According to a witness, on the day of the killing Mrs. Gilbert had said to her husband "I'm in pain. I want to die." Mr. Gilbert said later "Who's that somebody but me? I guess I got cold as ice. I took the gun off the shelf, put a bullet in it and shot her. Then I felt her pulse. I thought, 'Oh, my God, I loused it up.' I put in another bullet and shot her again."

Mr. Gilbert was sentenced to twenty-five years in prison with no chance of parole. As he left the courtroom, his daughter cried out, sobbing, "Daddy, Daddy, I don't want to see my daddy in jail—he'll die in jail."

Mr. Gilbert lost a chance for clemency when two of the members of the Florida Cabinet rejected the governor's recommendation that he be freed while the case was appealed. "The law does not give one person the right to kill another because of illness or age," said Gerald Lewis, one of those who voted against clemency.

In August 1990, Governor Bob Martinez petitioned the cabinet for clemency, citing Gilbert's failing health, and Gilbert was freed on probation.

1. *Compare the issues that are raised in these four cases. In what ways are the cases the same? In what ways different?*

2. *In which cases, if any, could the action taken be justified by Singer's arguments in favor of voluntary euthanasia?*

3. *In which cases, if any, could the action be justified by the reasoning in the* Cruzan *case?*

4. *Is it likely that the arguments presented by Rachels could be used to justify any of the actions taken?*

5. *Would Gaylin et al. condemn the actions in all these cases? Would Dworkin reject all attempts at regulation?*

Decision Scenario 6 . . . .

In 1984 the Netherlands Supreme Court held that an individual who suffers from a permanent mental or physical condition that he or she finds unendurable may request assistance in dying from a physician. The patient's decision to die must be informed and irrevocable, and there must be no other solution acceptable to the patient that would improve the situation.

The decision to help the patient die must involve the physician from whom help is sought and at least one other professional. The court also held that the time and manner of death should not cause avoidable misery to others.

1. *Can the arguments offered by Singer be used to support a public policy of this kind?*

2. *Are the procedural safeguards adopted in the Netherlands and those advocated by Singer adequate to prevent deliberate homicide? Are they adequate to prevent people who are temporarily depressed or irrational from harming themselves?*

3. *What danger does such a policy pose, according to Gay-Williams?*

4. *Does the right of an individual to refuse life-sustaining medical treatment imply that an individual has a right to terminate his life by active means? If so, does this mean that society has a duty to provide assistance?*

5. *On what grounds might Elizabeth Bouvia have been permitted to starve herself to death under medical supervision? On what grounds might her request have been refused?*

PART II
RIGHTS

CHAPTER 4
AIDS AND ITS ISSUES

CASE PRESENTATION:
Tod Thompson

Tod Thompson opened his sock drawer and took out a round, white enameled snuffbox. A green dragon breathing a jagged tongue of fire was painted on the lid. The box had been given to him almost five years ago by Alan Lauder as a memento of their trip to Cancun. Alan had always bought him a lot of presents; some were just tokens and others expensive, but all were in exquisite taste. In the note accompanying the snuffbox, Alan had said something clever and flattering about the dragon's fiery tongue.

As a matter of principle, Tod had never bought cocaine, but when somebody gave him a little he kept it in the dragon box. Those days now seemed as obscure and fragmentary as scenes from a movie watched in childhood. After Alan got sick, Tod never felt happy enough to risk doing drugs of any kind. He had never minded using them occasionally to intensify his pleasures, but he didn't want to come to depend on them to make life bearable.

After Alan died, he even stopped drinking. He had actually stopped a few months before that. That was now almost two years ago. Alan had been too sick even to eat, and Tod had no wish to drink alone. Now he drank only water and fruit juice, not even wine.

Tod opened the hinged lid of the snuffbox and looked at the blunt purple and gray capsules of Seconal inside. He dumped them into the palm of his hand and counted them, pushing each to one side with a fingertip.

Eight. Including the capsule Ken Heseltine had given him the day before, he had eight. Six was supposed to be enough, but with eight he felt much better. How ghastly it would be to wake up in a hospital feeling very sick and knowing you had failed. If you were going to do it, you should be sure you could pull it off. And he was sure he was going to do it. He had watched Alan, and nothing would make him want to go through that.

Tod put the snuffbox under his socks in the back corner and closed the drawer. He looked up at the mirror hanging above the dresser, and the reflection still shocked him. He couldn't believe how he had changed, and he always seemed to be looking at a stranger.

He was young, really—only twenty-seven. He looked young, but in the way photographs of children in concentration camps made them look young and old simultaneously. His gray eyes were abnormally large as they stared out of deep sockets, and his cheeks were drawn into dark hollows beneath sharp cheekbones. His blond hair was fine and wispy, barely hiding the pale skin of his scalp. His body was shrunken, and his thin shoulders hunched inward like the folded wings of a bat.

He pulled back one side of his shirt collar, exposing an edge of one of the bluish patches that ran across his chest and back and covered his arms and legs—the marks of Kaposi's sarcoma. They had been late in coming, at least compared to what he had heard about what had happened to other people. Maybe the AZT had helped slow down the process. The drug had appeared too late to do much for Alan, but maybe it had helped him.

He dropped his shirt collar and made himself smile. If he used his imagination, he could still catch a hint of the charm he used to work at developing. When he moved to Dallas from Tyler, his idea was to transfer his credits from Tyler Community College and finish his degree in English.

He would also have to work, though. His parents were barely making it themselves, and he couldn't count on them for support. The job he got with Bluffview Books was full time, but it had enough flexibility to allow him to take classes. That's just what he did for a semester. Then, when he met Alan at a party, they began doing so many things together that finishing his degree stopped being high on his list of priorities. He always planned to go back, but there had seemed plenty of time for that later. Alan was a lawyer, and he wanted Tod to train as a paralegal so they could work together. Tod had preferred the bookstore.

Alan introduced him to a world he never suspected existed. It was a world of glittering parties, long weekends on yachts, quick trips to Mexico, San Francisco, and New York, and above all, abundant and virtually unrestrained sex. Tod found himself the object of much attention, and he liked it. He and Alan had agreed that they wouldn't place any constraints on each other. Paradoxically, that was part of what kept them together.

He still missed Alan many times every day. When Alan first got sick, Tod had been angry and even blamed him for it, as though it were something Alan had done deliberately. He now knew that he had just been afraid then—afraid for Alan and for himself.

But that was long ago. Almost two years—two years that seemed like ten.

Hardly two months after Alan died, Tod got sick. First the night sweats started. He would wake up at three or four in the morning so drenched with sweat he would be freezing and burning up simultaneously. Then the mild but persistent fever had started, and diarrhea had come along with it.

He had put off seeing his doctor for almost a month. He hadn't taken the blood test, because he was sure he would test positive and then he wouldn't be able to deny that something so horrible was going to happen to him. When the symptoms finally started, it was almost a relief in a twisted way. Now he knew the worst and didn't have to fear it anymore.

He finally went to his doctor—to Alan's doctor—when he developed shingles on his legs. The rash was too painful to ignore. By then he had already lost a lot of weight. The diarrhea and the fever seemed to keep him tired. That and the lack of sleep. He was exhausted, but he felt too anxious to sleep. He would wake in the early morning hours while it was still dark and lie in bed and wonder what was going to happen to him.

He always asked for the early shift at the bookstore. Since he couldn't sleep, it was a relief to get up and have a place to go to. Also, few customers came in during the morning hours, and he didn't have to deal with people. Keeping up a normal front was very hard. He started the day by stocking the shelves, and usually he did as much as necessary before getting too exhausted. He was working only half-days now, but he was still tired all the time.

When he first got the diagnosis, he resolved to fight the disease and not give in. He wanted to try everything that people told him to try. He spent six weeks eating a macrobiotic diet, but it seemed to make his diarrhea worse. He tried smuggled doses of Compound Q, but he could tell no difference in what was happening to him. Eventually he simply took AZT.

It was the only drug he took for half a year. Then, when the first bruiselike Kaposi patch appeared on his leg, his doctor put him on alpha interferon. When he developed a cough and a fever and was found to have pneumonocystis pneumonia, he was given pentamidine spray. And now he was also trying one drug after another to try to control the diarrhea that had become chronic.

He knew he was lucky to be an employee of the bookstore. He was covered by the group Blue Cross policy, and so far it had paid for everything except 20% of his medical bills and medicines. He had tried to get a supplemental policy before Alan died, but he couldn't find a company willing to accept him without a blood test. So far he had been able to pay his part of the bills, but it wouldn't be long before he became so weak he would have to quit his job.

He couldn't ask his parents to help him. They knew the kind of life he had been living, and they didn't approve of it. But that's not why he couldn't turn to them. It was because they themselves had nothing, and he would become another burden for them. Besides, to be honest, he was afraid of their reaction to him. He couldn't stand the idea that they would treat him like a leper, not wanting to touch him or come near him. In sparing them, he was also sparing himself.

When he could no longer work, he knew what would happen, because he had seen it happen to other people. First they moved to a cheaper apartment, if they could find someone willing to rent to them. Then they sold their car. After that, they began to sell whatever furniture, stereo, or video equipment they had. Finally, they were forced to turn to Medicaid and the state welfare agencies for everything—medical care, medicine, rent money,

telephone, and even the food they didn't want to eat. Most people grew poorer faster than they grew sicker, and that guaranteed their dying in complete poverty.

He heard the sharp ding of the kitchen timer. The frozen pasta dinner he had put in the oven would be ready now. He would have to get it out before it burned. He picked up his cane from the bed and started to walk away.

Then he turned around and pulled open the drawer once more. He picked up the snuffbox and shook it. The capsules inside rattled reassuringly.

He put the box back inside and closed the drawer.

CASE PRESENTATION
The Inadvertent Infection of Kimberly Bergalis

In 1987 Kimberly Bergalis traveled from her hometown of Fort Pierce, Florida, to the nearby town of Stuart to keep an appointment with David J. Acer, her dentist. Bergalis had to have her wisdom teeth pulled, and Dr. Acer extracted one that day.

A month later Bergalis developed a rash on her face and a very sore throat. The symptoms eventually disappeared without any treatment, and she had no other medical problems until the spring of 1989, when she was about to graduate from the University of Florida in Gainesville. She was then plagued by fatigue, sore throats, and fits of coughing. White patches appeared inside her mouth. "I thought I was just stressed out," she later told reporter Felicity Barringer.

The first physician she consulted was puzzled by the white patches. He thought the infection might be thrush, but Bergalis was not a diabetic and was not taking any antibiotics. "That's funny," he told her. "Usually you only get thrush when you're a newborn, a diabetic, or on antibiotics. Or if you have AIDS." Over the following summer, Bergalis's health deteriorated. She continued to be fatigued; she lost weight; her hair fell out in clumps. In an effort to find out what was wrong with her, she consulted other physicians and submitted to a number of medical tests. The physicians presented her with a bewildering variety of possible diagnoses: flu, a particular kind of bone cancer, diabetes, hepatitis, and hysteria.

Bergalis denied being sexually active or using IV drugs, and she had never received any blood or blood products by transfusion. Her medical history seemed to rule out the only recognized modes of transmission of the AIDS virus. Hence, none of the physicians who examined her thought it necessary to test her for the presence of HIV, the virus that causes the disease.

A week after the 1989 Thanksgiving vacation with her family, when she had returned to Gainesville, Bergalis was hospitalized with pneumonia. Although the episode was life threatening, the disease was brought under control. Tests were then done that showed she had pneumocystis pneumonia—the variety typical of people with AIDS. Bergalis was finally tested for HIV, and the result was tentatively positive.

In January 1990 a second test confirmed that Kimberly Bergalis had AIDS. She didn't see how it was possible. "I thought maybe the government was wrong," she said. "Maybe you can get it by kissing. That's the only thing that made sense to me, an exchange of saliva."

Bergalis's mother, a nurse, told Kimberly it was essential that she tell the truth to her physicians. Otherwise, they might make the wrong diagnosis and treat her for the wrong disease. Bergalis insisted she was telling the truth.

Bergalis remained puzzled about how she could have become infected with the virus. Then she remembered that her dentist, Dr. Acer, had been canceling a lot of appointments. His staff said he had pneumonia or cancer, but she also recalled hearing the rumor that he had AIDS.

When she suggested to Florida health officials that she might have been infected by Dr. Acer, they told her they were not investigating that possibility. As it turned out, they were investigating her. Health officials asked her about her dates with her boyfriend and inquired in detail about the kinds of bodily contact they had had. They interviewed her friends and asked them about whether her father had ever shown any sexual interest in her.

No one was inclined to believe that Kimberly Bergalis had been infected by the AIDS virus in some previously unknown way. "They want to believe you were using IV drugs," she said later. "They want to believe you were sleeping around."

Then, in July 1990, the Centers for Disease Control released a report concluding that a young woman in Florida had been infected with the AIDS virus by her dentist. The CDC refused to identify her and later referred to her only as "Patient A."

David Acer died in September of AIDS-related cancer, and immediately after his death an open letter to his patients was printed in the *Stuart News*. "I am David J. Acer and I have AIDS," the letter began. It went on to advise his patients to be tested for the virus. Dr. Acer was a bisexual who treated an estimated 1,700 patients after becoming infected with the virus.

By the spring of 1991, 600 patients had been tested, and two more people were identified as likely to have been infected by Dr. Acer. The probability that Dr. Acer was the source of infection in the three cases was based primarily on the similarity of the viral DNA in all four cases.

When Kimberly Bergalis asked Florida officials whether she was the Patient A in the CDC report, they refused to tell her. After weighing the possible impact on her two younger sisters, Bergalis and her family decided to make the matter a public issue to warn others about what might happen to them. Bergalis entered a malpractice suit against Dr. Acer's insurance company.

The suit was settled out of court in January 1991 for $1 million. Kimberly Bergalis insisted that her interest was not in the money. "It's not going to buy me a cure," she said at the time of the settlement. Her main concern, she claimed, was to make HIV-positive health-care professionals either stop performing invasive procedures or inform patients of the risk they may be taking.

"I'm not asking that we be able to live in a risk-free world," she said in an interview. "I want people to choose their risks. I didn't have a choice to walk out of the office and seek another dentist."

SOCIAL CONTEXT: COMPOUND Q, DRUG TESTING, AND UNAPPROVED DRUGS

In April 1989, a group of AIDS activists and physicians in private practice agreed to conduct a test of the therapeutic effectiveness of a substance they called Compound Q. Until this time, drug trials had been the exclusive province of university- and hospital-based physicians and scientists working in cooperation with pharmaceutical companies and the Federal Drug Administration (FDA).

Compound Q, also known as trichosanthic, is a derivative of the root of the Chinese cucumber and had long been used in China to induce abortions and treat certain kinds of tumors. A study by Michael McGrath of San Francisco General Hospital had also suggested that, when the substance is added to cell cultures that include cells infected with the AIDS virus, infected cells are destroyed while formal cells are unaffected. Encouraged to hope by McGrath's results, some individuals infected with the AIDS virus had gone to great lengths and expense to secure Compound Q from China.

Compound Q seemed so promising as an AIDS treatment that Martin Delaney, head of the AIDS advocacy group Project Inform, decided it should be tested as quickly as possible. If it turned out to be effective, then it could be made available immediately to those needing it. The urgent need for action suggested to Delaney and his supporters that the complex and time-consuming mechanism for testing a drug and securing approval for its use from the FDA could not be followed. People with AIDS were dying daily, and the need for an effective drug was crucial.

Delaney got in touch with several private physicians in San Francisco, New York, Los Angeles, and Miami and assembled a group willing to administer Compound Q to volunteer AIDS patients, monitor their clinical signs, and send blood samples to laboratories for analysis.

The immediate problem then became one of obtaining a supply of Compound Q. Delaney turned to James Corti, a registered nurse who over the previous five years had been smuggling in from Mexico various drugs rumored to be effective in treating AIDS. Corti had established a smuggling network that extended into China. Corti and a Chinese friend obtained the label from a box of medicine containing Compound Q that had been processed at a factory in Shanghai, then flew to China. Paying bribes amounting to tens of thousands of dollars, they obtained 200 doses of Compound Q. Corti then made use of his smuggling network to get the drug into the United States.

Delaney and his associates drew up a set of rules for admitting patients into their program and for administering and evaluating the success of Compound Q. However, the procedures they laid out differed considerably from FDA guidelines. The stage of animal testing was omitted completely. Furthermore, instead of beginning human experimentation by employing low doses of the drug to test for its safety, the Delaney group began administering what they considered likely to be effective therapeutic doses. They then increased dosages from that point.

In addition, all patients in the Compound Q study received the drug. In standard drug testing, a control group would have received either a placebo or, more likely, some other drug with known therapeutic effects. Compound Q would then be compared in effectiveness with the established drug. The initial study involved about thirty patients and nine physicians, although the number of patients grew to around 100.

The Compound Q trials were intended to be conducted in complete secrecy. However,

when three patients participating in the study died, the experiment could no longer remain clandestine. Public attention focused on the last of the three, thirty-year-old Scott Sheaffer.

Sheaffer had a compromised immune system, but he had never taken AZT and seemed stable before taking Compound Q. He then declined rapidly, falling into a coma for three days and regaining consciousness only to die ten days later, at the end of August. Physicians at the two hospitals where Sheaffer received treatment were not told he was receiving Compound Q. Whether the drug caused his death has never been established, although some critics of the Delaney group believe it is likely.

The Delaney group's clandestine approach to testing Compound Q was condemned by a number of researchers and AIDS activists as soon as news of it became public. Mark Harrington, speaking for the AIDS Coalition to Unleash Power (or Act Up), said that, if advocates for people with AIDS wanted to conduct private studies, they would have to meet the same standards as scientific studies. He then called for an inquiry into Sheaffer's death and the Compound Q study. According to Paul Volberding, a respected AIDS researcher, "What they've done is a real disservice to volunteers in the study and to a drug that might be interesting. It doesn't take a genius to hand out drugs to people without controls, but it takes a certain amount of discipline to ask questions in a rigorous way."

The Federal Drug Administration halted the study, then conducted an investigation. In March 1990, to the surprise of many in the medical and scientific community, the agency announced that it was prepared to allow the trials of Compound Q by Delaney's group to continue, provided certain changes were made in the design of the experiments. Sandoz Pharmaceuticals agreed to supply the group with a synthetic form of Compound Q and, in addition, awarded the group a $250,000 grant to do its work. The new study will involve 100 patients.

The FDA decision attracted immediate criticism from hospital- and university-based AIDS researchers. The decision "grants carte blanche to people to do whatever they want to do," Donald Abrahams at San Francisco General Hospital said. "It opens a Pandora's box, and the only people who are going to be hurt are those we are trying to find an answer for." Paul Meier, a statistician at the University of Chicago, expressed the view that the FDA had been "pushed to do things that are not in the interest of the patient group. . . . For the agency simply to approve a study that was illegally conducted and that caused possibly unnecessary deaths shows a political weakness that is tragic for us all."

In the view of some observers, the FDA decision signaled an important change in attitude toward drug testing. For more than a decade, critics have charged that the machinery for testing drugs to determine whether they are safe and effective is much too slow in its operation. Furthermore, some have argued that the standards "safe and effective" are not even appropriate where fatal and quick-acting diseases are concerned.

Advocates for people with AIDS have repeatedly stressed that AIDS patients need immediate access to any drug that seems at all promising. Accordingly, they have been highly critical of federal laws and policies that have slowed the testing of potentially useful drugs. In taking this view, advocates for people with AIDS have repeated and reinforced the complaints of cancer patients, who have often denounced the FDA for its slowness in approving drugs already tested and available in Europe.

This point of view received a degree of support from the August 1990 recommendations of the nine-member National Committee to Review Current Procedures for Approval of New Drugs for Cancer and AIDS. The committee suggested that less evidence of the effectiveness of cancer and AIDS drugs should be required before the drugs are given approval for clinical use.

The committee recommended, in particular, that the FDA drop its requirement that drug companies provide evidence that an experimental drug can "prolong life." It is enough, the committee said, if the evidence shows that the drug improves the quality of a patient's life. As the report said, "For cancer and AIDS patients time is running out, and they are understandably impatient with the delays in obtaining the pharmacotherapy which represents their only hope." The FDA should approve new drugs "at the earliest possible point in their development" and certainly "earlier than has been true in the past."

The committee admitted that faster approval of experimental drugs will increase the risk of those using them. "Some of the drugs may turn out either to be ineffective or to present an unacceptable benefit-risk ratio." However, "Patients with life-threatening diseases who have no alternative therapy are entitled to make this choice."

The committee is only advisory, and there is no guarantee that its recommendations will be taken. Some observers believe that the FDA is not likely to go so far or so fast in altering its current policies.

Those opposed to speeding up the FDA's drug-approval process point to experiences with "expanded access program" involving the drug DDI (dideooxyinodine). The program, which was initiated in August 1989, allows patients to take experimental drugs under the supervision of private physicians even while the drugs are being tested in clinical trials. The "parallel track" approach was introduced to meet the criticisms of people with AIDS and their advocates that the slow process of testing denies useful drugs to those most in need of them.

Critics of the program claim that access to DDI has made it extremely difficult to recruit patients for clinical trials. Those wishing to try the drug must be unable to take AZT because of severe side effects, but they may receive DDI from their own physicians and not have to put up with the inconvenience and risks involved in participating in a controlled clinical trial. Specifically, those enrolled in a trial will have only a 50% chance of receiving the drug. Eight thousand patients are receiving DDI as part of the parallel-track approach, but fewer than half of the 1,500 needed for a clinical trial have volunteered.

Also, the way in which data are collected and monitored by private-practice physicians makes them less precise and reliable than data collected under study conditions. Hence, the expanded-access program undercuts the whole drug-testing effort. For the sake of satisfying the demands of a few people with AIDS now, the possibility of helping thousands more in the future is severely compromised.

Critics of the program also point to the risk of allowing a large group of people to use a drug before its safety has been adequately determined. The death rate among patients taking DDI was ten times higher than expected on the basis of the initial study. In the initial phase of the program, of 8,000 patients taking DDI, 290 died. Only 2 of 700 died in the pilot study. Speaking about the expanded-access program, Thomas C. Chalmers said "I think it's a painful way to learn the lesson, but maybe it's the only way to learn that, to my mind, they did the wrong thing."

For some advocates for people with AIDS or other lethal diseases, even the expanded-access program is too restrictive on patient autonomy. Even with lowered standards for approval and widened access, not every experimental drug is available to anyone who wishes to use it. The fact remains that the government still controls access to drugs and has the power to determine which ones are legally available for use.

The public first became aware that actor Rock Hudson had AIDS when his press representative announced that he was in Paris to seek treatment for the disease. A drug rumored to have some chance of success against AIDS was not legally available in the United States. After treatment, Hudson returned to his home in California, where he died a few weeks later.

Every year hundreds—perhaps even thousands—of Americans travel to foreign countries to seek medical treatments that are not available to them at home. They go to clinics in Mexico, West Germany, Switzerland, Brazil, Greece, the Bahamas, and a number of other places. In the past they were almost exclusively cancer patients, but now they include a growing number of AIDS patients. Most have learned that they can reasonably expect to live only a few more weeks or months. Whatever their disease, they all share a sense of desperation. They are trying to save their lives.

Furthermore, drugs they have heard might be helpful simply cannot be obtained legally in the United States. During the last few years, drugs like ribavirin, AL-721, and dextran sulfate, thought by some to be useful in treating AIDS, have been available only through illegal channels. Either they have been smuggled into the country by people like James Corti, or they have been produced in secret laboratories and sold on the black market.

Why are Americans required to travel to distant countries and spend large amounts of money just to get treatments they want? Why are they forced to resort to illegal means to secure access to drugs they believe will help them? Why should desperate and dying people be forced to make personal and financial sacrifices to gain access to therapies they wish to try?

One answer to these questions lies in the responsibilities assigned to the FDA. It has the task of approving for use all new drugs and medical devices. Even before a drug like Compound Q is used experimentally in clinical trials, it is supposed to have FDA approval for experimental use. Applications for approval must include data about the use of the drug in experimental animals. (This is the first requirement the Delaney group circumvented in its testing of Compound Q. The group took it for granted that, because the drug had been used for years, perhaps centuries, in China, it was safe to use in clinical trials.) Only after such approval can clinical studies of the drug be initiated.

Randomized clinical trials of the drug in patient populations are then conducted, and the significance of the results is established through statistical analysis. In general, an effort is made to design studies that possess the formal features of any good scientific experiment. (These are exactly the features that the critics claim are missing from the Compound Q study.)

The slow and rigorous process required in the past by the FDA has its advantages. Patients in the United States are provided with a great deal of protection from the harmful effects of new and poorly tested drugs. Perhaps the most dramatic instance of this is the FDA's refusal to approve the drug thalidomide. Even though it was widely prescribed as a tranquilizer in several European countries and some studies of its safety had been done, its effects when taken by pregnant women had not been studied. The tragic outcome was that the children born to women who had taken the drug were severely malformed, were blind or deaf, or had seriously defective internal organs. The United States was saved from having a "thalidomide generation" by FDA requirements.

Certainly no one wishes to run unknown risks from the effects of drugs under ordinary circumstances. However, those who have been told that they have a terminal disease for which approved therapies are of limited effectiveness can hardly be said to be in ordinary circumstances. Should they not be allowed access to whatever drug they might wish to try? Should they not be permitted to experiment on themselves if they choose to do so? Is it not paternalistic to the point of absurdity to attempt to protect people who believe themselves beyond protection and who wish only the freedom to attempt to save their lives?

It would be possible to pass laws that would allow anyone diagnosed as having AIDS or any illness expected to be terminal to request treatment of any sort. Thus, anyone who wished to use an untested drug merely rumored to be effective would have the freedom to do so.

Such legislation would promote individual freedom, but it would also have some serious negative consequences. Perhaps the most serious result would be that the integrity and effectiveness of the medical-care system would be threatened. The system is supported to a considerable extent by current drug regulations; if any and all drugs were legalized for even restricted therapeutic use, the way would be opened for the development of various forms of quackery. It is easy to imagine that clinics offering "new miracle drugs" and specializing in the treatment of "hopeless" patients would soon spring up.

The existence of such clinics would have the effect of encouraging patients to place their trust in worthless but well-publicized drugs. Patients who might derive benefits from established therapies would be likely to turn away from them in favor of unproved remedies. The very fact of legalization would serve to give an air of legitimacy to virtually any kind of treatment. Those desperately attempting to lengthen their lives might actually shorten them.

No one can deny that placing restrictions on the type of therapy an individual is free to choose can be construed as a form of paternalism. (For a discussion of paternalism, see Chapters 1 and 5.) We legitimately assume that individuals want to protect themselves from therapies judged by ordinary scientific standards as useless and potentially harmful. Thus, we are usually not inclined to regard drug regulations and standards of medical practice as paternalistic. However, from the point of view of someone with AIDS who is desperate enough to try any remedy, such restrictions may be viewed as blatantly paternalistic.

But can we make exceptions for such people without subjecting the rest of the population to unacceptable risks?

INTRODUCTION

The disorder now known as Acquired Immunodeficiency Syndrome, or AIDS, is a focus for a variety of pressing moral and social issues. AIDS faces us constantly with the question of what we should do about such matters as increasing the proportion of medical research funding allocated for AIDS, restricting individual freedom to protect society, balancing the need to protect confidentiality against the need to inform, making it easier for end-stage AIDS patients to die, and testing the effectiveness of AIDS drugs. The infectious, epidemic, and invariably fatal character of AIDS gives these issues an immediacy and urgency with few parallels in the history of medicine.

To understand how the issues connected with AIDS arise, it is helpful to put the disease in a historical and biomedical framework. Hence, we will begin with a sketch of the story of its discovery and the elucidation of its mode of operation, then look at its present social reality. Within that context, a number of moral and social issues will stand out clearly.

Because the ethical issues surrounding the AIDS epidemic are special cases of more general moral issues—confidentiality, distribution of resources, and so on—this chapter will not be structured like others in this book. The emphasis will be more on identifying issues and outlining responses to them, rather than sketching out ways particular moral principles and theories might be applied to them. That will be left to the readings and to the reader.

DISCOVERING THE DISEASE

In the spring of 1981, the federal Centers for Disease Control (CDC) began receiving reports from physicians in New York and Los Angeles that they were seeing patients with an unusual form of pneumonia caused by the protozoan *Pneumocystis carinii*. The patients also showed signs of having damaged immune systems, leaving them prey to opportunistic diseases that included bacterial and viral infections and rare forms of cancer. In fact, the CDC soon learned that a number of the reported cases of the unusual pneumonia, known as PCP, also had developed Kaposi's sarcoma, a rare form of cancer of the skin and internal organs. Until then Kaposi's sarcoma had been found almost exclusively in elderly Jewish and Mediterranean males.

The most striking aspect of the cases was that all the patients were homosexual males. When the CDC checked its records for similar cases in the past, it discovered ones in New York in 1978 and 1979 that also involved homosexual males. A rapid survey of several major cities led to the discovery of almost 100 cases. The almost exclusive occurrence of the disease—whatever it might be—among homosexual men led to the question "What characteristic do male homosexuals have that might be responsible for the disease they are getting?"

Out of the identified cases, investigators from the CDC intensively interviewed the thirty people known to be alive. The interviews produced information that led to the first hypothesis. Amyl and butyl nitrites, known as "poppers," are stimulants that when inhaled produce a temporary high. They are used almost exclusively by gay men, and more than 90% of those interviewed said that they had used them. This suggested that perhaps the nitrites might damage the immune system in some direct or indirect way. Or perhaps some bad batches of poppers had got on the market, and whatever was in them caused damage. The CDC began experiments with mice, collected samples of the various brands of nitrites, and conducted more interviews about their use.

Meanwhile, additional cases were being reported. The class of those affected grew to include intravenous drug users and Haitian immigrants. The fact that Haiti had a reputation for being a vacation spot for American homosexual men suggested that the disease might have spread from there, but not all the

Haitians with the disease were homosexuals. Some intravenous drug users were homosexuals, but by no means all of them. The facts were not falling into any neat and obvious pattern. The names that had been given to the disease, such as "the gay plague" and "gay-related immunological deficiency," or GRID, came to seem quite inappropriate.

Another syndrome that seemed connected with the disease was identified. Called lymphadenopathy, it was characterized by fatigue, sudden weight loss, swollen lymph nodes, fever, chills, and night sweats. The diseases that commonly cause such generalized symptoms were all absent. This led physicians and researchers to speculate that the syndrome might be the disease at an early stage.

Other hypotheses were proposed. An early one was the "immune system overload" theory. According to it, the frequency with which gay men engage in sexual activity and the nature of activity expose them to a great variety of foreign substances, and the immune systems of some simply break down from repeated assault. The obvious difficulty with the hypothesis was that such sexual activity had been going on for thousands of years, and there was no particular reason for such immunological assaults suddenly to produce a new disease.

Many researchers favored viewing the disorder as an infectious disease caused by a mutated virus or by an existing virus that was gaining wider circulation. The virus, according to the hypothesis, would in some way attack and destroy the immune system and leave its victims open to the opportunistic infections that people with an intact immune system are not prey to.

The hypothesis gained support when two cases of the disease were diagnosed in hemophiliacs. The only way they could have been exposed was through the injection of the blood factors required to control their hemophilia. Both had received injections of the blood-clotting protein called factor VIII. It is so chemically unstable that it cannot be subjected to the usual purification process of pasteurization without being destroyed. That, plus the fact that a single injection may contain the factor from as many as 2,500 people, means that hemophiliacs are exposed to an unusual extent to blood-borne viruses. It began to look more certain that the mysterious disease was caused by an infectious agent, probably a virus.

BIOMEDICAL ASPECTS OF AIDS

Identifying the Virus

The disease the CDC was sure it had found was given the more neutral name of Acquired Immunodeficiency Syndrome—AIDS—and laboratory work was pursued with speed and vigor. The research soon began to reveal some of the characteristics of AIDS at the biological and molecular level. Researchers discovered that, although AIDS patients may have a normal or elevated level of antibodies in their blood, they lack a normal number of white blood cells known as "helper T-cells" or T-4 lymphocytes, which play a crucial role in making antibodies effective. Furthermore, white blood cells known as "suppressor T-cells" or T-8 lymphocytes, which inhibit the antibody system, are present in increased numbers. The immune system is thus severely crippled. This was taken as more evidence that a viruslike organism that attacks the immune system might be responsible for the unknown disease.

In the spring of 1984, Robert C. Gallo of the National Cancer Institute and Luc Montagnier of the Pasteur Institute in Paris independently reported the identification of the virus that is the infectious agent causing AIDS. The virus is known as the human immunodeficiency virus, or HIV.

The HIV virus is now recognized as being one of several immunodeficiency viruses. The virus, designated as HIV-1, is known to cause AIDS. The consensus is that another virus, HIV-2, also causes AIDS but may have a longer incubation period. So far no evidence has been found to suggest that anyone has acquired an

HIV-2 infection in the United States. For this reason, references here to HIV and the AIDS virus will be to HIV-1.

Epidemiologists believe that AIDS may have originated in central Africa, most likely in Zaire, perhaps as the result of a gene mutation. The early view that the disease came from the AIDS-like disease caused by simian immuno-deficiency virus (SIV), which affects the African green monkey, is now considered wrong. Current evidence indicates that the similarities among SIV, HIV-1, and HIV-2 might be explained by their having had a common ancestor.

From Africa the disease spread in some way or other to the Caribbean, was acquired by American homosexuals in Haiti, then began to spread in the United States, probably from New York and then to San Francisco. Recent evidence indicates that the disease appeared several times as early as the late 1950s and 1960s in Britain, the United States, and elsewhere but failed to establish itself within the local population. That did not happen until the 1980s.

Cases in Europe now number in the thousands, and a few hundred cases have been reported in the USSR and the People's Republic of China. Very large numbers of cases have been reported in South America, and Brazil in particular is seen by some experts as a new frontier of the epidemic.

The spread of the disease is without doubt a worldwide phenomenon. The African continent has been hit particularly hard as educational programs have proved ineffective, and over the last few years AIDS has spread from the cities to the countryside. A very conservative estimate of the number of adults infected with the virus in Africa is 5 million. Considering that the number of HIV infections worldwide is thought to be around 8 million, Africa is in a bad situation that is likely to become worse.

AIDS Drugs and Vaccines

After the AIDS virus was identified, additional research soon identified major parts of the mechanism by which it works. The virus is known to be a retrovirus. When it is introduced into the body, it eventually enters a T-cell in the immune system and becomes incorporated into the DNA in the cell's nucleus. When the T-cell is activated in the presence of an infectious agent, the virus reproduces itself and kills the T-cell, and this releases new viruses to infect other T-cells.

That the virus is inside the cells of the immune system poses a major difficulty in developing a treatment for AIDS, because any drug likely to destroy the virus will also destroy the immune system. Researchers find it a daunting prospect to conceive of a drug that will eliminate immune cells containing the virus while leaving other cells untouched. AIDS itself compromises the immune system, and, when the immune system is further weakened or even destroyed by drugs, the body is without defense and even a minor infection can result in severe illness and death.

In September 1986, researchers announced results showing some success in treating AIDS with the drug AZT (azidothymidine). The investigators were quick to point out that this did not mean a cure for the disease was available. AZT halts the reproduction of the virus and prolongs the life of those infected with the AIDS virus, but it does not reverse the damage to the immune system caused by the virus. Also, because the drug itself interferes with the immune function, those with AIDS can still suffer from a variety of opportunistic infections that must be treated separately.

At first individuals who tested positive for HIV but were asymptomatic were not eligible to be treated with AZT, because it had been approved by the FDA only for use in patients with full-blown symptoms of AIDS. Then studies in 1989 established that AZT dramatically slows the replication of the AIDS virus in people with such mild symptoms of the disease as thrush (an infection of the lining of the mouth and throat), chronic rash, or diarrhea. Because of this, the FDA now permits the use of AZT in patients who are HIV positive but show no symptoms of AIDS. The hope now is that the onset of the disease may be significantly slowed in many patients by early intervention.

AZT remains the only drug established as effective in prolonging the lives of people with AIDS. Recently, however, the drug DDI (dideooxyinodine) has been found to delay the onset of the symptoms of AIDS for fifteen months or more. Like AZT, which has a similar molecular structure, DDI has toxic side effects, but early tests show it to be as effective as AZT. A 1990 study involved fifty-eight people with AIDS or AIDS-related complex (ARC); over eighteen months, only six (some 20%) died. Before the use of antiviral drugs, about 75% would have died. The T-cell count rose by 28%, although for patients who had been taking AZT the rise was significantly smaller. (For a discussion of the controversy over making DDI available as part of the FDA expanded-availability program, see the earlier Social Context section.)

The drug pentamidine in aerosol form is also commonly used in conjunction with AZT to prevent the growth of the organisms that cause pneumocystis pneumonia. In February 1989, the FDA decided to allow the use of pentamidine in seriously ill patients, although the drug had not gone through the approval process. Since PCP is a leading cause of death in people with AIDS, some viewed the FDA decision as a major victory.

The cost of AZT ranges from $5,600 to $6,400 a year per person, and at this time some 40,000 Americans are taking the drug. Only those with a large income or the right kind of insurance have been able to afford to pay for it. It has recently been shown, however, that the same results with fewer side effects can be obtained by using half the standard dose of AZT. As a result, the drug is more likely to be affordable by those who need it.

Not only have the antiviral drugs increased the life expectancy of people with AIDS, but with experience physicians have become more skilled at treating the opportunistic diseases that resulted in quick deaths during the early years of the AIDS epidemic. Now those with bacterial and fungal infections are treated early and aggressively. The pneumonia that first signaled the outbreak of the epidemic is now treated prophylactically, so that its significance as a cause of death has declined. As a result of this more aggressive treatment of secondary infections, AIDS patients are living longer, but they are also beginning to develop various forms of cancer. Developing effective treatment for these patients is seen by AIDS experts as a challenge for the coming years.

As soon as the AIDS virus was identified, the hope was that a vaccine for it would be developed immediately. AIDS would then join the ranks of diseases like smallpox and rabies that cannot be effectively treated but can be effectively prevented by vaccination. Unfortunately, HIV has turned out to be a virus that mutates rapidly and exists in many variant forms. Some researchers doubt it will be possible to get a vaccine that will prevent all forms of the disease. Nevertheless, work is underway, and at least seven vaccines are currently being tested in humans.

AIDS Transmission and Risks

The way in which the AIDS virus is transmitted is not completely understood. The virus is most concentrated in the blood and semen of those infected, and the introduction of the virus directly into the bloodstream seems the most certain mode of transmission. Thus, IV-drug users who share a syringe with an HIV carrier are at most risk of infection, as are those who receive blood or blood products contaminated with the virus. Health workers who get needle sticks with infected syringes or scalpel cuts during surgery on an HIV patient, or who come into contact with blood containing the virus, are at some risk.

The virus is also transmitted by sexual relations in which semen comes into contact with mucous membrane. Thus, in the case of male homosexuals or bisexuals, the virus may enter the bloodstream through the lining of the rectum during anal intercourse. In heterosexual intercourse, the vaginal membrane may be the means of entry. Anal sex seems to pose the greatest risk for both men and women, for the rectal membrane is delicate, and small tears may allow entry of the virus. Sores or cuts in the mouth may make oral sex a possible mode of infection.

Because of the presence of the virus in semen, transmission seems more likely from male to female than vice versa. (In Zaire, however, infection seems equally likely for men and women.) The mode of transmission of the virus from female to male during intercourse is not clear. An open sore or tear in the skin of the penis may offer a mode of entry. The presence of some other sexually transmitted disease—in particular, genital herpes or gonorrhea—seems to increase the likelihood of infection in both males and females. There is no evidence to show that the virus enters the body through the urethra.

Pregnant women who carry the virus may pass it on to the fetus through the maternal-fetal circulatory system. This seems to happen as much as 40–50% of the time.

Individuals most at risk are: intravenous-drug users, homosexual or bisexual males, those with multiple sexual partners, those with a history of sexually transmitted diseases, those receiving blood transfusions or blood products before 1985, and the sexual partners of anyone in one of these categories.

The AIDS virus has been discovered in low concentrations in the saliva and tears of those infected. Kissing in which saliva is exchanged is thought to be a slight risk, but sneezing, coughing, touching, and so on are not considered likely means of transmission. Even food handlers with AIDS are not thought to pose a risk to others.

Outside a host, the AIDS virus seems to be quite fragile, which means it is unlikely that anyone could become infected by using dishes, eating utensils, books, toilet seats, or other articles touched by a carrier. In short, there is strong evidence to believe that AIDS is not spread by means of ordinary social contact in the way that, for example, cold viruses are spread.

Blood Tests

An important development after the discovery of the AIDS virus was a blood test to determine its presence in individuals. ELISA (enzyme-linked immunosorbent assay), the most commonly used test, does not identify the virus directly but detects the presence of antibodies to the virus in a blood sample. The test is good on sensitivity—that is, it rarely fails to detect the presence of the virus. However, it is not so good on specificity; it shows many false positives (indicating that the virus is present when it is not). For this reason, anyone who tests positive for HIV should have the result confirmed by a test that is more specific. (The usual procedure is to use the ELISA test a second time and then, if the results are still positive, to use the Western blot.)

The antibodies to HIV typically develop about four weeks after infection, and the blood test now used cannot detect the presence of the virus before that time. This means that an individual may be infected for a four-week period without knowing it and without testing positive for HIV. Some evidence shows that the virus is most infectious before antibodies to it can be detected. Consequently, an individual may transmit the virus to others without being aware of it. (Additional evidence also suggests that the virus can sometimes stay inside a macrophage in a cell for three years or more. During that time, it does not infect the T-cells, and no antibodies to the virus are produced. The average time before the symptoms of AIDS appear (the latency period) is seven years.

A new test employing blood plasma, the part of blood free of red cells, can confirm the presence of the virus within two weeks of infection. The test works by directly detecting virus particles in the plasma before the immune system responds to the particles as antigens and produces antibodies. The FDA is expected to approve the test for diagnostic purposes.

Blood collection agencies routinely screen blood donors for the HIV virus. Yet because of the four-week period between an individual's becoming infected and developing antibodies, the usual test cannot eliminate all potential donors who might be carriers. However, the FDA probably will not require the use of the new test, because it would not add significantly to the safety of current screening procedures. Using present methods, out of 2,236 AIDS cases linked to blood transfusions, only two have occurred since current screening methods were introduced in 1985. (Blood plasma is also processed in a way that renders the virus harmless.) Public health officials claim that blood supplies are now safer than they have ever been.

Education and Personal Protection

No genuinely effective treatment for AIDS has been devised. Nor is a vaccine to protect against it available. Accordingly, experts agree, the most practical means to slow the spread of the virus and keep the number of cases from increasing is public education. Thus, people are advised to limit their sexual contacts, avoid anal intercourse, use condoms, avoid using unsterilized syringes, avoid unprotected sexual relations with anyone who might have AIDS, and make an effort to determine the sexual history of a potential sex partner. Those who think they might have been exposed to the virus should get a blood test; if it turns out positive, they should get another, more specific, test. Early detection is important, because recent studies show that the onset of AIDS can sometimes be significantly delayed. Also, the treatment of life-threatening secondary diseases like pneumonia is most successful when started early.

Current Statistics

Not only do statistics about AIDS change as more information accumulates, but most available statistics are considered untrustworthy to various degrees. The studies are usually based on small samples, and the samples themselves may be biased by such factors as deceit, denial, and an unwillingness to divulge private information. Nevertheless, here are some data that are considered established on the basis of information available as of November 1990:

• About 136,000 cases of AIDS have been reported in the United States. Some 83,000 people have died from the disease. No one has been known to recover.

• Each day there are 212 new cases. There is one new infection every 54 seconds, and one AIDS-related death occurs every 12 minutes.

• From 600,000 to 1 million people in the United States have been exposed to the virus and may be assumed to be able to pass on the virus to others.

• A statistical profile of reported cases of AIDS in 1989 was as follows:

Heterosexuals	5.0%
Homosexual male IV-drug users	5.8%
Other IV-drug users	23.2%
Other male homosexuals	55.3%
Others	10.7%

• The largest number of new cases of AIDS consists in IV-drug users. In 1981 they constituted only 11% of new cases, but by 1989 they made up more than twice that figure.

• The spread of AIDS to the heterosexual population is shown by the increase from the 1981 figure of 0.5% to the 1989 figure of 5%. Most of the increase is considered the result of unsafe sexual practices.

- During a six-month period in 1990, autopsies in New York City found 1 in 7 people infected with the AIDS virus. Black men of age 41–50 had the highest rates of infection (38%), and those of age 31–40 the second highest (31%). Women 31–40 had a rate of 35%. Males had a higher rate of infection than females, but the gap was not as wide as expected: 15.3% versus 11.7%.

- Worldwide, about 387,000 cases of AIDS have been reported from 151 countries. (The World Health Organization believes a more accurate figure is about 700,000.) The number of people infected is estimated to be 6–8 million. By the year 2000, the figure is expected to climb to 20 million.

ETHICAL AND SOCIAL ISSUES

Confidentiality and Notification

When New York City decided to keep autopsy statistics (see above) to determine what percentage of people were infected by the AIDS virus, the original plan announced by Health Commissioner S. C. Joseph was to record the names of the infected people and notify their spouses and sex and drug partners so they might get medical help if necessary.

Joseph's plan became the target of criticism by AIDS groups that objected to the violation of confidentiality that the partner-notification plan required. The plan would function without the consent of the deceased individual with AIDS and would involve revealing a significant fact about that person that he or she might not have wanted revealed. The matter became an issue in the mayoral campaign, and candidate David Dinkins suggested that if he were elected he would not reappoint Joseph. Dinkins was elected, and he appointed someone else as Commissioner of Health.

The issue of AIDS and confidentiality is politically volatile throughout the country.

Should AIDS tests be offered anonymously? Should physicians be required to report to health agencies the names of patients with AIDS? And, most controversial of all, should states and cities adopt notification policies requiring physicians or public health departments to notify the spouses and sex and drug partners of those who test HIV positive that they have been exposed to the virus?

The controversy over confidentiality involves a tangle of competing interests. On the one hand, individuals who test positive for HIV may not want this fact known to anyone. If it is, then however they acquired the virus, they may be thought to be drug abusers, sexually promiscuous, or, if male, homosexuals or bisexuals. They may fear discrimination or pity or may simply not wish something they consider intensely personal and private to be made public in any degree.

On the other hand, if people who are exposed to the virus without suspecting it are not notified, they may not recognize the need to be tested. Although anyone might choose to be tested for the AIDS virus, someone knowing of no reason to believe she or he has been put at risk for infection has no reason to seek the test. For example, a wife who does not know her husband is an IV-drug abuser does not know that she too is running a risk of infection when they have sex. If her husband consults a physician and tests positive for HIV, shouldn't the physician notify the wife that she also may be infected with the virus?

Knowing that one might be infected is important. A few years ago the question of notification may have been mostly abstract, but now that early treatment for those carrying the virus has been shown effective in delaying the onset of the disease, notification is of basic importance.

The potential conflict between the right to confidentiality of a person with AIDS and the welfare of those he or she may have exposed to the virus is obvious. It would remain potential if everyone testing HIV positive wished all partners notified or if partners never wished to be notified. However, these logical possibilities never hold in actuality. In fact, a 1988 study concluded that almost 25% of sexually active people tested for the AIDS virus said that, even if they tested positive for the virus, they would not inform casual sex partners that they were carriers. It is not likely that a larger percentage would voluntarily warn sex partners after the fact.

At present no national policy regulates notification, but a number of cities and states have formulated policies. Taken together, these policies do not offer a coherent approach. Almost every conceivable policy has been adopted somewhere, and the degree of enforcement is said to vary as widely as the policies themselves.

Voluntary notification programs permit those who test HIV positive to authorize health authorities to notify individuals named by those tested. By requiring consent, voluntary programs have the advantage of protecting the privacy and autonomy of those with AIDS.

Yet the obvious disadvantage is that they may fail to protect the interest of those whom the person with AIDS has exposed to the virus. The interest of those exposed is totally dependent on decisions made by others. Those at risk may be kept in ignorance of their danger and hence put into a position in which they do not have information relevant to making decisions about their own welfare or that of others. In this respect, their autonomy is violated without their knowledge or consent.

A mandatory notification program seems the ideal way to protect the welfare of a sex or drug partner of someone who tests HIV positive. One might reason that violating the confidentiality of the HIV-positive person is warranted by the partners' need to know. Although this may be so, an additional consequence of such a policy is that it discourages those who are at highest risk for AIDS from seeking testing.

Few people would be willing to risk such serious consequences as losing their jobs, not being able to find a place to live, or not being able to get insurance if information about their being HIV positive was deliberately or even accidentally made public. Of course, such possibilities can occur even in the absence of a mandatory notification program.

The lack of anonymity in testing is likely to discourage a large group of people from having a test and, hence, from receiving the treatment they may need. In addition, those who are actually infected with the AIDS virus but are ignorant of their condition may continue to spread the virus to others through sexual contacts.

Considerations such as these have encouraged the development of testing programs that permit anonymity. An individual submitting a blood sample is assigned a number and then can learn the results by using that number. Such a procedure protects the confidentiality of the individual tested and increases the likelihood that high-risk individuals will seek tests and treatment. Of course, the procedure leaves the matter of notifying a partner entirely to the individuals tested.

This outcome is not acceptable to all groups. In 1988 the House of Delegates of the American Medical Association broke with the tradition of presumptive confidentiality and passed a resolution urging physicians, if necessary, to take the step of warning the sex partners of patients carrying the AIDS virus. Physicians should encourage patients to take this step themselves, but, if they shirk the responsibility, the physicians should issue a warning. The AMA resolution expressed the view that state governments have the primary responsibility for tracing and warning sex partners, just as with other sexually transmitted diseases, and encouraged the adoption of laws to establish notification procedures.

The AMA position is reflected in a general movement by the states to treat AIDS more like any other communicable disease. By the end of 1988, 11 states had laws requiring the tracing of sex partners, and 15 had quarantine laws permitting authorities to detain people known to be spreading the disease. At least 15 states kept lists of people testing HIV positive, except for those tested anonymously. Those favoring such changes cite the value of early detection and early treatment of those infected with the virus. Both New York and California, which together have some 42% of AIDS cases, oppose this trend. Gay-rights groups in particular have spoken against it, citing their fear that violations of confidentiality will lead to discrimination. They also question the value of partner tracing by pointing to the lack of success it has produced in eliminating venereal diseases.

Advocates of more aggressive testing and tracing policies reply that violations of confidentiality have not occurred within the public health system. Hospitals and physicians have been the ones to blame. Furthermore, partner tracing is crucial in protecting unsuspecting people, such as the wife in our example above who does not know her husband is an IV-drug user. As Colorado Health Commissioner T. M. Vernon stated, "It's a real women's issue. The individuals least likely to be aware are the female mates of closet bisexual men or secret former intravenous drug users."

Confidentiality and Health-Care Providers

Suppose a physician, dentist, or other health-care provider has been tested and shown to be carrying the HIV virus. Does he or she have a duty to inform patients of that fact?

William H. Behringer was a staff physician at the Princeton Medical Center. When he was diagnosed with AIDS, he continued to practice there as an ear-nose-throat specialist. News of his illness spread, however, and the hospital asked him to give up performing surgery. He refused, and the hospital then required patients to sign consent forms saying that they were aware that Behringer had tested positive for the AIDS virus and that there was "a potential risk of transmission."

Behringer sued the hospital. His lawyers argued that the refusal of patients to sign the forms the hospital required constituted a de facto refusal to allow him to practice surgery. The hospital responded that the consent form was not unreasonable and that it had a duty to protect the interest of patients and itself.

Cases like this highlight the conflict between a patient's need to be informed adequately in order to assess his own risks and the health-care worker's claim to confidentiality about her own health.

Until the summer of 1990, there was no established case of the transmission of the HIV virus from a health worker to a patient. Then a case was documented by the Centers for Disease Control. (See the Bergalis Case Presentation.) Consequently, although the risk of transmission of the virus from a surgeon to a patient is quite small, it is now recognized as real. A 1991 study shows the probability of an HIV surgeon's infecting a patient to be 8.1%. Does even a small risk to the patient require a health worker to disclose relevant but private information? The American Medical Association and the American Dental Association have decided that it does. In 1991, both recommended that infected practitioners should inform patients or give up performing invasive procedures.

Behringer, who died of AIDS, believed that he had been infected with the virus when he performed an emergency tracheotomy on an infected patient while not properly masked. The infection may have occurred through contact with the patient's blood and saliva.

Behringer's own infection raises the same moral issue from the other perspective. Should a patient who knows that he is carrying the AIDS virus inform health-care workers of that fact? Most people would answer yes to this question, because an infected patient poses the threat of a fatal disease to those who are taking care of him.

A 1988 study showed that it is likely that hospitals do not rely on patients to volunteer such information about themselves, even if they possess it. Hospitals often regard patients as a potential source of HIV infection; to protect their staff, many hospitals routinely order an HIV test for each admission, even when it is not medically indicated. During the fifteen-month period of the 1988 study at the St. Paul-Ramsey Medical Center in St. Paul, Minnesota, 44% of the tests for AIDS had no medical justification. Furthermore, in these and in an additional 44% of tests for which there was justification, the patients' consent was not obtained. In only 10% of the tests was there both consent and a medical reason for the test.

Similar results were found in a 1990 study of 560 randomly selected hospitals. Many of the hospitals did not get patients' consent before testing them for AIDS—a practice illegal in many states, including New York, California, and Massachusetts. Also, despite federal guidelines on confidentiality, the test results were included in patients' charts. In 25% of the hospitals, patients who tested negative were never told. Even more surprising, in 2–3% of the hospitals, patients who tested positive were not told. Not only does this keep such patients from seeking early treatment, but they may unknowingly infect others.

Social Measures in AIDS Prevention

Many experts believe that the spread of AIDS could be slowed significantly if a federally funded "clean-needle" program was established. During the last decade, AIDS has spread faster among IV-drug users than in any other group. The number of those infected with HIV has more than doubled, from 11% to 22.3%. Countries that provide addicts with free sterile needles have evidence to show that such programs are successful in reducing the rate of infection.

Despite this experience, in the United States only a few small programs are in place, and some of them even operate in open defiance of the law. New York explicitly rejected a clean-needle program; on the federal level, so did the Bush administration. The only federally funded program directed to IV-drug users is an educational campaign to alert them that bleach can be used to sterilize needles.

The story is much the same regarding prevention through education. Leaving out IV-drug users, information about the sexual practices by which the virus is most likely to be transmitted is acknowledged by most public health experts as about the only means for bringing the disease under control in the population now at risk and soon to be at risk.

Public education, such as the informational brochure sent by Surgeon General Edward Koop to every household, plays an important role in reaching the population now sexually active. However, in order to prevent another generation from becoming infected with the AIDS virus, the education of teenagers about AIDS prevention is considered crucial.

This has become a highly contested political issue. Conservative politicians in particular object to the detailed discussion of sexual practices required in any effective AIDS-prevention program. Some believe that explicit discussions of sex encourage early or illicit sexual activity and that no form of sex education has a place in the public schools.

Not providing adequate funding for educational programs is likely to have serious health consequences for the nation. As writer Dick Thompson stated the issue, "If society is unwilling to expend the energy and resources necessary to teach its young people to avoid AIDS, then the epidemic could grow ever larger and ever more tragic well into the next century."

AIDS and Schools

An early issue about AIDS still remains a matter of controversy in several states: Should children with AIDS be allowed to attend public schools? A still-discussed case of conflict occurred in 1985 in Kokomo, Indiana, when thirteen-year-old Ryan White, a hemophiliac who acquired the virus from a blood transfusion, was allowed to enroll in the seventh grade only after a long court battle. Officials were afraid he would spread the disease to other children. Ryan White died in 1990, and no one in his school became infected.

School officials in most states have decided that children with AIDS should usually be allowed to attend regular classes. The City of New York set up a panel to review each child with the disease in a case-by-case fashion. Children with open sores, those who lack control over their bodily functions, or those who show a tendency to bite are dealt with under special programs and not allowed to enter ordinary classrooms. Most school districts now follow the Centers for Disease Control's recommendation that most children with AIDS be allowed in the classroom and that school officials do their best to protect the pupils' privacy.

The complete lack of transmission of the AIDS virus as the result of a child's attending school has muted early objection. However, despite the minuscule risk posed by HIV-positive children, some parents of unaffected children see any risk at all as too much. They point out that, because the disease in question is invariably fatal, then doing everything possible to minimize the risk is the only reasonable response. The courts have sometimes agreed, and in a 1989 Florida case a judge ruled that a child could attend school only if she were kept in an isolation booth.

AIDS Costs and Insurance

The cost for medical care for AIDS in 1990 was close to $3.75 billion. The cost by 1992 is expected to be twice as much. Federal and state programs currently pay 40% of the bill, while private insurance picks up another 40%; the remaining 20% is supposed to be paid by the individual. People who have group health insurance and are HIV positive (or worry that they might be) often try to get supplementary insurance policies to cover this additional amount.

If those who develop AIDS become unable to work or lose their jobs, they may also lose their group health insurance. They must then attempt to get individual coverage. Even if they are fortunate enough to keep their group health or to get an individual policy, if they don't also have a supplemental policy that pays in a timely way, they soon run out of money. In this event, their only resort is quite literally to impoverish themselves by expending their savings and selling their assets until they have a financial worth of less than $2,000. They then become eligible for Medicaid, the federal program for the indigent.

Given these circumstances, there is little wonder that insurance is a major issue generated by the AIDS epidemic. The issues of confidentiality and HIV testing are twined around the core problem of trying to get enough money to pay for needed drugs, physician visits, and hospitalizations. The cost of medical care for each AIDS patient has been estimated to be about $83,000.

Given the cost of treatment, insurance companies consider it important to determine how likely it is that an applicant will get the disease. Some companies have added a required blood test to the application procedure, while others are forbidden to require such a test by state laws or regulations. In these cases, they often rely on an applicant's medical and social history to indicate whether he is a higher-than-average risk.

Even when companies cannot use a blood test, homosexual-rights groups claim that the insurers use questions about AIDS to discriminate against male homosexuals in general. Further, they point out, such practices are likely to make it difficult for many other unmarried males to get insurance.

As an indication of this, Lincoln National issued a memo advising its underwriters to flag applications "if life style, habits or medical history suggest a person is in one of the AIDS risk groups." The memo also suggested using marital status as an indicator of possible homosexuality, particularly among those aged 20 to 49 who live in such cities as New York and Los Angeles. Major insurers like Blue Cross deny that they discriminate against people with AIDS. Smaller companies, though, are known to have directed their agents to employ information about an applicant's occupation, address, and domestic arrangements to determine the likelihood that he will develop AIDS.

The insurance industry contends that it should be able to use blood tests to determine whether an applicant is a carrier of the AIDS virus. "If we can't use the test, it will adversely affect our other applicants," an industry spokesperson said. That is, some who are not carriers of the virus will also be refused insurance on the grounds of suspicion alone. A number of states, such as California and Wisconsin, have forbidden the use of a blood test to determine insurability, as have several state regulatory agencies.

The industry does not believe it should be forced to insure individuals without attempting to determine whether they may be carriers of the AIDS virus. The industry would stand to increase its profits if it were able to refuse insurance to everyone likely to get AIDS. Critics point out, however, that the very notion of insurance involves spreading the cost of medical care over a large population, thus reducing the amount paid by an individual who needs expensive care. Hence, to allow insurers to eliminate people with AIDS from the insured population is to increase the profit to insurers at the expense of taxpayers, the ones who will have to bear the cost of those who are desperately sick but have no insurance.

Insurers respond that, although it is true that insurance involves spreading cost over a population, to be fair to individual buyers the risk must be similar for all members of the population. Otherwise, buyers with no special medical problems are put into the position of having to pay much more for their insurance than they should. For example, in 1987 actuarial figures showed that 200 out of 1,000 thirty-four-year-old males would die of AIDS within seven years but that only 7.5 in ordinary health would die of other causes. Carriers of the virus were 26.6 times more likely to die, so ignoring the difference between the two groups meant that those in ordinary health were subsidizing the medical care of those with AIDS.

AIDS and Discrimination

People with AIDS have often been made the lepers of our time. Some have been unable to rent apartments or renew their leases. Others have lost their jobs and been unable to find new ones. Some have been refused admission to health-care facilities, and even undertakers have sometimes been unwilling to accept the bodies of AIDS victims or have charged higher prices to bury them. In one case an entire jury refused to hear a case because the defendant was a person with AIDS. In another, because the defendant had AIDS, court officers refused to work unless they were permitted to wear masks and heavy rubber gloves during the trial.

In a special form of discrimination, a number of physicians have refused to accept people with AIDS as patients. Some physicians do not want to risk becoming infected themselves, while others do not want to bear the enormous psychological burden that caring for AIDS patients imposes. As a consequence, the growing number of people with AIDS must compete to receive treatment from the relatively small number of physicians willing to accept them.

In 1989 the AMA Council on Ethical and Judicial Affairs stated publicly that "A physician may not ethically refuse to treat a patient whose condition is within the physician's current realm of competence" only because the patient is infected with the AIDS virus. Physicians are obviously not bound in such matters to act in the way the AMA approves.

Discrimination against people with AIDS has also worked in the other direction. Hospitals have sometimes removed HIV-positive physicians from positions in which they come in contact with patients. In addition, a few private physicians have seen their practices dwindle as their patients learned they were carriers of the AIDS virus.

Acting out of fear, various municipalities have passed ordinances of doubtful legality that require a blood test for applicants for certain jobs, such as restaurant worker or school teacher, and that make testing positive for HIV grounds for refusing employment. The U.S. armed forces now require an HIV blood test for all new recruits and turn down those who test positive. A policy to extend testing to those who are already enlisted has recently been put into effect.

In addition, all people in federal prisons are tested for the virus when they enter an institution or finish their sentences. Some prisoners allege that infection with the virus is used as grounds to refuse parole. Foreign Service officers and applicants for the Job Corps are also among those required to take a blood test as a condition of employment.

No one doubts the obligation of government, through its laws and agencies, to protest the welfare of citizens. Protection from infectious disease sometimes requires restricting or abridging the rights of those likely to spread the disease. Thus, those with tuberculosis are not allowed to come into contact with schoolchildren or to hold jobs that may permit the bacillus to be passed on to others. We have many precedents for abridging liberties to keep disease from spreading and to protect the health of individuals.

Yet AIDS is not like tuberculosis or any similar disease. AIDS is undeniably an infectious disease, but it is not a highly infectious disease. Although many aspects of its modes of transmission remain obscure, infection apparently requires that a bodily fluid containing the virus come into contact with the bloodstream of a recipient. Infection is not at all a matter of casual contact. Except in extraordinary circumstances, to become infected with AIDS requires engaging in behavior that has high risk of exposing one to the virus.

These are the facts that must be borne in mind when considering controversies over whether a particular policy or practice is warranted by a legitimate concern for safety or whether it is no more than groundless discrimination.

Too Much for AIDS?

A decade has passed since AIDS became the name of a disease and an epidemic. At the start of the decade, the homosexual community had organized itself as a political force. Following the path taken by African Americans, women, and other disadvantaged groups, the homosexual community became a part of the civil rights movement. Homosexual males promoted "gay pride" and "gay rights" and called for an end to discrimination against homosexuals in jobs, housing, the armed forces, and the other institutions of society. They demanded the right to marry someone of the same gender and to adopt children. But most of all they insisted upon a change in social attitudes. They opposed the use of derisive and contemptuous terms applied to homosexuals. They emphasized "sexual preference" as a free choice and rejected the notion that homosexuality was abnormal or unnatural and morally wrong. With equal emphasis, they rejected the idea that it was a disease or disorder to be treated and eliminated.

Many of the changes sought required that existing laws be rewritten or overturned and that laws be passed acknowledging and protecting the civil rights of homosexuals. The same nondiscriminatory legislation applicable to African Americans, women, and other groups should be interpreted as applicable to homosexuals. To achieve these ends, for the first time homosexuals publicly joined the political process, and politicians perceived as sympathetic to the aims of the homosexual community were supported. As part of its political activism, the homosexual community began to prize and celebrate openness about being gay. Gay pride encouraged homosexuals to stand up to others to demand their rights and improve their status within society.

Behind the political activism, however, the homosexual subculture continued much as it had before. Many homosexual males in large cities like New York and San Francisco continued to live a life in which having multiple sex partners, often completely anonymous ones, was a way of life. It was not unusual for men to have a hundred or more—sometimes many more—sexual contacts a year.

In the new atmosphere of assertiveness and exuberance, pride and self-acceptance, the mid-1970s were generally happy and hopeful years for homosexuals. The gay-rights movement had raised public awareness and accomplished many of its aims, and homosexuals seemed closer than ever to winning full membership in society.

Then, at the beginning of the new decade, AIDS came along to destroy the lives and shatter the personal and political dreams of those in the gay-rights movement. The promiscuity so recently celebrated as part of the gay lifestyle became the instrument of its destruction. The threat to homosexual males was suddenly not just one of discrimination, but one of life itself. This realization grew only slowly, however. During a period of denial, the traditional life-style continued with little change, and promiscuous sex with multiple anonymous partners remained a practice in the cities.

Eventually the spread of the disease could not be ignored. Almost everyone in the homosexual community knew someone who had died of the mysterious disease. As the threat became recognized, those in the gay-rights movement switched their attention to AIDS. Groups worked to raise awareness of the danger from the disease within the homosexual community and promoted safer sexual practices. They conducted educational campaigns and raised money for clinics and support services.

Advocacy groups also turned their attention to the broader issues. From the beginning, group leaders rightly charged that society was not moving fast enough to cope with the rising epidemic. Research institutions were not doing enough research related to AIDS and not testing enough drugs; the FDA was not approving potentially useful drugs fast enough, and the country was not spending enough money to do all that needed to be done.

A frequently repeated assertion was that, if the group most affected by AIDS was a socially accepted one—like heterosexual male legislators—then everything that needed to be done would be done at top speed and with all the resources needed. AIDS would be perceived as and treated as a genuine national emergency. Only the fact that such "undesirables" as homosexual males and IV-drug abusers were most likely to get the disease kept it from being taken seriously. Even at the distance of almost a decade, few doubt the truth of this assertion.

AIDS advocacy groups began to pressure the federal government to change its policies toward AIDS. Using political techniques developed during the gay-rights movement, the groups began to lobby legislators and other public officeholders. They began to make public their demands and their criticisms of the way AIDS research and treatment were being dealt with. Enlisting celebrities to help attract attention to their cause, they demanded that more be done in response to the AIDS crisis.

Members of the advocacy groups tend to be white, educated, middle-class men with substantial incomes. They include many people in the arts, fashion, law, medicine, education, and business. With members having these social characteristics, in addition to strong personal commitments and concerns, the advocacy groups became a strong force and have remained so over the decade. They have also gained additional power by forming umbrella organizations. NORA, or National Organizations Responding to AIDS, for example, represents 150 health and civil-rights groups.

Through their efforts, the advocacy groups substantially increased public awareness of AIDS, pressured the FDA into altering its drug-approval system, and convinced Congress to increase the proportion of the budget related to AIDS. Many, if not most, of the goals of the AIDS advocates were met, although perhaps not as soon as they ought to have been.

During the decade, AIDS advocates have often warned of a universal plague spreading throughout the heterosexual population and across the nation. The immediate aim was to get society to take the threat of AIDS seriously and respond appropriately. This was not just a rhetorical strategy, however. The statistics describing the disease's manifestation in the population and the projections of its increases supported the scenario of a deadly and virtually untreatable disease devastating the society. The statistics showed that perhaps 2 million were carrying the virus, and, if steps were not taken, the number would increase geometrically.

Recent figures show that AIDS has not spread to the extent that was predicted. The official estimates put the figure of infection at around 650,000, although other estimates put it closer to 1 million. In either case, the number is significantly less than earlier estimates. Also, the disease has not spread within the heterosexual population (5% of reported cases) to the extent expected. Although IV-drug users represent the largest increase in infection, more than 60% of reported AIDS cases are homosexual males.

In the face of newer statistics, some critics are beginning to suggest that society's response to the disease has been distorted. The pressure exerted by the AIDS advocacy groups has led to changes that may have damaged the entire health-care system. In a review of the situation, Dick Thompson lists three areas of concern.

1. *Spending.* Current AIDS funding is $1.6 billion, compared to $1.5 billion for cancer. However, cancer killed twelve times more people in 1989 (500,000 compared to the 40,000 who died from AIDS). Heart disease, the leading cause of death in the United States, has a budget of only $610 million.

2. *Treatment emphasis.* The traditional way of controlling epidemics is to focus on those who are not infected and devise measures to protect them. The emphasis in the AIDS epidemic has been on the development of effective treatments for those already infected. The outcome is that twice as much money has been spent to discover treatments for AIDS as has been spent to prevent it. This strategy has left vulnerable populations like IV-drug users and their sex partners particularly at risk. These individuals are mostly black or Hispanic inhabitants of inner-city neighborhoods.

    The emphasis on treatment has also distorted the funding pattern of science. Because the money is targeted specifically for AIDS research, other forms of basic research go unfunded.

3. *Lowered standards for drugs.* AIDS advocacy groups, citing the need for immediate treatments, forced changes in the drug approval system. Drugs that would have taken years to approve were approved in a matter of months. Experimental drugs that would not have been available were accepted for use as part of programs of special exemption and testing. (See Social Context: Compound Q, at the beginning of this chapter, for more details.) In the future, this may mean that the system of drug approval that protects the population, even at the cost of denying potentially helpful drugs to those who wish them, will be weakened; as a result, we may lose the protection from harmful and useless drugs it has afforded us.

The AIDS lobby has been able to secure support for work on the disease in a way that advocates for diseases that affect even more people have not. As the executive director of

NORA explained the difference, "The un-levelness of the playing field is a result of the gay community's initial articulateness and money." The Reagan administration was slow to respond to the problems presented by AIDS, and the current situation is perhaps the result of the pressure applied constantly to Congress over the years.

Critics who charge that AIDS is getting more resources than is fair are quick to point out that they are not suggesting the money is being wasted. They admit the disease is epidemic and requires appropriate scientific, medical, educational, and public health responses. Thousands have died of AIDS, and thousands more seem almost certain to die.

AIDS, Gays, and State Coercion

Richard D. Mohr

Richard D. Mohr emphasizes the independence (autonomy) of the individual as a value threatened by AIDS policies. Mohr claims that, since most cases of AIDS are the result of self-exposure by sexual practices and the use of IV drugs, "direct coercive acts by government" are inappropriate to control the disease. Nor is coercion justifiable because of indirect harm (for example, higher taxes and insurance rates) caused by AIDS.

Coercion is warranted, Mohr says, only when the harm becomes great enough to violate another's rights, and increases in taxes or insurance don't violate rights. Also, Mohr rejects state paternalism, because it "denies independence as a value."

Finally, for Mohr it is justifiable to coerce selected individuals for the sake of public health only to prevent harm to others or to secure a "necessary end" such as the survival of the country. AIDS does not present such a situation.

Alarums and Excursions

Of those dead and dying from AIDS three-quarters are gay men. Government funding for AIDS research was at best sluggish till the disease appeared to the dominant non-gay culture as a threat. That perceived threat has spawned state-mandated discrimination against groups at risk for AIDS in employment and access to services, allegedly on medical grounds but in pointed contradiction to the judgments of the very medical institutions to which society has entrusted the determination of such grounds (the US Department of Health and Human Services, the Centers for Disease Control, and the National Institutes of Health).[1]

Government's disregard for medical opinion and for the lives of gays strongly suggests that prej-

udicial forces are at work. There is of course nothing new in this, but the stakes here are high. The armed forces have already established quarantines of those at risk for AIDS on some bases (*The Washington Post*, 19 October 1985, A12; *The Advocate*, #442, 18 March 1986, p. 14). With state-mandated discriminations installed and calls for civilian quarantines circulating, it is clear that the AIDS crisis is going to test the country's mettle. Not since the Supreme Court affirmed the internments of Japanese-Americans in World War II has so live a danger existed to America's traditional commitment to civil liberties. And again the danger is created by hysteria and not a reasoned necessity.

The hysteria, when not simply an expression of old anti-gay prejudices, is based on the presumption that the disease is spread indiscriminately. This

Abridged and reprinted by permission of the author from Bioethics, *Vol. 1, No. 1, 1987, pp. 35–50.*
© *Richard D. Mohr, 1987.*

presumption permitted Jeane Kirkpatrick to begin a syndicated column by using AIDS as a metaphor for international terrorism—"it can affect anyone"—in the serene belief that her audience, educated America, already thought this about AIDS and might even be ready for extreme measures (*The Washington Post*, 13 October 1985, B8).

Alleged Harms to Others

For public policy purposes, the most important fact about AIDS is not that it is deadly but that it, like hepatitis B, is caused by a blood-transmitted virus. For the disease to spread, body fluids of someone with the virus must *directly enter the bloodstream of another;* "It appears that, in order to infect, this virus must be virtually injected into the blood stream."[2] But not just any bodily fluid will do. Only blood and semen have been implicated in the transmission of the virus (*MMWR* 34:45, p. 682).

That the virus is blood transmitted means first and foremost that, in countries with reasonable sanitation, groups at risk for the disease are clearly definable—more so than for virtually any other disease known—with 96 per cent of cases having clearly demarcated modes of transmission and cause. And now that blood supplies are screened with a test for antibodies to the AIDS virus, the number of these groups is indeed dropping. Hemophiliacs not already exposed and blood transfusion recipients are now no longer groups at risk. . . .

The July 1985 cover of *Life* informed the nation in three-inch red letters that "NOW NO ONE IS SAFE FROM AIDS." The magazine used as its allegedly compelling example a seemingly typical Pennsylvania family all but one of whose members has the disease. But it turns out that all those members with the disease were indeed in high risk groups. The father was a hemophiliac, his wife had sex with him, and she conveyed the virus to a child in the process of giving birth. No one got the disease either mysteriously or through casual contact, The family example in fact was evidence *against* the article's generic contagion thesis. Equally irresponsible journalists, lobbyists, and elected officials have compared AIDS to air-borne viral diseases like influenza and the common cold.

The case for general contagion cannot be made. In consequence government policy which is based on that fear is unwarranted. The extraordinary measures—including the suspension of civil liberties—which government might justifiably take, as in war, to prevent wholesale slaughter simply do not apply here. In particular, quarantining the class of AIDS-exposed persons in order to protect society from indiscriminate harm is unwarranted.

Harm to Self

The disease's mode of contagion assures that those at risk are those whose actions contribute to their risk of infection, chiefly through intimate sexual contact and shared hypodermic needles. In the transmission of AIDS, it is the general feature of self-exposure to contagion that makes direct coercive acts by government—like bathhouse closings—particularly inappropriate as efforts to abate the disease.

If independence—the ability to guide one's life by one's own lights to an extent compatible with a like ability on the part of others—is, as it is, a major value, one cannot respect that value while preventing people from putting themselves at risk through voluntary associations. Voluntary associations are star cases of people acting in accordance with the principle of independence, for mutual consent guarantees that the "compatible extent" proviso of the principle is fulfilled. But the state and even the courts have not been very sensitive to the distinction between one harming oneself and one harming another—nor has the medical establishment.[3] It appears to all of them that a harm is a harm, a disease a disease, however caused or described. The moral difference, however, is enormous. Preventing a person from harming another is required by the principle of independence, but preventing someone from harming himself is incompatible with it. While no further justification is needed for the state to protect a person from others, a rather powerful justification is needed if the state is to be warranted in protecting a person from himself.

In the absence of such a justification, the state sometimes tries to split the moral difference and argues that state coercion *may* be used when the harm to others is remote and indirect. Such an argument from indirect harms runs to the effect that state-coerced use of, say, seatbelts and motorcycle helmets is warranted, for helmetless motorcycle crashes and seatbeltless car accidents harm even those not involved in the accidents, by raising everyone's insurance costs and burdening the public purse when victims end up in county hospitals. Here state coercion comes in through the backdoor.

This line of argument has been used with increasing frequency even by self-described liberals like New York's Governor Cuomo, and it is beginning to be heard in AIDS discussions. This is not surprising, for the cost of AIDS patient care from diagnosis to death is somewhere between $35,000 and $150,000. Private funds are often quickly exhausted, and the patient ends up on the dole—harming everyone, and so allegedly warranting state coercion of the means of possible AIDS transmission.

J. S. Mill's rule-of-thumb for appraising such appeals to indirect harms is exactly on target: an indirect harm counts toward justifying state coercion only when the harm grows large enough to be considered a violation of another person's right. This understanding of harm to others is necessary so that independence is not rendered nugatory and, *as a right*, is only outweighed by something comparable to it. Now, while it is nice if products (like insurance) are cheap and taxes low, the considered opinion of our society is not that one's rights have been violated when taxes or the price of milk goes up. Indeed, in the case of taxes, the considered opinion is cast as a Constitutional provision. So arguments that smuggle coercion in through the backdoor of indirect harms are not successful. . . .

State Paternalism Considered

The important question remains whether AIDS warrants paternalistic state coercion to prevent those not-exposed from harming themselves, through banning or highly regulating the means of possible viral transmission. Usually paternalistic arguments cannot be made sensible and consistent. For example: federal AIDS funding for FY 1986 in the House came with a paternalistic rider giving the surgeon general a power he already has—to close bathhouses, gay social institutions, if they are determined to facilitate the transmission or spread of the disease, which indeed they do. (So do parks and bedrooms.) The sponsor of the rider argued that it was "a small step to help those who are unable or unwilling to help themselves" (*The Washington Blade*, 4 October 1985, p. 1). Cast *so* baldly, the argument simply denies independence as a value. For it is consistent with the presumption that the majority gets to determine both what the good life is and to enforce it coercively. The argument could as well be used to justify compulsory religious con-

version—those who are unable or unwilling to see the light are helped to see it. . . .

Public Health and Totalitarianism

Arguments offered so far by the medical community against quarantines and bathhouse closings have largely adopted the terms of mere practicality, appealing to such facts as the large number of people involved, the permanence of the virus in those exposed, and the possibility that the sexual arena may simply shift away from bathhouses where some educational efforts may be possible. I have suggested to the contrary that quarantines and closings should be opposed, not because they are impractical (though they may be), but because they are immoral.

Doctors tend to hold their unrefined view that health policy is merely a matter of strategy because they, not surprisingly, tend to see health itself as a trumping good, second to none in importance. This is a dangerous view, especially when coupled with their idea that health is an undifferentiated good. They fail to distinguish between my harming my health and my harming your health. Behind this oversight lies the further (sometimes unarticulated) presumption that you and I both are absorbed into and subordinated under something called the public health—a concept that tends to be analyzed in inverse proportion to the frequency with which it is used when trying to justify coercive acts.

No literal sense exists in which there could be such thing as a public health. To say the public has a health is like saying the number seven has a color: such a thing cannot have such a property. You have health or you lack it and I have health or lack it, because we each have a body with organs that function or do not function. But the public, an aggregate of persons similarly disposed as persons, has no such body of organs with functions which work or fail. There are, however, two frequently used metaphoric senses of public health that do have a reference: one, is a legitimate use but largely inapplicable to the AIDS crisis; the other, when used normatively, is the pathway to totalitarianism.

The legitimate sense places public health in the same conceptual scheme as national defense and water purification. These are types of public goods in a technical sense—not what most people want and thus what democratic governments give them nor what tend to maximize by state means some type of good (pleasure, happiness, beauty), but what everyone wants but cannot get or get efficiently through voluntary arrangements and which thus require coercive coordinations from the state, so that *each* person gets what he wants. Thus, the private or voluntary arrangements of the market system do not seem likely to provide adequate national security, because a defense system that protects those who pay for it will also protect those who do not; everyone (reasonably enough) will tend to wait for someone else to pay for it, so that national security ends up not being purchased at all, or at least far less of it is purchased than everyone would agree to pay for if there were some means to manifest that agreement. The coercive actions of the state through taxation are then required to achieve the public good of national defense.

For exactly the same reason, the state is warranted in using coercive measures to drain swamps and provide vaccines against air-borne viruses. But the state is not warranted by appeal to the public good in coercing people to take the vaccine once it is freely available, for then *each* person is capable on his own—without further state coercion—of getting the protection from the disease he wants. The mode of AIDS contagion makes it relevantly like this latter case. Each person on his own—without state coercion—can get the protection from the disease that he wants through his own actions, and indeed can get it by doing himself what he might be tempted to try to get the state to force upon others, say, avoiding bathhouses. As far as the good of protection is concerned, it can be achieved with no state coercion.

Is there a public good involved simply in reducing the size of the pool of AIDS-exposed people? I see just one, the one I argued for—the ability to have a robust sex life, without fear of death. But this good does not permit every form of state coercion. Not every public good motivates every form of coercion. The public goods mentioned so far could all be achieved by *equitable* coercion (e.g., universal conscription, taxation, compensated taking of property). When equitable coercion is the means, the public good can be quite slight and still be justified (as in government support for the arts). But when the coercion is inequitably dispersed, the public good served must be considerably more compelling than the means are intrusive. Thus, dispersed coercion against select individuals that involves restricted motion and physical suffering is warranted

only by unqualifiedly necessary ends: when the individuals coerced have harmed others (as in punishment) or when it is necessary to the very existence of the country (as a partial military draft may be for a nation at defensive war). And thus too, the substantial good of civil rights protections is advanced only through the considerably weak intrusion of barring the desire of employers to indulge in whimsical and arbitrary hiring practices. The public good of an unencumbered sex life however fails this weighted ends-to-means test if the means are a dispersedly coerced sex life. For the intrusion and the good are on a par—on the one hand encumbered sex, on the other unencumbered sex. And so it appears that only equitably coercive means are available to achieve the end of reducing the pool of AIDS-exposures—taxation for preventive measures like vaccine development, but not coercive measures that effect some but not others, like closing bathhouses or banning or regulating sex practices selectively.

Those who do not find the possibility of carefree sex a public good—probably the bulk of those actually calling for state coercion—will find no legitimate help in the notion of public health for state coercion here. Those who do will find it justifies only equitable measures.

The other metaphoric sense of public health takes the medical model of the healthy body and unwittingly transfers it to society—the body politic. But this transfer (when it has any content at all) bears hidden and extremely dangerous assumptions. Plato in the *Republic* was the first thinker systematically to press the analogy of the good society to the healthy body. The state stands to the citizenry and its good, as a doctor stands to the body and its health. Society, so it is claimed, is an organism in which people are mere functional parts, ones that are morally good and emotionally well-off only insofar as they act for the sake of the organism. The analogy is alive and well today and calling out for extreme measures now: 'Much as a physician treating one organ must consider the effects on the entire organism, a public official has the community as the patient and must attend to all factors in seeking the greatest overall good' (Silverman and Silverman, p. 22). On this view, the individual however harmed cannot fulfill his role. A damaged organ, the spleen for example, can be, to continue the analogy, simply cut out. By comparison, quarantines and coerced sex lives might appear as mild remedies on this analogy, But something has been lost here—persons.

The medical model of society is the conceptual engine of totalitarianism. It presumes not that the goods of individuals are final goods but that individuals are good only as they serve some good beyond themselves, that of the state or body politic. The state exists not for the sake of individuals—to protect and enhance their prospects as rational agents—but rather individuals exist for the state and are subordinated to society as a whole, the worth of which is to be determined only from the perspective of the whole. The individual, thus, is not an end in himself but exists for some social good—whether that good be some hoped-for overall happiness or some social ideal—like, purity, wholesomeness, decency, or "traditional values." Unconscious obedient servicing is dressed up as virtue.

The worst political consequence of the AIDS crisis would not be simply the further degradation of gays. Gay internments would not be anything new to this century. In the European internment camps of World War II, gypsies wore brown triangle identifying badges, Jehovah's Witnesses purple, political prisoners red, race defilers black, and gays pink triangles. Worse than the further degradation of gays in America would be a general, and not easily reversed, shift in the nation's center of gravity toward the medical model and away from the position, acknowledged in America's Constitutional tradition, that individuals have broad yet determinate claims against both general welfare and social ideals. The consequence of such a shift would be that people would come to be treated essentially as resources, sometimes expendable—a determination no less frightening when made by a combined father, colonel, and doctor than by a fearful mob.

Notes

1. See particularly the CDC's guidelines for preventing transmission in the workplace, "Recommendations for Preventing Transmission of Infection with Human T-Lymphotrophic Virus Type III/Lymphadenopathy-Associated Virus in the Workplace," *Morbidity and Mortality Weekly Report (MMWR)*, 15 November 1985, 34:45, 682–95.

2. Krim, Mathilde. 1985. "AIDS: The Challenge to Science and Medicine." *AIDS: The Emerging Ethical Dilemmas. A Hastings Center Report Special Supplement*, p. 4.

3. For instance, Mervyn F. Silverman, former Director of Health for San Francisco, shows no cognizance of the distinction in his argument for his unsuccessful 1984 attempt to close that city's bathhouses: Silverman, Mervyn F. and Silverman, Deborah B. "AIDS and the Threat to Public Health," *Special Supplement* (see n. 2 above), pp. 21–2.

Harming, Wronging, and AIDS

Bonnie Steinbock

Bonnie Steinbock considers the implications of the harm principle as a basis for legitimate state intervention in the AIDS crisis. She first examines the kind of harm the principle might prohibit and argues that in some circumstances deliberately infecting another person with the AIDS virus could be considered the moral equivalent of second-degree murder.

She next considers what state interventions to stop AIDS are legitimate. She argues that restricting behavior to halt the spread of AIDS may be consistent with the harm principle when those restrictions are likely to be effective and are the least restrictive ways available. She also argues the financial cost can be a justification for restricting behavior and rejects Mohr's claim that cost is irrelevant in applying the harm principle.

Finally, Steinbock argues that the danger of discrimination to people with AIDS does not outweigh the right of their contacts to knowledge necessary for informed consent. Rather than not engaging in contact tracing, the government should enforce rules against discrimination.

The AIDS crisis poses a number of tough questions for society. Some are medical: for example, how can we stop the spread of the disease? Others are political: what measures will people be willing to accept? But there are also moral and philosophical issues raised about the legitimacy of measures that might be taken to prevent the spread of this fatal disease. Measures designed to protect some people may adversely affect the interests of others. I will examine the implications of one theory regarding legitimate state intervention—Mill's harm principle—for the AIDS crisis.

In *On Liberty*, John Stuart Mill argued that "the only purpose for which power can be rightfully exercised over any member of a civilized community, against his will, is to prevent harm to others."[1] Forcibly restricting one's behavior for one's *own* good (legal paternalism) is never justified, nor is the prohibition of behavior simply on the grounds that it is widely regarded as sinful or wicked (legal moralism). The harm principle, as it has come to be known, absolutely rejects any grounds for social or legal coercion except harm to others.

Not everyone agrees that harm to others is the sole justification for restricting freedom. It has been argued that some paternalistic intervention is not only justified, but consistent with Mill's emphasis on liberty.[2] Others maintain that upholding a certain standard of morality is a proper function of the state.[3] I do not intend to discuss the merits of legal paternalism or legal moralism in this paper. I propose to assume that Mill was right: harm to others is the sole justification for limiting individual freedom. However, as we will see, acceptance of the harm principle raises as many questions as it answers.

In the first section, I shall discuss briefly the kind of harm that might plausibly be prohibited by the harm principle. Whereas disease cannot be outlawed, behavior that infects others may be. AIDS is a fatal disease. Should we regard infecting a person with AIDS as a criminal act, possibly even murder?

I shall argue that, although practical difficulties regarding proximate cause would make criminal charges nearly impossible to sustain, nevertheless, infecting another person with AIDS might be considered in some cases to evidence a "depraved indifference to human life" and so be the moral equivalent of second-degree murder.

The second section discusses legitimate governmental intervention to halt the spread of AIDS. The criminal law is only one way that the state can intervene to influence behavior. Another way to restrict behavior is to limit opportunities to engage in it: e.g., closing gay bathhouses. Would such measures necessarily be a reflection of legal moralism or legal paternalism? I shall argue that this need not be the case. However, to be consistent with the harm principle, it would have to be shown both that closing the baths is likely to be effective in halting the spread of disease, and that this is the least restrictive effective method of doing so.

Another possible justification for governmental coercion is the financial cost to society as a whole. AIDS is a terribly expensive disease. I will reject the claim that the harm principle rules out consideration of the cost of AIDS and instead suggest that it calls for the least restrictive measures necessary to contain costs.

Lastly, I shall turn to the question of whether the potential harm to AIDS victims resulting from "contact-notification" is a decisive argument against it. Although the danger to AIDS victims cannot be ignored, it does not outweigh the right of their contacts to the knowledge necessary for fully informed consent to sexual activity. Instead, the state should take vigorous measures to protect AIDS victims from discrimination.

The Harm Principle and the Obligations of Individuals

In its broadest sense, harm is any adverse affecting of an individual's interests. One can be

Reprinted by permission from Biomedical Ethics: 1988, *ed. James M. Humber and Robert F. Almeder (Clifton, N.J.: Humana Press, 1989), pp. 27–43. An earlier version of this paper was commissioned by the The Hastings Center Project on AIDS and the Ethics of Public Health.*

harmed by natural events, such as storms, or even nonevents, such as drought, as well as by human actions. The harm principle, which justifies the restriction of human freedom, must concern harm brought about by human action. Joel Feinberg suggests that we think of harming as having two components: (1) It must lead to some kind of adverse effect, or create the danger of such an effect, on its victim's *interests*; and, (2) It must be inflicted wrongfully in violation of the victim's rights.[4]

The first component makes the harm principle sufficiently broad, enabling us to recognize that people can be harmed in nonphysical ways. People have all kinds of interests, in their lives and health, in property, in their reputations, in their emotional well-being. Although certain kinds of injuries might count more heavily than others, an adequate conception of harm should do justice to the variety of kinds of harm.

The second condition is necessary to restrict the harm principle. The interests of one person may be adversely affected by the actions of another in many cases where this provides little or no reason for restricting the behavior. My taking a job that would otherwise have been offered to you does adversely affect your interests, but that is no reason for me to turn it down, much less for the state to prevent me from taking it. Another example would be a person who freely consents to plastic surgery that turns out badly, but not because of any negligence on the part of the surgeon. (That can happen, though Americans may find it difficult to believe.) The disfigured person has been harmed, but not wronged, because the physician was not at fault. There would be, on this understanding of harming, no grounds for civil, much less criminal liability.

To give someone a painful and inevitably fatal disease is clearly adversely to affect that person's interests, but is the second condition met? Do I wrong you, and do I violate your rights, if I give you AIDS? Certainly I do if I deliberately try to infect you. Although this is an unlikely scenario, it is not impossible. Two Florida inmates were charged with conspiracy to commit murder after a third inmate alleged that they had put AIDS-infected blood serum in a correction officer's coffee.[5] (Since it is extremely unlikely that anyone could contract AIDS this way, it is questionable whether putting AIDS-infected blood serum in coffee constitutes a real attempt. This issue belongs to the fascinating area of "inchoate attempts," a discussion of which would take us too far afield.)

Few people deliberately try to infect others with fatal diseases, but carriers of disease may unknowingly infect others: Typhoid Mary is a classic example. Society must protect people from unintentional infection—a topic to which I shall return in the next section—but the unknowing carrier is not to blame (unless she is to blame for not knowing). What about the person who does know that she poses a risk to others, but does not mean to infect them? Could Typhoid Mary escape condemnation by employing double effect reasoning, and saying, "I don't mean to infect these people, just prepare their meals for them"? Certainly not. Although knowingly exposing people to harm is not usually regarded as being as bad as deliberately exposing them, it is still wrong and a violation of their right not to be exposed to serious health hazards. Indeed, where such exposure is not merely negligent, but reckless, and evidence of a "depraved indifference" to human life, it may even be considered to be murder in the second-degree. Causing death by drunk driving has sometimes come under this category.[6]

A dramatic example of a murder conviction for knowingly exposing people to the risk of death occurred in June, 1985, when three executives of Film Recovery Systems, Inc. were convicted of murder, and sentenced to 25 years in prison, for the death of an employee from cyanide poisoning. The murder conviction, alleged to be the first in an industrially related death, was based on the fact that the company executives were "totally knowledgeable" of the plant's hazardous conditions, and did nothing to protect, or even warn, the workers. The judge who sentenced the defendants likened their actions to leaving a time bomb on an airplane. "Every day people worked there," he said, "it kept ticking, it kept ticking."[7]

Individuals have a legal as well as moral duty not to engage in activity likely to cause the death of others. The mere fact that one did not mean to cause the death or serious bodily harm does not necessarily absolve one from criminal liability. What are the implications for the person who knows he is seropositive, but nevertheless engages in activity capable of infecting others, such as anal sex and sharing contaminated needles? If he infects someone with AIDS, which is always fatal, is that murder?

Admittedly, in most cases of AIDS, the "victim" has had numerous contacts, and so establishing the proximate causation necessary for criminal, or even civil, liability would be nearly impossible. Still, there could be cases in which the causal connection was clear. Is that murder?

Many people will be offended by the very suggestion. Seropositive individuals, if not already ill, are themselves at risk of developing AIDS. It seems very harsh to accuse the victims of a terrible disease of murder. Moreover, how can we persuade those who may be infected to submit to a test, if the result is that they are exposed to criminal liability? Is not the whole discussion of AIDS and murder entirely wrongheaded?

I am not suggesting criminal or civil liability as a practical way to deal with the AIDS crisis. However, if we think that the individual who knowingly risks infecting others seriously wrongs them, that has implications for behavior on the part of others, such as physicians and public health officials. It may be justified to infringe the rights of one person to prevent a more serious violation of the rights of another. If, on the other hand, the AIDS carrier who has sex with others does not wrong them, then violating the carrier's confidentiality will be unjustified. For this reason, we need to take seriously the charge that having sex or sharing needles with others, knowing you are seropositive, is immoral, comparable to shooting a gun into an occupied building, or driving while intoxicated.

Although AIDS carriers may be deserving of our sympathy, that fact by itself does not make their behavior in infecting others less culpable. A sick person can be as guilty of murder as a well one. Illness is relevant only if it diminishes the capacity for responsible behavior. AIDS can do this, in the later stages, and thus might affect the "capacity-responsibility"[8] of a person with AIDS, although this would not be the case for carriers who do not themselves have the disease.

Another possibility for diminishing responsibility for causing harm is when harm results from less than fully voluntary behavior. Sexual behavior is often less than fully voluntary, because it stems from strong feelings and drives. Still, although we may blame less the person driven by passion to do something that harms another than we would the person who does it "in cold blood," this factor does not completely exonerate. People who have the ability to conform their behavior to the requirements of morality or law have an obligation not to get into situations in which their passions are likely to rule. If they do anyway, they cannot excuse their harmful behavior by saying, "I couldn't help it." The alcoholic who cannot control his or her drinking may not be to blame for drinking, but is to blame for driving to a bar, knowing that he or she will become intoxicated and then drive home. What are the implications for seropositive individuals? In my view, they are morally required to do two things: reduce the risk of infection by practicing "safer sex" techniques, and inform their sexual contacts of their seropositive status. Are both necessary to escape moral liability? Cannot seropositive individuals fulfill their duty not to harm others simply by taking steps likely to protect them? I do not think so. Consider the case of Rock Hudson and Linda Evans, a star of the television series, *Dynasty*. Hudson, who was dying of AIDS, was scheduled to shoot a romantic scene with Evans, which required him to kiss her. At that time, neither his disease nor his homosexuality was widely known. Fearing the effect on his career if the news got out, Hudson decided to go ahead with the kiss and not tell Linda Evans.

There was little, if any, objective risk of infection to Linda Evans from that kiss. AIDS is transmitted through the direct introduction of bodily fluids, such as blood and semen, into the bloodstream of another. Does that fact make Rock Hudson's decision morally permissible? No. This is partly because Rock Hudson was not in a position to know that he was not exposing Linda Evans to the risk of death; at that time hemophiliacs were being advised to avoid "deep kissing," because it was feared that AIDS might be transmitted through saliva. It is wrong to be willing to expose another to the risk of harm, even where there is no objective risk. Suppose Hudson had known that his kissing was extremely unlikely to infect her. Would that make kissing and not telling morally all right?

Not in my view. Intimate contact is permissible only when voluntary. When Linda Evans agreed to kiss Rock Hudson, she did not agree to kiss someone with a potentially communicable fatal disease. She could agree to that only if she knew about it. Even if the risk of catching AIDS from kissing is low, the decision whether to take that risk is hers, and hers alone. No one else, including Rock Hudson, has the right to make that decision for her. He could explain to her that there was very little danger. He could reassure her that there would be no exchange of saliva. He could press on her the damage to his career if the story got out. But to conceal from her the fact of his AIDS is to lie to her. That is a serious wrong even if his kissing her did not, as it turns out, harm her, or even run a significant risk of harming her. I do not believe that it is morally permissible to lie to someone about a matter of vital concern to avoid adverse effects on one's career.

If this is right, and Rock Hudson had a moral duty to inform Linda Evans of his condition before engaging in an activity unlikely to do her harm, how much stronger is the obligation of the seropositive individual to inform others of his or her condition before engaging in activities that may well cause them harm. The use of safer sex techniques may protect them from harm but does not meet the condition that they not be wronged. Although it is less bad to wrong but not harm than to wrong and harm, wronging is still—wrong.

Is it morally permissible merely to inform and not use safer sex techniques? It might be thought that respect for the other person's autonomy requires a mutual decision on the use of safer sex techniques, and that it would be paternalistic for the AIDS carrier to decide unilaterally to use safer sex techniques. This has more plausibility regarding sex than it does, say, regarding the sharing of needles, because it is hard to imagine anyone who would knowingly choose to take the risk of getting AIDS from sharing an unsterilized needle. By contrast, someone might value certain unsafe sexual practices (in which semen enters the body) so highly that he or she is willing to take the risk of contracting AIDS. Nevertheless, I do not regard depriving such a person of the opportunity to take the risk as objectionably paternalistic. Respect for the autonomy of others does not require us to provide them with opportunities to hurt themselves, much less require us to inflict the harm ourselves. Your right to risk your life imposes no corresponding obligation on me to inflict harm. So although I have no right to force *you* to use safer sex techniques, or to prevent you from having sex with others who choose not to use them, neither do you have the right to a say in my use of such techniques. Moreover, concern for the lives of others should make the seropositive person engage only in safer sex.

To sum up, merely taking precautions probably avoids harming others, but is still morally objection-

able, because the failure to disclose one's status as seropositive deprives one's sexual partners of information they have a right to know. Having unprotected sex with informed and willing partners respects their autonomy, but, given the seriousness of the risk, shows insufficient concern for their welfare. Someone who neither informs nor takes precautions, but has sex with others, knowing that he or she is seropositive, wrongs and harms, or runs the risk of harming. This displays reckless indifference to the value of human life, and, when it results in the death of a person, might reasonably be seen as the moral equivalent of murder.

Governmental Coercion to Prevent the Spread of Disease

What are the implications of the above section for legitimate coercive activity on the part of the state? What measures may the state take to protect people from being infected with AIDS? In discussing justifiable coercive measures to stop the spread of AIDS, we must remember first that most of the people at risk can protect themselves by taking certain precautions. This is precisely what has happened among homosexuals, resulting in a leveling off of the exponential increase in the disease.[9] Unfortunately, this is unlikely to happen with heroin addicts who are now most threatened with the massive spread of the disease. Second, although changes in voluntary behavior can protect most of those at risk, even those who are not "voluntary risk-takers" may be at risk, namely, women who have sex with men whom they do not know are homosexual or intravenous drug users, and their fetuses. What should be done to protect them? Finally, AIDS is an extremely expensive disease. Are coercive measures, which go beyond mere education, justifiable if likely to contain costs?

Obviously, the first thing the government ought to do is educate. That violates no one's rights, and is likely to be very effective in halting the spread of AIDS. The refusal to disseminate information about safer sex in places where AIDS is rampant, such as prisons, because of a moralistic and unrealistic attitude about sex, is unconscionable. Is there anything else the state would be justified in doing, along with education? Are measures that restrict the freedom of AIDS carriers ever justified? A clear requirement of justifiable coercive measures is that they are likely to be effective, since it would obviously be illegitimate, on the harm principle, to restrict freedom without good reason to believe that such restrictions protected others. Further, the protection we gain has to be significant enough to outweigh the costs of the restriction, including loss of liberty and expense.

Some of the recent proposals to combat AIDS would be unjustified, on grounds of inefficacy, even if they were not also outrageous violations of civil rights; for example, the ludicrous suggestion that those who test seropositive to AIDS be quarantined. Since AIDS carriers do not pose a danger to others through casual contact, segregation from the general population is unnecessary to prevent the spread of AIDS. Quarantine might be intended to prevent those who have been exposed to the AIDS virus from having sex or sharing needles with those who have not been exposed. However, HIV-positive individuals have the ability to infect others *forever*, whether or not they ever develop the disease themselves. To prevent those who have been exposed to AIDS from having sexual contact with others, those who test seropositive—a predicted 70% of the homosexual population of New York and San Francisco—would have to be quarantined forever—or until a vaccine or treatment is found. The idea is absurd, yet apparently was required by Proposition 64, a Lyndon LaRouche sponsored initiative that appeared on the California ballot in November, 1986.[10] This sort of hysterical reaction makes gay activists and civil libertarians alike believe that the motivation for such legislation is not a serious attempt to control the spread of the disease, but rather antipathy to homosexuals: the worst kind of legal moralism.

Less restrictive than quarantining those who test seropositive is closing places where sexual practices that spread AIDS occur, such as gay bathhouses. This was done in New York in 1985. Some people opposed this on purely pragmatic grounds: it won't stop homosexual activity, and so won't stop the spread of AIDS. In fact, it has been argued, it is counterproductive, as the baths offer an opportunity for education about techniques for avoiding the disease.

A different sort of argument against the closing of the baths is offered by philosopher Richard Mohr in "AIDS, Gays, and State Coercion."[11] Mohr maintains that it is morally unjustified to close them down, even if this would retard the spread of disease, because it would be paternalistic. The reason

for this is that the disease's mode of contagion assures that those at risk are those whose actions contribute to their risk of infection, chiefly through intimate sexual contact and shared hypodermic needles. If gay men choose to take risks with their health by frequenting the baths, that is their prerogative. Preventing competent adults from voluntarily taking risks with their health is paternalistic. It would no more be justified to close the baths, according to Mohr, than it would be to ban race car driving or mountain climbing.

There are two flaws in Mohr's argument. The first is that not only voluntary risk-takers are threatened by AIDS. According to a report in *The New York Times*:

> . . . drug users are a main conduit for the AIDS virus into the heterosexual population. In addition, drug-related infections passed on at birth account for most AIDS cases in children, projected to surpass 3,000 by 1991. AIDS spread by needles has been especially prevalent among minorities in New York and New Jersey, giving black and Hispanic people a disproportionate share of the country's total cases.[12]

Are women who sleep with, or are even married to, gay men, unaware that they are gay, voluntary risk-takers? This is plausible only if one adopts the view that sex *per se* is a risky activity these days, so that anyone who has sex, even in an ostensibly heterosexual, monogamous marriage, must be considered to be voluntarily undergoing the risk of catching AIDS. I submit that this is implausible. A person who has sex with multiple partners, refusing to use safer sex techniques, might be regarded as a "volunteer," but not the woman unknowingly married to a bisexual. The notion of voluntary risk-taking is even more implausible when applied to the fetus who contracts the disease *in utero*, who does not act at all, much less act voluntarily. If these nonvoluntary risk-takers could be protected from getting AIDS by closing the baths, the motivation would not be paternalistic, for it is paternalism only to forcibly prevent people from doing what they wish to do and to protect them from risks they willingly undergo. To justify closing the baths on harm principle grounds, then, it remains to be shown that this is both likely to be effective and the least restrictive measure to prevent the spread of fatal disease.

The second flaw in Mohr's argument is his denial that cost may be considered on the harm principle.

By 1991, when a projected 74,000 new AIDS cases will be diagnosed in a single year and a total of 145,000 patients will still be alive, the direct medical expenses of AIDS will be $8 billion to $16 billion. While this will amount to only about 2 percent of total national medical expenses, cities where AIDS is concentrated will be dramatically affected. Moreover, the projections do not include the expenses of the hundreds of thousands who will not be diagnosed with AIDS but will suffer related disorders. [13]

Astonishingly, Mohr believes that these costs may not be even considered in justifying coercive measures. Referring to such costs as "indirect harm," he invokes Mill as maintaining that an indirect harm counts toward justifying state coercion only when the harm grows large enough to be considered the violation of a right. Also, although it is nice if taxes are low, no one's rights are violated when taxes go up. So we may not close the baths, forcibly preventing people from using them, even if it could be shown that this would reduce AIDS and save money.

A more antiutilitarian approach can scarcely be imagined. But one need not be a utilitarian to reject this cavalier approach toward the spending of public funds. Instead, we can recognize that an individual's right to pursue his or her life-style in the manner he or she prefers, including the taking of certain risks, is not an absolute right. If personal choices of some members of society place an enormous financial burden on others, and they cannot be persuaded by noncoercive means to change their ways, coercive measures may be justifiable. However, the least restrictive measures should be adopted. For example, we do not entirely ban mountain climbing, even though we can foresee the inevitable expensive rescues that will result from allowing it, because we acknowledge the legitimacy of an activity many people find extremely pleasurable and meaningful. Our respect for their freedom to engage in mountain climbing does not require us to let people go wherever they choose. It is legitimate to close the riskiest routes, in order to contain costs. An alternative would be to warn people in advance that, should they get in trouble, they could expect not to get rescued. Whereas this policy has the merit of respecting autonomy, it would require callousness to carry out, and should on that ground be rejected. Instead, it is legitimate to restrict somewhat, but not entirely ban, risky behavior. Unsafe sex, with multiple partners, is risky, but attempting to legislate against it is both impractical and too great

an invasion of privacy and self-determination. However, public health officials might justifiably close the riskiest places (like the notorious Mineshaft), if this were likely to halt the spread of a deadly and expensive disease, both to protect nonvolunteers at risk, and to contain costs. The freedom to have sex with anonymous, multiple partners does not seem important enough to justify great public expense.

Other possible government action includes warning the sexual partners of those who test seropositive, or "contact-notification," a program that is being carried out in San Francisco. Such programs may be objected to on the ground that the individual's right to privacy and confidentiality is violated by revealing medical information without consent. The question of how doctors should weigh their obligation of confidentiality to the patient against their obligation of protection to members of the public, especially in light of *Tarasoff*,[14] is a large and difficult one; I do not propose to undertake it here. Instead, I will address the question of whether the adverse effects on AIDS carriers should be considered in deciding whether to reveal their seropositivity to sexual partners.

The harm done to an individual by disclosure may be private and personal, or public and institutional. An example of the first kind would be the breakup of a marriage resulting from a wife learning that her husband is gay. Examples of the second include denying infected individuals insurance, jobs, and housing.

One way to safeguard individuals from harm from disclosure is to promise confidentiality. Contacts are told that they have been exposed, but not by whom. Some are worried that confidentiality simply cannot be assured, and that if official lists are created, this will lead to discrimination. In some settings (for example, prisons), this may be the case, but it seems unduly pessimistic in general. All steps should be taken to ensure confidentiality where possible.

However, confidentiality cannot be assured where there is only one sexual contact. A monogamous woman who is told that she has been exposed to AIDS will not only figure out who has infected her, but is also likely to conclude that her husband may be gay. Unfortunately, this is also the situation in which contact-notification is most clearly justified, because the woman is not a voluntary risk-taker. Some have argued against her being informed of her exposure, on the grounds that this will likely result in great harm to him, while offering her little or no protection. She has probably already been infected, nor is there presently a cure or treatment for AIDS. Isn't this a bit like closing the barn door after the horse is gone? It has even been suggested that the real motivation for informing her that she has been exposed to AIDS is to provide her with information about her husband's possible sexual orientation, something the state has no business doing.

However, there is evidence that repeated exposure to the AIDS virus increases the chance of infection. If she is informed, she can undergo testing to see if she has been infected. She can then decide whether to continue the relationship, and what precautions to take. She can make an informed decision about whether to become pregnant. These health considerations, combined with her right to make informed decisions regarding her own welfare, make entirely reasonable "contact-notification" programs.

There is little anyone can do about the private and personal fall-out resulting from such notification. Nor does it seem to me to have much weight in this sort of scenario. The harm that befalls the husband he has brought on himself, through his own deception. He is not entitled to compound that deception now by keeping his wife uninformed of risks to her own life and health.

Considerably more can and should be done to protect AIDS carriers from discrimination. This is another example of justifiable coercion, only here the coercion is directed at those who would discriminate against AIDS victims. AIDS victims are especially vulnerable to discrimination, "irrationally ostracized by their communities because of medically baseless fears of contagion." Therefore, they come under Section 504 of the Rehabilitation Act of 1973, according to a draft opinion prepared in April 1986 by a member of the Justice Department's Civil Rights Division. However, in June 1986 the Justice Department's Office of Legal Counsel issued a ruling, permitting the dismissal of AIDS victims based on "fear of contagion." Assistant Attorney General Charles J. Cooper held that, although the "disabling effects" of AIDS were indeed a handicap, and could not be used as a basis for discrimination by employers, the ability to transmit the disease to others is not a handicap. Mr. Cooper concluded that the law did not prohibit the dismissal of AIDS victims based on

fear of contagion, however irrational. Mr. Cooper said that the Rehabilitation Act is "certainly not a general prohibition against irrational decision making by employers." Employers who discriminate against people who are left-handed or red-haired may be acting irrationally, but Congress has not yet made such discrimination illegal.

According to Mr. Cooper's interpretation of the law, a sincere belief in contagion, however irrational, is sufficient to protect the employer. On this analysis, presumably an employer who sincerely believed cancer to be catching could fire a worker with leukemia with impunity. The analysis is bogus, and so is the protection it affords handicapped people. Fortunately, a number of states have rejected the interpretation and protect AIDS victims from discrimination under state law. In June 1988, a Presidential Commission urged a Federal ban against AIDS discrimination. So far, neither the President nor Congress has acted.[15]

Conclusion

Individuals have a moral and legal duty not to inflict serious harms on others. Reckless infliction of harm on those who do not willingly consent is seriously wrong: indeed, it may be the moral equivalent of murder. To protect nonvolunteers from fatal disease, the government is entitled to use coercive measures, so long as these are reasonably expected to be effective and as unrestrictive as possible. However, most coercive measures so far proposed are unlikely to be effective in controlling AIDS. Many seem motivated either by panic or hatred of gays or both. A government serious about stopping the AIDS epidemic would use resources in educational campaigns and treatment programs for heroin addicts. In addition, compassion and fairness require the use of legal coercion to protect AIDS victims from discrimination.

Notes and References

1. Mill, *On Liberty*, Chap. 1, para. 9.

2. Gerald Dworkin, "Paternalism," in *Morality and the Law* (Richard A. Wasserstrom, ed.), Wadsworth Publishing Company Inc., California, 1971.

3. Irving Kristol, "Pornography, Obscenity, and the Case for Censorship," *The New York Times Magazine*, March 28, 1971. Reprinted in *Philosophy of Law*, 3rd edition, by Joel Feinberg and Hyman Gross, Wadsworth Publishing Company Inc., California, 1986.

4. Joel Feinberg, "Wrongful Life and the Counterfactual Element in Harming," *Social Philosophy & Policy*, vol. 4, no. 1, 1986, 145–178. See also Feinberg, *Harm to Others*, Oxford University Press, New York, 1984, Chap. 1.

5. *Newsweek*, August 11, 1986, p. 24.

6. Bonnie Steinbock, "Drunk Driving," *Philosophy and Public Affairs*, Summer 1985, 278–295.

7. *The New York Times*, Tuesday, July 2, 1985, A11.

8. The term is H. L. A. Hart's, "Postscript: Responsibility and Retribution," in *Punishment and Responsibility*, Chap. 9, Oxford University Press, 1968.

9. John Kaplan, "AIDS and the Heroin Connection," *The Wall Street Journal*, Tuesday, September 11, 1986, A28.

10. *The New York Times*, Thursday, September 11, 1986, A27.

11. *Bioethics*, vol. 1, no. 1, January 1987, 35–50.

12. *The New York Times*, Tuesday, June 17, 1986, C3.

13. *Ibid.*

14. *17 Cal.* 3d, 425, 131, *Cal. Rep.* 14, 551, p. 2d, 334 (1976).

15. Federal Policy Against Discrimination Is Sought for AIDS Victims," *The New York Times*, Thursday, September 22, 1988, A35.

Nonvalidated Therapies and HIV Disease

Benjamin Freedman and the McGill/Boston Research Group

Freedman addresses the problem of treatments that are potentially useful but clinically untested—"nonvalidated therapies," or NTs. He argues against permitting AIDS patients free access to just any treatment. Not only might this make controlled trials impossible, but trying to distinguish AIDS from early forms of HIV infection is "medically inappropriate." An AIDS patient who is beyond help is not beyond hurt, and both these conditions must be met.

Freedman examines a new FDA regulation permitting the use of investigational drugs and points to several practical and conceptual difficulties in interpreting it. Rejecting the radical proposals, he comes down in favor of the basics of current drug regulation: testing for safety and effectiveness, leaving the decisions to experts, and forbidding drug companies to charge for test drugs. He does believe the approval process should be streamlined. In a conflict between a patient's wish to use a test drug and a "sound ethical trial," for Freedman the trial takes precedence. A patient's right to medical treatment is not impaired, for "medical treatment" must be defined by medical expertise, not by a patient's beliefs about what he or she needs.

Freedman closes with a proposal to institute Authorized Investigational Units that are granted authority to use investigational drugs on a "compassionate use" basis. Such an approach permits sound science while meeting the pressing needs of patients.

The introduction of potential treatments for HIV disease has, in almost every instance, engendered controversy. The speedy approval of AZT (Zidovudine) has led to charges that FDA was inappropriately influenced by political considerations, and the current extensive studies on AZT are pointed out as evidence that the drug was granted approval before adequate testing had been completed.[1] The initial tests of ribavirin were criticized by some for their supposed inappropriate and un-

Reprinted by permission of the authors and The Hastings Center from Hastings Center Report, *May/June 1989, pp. 14–18, 20.*

ethical use of a placebo control group. Organized demonstrations have been held and legal action taken to rectify perceived delays in providing aerosolized pentamidine as prophylaxis against *pneumocystis carinii* pneumonia (PCP).[2]

The controversies that have swirled about nonvalidated treatments (NTs) for HIV disease touch upon crucial questions of ethics and public policy. These questions are unresolved within the communities professionally concerned—physicians, researchers, and government officials—as they are unresolved among patients and in society at large.

Scope and Context of the Problem

The definition of nonvalidated therapies has been itself a matter of some controversy in the literature.[3] In what follows, I shall mean by nonvalidated therapies those drugs, medical and surgical interventions, and regimens that are offered to and accepted by a patient on the basis of potential benefit, and that have neither been accepted nor discredited by the expert clinical community. Nonvalidated therapies are distinct from, on the one hand, customary and accepted treatments; and, on the other, quack remedies. Because of the uncertainty surrounding them, the ethics of practice in providing nonvalidated therapies cannot be subsumed under the general ethics of clinical practice; nor are such therapies uniformly provided pursuant to an approved protocol, and in those instances are not subjected to the moral canons of clinical research. What treatments currently fall within this rubric? And what are the characteristics of the population seeking NTs?

Discussions of policy and ethics regarding NTs tend to focus on investigational new drugs (INDs), which are novel pharmacologically active substances under testing for anti-viral, immunomodulating, or other beneficial effect.[4] AZT stands as the paradigm case, a drug whose only previous presumed use, as an anti-cancer agent, had been discredited in early trials.

Investigational new drugs are under the close control of regulatory bodies, such as FDA (in the United States) or Health Protection Branch (in Canada). The view that equates nonvalidated treatments with INDs, therefore, leads naturally to the presumption that reform of the policy and rules governing NTs must focus upon the conduct of such regulatory bodies. The scope of NTs is, however, much broader than that; and the power of regulatory agencies correspondingly limited.

Nonvalidated therapies without IND status fall into several categories; each shares the qualities of uncertainty, therapeutic intention, and immunity from regulatory control:

Licensed Drugs Offered for an Unapproved Use. Whereas a drug receives marketing approval after demonstrated safety and effectiveness under defined conditions of use, once approved, a licensed drug may be prescribed by a physician, exercising his or her clinical discretion, for other conditions.[5] U.S. regulations, for example, state that "the physician may, as part of the practice of medicine, lawfully prescribe a different dosage for his patient or may otherwise vary the conditions of use from those approved in the package insert without informing or obtaining the approval of the Food and Drug Administration."[6] Antabuse is an example of a drug licensed for one condition that is currently taken by many persons infected with HIV. Regulatory agencies have taken the stance that enforcing the restriction of licensed drugs to approved uses is beyond their jurisdiction. The point is not always appreciated. The expert panel FDA assembled on AZT, for example, had recommended that the drug be approved only as a treatment for AIDS patients who had had an episode of PCP.[7] In licensing the drug for marketing, however, FDA cannot enforce such a restriction.

Non-Drugs and Not-Necessarily-Drugs. Among the treatments touted for HIV are dietary and life-style changes, which are obviously beyond regulatory control. One interesting case is AL-721. This substance, with suspected anti-viral properties, is a special preparation of common foodstuffs. It is being marketed as a prescription drug in Great Britain, but because of the cost and delay involved in receiving U.S. regulatory approval, and under pressure from generic competitors, its manufacturer now plans to market it as a "food supplement" in the United States.[8] Other possible inclusions within this category would be substances such as dextran sulfate or DTC (Imuthiol), which are under clinical investigation but may be obtained by the public from nonpharmaceutical sources such as chemical supply houses and which the patient may then self-administer.

New Combinations of Treatments.   As with the first category of unapproved use of licensed substances, attempting new combinations of treatments reproduces the combination of therapeutic intent and scientific uncertainty. Current AIDS research is largely preoccupied with testing new combinations of drugs and other treatments (for example, AZT in combination with interferon or acyclovir), and this category will necessarily grow as new drugs are included within the validated AIDS pharmacopoeia.

Smuggled Substances.   The growing use of drugs smuggled from Europe and Mexico by AIDS patients or their doctors has been widely noted; FDA has in fact recently informed its agents in writing to ignore the importation of unapproved drugs by patients for their own use.[9]

In the light of these categories of nonvalidated therapies, it is clear that the role of regulators, though crucial, is limited. By the same token, the central importance of the doctor-patient relationship in confronting these issues is brought to the fore. Only in the clinical setting can much use of NTs in HIV be monitored (if indeed it can be done there); only in that setting can such use be influenced by informed judgment. At the same time, it must be acknowledged that the controversies to date have largely swirled about IND treatments, and that IND policy is the element most given to rapid reform.

Previous experience with treatments for other conditions, notably tuberculosis, indicates that unproven therapy remains popular until such point as an effective therapy is developed; thus, the issue in HIV treatment is likely to persist for some time to come. Current research on those being treated for cancer by unorthodox means also has some lessons to teach us. Among cancer patients, there is a strong direct relationship between experienced toxicity from standard treatment and the subsequent use of unorthodox treatments. In addition, contrary to the stereotype of the uneducated, credulous patient victimized by the unscrupulous practitioner, "[t]he evidence seems overwhelming that socioeconomic status is either independent of the use of such therapies or that higher status and better educated individuals are overrepresented among the patients of unorthodox practitioners."[10]

These characteristics have expressed themselves in our context of HIV disease in a way that raises an urgent ethical problem of equity.[11] In the United States, the bulk of the infected population is increasingly bifurcated, being composed of gay men on the one hand, and, on the other, intravenous drug users and their sexual partners. The latter group has little in the way of education, information, or resources to deploy toward novel therapies. Gay infected men, on the other hand—particularly as their illness progresses—have voted with their feet, vigorously gathering information about potential therapies and aggressively pursuing access to them. Within this group, motivated by desperation, the use of nonvalidated therapies with or without a physician's assistance may yet become the rule rather than the exception. At one meeting of Body Positive in 1987, for example, more than three-quarters of the audience of 400 raised their hands when asked how many were taking experimental or alternative drug treatment.[12]

In part their efforts are expressed in unprecedented activity providing information about current clinical trials directly to infected persons. The American Foundation for AIDS Research publishes a pamphlet with regular updates listing the protocols of clinical trials currently underway, together with their operative criteria of inclusion and exclusion.[13] This publication is distributed gratis upon request to persons who have tested positive for HIV antibodies. Groups such as Project Inform in San Francisco and Treatment AIDS in Toronto gather information about the clinical use of NTs and distribute it to persons with AIDS via newsletters. Some sources will inform persons about means of preparation and self-administration of experimental substances, and how they may be smuggled into the country.

These facts raise some clear challenges to any proposal for reform of the process regarding NTs. Overall, the number of persons prepared to take the risks involved in receiving nonvalidated treatment far outnumber those who may be admitted to controlled scientific trials. The regulatory authorities are increasingly in danger of becoming irrelevant; as I will suggest below, the response to this adopted by FDA—strategic retreat in the form of the treatment IND exemption—only hastens this mounting irrelevancy, with added unfortunate precedential value for other conditions. In turn, the gay male community is left to self-help resources; without a counterbalance, this leaves it potential prey to rumor fostered by hope and nourished by companies who see a profit opportunity in the manufacture of nonvalidated therapies. Finally, the other major group of infected persons—inner-city IV drug users and their sexual partners—has no entrée to the system. Often excluded from trials because of supposed unreliability, or dropping out because of actual unreliability, and lacking the knowledge or resources to pursue NTs on an off-protocol basis, they are denied any potential benefits that may accrue to those receiving drugs prior to conclusion of the validating process.

Some Policy Options

Proposals for reforming the process for dealing with NTs fall along a continuum of change. The least radical changes involve reform of the manner in which the drug agencies operate under current regulations and statutory authority. Much remains to be done along these lines. "Compassionate use" exemptions, for example, could be interpreted broadly rather than narrowly; queuing and consequent delays in reviewing could be managed better than in noncrisis times; traditional cautious practices, such as requiring the replication of well-designed double blind randomized trials, could be amended. However, most attention has been focused upon radical proposed changes to the process altering the underlying philosophy of drug regulation.

An early proposal by Mathilde Krim may be the most familiar.[14] She had proposed maintaining the bureaucratic *status quo* with respect to asymptomatic infected persons, or those in the early stages of HIV disease (AIDS-Related Complex), but eliminating all restrictions to free access, via their physician, to any substance proposed for treatment of a person with full-blown AIDS. In exempting an entire class of patients from regulatory restraints on the basis of the severity of their illness, Krim's proposal represents a radical departure from traditional drug regulation philosophy, which held the critically ill to be in at least as great need of protection through regulation as any other patient.

Were Krim's proposal to be implemented, it might become impossible to conduct controlled trials on AIDS patients since they would all have unrestricted access to experimental substances. This consequence does not concern her, for in her view "[t]he most valuable proof of the efficacy of the drugs will be studies conducted on patients in the earlier stages of illness." The ravages involved in the progression to AIDS make it unlikely in her view

that treatment would help, but nevertheless she believes that offering such treatment is ethically imperative:

> Permitting physicians to use experimental drugs to treat patients whose lives are in immediate jeopardy should not be done out of a wishful belief that the treatment would work. It should be done out of respect for the patient's right to fight for life with whatever tools we can offer.

AZT itself demonstrates several problems with her proposal. As AZT shows, AIDS patients can receive significant therapeutic benefit; meaningful controlled results can be obtained in tests upon a population with full-blown AIDS; and, the harm-benefit ratio associated with a drug changes over the course of disease, rendering drug toxicity that may be excessive early on acceptable as the patient's options shrink. Moreover, persons with AIDS die of opportunistic infections, not HIV, and treatments specific to these infections cannot be tested before they occur, whether early or late in the progressive breakdown of the immune system. In general, our growing knowledge of the erratic continuum of HIV disease makes a hard division between AIDS itself and everything up to it medically inappropriate.

One final point is most troubling. Even were it the case that an AIDS patient is beyond help, it does not follow that he or she is beyond being hurt as well—and both must be true if drugs are to be made available that have satisfied neither norms of safety or of efficacy. For example, the early experimental treatment suramin proved in tests to be both toxic and, in some instances, to contribute itself to worsening immune disorders. The death of an AIDS patient is not so imminent that it cannot be hastened by misguided treatment, nor is the disease so dreadful that the quality of life of its sufferers cannot be worsened by inappropriate treatments. As Oliver Wendell Holmes, Sr., once said, if all of the unproven remedies doctors carry in their saddle bags were to be dumped in to the ocean, it would be so much the better for their patients and so much the worse for the fish.

A second radical proposal that has been implemented by FDA, the introduction of the category of the treatment IND, responds to some of these points.[15] The new category was adopted under the obvious impetus and avowed influence of the AIDS crisis, although since its recent adoption its most frequent use has been for non-AIDS drugs. The treatment IND category is intended to weaken substantially, without abandoning altogether, the requirement that a drug be demonstrably effective before being allowed into clinical practice. In brief, it requires that a drug for an immediately life-threatening condition be approved provided FDA is satisfied that it "may be effective" and the risk of its use is not "unreasonable and significant"; if a drug is intended for use on a serious but not immediately life-threatening condition, it shall be approved for clinical use upon demonstration of safety and preliminary evidence of effectiveness.[16]

It is still uncertain how this amended regulation will be interpreted and work out in practice. For example, a broad reading of the regulation would include asymptomatic HIV infection under the "immediately life-threatening" rubric, defined as "a stage of a disease in which there is a reasonable likelihood that death will occur within a matter of months *or in which premature death is likely without early treatment*" (emphasis added). The financial implications for drug companies are also unclear at this point. It appears that while the preparation of applications for treatment IND status will be fairly expensive, they will nonetheless still be much cheaper than the ordinary cost of drug development is currently;[17] and treatment IND status is granted prior to completion of Phase III trials, which represent by far the most expensive phase of drug testing for companies. Until the treatment IND category was introduced, drug companies were not permitted to charge for drugs in clinical trials without special approval. Supplying drugs for trials was considered part of the normal costs of doing business. Drug companies by contrast are automatically permitted to charge for the use of drugs with treatment IND status, at a rate that permits them "to recover costs of manufacture, research, development, and handling" of the drug. The companies are nonetheless forbidden to "commercialize" treatment INDs, a prohibition whose force and meaning remains uncertain.

The Pharmaceutical Manufacturers Association has warned that a company that can charge for its drug will have no incentive to complete the expensive testing necessary to achieve regular marketing approval.[18] In response, the regulations require that the companies whose product has been granted this status be vigorously engaged concurrently in completing testing and the approval process. As a matter of structural public policy, however, this seems an inadequate response. Heretofore, the drug companies' vigorous pursuit of testing was motivated by the pull toward potential drug profits, which could not be realized without FDA approval. Henceforward, rather than being pulled by natural market forces, testing will be pushed by FDA pressure. It is economically wasteful to substitute artificial regulatory pressure for natural market forces, and it is particularly doubtful that in the current context of scarce regulatory resources the money needed will be found—money that must be carved out of the same budget that is already failing to keep up with IND and other new drug (NDA) applications.

Other practical concerns stated by university researchers and the American Medical Association express fear that controlled clinical trials of drugs granted this status will become impossible due to a failure of enrollment of subjects. Patients may not agree to be randomized into treatment or placebo control groups if they have guaranteed access to the treatment by clinical prescription. Clamor to receive the "new treatment" may prove to be intensified by a now-unjustified reliance by patients upon regulators, for patients have become accustomed to the idea that a drug cannot be legally sold unless it is safe and effective. But the failure to complete these trials will serve neither those patients themselves—who serve as guinea pigs for treatments of unproved efficacy, and pay for the privilege—nor future patients, who are denied the advantage of prior validation of treatments.

One final conceptual difficulty of the regulations should be noted. It treats safety and efficacy as two separate categories. As long as a drug is shown to be safe (more precisely, not unreasonably risky) its treatment use may be authorized pending a finding of efficacy. But safety, and efficacy must nearly always be judged in relative rather than absolute terms, and nearly always as a balance rather than as independent factors—a function rather than a conjunction. The bottom line—Is this drug worth prescribing or not?—is affected by knowledge concerning systemic or symptomatic benefit, side effects, and other factors, and safety and efficacy may only be understood as elements within this function. To make the same point in other words, a drug's pharmacologic activity is the basis of both positive and negative effects (that is, "efficacy" as well as "risk"). The only perfectly safe drug is a perfectly inert—hence, perfectly useless—drug. A regulation presuming the contrary will yield either limited or distorted application.

Libertarians have seen in AIDS an opportunity to further their anti-regulationist agenda. Dale Gieringer, on behalf of the Cato Institute, has suggested that the informed consent of the patient, rather than regulation, be the determinant of access to investigational drugs.[19] Any patient who, being fully informed about any new substance, chooses to risk his life and health by taking it, should be granted that option.

Confidence in consent is misplaced in this instance. By definition of nonvalidated therapies, the consent would be minimally informed at best. It would be consent granted under desperation, and consent that is likely fostered by drug company promotion. Adherence to such a consent in the form of administering such a drug also professionally impugns the responsible physician, who is trained to use his or her own educated judgment rather than simply complying with patient's requests. The testing and medical research upon which this professional judgment relies would be entirely undercut by Gieringer's proposal.

What Constitutes a Desirable Policy?

The elements of desirable changes in policy toward nonvalidated treatments used for HIV disease have emerged from the above critique. The central points of the current philosophy of drug regulation should be conserved. In particular, drugs should not be licensed for marketing until they have been proved safe and effective under proposed conditions of use, a judgment that should be arrived at by a panel with comprehensive expertise rather than by private practitioners and their patients alone. (It may, however, be argued that "comprehensive expertise" requires representation from the points of view of patients and private physicians.) Finally, it is critically important that drug companies should not be permitted to reap any economic benefit from a drug until this process has been completed.

One additional desideratum is implicit in the above discussion: Any change in the process must be at least consistent with, if not positively enhancing of, the ability to speedily conclude sound scientific evaluations of any new treatments. Because of the ever-growing numbers of infected persons,

practices and procedures within the context of the regulations should be streamlined to the maximum extent. Equally, however, the growing number of cases argues for the early resolution of the question of safety and effectiveness.

This double-edged character of the epidemic factor in AIDS may be illustrated by a simple analogy. A large boulder is rolling down a cliff, toward a populated area. An early nudge will achieve the largest alteration of its path with the minimum effort. But you want to be sure that you're nudging it in the right direction: because you don't want to waste your effort; because there may not be time to mount a second effort; because a misguided nudge might endanger a still-more-populated region. For AIDS, as for the boulder, the message is: Hurry up—carefully. More lives will be saved, in the end, by aiming accurately than by aiming early. Applied to the specific issue of drug licensure, the metaphor cautions us not to jeopardize the conclusion of needed clinical trials in the interest of satisfying patient demands for access to an NT.

This point requires some further discussion. It entails that, when conflict between a patient or treating physician's desire for access to a nonvalidated treatment and the pursuit and early conclusion of a sound, ethical trial is unavoidable, the latter may be allowed to take precedence. If, for example, it is only possible to recruit sufficient subjects by restricting access to the drug to those eligible persons who agree to enroll, we would be expressing such a preference. Yet seemingly, to do this would grant the progress of science priority over patient rights.

The justification depends upon establishing that the patient's right to medical treatment is unimpaired by denying the patient access to an unvalidated intervention. The ethics of a controlled clinical trial require that throughout its conduct a state of clinical equipoise exist between the experimental and control arm(s) (including placebo control, if any); in other words, that the relative therapeutic merit of the proposed innovation remains a genuinely undecided question amongst the community of expert practitioners.[20] It is this state of equipoise, of clinical uncertainty, that serves to justify the withholding of the innovation from the control population, because as long as this state of uncertainty persists, the innovation cannot be classified for normative purposes as a medical treatment. Once the uncertainty has been resolved, however, the trial must ethically be terminated, and the now-validated treatment offered to all eligible patients.

The same ethical analysis concerning the right to treatment that applies to the control population applies to the patient population outside of the trial as well. A patient, within a trial as without, is unconditionally entitled to receive medical treatment. "Medical treatment" as a normative concept, however, must be defined and delimited by medical expertise rather than by a patient's beliefs. The right to medical treatment does not encompass every drug or intervention that a patient considers therapeutically worthwhile, on whatever evidence he or she has found convincing. Until the therapeutic advantage of an innovation has been demonstrated to the satisfaction of the community of expert practitioners, an innovation is no medical treatment, and so is not covered by a patient's right to access to medical treatments. Consistent with the above, however, we may add that to the extent that a patient's desire to receive an innovation may be satisfied without jeopardizing the conduct of a clinical trial, then, consistent with good clinical judgment, the desire of the patient should be allowed to prevail.

A reform that might satisfy these various desiderata would focus upon the factor missing from other proposals, the physician-researcher treating persons with HIV infection. The proposal builds upon the growing development of specialized research and treatment units for AIDS—for example, AIDS Clinical Trial Limits (ACTUs)—which combine substantial expertise in AIDS diagnosis, treatment, and research, together with sophisticated laboratory support. Clinicians in these units are active collaborators in treatment protocols granted high priority by the AIDS Clinical Drug Development Committee, and play an important role in developing treatment protocols and in their accelerated evaluation.[21] They have not yet been assigned any formal role, however, in expediting the evaluation of NTs, nor have other similarly designated expert units.[22]

The proposal is to institute similar units (or specified investigators), in the United States and Canada, which are formally granted the authority to utilize restricted investigational drugs on a compassionate use basis.[23] The regulatory authorities would be notified about such use, and would be able to monitor these Authorized Investigational Units (AIUs) and provide retrospective control, but their prior approval for individual use would not be needed. In effect, any drug having IND status would be available for the testing and clinical use of the designated AIDS facilities; something resembling "treatment IND" status would be granted at the (monitored) discretion of the expert practitioners of these units. Consistent with previous practice, drug companies would not be permitted to charge for drugs employed within protocols. For those drugs used on an "off-protocol" basis, they would be permitted to recover the direct marginal cost of production and handling only. Charges allowing amortization of other costs of research and development would not be permitted until the drug had completed the approval process, so that the natural incentives for completion of testing would be retained. . . .

Acknowledgments

The ideas in this paper were discussed at workshops of the McGill University/Boston University Cooperative Research Group on Ethics, Law and Policy on HIV. Major support for this work was provided by Grant #6605-2897, National Health Research and Development Program, Ministry of Health, Government of Canada. While it is not possible to acknowledge all who contributed, special thanks must be given to Margaret Sommerville, George J. Annas, Norbert Gilmore, and Julie Hamblin.

References

1. "Are Experimental Drugs Moving Through System Too Slowly?" *AIDS Alert* 3:1 (1988), 1–6.

2. George J. Annas, "AIDS, Judges, and the Right to Medical Care," *Hastings Center Report* 18:4 (1988), 20–22.

3. Dale H. Cowan and Eva Bertch, "Innovative Therapy: The Responsibility of Hospitals," *Journal of Legal Medicine* 5:2 (1984), 219–51.

4. Mathilde Krim, "Making Experimental Drugs Available for AIDS Treatment," *AIDS and Public Policy Journal* 2:2 (1987), 1–5.

5. Lynn McMonagle, "Private Rights to Adulterated/Misbranded Articles," *AIDS and Public Policy Journal* 2:2 (1987), 33–49.

6. 37 *Fed. Reg.* 16,503 (1972).

7. David J. Rothman, "Ethical and Social Issues in the Development of New Drugs and Vaccines," *Bulletin of the New York Academy of Medicine* 63:6 (1987), 557–68.

8. "Makers of AL-721 to Market Compound as Food Supplement," *AIDS and Policy Law* 3:6 (1988), 6.

9. "In Brief: Unapproved Drugs," *Rx Ipsa Loquitur* 15:8 (1988), 3.

10. B. R. Cassileth and H. Brown, "Unorthodox Cancer Medicine," *CA-Cancer Journal for Clinicians* 38:3 (1988), 176–86.

11. I am grateful to Gary Freedman for raising this important point.

12. J. A. Revson, "HIV Positive: Living Under the Shadow," *Newsday*, 18 Feb. 1988, Part II, 4–5, 11.

13. American Foundation for AIDS Research, *AIDS/HIV Experimental Treatment Directory*, (NY: AmFAR).

14. Mathilde Krim, "A Chance for Life for AIDS Sufferers," *New York Times*, 8 August 1986, A-27.

15. Frank E. Young *et al.*, "The FDA's New Procedures for the Use of Investigational Drugs in Treatment," *Journal of the American Medical Association* 259:15 (1988), 2267–70.

16. 52 *Fed. Reg.* no. 99, May 22, 1987, 19467-77.

17. Robert E. Wittes, "Noninvestigational Uses of Investigational Drugs: Some Implications of FDA's Revised Regulations," *Journal of the National Cancer Institute* 80:5 (1988), 301–304.

18. "Proposal to Make Investigational New Drugs Available Without Clinical Trial Participation in Certain Cases is Receiving Mixed Responses," *Journal of the American Medical Association* 257:22 (1987), 3020.

19. Dale Gieringer, "Twice Wrong on AIDS," *New York Times*, 12 January 1987, A-21.

20. Benjamin Freedman, "Equipoise and the Ethics of Clinical Research," *New England Journal of Medicine* 317 (1987), 141–45.

21. *Dateline: NIAID*, November 1987 (AIDS Research Issue), 7 ff.

22. I. Feldman *et al.*, "AIDS Center Designation/AIDS Intervention Management System," *AIDS and Public Policy Journal* 3:1 (1988), 29–31.

23. Currently, the open trial of long-term effects of AZT run by Burroughs-Wellcome in selected Canadian centers bears some resemblance to the system described herein, but differs in the degree of control granted to the drug company, in conformity with Canadian regulations on the control of investigational drugs. The designated center approach has also been utilized in the introductory period of some medical devices and surgical procedures (for example, major organ transplants), but this has commonly been under the direction of insurers, governmental or private.

Insurers Are Right on AIDS Testing

Bob Hunter and Jay Angoff

Hunter and Angoff assert that the principle of an individual's sharing the risk with *similar* individuals warrants testing, because otherwise the cost of insurance is unfair to those who do not carry the AIDS virus. They admit that other considerations might override this principle, but they do not regard any of the four factors they examine as sufficient. In their view, national health insurance offers the best solution of paying for the care of AIDS patients.

The insurance industry has filed suit to block a regulation proposed by the New York Insurance Department that would prohibit insurance companies from testing applicants for health insurance for exposure to the AIDS virus. The insurance industry has a valid point.

Insurance companies are supposed to charge insurance buyers a price that reflects the risk presented by an individual buyer or by a group of similarly situated buyers.

In seeking to test insurance applicants for exposure to the AIDS virus, life and health insurers are trying to abide by this principle. For example, out of 1,000 34-year-males who test positive for the presence of the AIDS antibody, which indicates infection by the virus, at least 200 will die of AIDS within seven years, according to the National Centers for Disease Control.

By contrast, actuarial tables tell us that of 1,000 34-year-old males in standard health, 7.5 will die within seven years. Those who test positive, therefore, are 26.6 times more likely to die within seven years than 34-year-old males in standard health. To ignore the risk factor responsible for this 2,666 percent risk differential is bad insurance policy.

However, other factors must be considered in assessing whether a particular restriction on AIDS testing might nevertheless be good social policy. They include the following:

• *The magnitude of the impact of a particular restriction on the insurance industry.*

People who apply for insurance as individuals are tested to determine the likelihood of their developing various diseases, such as diabetes and heart disease, but those who buy insurance as a group are not.

Because group insurance accounts for 90 percent of all health insurance, but less than 50 percent of all life insurance, prohibiting AIDS testing for health insurance would have a relatively minor impact on the health insurance business, while prohibiting testing for life insurance would have a more substantial effect.

• *The effect of permitting testing on those at risk for AIDS.*

The gay community argues that insurers cannot possibly guarantee confidentiality and that a breach of it to someone who tests positive can be devastating. A proposed Massachusetts regulation, however, if enforced, would seem to offer true confidentiality: It sets up a "need to know" standard for disclosing the results of an AIDS test even to other individuals in an insurance company.

• *The effect of prohibiting testing on those not at risk for AIDS.*

If testing for AIDS is prohibited, people in standard health and people at risk for other diseases will subsidize those at risk for AIDS. Whether lawmakers are willing to accept such a subsidy would seem to depend on its cost for each policy holder, which insurers could easily calculate. So far, however, they have failed to do so.

• *The alternatives to permitting testing.*

If insurers are prohibited from testing, they will use less accurate, and more offensive, methods of determining who is at risk for AIDS. For example, they may seek to charge higher rates to all unmarried males living in zip code areas with a large proportion of gay men.

States may prohibit insurers from either testing for AIDS or using sexual preference or any surrogate for sexual preference as a risk factor, as the District of Columbia has done. But they cannot force insurers to write insurance under those conditions. The heavy-handed but not entirely unjustified response of several insurers to the District's AIDS law has been to stop doing business there.

The best solution to providing health insurance for those at risk for AIDS is national health insurance. By spreading the cost of AIDS as widely as possible throughout society, the burden on any individual will be minimal.

Unless such a system is enacted, any "solution" will be a compromise. The compromise reached by the New York Insurance Department may be reasonable. But we should recognize that insurers that want to test for infection by the AIDS virus—and to decline to insure those testing positive—have sound insurance principles on their side.

An Insidious Test for AIDS

William C. Gifford III

William Gifford explains why he refused to consent to be tested for the AIDS virus as part of an insurance application. Anyone testing positive would be "uninsurable," and the results might become known to prospective employers, the federal government, or others. Also, those who are seropositive must then rely on public clinics, rather than private physicians. Most important, in Gifford's view, "the test not only amounts to a subsidy of the insurance industry, it could also create a vast class of young people who are uninsurable." At the same time as it wants to avoid insuring those who might have AIDS, the industry campaigns against national health insurance.

One morning not long ago, a young woman came to my apartment to take blood and urine samples, as required by the company to which I had applied for an individual health insurance policy. She opened her briefcase and began arranging needles, vials and bandages on the kitchen table.

Then she asked me to sign a form. In very fine print, it said that my blood and urine would be tested for the presence of HIV, the virus that causes AIDS, and for cocaine and other drugs. The results would determine my eligibility for insurance.

For a straight, white, young middle class male like me, AIDS remains a remote possibility. And I don't use drugs. Though my sense of civil liberties was a bit ruffled, my first instinct was to sign and get the test over with.

But as I reread the statement, its implications became clear. If the test showed I carry HIV, then I would be denied insurance—and not just by one company. A call to the company's agent revealed I would be "uninsurable."

In addition, this information would be recorded in a medical information bank. I asked who else would see my test results. Prospective employers? The Federal Government? What if the confidentiality rules changed, and drug users or HIV carriers were reported?

The company agent was annoyed that I would bother to ask these questions. Such a climate of hysteria surrounds both AIDS and drugs, however, that I needed to know how this sensitive information would be used.

I couldn't sign the form. The unlikely scenario played in my head: What if I did test positive? With HIV, and thus without insurance, I would have to pay all my health care expenses—even the podiatrist's bills. That would mean going to public clinics rather than a private physician. If and when I developed the disease, I would become dependent on Medicare and would qualify for some treatments, like AZT, but not others. I would get by, a burden to the taxpayers rather than the private sector.

The AIDS test not only amounts to a subsidy of the insurance industry, it also could create a vast class of young people who are uninsurable.

According to a recent news article, teen-agers are becoming infected at very high rates. Unlike the situation in the adult population, the article pointed out, among teen-agers the disease is spread equally between males and females. That means the Government will soon be picking up the medical expenses of many more young people with AIDS who are ineligible for private insurance, thereby absorbing much of the risk and the losses that would ordinarily belong to the insurance companies.

Typically, insurance works by spreading the health care costs of very sick people around the general insured population. The insurance company gambles that its premiums will be greater than its outlays, and takes steps, like raising premiums, to improve the odds.

Excluding carriers of HIV keeps down premiums for most people, the company agent informed me. But this is an illusory savings. First, according to an article in The New England Journal of Medicine the actual cost of treating a person with AIDS has turned out to be much lower than the initial estimates cited by insurance companies. Second, we all end up paying for AIDS care through taxes.

These companies and their political spokesmen squeal in agony at the mention of national health insurance. Nevertheless, insurance companies that require an AIDS test seem to be quite willing to let the Government pick up the tab for people with HIV.

They can get away with it because AIDS remains largely a disease of homosexuals, drug users, blacks and Hispanics. But as AIDS slowly seeps into the straight, white majority, discrimination against HIV carriers will no longer be acceptable.

It shouldn't be acceptable now, when between one million and 1.5 million Americans are estimated to carry the AIDS virus. If insurance companies are going to campaign against national health care, they should be held to their argument. The private sector must accept full responsibility for the nation's health, or step aside.

A "Manhattan Project" for AIDS

Larry Kramer

Larry Kramer calls upon the federal government to establish a biomedical equivalent of the Manhattan Project. If the government does not marshal all needed resources into a single organized effort to a cure for AIDS as quickly as possible, thousands will die needlessly. (Kramer seems to believe that measures to control the spread of AIDS have not worked.) In current efforts, he sees disorganization, lack of focus, in-fighting, inadequate funding, and a lack of serious commitment.

I am so frightened that the war against AIDS has already been lost.

It is beyond comprehension why, in a presumably civilized country, in the modern era, such a continuing, extraordinary destruction of life is being attended to so tentatively, so meekly and in such a cowardly fashion.

The armies of the infected, their families, loved ones and friends no longer know how to deliver their pleas for help. Every conceivable method has been attempted, from quietly working from within to noisily demonstrating without.

Millions of people who need not die so young will die so young. As things stand now, everyone who is presently infected can reasonably expect to die. So desperate is the situation that Dr. David Baltimore, president of Rockefeller University, has called for a "Manhattan Project" for AIDS, an equivalent of the scientific effort that projected the atomic bomb. He's right. Only the Federal Government can manage the project to find, as quickly as possible, the cure that top scientists believe is there and that could stem the ocean of death.

The number of those infected with AIDS is now so terrifyingly large that, even if a satisfactory treatment or cure were found tomorrow, there is no system in existence anywhere in the world that could deliver it in time to save so many people. The numbers of those facing death from AIDS are so large that the eyes should glaze—with tears.

In America, 212 new cases of full-blown AIDS are diagnosed every day; there is one AIDS death every 12 minutes, and a new case of infection every 54 seconds. At a minimum, one to one and a half million Americans are infected.

A report by the American Council on Science and Health predicted that one in every 25 New York City residents will have AIDS in the next 10 years. Last week, another study revealed that AIDS is already the leading cause of death among black women between the ages of 15 and 44.

Worldwide, 386,588 cases have been reported in 151 countries. The World Health Organization estimates that this number is now at least 700,000, and that six to eight million people have the virus that causes fullblown AIDS. By the year 2000, the infected population will approach 20 million.

All of these figures, which are known to be imprecise, are also known to be low. They are mostly based on extrapolations from small samplings from isolated areas or from cases that doctors report to authorities. We know that many doctors and patients do not report their cases, and that large numbers of those infected never see a doctor.

A transmissible virus is loose in the world. It may be one or several. It is completely out of control. Short of a cure, there is no way it can be stopped—not by mandatory or volunteer contact tracing, partner notification, quarantining, incarceration or legislation. It is out there, everywhere, and it is rampant.

We are living in a time of plague, and two Presidents in a row have refused to stem it. Their refusal to act will cost taxpayers a fortune—easily more than the entire cost of the savings and loan bailout.

Six Federal studies and more than 50 Congressional oversight hearings have all concluded the same thing: The research on AIDS is uncoordinated and the funding cycles are inefficient. No one is in charge.

President Bush has done as little about AIDS as President Reagan. Twenty-four thousand Americans have died from AIDS since he took office. After stumbling on abortion, the Secretary of Health and Human Services, Dr. Louis Sullivan, has meekly followed the lead of the White House on AIDS, even though many sense he would like to perform adequately.

It is suspected that the real villain of the piece is John Sununu, the White House chief of staff, whose mission seems to be appeasing the conservative right. The result is the perpetuation of a Federal policy on AIDS that was crafted by Ronald Reagan's AIDS adviser, Gary Bauer, who is now more visibly displaying his rhetoric of hate as head the Family Research Council.

Tens years into this plague, the Federal agencies dealing with AIDS are mired in such bureaucracy that is is next to impossible for them to respond to the crisis. There are so many committees and committees within committees, peer reviews and inter-agency task forces that few can sort them all out.

Paths of least resistance are the chosen norm. Imagination is not encouraged and exchange of vital information is often nonexistent. The two most important agencies, the National Institutes of Health and the Food and Drug Administration, are both still lacking a permanent director. Rivalries and distrust between them are embarrassingly, visibly rife. International fist fights over who should get the Nobel Prize for AIDS research has destroyed trust universally. Pharmaceutical companies now test their drugs abroad rather than confront the American maze.

The bureaucracy is so byzantine, nobody can or has to make a decision.

Research is delayed not only by a lack of any coherent plan and mature guidance, but also by a lack of first-rate personnel. The chief N.I.H. laboratories have 27 vacancies for AIDS scientists. Vital studies that many assume are being done are not.

Conflict of interest is rampant. Just about every major AIDS researcher with a Government grant is also on the payroll of a major pharmaceutical manufacturer as a "consultant." Thus, the only drugs that are being tested are ones controlled by these same manufacturers. Hundreds of promising treatments developed by the less well-connected are simply ignored—and people continue to suffer and die.

President Bush and Dr. Anthony Fauci of the N.I.H. have constantly assured us that more has been learned in record time about AIDS than any disease in history, that everything that can be done is being done. Dr. Fauci, a dedicated and overburdened scientist, is no doubt trying to calm the waters for his boss, the President, who once called him a "hero." But a real hero must tell the truth, even when it is unpopular.

Huge areas of AIDS still aren't understood. Yet Government grants that would locate and assign a researcher to a specific AIDS problem are prohibited by some funding regulations.

Dr. Fauci's $500 million program for conducting experimental drug trials at local hospital sites around the country, the AIDS Clinical Trials Group, has fallen tragically short of its goals. Slots for tens of thousands of patients attract only hundreds, mainly because most people with AIDS are excluded from the trials by a battery of illogical and murderous clinical restrictions.

And recent editorials in The Lancet and the Journal of the American Medical Association seriously questioned the usefulness of AZT, a 25-year-old, exceedingly toxic anti-viral treatment on which the N.I.H. spends billions of dollars. AIDS doctors and patients desperately need something more effective, but they won't get it until the AIDS drug pipeline is rerouted and streamlined.

Stopping the tragic delays in research and treatment—delays which are mostly bureaucratic, not scientific—seems impossible. The President is not interested, and while Congress votes money for the war, it abdicates its responsibility to see that these precious funds are spent wisely.

To top it all off, the media have yet to expose most, if not all, of the wrongs enumerated above. They reserve their energies for criticizing the tactics activists have used to compensate for their shameful silence.

Only an all-out effort by the Federal Government can defeat AIDS. It alone has the resources and authority to win. President Bush must put one person in charge of all aspects of AIDS and grant this person emergency powers to cut through the red tape. And the President must take up Dr. Baltimore's call for a "Manhattan Project" to find that cure.

Anything less will condemn millions to death, and the war against AIDS will indeed by irrevocably lost. And history will record that it was lost because two U.S. Presidents and the entire Federal Government surrendered.

AIDS: Getting More Than Its Share?

Charles Krauthammer

Charles Krauthammer argues that the idea that government or society "has been inattentive or unresponsive to AIDS is quite simply absurd." He points to the special treatment given AIDS in funding research and in approving new drugs, due in part to the youth of AIDS victims and the power of the AIDS lobby. AIDS activists initially appealed to the idea that AIDS threatens everyone, but when this turned out to be false they appealed to guilt. Yet, because advocates for every disease can claim society is not doing enough, activists now claim that AIDS is an act of God and the government must do more.

Krauthammer points out that, except for special cases and people infected more than six years ago, AIDS is a result of certain kinds of behavior, not an act of God. AIDS sufferers deserve our help, but in Krauthammer's view they have no basis for claiming more resources and compassion than those dying of other diseases.

Last month a thousand demonstrators camped outside the National Institutes of Health near Washington and with a talented display of street theater protested governmental and scientific neglect of AIDS. If not the angriest demonstration Washington has seen in a long time, it was certainly the most misdirected. The idea that American government or American society has been inattentive or unresponsive to AIDS is quite simply absurd. Consider:

Treatment. Congress is about to do something extremely rare: allocate money specifically for the treatment of one disease. The Senate voted $2.9 billion, the House $4 billion over five years for treating AIDS. And only AIDS. When Senator Mal-colm Wallop introduced an amendment allowing rural districts with few AIDS patients to spend the money on other diseases, the amendment was voted down, 2 to 1.

Research. Except for cancer, AIDS now receives more Government research money than any other illness in America. AIDS gets $1.2 billion to $1.3 billion. Heart disease, for example, receives about half as much, $700 billion. The AIDS research allocation is not just huge, it is hugely disproportionate. AIDS has killed 83,000 Americans in nine years. Heart disease kills that many every six weeks.

Testing. Under pressure from AIDS activists, the FDA has radically changed its regulations for testing new drugs. The Administration has proposed "parallel track" legislation that would make drugs available to certain patients before the usual testing process is complete. Nothing wrong with this. But this exception is for AIDS patients only—a fact that hardly supports the thesis that government is holding back an AIDS cure or discriminating against AIDS patients.

The suffering caused by AIDS is enormous. Sufferers deserve compassion, and their disease deserves scientific inquiry. But AIDS has got far more. AIDS has become the most privileged disease in America. Why? Mainly because its victims are young, in many cases creative and famous. Their deaths are therefore particularly poignant and public. And because one of the two groups that AIDS disproportionately affects (gay men) is highly organized. This combination of conspicuousness and constituency has allowed AIDS activists to get more research funding, more treatment money and looser drug-testing restrictions than any comparable disease.

Nothing wrong with that. The system for allocating research and treatment money in American medicine is archaic, chaotic and almost random anyway. Under the "Disease of the Month Club" syndrome, any disease that has in some way affected a Congressman or some relation gets special treatment. There is a rough justice in this method of allocation because after a while Congressmen and their kin get to experience most of the medical tragedies that life has to offer. At the end of the day, therefore, funds tend to get allocated in a fairly proportionate way.

AIDS is now riding a crest of public support, won in the rough and tumble of politics. All perfectly legitimate, and a tribute to the passion and commitment of AIDS activists. But that passion turns to mere stridency when they take to the streets to protest that a homophobic society has been ungenerous and stinting in its response to the tragedy of AIDS. In fact, American society is giving overwhelming and indeed disproportionate attention and resources to the fight.

At first the homosexual community was disoriented and defensive in reaction to AIDS. In the quite understandable attempt to get public support, it fixed on a strategy of claiming that AIDS was everyone's problem. Since we were all potential sufferers—anyone can get AIDS, went the slogan—

society as an act of self-protection should go all out for cure and care.

This campaign was initially successful. But then it ran into an obstacle. It wasn't true. AIDS is not everyone's problem. It is extremely difficult to get AIDS. It requires the carrying out of specific and quite intentional acts. Nine out of ten people with AIDS have got it through homosexual sex and/or intravenous drug use. The NIH demonstrators, therefore, now appeal less to solidarity than to guilt: every person who dies is more blood on the hands of a society unwilling to give every dollar demanded for a cure.

But society has blood on its hands every time it refuses to give every dollar demanded by the cancer lobby, the heart disease lobby, the diabetes lobby. So now a different tack: the claim that the AIDS epidemic is, of course, not an act of government but an act of God—and government has not done enough to help its helpless victims.

In fact, AIDS is far less an act of God than is, say, cancer or diabetes. Apart from a small number of relentlessly exploited Ryan White–like exceptions, the overwhelming majority of sufferers get AIDS through some voluntary action: sex or drug abuse. You don't get AIDS the way you used to get TB, by having someone on the trolley cough in your face. You don't get it the way you get, say, brain cancer, which is through some act of God that we don't understand at all.

AIDS is in the class of diseases whose origins we understand quite well. It is behaviorally induced and behaviorally preventable. In that sense it is in the same moral class as lung cancer, the majority of whose victims get it through voluntary behavior well known to be highly dangerous. For lung cancer the behavior is smoking; for AIDS, unsafe sex (not, it might be noted, homosexuality) and IV drug use.

As a society we do not refuse either to treat or research lung cancer simply because its sufferers brought it on themselves. But we would find it somewhat perverse and distasteful if lung cancer sufferers began demonstrating wildly, blaming society and government for their problems, and demanding that they be first in line for a cure.

Many people contracted AIDS before its causes became known, about six years ago. For them it is truly an act of God. For the rest (as the word has gone out, an ever increasing percentage), it is an act of man. They, of course, deserve our care and treatment. But it is hard to see from where they derive the claim to be first in line—ahead of those dying of leukemia and breast cancer and stroke—for the resources and compassion of a nation.

Decision Scenario 1 •

"I couldn't believe what he was saying," Lorenzo Owens kept repeating to the police in Hempstead, New York. Owens, nineteen years old, was charged with killing his twenty-two-year-old friend Kenneth Grice. Grice was the person who said something Owens couldn't believe. What Grice said, immediately after the two men had sex at Grice's house, was that he had AIDS.

In a handwritten confession, Owens admitted killing Grice. "Obviously he killed that man in a fit of extreme emotional distress," said John Lewis, Owens's attorney. The Owens case may be the first to use the classic "heat of passion" defense in an AIDS-related murder.

This approach is condemned by gay-rights activists. "Where does it all lead?" asked Leonard Graff of the Gay Rights Advocates. "What if someone who finds out they have been working close to someone who has AIDS gets violent? Isn't that just a step away from this circumstance?"

1. *What answer can be given to Graff's question? Is there any significant and relevant difference between the Owens case and the case he describes?*

2. *Are the circumstances in the case such that Steinbock might consider Grice's behavior in failing to inform Owens the moral equivalent of second-degree murder?*

Decision Scenario 2 •

"When we had a problem with polio in the 1940s and 1950s, we closed the swimming pools, movie theaters, and every other place we thought kids might become infected," Margaret Sank said. "It's just as reasonable to close bathhouses and other public places likely to encourage male homosexuals to engage in sex."

"You're talking about another age," Sandra Kline said. "Nowadays no one thinks it's justifiable to interfere with individual freedom to such an extent."

"Sometimes public health measures have to place restrictions an individual freedom to be effective," Sank said.

"I don't think so," Kline said. "You can't legitimately keep people from doing what they want, so long as they know the risk."

"You can when all of us must pay for it," Sank responded.

1. *On what grounds might Mohr object to closing public places that permit homosexual contact?*

2. *Would Steinbock agree with the position taken by Sank?*

3. *Why does Mohr consider the indirect cost of AIDS an inappropriate justification for restricting the behavior of individuals?*

4. *When does Steinbock consider indirect consequences, including financial costs, to be relevant to justifying placing controls on behavior?*

Decision Scenario 3 •

"Now, if you'll just give me the names of people you've shared needles with," Beth Adderly said, "I'll arrange to have them contacted."

"Man, what are you talking about?" Claude Williams asked. "I'm not about to tell you the peoples I've shot up with."

"But I've already explained to you—you're carrying the AIDS virus. That means people you

shared needles with may have the virus too. You may have given it to them."

"I'm still not going to say they names. I don't want to get them in trouble, for one thing."

"I see what's bothering you. I can promise you complete confidentiality. That means we'll just talk to the people you tell us to, and nobody else will know."

"Ma'am, excuse me, but they ain't no such thing as complete anything. If I was to give you some names, I might see them people get arrested tomorrow. And somebody else might hear I turned him in and just might shoot me dead. It's just too risky."

1. In Mohr's view, does Williams have a duty to turn over the names of those he has shared needles with so those people can be traced?

2. According to Steinbock, Williams does have such a duty, despite a risk to himself. What basis does she offer for this claim?

3. Suppose Williams is right about risking death if he turns over the names. Has Steinbock provided enough justification for holding that Williams is morally obliged to name his contacts?

Decision Scenario 4 •

"I believe it is wrong to have to submit to a blood test to get health insurance," John Tshe said. "If I test positive for the AIDS virus, which I'm virtually certain I will not do, then nobody will give me any insurance."

"That's the way it should be," Aerial Stipps said. "No insurance company should have to accept people who have an existing disease. Otherwise, you could just not pay any premiums until you got sick, and then an insurance company would be forced to accept your application and pay your bills."

"But not everyone who tests positive for the AIDS virus has AIDS," Tshe said.

"That may be true at the moment, but, let's face it, people who carry the virus develop the disease."

"All right, but I thought insurance companies were supposed to spread the risk around."

1. Why does Gifford believe a blood test for the HIV virus should not be part of an insurance application?

2. Why do Hunter and Angoff believe it is a mistake not to allow insurance companies to test for the AIDS virus?

3. Explain the conflict between Tshe and Stipps on the matter of having an insurance company take the financial risk of paying the medical costs of someone with the AIDS virus.

4. How do Hunter and Angoff answer the charge of Gifford and Tshe that, by its very nature, insurance is supposed to spread the risk of financial loss?

Decision Scenario 5 •

"So far as I'm concerned, if I want to drink frog's eyes boiled in bat's blood, that's my prerogative," Mike Bruder said.

"Maybe so," Dr. Malley told him." But I can't prescribe Compound Q for you. The drug is classified as investigational, and the only way to get it is to be part of a controlled clinical trial."

"But then you may not get it anyway," Bruder said. "You might be in a group that gets fake medicine or some other drug." He shook his head. "I've heard that Compound Q has really helped some people, and I want to try it. Isn't it bad enough to have AIDS, without some bureaucracy denying you access to the drugs you want?"

"I can see why you feel that way," Dr. Malley said. "But we have to consider everyone with your

disease, not just now but those in the future as well."

1. Should people with fatal diseases be legally permitted to take any drug they think might be helpful to them?

2. Does Freedman believe that a patient has a right to any drug he wishes to take? If a patient is denied access to a drug he wishes, has his right to medical care been violated?

3. If allowing Bruder the drug he wants will interfere with a clinical trial of the drug, according to Freedman, should the clinical trial or the patient's wishes take precedence?

4. How might a utilitarian formulate a policy to deal with situations like the one depicted here?

5. *Could a Kantian justify denying Bruder access to Compound Q?*

6. *How might Freedman's Authorized Investigational Units deal with the problem represented here?*

Decision Scenario 6 •

In 1986 the Texas Department of Public Health supported legislation empowering it to quarantine individuals with AIDS whom it considered to be a threat to the health of the public. Those supporting the bill pointed to the case of a Houston man with AIDS who continued to work as a prostitute after being diagnosed and informed that he could infect others by sexual contact. Public health officials were powerless to take any steps against him.

Critics objected, maintaining that the legislation would make it possible for the health department to deprive a person with AIDS of his freedom of movement and action, even though he had committed no crime and never been tried for one. Further, the rare case of someone with AIDS acting irresponsibly would not be adequate to justify handing over such power to a health department.

After hearings, the bill was dropped.

1. *To what extent does such legislation appear to be a reflection of "homophobia," and to what extent does it represent a legitimate response to a genuine problem?*

2. *If quarantine controls can be justified in the case of other infectious diseases (tuberculosis, for example), is there any reason why AIDS should be viewed any differently?*

3. *According to Steinbock, should the male prostitute described above be considered guilty of some crime?*

Decision Scenario 7 •

Archbishop Roger Mahony sent a letter in February 1990 to the 3,500 nuns and priests in the Archdiocese of Los Angeles. The archbishop explained that he was seeking ten volunteers, aged sixty-five or older, to serve as subjects in the test of an experimental AIDS vaccine. The volunteers did not have to be priests or nuns, although they were the recipients of the letter. The vaccine to be tested was one developed by Jonas Salk.

In a letter accompanying the archbishop's letter, Salk's associate B. E. Henderson said that the research group was "looking for individuals who would find a role as such a volunteer a meaningful part of their life."

Some scientists expressed doubts about the safety of the vaccine, because it is made with the whole AIDS virus.

1. *Is it likely that nuns and priests sixty-five or older will gain any direct benefit from participating in the vaccine trial? If not, is it morally legitimate to ask them to participate?*

2. *The letter is from an archbishop to nuns and priests under his control asking for volunteers in an experimental investigation that may have a lethal outcome for participants. Does the archbishop's position of power make the free consent of nuns and priests impossible?*

Decision Scenario 8 •

John Johnson, as we will call him, was offered a job as a pharmacist in the Westchester County Medical Center. While taking a preemployment physical, a nurse recognized him as having taken an HIV test. She told the examining physician, who checked Johnson's confidential records and learned that the test was positive. The physician expressed concern that if Johnson worked in the pharmacy, he might accidentally prick himself and contaminate IV medications with his blood.

The directors of the medical center later announced that, for "medical reasons" that were "compelling," they were not hiring Johnson. They expressed the view that he posed "an unnecessary and unacceptable risk" to patients. Johnson filed a claim with a New York state agency alleging that he had been discriminated against in hiring because he was HIV positive.

1. *Would Mohr consider it appropriate to appeal to the harm principle in this case?*

2. *According to Steinbock, should the government enforce antidiscrimination rules and protect Johnson?*

3. *Should those diagnosed as HIV positive be forbidden by law from holding jobs that put other people at any degree of risk?*

CHAPTER 5

PHYSICIANS, PATIENTS, AND OTHERS ⬜

SOCIAL CONTEXT:
DOES A PREGNANT WOMAN
HAVE AN OBLIGATION TO
PROTECT THE FETUS?

Pamela Rae Stewart Monson was a twenty-seven-year-old mother of two, living in San Diego, California. In 1985 she became pregnant again, but things did not go well. Toward the end of her term, she began to experience vaginal bleeding. The cause was diagnosed as placenta previa, and her physician advised her to stay off her feet as much as possible and to get immediate medical treatment if she began to bleed again. She was also told not to engage in sexual intercourse and not to use amphetamines.

Monson disregarded virtually all these instructions. On November 23, 1985, she began to bleed, but instead of seeking medical treatment she stayed home, took amphetamines, and had sex with her husband. Later that day, she began to have contractions, and several hours after they began, she finally went to a hospital. She gave birth that evening to a boy who suffered from massive brain damage. He lived for six weeks.

Although the San Diego police wanted Monson prosecuted for homicide, the district attorney charged her with a misdemeanor under a child-support statute. Under the law, a parent must provide "medical attendance" to a child who requires it. However, the judge threw out the case, on the ground that an appeals Court had already ruled that a conceived but unborn child is not to be considered a person within the intended scope of the child-abuse law.

Despite the legal outcome, the Monson case received much national publicity. The case suggested to prosecutors in various states and cities that they might use the law to punish pregnant women for acting in ways that cause harm to the fetuses they are carrying. For example:

- In May 1989 a woman in Rockford, Illinois, who used cocaine during her pregnancy and just a few hours before giving birth, was found guilty in a juvenile court of prenatal child abuse and neglect. The woman was not punished, but a hearing was held to determine whether the state should take custody of the child.

- In the same city during the same month, twenty-four-year-old Melanie Green was charged with involuntary manslaughter in the death of her child Bianca. The child died on February 4, and an autopsy showed the cause of death to be oxygen starvation due to the use of cocaine late in pregnancy.

- In Laramie, Wyoming, in February 1990, Diane Pfannensteil, twenty-nine years old, was charged with felony child abuse because she drank alcohol while pregnant. A blood test had earlier determined that Pfannensteil was legally intoxicated, and a judge had ordered her to remain alcohol-free to protect the fetus. The charge against her was dismissed by a judge who ruled that, according to the law, "the child already has to have suffered," and it might be years before it could be determined whether Pfannensteil's child was damaged.

- In May 1990 a New York State appeals court ruled that the presence of cocaine in the blood of a newborn infant and admission of drug use by the mother were grounds enough to hold a child-neglect hearing to consider what action should be taken for the best interest of the child.

Civil liberties groups have been highly critical of the prosecutorial approach toward pregnant women taken by some cities and states. Some thirty-five cases have been brought throughout the country, but so far only one woman has been convicted and sentenced. In a Florida trial, Jennifer Johnson, twenty-three, was found guilty of delivering cocaine to her newborn through the umbilical cord and sentenced to fifteen years' probation.

The case is being appealed with the support of fourteen public health and women's groups. Even prosecutors admit that the cases they bring are on novel legal grounds, but they claim that something must be done to protect developing fetuses and newborns. "We're really not interested in arresting women and sending them to jail," the Solicitor of Charleston said in a *New York Times* interview. "We're just interested in getting them to stop using drugs before they do something horrible to their babies."

Everyone agrees the problem of infants damaged or put at risk by drug use is enormous. By some estimates, as many as 375,000 newborns a year may be affected by drug abuse by pregnant women. Alcohol is estimated to cause harm in about two of every thousand fetuses.

Babies whose mothers use cocaine or crack cocaine during pregnancy face severe risks. Because the drug triggers spasms in the fetus's blood vessels, oxygen and nutrients can be severely restricted for long periods. Prenatal strokes and seizures may occur, and malformations of the kidneys, genitals, intestines, and spinal cord may develop. "Crack babies" are often premature and suffer from a high incidence of irreversible brain damage.

Pregnant women who consume alcohol put their developing fetuses at risk for the same kind of damage. Fetal alcohol syndrome includes growth retardation before and after birth, facial malformations, such abnormal organ development as heart and urinary-tract defects and underdeveloped genitals, and various degrees of brain damage. Alcohol use is believed to be one of the leading causes of retardation. The damage done by alcohol seems permanent, so that even excellent postnatal nutrition and compassionate care cannot alter the growth retardation or the brain damage.

At least one study shows a racial bias in the prosecution of pregnant woman addicted to illegal drugs. In Florida all drug use during pregnancy must be reported to health departments and pregnant women using illegal drugs prosecuted. A study of urine collected during a one-month period in public health clinics and obstetricians' offices showed a 15% incidence of drug use by both blacks and whites. However, blacks were ten times more likely to be prosecuted than whites, and poor women were more likely than middle-class women.

Although the incidence of illegal drug use is about the same for black and white women, the frequency of cocaine use is much higher among black women. White women use marijuana more frequently, and, although it is associated with fetal harm, the harm is much less than that caused by cocaine.

Cases against pregnant women are usually based on the notion that the fetus has legally recognizable interests apart from the woman. However, the pregnant woman is also acknowledged to have a legally recognizable right to seek an abortion. The basic idea is that, if a woman decides not to have an abortion, then she acquires a duty to protect the fetus.

This position faces a number of problems. First, the legal basis is at best murky. Most courts do not consider a fetus a child, so child-abuse laws do not apply in any obvious way. Similarly, the notion of "delivering" drugs by maternal-fetal circulation is an apparently significant departure from the notion of delivering that lies behind antidrug legislation.

Second, the notion of what might count as "fetal abuse" is unclear and elastic. Should a pregnant woman who has two drinks be considered as endangering the fetus? Since there is no safe level of alcohol consumption, the answer might be yes. But what about making sure she eats a proper diet to nourish the developing fetus? Should the woman be charged with a crime if she fails to provide whatever the medical profession believes to be proper prenatal care? Should she be prosecuted even though she cannot afford to provide the right care?

Third, what about the interests of the pregnant woman herself? Does becoming pregnant and not having an abortion commit her to subordinating her own welfare to that of the fetus? Does she have an obligation to avoid using drugs and alcohol, even though no one else—woman or man—may have such an obligation?

Does she have an obligation to avoid engaging in any activities likely to cause a miscarriage?

In general, does the pregnant woman have a duty to live in such a way that, whenever there is a conflict of interest between what she wishes to do and what others consider the best interest of the fetus, the conflict must be resolved in favor of the fetus?

The epidemic of crack cocaine use has been accompanied by an epidemic of crack-damaged children. In 1984 about 5% of the newborns at Oakland's Highland Hospital showed the effects of the drug, but by 1988 the number was close to 20%. The prospect of a continuing generation of children damaged by a preventable cause is appalling. No one believes that the punishment of pregnant women is a solution. It is more an act of frustration and desperation.

But what is the solution?

CASE PRESENTATION
The Death of Robyn Twitchell

On April 3, 1986, two-year-old Robyn Twitchell ate very little for dinner. Then, shortly after eating, he began to cry. The crying was then replaced by vomiting and screaming.

Robyn lived in Boston, the city where the Christian Science religion was founded, and both his parents, David and Ginger Twitchell, were devout Christian Scientists. The tenets of the religion hold that disease has no physical being or reality but, rather, is the absence of being. Because God is complete being, disease is an indication of the absence of God, of being away from God. Healing must be mental and spiritual, for it consists in bringing someone back to God, of breaking down the fears, misperceptions, and disordered thinking that keep someone from having the proper relationship with God. When someone is ill, the person may need help getting to the root cause of the estrangement from God. The role of a Christian Science practitioner is to employ teaching, discussion, and prayer to assist someone suffering from an illness to discover its spiritual source.

Acting on the basis of their beliefs, the Twitchells called in Nancy Calkins, a Christian Science practitioner, to help Robyn. She prayed for Robyn and sang hymns, and, although she visited him three times during the next five days, he showed no signs of getting better. A Christian Scientist nurse was brought in to help feed and bathe Robyn, and on her chart she described him as "listless at times, rejecting all food, and moaning in pain" and as "vomiting." On April 8, Robyn began to have spasms, and his eyes rolled up into his head. He finally lost consciousness, and that evening he died.

Robyn was found to have died of a bowel obstruction that could have been treated by medicine and surgery. Medical experts were sure that he wouldn't have died had his parents sought medical attention for him.

David and Ginger Twitchell were charged with involuntary manslaughter. In a trial lasting two months, the prosecution and defense both claimed rights had been violated. The Twitchells' attorneys appealed, in particular, to the First Amendment guarantee of the free exercise of religion and claimed that the state was attempting to deny it to them.

Prosecutors responded by pointing out that courts have repeatedly held that not all religious practices are protected. For example, laws against polygamy, as well as laws requiring vaccinations or blood transfusions for minors, have all been held to be constitutional.

The prosecutors also claimed that Robyn's rights had been violated by his parents' failure to seek care for him as required by law. In addition, they cited the 1923 Supreme Court ruling in *Prince v. Massachusetts* that held that "Parents may be free to become martyrs of themselves, but it does not follow they are free to make martyrs of their children."

The jury found the Twitchells guilty of the charge, and the judge handed down a sentence of ten years' probation. John Kiernan, the prosecutor, did not recommend a jail sentence but asked for "a lengthy period" of probation. "The intent of our recommendation was to protect the other Twitchell children." Judge Sandra Hamlin instructed the Twitchells that they must seek medical care for their three children, if they showed signs of needing it, and they must take the children to a physician for regular checkups.

"This has been a prosecution against our faith," David Twitchell said. Although, speaking of Robyn, at one point he also said most sadly, "If medicine could have saved him, I wish I had turned to it."

The prosecutor called the decision "a victory for children." However, Stephen Lyons, one of the defense attorneys, said it was wrong to "substitute the imperfect and flawed judgment of medicine for the judgment of a parent." Along the same lines, a spokesman for the Christian Science church said it was not possible to combine spiritual and medical healing as the ruling required. "They're trying to prosecute out of existence this method of treatment," he said. "You cannot untangle spiritual healing from Christian Science."

During the last two years a number of children have died because religious beliefs kept their parents from getting them necessary medical care. Christian Science parents have been convicted of involuntary manslaughter, felony child abuse, or child endangerment in two California cities, as well as in Arizona and Florida. Charges have been brought, but dismissed, in Santa Monica, California, and Minneapolis.

The Twitchell case is one of several successful prosecutions, although it is considered to be nationally important. The case directly challenged the First Church of Christ Scientist (the proper name of the church) in the city where it was founded and has its headquarters, and the church recognized the challenge and helped in providing leading attorneys to defend the case. "The message has been sent," John Kiernan is quoted as saying after the Twitchells were sentenced. "Every parent of whatever religious belief or persuasion is obligated to include medical care in taking care of his child."

The Twitchells' attorneys immediately announced that they would appeal the decision on the grounds that the ruling rests on the judge's misinterpretation of a Massachusetts child-neglect law. The statute explicitly creates a legal exemption for those who believe in spiritual healing. Because of this exemption, legal authorities consider it likely that the Twitchell decision will be overturned on appeal.

A spiritual-healing exemption is found in similar laws in forty-four states. Such exclusions make it difficult to successfully prosecute Christian Scientists on the grounds of child neglect or abuse. The American Academy of Pediatrics is one group that has campaigned to eliminate spiritual-healing exceptions from child-protection laws, but so far only South Dakota has actually changed its laws.

Despite legal exemptions, parents belonging to religious groups like the Church of the First Born, Faith Assembly, and True Followers of Christ have been convicted and imprisoned for failing to provide their children with medical care. However, so far no Christian Scientist has gone to jail. When a Christian Scientist has been convicted, the sentence has been suspended or has involved probation or community service and the promise to seek medical care for their children in the future.

In the view of some critics, Christian Scientists have been treated more leniently than members of more fundamentalist groups, because a high proportion of church members are middle to upper-middle class and occupy influential positions in business, government, and the law. It has also been suggested that the legal exceptions for spiritual healing in child-protection laws are there because of the social and lobbying power of the Christian Science church and its members.

Some legal observers think that, if the Twitchell conviction is overturned, this will spur wider and more intense efforts to eliminate the spiritual-healing exception. Groups representing the rights of children believe such a change is long overdue.

"We're interested not just in the kids who die," said Norman Fost, former head of the bioethics committee of the American Academy of Pediatrics. "What we're concerned about are the hundreds and hundreds more who suffer from inadequate medical treatment."

CASE PRESENTATION

Juan Gonzalez and the Prediction of Dangerousness

In July of 1986, while the Staten Island ferry was making its run across New York harbor, Juan Gonzalez unsheathed a two-foot souvenir sword and began slashing and stabbing the people around him. Shouting incoherently, Gonzalez continued his attack until Edward del Pino, a retired police officer, fired a shot into the air and ordered Gonzalez to drop to the deck. By that time, two people were dead and nine others were wounded.

"The Father, the Son, and the Holy Spirit made me do it," Mr. Gonzalez told the police as he was charged with murder and assault. He was later taken to a hospital for a psychiatric evaluation. Only a few days before, Gonzalez had undergone another evaluation. Police had taken him into custody after he had been reported wandering the streets and making threats like "I'm going to kill! God told me so." At Presbyterian Hospital, psychiatrists had diagnosed his illness as a psychotic paranoid disorder and released him after two days.

After events aboard the ferry, the question asked by the mayor, physicians, and ordinary citizens was, Why was such an obviously dangerous person released? A brief investigation showed that Mr. Gonzalez had responded well to treatment, that no hospital space was available, and that he had been given antipsychotic drugs to take. He had also agreed to report as an outpatient, although he never did.

The Gonzalez case raised in combination two issues that have been the subjects of dispute in recent years—the right of the state to restrict the liberties of mentally ill individuals and the ability of psychiatry to predict dangerous behavior.

For almost thirty years, in response to court decisions, states have moved away from forcibly confining the mentally ill. More effective drugs to control psychoses and the movement to protect the civil rights of the mentally ill are two major factors responsible for this change in legal and social policies. In most states, the grounds for involuntary civil commitment and psychiatric treatment require that an individual be shown to be dangerous to himself or to others or to suffer from a condition that renders him mentally disabled. After a period of time, typically amounting to only a few days, a court hearing is then required to determine whether commitment and treatment may legitimately continue.

Some critics are of the opinion that the movement to keep the majority of mentally ill people out of institutions has gone too far. By some estimates, more than 30% of the homeless people on the streets of larger cities suffer from some kind of psychiatric illness that would warrant their being confined to an institution. The liberty of these people has been protected only by imposing on them a burden of responsibility they are unable to bear.

Furthermore, critics charge, a new standard of involuntary commitment and treatment is needed to prevent incidents like the one on the Staten Island ferry. Those who are judged to pose a *potential*, as well as an immediate, threat to others should be institutionalized and treated. The safety of the public demands no less.

However, the difficulty with adopting such a standard is that it is not possible to make reliable predictions about the dangerousness of an individual. This is a matter on which psychiatric experts are in general agreement. John Monahan, the author of *Predicting Violent Behavior*, points out that "No psychological test has any proven ability, not even the crudest accuracy, in forecasting violence." Furthermore, there is no apparent connection between a particular psychiatric diagnosis and violent behavior. For example, schizophrenics as a group are no more likely to be violent than are other people. Violence is associated with a wide range of both chronic and acute mental problems.

Whether an individual has been violent in the past is something of an indicator of how he is likely to behave in the future. But unless the individual is able to reveal this information and chooses to do so, it is often not known to the psychiatrist who is called upon to make an evaluation. Also, an individual who has "command hallucinations," voices that command him to act in certain ways, may be presumed to be more inclined to violence than others, if the hallucinations have a violent content. (It was the manifestation of command hallucinations that led Mr. Gonzalez to be taken to Presbyterian Hospital for his first psychiatric evaluation.) However, not all who have such hallucinations will admit to them, and a psychiatrist may have little or no objective reason to believe that such a patient may be dangerous.

The dilemma facing the psychiatrist is neatly summed up by Samuel Perry of the Payne-Whitney Clinic. "The decision to hold someone because he is dangerous is psychiatry's Scylla and Charybdis. On one hand, if you hold a patient against his will and there is no good medical reason, you are violating his civil rights. On the other hand, if you fail to keep someone who is disturbed and dangerous, and he harms someone, the victim can sue you for negligence."

INTRODUCTION

Consider the following cases:

1. A state decides to require that all behavioral therapists (that is, all who make use of psychological conditioning techniques to alter behavior patterns) be either licensed psychologists or psychiatrists.

2. A member of the Jehovah's Witnesses religion, which is opposed to the transfusion of blood and blood products, refuses to consent to a needed appendectomy. But when his appendix ruptures and he lapses into unconsciousness, the surgical resident operates and saves his life.

3. A physician decides not to tell the parents of an infant who died shortly after birth that the cause of death was an un-

predictable birth defect, because he does not wish to influence their desire to have a child.

4. A janitor employed in an elementary school consults a psychiatrist retained by the school board and tells her that he has on two occasions molested young children; the psychiatrist decides that it is her duty to inform the school board.

5. A six-year-old girl develops a high fever accompanied by violent vomiting and convulsions while at school. The child is rushed to a nearby hospital. The attending physician makes a diagnosis of meningitis and telephones the parents for permission to initiate treatment. Both parents are Christian Scientists, and they insist that no medical treatment be given to her. The physician initiates treatment anyway, and the parents later sue the physician and the hospital.

6. A thirty-year-old woman who is twenty-four weeks' pregnant is involved in an automobile accident that leaves her with a spinal cord injury. Her physician tells her that she would have had a greater chance of recovery had she not been pregnant. She then requests an abortion. The hospital disagrees with her decision and gets a court order forbidding the abortion.

There is perhaps no single moral issue that is present in all these cases. Rather, there is a complex of related issues. Each case involves acting on the behalf of someone else—another individual, the public at large, or a special group. And each action comes into conflict with the autonomy, wishes, or expectations of some person or persons. Even though the issues are related, it is most fruitful to discuss them under separate headings. We will begin with a brief account of autonomy, then turn to a discussion of paternalism and imposed restrictions on autonomy.

AUTONOMY

We are said to act autonomously when our actions are the outcome of our deliberations and choices. To be autonomous is to be self-determining. Hence, autonomy is violated when we are coerced to act by actual force or by explicit and implicit threats or when we act under misapprehension or under the influence of factors that impair our judgment.

We associate autonomy with the status we ascribe to rational agents as persons in the moral sense. Moral theories are committed to the idea that persons are by their nature uniquely qualified to decide what is in their own best interest. This is because they are ends in themselves, not means to some other end. As such, persons have inherent worth, rather than instrumental worth. Others have a duty to recognize this worth and to avoid treating persons as though they were only instruments to be employed to achieve a goal chosen by someone else. To treat someone as if she lacks autonomy is thus to treat her as less than a person.

All the cases above may be viewed as involving violations of the autonomy of the individuals concerned. Consider: (1) laws requiring a license to provide therapy restrict the actions of individuals who do not qualify for a license; (2) the Jehovah's Witness is given blood he does not want; (3) information crucial to decision making is withheld from the parents of the child with the genetic disease, so their future decision cannot be a properly informed one; (4) by breaking confidentiality, the psychiatrist is usurping the prerogative of the janitor to keep secret information that may harm him; (5) by treating the girl with meningitis, the physician is violating the generally recognized right of parents to make decisions concerning their child's welfare; (6) by refusing the woman's request for an abortion, the hospital and the court are forcing her to remain pregnant against her will.

The high value we place on autonomy is based on the realization that without it we can make very little of our lives. In its absence, we become the creatures of others, and our lives assume the forms they choose for us. Without being able to act in ways to shape our own destiny by pursuing our aims and making our own decisions, we are not realizing the potential we have as rational agents. Autonomy permits us the opportunity to make ourselves; even if we are dissatisfied with the result, we have the satisfaction of knowing that the mistakes were our own. We at least acted as rational agents.

One of the traditional problems of social organization is to structure society in such a way that the autonomy of individuals will be preserved and promoted. However, autonomy is not an absolute or unconditional value, but just one among others. For example, few would wish to live in a society in which you could do what you wanted only if you had enough physical power to get your way. Because one person's exercise of autonomy is likely to come into conflict with another's, we are willing to accept some restrictions to preserve as much of our own freedom as possible. We value our own safety, the opportunity to carry out our plans in peace, the lives of other rational beings, and perhaps even their welfare.

Because autonomy is so basic to us, we usually view it as not requiring any justification. However, this predisposition in favor of autonomy means that to violate someone's autonomy, to set aside that person's wishes and render impotent her power of action, requires that we offer a strong justification. Various principles have been proposed to justify conditions under which we are warranted in restricting autonomy.

The one most relevant in discussing the relationships among physicians, patients, and society is the principle of paternalism. The connection of paternalism with the physician-patient relationship and with truth telling and confidentiality in the medical and social context will be discussed in the following section. (For a fuller account of autonomy, as well as the principles invoked to justify restricting its exercise, see Chapter 1. The harm principle is of particular relevance to the topics presented here.)

PATERNALISM

Exactly what paternalism is, is itself a matter of dispute. Roughly speaking, we can say that paternalism consists in acting in a way that is believed to protect or advance the interest of a person, although acting in this way goes against the person's own immediate desires or limits the person's freedom of choice. Oversimplifying, paternalism is the view that "Father knows best." (The word "parentalism" is now often preferred to "paternalism," because of the latter's gender association. See Chapter 1 for the distinction between the weak and strong versions of the principle of paternalism.) Thus, the first three cases presented above are instances of paternalistic behavior.

It is useful to distinguish what we can call "state paternalism" from "personal paternalism." State paternalism, as the name suggests, is the control exerted by a legislature, agency, or other governmental body over particular kinds of practices or procedures. Such control is typically exercised through laws, licensing requirements, technical specifications, and operational guidelines and regulations. (The first case above is an example of state paternalism.)

By contrast, personal paternalism consists in an individual's deciding, on the basis of his own principles or values, that he knows what is best for another person. The individual then acts in a way that deprives the other person of genuine and effective choice. (Cases two and three are examples of this.) Paternalism is personal when it is not a matter of public or semipublic policy but is a result of private, moral decision making.

The line between public and private paternalism is often blurred. For example, suppose a physician on the staff of a hospital believes a pregnant patient should have surgery to improve the chances for the normal development of the fetus. The physician presents his view to the hospital's attorney, and, agreeing with him, the attorney goes to court to request a court order for the surgery. The judge is persuaded and issues the order. Although the order is based on arguments that certain laws are applicable in the case, the order itself is neither a personal decision nor a matter of public policy. The order reflects the judgment of a physician who has succeeded in getting others to agree.

Despite the sometimes blurred distinction between state and personal paternalism, the distinction is useful. Most important, it permits us to separate issues associated with decisions about public policies affecting classes of individuals (for example, people needing medication) from issues associated with decisions by particular people affecting specific individuals (for example, a Dr. Latvia explaining treatment options to a Mr. Zonda).

State Paternalism in Medical and Health Care

At first sight, state paternalism seems wholly unobjectionable in the medical context. We are all certain to feel more confident in consulting a physician when we know that she or he has had to meet the standards for education, competence, and character set by a state licensing board and medical society. We feel relatively sure that we aren't putting ourselves in the hands of an incompetent quack.

Indeed, that we can feel such assurance can be regarded as one of the marks of the social advancement of medicine. As late as the early twentieth century in the United States, the standards for physicians were low, and licensing laws were either nonexistent or poorly enforced. It was possible to qualify as a physician with as little as four months' formal schooling and a two-year apprenticeship.

Rigorous standards and strictly enforced laws have undoubtedly done much to improve medical care in this country. At the very least, they have made it less dangerous to consult a physician. At the same time, however, they have also placed close restrictions on individual freedom of choice. In the nineteenth century, a person could choose among a wide variety of medical viewpoints. That is no longer so today.

We now recognize that some medical viewpoints are simply wrong and, if implemented, may endanger a patient. At the least, people treated by those who espouse such views run the risk of not getting the best kind of medical care available. Unlike people in the nineteenth century, we are confident that we know (within limits) what kinds of medical therapies are effective and what kinds are useless or harmful. The scientific character of contemporary medicine gives us this assurance.

Secure in these beliefs, our society generally endorses paternalism by the state in the regulation of medical practice. We believe it is important to protect sick people from quacks and charlatans, from those who raise false hopes and take advantage of human suffering. We generally accept, then, that the range of choice of health therapy ought to be limited to what we consider to be legitimate and scientific.

This point of view is not one that everyone is pleased to endorse. In particular, those seeking treatment for cancer or for AIDS have sometimes wanted to try drugs rumored to be effective but not approved by the Food and Drug Administration. Such drugs cannot be legally prescribed in the United States, and those wishing to gain access to them must travel to foreign clinics, often at considerable discomfort and expense. (See the Social Context in Chapter 4 for additional discussion of the situation.) Some have claimed that FDA regulations make it impossible for them to choose the therapy they wish and that this is an unwarranted restriction of their rights. It should be enough, they claim, for the government to issue a warning if it thinks one is called for. But after that, people should be free to act as they choose.

The debate about unapproved therapies raises a more general question: To what extent is it legitimate for a government to restrict the actions and choices of its citizens for their own good? It is perhaps not possible to give a wholly satisfactory general answer to this question. People don't object that they are not permitted to drink polluted water from the city water supply or that they are not able to buy candy bars contaminated with insect parts. Yet some do object if they have to drink water that contains fluorides or if they cannot buy candy bars that contain saccharine. But all such limitations result from governmental attempts to protect the health of citizens.

Seeing to the well-being of its citizens certainly must be recognized as one of the legitimate aims of a government. And this aim may easily include seeing to their physical health. State paternalism with respect to health seems, in general, to be justifiable. Yet the laws and regulations through which the paternal concern is expressed are certain to come into conflict with the exercise of individual liberties. Perhaps the only way in which conflicts can be resolved is on an issue-by-issue basis. Later, we will discuss some of the limitations that moral theories place on state paternalism.

It is worth noticing that state paternalism in medical and health-care matters may be more pervasive than it seems at first sight. Laws regulating medical practice, the licensing of physicians and medical personnel, regulations governing the licensing and testing of drugs, and guidelines that must be followed in scientific research are some of the more obvious expressions of paternalism. Less obvious is the fact that government research funds can be expended only in prescribed ways and that only certain approved forms of medical care and therapy will be paid for under government-sponsored health programs. For example, it was a political and social triumph for chiropractors and Christian Science Readers when some of their services were included under Medicare coverage. Thus, government money, as well as laws and regulations, can be used in paternalistic ways.

Personal Paternalism in Medical and Health Care

That patients occupy a dependent role with respect to their physicians seems to be true historically, sociologically, and psychologically. The patient is sick, the physician is well. The patient is in need of the knowledge and skills the physician possesses, but the physician does not need those possessed by the patient. The patient seeks out the physician to ask for help, but the physician does not seek out the patient. The patient is a single individual, while the physician represents the institution of medicine with its hospitals, nurses, technicians, consultants, and so on.

In his dependence on the physician, the patient willingly surrenders some of his autonomy. Explicitly or implicitly, he agrees to allow the physician to make certain decisions for him that he would ordinarily make for himself. The physician tells him what to eat and drink and what to avoid, what medicine he should take and when to take it, how much exercise he should get and what kind it should be. The patient consents to run at least part of his life by "doctor's orders" in the hope that he will regain his health or at least improve his condition.

The physician acquires a great amount of power in this relationship. But she also acquires a great responsibility. It has been recognized at least since the time of Hippocrates that the physician has an obligation to act in the best interest of the patient. The patient is willing to transfer part of his autonomy because he is confident that the physician will act in this way.

If this analysis of the present form of the physician-patient relationship is roughly correct, two questions are appropriate.

First, should the relationship be one in which the patient is so dependent on the paternalism of the physician? Perhaps it would be better if patients did not think of themselves as transferring *any* of their autonomy to physicians. Physicians might better be thought of as people offering advice, rather than as ones issuing orders. Thus, patients, free to accept or reject advice, would retain fully their power to govern their own lives. If this is a desirable goal, it is clear that the present nature of the physician-patient relationship needs to be drastically altered.

The problem with this point of view is that the patient is ordinarily not in a position to judge the advice that is offered. The reason for consulting a physician in the first place is to gain the advantage of her knowledge and judgment. Moreover, courses of medical therapy are often complicated ones involving many interdependent steps. A patient could not expect the best treatment if he insisted on accepting some of the steps and rejecting others. As a practical matter, a patient who expects good medical care must pretty much put himself in the hands of his physician.

For this reason, the second question is perhaps based on a more realistic assessment of the nature of medical care: How much autonomy must be given up by the patient? The power of the physician over the patient cannot be absolute. The patient cannot become the slave or creature of the physician—this is not what a patient consents to when he agrees to place himself under the care of a physician. What, then, are the limits of the paternalism that can be legitimately exercised by the physician?

TRUTH TELLING IN MEDICINE

This question arises most forcefully when physicians deceive patients. When, if ever, is it justifiable for a physician to deceive her or his patient?

The paternalistic answer, of course, is that deception by the physician is justified when it is in the best interest of the patient. Suppose, for example, that a transplant surgeon detects signs of tissue rejection in a patient who has just received a donor kidney. The surgeon is virtually certain that within a week the kidney will have to be surgically removed and the patient transferred to dialysis equipment again. Although in no immediate clinical danger, the patient is suffering from postoperative depression. It is altogether possible that, if the patient is told at this time that the transplant appears to be a failure, his depression will become more severe. This, in turn, might lead to a worsening of the patient's physical condition, perhaps even to a life-threatening extent.

Eventually the patient will have to be told of the need for another operation. But by the time that need arises, his psychological condition may have improved. Is the surgeon justified in avoiding giving a direct and honest answer to the patient when he asks about his condition? In the surgeon's assessment of the situation, the answer is likely to do the patient harm. His duty as a physician, then, seems to require that he deceive the patient, either by lying to him (an act of commission) or by allowing him to believe (an act of omission) that his condition is satisfactory and the transplant was successful.

Yet doesn't the patient have a right to know the truth from his physician? After all, it is his life that is being threatened. Should he not be told how things stand with him so that he will be in a position to make decisions that affect his own future? Is the surgeon not exceeding the bounds of the powers granted to him by the patient? The patient surely had no intention of completely turning over his autonomy to the surgeon.

This issue is one of "truth telling." Does the physician always owe it to the patient to tell the truth? Some writers make a distinction between lying to the patient and merely being nonresponsive or evasive. But is this really a morally relevant distinction? In either case, the truth is being kept from the patient. Both are instances of medical paternalism.

The use of placebos (from the Latin *placebo*, meaning "I shall please") in medical therapy is another issue that raises questions about the legitimate limits of paternalism in medicine. The "placebo effect" is a well-documented psychological phenomenon: even patients who are seriously ill will sometimes show improvement when they are given *any* kind of medication (a sugar pill, for example) or treatment. This can happen even when the medication or treatment is irrelevant to their condition.

The placebo effect can be exploited by physicians for the (apparent) good of their patients. Many patients cannot accept a physician's well-considered judgments. When they come to a physician with a complaint and are told that there is nothing organically wrong with them, that no treatment or medication is called for, they continue to ail. They may then lose confidence in their physician or be less inclined to seek medical advice for more serious complaints.

One way to avoid these consequences is for the physician to prescribe a placebo for the patient. Since the patient (we can assume) suffers from no organic disease condition, he is not in need of any genuine medication. And because of the placebo effect, he may actually find himself relieved of the symptoms that caused him to seek medical help. Moreover, the patient feels satisfied that he has been treated, and his confidence in his physician and in medicine in general remains intact.

Since the placebo effect is not at all likely to be produced if the patient knows he is being given an ineffective medication, the physician cannot be candid about the "treatment" prescribed. She must either be silent, say something indefinite like "I think this might help your condition," or lie. Since the placebo effect is more likely to be achieved if the medication is touted as being amazingly effective against complaints like those of the patient, there is a reason for the physician to lie outright. Because the patient may stand to gain a considerable amount of good from placebo therapy, the physician may think of herself as acting in the best interest of her patient.

Despite its apparent advantages, placebo therapy may be open to two ethical criticisms. First, we can ask whether giving placebos is really in the best interest of a patient. It encourages many patients in their belief that drugs can solve their problems. Patients with vague and general complaints may need some kind of psychological counseling, and giving them placebos merely discourages them from coming to grips with their genuine problems. Also, not all placebos are harmless (see the discussion in the introduction to Chapter 6). Some contain active chemicals that produce side effects (something likely to enhance the placebo effect) so the physician who prescribes placebos may be subjecting her patient to some degree of risk.

Second by deceiving her patient, the physician is depriving him of the chance to make genuine decisions about his own life. Because the person is not genuinely sick, it does not seem legitimate to regard him as having deputized his physician to act in his behalf or as having transferred any of his power or autonomy to the physician. In Kant's terms, the physician is not acknowledging the patient's status as an autonomous rational agent. She is not according him the dignity that he possesses simply by virtue of being human. (A utilitarian who wished to claim that telling the truth to patients is a policy that will produce the best overall benefits could offer essentially the same criticism.)

Deception is not the only issue raised by the general question of the legitimacy of medical paternalism. Another of some importance is difficult to state precisely, but it has to do with the general attitude of physicians toward their patients. Patients often feel that physicians deal with them in a way that is literally paternalistic—that physicians treat them like children.

The physician, like the magician or shaman, is often seen as a figure of power and mystery, one who controls the forces of nature and, by doing so, relieves suffering and restores health. Some physicians like this role and act in accordance with it. They resent having their authority questioned and fail to treat their patients with dignity and respect.

For example, many physicians call their patients by their first names while expecting patients to refer to them as "Dr. X." In our society, women in particular have been most critical of such condescending attitudes displayed by physicians.

More serious is the fact that many physicians do not make a genuine effort to educate patients about the state of their health, the significance of laboratory findings, or the reasons why medication or other therapy is being prescribed. Patients are not only expected to follow orders, but they are expected to do so blindly.

The issue here is not one of informed consent (which we will discuss in detail in the next chapter). For in informed consent, a patient must give permission for a procedure of a special sort to be performed. Here we are talking only about the ordinary medical situation—someone consults a physician because of a shoulder pain or just to get a yearly checkup.

The amount of time that it takes to help a patient understand his medical condition and the reason for the prescribed therapy is, of course, one reason why physicians do not attempt to provide such information. A busy physician in an office practice might see thirty or forty patients a day, and it is difficult to give each of them the necessary amount of attention. Also, patients without a medical background obviously can find it hard to understand medical explanations—particularly in the ways in which they are often given.

The result, for whatever reasons, is a situation in which physicians make decisions about patients without allowing patients to know the basis for them. Explanations are not given, it is sometimes said, because patients "wouldn't understand" or "might draw the wrong conclusions about their illness" or "might worry needlessly." Patients are thus not only *not* provided information, but they are discouraged from asking questions or revealing their doubts.

The moral questions here concern the responsibility of the physician. Is it ultimately useful for patients that physicians should play the role of a distant and mysterious figure of power? If so, then it may be that physicians should cultivate the role. Do patients have a right to ask that physicians treat them with the same dignity as physicians treat one another? Should a physician attempt to educate her or his patients about their illnesses? Or is a physician's only real responsibility to provide patients with needed medical treatment?

Furthermore, is it always obvious that the physician knows what will count as the all-around best treatment for a patient? Patients, being human, have values of their own, and they may well not rank their best chance for effective medical treatment above all else. A woman with breast cancer, for example, may wish to avoid having a breast surgically removed (mastectomy) and so prefer another mode of treatment, even though her physician may consider it less effective. Can her physician legitimately withhold from her knowledge of alternative modes of treatment and so allow her no choice? Can he make the decision about treatment himself on the grounds that it is a purely medical matter, one about which the patient has no expert knowledge?

CONFIDENTIALITY

"Whatever I see or hear, professionally or privately, which ought not to be divulged, I will keep secret and tell no one," runs one of the pledges in the Hippocratic Oath.

The tradition of medical practice in the West has taken this injunction very seriously. That it has done so is not entirely due to the high moral character of physicians, for the pledge to secrecy also serves an important practical function. Physicians need to have information of an intimate and highly personal sort in order to make diagnoses and prescribe

courses of therapy. If physicians were known to reveal such personal information, then patients would be reluctant to cooperate, and the practice of medicine would be adversely affected. Furthermore, because psychological factors play a role in medical therapy, the chances of success in medical treatment are improved when patients can place trust and confidence in their physicians. This aspect of the physician-patient relationship actually forms a part of medical therapy. Of course, this is particularly so of the "talking cures" characteristic of some forms of psychiatry.

A number of states recognize the need for "privileged communication" between physician and patient and have laws to protect physicians from being compelled to testify about their patients in court. Yet physicians are also members of a society, and the society must attempt to protect the general interest. This sometimes places the physician in the middle of a conflict between the interest of the individual and the interest of society.

For example, physicians are often required by law to act in ways that force them to reveal certain information about their patients. The best instance of this is perhaps the legal obligation to report to health departments the names of those patients who are carriers of such communicable diseases as syphilis and tuberculosis. This permits health authorities to warn those with whom the carriers have come into contact and to guard against the spread of the diseases. Thus, the interest of the society is given precedence over physician-patient confidentiality.

Few people would question society's right to demand that physicians violate a patient's confidence when the issue is that of protecting the health of great numbers of people. More open to question are laws that require physicians to report gunshot wounds or other injuries that might be connected with criminal actions. (In some states, before abortion became legal, physicians were required to report cases of attempted abortion.) Furthermore, physicians as citizens have a legal duty to report any information they may have about a crime unless they are protected by a privileged-communication law.

Thus, the physician is placed in a position of conflict. If he acts to protect the patient's confidences, then he runs the risk of acting illegally. If he acts in accordance with the law, then he must violate the confidence of his patients. What needs to be decided from a moral point of view is to what extent the laws that place a physician in such a situation are justified.

The physician who is not in private practice but is employed by a government agency or a business organization also encounters similar conflicts. Her obligations run in two directions: to her patients and to her employer. Should a physician who works for a government agency tell her superiors that an employee has confided in her that he is a drug addict? If she does not, the man may be subject to blackmail or bribery. If she does, then she must violate the patient's confidence. Or what if a psychiatrist retained by a company decides that one of the employees is so psychologically disturbed that she cannot function effectively in her job? Should the psychiatrist inform the employer of this, even if it means going against the wishes of the patient? (Consider also the fourth case cited at the beginning of this Introduction.)

Even more serious problems arise in psychiatry. Suppose that a patient expresses to his psychiatrist feelings of great anger against someone and even announces that he intends to go out and kill that person. What should the psychiatrist do? Is it his obligation to warn the person being threatened? Should he report the threat to the police? This is fundamentally the issue that was dealt with by the California Supreme Court in the case of *Tarasoff* v. *Regents of the University of California*. (See the selection in this chapter by William J. Curran for a discussion.)

The basic question about confidentiality concerns the extent to which we are willing to go to protect it. It is doubtful that anyone would want to assert that confidentiality should be absolutely guaranteed. But, if not, then under what conditions is it better to violate it than to preserve it?

AUTONOMY AND THE INTERESTS OF OTHERS

Patients do not always choose to do as they are advised by their physicians. Some people refuse to take needed medications, change their diets, quit smoking, exercise more, or undergo surgical procedures that promise to improve the quality of their lives, if not lengthen them. Valuing autonomy requires recognizing that people do not always do what is good for them in a medical way, and accepting this as a consequence. Over the years, the courts have recognized repeatedly and explicitly that the right to refuse or discontinue medical treatment has a basis in the Constitution and in the common law.

Most public and legal attention on the matter of rejecting therapy has focused recently on cases in which terminally ill patients wish to have respirators disconnected or in which the guardians of patients in chronic vegetative states want their nutrition and hydration to be discontinued. The issues have concerned the rights of patients themselves, and in this respect the questions were more or less straightforward.

The matter of refusing treatment becomes more complicated when the interest of someone other than or in addition to the patient is involved. Two sorts of cases, in particular, present difficulties: cases in which parents' beliefs cause them to deny their children necessary medical attention and cases in which a pregnant woman's behaviors result in damage to her fetus.

First is the situation in which parents, acting on the basis of their beliefs, refuse to authorize needed medical treatment for their child. The duty of the physician is to provide the child the best medical care possible. The duty of the parent is to protect and promote the welfare of the child. Ordinarily, in the medical context, these two duties are convergent with respect to the line of action they lead to. The parents ask the physician to "do what is best" for their child, and the physician discusses the options and risks with the parents and secures their consent on behalf of the child. (See the discussion of informed consent in the next chapter.)

However, this convergence of duties leading to agreement about action is dependent on physicians and parents sharing some fundamental beliefs about the nature of disease and the efficacy of medical therapy in controlling it. When these beliefs are not shared, then the outcome is a divergence of opinion about what should be done in the best interest of the child. The actions favored by the physician will be incompatible with the actions favored by the parents.

As in the Case Presentation about Robyn Twitchell and example five above, some parents are adherents of religions like Christian Science that teach that disease has no reality but is a manifestation of incorrect or disordered thinking. People with such beliefs think that the appropriate response to illness is to seek spiritual healing, rather than to employ medical modalities.

What about the children of those with such beliefs? Their parents can legitimately claim that by refusing to seek or accept medical treatment for their children they are doing what they consider best. It is a recognized principle that parents should decide the best interest of their children, except in very special circumstances. We don't think, for example, that a psychotic or clinically depressed parent should be allowed to decide about a child's welfare. Should Christian Scientists and others with similar beliefs be put in the category of incompetent parents and forced to act against their beliefs and seek medical care for their children?

A strong case can be made for answering yes. If mentally competent adults wish to avoid or reject medical treatment for themselves, the principle of autonomy supports a public policy permitting this. However, when the interest of someone who lacks the abilities to deliberate and decide for himself is concerned, it is reasonable to favor a policy that will protect that person from harm. This is particularly so when matters as basic as the person's health and safety are at stake.

Hence, to warrant restricting the generally recognized right of parents to see to the welfare of their children, we can appeal to the harm principle. We might say that, if a parent's action or failure to take action tends to result in harm to a child, then we are justified in restricting his or her freedom to make decisions on behalf of the child. We could then look to someone else—a court or appointed guardian—to represent the child's best interest.

In general, we consider a legitimate function of the state to be the protection of its citizens. When parents fail to take reasonable steps to secure the welfare of their children, then doing so becomes a matter of interest to the state.

The second kind of case is one that involves an actual or potential conflict between the actions of a pregnant woman and the interest of the fetus she is carrying. This kind of case is illustrated in example six above and discussed in the Social Context section at the beginning of the chapter.

An obvious way of dealing with an alleged conflict between what a pregnant woman wants or does and the interest of her fetus is to deny that conflict is possible. If one holds that the fetus, at every developmental stage, is a part of the woman's body and that she is free to do with her body as she pleases, then there can be no conflict. The woman is simply deciding for herself, and it would be an unjustifiable violation of her autonomy to regulate her actions in ways that those of men or nonpregnant women are not regulated.

However, a number of difficulties are associated with this position. The most significant difficulty is that as a fetus continues to develop it becomes increasingly implausible to hold that it is no different from any other "part" of a woman's body. The problem of when the fetus is a person in the moral sense is one that plagues the abortion dispute (see Chapter 1), and it is no less relevant to this issue.

Furthermore, even if one is not prepared to say that the fetus can claim any serious consideration to life, particularly at the very early stages of pregnancy, it seems prima facie wrong to act as though the fetus (barring miscarriage or abortion) is not going to develop into a child. Suppose a woman knows that she is pregnant and knows that continuing to drink alcohol even moderately is likely to cause the child who will be born to suffer from birth defects. Most people would consider it wrong for her to disregard the consequences of her actions. Once she has decided against (or failed to secure) an abortion, then it seems she must accept the responsibility that goes with carrying a child to term. On even a moderate view, this would imply avoiding behavior she knows will be likely to cause birth defects.

However, another aspect of the question of whether a pregnant woman has any responsibility to protect the welfare of the fetus is to what extent, if any, we are justified in regulating the actions of a pregnant woman. Should a pregnant woman retain her autonomy intact? Or is it legitimate for us to require her, by virtue of being pregnant, to follow a set of rules or laws not applicable to other people?

Once again, the status of the fetus as a person makes such a question hard to answer. Should we regard cases of "fetal neglect" or "fetal abuse" as no different from cases of child neglect or abuse? If the answer is yes, then the pregnant woman is no different from the parent of a minor child. In the same way that the state might order a Christian Science parent to seek medical help for a sick child, we might consider ourselves justified in insisting that a pregnant woman get prenatal care and avoid drugs and alcohol. Just as parents are subject to laws and rules that other people are not, then so are pregnant women.

Assuming this answer is accepted, then the question becomes one of how far we should go in prescribing behavior for a pregnant woman. Should we require a basic minimum, or should we establish an obtainable ideal?

Even the basic questions surrounding the issue of pregnancy and responsibility remain unanswered by our society. We have yet to develop a social policy to reduce the incidence of fetal alcohol syndrome and drug-damaged babies while also protecting the autonomy of pregnant women.

ETHICAL THEORIES: PATERNALISM, TRUTH TELLING, CONFIDENTIALITY

What we have called state paternalism and personal paternalism are compatible with utilitarian ethical theory. But whether they are justifiable is a matter of controversy. If the principle of utility shows that governmental laws, policies, practices, or regulations increase the general happiness, then they are justified. It can be argued that they are justified even if they restrict the individual's freedom of choice or action because for utilitarianism such freedom has no absolute value. Personal paternalism is justified in a similar way. If a physician believes that she can protect her patient from unnecessary suffering or can relieve his pain by keeping him in ignorance, by lying to him, by giving him placebos, or by otherwise deceiving him, then these actions are morally legitimate.

However, John Stuart Mill did not take this view of paternalism. Mill argued that freedom of choice is of such importance that it can be justifiably restricted only when it can be shown that unregulated choice would cause harm to other people. Mill claimed that compelling people to act in certain ways "for their own good" is never legitimate. This position, Mill argued, is one that is justified by the principle of utility. Gerald Dworkin, in the selection included in this chapter, provides an analysis of

Mill's position, and there is no need for us to repeat it here. We should note, however, that utilitarianism does not offer a straightforward answer to the question of the legitimacy of paternalism.

What we have said about paternalism also applies more or less to the issue of confidentiality. Generally speaking, if violating confidentiality seems necessary to produce a state of affairs in which happiness is increased, then the violation is justified. This might be the case when, for example, someone's life is in danger or someone is being tried for a serious crime and the testimony of a physician is needed to help establish her innocence. Yet it also might be argued from the point of view of rule utilitarianism that confidentiality is such a basic ingredient in the physician-patient relationship that, in the long run, more good will be produced if confidentiality is never violated.

The Kantian view of paternalism, truth telling, and confidentiality is more clear-cut. Every person is a rational and autonomous agent. As such he or she is entitled to make decisions that affect his or her own life. This means that a person is entitled to receive information relevant to making such decisions and is entitled to the truth, no matter how painful it might be. The use of placebos or any other kind of deception in medicine is morally illegitimate because this would involve denying a person the respect and dignity to which he or she is entitled. The categorical imperative also rules out lying, for the maxim involved in such an action produces a contradiction. (There are special difficulties in applying the categorical imperative that we discussed in the introductory chapter. When these are taken into account, Kant's view is perhaps not quite so straightforward and definite as it first appears.)

It can be argued that Kant's principles also establish that confidentiality should be regarded as absolute. When a person becomes a patient, she does so with the expectation that what she tells her physician will be kept confidential. Thus, in the physician-patient relationship there is an implicit promise. The physician implicitly promises that he will not reveal any information about his patient, either what he has been told or what he has learned for himself. If this analysis is correct, then the physician is under an obligation to preserve confidentiality because keeping promises is an absolute duty, (Here, as in the case of lying, there are difficulties connected with the way in which a maxim is stated. See the introductory chapter for a discussion.)

Ross's principles recognize that everyone has a moral right to be treated as an autonomous agent who is entitled to make decisions affecting his own life. Also, everyone is entitled to know the truth and to be educated in helpful ways. Similarly, if confidentiality is a form of promise keeping, everyone is entitled to expect that it will be maintained. Thus, paternalism, lying, and violation of confidence are prima facie morally objectionable. But, of course, it is possible to imagine circumstances in which they would be justified. The right course of action that a physician must follow is one that can be determined only on the basis of the physician's knowledge of the patient, the patient's problem, and the general situation. Thus, Ross's principles rule out paternalism, deception, and violations of confidence as general policies, but they do not make them morally illegitimate in an absolute way.

Rawls's theory of social and political morality is compatible with state paternalism of a restricted kind. No laws, practices, or policies can legitimately violate the rights of individuals. At the same time, however, a society, viewing arrangements from the original position, might decide to institute a set of practices that would promote what they agreed to be their interests. If, for example, health is agreed to be an interest, then they might be willing to grant to the state the power to regulate a large range of matters connected with the promotion of health. Establishing standards for physicians would be an example of such regulation. But they might also go so far as to give the state power to decide (on the advice of experts) what medical treatments are legitimate, what drugs are safe and effective to use, what substances should be controlled or prohibited, and so on. So long as the principles of justice are not violated and so long as the society can be regarded as imposing these regulations on itself for the promotion of its own good, then such paternalistic practices are unobjectionable. With respect to personal paternalism, deception, and confidentiality, Rawls's general theory offers no specific answers. But since Rawls endorses Ross's account of prima facie duties (while rejecting Ross's intuitionism), it seems reasonable to believe that Rawls's view on these matters would be the same as Ross's.

The natural law doctrine of Roman Catholicism suggests that paternalism in both of its forms is legitimate. When the state is organized to bring about such "natural goods" as health, then laws and practices that promote those goods are morally right. Individuals do have a worth in themselves and should be free to direct and organize their own lives. But at the same time, individuals may be ignorant of relevant information, lack the intellectual capacities to determine what is really in their best interest, or be moved by momentary passions and circumstances. For these reasons, the state may act so that people are protected from their own shortcomings, and yet their genuine desires, their "natural ends," are satisfied.

Thus, natural law doctrine concludes that because each individual has an inherent worth, she is entitled to be told the truth in medical situations (and others) and not deceived. But it reasons too that because a physician has superior knowledge, he may often perceive the interest of the patient better than the patient herself. Accordingly, natural law doctrine indicates that, although he should avoid lying, a physician is still under an obligation to act for the best interest of his patient. This may mean allowing the patient to believe something that is not so (as in placebo therapy)

or withholding information from the patient. In order for this to be morally legitimate, however, the physician's motive must always be that of advancing the welfare of the patient.

In the matter of confidentiality, the natural law doctrine of Roman Catholicism recognizes that the relationship between physician and patient is one of trust, and a physician has a duty not to betray the confidences of her patients. But the relationship is not sacrosanct and the duty is not absolute. When the physician finds herself in a situation in which a greater wrong will be done if she does not reveal a confidence entrusted to her by a patient, then she has a duty to reveal the confidence. If, for example, the physician possesses knowledge that would save someone from death or unmerited suffering, then it is her duty to make this knowledge available, even if by doing so she violates a patient's trust.

We have been able merely to sketch an outline of possible ways in which our ethical theories might deal with the issues involved in paternalism, truth telling, and confidentiality. Some of the views presented are open to challenge, and none of them has been worked out in a completely useful way. That is one of the tasks that remains to be performed.

No ethical theory would justify, under ordinary circumstances, a pregnant woman's knowingly behaving in a way that would cause birth defects in a child she intends to carry to term. If the woman acts out of ignorance or under various psychological or social pressures, or if she would have to engage in extraordinary sacrifices, there may be reason to excuse her actions, should they result in preventable impairments.

However, it remains to be seen exactly how any moral theory can resolve the issue of to what extent, if any, a pregnant woman is responsible for a fetus she is carrying to term. Relevant to dealing with the problem is the matter of whether the woman intends to carry the fetus to term by choice, whether she has merely neglected to secure an abortion, or whether the unavailability of abortion forces her to remain pregnant. The woman's wishes and circumstances may result in our giving different answers to the basic question.

On the final matter of restricting the autonomy of adults in order to protect the health and safety of their minor children, each ethical theory considered can be interpreted as regarding such restrictions as justified. In terms of each theory, children occupy a special status that must be protected. If a parent acts in ways that cause danger to his child, then the state may legitimately restrict his action. If the parent fails in his basic duty to protect the well-being of his children, the state must assume this function. A state that fails to guarantee protection to a child is open to moral condemnation.

John Stuart Mill, in the final chapter of *On Liberty*, explicitly addresses the issue of whether the state can require parents to act to protect or promote the interest of their children. In accord with his general position that violating the harm principle is the only ground that warrants restricting individual autonomy, Mill observes that, although individuals may do as they choose to themselves, when someone exercises power over someone else the state is "bound to maintain a vigilant control" over that power. However, this is an obligation "almost entirely disregarded in family relations." People tend to treat children as though they were literally a part of themselves, and the state ordinarily does nothing to interfere with the actions of parents. But, Mill observes, such "misapplied notions of liberty are a real obstacle to the fulfillment by the state of its duties."

Education is Mill's example of a parental responsibility that must be enforced by the state. In his view, the state must see to it that families educate children, because to fail to educate a child is to deprive her of "at least the ordinary chance of a desirable existence" and so is "a crime against that being." If the family does not provide the education, then the state must assume the task.

It seems reasonable to believe that a failure to provide a child with needed health care is at least as serious a deprivation as a failure to provide a child an education. Hence, Mill's arguments in *On Liberty* can be employed to support the view that parents should be required to provide needed medical care for dependent children. If the parents fail in their duty, then the state must assume responsibility.

Autonomy, paternalism, truth telling, and confidentiality are bound together in a complicated web of moral issues. We have not identified all of the strands of the web, nor have we traced out their connections with one another. We have, however, mentioned enough difficulties to reveal the seriousness of the issues.

Some of the issues are social ones and require that we decide about the moral legitimacy of certain kinds of laws, practices, and policies. Others are matters of personal morality, ones that concern our obligations to society and to other people. Our ethical theories, we can hope, will provide us with the means of arriving at workable and justifiable resolutions of the issues. But before this point is reached, much intellectual effort and ingenuity will have to be invested.

Paternalism

Gerald Dworkin

Gerald Dworkin attempts to show that, even if we place an absolute value on individual choice, a variety of paternalistic policies can still be justified. In consenting to a system of representative government, we understand that it may act to safeguard our interests in certain ways. But, Dworkin asks, what are the "kinds of conditions which make it plausible to suppose that rational men could reach agreement to limit their liberty even when other men's interests are not affected?"

Dworkin suggests that such conditions are satisfied in cases in which there is a "good" such as health involved—one that everybody needs to pursue other goods. Rational people would agree that attaining such a good should be promoted by the government even when individuals don't recognize it as a good at a particular time. There is a sense, Dworkin argues, in which we are not really imposing such a good on people. What we are really saying is that, if everyone knew the facts and assessed them properly, this is what they would choose. Also, we are sometimes influenced by immediate alternatives that look more attractive, or we are careless or depressed and so do not act for what we acknowledge as a good. Thus, we might approve of laws such as ones against cigarette smoking because we know we should not smoke cigarettes.

It is plausible, Dworkin suggests, that rational people would grant to a legislature the right to impose such restrictions on their conduct. But the government has to demonstrate the exact nature of the harmful effects to be avoided. Also, if there is an alternative way of accomplishing the end without restricting liberty, then the society should adopt it.

Neither one person, nor any number of persons, is warranted in saying to another human creature of ripe years, that he shall not do with his life for his own benefit what he chooses to do with it. *Mill*

I do not want to go along with a volunteer basis. I think a fellow should be compelled to become better and not let him use his discretion whether he wants to get smarter, more healthy or more honest. *General Hershey*

I take as my starting point the "one very simple principle" proclaimed by Mill in *On Liberty* . . . "That principle is, that the sole end for which mankind are warranted, individually or collectively, in interfering with the liberty of action of any of their number, is self-protection. That the only purpose for which power can be rightfully exercised over any member of a civilized community, against his will, is to prevent harm to others. He cannot rightfully be compelled to do or forbear because it will be better for him to do so, because it will make him happier, because, in the opinion of others, to do so would be wise, or even right."[1]

This principle is neither "one" nor "very simple." It is at least two principles; one asserting that self-protection or the prevention of harm to others is sometimes a sufficient warrant and the other claiming that the individual's own good is *never* a sufficient warrant for the exercise of compulsion either by the society as a whole or by its individual members. I assume that no one with the possible exception of extreme pacifists or anarchists questions the correctness of the first half of the principle. This essay is an examination of the negative claim embodied in Mill's principle—the objection to paternalistic interferences with a man's liberty.

I

By paternalism I shall understand roughly the interference with a person's liberty of action justified by reasons referring exclusively to the welfare, good, happiness, needs, interests or values of the person being coerced. One is always well-advised to illustrate one's definitions by examples but it is not easy to find "pure" examples of paternalistic interferences. For almost any piece of legislation is justified by several different kinds of reasons and even if historically a piece of legislation can be shown to have been introduced for purely paternal-

Reprinted from The Monist, *LaSalle, IL, Vol. 56, no. 1, with the permission of the author and the publisher.*

istic motives, it may be that advocates of the legislation with an anti-paternalistic outlook can find sufficient reasons justifying the legislation without appealing to the reasons which were originally adduced to support it. Thus, for example, it may be that the original legislation requiring motorcyclists to wear safety helmets was introduced for purely paternalistic reasons. But the Rhode Island Supreme Court recently upheld such legislation on the grounds that it was "not persuaded that the legislature is powerless to prohibit individuals from pursuing a course of conduct which could conceivably result in their becoming public charges," thus clearly introducing reasons of a quite different kind. Now I regard this decision as being based on reasoning of a very dubious nature but it illustrates the kind of problem one has in finding examples. The following is a list of the kinds of interferences I have in mind as being paternalistic.

II

1. Laws requiring motorcyclists to wear safety helmets when operating their machines.
2. Laws forbidding persons from swimming at a public beach when lifeguards are not on duty.
3. Laws making suicide a criminal offense.
4. Laws making it illegal for women and children to work at certain types of jobs.
5. Laws regulating certain kinds of sexual conduct, e.g. homosexuality among consenting adults in private.
6. Laws regulating the use of certain drugs which may have harmful consequences to the user but do not lead to anti-social conduct.
7. Laws requiring a license to engage in certain professions with those not receiving a license subject to fine or jail sentence if they do engage in the practice.
8. Laws compelling people to spend a specified fraction of their income on the purchase of retirement annuities. (Social Security)
9. Laws forbidding various forms of gambling (often justified on the grounds that the poor are more likely to throw away their money on such activities than the rich who can afford to).
10. Laws regulating the maximum rates of interest for loans.
11. Laws against duelling.

In addition to laws which attach criminal or civil penalties to certain kinds of action there are laws, rules, regulations, decrees, which make it either difficult or impossible for people to carry out their plans and which are also justified on paternalistic grounds. Examples of this are:

1. Laws regulating the types of contracts which will be upheld as valid by the courts, e.g. (an example of Mill's to which I shall return) no man may make a valid contract for perpetual involuntary servitude.
2. Not allowing as a defense to a charge of murder or assault the consent of the victim.
3. Requiring members of certain religious sects to have compulsory blood transfusions. This is made possible by not allowing the patient to have recourse to civil suits for assault and battery and by means of injunctions.
4. Civil commitment procedures when these are specifically justified on the basis of preventing the person being committed from harming himself. (The D.C. Hospitalization of the Mentally Ill Act provides for involuntary hospitalization of a person who "is mentally ill, and because of that illness, is likely to injure *himself* or others if allowed to remain at liberty." The term injure in this context applies to unintentional as well is intentional injuries.)
5. Putting fluorides in the community water supply.

All of my examples are of existing restrictions on the liberty of individuals. Obviously one can think of interferences which have not yet been imposed. Thus one might ban the sale of cigarettes, or require that people wear safety-belts in automobiles (as opposed to merely having them installed) enforcing this by not allowing motorists to sue for injuries even when caused by other drivers if the motorist was not wearing a seat-belt at the time of the accident.

I shall not be concerned with activities which though defended on paternalistic grounds are not interferences with the liberty of persons, e.g. the giving of subsidies in kind rather than in cash on the grounds that the recipients would not spend the money on the goods which they really need, or not including a $1000 deductible provision in a basic protection automobile insurance plan on the ground that the people who would elect it could least afford it. Nor shall I be concerned with measures such as "truth-in-advertising" acts and the Pure Food and Drug legislation which are often attacked as paternalistic but which should not be considered so. In these cases all that is provided—it is true by the use of compulsion—is information which it is presumed that rational persons are interested in having in order to make wise decisions. There is no interference with the liberty of the consumer unless one wants to stretch a point beyond good sense and say that his liberty to apply for a loan without knowing the true rate of interest is diminished. It is true that sometimes there is sentiment for going further than providing information, for example when laws against usurious interest are passed preventing those who might wish to contract loans at high rates of interest from doing so, and these measures may correctly be considered paternalistic.

III

Bearing these examples in mind let me return to a characterization of paternalism. I said earlier that I meant by the term, roughly, interference with a person's liberty for his own good. But as some of the examples show the class of persons whose good is invoiced is not always identical with the class of persons whose freedom is restricted. Thus in the case of professional licensing it is the practitioner who is directly interfered with and it is the would-be patient whose interests are presumably being served. Not allowing the consent of the victim to be a defense to certain types of crime primarily affects the would-be aggressor but it is the interests of the willing victim that we are trying to protect. Sometimes a person may fall into both classes as would be the case if we banned the manufacture and sale of cigarettes and a given manufacturer happened to be a smoker as well.

Thus we may first divide paternalistic interferences into "pure" and "impure" cases. In "pure" paternalism the class of persons whose freedom is restricted is identical with the class of persons whose benefit is intended to be promoted by such restrictions. Examples: the making of suicide a crime, requiring passengers in automobiles to wear seat-belts, requiring a Christian Scientist to receive a blood transfusion. In the case of "impure" paternalism in trying to protect the welfare of a class of persons we find that the only way to do so will involve restricting the freedom of other persons besides those who are benefitted. Now it might be thought that there are no cases of "impure" paternalism since any such case could always be justified on non-paternalistic grounds, i.e. in terms of preventing harm to others. Thus we might ban cigarette manufacturers from continuing to manufacture their product on the grounds that we are preventing them from causing illness to others in the same way that we prevent other manufacturers from releasing pollutants into the atmosphere, thereby causing danger to the members of the community. The difference is, however, that in the former but not the latter case the harm is of such a nature that it could be avoided by those individuals affected if they so chose. The incurring of the harm requires, so to speak, the active co-operation of the victim. It would be mistaken theoretically and hypocritical in practice to assert that our interference in such cases is just like our interference in standard cases of protecting others from harm. At the very least someone interfered with in this way can reply that no one is complaining about his activities. It may be that impure paternalism requires arguments or reasons of a stronger kind in order to be justified since there are persons who are losing a portion of their liberty and they do not even have the solace of having it be done "in their own interest." Of course in some sense, if paternalistic justifications are ever correct then we are protecting others, we are preventing some from injuring others, but it is important to see the differences between this and the standard case.

Paternalism then will always involve limitations on the liberty of some individuals in their own interest but it may also extend to interferences with the liberty of parties whose interests are not in question.

IV

Finally, by way of some more preliminary analysis, I want to distinguish paternalistic interferences with liberty from a related type with which it is often confused. Consider, for example, legislation which forbids employees to work more than, say, 40 hours per week. It is sometimes argued that such legislation is paternalistic for if employees desired such a restriction on their hours of work they could agree among themselves to impose it voluntarily. But because they do not the society imposes its own conception of their best interests upon them by the use of coercion. Hence this is paternalism.

Now it may be that some legislation of this nature is, in fact, paternalistically motivated. I am not denying that. All I want to point out is that there is another possible way of justifying such measures which is not paternalistic in nature. It is not paternalistic because as Mill puts it in a similar context such measures are "required not to overrule the judgment of individuals respecting their own interest, but to give effect to that judgment: they being unable to give effect to it except by concert, which concert again cannot be effectual unless it receives validity and sanction from the law."[2]

The line of reasoning here is a familiar one first found in Hobbes and developed with great sophistication by contemporary economists in the last decade or so. There are restrictions which are in the interests of a class of persons taken collectively but are such that the immediate interest of each individual is furthered by his violating the rule when others adhere to it. In such cases the individuals involved may need the use of compulsion to give effect to their collective judgment of their own interest by guaranteeing each individual compliance by the others. In these cases compulsion is not used to achieve some benefit which is not recognized to be a benefit by those concerned, but rather because it is the only feasible means of achieving some benefit which *is* recognized as such by all concerned. This way of viewing matters provides us with another characterization of paternalism in general. Paternalism might be thought of as the use of coercion to achieve a good which is not recognized as such by those persons for whom the good is intended. Again while this formulation captures the heart of the matter—it is surely what Mill is objecting to in *On Liberty*—the matter is not always quite like that. For example when we force motorcyclists to wear helmets we are trying to promote a good—the protection of the person from injury—which is surely recognized by most of the individuals concerned. It is not that a cyclist doesn't value his bodily integrity; rather, as a supporter of such legislation would put it, he either places, perhaps irrationally, another value or good (freedom from wearing a helmet) above that of physical well-being or, perhaps, while recognizing the danger in the abstract, he either does not fully appreciate it or he underestimates the likelihood of its occurring. But now we are approaching the question of possible justifications of paternalistic measures and the rest of this essay will be devoted to that question.

V

I shall begin for dialectical purposes by discussing Mill's objections to paternalism and then go on to discuss more positive proposals.

An initial feature that strikes one is the absolute nature of Mill's prohibitions against paternalism. It is so unlike the carefully qualified admonitions of Mill and his fellow Utilitarians on other moral issues. He speaks of self-protection as the *sole* end warranting coercion, of the individual's own goals as *never* being a sufficient warrant. Contrast this with his discussion of the prohibition against lying in *Util[itarianism]*.

> Yet that even this rule, sacred as it is, admits of possible exception, is acknowledged by all moralists, the chief of which is where the with-holding of some fact . . . would save an individual . . . from great and unmerited evil.[3]

The same tentativeness is present when he deals with justice.

> It is confessedly unjust to break faith with any one: to violate an engagement, either express or implied, or disappoint expectations raised by our own conduct, at least if we have raised these expectations knowingly and voluntarily. Like all the other obligations of justice already spoken of, this one is not regarded as absolute, but as capable of being overruled by a stronger obligation of justice on the other side.[4]

This anomaly calls for some explanation. The structure of Mill's argument is as follows:

1. Since restraint is an evil the burden of proof is on those who propose such restraint.

2. Since the conduct which is being considered is purely self-regarding, the normal appeal to the protection of the interests of others is not available.

3. Therefore we have to consider whether reasons involving reference to the individual's own good, happiness, welfare, or interests are sufficient to overcome the burden of justification.

4. We either cannot advance the interests of the individual by compulsion, or the attempt to do so involves evil which outweighs the good done.

5. Hence the promotion of the individual's own interests does not provide a sufficient warrant for the use of compulsion.

Clearly the operative premise here is 4 and it is bolstered by claims about the status of the individual as judge and appraiser of his welfare, interests, needs, etc.

> With respect to his own feelings and circumstances, the most ordinary man or woman has means of knowledge immeasurably surpassing those that can be possessed by any one else.[5]
>
> He is the man most interested in his own well-being: the interest which any other person, except in cases of strong personal attachment, can have in it, is trifling, compared to that which he himself has.[6]

These claims are used to support the following generalizations concerning the utility of compulsion for paternalistic purposes.

> The interferences of society to overrule his judgment and purposes in what only regards himself must be grounded in general presumptions; which may be altogether wrong, and even if right, are as likely as not to be misapplied to individual cases.[7]
>
> But the strongest of all the arguments against the interference of the public with purely personal conduct is that when it does interfere, the odds are that it interferes wrongly and in the wrong place.[8]
>
> All errors which the individual is likely to commit against advice and warning are far outweighed by the evil of allowing others to constrain him to what they deem his good.[9]

Performing the utilitarian calculation by balancing the advantages and disadvantages we find that:

> Mankind are greater gainers by suffering each other to live as seems good to themselves, than by compelling each other to live as seems good to the rest.[10]

From which follows the operative premise 4.

This classical case of a utilitarian argument with all the premises spelled out is not the only line of reasoning present in Mill's discussion. There are asides, and more than asides, which look quite different and I shall deal with them later. But this is clearly the main channel of Mill's thought and it is one which has been subjected to vigorous attack from the moment it appeared—most often by fellow Utilitarians. The link that they have usually seized on is, as Fitzjames Stephen put it, the absence of proof that the "mass of adults are so well acquainted with their own interests and so much disposed to pursue them that no compulsion or restraint put upon them by any others for the purpose of promoting their interest can really promote them."[11] Even so sympathetic a critic as Hart is forced to the conclusion that:

> In Chapter 5 of his essay Mill carried his protests against paternalism to lengths that may now appear to us as fantastic. . . . No doubt if we no longer sympathise with this criticism this is due, in part, to a general decline in the belief that individuals know their own interest best.[12]
>
> Mill endows the average individual with "too much of the psychology of a middle-aged man whose desires are relatively fixed, not liable to be artificially stimulated by external influences; who knows what he wants and what gives him satisfaction or happiness, and who pursues these things when he can."[13]

Now it is interesting to note that Mill himself was aware of some of the limitations on the doctrine that the individual is the best judge of his own interests. In his discussion of government intervention in general (even where the intervention does not interfere with liberty but provides alternative institutions to those of the market) after making claims which are parallel to those just discussed, e.g.

> People understand their own business and their own interests better, and care for them more, than the government does, or can be expected to do.[14]

He goes on to an intelligent discussion of the "very large and conspicuous exceptions" to the maxim that:

> Most persons take a juster and more intelligent view of their own interest, and of the means of promoting it than can either be prescribed to them by a general enactment of the legislature, or pointed out in the particular case by a public functionary.[15]

Thus there are things

> of which the utility does not consist in ministering to inclinations, nor in serving the daily uses of life, and the want of which is least felt where the need is greatest. This is peculiarly true of those things which are chiefly useful as tending to raise the character of human beings. The uncultivated cannot be competent judges of cultivation. Those who most need to be made wiser and better, usually desire it least, and, if they desired it, would be incapable of finding the way to it by their own lights.

. . . . A second exception to the doctrine that individuals are the best judges of their own interest, is when an individual attempts to decide irrevocably now what will be best for his interest at some future and distant time. The presumption in favor of individual judgment is only legitimate, where the judgment is grounded on actual, and especially on present, personal experience; not where it is formed antecedently to experience, and not suffered to be reversed even after experience has condemned it.[16]

The upshot of these exceptions is that Mill does not declare that there should never be government interference with the economy but rather that

. . . in every instance, the burden of making out a strong case should be thrown not on those who resist but on those who recommend government interference. Letting alone, in short, should be the general practice: every departure from it, unless required by some great good, is a certain evil.[17]

In short, we get a presumption not an absolute prohibition. The question is why doesn't the argument against paternalism go the same way?

I suggest that the answer lies in seeing that in addition to a purely utilitarian argument Mill uses another as well. As a Utilitarian Mill has to show, in Fitzjames Stephen's words, that:

Self-protection apart, no good object can be attained by any compulsion which is not in itself a greater evil than the absence of the object which the compulsion obtains.[18]

To show this is impossible; one reason being that it isn't true. Preventing a man from selling himself into slavery (a paternalistic measure which Mill himself accepts as legitimate), or from taking heroin, or from driving a car without wearing seat-belts may constitute a lesser evil than allowing him to do any of these things. A consistent Utilitarian can only argue against paternalism on the grounds that it (as a matter of fact) does not maximize the good. It is always a contingent question that may be refuted by the evidence. But there is also a non-contingent argument which runs through *On Liberty*. When Mill states that "there is a part of the life of every person who has come to years of discretion, within which the individuality of that person ought to reign uncontrolled either by any other person or by the public collectively" he is saying something about what it means to be a person, an autonomous agent.

It is because coercing a person for his own good denies this status as an independent entity that Mill objects to it so strongly and in such absolute terms. To be able to choose is a good that is independent of the wisdom of what is chosen. A man's "mode of laying out his existence is the best, not because it is the best in itself, but because it is his own mode."[19]

It is the privilege and proper condition of a human being, arrived at the maturity of his faculties, to use and interpret experience in his own way.[20]

As further evidence of this line of reasoning in Mill consider the one exception to his prohibition against paternalism.

In this and most civilised countries, for example, an engagement by which a person should sell himself, or allow himself to be sold, as a slave, would be null and void; neither enforced by law nor by opinion. The ground for thus limiting his power of voluntarily disposing of his own lot in life, is apparent, and is very clearly seen in this extreme case. The reason for not interfering, unless for the sake of others, with a person's voluntary acts, is consideration for his liberty. His voluntary choice is evidence that what he so chooses is desirable, or at least endurable, to him, and his good is on the whole best provided for by allowing him to take his own means of pursuing it. But by selling himself for a slave, he abdicates his liberty; he foregoes any future use of it beyond that single act.

He therefore defeats, in his own case, the very purpose which is the justification of allowing him to dispose of himself. He is no longer free; but is thenceforth in a position which has no longer the presumption in its favour, that would be afforded by his voluntarily remaining in it. The principle of freedom cannot require that he should be free not to be free. It is not freedom to be allowed to alienate his freedom.[21]

Now leaving aside the fudging on the meaning of freedom in the last line it is clear that part of this argument is incorrect. While it is true that *future* choices of the slave are not reasons for thinking that what he chooses then is desirable for him, what is at issue is limiting his immediate choice; and since this choice is made freely, the individual may be correct in thinking that his interests are best provided for by entering such a contract. But the main consideration for not allowing such a contract is the need to preserve the liberty of the person to make future choices. This gives us a principle—a very narrow one—by which to justify some paternalistic interferences. Paternalism is justified only to preserve a wider range of freedom for the individual in question. How far this principle could be extended, whether it can justify all the cases in which we are inclined upon reflection to think paternalistic measures justified remains to be discussed. What I have tried to show so far is that there are two strains of argument in Mill—one a straight-forward Utilitarian mode of reasoning and one which relies not on the goods which free choice leads to but on the absolute value of the choice itself. The first cannot establish any absolute prohibition but at most a presumption and indeed a fairly weak one given some fairly plausible assumptions about human psychology; the second while a stronger line of argument seems to me to allow on its own grounds a wider range of paternalism than might be suspected. I turn now to a consideration of these matters.

VI

We might begin looking for principles governing the acceptable use of paternalistic power in cases where it is generally agreed that it is legitimate. Even Mill intends his principles to be applicable only to mature individuals, not those in what he calls "non-age." What is it that justifies us in interfering with children? The fact that they lack some of the emotional and cognitive capacities required in order to make fully rational decisions. It is an empirical question to just what extent children have an adequate conception of their own present and future interests but there is not much doubt that there are many deficiencies. For example it is very difficult for a child to defer gratification for any considerable period of time. Given these deficiencies and given the very real and permanent dangers that may befall the child it becomes not only permissible but even a duty of the parent to restrict the child's freedom in various ways. There is however an important moral limitation on the exercise of such parental power which is provided by the notion of the child eventually coming to see the correctness of his parent's interventions. Parental paternalism may be thought of as a wager by the parent on the child's subsequent recognition of the wisdom of the restrictions. There is an emphasis on what could be called future-oriented consent—on what the child will come to welcome, rather than on what he does welcome.

The essence of this idea has been incorporated by idealist philosophers into various types of "real-will" theory as applied to fully adult persons. Extensions of paternalism are argued for by claiming that in various respects, chronologically mature individuals share the same deficiencies in knowledge, capacity to think rationally, and the ability to carry out decisions that children possess. Hence in interfering with such people we are in effect doing what they would do if they were fully rational. Hence we are not really opposing their will, hence we are not really interfering with their freedom. The dangers of this move have been sufficiently exposed by Berlin in his Two Concepts of Liberty. I see no gain in theoretical clarity nor in practical advantage in trying to pass over the real nature of the interferences with liberty that we impose on others. Still the basic notion of consent is important and seems to me the only acceptable way of trying to delimit an area of justified paternalism.

Let me start by considering a case where the consent is not hypothetical in nature. Under certain conditions it is rational for an individual to agree that others should force him to act in ways in which, at the time of action, the individual may not see as desirable. If, for example, a man knows that he is subject to breaking his resolves when temptation is present, he may ask a friend to refuse to entertain his requests at some later stage.

A classical example is given in the Odyssey when Odysseus commands his men to tie him to the mast and refuse all future orders to be set free, because he knows the power of the Sirens to enchant men with their songs. Here we are on relatively sound ground in later refusing Odysseus' request to be set free. He may even claim to have changed his mind but since it is just such changes that he wished to guard against we are entitled to ignore them.

A process analogous to this may take place on a social rather than individual basis. An electorate may mandate its representatives to pass legislation which when it comes time to "pay the price" may be unpalatable. I may believe that a tax increase is necessary to halt inflation though I may resent the lower pay check each month. However in both this case and that of Odysseus the measure to be enforced is specifically requested by the party involved and at some point in time there is genuine consent and agreement on the part of those persons whose liberty is infringed. Such is not the case for the paternalistic measures we have been speaking about. What must be involved here is not consent to specific measures but rather consent to a system of government, run by elected representatives, with an understanding that they may act to safeguard our interests in certain limited ways.

I suggest that since we are all aware of our irrational propensities, deficiencies in cognitive and emotional capacities and avoidable and unavoidable ignorance it is rational and prudent for us to in effect take out "social insurance policies." We may argue for and against proposed paternalistic measures in terms of what fully rational individuals would accept as forms of protection. Now, clearly since the initial agreement is not about specific measures we are dealing with a more-or-less blank check and therefore there have to be carefully defined limits. What I am looking for are certain kinds of conditions which make it plausible to suppose that rational men could reach agreement to limit their liberty even when other men's interests are not affected.

Of course as in any kind of agreement schema there are great difficulties in deciding what rational individuals would or would not accept. Particularly in sensitive areas of personal liberty, there is always a danger of the dispute over agreement and rationality being a disguised version of evaluative and normative disagreement.

Let me suggest types of situations in which it seems plausible to suppose that fully rational individuals would agree to having paternalistic restrictions imposed upon them. It is reasonable to suppose that there are "goods" such as health which any person would want to have in order to pursue his own good—no matter how that good is conceived. This is an argument that is used in connection with compulsory education for children but it seems to me that it can be extended to other goods which have this character. Then one could agree that the attainment of such goods should be promoted even when not recognized to be such, at the moment, by the individuals concerned.

An immediate difficulty that arises stems from the fact that men are always faced with competing goods and that there may be reasons why even a value such as health—or indeed life—may be overridden by competing values. Thus the problem with the Christian Scientist and blood transfusions. It may be more important for him to reject "impure substances" than to go on living. The difficult problem that must be faced is whether one can give sense to the notion of a person irrationally attaching weights to competing values.

Consider a person who knows the statistical data on the probability of being injured when not wearing seat-belts in an automobile and knows the types and gravity of the various injuries. He also insists that the inconvenience attached to fastening the belt every time he gets in and out of the car outweighs for him the possible risks to himself. I am inclined in this case to think that such a weighing is irrational. Given his life-plans which we are assuming are those of the average person, his interests and commitments already undertaken, I think it is safe to predict that we can find inconsistencies in his calculations at some point. I am assuming that this is not a man who for some conscious or unconscious reasons is trying to injure himself nor is he a man who just likes to "live dangerously." I am assuming that he is like us in all the relevant respects but just puts an enormously high negative value on inconvenience—one which does not seem comprehensible or reasonable.

It is always possible, of course to assimilate this person to creatures like myself. I, also, neglect to fasten my seat-belt and I concede such behavior is not rational but not because I weigh the inconvenience differently from those who fasten the belts. It is just that having made (roughly) the same calculation as everybody else I ignore it in my actions. [Note: a much better case of weakness of the will than those usually given in ethics texts.] A plausible explanation for this deplorable habit is that although I know in some intellectual sense what the probabilities and risks are I do not fully appreciate them in an emotionally genuine manner.

We have two distinct types of situation in which a man acts in a non-rational fashion. In one case he attaches incorrect weights to some of his values; in the other he neglects to act in accordance with his actual preferences and desires. Clearly there is a stronger and more persuasive argument for paternalism in the latter situation. Here we are really not—by assumption—imposing a good on another person. But why may we not extend our interference to what we might call evaluative delusions? After all in the case of cognitive delusions we are prepared, often, to act against the expressed will of the person involved. If a man believes that when he jumps out the window he will float upwards—Robert Nozick's example—would not we detain him, forcibly if necessary? The reply will be that this man doesn't wish to be injured and if we could convince him that he is mistaken as to the consequences of his action he would not wish to perform the action. But part of what is involved in claiming that a man who doesn't fasten his seat-belts is attaching an irrational weight to the inconvenience of fastening them is that if he were to be involved in an accident and severely injured he would look back and admit that the inconvenience wasn't as bad as all that. So there is a sense in which if I could convince him of the consequences of his action he also would not wish to continue his present course of action. Now the notion of consequences being used here is covering a lot of ground. In one case it's being used to indicate what will or can happen as a result of a course of action and in the other it's making a prediction about the future evaluation of the consequences—in the first sense—of a course of action. And whatever the difference between facts and values—whether it be hard and fast or soft and slow—we are genuinely more reluctant to consent to interferences where evaluative differences are the issue. Let me now consider another factor which comes into play in some of these situations which may make an important difference in our willingness to consent to paternalistic restrictions.

Some of the decisions we make are of such a character that they produce changes which are in one or another way irreversible. Situations are created in which it is difficult or impossible to return to anything like the initial stage at which the decision was made. In particular some of these changes will make it impossible to continue to make reasoned choices in the future. I am thinking specifically of decisions which involve taking drugs that are physically or psychologically addictive and those which are destructive of one's mental and physical capacities.

I suggest we think of the imposition of paternalistic interferences in situations of this kind as being a kind of insurance policy which we take out against making decisions which are far-reaching, potentially dangerous and irreversible. Each of these factors is important. Clearly there are many decisions we make that are relatively irreversible. In deciding to learn to play chess I could predict in view of my general interest in games that some portion of my free-time was going to be preempted and that it would not be easy to give up the game once I acquired a certain competence. But my whole life-style was not going to be jeopardized in an extreme manner. Further it might be argued that even with addictive drugs such as heroin one's normal life plans would not be seriously interfered with if an inexpensive and adequate supply were readily available. So this type of argument might have a much narrower scope than appears to be the case at first.

A second class of cases concerns decisions which are made under extreme psychological and sociological pressures. I am not thinking here of the making of the decision as being something one is pressured into—e.g. a good reason for making duelling illegal is that unless this is done many people might have to manifest their courage and integrity in ways in which they would rather not do so—but rather of decisions such as that to commit suicide which are usually made at a point where the individual is not thinking clearly and calmly about the nature of his decision. In addition, of course, this comes under the previous heading of all-too-irrevocable decision. Now there are practical steps which a society could take if it wanted to decrease the possibility of suicide—for example not paying social security benefits to the survivors or as religious institutions do, not allowing such persons to be buried with the same status as natural deaths. I think we may count these as interferences with the liberty of persons to attempt suicide and the question is whether they are justifiable.

Using my argument schema the question is whether rational individuals would consent to such limitations. I see no reason for them to consent to an absolute prohibition but I do think it is reasonable for them to agree to some kind of enforced waiting period. Since we are all aware of the possibility of temporary states, such as great fear or depression, that are inimical to the making of well-informed and rational decisions, it would be prudent for all of us if there were some kind of institutional arrangement whereby we were restrained from making a decision which is (all too) irreversible. What this would be like in practice is difficult to envisage and it may be that if no practical arrangements were feasible then we would have to conclude that there should be no restriction at all on this kind of action. But we might have a "cooling off" period, in much the same way that we now require couples who file for divorce to go through a waiting period. Or, more far-fetched, we might imagine a Suicide Board composed of a psychologist and another member picked by the applicant. The Board would be required to meet and talk with the person proposing to take his life, though its approval would not be required.

A third class of decisions—these classes are not supposed to be disjoint—involves dangers which are either not sufficiently understood or appreciated correctly by the persons involved. Let me illustrate, using the example of cigarette smoking, a number of possible cases.

1. A man may not know the facts—e.g. smoking between 1 and 2 packs a day shortens life expectancy 6.2 years, the costs and pain of the illness caused by smoking, etc.

2. A man may know the facts, wish to stop smoking, but not have the requisite willpower.

3. A man may know the facts but not have them play the correct role in his calculation because, say, he discounts the danger psychologically because it is remote in time and/or inflates the attractiveness of other consequences of his decision which he regards as beneficial.

In case 1 what is called for is education, the posting of warnings, etc. In case 2 there is no theoretical problem. We are not imposing a good on someone who rejects it. We are simply using coercion to enable people to carry out their own goals. (Note: There obviously is a difficulty in that only a subclass of the individuals affected wish to be prevented from doing what they are doing.) In case 3 there is a sense in which we are imposing a good on someone since given his current appraisal of the facts he doesn't wish to be restricted. But in another sense we are not imposing a good since what is being claimed—and what must be shown or at least argued for—is that an accurate accounting on his part would lead him to reject his current course of action. Now we all know that such cases exist, that we are prone to disregard dangers that are only possibilities, that immediate pleasures are often magnified and distorted.

If in addition the dangers are severe and far-reaching we could agree to allowing the state a certain degree of power to intervene in such situations. The difficulty is in specifying in advance, even vaguely, the class of cases in which intervention will be legitimate.

A related difficulty is that of drawing a line so that it is not the case that all ultra-hazardous activities are ruled out, e.g. mountain-climbing, bull-fighting, sports-car racing, etc. There are some risks—even very great ones—which a person is entitled to take with his life.

A good deal depends on the nature of the deprivation—e.g. does it prevent the person from engaging in the activity completely or merely limit his participation—and how important to the nature of the activity is the absence of restriction when this is weighed against the role that the activity plays in the life of the person. In the case of automobile seatbelts, for example, the restriction is trivial in nature, interferes not at all with the use or enjoyment of the activity, and does, I am assuming, considerably reduce a high risk of serious injury. Whereas, for example, making mountain-climbing illegal prevents completely a person engaging in an activity which may play an important role in his life and his conception of the person he is.

In general the easiest cases to handle are those which can be argued about in the terms which Mill thought to be so important—a concern not just for the happiness or welfare, in some broad sense, of the individual but rather a concern for the autonomy and freedom of the person. I suggest that we would be most likely to consent to paternalism in those instances in which it preserves and enhances for the individual his ability to rationally consider and carry out his own decisions.

I have suggested in this essay a number of types of situations in which it seems plausible that rational men would agree to granting the legislative powers of a society the right to impose restrictions on what Mill calls "self-regarding" conduct. However, rational men knowing something about the resources of ignorance, ill-will and stupidity available to the lawmakers of a society—a good case in point is the history of drug legislation in the United States—will be concerned to limit such intervention to a minimum. I suggest in closing two principles designed to achieve this end.

In all cases of paternalistic legislation there must be a heavy and clear burden of proof placed on the authorities to demonstrate the exact nature of the harmful effects (or beneficial consequences) to be avoided (or achieved) and the probability of their occurrence. The burden of proof here is two-fold—what lawyers distinguish as the burden of going forward and the burden of persuasion. That the authorities have the burden of going forward means that it is up to them to raise the question and bring forward evidence of the evils to be avoided.

Unlike the case of new drugs where the manufacturer must produce some evidence that the drug has been tested and found not harmful, no citizen has to show with respect to self-regarding conduct that it is not harmful or promotes his best interests. In addition the nature and cogency of the evidence for the harmfulness of the course of action must be set at a high level. To paraphrase a formulation of the burden of proof for criminal proceedings—better 10 men ruin themselves than one man be unjustly deprived of liberty.

Finally I suggest a principle of the least restrictive alternative. If there is an alternative way of accomplishing the desired end without restricting liberty then although it may involve great expense, inconvenience, etc. the society must adopt it.

Notes

1. J. S. Mill, *Utilitarianism* and *On Liberty* (Fontana Library Edition, ed. by Mary Warnock, London, 1962), p. 135. All further quotes from Mill are from this edition unless otherwise noted.

2. J. S. Mill, *Principles of Political Economy* (New York: P. F. Collier and Sons, 1900), p. 442.

3. Mill, *Utilitarianism* and *On Liberty*, p. 174.

4. *Ibid.*, p. 299.

5. *Ibid.*, p. 207.

6. *Ibid.*, p. 206.

7. *Ibid.*, p. 207.

8. *Ibid.*, p. 214.

9. *Ibid.*, p. 207.

10. *Ibid.*, p. 138.

11. J. F. Stephen, *Liberty, Equality, Fraternity* (New York: Henry Holt & Co., n.d.), p. 24.

12. H. L. A. Hart, *Law, Liberty and Morality* (Stanford: Stanford University Press, 1963), p. 32.

13. *Ibid.*, p. 33.

14. Mill, *Principles*, II, 448.

15. *Ibid.*, II, 458.

16. *Ibid.*, II, 459.

17. *Ibid.*, II, 451.

18. Stephen, p. 49.

19. Mill, *Utilitarianism* and *On Liberty*, p. 197.

20. *Ibid.*, p. 186.

21. *Ibid.*, pp. 235–236.

On Telling Patients the Truth

Mack Lipkin

Mack Lipkin provides a defense of the paternalistic practice of withholding information from patients. Lipkin claims it is usually a practical impossibility to tell patients "the whole truth." They usually simply do not possess enough information about how their bodies work to understand the nature of their disease, and their understanding of the terms used by a physician is likely to be quite different from the meaning intended. Besides, some patients do not wish to be told the truth about their illness. Whether it is a matter of telling the truth or of deceiving patients by giving them placebos, the crucial question, according to Lipkin, is "whether the deception was intended to benefit the patient or the doctor."

Should a doctor always tell his patients the truth? In recent years there has been an extraordinary increase in public discussion of the ethical problems involved in this question. But little has been heard from physicians themselves. I believe that gaps in understanding the complex interactions between doctors and patients have led many laymen astray in this debate.

It is easy to make an attractive case for always telling patients the truth. But as L. J. Henderson, the great Harvard physiologist-philosopher of decades ago, commented:

Reprinted by permission from Newsweek, *4 June 1979, p. 13.*

To speak of telling the truth, the whole truth and nothing but the truth to a patient is absurd. Like absurdity in mathematics, it is absurd simply because it is impossible. . . . The notion that the truth, the whole truth, and nothing but the truth can be conveyed to the patient is a good specimen of that class of fallacies called by Whitehead "the fallacy of misplaced concreteness." It results from neglecting factors that cannot be excluded from the concrete situation and that are of an order of magnitude and relevancy that make it imperative to consider them. Of course, another fallacy is also often involved, the belief that diagnosis and prognosis are more certain than they are. But that is another question.

Words, especially medical terms, inevitably carry different implications for different people. When these words are said in the presence of anxiety-laden illness, there is a strong tendency to hear selectively and with emphases not intended by the doctor. Thus, what the doctor means to convey is obscured.

Indeed, thoughtful physicians know that transmittal of accurate information to patients is often impossible. Patients rarely know how the body functions in health and disease, but instead have inaccurate ideas of what is going on; this hampers the attempts to "tell the truth."

Take cancer, for example. Patients seldom know that while some cancers are rapidly fatal, others never amount to much; some have a cure rate of 99 percent, others less than 1 percent; a cancer may grow rapidly for months and then stop growing for years; may remain localized for years or spread all over the body almost from the beginning; some can be arrested for long periods of time, others not. Thus, one patient thinks of cancer as curable, the next thinks it means certain death.

How many patients understand that "heart trouble" may refer to literally hundreds of different abnormalities ranging in severity from the trivial to the instantly fatal? How many know that the term "arthritis" may refer to dozens of different types of joint involvement? "Arthritis" may raise a vision of the appalling disease that made Aunt Eulalee a helpless invalid until her death years later; the next patient remembers Grandpa grumbling about the damned arthritis as he got up from his chair. Unfortunately but understandably, most people's ideas about the implications of medical terms are based on what they have heard about a few cases.

The news of serious illness drives some patients to irrational and destructive behavior; others handle it sensibly. A distinguished philosopher forestalled my telling him about his cancer by saying, "I want to know the truth. The only thing I couldn't take and wouldn't want to know about is cancer." For two years he had watched his mother die slowly of a painful form of cancer. Several of my physician patients have indicated they would not want to know if they had a fatal illness.

Most patients should be told "the truth" to the extent that they can comprehend it. Indeed, most doctors, like most other people, are uncomfortable with lies. Good physicians, aware that some may be badly damaged by being told more than they want or need to know, can usually ascertain the patient's preferences and needs.

Discussions about lying often center about the use of placebos. In medical usage, a "placebo" is a treatment that has no specific physical or chemical action on the condition being treated, but is given to affect symptoms by a psychologic mechanism, rather than a purely physical one. Ethicists believe that placebos necessarily involve a partial or complete deception by the doctor, since the patient is allowed to believe that the treatment has a specific effect. They seem unaware that placebos, far from being inert (except in the rigid pharmacological sense), are among the most powerful agents known to medicine.

Placebos are a form of suggestion, which is a direct or indirect presentation of an idea, followed by an uncritical, i.e., not thought-out, acceptance. Those who have studied suggestion or looked at medical history know its almost unbelievable potency; it is involved to a greater or lesser extent in the treatment of every conscious patient. It can induce or remove almost any kind of feeling or thought. It can strengthen the weak or paralyze the strong; transform sleeping, feeding, or sexual patterns; remove or induce a vast array of symptoms; mimic or abolish the effect of very powerful drugs. It can alter the function of most organs. It can cause illness or a great sense of well-being. It can kill. In fact, doctors often add a measure of suggestion when they prescribe even potent medications for those who also need psychologic support. Like all potent agents, its proper use requires judgment based on experience and skill.

Communication between physician and the apprehensive and often confused patient is delicate and uncertain. Honesty should be evaluated not only in terms of a slavish devotion to language often misinterpreted by the patient, but also in terms of intent. *The crucial question is whether the deception was intended to benefit the patient or the doctor.*

Physicians, like most people, hope to see good results and are disappointed when patients do poorly. Their reputations and their livelihood depend on doing effective work; purely selfish reasons would dictate they do their best for their patients. Most important, all good physicians have a deep sense of responsibility toward those who have entrusted their welfare to them.

As I have explained, it is usually a practical impossibility to tell patients "the whole truth." Moreover, often enough, the ethics of the situation, the true moral responsibility, may demand that the naked facts not be revealed. The now popular complaint that doctors are too authoritarian is misguided more often than not. Some patients who insist on exercising their right to know may be doing themselves a disservice.

Judgment is often difficult and uncertain. Simplistic assertions about telling the truth may not be helpful to patients or physicians in times of trouble.

Lies to the Sick and Dying

Sissela Bok

Sissela Bok reviews three arguments that physicians frequently use to justify not telling the truth to their patients. Bok finds each of them faulty and unpersuasive.

Bok points out that the first of the arguments trades on a confusion between telling "the truth" (that is, everything that is true about a situation) and "truthfulness" (being honest). In effect, the argument asserts that since it is impossible to tell "the truth" to people who are not medical experts, then there is no clear distinction between what is true and what is false. Anything medical said to them is, at best, partially true. When this argument is accepted, Bok claims, the way is open for the physician to decide just how much of "the truth" will be revealed to serve the best interest of the patient.

Are physicians correct in claiming that patients don't want to know the truth? This is an issue that is open to empirical tests. Bok cites studies showing that a large majority of people say they want to be told the truth about themselves, even if they should be diagnosed as having a catastrophic illness.

The last argument examined by Bok holds that information given to a patient might damage the patient (or at least not help the patient); thus, proper health care demands that information not be supplied. This argument also has an empirical aspect and is open to challenge on factual grounds. As Bok observes, the harm associated with the disclosure of bad news and risks is probably greatly overestimated. What is more, very real benefits (such as increased cooperation) are never mentioned.

Bok is not willing to go so far as to say that lying to a patient is never justified. She is primarily concerned with showing that withholding the truth is a serious matter that requires justification in each case.

Deception as Therapy

A forty-six-year-old man, coming to a clinic for a routine physical checkup needed for insurance purposes, is diagnosed as having a form of cancer likely to cause him to die within six months. No known cure exists for it. Chemotherapy may prolong life by a few extra months, but will have side effects the physician does not think warranted in this case. In addition, he believes that such therapy should be reserved for patients with a chance for recovery or remission. The patient has no symptoms giving him any reason to believe that he is not perfectly healthy. He expects to take a short vacation in a week.

For the physician, there are now several choices involving truthfulness. Ought he to tell the patient what he has learned, or conceal it? If asked, should he deny it? If he decides to reveal the diagnosis, should he delay doing so until after the patient returns from his vacation? Finally, even if he does reveal the serious nature of the diagnosis, should he mention the possibility of chemotherapy and his reasons for not recommending it in this case? Or should he encourage every last effort to postpone death?

In this particular case, the physician chose to inform the patient of his diagnosis right away. He did not, however, mention the possibility of chemotherapy. A medical student working under him disagreed; several nurses also thought that the patient should have been informed of this possibility. They tried, unsuccessfully, to persuade the physician that this was the patient's right. When persuasion had failed, the student elected to disobey the doctor by informing the patient of the alternative of chemotherapy. After consultation with family members, the patient chose to ask for the treatment.

Doctors confront such choices often and urgently. What they reveal, hold back, or distort will matter profoundly to their patients. Doctors stress with corresponding vehemence their reasons for the distortion or concealment: not to confuse a sick person needlessly, or cause what may well be unnecessary pain or discomfort, as in the case of the cancer patient; not to leave a patient without hope, as in those many cases where the dying are not told

the truth about their condition; or to improve the chances of cure, as where unwarranted optimism is expressed about some form of therapy. Doctors use information as part of the therapeutic regimen; it is given out in amounts, in admixtures, and according to timing believed best for patients. Accuracy, by comparison, matters far less.

Lying to patients has, therefore, seemed an especially excusable act. Some would argue that doctors, and *only* doctors, should be granted the right to manipulate the truth in ways so undesirable for politicians, lawyers, and others.[1] Doctors are trained to help patients; their relationship to patients carries special obligations, and they know much more than laymen about what helps and hinders recovery and survival.

Even the most conscientious doctors, then, who hold themselves at a distance from the quacks and the purveyors of false remedies, hesitate to forswear all lying. Lying is usually wrong, they argue, but less so than allowing the truth to harm patients. B. C. Meyer echoes this very common view:

> [O]urs is a profession which traditionally has been guided by a precept that transcends the virtue of uttering truth for truth's sake, and that is, "so far as possible, do no harm."[2]

Truth, for Meyer, may be important, but not when it endangers the health and well-being of patients. This has seemed self-evident to many physicians in the past—so much so that we find very few mentions of veracity in the codes and oaths and writings by physicians through the centuries. This absence is all the more striking as other principles of ethics have been consistently and movingly expressed in the same documents.

The two fundamental principles of doing good and not doing harm—of beneficence and nonmaleficence—are the most immediately relevant to medical practitioners, and the most frequently stressed. To preserve life and good health, to ward off illness, pain, and death—these are the perennial tasks of medicine and nursing. These principles have found powerful expression at all times in the history of medicine. In the Hippocratic Oath physicians promise to:

use treatment to help the sick . . . but never with a view to injury and wrong-doing.[3]

And a Hindu oath of initiation says:

> Day and night, however thou mayest be engaged, thou shalt endeavor for the relief of patients with all thy heart and soul. Thou shalt not desert or injure the patient even for the sake of thy living.[4]

But there is no similar stress on veracity. It is absent from virtually all oaths, codes, and prayers. The Hippocratic Oath makes no mention of truthfulness to patients about their condition, prognosis, or treatment. Other early codes and prayers are equally silent on the subject. To be sure, they often refer to the confidentiality with which doctors should treat all that patients tell them; but there is no corresponding reference to honesty toward the patient. One of the few who appealed to such a principle was Amattis Lusitanus, a Jewish physician widely known for his skill, who, persecuted, died of the plague in 1568. He published an oath which reads in part:

> If I lie, may I incur the eternal wrath of God and of His angel Raphael, and may nothing in the medical art succeed for me according to my desires.[5]

Later codes continue to avoid the subject. Not even the Declaration of Geneva, adopted in 1948 by the World Medical Association, makes any reference to it. And the Principles of Medical Ethics of the American Medical Association[6] still leave the matter of informing patients up to the physician.

Given such freedom, a physician can decide to tell as much or as little as he wants the patient to know, so long as he breaks no law. In the case of the man mentioned at the beginning of this chapter, some physicians might feel justified in lying for the good of the patient; others might be truthful. Some may conceal alternatives to the treatment they recommend, others not. In each case, they could appeal to the AMA Principles of Ethics. A great many would choose to be able to lie. They would claim that not only can a lie avoid harm for the patient, but that it is also hard to know whether they have been right in the first place in making their pessimistic diagnosis; a "truthful" statement could therefore turn out to hurt patients unnecessarily. The concern for curing and for supporting those who cannot be cured then runs counter to the desire to be completely open. This concern is especially strong where the prognosis is bleak; even more so when patients are so affected by their illness or their medication that they are more dependent than usual, perhaps more easily depressed or irrational.

Physicians know only too well how uncertain a diagnosis or prognosis can be. They know how hard it is to give meaningful and correct answers regarding health and illness. They also know that disclosing their own uncertainty or fears can reduce those benefits that depend upon faith in recovery. They fear, too, that revealing grave risks, no matter how unlikely it is that these will come about, may exercise the pull of the "self-fulfilling prophecy." They dislike being the bearers of uncertain or bad news as much as anyone else. And last, but not least, sitting down to discuss an illness truthfully and sensitively may take much-needed time away from other patients.

These reasons help explain why nurses and physicians and relatives of the sick and dying prefer not to be bound by rules that might limit their ability to suppress, delay, or distort information. This is not to say that they necessarily plan to lie much of the time. They merely want to have the freedom to do so when they believe it wise. And the reluctance to see lying prohibited explains, in turn, the failure of the codes and oaths to come to grips with the problems of truth-telling and lying.

But sharp conflicts are now arising. Doctors no longer work alone with patients. They have to consult with others much more than before; if they choose to lie, the choice may not be met with approval by all who take part in the care of the patient. A nurse expresses the difficulty which results as follows:

> From personal experience I would say that the patients who aren't told about their terminal illness have so many verbal and mental questions unanswered that many will begin to realize that their illness is more serious than they're being told. . . .
>
> Nurses care for these patients twenty-four hours a day compared to a doctor's daily brief visit, and it is the nurse many times that the patient will relate to, once his underlying fears become overwhelming. . . . This is difficult for us nurses because being in constant contact with patients we can see the events leading up to this. The patient continually asks you, "Why isn't my pain decreasing?" or "Why isn't the radiation treatment easing the pain?" . . . We cannot legally give these patients an honest answer

as a nurse (and I'm sure I wouldn't want to) yet the problem is still not resolved and the circle grows larger and larger with the patient alone in the middle.[7]

The doctor's choice to lie increasingly involves co-workers in acting a part they find neither humane nor wise. The fact that these problems have not been carefully thought through within the medical profession, nor seriously addressed in medical education, merely serves to intensify the conflicts.[8] Different doctors then respond very differently to patients in exactly similar predicaments. The friction is increased by the fact that relatives often disagree even where those giving medical care to a patient are in accord on how to approach the patient. Here again, because physicians have not worked out to common satisfaction the question of whether relatives have the right to make such requests, the problems are allowed to be haphazardly resolved by each physician as he sees fit.

The Patient's Perspective

The turmoil in the medical profession regarding truth-telling is further augmented by the pressures that patients themselves now bring to bear and by empirical data coming to light. Challenges are growing to the three major arguments for lying to patients: that truthfulness is impossible; that patients do not want bad news; and that truthful information harms them.

The first of these arguments . . . confuses "truth" and "truthfulness" so as to clear the way for occasional lying on grounds supported by the second and third arguments. At this point, we can see more clearly that it is a strategic move intended to discourage the question of truthfulness from carrying much weight in the first place, and thus to leave the choice of what to say and how to say it up to the physician. To claim that "since telling the truth is impossible, there can be no sharp distinction between what is true and what is false"[9] is to try to defeat objections to lying before even discussing them. One need only imagine how such an argument would be received, were it made by a car salesman or a real estate dealer, to see how fallacious it is.

In medicine, however, the argument is supported by a subsidiary point: even if people might ordinarily understand what is spoken to them, patients are often not in a position to do so. This is

where paternalism enters in. When we buy cars or houses, the paternalist will argue, we need to have all our wits about us; but when we are ill, we cannot always do so. We need help in making choices, even if help can be given only by keeping us in the dark. And the physician is trained and willing to provide such help.

It is certainly true that some patients cannot make the best choices for themselves when weakened by illness or drugs. But most still can. And even those who are incompetent have a right to have someone—their guardian or spouse perhaps—receive the correct information.

The paternalistic assumption of superiority to patients also carries great dangers for physicians themselves—it risks turning to contempt. The following view was recently expressed in a letter to a medical journal:

> As a radiologist who has been sued, I have reflected earnestly on advice to obtain Informed Consent but have decided to "take the risks without informing the patient" and trust to "God, judge, and jury" rather than evade responsibility through a legal gimmick. . . .
> [I]n a general radiologic practice many of our patients are uninformable and we would never get through the day if we had to obtain their consent to every potentially harmful study.
> . . . We still have patients with language problems, the uneducated and the unintelligent, the stolid and the stunned who cannot form an Informed Opinion to give an Informed Consent; we have the belligerent and the panicky who do not listen or comprehend. And then there are the Medicare patients who comprise 35 percent of general hospital admissions. The bright ones wearily plead to be left alone.
> . . . As for the apathetic rest, many of them were kindly described by Richard Bright as not being able to comprehend because "their brains are so poorly oxygenated."[10]

The argument which rejects informing patients because adequate truthful information is impossible in itself or because patients are lacking in understanding must itself be rejected when looked at from the point of view of patients. They know that liberties granted to the most conscientious and altruistic doctors will be exercised also in the "Medicaid Mills"; that the choices thus kept from patients will be exercised by not only competent but incompetent physicians; and that even the best doctors can make choices patients would want to make differently for themselves.

The second argument for deceiving patients refers specifically to giving them news of a frightening or depressing kind. It holds that patients do not, in fact, generally want such information. That they prefer not to have to face up to serious illness and death. On the basis of such a belief, most doctors in a number of surveys stated that they do not, as a rule, inform patients that they have an illness such as cancer.

When studies are made of what patients desire to know, on the other hand, a large majority say that they *would* like to be told of such a diagnosis.[11] All these studies need updating and should be done with larger numbers of patients and nonpatients. But they do show that there is generally a dramatic divergence between physicians and patients on the factual question of whether patients want to know what ails them in cases of serious illness such as cancer. In most of the studies, over 80 percent of the persons asked indicated that they would want to be told.

Sometimes this discrepancy is set aside by doctors who want to retain the view that patients do not want unhappy news. In reality, they claim, the fact that patients say they want it has to be discounted. The more someone asks to know, the more he suffers from fear which will lead to the denial of the information even if it is given. Informing patients is, therefore, useless; they resist and deny having been told what they cannot assimilate. According to this view, empirical studies of what patients say they want are worthless since they do not probe deeply enough to uncover this universal resistance to the contemplation of one's own death.

This view is only partially correct. For some patients, denial is indeed well established in medical experience. A number of patients (estimated at between 15 percent and 25 percent) will give evidence of denial of having been told about their illness, even when they repeatedly ask and are repeatedly informed. And nearly everyone experiences a period of denial at some point in the course of approaching death.[12] Elisabeth Kübler-Ross sees denial as resulting often from premature and abrupt information by a stranger who goes through the process quickly to "get it over with." She holds that denial functions as a buffer after unexpected shocking news, permitting individuals to collect themselves and to mobilize other defenses. She describes prolonged denial in one patient as follows:

She was convinced that the x-rays were "mixed up"; she asked for reassurance that her pathology report could not possibly be back so soon and that another patient's report must have been marked with her name. When none of this could be confirmed, she quickly asked to leave the hospital, looking for another physician in the vain hope "to get a better explanation for my troubles." This patient went "shopping around" for many doctors, some of whom gave her reassuring answers, others of whom confirmed the previous suspicion. Whether confirmed or not, she reacted in the same manner, she asked for examination and reexamination. . . .[13]

But to say the denial is universal flies in the face of all evidence. And to take any claim to the contrary as "symptomatic" of deeper denial leaves no room for reasoned discourse. There is no way that such universal denial can be proved true or false. To believe in it is a metaphysical belief about man's condition, not a statement about what patients do and do not want. It is true that we can never completely understand the possibility of our own death, any more than being alive in the first place. But people certainly differ in the degree to which they can approach such knowledge, take it into account in their plans, and make their peace with it.

Montaigne claimed that in order to learn both to live and to die, men have to think about death and be prepared to accept it.[14] To stick one's head in the sand, or to be prevented by lies from trying to discern what is to come, hampers freedom—freedom to consider one's life as a whole, with a beginning, a duration, an end. Some may request to be deceived rather than to see their lives as thus finite; others reject the information which would require them to do so; but most say that they want to know. Their concern for knowing about their condition goes far beyond mere curiosity or the wish to make isolated personal choices in the short time left to them; their stance toward the entire life they have lived, and their ability to give it meaning and completion, are at stake.[15] In lying or withholding the facts which permit such discernment, doctors may reflect their own fears (which, according to one study,[16] are much stronger than those of laymen) of facing questions about the meaning of one's life and the inevitability of death.

Beyond the fundamental deprivation that can result from deception, we are also becoming increasingly aware of all that can befall patients in the course of their illness when information is denied or distorted. Lies place them in a position where they no longer participate in choices concerning their own health, including the choice of whether to be a "patient" in the first place. A terminally ill person who is not informed that his illness is incurable and that he is near death cannot make decisions about the end of his life; about whether or not to enter a hospital, or to have surgery; where and with whom to spend his last days; how to put his affairs in order—these most personal choices cannot be made if he is kept in the dark, or given contradictory hints and clues. . . .

The reason why even doctors who recognize a patient's right to have information might still not provide it brings us to the third argument against telling all patients the truth. It holds that the information given might hurt the patient and the concern for the right to such information is therefore a threat to proper health care. A patient, these doctors argue, may wish to commit suicide after being given discouraging news, or suffer a cardiac arrest, or simply cease to struggle, and thus not grasp the small remaining chance for recovery. And even where the outlook for a patient is very good, the disclosure of a minute risk can shock some patients or cause them to reject needed protection such as a vaccination or antibiotics.

The factual basis for this argument has been challenged from two points of view. The damages associated with the disclosure of sad news or risks are rarer than physicians believe; and the *benefits* which result from being informed are more substantial, even measurably so. Pain is tolerated more easily, recovery from surgery is quicker, and cooperation with therapy is greatly improved. The attitude that "what you don't know won't hurt you" is proving unrealistic; it is what patients do not know but vaguely suspect that causes them corrosive worry.

It is certain that no answers to this question of harm from information are the same for all patients. If we look, first, at the fear expressed by physicians that informing patients of even remote or unlikely risks connected with a drug prescription or operation might shock some and make others refuse the treatment that would have been best for them, it appears to be unfounded for the great majority of patients. Studies show that very few patients respond to being told of such risks by withdrawing their consent to the procedure and that those who

do withdraw are the very ones who might well have been upset enough to sue the physician had they not been asked to consent beforehand.[17] It is possible that on even rarer occasions especially susceptible persons might manifest physical deterioration from shock; some physicians have even asked whether patients who die after giving informed consent to an operation, but before it actually takes place, somehow expire because of the information given to them.[18] While such questions are unanswerable in any one case, they certainly argue in favor of caution, a real concern for the person to whom one is recounting the risks he or she will face, and sensitivity to all signs of distress.

The situation is quite different when persons who are already ill, perhaps already quite weak and discouraged, are told of a very serious prognosis. Physicians fear that such knowledge may cause the patients to commit suicide, or to be frightened or depressed to the point that their illness takes a downward turn. The fear that great numbers of patients will commit suicide appears to be unfounded.[19] And if some do, is that a response so unreasonable, so much against the patient's best interest that physicians ought to make it a reason for concealment or lies? Many societies have allowed suicide in the past; our own has decriminalized it; and some are coming to make distinctions among the many suicides which ought to be prevented if at all possible, and those which ought to be respected.[20]

Another possible response to very bleak news is the triggering of physiological mechanisms which allow death to come more quickly—a form of giving up or of preparing for the inevitable, depending on one's outlook. Lewis Thomas, studying responses in humans and animals, holds it not unlikely that:

> . . . there is a pivotal movement at some stage in the body's reaction to injury or disease, maybe in aging as well, when the organism concedes that it is finished and the time for dying is at hand, and at this moment the events that lead to death are launched, as a coordinated mechanism. Functions are then shut off, in sequence, irreversibly, and, while this is going on, a neural mechanism, held ready for this occasion, is switched on. . . .[21]

Such a response may be appropriate, in which case it makes the moments of dying as peaceful as those who have died and been resuscitated so often testify. But it may also be brought on inappropriately, when the organism could have lived on, perhaps even induced malevolently, by external acts intended to kill. Thomas speculates that some of the deaths resulting from "hexing" are due to such responses. Levi-Strauss describes deaths from exorcism and the casting of spells in ways which suggest that the same process may then be brought on by the community.[22]

It is not inconceivable that unhappy news abruptly conveyed, or a great shock given to someone unable to tolerate it, could also bring on such a "dying response," quite unintended by the speaker. There is every reason to be cautious and to try to know ahead of time how susceptible a patient might be to the accidental triggering—however rare—of such a response. One has to assume, however, that most of those who have survived long enough to be in a situation where their informed consent is asked have a very robust resistance to such accidental triggering of processes leading to death. . . .

Apart from the possible harm from information, we are coming to learn much more about the benefits it can bring patients. People follow instructions more carefully if they know what their disease is and why they are asked to take medications; any benefits from those procedures are therefore much more likely to come about. Similarly, people recover faster from surgery and tolerate pain with less medication if they understand what ails them and what can be done for them.

Respect and Truthfulness

Taken all together, the three arguments defending lies to patients stand on much shakier ground as a counterweight to the right to be informed than is often thought. The common view that many patients cannot understand, do not want, and may be harmed by, knowledge of their condition, and that lying to them is either morally neutral or even to be recommended, must be set aside. Instead, we have to make a more complex comparison. Over against the right of patients to knowledge concerning themselves, the medical and psychological benefits to them from this knowledge, the unnecessary and sometimes harmful treatment to which they can be subjected if ignorant, and the harm to physicians, their profession, and other patients from deceptive practices, we have to set a severely restricted and narrowed paternalistic view—that *some* patients cannot understand, *some* do not want, and *some* may be harmed by, knowledge of their condition, and that they ought not to have to be treated like everyone else if this is not in their best interest.

Such a view is persuasive. A few patients openly request not to be given bad news. Others give clear signals to that effect, or are demonstrably vulnerable to the shock or anguish such news might call forth. Can one not in such cases infer implied consent to being deceived?

Concealment, evasion, withholding of information may at times be necessary. But if someone contemplates lying to a patient or concealing the truth, the burden of proof must shift. It must rest, here, as with all deception, on those who advocate it in any one instance. They must show why they fear a patient may be harmed or how they know that another cannot cope with the truthful knowledge. A decision to deceive must be seen as a very unusual step, to be talked over with colleagues and others who participate in the care of the patient. Reasons must be set forth and debated, alternatives weighed carefully. At all times, the correct information must go to *someone* closely related to the patient.

The law already permits doctors to withhold information from patients where it would clearly hurt their health. But this privilege has been sharply limited by the courts. Certainly it cannot be interpreted so broadly as to permit a general practice of deceiving patients "for their own good." Nor can it be made to include cases where patients might calmly decide, upon hearing their diagnosis, not to go ahead with the therapy their doctor recommends.[23] Least of all can it justify silence or lies to large numbers of patients merely on grounds that it is not always easy to tell what a patient wants.

For the great majority of patients, on the contrary, the goal must be disclosure, and the atmosphere one of openness. But it would be wrong to assume that patients can therefore be told abruptly about a serious diagnosis—that, so long as openness exists, there are no further requirements of humane concern in such communication. Dr. Cicely Saunders, who runs the well-known St. Christopher's Hospice in England, describes the sensitivity and understanding which are needed:

> Every patient needs an explanation of his illness that will be understandable and convincing to him if he is to cooperate in his treatment or be relieved of the burden of unknown fears. This is true whether it is a question of giving a diagno-

sis in a hopeful situation or of confirming a poor prognosis.

The fact that a patient does not ask does not mean that he has no questions. One visit or talk is rarely enough. It is only by waiting and listening that we can gain an idea of what we should be saying. Silences and gaps are often more revealing than words as we try to learn what a patient is facing as he travels along the constantly changing journey of his illness and his thoughts about it.

. . . So much of the communication will be without words or given indirectly. This is true of all real meeting with people but especially true with those who are facing, knowingly or not, difficult or threatening situations. It is also particularly true of the very ill.

The main argument against a policy of deliberate, invariable denial of unpleasant facts is that it makes such communication extremely difficult, if not impossible. Once the possibility of talking frankly with a patient has been admitted, it does not mean that this will always take place, but the whole atmosphere is changed. We are then free to wait quietly for clues from each patient, seeing them as individuals from whom we can expect intelligence, courage, and individual decisions. They will feel secure enough to give us these clues when they wish.[24]

Above all, truthfulness with those who are suffering does not mean that they should be deprived of all hope: hope that there is a chance of recovery, however small; nor of reassurance that they will not be abandoned when they most need help.

Much needs to be done, however, if the deceptive practices are to be eliminated, and if concealment is to be restricted to the few patients who ask for it or those who can be shown to be harmed by openness. The medical profession has to address this problem.

Notes

1. Plato, *The Republic,* 389 b.

2. B. C. Meyer, "Truth and the Physician," *Bulletin of the New York Academy of Medicine* 45 (1969): 59–71.

3. W. H. S. Jones, trans., *Hippocrates,* Loeb Classical Library (Cambridge, Mass.: Harvard University Press, 1923), p. 164.

4. Reprinted in M. B. Etziony, *The Physician's Creed: An Anthology of Medical Prayers. Oaths and Codes of Ethics* (Springfield, Ill.: Charles C Thomas, 1973), pp. 15–18.

5. See Harry Friedenwald, "The Ethics of the Practice of Medicine from the Jewish Point of View," *Johns Hopkins Hospital Bulletin,* no. 318 (August 1917), pp. 256–61.

6. "Ten Principles of Medical Ethics," *Journal of the American Medical Association* 164 (1957): 1119–20.

7. Mary Barrett, letter, *Boston Globe,* 16 November 1976, p. 1.

8. Though a minority of physicians have struggled to bring them to our attention. See Thomas Percival, *Medical Ethics,* 3d ed. (Oxford: John Henry Parker, 1849), pp. 132–41; Worthington Hooker, *Physician and Patient* (New York: Baker and Scribner, 1849), pp. 357–82; Richard C. Cabot, "Teamwork of Doctor and Patient Through the Annihilation of Lying," in *Social Service and the Art of Healing* (New York: Moffat, Yard & Co., 1909), pp. 116–70; Charles C. Lund, "The Doctor, the Patient, and the Truth," *Annals of Internal Medicine* 24 (1946): 955; Edmund Davies, "The Patient's Right to Know the Truth," *Proceedings of the Royal Society of Medicine* 66 (1973): 533–36.

9. Lawrence Henderson, "Physician and Patient as a Social System," *New England Journal of Medicine* 212 (1955).

10. Nicholas Demy, Letter to the Editor, *Journal of the American Medical Association* 217 (1971): 696–97.

11. For the views of physicians, see Donald Oken, "What to Tell Cancer Patients," *Journal of the American Medical Association* 175 (1961): 1120–28; and tabulations in Robert Veatch, *Death, Dying, and the Biological Revolution* (New Haven and London: Yale University Press, 1976), pp. 229–38. For the view of patients, see Veatch, ibid; Jean Aitken-Swan and E. C. Easson, "Reactions of Cancer Patients on Being Told Their Diagnosis," *British Medical Journal,* 1959, pp. 779–83; Jim McIntosh, "Patients' Awareness and Desire for Information About Diagnosed but Undisclosed Malignant Disease," *The Lancet* 7 (1976): 300–303; William D. Kelly and Stanley R. Friesen, "Do Cancer Patients Want to Be Told?," *Surgery* 27 (1950): 822–26.

12. See Avery Weisman, *On Dying and Denying* (New York: Behavioral Publications, 1972); Elisabeth Kübler-Ross, *On Death and Dying* (New York: The Macmillan Co., 1969); Ernest Becker, *The Denial of Death* (New York: Free Press, 1973); Philippe Ariès, *Western Attitudes Toward Death,* trans. Patricia M. Ranum (Baltimore and London: Johns Hopkins University Press, 1974); and Sigmund Freud, "Negation," *Collected Papers,* ed. James Strachey (London: Hogarth Press, 1950), 5: 181–85.

13. Kübler-Ross, *On Death and Dying,* p. 34.

14. Michel de Montaigne, *Essays,* bk. 1, chap. 20.

15. It is in literature that these questions are most directly raised. Two recent works where they are taken up with striking beauty and simplicity are

May Sarton, *As We Are Now* (New York: W. W. Norton & Co., 1973); and Freya Stark, *A Peak in Darien* (London: John Murray, 1976).

16. Herman Feifel *et al.*, "Physicians Consider Death," *Proceedings of the American Psychoanalytical Association*, 1967, pp. 201–2.

17. See Ralph Alfidi, "Informed Consent: A Study of Patient Reaction," *Journal of the American Medical Association* 216 (1971): 1325–29.

18. See Steven R. Kaplan, Richard A. Greenwald, and Arvey I. Rogers, Letter to the Editor, *New England Journal of Medicine* 296 (1977): 1127.

19. Oken, "What to Tell Cancer Patients"; Veatch, *Death, Dying, and the Biological Revolution*; Weisman, *On Dying and Denying*.

20. Norman L. Cantor, "A Patient's Decision to Decline Life-Saving Treatment: Bodily Integrity Versus the Preservation of Life," *Rutgers Law Review* 26: 228–64; Danielle Gourevitch, "Suicide Among the Sick in Classical Antiquity," *Bulletin of the History of Medicine* 18 (1969): 501–18; for bibliography, see Bok, "Voluntary Euthanasia."

21. Lewis Thomas, "A Meliorist View of Disease and Dying," *The Journal of Medicine and Philosophy* 1 (1976): 212–21.

22. Claude Lévi-Strauss, *Structural Anthropology* (New York: Basic Books, 1963), p. 167; see also Eric Cassell, "Permission to Die," in John Behnke and Sissela Bok, eds., *The Dilemmas of Euthanasia* (New York: Doubleday, Anchor Press, 1975), pp. 121–31.

23. See Charles Fried, *Medical Experimentation: Personal Integrity and Social Policy* (Amsterdam and Oxford: North Holland Publishing Co., 1974), pp. 20–24.

24. Cicely M. S. Saunders, "Telling Patients," in S. J. Reiser, W. J. Dyck, A. J. Curran, *Ethics in Medicine* (Cambridge, Mass.: M.I.T. Press, 1977), pp. 238–40.

Confidentiality in Medicine—A Decrepit Concept

Mark Siegler

Mark Siegler calls attention to the impossibility of preserving the confidentiality traditionally associated with the physician-patient relationship. In the modern hospital, a great many people have legitimate access to a patient's chart and so to all medical, social, and financial information the patient has provided. Yet the loss of confidentiality is a threat to good medical care. Confidentiality protects a patient at a time of vulnerability and promotes the trust that is necessary for effective diagnosis and treatment. Siegler concludes by suggesting some possible solutions for preserving confidentiality while meeting the needs of others to know certain things about the patient.

Medical confidentiality, as it has traditionally been understood by patients and doctors, no longer exists. This ancient medical principle, which has been included in every physician's oath and code of ethics since Hippocratic times, has become old, worn-out, and useless; it is a decrepit concept. Efforts to preserve it appear doomed to failure and often give rise to more problems than solutions. Psychiatrists have tacitly acknowledged the impossibility of ensuring the confidentiality of medical records by choosing to establish a separate, more secret record. The following case illustrates how the confidentiality principle is compromised systematically in the course of routine medical care.

Supported by a grant (OSS-8018097) from the National Science Foundation and by the National Endowment for the Humanities. The views expressed are those of the author and do not necessarily reflect those of the National Science Foundation or the National Endowment for the Humanities.

Reprinted by permission from The New England Journal of Medicine, *Vol. 307, No. 24 (9 Dec. 1982), 518–521. Copyright 1982 by the Massachusetts Medical Society.*

A patient of mine with mild chronic obstructive pulmonary disease was transferred from the surgical intensive-care unit to a surgical nursing floor two days after an elective cholecystectomy. On the day of transfer, the patient saw a respiratory therapist writing in his medical chart (the therapist was recording the results of an arterial blood gas analysis) and became concerned about the confidentiality of his hospital records. The patient threatened to leave the hospital prematurely unless I could guarantee that the confidentiality of his hospital record would be respected.

This patient's complaint prompted me to enumerate the number of persons who had both access to his hospital record and a reason to examine it. I was amazed to learn that at least 25 and possibly as many as 100 health professionals and administrative personnel at our university hospital had access to the patient's record and that all of them had a legitimate need, indeed a professional responsibility, to open and use that chart. These persons included 6 attending physicians (the primary physician, the surgeon, the pulmonary consultant, and others); 12 house officers (medical, surgical, intensive-care unit, and "covering" house staff); 20 nursing personnel (on three shifts); 6 respiratory therapists; 3 nutritionists; 2 clinical pharmacists; 15 students (from medicine, nursing, respiratory therapy, and clinical pharmacy); 4 unit secretaries; 4 hospital financial officers; and 4 chart reviewers (utilization review, quality assurance review, tissue review, and insurance auditor). It is of interest that this patient's problem was straightforward, and he therefore did not require many other technical and support services that the modern hospital provides. For example, he did not need multiple consultants and fellows, such specialized procedures as dialysis, or social workers, chaplains, physical therapists, occupational therapists, and the like.

Upon completing my survey I reported to the patient that I estimated that at least 75 health professionals and hospital personnel had access to his medical record. I suggested to the patient that these people were all involved in providing or supporting his health-care services. They were, I assured him, working for him. Despite my reassurances the patient was obviously distressed and retorted, "I always believed that medical confidentiality was part of a doctor's code of ethics. Perhaps you should tell me just what you people mean by 'confidentiality'!"

Two Aspects of Medical Confidentiality

Confidentiality and Third-Party Interests

Previous discussions of medical confidentiality usually have focused on the tension between a physician's responsibility to keep information divulged by patients secret and a physician's legal and moral duty, on occasion, to reveal such confidences to third parties, such as families, employers, public-health authorities, or police authorities. In all these instances, the central question relates to the stringency of the physician's obligation to maintain patient confidentiality when the health, well-being, and safety of identifiable others or of society in general would be threatened by a failure to reveal information about the patient. The tension in such cases is between the good of the patient and the good of others.

Confidentiality and the Patient's Interest

As the example above illustrates, further challenges to confidentiality arise because the patient's personal interest in maintaining confidentiality comes into conflict with his personal interest in receiving the best possible health care. Modern high-technology health care is available principally in hospitals (often, teaching hospitals), requires many trained and specialized workers (a "health-care team"), and is very costly. The existence of such teams means that information that previously had been held in confidence by an individual physician will now necessarily be disseminated to many members of the team. Furthermore, since health-care teams are expensive and few patients can afford to pay such costs directly, it becomes essential to grant access to the patient's medical record to persons who are responsible for obtaining third-party payment. These persons include chart reviewers, financial officers, insurance auditors, and quality-of-care assessors. Finally, as medicine expands from a narrow, disease-based model to a model that encompasses psychological, social, and economic problems, not only will the size of the health-care team and medical costs increase, but more sensitive information (such as one's personal habits and financial condition) will now be included in the medical record and will no longer be confidential.

The point I wish to establish is that hospital medicine, the rise of health-care teams, the existence of third-party insurance programs, and the expanding limits of medicine all appear to be responses to the wishes of people for better and more comprehensive medical care. But each of these developments necessarily modifies our traditional understanding of medical confidentiality.

The Role of Confidentiality in Medicine

Confidentiality serves a dual purpose in medicine. In the first place, it acknowledges respect for the patient's sense of individuality and privacy. The patient's most personal physical and psychological secrets are kept confidential in order to decrease a sense of shame and vulnerability. Secondly, confidentiality is important in improving the patient's health care—a basic goal of medicine. The promise of confidentiality permits people to trust (i.e., have confidence) that information revealed to a physician in the course of a medical encounter will not be disseminated further. In this way patients are encouraged to communicate honestly and forthrightly with their doctors. This bond of trust between patient and doctor is vitally important both in the diagnostic process (which relies on an accurate history) and subsequently in the treatment phase, which often depends as much on the patient's trust in the physician as it does on medications and surgery. These two important functions of confidentiality are as important now as they were in the past. They will not be supplanted entirely either by improvements in medical technology or by recent changes in relations between some patients and doctors toward a rights-based, consumerist model.

Possible Solutions to the Confidentiality Problem

First of all, in all nonbureaucratic, noninstitutional medical encounters—that is, in the millions of doctor-patient encounters that take place in physicians' offices, where more privacy can be preserved—meticulous care should be taken to guarantee that patients' medical and personal information will be kept confidential.

Secondly, in such settings as hospitals or large-scale group practices, where many persons have opportunities to examine the medical record, we should aim to provide access only to those who have "a need to know." This could be accomplished through such administrative changes as dividing the entire record into several sections—for example, a medical and financial section—and permitting only health professionals access to the medical information.

The approach favored by many psychiatrists—that of keeping a psychiatric record separate from the general medical record—is an understandable strategy but one that is not entirely satisfactory and that should not be generalized. The keeping of separate psychiatric records implies that psychiatry and medicine are different undertakings and thus drives deeper the wedge between them and between physical and psychological illness. Furthermore, it is often vitally important for internists or surgeons to know that a patient is being seen by a psychiatrist or is taking a particular medication. When separate records are kept, this information may not be available. Finally, if generalized, the practice of keeping a separate psychiatric record could lead to the unacceptable consequence of having a separate record for each type of medical problem.

Patients should be informed about what is meant by "medical confidentiality." We should establish the distinction between information about the patient that generally will be kept confidential regardless of the interest of third parties and information that will be exchanged among members of the health-care team in order to provide care for the patient. Patients should be made aware of the large number of persons in the modern hospital who require access to the medical record in order to serve the patient's medical and financial interests.

Finally, at some point most patients should have an opportunity to review their medical record and to make informed choices about whether their entire record is to be available to everyone or whether certain portions of the record are privileged and should be accessible only to their principal physician or to others designated explicitly by the patient. This approach would rely on traditional informed-consent procedural standards and might permit the patient to balance the personal value of medical confidentiality against the personal value of high-technology, team health care. There is no reason that the same procedure should not be used with psychiatric records instead of the arbitrary system now employed, in which everything related to psychiatry is kept secret.

Afterthought: Confidentiality and Indiscretion

There is one additional aspect of confidentiality that is rarely included in discussions of the subject. I am referring here to the wanton, often inadvertent, but avoidable exchanges of confidential information that occur frequently in hospital rooms, elevators, cafeterias, doctors' offices, and at cocktail parties. Of course, as more people have access to medical information about the patient the potential for this irresponsible abuse of confidentiality increases geometrically.

Such mundane breaches of confidentiality are probably of greater concern to most patients than the broader issue of whether their medical records may be entered into a computerized data bank or whether a respiratory therapist is reviewing the results of an arterial blood gas determination. Somehow, privacy is violated and a sense of shame is heightened when intimate secrets are revealed to people one knows or is close to—friends, neighbors, acquaintances, or hospital roommates—rather than when they are disclosed to an anonymous bureaucrat sitting at a computer terminal in a distant city or to a health professional who is acting in an official capacity.

I suspect that the principles of medical confidentiality, particularly those reflected in most medical codes of ethics, were designed principally to prevent just this sort of embarrassing personal indiscretion rather than to maintain (for social, political, or economic reasons) the absolute secrecy of doctor-patient communications. In this regard, it is worth noting that Percival's Code of Medical Ethics (1803) includes the following admonition: "Patients should be interrogated concerning their complaint in a tone of voice which cannot be overheard" [Leake, C. D., ed., *Percival's Medical Ethics*. Baltimore: Williams and Wilkins, 1927]. We in the medical profession frequently neglect these simple courtesies.

Conclusion

The principle of medical confidentiality described in medical codes of ethics and still believed in by patients no longer exists. In this respect, it is a decrepit concept. Rather than perpetuate the myth of confidentiality and invest energy vainly to preserve it, the public and the profession would be better served if they devoted their attention to determining which aspects of the original principle of confidentiality are worth retaining. Efforts could then be directed to salvaging those.

Confidentiality and the Prediction of Dangerousness in Psychiatry: The Tarasoff Case

William J. Curran

William J. Curran discusses a case decided by the California Supreme Court that has been of particular concern to psychiatrists and psychotherapists. The court ruled that therapists at the student health service of the University of California at Berkeley were negligent in their duty to warn Tatiana Tarasoff that Prosenjit Poddar, one of their patients, had threatened her life. Although the therapists reported the threat to the police, Tarasoff herself was not warned, and she was murdered by Poddar.

The question that Curran addresses is whether or not the therapists had done all they were obligated to do to protect both their patient and the community (including Tarasoff) by reporting the case to the police.

The case also raises more general issues: Does a therapist have a duty to warn at all? Should a patient be told that not everything he tells his psychiatrist will beheld in confidence? Is a therapist obliged to seek a court order committing a patient involuntarily to an institution if the patient utters a threat that the psychiatrist judges to be seriously motivated? (See the Juan Gonzalez Case Presentation for a recent example of these issues.)

Poddar was convicted of second-degree murder. The conviction was overturned on appeal, on the grounds that the jury had not been properly instructed. The state decided against a second trial, and Poddar was released on condition that he return to India.

The California Supreme Court continues to make financial awards to patients in suits against physicians with seemingly little regard for the effect of these awards and decisions upon the practice of medicine and the availability of insurance to cover this largesse of the judiciary, and without regard for the social consequences of this "money-for-everything" attitude.

The particular case, *Tarasoff vs. Regents of the University of California*,[1] has already become infamous among mental-health programs in California and among college and university student medical programs all over the country as it has taken its course through the various levels of trial and appeals courts in the Golden State.

The facts of the situation are undisputed. A student at the University of California's Berkeley campus was in psychotherapy with the student health service on an outpatient basis. He told his therapist, a psychologist, that he wanted to kill an unmarried girl who lived in Berkeley but who was then on a summer trip to Brazil. The psychologist, with the concurrence of another therapist and the assistant director of the Department of Psychiatry, reported the matter orally to the campus police and on their suggestion sent them a letter requesting detention of the student and his commitment for observation to a mental hospital. The campus police picked up the student for questioning but "satisfied" that he was "rational," released him on his "promise to stay away" from Miss Tarasoff. The police reported back to the director of psychiatry, Dr. Powelson. Dr. Powelson asked for the return of the psychologist's letter to the police and directed that all copies of the letter be destroyed. Nothing more was done at the health service about the matter. Two months later, shortly after Miss Tarasoff's return, the student went to her home and killed her.

The parents of Miss Tarasoff brought suit for damages against the University and against the therapists and the campus police, as employees of the University and individually. In suing Dr. Powelson, the plaintiffs sought not only general money damages for negligence in failure to warn the girl and her parents and to confine the student, but exemplary or punitive damages (which could be assessed in huge amounts as multiples of the general damages or in any amount at the determination of the jury) for malicious and oppressive abandonment of a dangerous patient.

The Superior Court dismissed all these grounds for legal action against the defendants. The Supreme Court, in a four-to-two decision, reversed the decision and found that on these facts a cause of action was stated for general damages against all the therapists involved in the case and the assistant director and the director of psychiatry and against the University as their employer for breach of the duty to warn Miss Tarasoff. The Court dismissed the claim for exemplary damages against the therapists. It also dismissed the action against the police as protected from a suit by a statutory immunity, as well as the suit against the therapists for failure to confine the student under a commitment order, again because of a statutory immunity. The Court implied that without the immunity, both these actions might have been meritorious.

It seems to me most physicians would throw up their hands in dismay over this result and the massive contradictions in the assessment of who was and who was not legally responsible for this death. If I were to describe in detail the reasoning of the court, the confusion of the medical mind would be compounded a thousand times.

The Court asserted that the *Principles of Medical Ethics of the American Medical Association*, Section 9,

Reprinted by permission from the New England Journal of Medicine 293 (August 7, 1975): 285–286.

did not bar breaching the confidentiality of this patient "in order to protect the welfare of this individual [the patient] or the community." From this premise the Court jumped wholeheartedly to a positive duty to warn Miss Tarasoff. This is not what the *Principles* said. The traditional code of medical ethics allows a physician in his sound discretion to breach the confidentiality, but does not require it. It is almost impossible to draft an ethical principle to force a duty on physicians to breach confidences. Must they always warn of death threats, but have discretion on less dangerous threats? Must they warn if the patient is psychotic, but not if he is less disturbed? Does this case mean that every time a patient makes a threat against an unnamed person, the therapist must take steps to find out who it is and warn him (of anything at all, from vague threats to murder) or suffer money damages in the thousands or tens of thousands if the threat, or an aspect of the threat, is carried out?

This case was greatly confused by the array of immunities from suits created under California law. It can be strongly argued that the thrust of these immunity statutes regarding the duty to warn should also have been applied to the therapists, since the statutes were intended to encourage police and mental-health personnel to release patients and not confine them on the basis of unreliable diagnoses of dangerousness. In the past it was thought that too many mental patients were confined for years and years because of their threats to other people, rarely carried out, and because of the conservatism of mental-health personnel in exercising any doubt about dangerousness in favor of confinement as the safest way to prevent harm to third parties.

It seems clear that the therapists here thought that they had done all they could to protect their patient and the community by reporting the case to the police. They had exercised their discretion to warn the community and to breach the confidence of the patient, for his own sake, and that of the unknown girl. They could hardly warn her, since she was not even in the country at the time. Also, the threat to Miss Tarasoff might actually have been vaguely directed. The student could well have turned his anger and violence toward another person or toward himself. The only basic recourse was to recommend temporary observational commitment. The practice was to [t]ake this to the campus police. It was the police who acted, and they decided to release the student with a warning and a promise to stay away from the girl. How many thousands of such warnings—and releases—do police departments make every year? How many people then proceed to kill? The immunity statute was established to encourage release in these circumstances. But the statutory armor had a hole in it. The director of psychiatry was found by the Court to have a "duty" to warn the girl, irrespective of the police action. The Court utilized some precedents, none clearly applicable to this case, to justify its decision. It seems, however, that the real rationale was the aggravated nature of the case—a killing—in which the family was left without someone else to sue. The therapists, particularly Dr. Powelson, could have warned the girl if they had wanted to go against the police action and if they had thought the specific threat to Miss Tarasoff so serious as to warrant that action. The Court did not apply any test to ascertain the custom of psychiatrists and mental-health programs actually in such situations. The Court declared the duty as a matter of law, regardless of the accepted practices of the profession. As in the *Helling* decision[2] discussed in an earlier column,[3] the Court made the physician a guarantor against harm to this party, here not even a patient, on the basis of its own concept of monetary justice.

Notes

1. 529 P. 2d 553.
2. *Helling vs. Carey and Laughlin*, 519 P. 2d 981.
3. Curran W. J. Glaucoma and streptococcal. Pharyngitis: diagnostic practices and malpractice liability. *N Engl J Med* 291:508–509, 1974.

Pregnant Women as Fetal Containers

George J. Annas

George J. Annas uses the Pamela Stewart Monson case to illustrate his argument that to prosecute pregnant women for fetal neglect is to treat women as less important than the fetuses they carry. It deprives women of their status as persons in their own right and relegates them to the role of fetal containers. Annas claims that the child-neglect laws were not written to be applied to fetuses and that applying them in this way has unacceptable consequences. Nor is Annas convinced by the argument that a woman who has "waived" her right to an abortion can be held responsible for fetal neglect.

In Margaret Atwood's *The Handmaid's Tale,* most women are sterile, and the few who retain the capacity to bear children have reproduction as their exclusive function. As one handmaid describes her station: "We are two-legged wombs, that's all; sacred vessels, ambulatory chalices." This future scenario strikes many as unlikely, but a recent criminal indictment directly raises the issue of when it is legally acceptable to treat a pregnant woman as a container, while treating the welfare of the fetus she contains as more significant than hers.

Mrs. Pamela Monson is the subject of what may be the first criminal charge ever brought against a woman for acts and omissions during pregnancy. Criminal charges were filed against her in California in October 1986. The available reports suggest that sometime very late in her pregnancy Mrs. Monson was advised by her physician not to take amphetamines, to stay off her feet, to avoid sexual intercourse, and, because of a placenta previa, to seek immediate medical treatment if she began to hemorrhage.

According to the police, Mrs. Monson noticed some bleeding the morning of November 23, 1985. Nevertheless, she remained at home, took some amphetamines, and had intercourse with her husband. She began bleeding more heavily, and contractions began sometime during the afternoon. It was only later, perhaps "many hours" later, that she went to the hospital. Her son was born that evening. He had massive brain damage, and died about six weeks thereafter.

Police lieutenant Randy Narramore has said, "We contend that she willfully disobeyed instructions (of the doctor) and as a direct result the child was born brain dead [sic] and later died" (*Washington Post,* October 2, 1986). District Attorney Harry Elias says simply that she "did not follow through on the medical advice she was given" (*New York Times,* October 9, 1986). Police officials wanted Mrs.

Monson prosecuted for murder, but the District Attorney has decided to proceed with a prosecution under a California child support statute.

The support statute itself has been amended many times since it was first passed in 1872, and during much of the subsequent time applied only to fathers. The relevant part of the current version reads:

> If a parent of a minor child *willfully omits,* without lawful excuse, *to furnish* necessary clothing, food, shelter or *medical attendance, or other remedial care* for his or her child, he or she is guilty of a misdemeanor punishable by a fine not exceeding two thousand dollars, or by imprisonment [for one year] (emphasis added) (Cal. Penal Code, Sec. 270 [West, 1986]).

A later provision decrees that "a child conceived but not yet born is to be deemed an existing person insofar as this section is concerned."

Use of this statute, instead of a homicide charge, avoids the issue of causation, since violation of the duty itself violates the statute regardless of the consequences to the fetus or child. Thus, for example, a father's failure to provide food for his children would violate the statute, even if the mother was able to provide her children with food from another source. Why the father hasn't been charged in this case is puzzling.

Very few cases have attempted to define the scope of the statute, and the only cases that deal with its application to fetuses were decided during the Depression. These cases hold that a father can fail to provide food, clothing, and shelter to the "unborn child" and that because these needs are "common to all mankind," proof of their "necessity" is not required. In regard to "medical attendance and other remedial care," however, "in a prosecution based on failure to furnish them, it would be incumbent on the prosecution to make affirmative proof of their necessity" (*People v. Yates,* 298 p. 961, 962 [(LA. Sup.

From the Hastings Center Report, *December 1986, pp 13–14. Reprinted by permission of the author.*

1931]). Such proof would, of course, require medical testimony. Mrs. Monson did provide "medical attendance" by seeking prenatal care and by seeking assistance in childbirth at a hospital.

Fetal Neglect

The District Attorney's use of this provision is an attempt to extend child support statutes to create a crime of "fetal neglect." Does it mean that the pregnant woman must, in effect, live for her fetus? That she must legally "stay off her feet" if walking or working might induce contractions? That she commits a crime if she does not eat only healthy foods; smokes or drinks alcohol; takes any drugs (legal or illegal); has intercourse with her husband?

And how does such a criminal law change the nature of the doctor-patient relationship? It seems evident that, to the police, the doctor's patient was not Mrs. Monson at all, but her fetus. It also seems evident that although the police spoke of "advice" and "instructions," they believed that the physician was giving the fetal container, Mrs. Monson, orders—orders that she *must* follow or face criminal penalties, including jail.

In this case, for example, the doctor had instructed Mrs. Monson not to have intercourse with her husband during the remainder of her pregnancy, because it might induce contractions and a premature delivery. She nonetheless engaged in intercourse. The prosecution alleges that such "disobeying instructions" or "failure to follow through on medical advice" is grounds for criminal action. This strikes me as both silly and dangerous. Silly because medical *advice* should remain *advice*: physicians are neither law makers nor seers.

After the fact prosecutions would not help individual fetuses. Dangerous because medical advice is a vague term that can cover almost anything. Effectively monitoring compliance would require confining pregnant women to an environment in which eating, exercise, drug use, and sexual intercourse could be controlled. This could, of course, be a maximum security country club, but such massive invasions of privacy can only be justified by treating pregnant women during their pregnancy as nonpersons. Like Margaret Atwood's handmaids, they have only one function: to have the healthiest children we can make them have.

Other quandaries arise if we apply child neglect statutes to fetuses. Unlike a child, the fetus is absolutely dependent upon its mother and cannot itself be "treated" without in some way invading the mother. The "fetal protection" policy enunciated by the prosecution seems to assume that like mother and child, mother and fetus are two separate individuals, with separate lights. But treating them separately before birth can only be done by favoring one over the other in disputes. Favoring the fetus radically devalues the pregnant woman and treats her like an inert incubator, or a culture medium for the fetus.

This view makes women unequal citizens, since only they can have children, and relegates them to performing one main function: childbearing. It is one thing for the state to view the fetus as a patient; it is another to assume that the fetus's interests are in opposition to its mother, and to require the mother to be the fetus's servant.

Child neglect covers a wide variety of activities, but generally involves failure to provide necessities like clothing, food, housing, or medical attention to the child. Such laws *do not*, however, require parents to provide optimal clothing, food, housing, or medical attention to their children; and do not even forbid taking risks with children (such as permitting them to engage in dangerous sports) or affirmatively injuring children (corporal punishment to teach them a lesson). None forbid mothers to smoke, take dangerous drugs, or to consume excessive amounts of alcohol, even though these activities may have a negative effect on their children.

While it seems draconian to apply the child neglect standards to the mother's life style during pregnancy, the California statute could be interpreted to apply to fetuses in a way never envisioned by the legislature. Certainly the legislature never intended that women must provide any more "clothing, food or shelter" to their fetuses than they provide for themselves. But what about the terms "medical attendance" and "remedial care"? Historically, medical attendance for the fetus meant medical attendance for the mother. If fetal surgery becomes an accepted procedure sometime in the future, however, "remedial care" may be applicable. Suppose, for example, that instead of the instructions the doctor gave Mrs. Monson, he had diagnosed her fetus as suffering from blocked ureters, and "recommended" surgery on the fetus to attempt to correct the problem. Would her failure to agree to this surgery be tantamount to "fetal neglect" for failure to provide her fetus with "necessary remedial care"?

This carries us into even more problematic waters. If women *must* "consent" to such "care" of their fetuses, they are relegated to the role of containers. Moreover their own rights are made so subordinate that the container may be opened to gain access to the fetus, even when the container may be damaged. (G. J. Annas, "Forced Caesareans: The Most Unkindest Cut of All," *Hastings Center Report*, June 1982, 16–17).

Waiving One's Right to Abortion

Some have argued that it is nonetheless fair to subject pregnant women to fetal neglect statutes because after they waive their right to abortion and decide to have a child, they take on added obligations to the future child, including providing it with such things as "necessary medical attendance." This argument seems misplaced for at least two reasons. First, such a "waiver" never in fact takes place. Women do not appear before judges or even notaries to waive their rights at any time during the pregnancy. Indeed, the vast majority of pregnancies in marriage are planned and welcomed, and viewing all pregnant women as potential aborters seems bizarre. Moreover, insofar as the right to terminate one's pregnancy is constitutionally protected, it remains a woman's legal right to the time of birth, at least when her life or health is at stake.

Second, and more important, women have a constitutional right to bear children if they are physically able to do so. To have a legal rule that there are no restrictions on a woman's decision to have an abortion, but if she elects childbirth instead, then the state will require her to surrender her basic rights of bodily integrity and privacy, creates a state-erected penalty on her exercise of her right to bear a child (D. E. Johnsen, "The Creation of Fetal Rights: Conflicts with Women's Constitutional Rights to Liberty, Privacy and Equal Protection," 95 *Yale Law Journal* 599, 618 [1986]). Such a penalty would (or at least should) be unconstitutional.

Attempts to define fetal neglect and to establish a prenatal police force to protect fetuses from their mothers, are steps backwards in terms of both women's rights and fetal protection. Women's rights will only be fostered when we treat women equally. The best chance the state has to protect fetuses is through actions to enhance the status of all women by fostering reasonable pay for the work they do and equal employment opportunities, and providing a reasonable social safety net, quality prenatal services, and day care programs. It is probably not coincidental that government is trying to blame the pregnant victims of poverty for their problems at the same time it is cutting funds for maternal and child health care and nutrition. If the state really wants to protect fetuses it should do so by improving the welfare of pregnant women—not by oppressing them.

Decision Scenario 1 . . . .

"I find it incredible that you plan on allowing yourself to be treated by a chiropractor," Martha Redpath said.

"What's the matter with going to a chiropractor?" Roger Smith asked. "I went to an M.D. and that didn't do any good. I haven't felt really good in years, but he told me there wasn't anything wrong with me."

"Chiropractors are frauds," Martha said. "They work on the basis of a false theory because they claim that all illnesses are caused either directly or indirectly by misalignments of the vertebrae. That is just sheer nonsense."

"Maybe so," said Roger. "But why shouldn't I go if it makes me feel better? I think they help a lot of people."

"Maybe they won't do you any harm. But in general they're dangerous. They keep a lot of people from getting competent medical treatment, because the people go see a chiropractor instead of a physician. Also, chiropractors often give a lot of X-rays, even though most of them aren't trained to do that, and that means that a great number of people receive massive doses of harmful radiation."

Ralph shook his head. "I don't say that you're wrong. But it seems to me that everybody ought to be free to choose the kind of treatment that he wants to get. If he thinks a chiropractor can do him some good, then he ought to be able to consult one."

"Look," Martha said, "I'm as much in favor of individual freedom as you are. But a lot of people just aren't well-enough informed to make good choices about their own medical care. I think that we should have laws that make chiropractic medicine illegal. We need to protect people from their own ignorance and from those who take advantage of it."

1. *Using the principles argued for by Dworkin, construct an argument in support of Martha's position.*

2. *Is regulation of the sort advocated by Martha compatible with Rawls's theory?*

3. *Do such regulations or laws violate the notion of the individual as an autonomous rational agent?*

Decision Scenario 2 ●

"I really don't understand you," Dr. Lowell said. "You definitely have cancer of the bladder. We may be able to remove it all surgically, but even if we can't, chemotherapy or radiation treatments have a good chance of success."

"I want none of those," Patricia Jenkins said. "I believe that a high-fiber diet and pure, filtered water are more likely to help me. I don't want to be cut or poisoned or burned."

"You're crazy," Dr. Lowell said. "That won't do anything."

"I intend to try it. Even if I'm wrong, it's my life."

"I won't let you," said Dr. Lowell. "Anybody who thinks the way you do about cancer is out of touch with reality. That's one of the marks of mental illness. And I intend to have you declared mentally incompetent to make decisions about your own welfare. I shall speak to the psychiatrists on our staff and ask the hospital lawyer to arrange for a sanity hearing."

"That's fascism!"

"Call it anything you like. But my duty as a physician is to give you the best medical care possible. If that means having you declared mentally incompetent, then so be it."

Dr. Lowell picked up the telephone.

1. *State and evaluate the argument Dr. Lowell offers to justify her intended course of action.*

2. *Dr. Lowell claims that it is her duty as a physician to provide Ms. Jenkins with the best medical care possible. If this is so, is it her only duty as a physician? Is there some other duty that conflicts with this one?*

3. *On what grounds might Dr. Lowell be accused of paternalism?*

4. *Suppose that Dr. Lowell is successful in her aims and that Ms. Jenkins has surgery and makes a good recovery. Would such an outcome justify her actions? If not, why not?*

Decision Scenario 3 ●

Angela Carter was diagnosed as having bone cancer when she was thirteen. Over the following years she received a variety of treatments and underwent surgery several times. In one operation, her leg was amputated. By the time she was twenty-seven the cancer had been in remission for three years, and she became pregnant. Twenty-five weeks into the pregnancy, she went for a routine checkup, and her physician discovered a large tumor in a lung. She was told she might have only days to live.

She was admitted to George Washington Hospital, and five days later her condition worsened. Despite the objections of Angela Carter, her family, and even her physicians, the hospital decided to

attempt to save the developing child. The hospital went to court, and at a hearing staff physicians stated that, despite the fact that the fetus was only twenty-six weeks old, there was a 50–60% chance that it would survive if a Caesarean section was performed. Furthermore, they estimated that there was a less than 20% chance that the child would be handicapped. The physicians also testified that the surgery would increase the chances of Angela Carter's death.

The hospital obtained a court order, which was immediately appealed. Because the case demanded a quick resolution, the three judges on appeals court consulted by telephone. The whole process, hearing and appeal, took less than six hours. During this time, the hospital had ordered Angela prepared for surgery.

The appeals court let the lower court ruling stand, and Angela underwent the court-ordered surgery. The child, a girl, lived for only two hours. Angela lived for two days. The surgery was listed as a contributing cause to her death.

1. *On what grounds might Annas object to the court-ordered surgery?*

2. *Is there any reason to view this case any differently than cases involving drug abuse by a pregnant woman? That is, are the issues the same in both kinds of cases?*

3. *Suppose Angela Carter had been further along in her pregnancy so that the chance of her child's surviving was virtually certain. If she refused to have a Caesarian, would it be justifiable to subject her to one anyway?*

4. *Is it possible, without inconsistency, to recognize that a woman has a right to seek an abortion, yet also hold that a woman has a duty to act in the best interest of the developing fetus?*

Decision Scenario 4 . . . .

"You realize that I talked to him for only fifteen or twenty minutes," said Dr. Susan Beck.

"Yeah, but you psychiatrists are supposed to be able to size up a guy just by listening to how he says hello," Dr. Mark Brunetti said.

"Now that I've talked to him, tell me more about him," Beck said.

"I presume you learned his name is T. D. Chang?"

"That was written down for me."

"Fine," said Brunetti. "He's fifty-two years old, a professor of Asian History at Southwestern University. He's married, has two children in college, and has a solid scholarly reputation."

"What was his complaint?" asked Beck.

"About a month ago he began to experience difficult and painful urination. His attending examined him, found that he had an enlarged prostate, and treated with sulfa. No joy. So the attending sent him here. We're doing an X-ray scan and a punch biopsy in the morning."

"And you want me to tell you how I think he'll take it if you tell him you suspect cancer?"

"Right," said Brunetti. "I don't like to scare people unless I have to. My inclination here is just to keep quiet until we know for sure."

"I think he would take it all right. He shows no tendency toward hysteria, and his background reveals him to be a person who functions well under normal conditions of stress."

"Good, then if I have to tell him, I won't worry about it."

"Mark, do you mean you're not going to tell him?"

"That's right. Not until I know for sure. It's a kindness to him. What he doesn't know won't hurt him, and there's no reason to cause him unnecessary anxiety."

"I don't think I agree with that decision," Beck said. "I think a man like Mr. Chang has a right to know as much about his condition as you do. "

"That's silly," Brunetti said. "He can't possibly know as much as I do, and he wouldn't know what to make of the information even if I gave it to him. He would probably figure he's going to die in the next hour."

"So you aren't going to tell him what you suspect or why you're doing the biopsy?"

"I'm not that cruel, even if I am a surgeon."

1. *Do the arguments presented by Lipkin support Brunetti's views? State the arguments explicitly and, if possible, relate them to this example.*

2. *Using Bok's line of reasoning, what criticisms might be made of the position taken by Brunetti?*

3. *Is it reasonable to believe that Mr. Chang might be able to understand and assess the significance of the medical information relevant to the procedures planned?*

4. *What might an act or rule utilitarian say about this situation?*

Decision Scenario 5 ••••••••••••••••••••••••••••••

Multiple sclerosis is a chronic, progressive, neurological disease with symptoms that include loss of coordination, blurred vision, speech difficulties, and severe fatigue. It is most frequent among young adults. A study at Albert Einstein Medical College revealed that MS patients typically had a very hard time getting an explicit diagnosis and explanation from their physicians. Yet the physicians surveyed reported overwhelmingly that they always or usually tell patients the diagnosis.

The researchers learned that a variety of factors account for this discrepancy. Physicians find many reasons for delay—the patient may be under twenty, emotionally unstable, or apparently incapable of understanding the diagnosis. Also, the patient may not ask specifically, a relative may ask that the patient not be told, the patient may be medically unsophisticated or in the midst of an emotional crisis. Most important, there is no cure or wholly effective therapy for MS, and emotional stress seems to aggravate its symptoms. Telling a patient that she or he has a progressive, incurable disease may do no good and may do harm.

Patients are frequently told that they have "a chronic virus infection," "neuritis," and "inflammation of the nervous system," instead of being told they have MS. This sometimes leads patients to consult several physicians and to undergo expensive and unnecessary diagnostic tests in the attempt to get a diagnosis.

1. *Are the physicians who claim they believe in telling MS patients the diagnosis but then don't do so necessarily being hypocritical?*

2. *What sort of arguments or considerations might Lipkin offer in their defense?*

3. *In what sort of cases, according to Bok's arguments, would it be justifiable to withhold a diagnosis from a patient?*

4. *If there is a chance that knowing the diagnosis will make the symptoms of an MS patient worse and if there is no wholly effective therapy for MS, why is it not the duty of a physician to withhold the diagnosis? After all, "Do no harm" is perhaps the most important of the Hippocratic maxims.*

Decision Scenario 6 •••••••••••••••••••••••••••••

Charles Lofton was a thirty-four-year-old systems analyst who was admitted to Towson Memorial Hospital with a diagnosis of testicular cancer. An intensely private man, Lofton seemed to be as embarrassed by his disease as he was frightened by the impending surgery.

"I want you to guarantee me that an absolute minimum number of people will be told what's wrong with me," he said to Dr. Samuel Shem. "I know the surgeon and the surgical team have to find out, obviously, and maybe three or four nurses, but I would like for that to be all. I don't want people on the staff talking about me."

"I understand how you must feel," Dr. Shem said. "But I have to be honest with you and tell you that a fairly large number of people will have to know about the disease and the surgery."

"How many are you talking about?"

"I don't know for sure. But there are three nursing shifts with eight nurses on each shift. I can't be here all the time so we're talking about the house staff, and that's another two or three people. Then there are some committee reviews involving several people."

"You must be talking about fifty people," Lofton said.

"I wouldn't be surprised."

"Isn't there anything that can be done to protect my privacy?" Lofton asked.

1. *Why is confidentiality important to good medical practice?*

2. *What are some of the more serious threats posed to confidentiality in contemporary medicine?*

3. *Does confidentiality have a different meaning in the current medical setting? That is, does it have to be understood as involving something other than a personal and private relationship with a physician?*

4. *What proposals does Siegler make in order to resolve some of the problems of maintaining a patient's confidentiality?*

5. *If Siegler's proposals were adopted, would confidentiality of the traditional sort be preserved?*

Decision Scenario 7 · · · · · · · · · · · · · · ·

Jane Montrose told herself that it was just one of the things you had to do if you wanted to get promoted. Talking to eleven department heads might be a bore, but so far they had all been quite nice. And it wasn't even a bad idea. If she were going to be working as an assistant vice-president, she would have to deal with all of these people frequently. It made sense for them to have an opportunity to say whether they would feel comfortable working with her.

"How did you learn so much about computers?" Art Davis asked her.

It was a question people always asked. For some reason, they invariably seemed surprised to learn that a woman was comfortable dealing with the mysteries of data processing.

"I have a degree in computer science," she said. "Besides, I've been working with computers for about eight years now. You get to know their ways."

Davis nodded and smiled at her. She was somewhat surprised that he would ask such a naive question. As head of personnel, he more than anyone knew about her educational background and her work history. She wondered if he wasn't just stalling, making polite conversation until he could ask what really interested him.

"How are you doing with your psychiatrist?" Davis asked.

Jane was totally surprised by the question. She had assumed that only her closest friends knew she had been going to a psychiatrist.

"Fine," she said. "I mean, I've been able to work through a lot of problems that were bothering me."

She didn't really want to talk to Davis about her feelings of depression and lack of self-worth that had been troubling her for the last few years. None of it was any of his business.

"Do you think you'll be able to handle new responsibilities? This is a pretty important job you're being considered for, you know."

"I can handle them. I've always done very well at whatever job I've worked at."

"I know you have," Davis said. "But when we see that an employee has been going to a psychia-

trist . . . well, that makes us wonder if that person is really to be trusted with a lot of responsibility. I'm sure you understand."

"I don't really. I don't see what my personal problems have to do with my work, assuming they don't get in the way of my doing it. And they never have."

Davis smiled at her in a way that made her very angry. It was the kind of tolerant but superior smile adults usually reserve for children who are talking about things they don't understand.

"What I want to know," Jane said, "is how you knew about my seeing a psychiatrist. I thought my medical records were all confidential."

"They are, so far as I know. But you did put in an insurance claim for payment, and I have to sign off on all the claims. When I did that, I saw you were getting psychiatric help."

"Are you going to make that public?"

"Not public," Davis said. "But I do feel obliged to mention it to the Executive Planning Group. If they're thinking about promoting you, then that's something they ought to know. I'm surprised you didn't volunteer the information yourself."

"I didn't think it was relevant," Jane said. "I didn't tell them I also suffer from hemorrhoids."

"Well, we'll let them judge whether it's relevant."

1. *Does Davis have an obligation to inform the Executive Planning Group that Jane Montrose is receiving psychiatric treatment?*

2. *In New York, employees of the state government have the right to send medical claims for psychiatric or psychological services directly to the insurance company. Should this be made a legal right for all employees in all states?*

3. *The so-called Privacy Protection Act of 1980 permits federal law-enforcement agencies to secure search warrants and gain access to all private records, except those of the media. Should the Act be restricted to exclude medical and mental-health records?*

Decision Scenario 8 · · · · · · · · · · · · · · ·

In 1985 investigators from the Massachusetts Attorney General's office secured permission from the

state courts to examine the notes taken during patient sessions by psychiatrist Kennard C. Kobrin of

Fall River, Massachusetts. Dr. Kobrin was suspected of Medicaid fraud, and the state's Assistant Attorney General Michelle Kacynski argued before the Supreme Judicial Court that the patient's rights to privacy must be set aside in favor of the public's need to know. "We believe that the state should have access to records which may or may not verify that Dr. Kobrin has provided certain services to certain patients on certain dates," she said.

Dr. Kobrin's patients openly protested the violation of their privacy and the fact that some of their records are now in open court files. "I feel kind of humiliated and upset," one of them said. "If you go to see a doctor, and it's supposed to be confidential, that's why you go. If it wasn't, you could tell a friend, and they could blab it all over the city." Although last names have been deleted from the public records, Fall River is a city of only 92,500, and

some of the information in the records would make it possible to identify the patients by name.

Massachusetts state laws protect private conversations between patients and therapists, but the laws regulating Medicaid are federal laws. There are no federal laws protecting a confidential privilege for patient communication.

1. *Is there a solution to the problem posed by Ms. Kacynski? If the public's interest is to be protected, isn't it necessary to set aside the individual's right to privacy?*

2. *If it is possible that a therapist's notes might be made part of a public record, what effect is this likely to have on therapy?*

3. *Should there be a federal law guaranteeing confidentiality for patient communication?*

Decision Scenario 9 . . . .

"Sometimes I think that what I really want to do is to kill people and drink their blood."

Dr. Allen Wolfe looked at the young man in the chair across from him. The face was round and soft and innocent looking, like that of a large baby. But the body had the powerful shoulders of a college wrestler. There was no doubt that Hal Crane had the strength to carry out his fantasies.

"Any people in particular?" Dr. Wolfe asked.

"Women. Girls about my age. Maybe their early twenties."

"But no one you're personally acquainted with."

"That's right. Just girls I see walking down the street or getting off a bus. I have a tremendous urge to stick a knife into their stomachs and feel the blood come out on my hands."

"But you've never done anything like that?"

Crane shook his head. "No, but I'm afraid I might."

Dr. Wolfe considered Crane a paranoid schizophrenic with compulsive tendencies, someone who might possibly act out his fantasies. He was a potentially dangerous person.

"Would you be willing to take my advice and put yourself in a hospital under my care for a while?"

"I don't want to do that," Crane said. "I don't want to be locked up like an animal."

"But you don't really want to hurt other people, do you?"

"I guess not," Crane said. "But I haven't done anything yet."

"But you might," Dr. Wolfe said. "I'm afraid you might let yourself go and kill someone."

Crane smiled. "That's just the chance the world will have to take, isn't it? I told you I'm not going to let myself be locked up."

1. *Suppose that you are Dr. Wolfe. To take the legal steps necessary to have Mr. Crane committed against his will requires that you violate confidentiality. What justification might a utilitarian offer for doing this?*

2. *Might a Kantian oppose commitment on the grounds that it would violate Crane's dignity as a person?*

3. *As a physician, how would you justify acting to protect others while going against the wishes of your patient?*

4. *Should a physician be required by law to act to protect the welfare of others?*

5. *How does this case compare with the Tarasoff case discussed by Curran? What actions, on Curran's view, should be taken by Dr. Wolfe?*

CHAPTER 6

MEDICAL EXPERIMENTATION AND ☐
INFORMED CONSENT

CASE PRESENTATION
Baby Fae

On October 14, 1984, a baby was born in a community hospital in southern California with a malformation known as hypoplastic left-heart syndrome. In such a condition, the mitral valve or aorta on the left side of the heart is underdeveloped, and essentially only the right side of the heart functions properly. Some 300 to 2,000 infants a year are born with this defect, and most die from it within a few weeks.

The infant, who became known to the public as Baby Fae, was taken to the Loma Linda University Hospital Center. There, on October 26, a surgical team headed by Dr. Leonard Bailey performed a heart transplant; Baby Fae became the first human infant to receive a baboon heart. She died twenty days later.

Baby Fae was not the first human to receive a so-called xenograft, or cross-species transplant. In early 1964, a sixty-eight-year-old man was transplanted with a chimpanzee heart at the University of Mississippi Medical Center. The heart failed after only an hour, and the patient died. Before Baby Fae, three other cross-species transplants had also ended in a quick death.

In the case of Baby Fae, questions about the moral correctness and scientific legitimacy of the transplant were raised immediately. Hospital officials revealed that no effort had been made to find a human donor before implanting the baboon heart, and this led some critics to wonder if research interests were not being given priority over the welfare of the patient. Others questioned whether the parents were adequately informed about alternative corrective surgery, the Norwood procedure, available in Boston and Philadelphia.

Other observers wondered whether the nature of the surgery and its limited value had been prop-

erly explained to the parents. Also, some critics raised objections to sacrificing a healthy young animal as part of an experiment not likely to bring any lasting benefit to Baby Fae.

Scientific critics charged that not enough is known about crossing the species barrier to warrant the use of transplant organs at this time. The previous record of failures, with no major advances in understanding, did not make the prospect of another such transplant reasonable. Furthermore, critics said, chimpanzees and gorillas are genetically more similar to humans than baboons, so the choice of a baboon heart was not a wise one. The only advantage of baboons is that they are easier to breed in captivity. Also, one critic suggested that Dr. Bailey was merely engaged in "wishful thinking" in believing that Baby Fae's immune system would not produce a severe rejection response because of its immaturity.

An autopsy on Baby Fae showed that her death was caused by the incompatibility of her blood with that of the baboon heart. Baby Fae's blood was type O, the baboon's type AB. This resulted in the formation of blood clots and the destruction of kidney function. The heart showed mild signs of rejection.

In an address before a medical conference after Baby Fae's death, Dr. Bailey commented on some of the criticisms. He is reported to have said that it was "an oversight on our part not to search for a human donor from the start." Dr. Bailey also told the conference that he and his team believed that the difference in blood types between Baby Fae and the baboon would be less important than other factors and that the immunosuppressive drugs used to prevent rejection would also solve the problem of blood incompatibility. "We came to regret those assumptions," Dr. Bailey said. The failure to match blood types was "a tactical error that came back to haunt us."

On other occasions Dr. Bailey reiterated his view that, because infant donors are extremely scarce, animal-to-human transplants offer a realistic hope for the future. Before the Baby Fae operation, Dr. Bailey had transplanted organs in more than 150 animals. He indicated that he would use the information obtained from Baby Fae to conduct additional animal experiments before attempting another such transplant.

In March of 1985 the National Institutes of Health released a report of a committee that made a site visit to Loma Linda to review the Baby Fae matter. The committee found that the informed-consent process was generally satisfactory, in that "the parents were given an appropriate and thorough explanation of the alternatives available, the risks and benefits of the procedure and the experimental nature of the transplant." Moreover, consent was obtained in an "atmosphere which allowed the parents an opportunity to carefully consider, without coercion or undue influence, whether to give permission for the transplant."

The committee also pointed out certain flaws in the consent document. First, it "did not include the possibility of searching for a human heart or performing a human heart transplant." Second, the expected benefits of the procedure "appeared to be overstated," because the consent document "stated that 'long-term survival' is an expected possibility with no further explanation." Finally, the document did not explain "whether compensation and medical treatment were available if injury occurred."

The committee did not question the legitimacy of the cross-species transplant. Moreover, it made no mention of the Norwood procedure, except to say that it had been explained to the mother at the community hospital at the birth of the infant. (The consent document described the procedure as a generally unsuccessful "temporizing operation.")

Although the committee was generally critical of the university's Institutional Review Board in "evaluating the entire informed-consent process," it reached the conclusion that "the parents of Baby Fae understood the alternative available as well as the risks and reasonably expected benefits of the transplant."

Officials at Loma Linda University Medical Center promised that before performing another such transplant they would first seek a human infant heart donor.

CASE PRESENTATION
The Willowbrook Hepatitis Experiments

The Willowbrook State School in Staten Island, New York, is an institution devoted to housing and caring for mentally retarded children. In 1956 a research group led by Saul Krugman and Joan P. Giles of the New York University School of Medicine initiated a long-range study of viral hepatitis at Willowbrook. The children confined there were made experimental subjects of the study.

Hepatitis is a disease affecting the liver that is now known to be caused by one of two (possibly more) viruses. Although the viruses are distinct, the results they produce are the same. The liver becomes inflamed and increases in size as the invading viruses replicate themselves. Also, part of the tissue of the liver may be destroyed and the liver's normal functions impaired. Often the flow of bile through the ducts is blocked, and bilirubin (the major pig-

ment in bile) is forced into the blood and urine. This produces the symptom of yellowish or jaundiced skin.

The disease is generally relatively mild, although permanent liver damage can be produced. The symptoms are ordinarily flulike—mild fever, tiredness, inability to keep food down. The viruses causing the disease are transmitted orally through contact with the feces and bodily secretions of infected people.

Krugman and Giles were interested in determining the natural history of viral hepatitis—the mode of infection and the course of the disease over time. They also wanted to test the effectiveness of gamma globulin as an agent for inoculating against hepatitis. (Gamma globulin is a protein complex extracted from the blood serum that contains antigens, substances that trigger the production of specific antibodies to counter infectious agents.)

Krugman and Giles considered Willowbrook to be a good choice for investigation because viral hepatitis occurred more or less constantly in the institution. In the jargon of medicine, the disease was endemic. That this was so was recognized in 1949, and it continued to be so as the number of children in the school increased to over 5,000 in 1960. Krugman and Giles claimed that "under the chronic circumstances of multiple and repeated exposure . . . most newly admitted children became infected within the first six to twelve months of residence in the institution."

Over a fourteen-year period, Krugman and Giles collected over 25,000 serum specimens from more than 700 patients. Samples were taken before exposure, during the incubation period of the virus, and for periods after the infection. In an effort to get the kind of precise data they considered most useful, Krugman and Giles decided to deliberately infect some of the incoming children with the strain of the hepatitis virus prevalent at Willowbrook.

They justified their decision in the following way:

> It was inevitable that susceptible children would become infected in the institution. Hepatitis was especially mild in the 3- to 10-year age group at Willowbrook. These studies would be carried out in a special unit with optimum isolation facilities to protect the children from other infectious diseases such as shigellosis [dysentery caused by a bacillus], and parasitic and respiratory infections which are prevalent in the institution.

Most important, Krugman and Giles claimed that being an experimental subject was in the best medical interest of the child, for not only would the child receive special care, but infection with the milder form of hepatitis would provide protection against the more virulent and damaging forms. As they say: "It should be emphasized that the artificial induction of hepatitis implies a 'therapeutic' effect because of the immunity which is conferred."

Krugman and Giles obtained what they considered to be adequate consent from the parents of the children used as subjects. Where they were unable to obtain consent, they did not include the child in the experiment. In the earlier phases of the study, parents were provided with relevant information either by letter or orally, and written consent was secured from them. In the later phases, a group procedure was used:

> First, a psychiatric social worker discusses the project with the parents during a preliminary interview. Those who are interested are invited to attend a group session at the institution to discuss the project in greater detail. These sessions are conducted by the staff responsible for the program, including the physician, supervising nurses, staff attendants, and psychiatric social workers. . . . Parents in groups of six to eight are given a tour of the facilities. The purposes, potential benefits, and potential hazards of the program are discussed with them, and they are encouraged to ask questions. Thus, all parents can hear the response to questions posed by the more articulate members of the group. After leaving this briefing session parents have an opportunity to talk with their private physicians who may call the unit for more information. Approximately two weeks after each visit, the psychiatric social worker contacts the parents for their decision. If the decision is in the affirmative, the consent is signed but parents are informed that signed consent may be withdrawn any time before the beginning of the program. It has been clear that the group method has enabled us to obtain more thorough informed consent. Children who are wards of the state or children without parents have never been included in our studies.

Krugman and Giles point out that their studies have been reviewed and approved by the New York State Department of Mental Hygiene, the New York State Department of Mental Health, the Armed Forces Epidemiological Board, and the human-experimentation committees of the New York University School of Medicine and the Willowbrook School. They also stress that, although they were under no obligation to do so, they chose to meet the World Medical Association's Draft Code on Human Experimentation.

The value of the research conducted by Krugman and Giles has been recognized as significant in furthering a scientific understanding of viral hepatitis and methods for treating it. Yet serious moral doubts have been raised about the nature and conduct of the experiments. In particular, many have questioned the use of retarded children as experimental subjects, some claiming that children should never be experimental subjects in investigations that are not directly therapeutic. Others have raised questions about the ways in which consent was obtained from the parents of the children, suggesting that parents were implicitly blackmailed into giving their consent. The letters to the British medical journal *Lancet* and the selection from Paul Ramsey's *The Patient as Person* presented in this chapter discuss these issues.

CASE PRESENTATION
The Detroit Psychosurgery Case

Lafayette Clinic is a research facility in Detroit that is part of the Michigan Department of Mental Health. In 1972, the director of the clinic was Dr. J. S. Gottlieb, a psychiatrist, and its chief of neurology was Dr. Ernst Rodin. Both Rodin and Gottlieb had read the book *Violence and the Brain*, by V. H. Mark and F. R. Ervin, shortly after its publication in 1970. They discussed the work and agreed that some of the techniques it described might be useful in treating patients suffering from uncontrollable sexual and aggressive impulses.

Rodin wrote a description of a research project they might conduct: "Proposal for the Study of the Treatment of Uncontrollable Aggression at Lafayette Clinic." The research was to involve a comparative study of the value of surgical versus drug treatment of aggressive patients. The surgical part of the project proposed implanting depth-electrodes in the brains of twelve subjects to study their brain activity and to attempt to locate areas of electrical abnormality. If such an area was found and if, by brain stimulation, it could be linked to aggressive behavior, then stereotactic surgery would be performed. (Stereotactic surgery involves locating relatively precise areas by using careful measurements.) The target areas would then be either resectioned (cut out) or destroyed by electrocoagulation. The ultimate aim of the project was said to be to restore patients to a "useful life" in the community.

The proposal, which requested $164,000, was submitted to the State Department of Mental Health. It was approved and included in the Department's legislative budget request. Although the state legislature held two hearings, no questions were raised about the Rodin proposal. The money was made available in July 1972.

Even before the allocation of funds, a search was being conducted for suitable subjects. The candidates were those confined in state institutions under the Michigan "Criminal Sexual Psychopath" law. These were people charged with serious sex crimes who were not prosecuted but confined involuntarily for an indeterminate period of time until considered sufficiently "cured" for release.

One such person, identified for the record only as John Doe, was approached by Dr. E. G. Yudashkin, the director of Ionia State Hospital, where Doe was confined. Yudashkin described the project to Doe and told him he would probably be released within six months or a year whether or not he participated. But he also pointed out that successful treatment in the research project would lead to an even speedier release.

Doe was not interested in the drug part of the research program but thought he might volunteer for the surgical part. Yudashkin and two staff physicians explained to him on three occasions what this might involve. But the knowledge of the physicians on this topic was not extensive, and Doe later testified that they gave him a misleadingly simple account. But, at the time, Doe decided to consent to becoming a subject, and Rodin was informed of this.

Rodin had decided that it was necessary to broaden the population of candidates from which subjects were to be selected. He had gone to Boston and talked with Vernon Mark about the project, and Mark had been critical of the ethical aspects. Rodin wrote in a memo to Gottlieb:

> When I informed Mr. Mark of our project, namely doing amygdalotomies on patients who do not have epilepsy, he became extremely concerned and stated we had no ethical right in so doing. . . . I then retorted that he was misleading us with his previously cited book and he had no right at all from a scientific point of view to state that in the human, aggression is accompanied by seizure discharges in the amygdala, because he is dealing only with patients who have susceptible brains, namely, temporal lobe epilepsy. . . .
>
> He stated categorically that as far as present evidence is concerned, one has no right to make

lesions in a "healthy brain" when the individual suffers from rage attacks only.

Rodin discussed this matter with colleagues, and they decided not to do surgery on patients without verifiable organic brain dysfunctions. They expanded the population to be considered to include retarded, epileptic, and self-mutilating patients.

Lafayette Clinic's Human and Animal Experimentation Committee reviewed the project description and procedures and a draft of the informed-consent form. The committee, charged with protecting the rights and welfare of experimental subjects, raised no questions about the moral issues in the project. They approved it in October of 1972.

The project, as approved, required establishing two review committees to supervise patient selection and to protect patients from unethical practices. The three-member Medical Review Committee was to consider the medical condition and history of potential subjects recommended by Rodin. They were to eliminate patients unsuitable from a medical standpoint. After screening, a three-member Human Rights Review Committee was to determine for each patient whether informed consent was adequate and whether any rights were being infringed. After approval by both committees, a patient would then be given a consent form and a detailed explanation of the procedure to be performed on him. Then he and his family would have a week to consider whether they wished to sign the consent form.

None of this procedure was followed in the case of John Doe. Rodin met with John Doe on October 27. They discussed Doe's medical history for an hour, and at the end Doe indicated that he still wanted to participate in the project as a subject. Rodin read him the consent form, which read in part:

> Since conventional treatment efforts over a period of several years have not enabled me to control my outbursts of rage and anti-social behavior, I submit an application to be a subject in a research project which may offer me a form of effective therapy. This therapy is based upon the idea that episodes of anti-social rage and sexuality might be triggered by a disturbance in certain portions of my brain. I understand that in order to be certain that a significant brain disturbance exists, which might relate to my anti-social behavior, an initial operation will have to be performed. This procedure consists of placing

fine wires into my brain, which will record the electrical activity from those structures which play a part in anger and sexuality. These electrical waves can then be studied to determine the presence of an abnormality.

> In addition electrical stimulation with weak currents passed through these wires will be done in order to find out if one or several points in the brain can trigger my episodes of violence or unlawful sexuality. In other words this stimulation may cause me to want to commit an aggressive or sexual act, but every effort will be made to have a sufficient number of people present to control me. If the brain disturbance is limited to a small area, I understand that the investigators will destroy this part of my brain with an electrical current. If the abnormality comes from a larger part of my brain, I agree that it should be surgically removed, if the doctors determine that it can be done so, without risk of side effects. Should the electrical activity from the parts of my brain into which the wires have been placed reveal that there is no significant abnormality, the wires will simply be withdrawn.

Rodin talked about the meanings of the terms in the form and explained the risks of the surgical procedures.

Later, John Doe was allowed to call his parents. The only explanation they received before signing the consent form was from him. Doe believed that he was agreeing only to implantation of depth-electrodes and not to stereotactic surgery. He thought that additional consent would be required for surgery. He and his parents signed the form.

Eventually, after the signing, both committees were given materials relating to John Doe. The members of the committees were all picked by Rodin. The medical committee never met, but each member considered the materials submitted by Rodin. The Human Rights Committee also examined the materials individually. Thus, neither committee ever met to discuss Doe's case, nor did any member of either committee talk with Doe.

John Doe was the only patient located to participate in the entire research program. Yet by the end of December, all the committee reviews were completed, and plans were made to implant the electrodes in John Doe's brain in early January.

Before this could happen, the process was brought to a halt. A psychiatric resident at Lafayette Clinic was bothered by the secret way in which the project was being run. He expressed these concerns to Gabe Kaimowitz, an attorney for the Michigan

Medical Committee for Human Rights. In early January, Kaimowitz filed a petition and complaint with the Wayne County Circuit Court that asked that the state Department of Mental Health be required to "show cause . . . why they should not be enjoined from performing psychosurgery or using chemotherapy on persons involuntarily confined in the state hospital system in order to study 'uncontrollable aggression' or for any other similar purpose." Kaimowitz also asked that a writ of habeas corpus be issued to release John Doe and others from state hospitals because they were not receiving treatment.

Soon afterward, the Department of Mental Health decided to cancel funding for the Rodin project. But the court decided that the legal issues were not moot and that the case should be heard. On March 23, the court also decided that the Criminal Sexual Psychopath law, under which John Doe had been committed, was unconstitutional. The court ordered him released, and John Doe was freed from Ionia State Hospital after eighteen years of confinement.

The court then heard arguments on the major legal and moral issues of the complaint. For the first time, a court was being asked to give an opinion on the legitimacy of psychosurgery and other experimental treatment methods involving people involuntarily confined to institutions.

On July 10, 1973, the court ruled that an involuntarily detained adult in a facility of the State Department of Mental Health cannot give legally adequate consent to "an innovative or experimental surgical procedure on the brain." The court was careful to point out that its ruling was based upon the state of knowledge about psychosurgery at the time of the decision. Furthermore, the court emphasized that an involuntary mental patient can give adequate consent to accepted neurological procedures. In the court's view, then, the type of neurosurgery proposed for Doe was not of the character to which he could give proper consent.

SOCIAL CONTEXT: THE ARTIFICIAL HEART: CONSENT TO DISASTER?

On April 4, 1969, Haskell Karp, a forty-seven-year-old printing estimator from Illinois, be-came the first patient in history to receive an artificial heart. For sixty-three hours the device maintained Karp's blood pressure and circulation; then a transplanted heart was put in its place. Karp died some twenty hours after receiving the transplant.

The surgery was performed at St. Luke's Hospital in Houston by Denton Cooley. Cooley claimed in television interviews after the surgery that he had implanted the artificial device as a desperate measure, because Mr. Karp was dying on the operating table and a donor heart was not available. During the interviews, Cooley made a plea for the donation of a heart to transplant into Mr. Karp.

Almost immediately Cooley's actions became the center of a storm of controversy. In deciding to use the artificial heart, Cooley had consulted no one but his patient. Although a member of the faculty of Baylor University, Cooley had not sought permission from Michael DeBakey, the head of the artificial heart program, nor had he brought the issue before the university's human-subjects committee.

In hearings held before various committees charged with investigating the matter, other charges and criticisms emerged. Most seriously, Cooley was said to have acted unethically by implanting "an unproved device . . . into a human being for primary experimentation before its safety and effectiveness" had been "proved scientifically in animal experiments." Cooley replied that the device had been tested in seven calves; although all had died, one had lived for forty-four hours. That, Cooley claimed, was enough to justify going forward with using the device in humans. Besides, he said, the device was used because his patient was dying, and no other option was available. The artificial heart was there and ready to use. "Everything came together at once," Cooley said.

Cooley insisted that his experience in heart surgery was the only real grounds for his decision: "Based on this experience, I believe I am qualified to judge what is right and proper for my patients. The permission I receive to do what I do, I receive from my patients. It is not received from a government agency or from one of my seniors."

Critics charged that Cooley had actually engineered the whole episode to seek publicity for himself. DeBakey claimed that Cooley had not made an appeal for a donor heart until after he had performed the operation and gone on television. Furthermore, the situation was not the life-or-death one that Cooley claimed. One surgeon said that Cooley had asked him to participate in the surgery days before it took place. Also, Cooley had planned enough in advance to have the console power source for the heart available and to have movie cameras in place to make a complete record of the operation.

At the end of the inquiry, Cooley was found guilty by the local medical society on eight counts of seeking publicity, but no other disciplinary actions were taken against him. He resigned from Baylor because of his unwillingness to sign National Institutes of Health guidelines on experimental human surgery. He explained that if he did so he would feel that he was giving in to DeBakey, his major critic.

Cooley continued to practice surgery at his Texas Heart Institute, and at medical meetings he was in much demand as a speaker on the Karp operation. Although Karp's widow sued Cooley on the grounds that he had failed to secure a proper consent form for the unprecedented procedure, the courts held that the procedure was primarily therapeutic and not experimental.

The artificial heart program at Baylor was part of a research effort initiated in 1964 by the National Heart, Lung, and Blood Institute of NIH. The head of NIH, James Shannon, had opposed the program on the grounds that not enough was known to make the technology workable and reliable. Michael DeBakey was a strong advocate of the research, however, and convinced Congress that it should be funded. As DeBakey recalled almost fifteen years later: "Jim Shannon was opposed to the concept and NIH's involvement in it, because he thought there wasn't enough basic knowledge and it wasn't scientifically sound. I went over his head to Congress."

The initial aim of the new federal program was to develop a completely implantable artificial heart by 1970, but this goal turned out to be unrealistic. Research then focused on the development of a reliable, externally powered device as a necessary first step.

The controversy around the Cooley affair had subsided before the next major event occurred. In 1982 Barney Clark, a retired dentist, became the first person to receive an implanted artificial heart intended to be permanent. The surgery was performed with federal Food and Drug Administration approval and only after extensive animal testing had taken place. William C. DeVries of the University of Utah Medical Center was the head of the surgical team. Clark received the Jarvik-7 heart, and despite numerous complications he lived for 112 days.

After Barney Clark's, DeVries performed three more permanent implants. An additional implant was made in Sweden so that a total of five were done. Everyone given a permanent implant died. The major problem appeared to be that small blood clots formed on the surface or valves of the artificial heart; when these clots broke off, they blocked blood flow to the brain and caused disabling strokes.

William J. Schroeder lived longer than anyone else with an artificial heart—620 days. However, he suffered three strokes, was often in a coma-like state, and, when aroused, was able to say only a few words. Other medical problems, such as recurrent infections due to the suppression of the immune system, internal bleeding, and respiratory difficulties, affected Mr. Schroeder and all other implant recipients.

The very poor quality of life that the artificial heart provided to patients did not make it a realistic alternative to heart transplants. As DeVries himself remarked, "There is no question that if you have a choice, you have a transplant. Transplants are therapeutic reality and they are good, whereas the artificial heart is still a very highly experimental thing."

DeVries also pointed out that for patients not eligible for transplants because of their age or because they had diseases like pulmonary hypertension, the artificial heart offered the only therapy possible. He mentioned William Schroeder as an example of someone who had a poor quality of life but was at least alive and capable of having experiences that otherwise he would have missed. He was able to enjoy the birth of his grandson, celebrate birthdays, and be present at family gatherings. "We lose track of the fact that he would have been dead" without the artificial heart, DeVries pointed out.

Even at the height of its public acclaim, critics of the artificial heart program charged that the device should not be used as a permanent implant. In their view, even when the surgery was successful and the device functions properly, the quality of life that it provided was so poor that there was no justification for keeping people alive by such means. The device should be used only as a temporary measure to keep patients alive until a donor heart for transplant could be secured.

Other critics were even more severe in their strictures and argued for a moratorium on the use of the artificial heart. They pointed out that even when the device was used as a temporary bridge to a transplant, results were mixed and a significant number of patients died. Strong evidence suggested that, the longer a patient had an implant, the worse his physical condition became.

Furthermore, the cost of using the artificial heart was staggeringly high. Even when the device was used as a temporary bridge, treatment cost tens of thousands of dollars per patient. If complications developed or if the patient had to remain on the device for an extended period of time, the costs then mounted to hundreds of thousands of dollars. Far more lives could be saved, critics said, by using these resources to prevent heart disease through the funding of programs aimed at improving diet, promoting exercise, or eliminating smoking.

In May 1988, Claude Lenfant, Director of NIH, announced that he was canceling federal funds for research on the artificial heart. "The human body just couldn't seem to tolerate it," he said, citing the many medical problems mentioned by critics. Lenfant did not eliminate money for the support of the left-ventricular assist device or other heart-related technology.

William DeVries, who had now moved to Humana Hospital in Louisville, Kentucky, objected to the cancellation on the grounds that it would halt or interrupt the work of many outstanding researchers who had made long-term commitments to developing the artificial heart. DeVries claimed that he would continue his work without federal funding, although the lack of NIH approval would make it difficult to raise private money.

Others saw the cancellation of federal support as long overdue. During its twenty-four years, the program consumed $240 million in research funds. Important devices like the intra-aortic balloon pump, blood-flow meters, and oxygenators came from the research program, but in the view of critics the costs were completely out of line with the value.

The artificial heart program has strong defenders who would like to see it revived. Whether it should be remains a serious social question. In addition, while research was in progress, the use of the device was morally controversial in a number of respects. As an experimental therapy it raised serious questions about consent, participation, and termination. The questions remain genuine, even though the program is no longer supported. In the debate over whether the research program should be reinstituted, the moral questions are particularly relevant. If the research itself is ethically objectionable, this is a powerful—perhaps even decisive—argument against it. We may look to the past to help guide us in the future.

When should an experimental therapy be ended? In the case of the artificial heart, this question is especially relevant, because it may involve turning off the power supply and allowing the patient to die. Barney Clark was given a key to turn off his power source; in principle, he would have been able to terminate the experiment at any time of his choosing. However, because of his stroke and his deteriorated physical condition, very soon after the implant he was not considered mentally competent to make decisions about his own treatment. Decisions involving consent were made by his wife. In practice, Clark's case, as well as the others, suggests that, once a person has agreed to a permanent implant, he is likely to be incapable of exercising any control over the future course of his life.

If this is so, then who should decide when the experiment is to be stopped? Should the patient be allowed to stipulate before the surgery under what conditions he would want the experiment discontinued? Should the physician be allowed to continue the experiment against the wishes of a family member? Furthermore, is turning off an artificial heart no different from turning off a respirator? Or does the certainty of death in the case of the heart make the action different in a morally relevant way? These and others like them are basic questions that were never resolved by researchers in the artificial heart program.

Since the artificial heart was a therapy involving so many risks and uncertainties, it was made available only to those not likely to benefit from established therapies. It was a therapy of last resort. This alone meant that candidates who nominated themselves to become recipients were likely to agree to accept any risks spelled out for them. Dr. DeVries reported that all four of his implant patients "told me in their own way that they didn't care" whether they read the consent form or not. "They were not really interested in listening to the long list of horrors that could happen to them," he said. "They didn't want to hear that they may have a stroke and be unable to use all mental capabilities. Those are issues that they would rather be left unsaid."

In a sense, such people can be regarded as coerced by their own diseases and their own desperation. In such a circumstance, the very notion of informed consent seems to lose the significance ordinarily attached to it. Given that this is so and given the dismal record of outcomes from permanent implant surgery, should we as a society even allow people to agree to become subjects in an experimental therapy that promises so little?

One might argue that the benefits of an artificial heart implant are so meager that individuals ought not be allowed to consent to it. Certainly, then, we should not support the program until enough basic scientific and clinical research has been done to improve the benefits to potential recipients far beyond those of the five people who received the devices. Indeed, perhaps our society should not just refuse to support with federal funds the use of the device; perhaps we should also declare a moratorium on such surgery. Thus, even if DeVries and other researchers secure private funding and find willing and consenting volunteers, perhaps they should not be allowed to implant an artificial heart into their patients.

On the other side, though, how far are we as a society willing to go in refusing to allow individuals to take whatever risks with their own lives that they choose? If an artificial heart offers some additional life, even of poor quality, should we refuse to allow a person to choose this as an option? Further, what if the patient is aware of the consequences but also believes that by participating he is making a contribution to the development of a device that might eventually save the lives of millions?

As DeVries points out, the first twelve dialysis patients died. Presumably he wants us to see that every significant medical advancement typically involves an unavoidable loss of life. Although this may be true, other factors must also be considered. For example, from ancient times until the end of the last century, hundreds of attempts were made to transfuse blood from human to human and from animal to human. Virtually all were disastrous for the recipients, and little or nothing was learned from the attempts. When Karl Landsteiner, building on the work of a number of people, developed blood typing in 1900, successful transfusion become a reality.

Can we say whether someone who consents to receive a heart is contributing to the advancement of medicine and science? That depends upon what stage of research we think the artificial heart has reached. If it is in a pre-Landsteiner phase, then one may be contributing very little. But perhaps even a little is enough.

These are questions to answer about any artificial heart program, past or future.

INTRODUCTION

In 1947, an international tribunal meeting in Nuremberg convicted fifteen German physicians of "war crimes and crimes against humanity." The physicians were charged with taking part in "medical experiments without the subjects' consent." But the language of the charge fails to indicate the cruel and barbaric nature of the experiments. Here are just some of them:

> At the Ravensbrueck concentration camp, experiments were conducted to test the effectiveness of the drug sulfanilamide. Cuts were deliberately made on the bodies of people; then the wounds were infected with bacteria. The infection was worsened by forcing wood shavings and ground glass into the cuts. Then sulfanilamide and other drugs were tested for their effectiveness in combatting the infection.
>
> At the Dachau concentration camp, healthy inmates were injected with

extracts from the mucous glands of mosquitos to produce malaria. Various drugs were then used to determine their relative effectiveness.

> At Buchenwald, numerous healthy people were deliberately infected with the spotted-fever virus merely for the purpose of keeping the virus alive. Over 90% of those infected died as a result.
>
> Also at Buchenwald, various kinds of poisons were secretly administered to a number of inmates to test their efficacy. Either the inmates died or they were killed at once so that autopsies could be performed. Some experimental subjects were shot with poisoned bullets.
>
> At Dachau, to help the German Air Force, investigations were made into the limits of human endurance and existence at very high altitudes. People were placed in sealed chambers, then subjected to very high and very low atmospheric pressures. As the indictment puts it, "Many victims died as a result of these experiments and others suffered grave injury, torture, and ill-treatment."

Seven of the physicians convicted were hanged, and the other eight received long prison terms. From the trial there emerged the Nuremberg Code, a statement of the principles that should be followed in conducting medical research with human subjects. (The principles of the code appear as a selection in this chapter.)

Despite the moral horrors that were revealed at Nuremberg, few people doubt the need for medical experimentation involving human subjects. The extent to which contemporary medicine has become effective in the treatment of disease and illness is due almost entirely to the fact that it has become scientific medicine. This means that contemporary medicine must conduct inquiries in which data are gathered to test hypotheses and general theories related to disease processes and their treatment. Investigations involving nonhuman organisms are essential, but ultimate tests of the correctness and effectiveness of medical treatments must involve human beings as research subjects. Human physiology and psychology are sufficiently different to make animal studies alone inadequate.

The German physicians tried at Nuremberg were charged with conducting experiments without the consent of their subjects. The notion that consent must be given before a person becomes an experimental subject is still considered to be the basic requirement that must be met for an experiment to be morally legitimate. Ordinarily, it is not merely consent—saying yes—but *informed consent* that is demanded. The basic idea is simply that a person decides to participate in research after he or she has been provided with background information relevant to making the decision.

This same notion of informed consent is also considered a requirement that has to be satisfied before a person can legitimately be subjected to medical treatment. Thus, people are asked to agree to submit themselves to such ordinary medical procedures as blood transfusion or to other procedures such as surgical operations or radiation therapy.

The underlying idea of informed consent in both research and treatment is that people have a right to control what is done to their bodies. The notion of informed consent is thus a recognition of an individual's autonomy—of the right to make decisions governing one's own life. This right is recognized both in practice and in the laws of our society. (Quite often, malpractice suits turn on the issue of whether a patient's informed consent was valid.)

In the abstract, informed consent seems a clear and straightforward notion. After all, we all have an intuitive grasp of what it is to make a decision after we have been supplied with information. Yet in practice informed consent has proved to be a slippery and troublesome concept. In this introduction, we will attempt to identify some of the moral and practical difficulties that make the concept controversial and hard to apply. Our focus will be on informed consent in the context of human experimentation. But most of the issues that arise here also arise in connection with giving and securing informed consent for the application of medical therapies. (They also arise in special forms in abortion and euthanasia.) In effect, then, we will be considering the entire topic.

Before starting our discussion of informed consent, it will be useful to have some idea of what takes place in a typical medical experiment. Perhaps the most common type of research involves the testing of new drugs. Let us consider, then, a sketch of what is involved in such testing.

DRUG TESTING

Traditions of medical research and regulations of the U.S. Food and Drug Administration more or less guarantee that the development of new drugs follows a set procedure. The procedure consists of two major parts: preclinical and clinical testing.

When it is thought likely that a chemical substance might be useful, animal experiments are conducted to determine how toxic it is. These tests are also used to estimate the drug's therapeutic index (the ratio of a dose producing toxic effects to a dose producing desired effects). The effects of the substance on particular organs and tissues, as well as on the whole animal, are studied. Efforts are made to determine the drug's potential side effects and hazards (whether, for example, it is carcinogenic).

Clinical testing of the substance occurs in three phases. In phase one, normal human volunteers are used to determine whether the drug produces any toxic effects. If these results are acceptable, then in phase two the drug is administered to a limited number of patients who might be expected to benefit from it. If the drug produces desirable results and has no serious side effects, then phase three studies are initiated. The drug is administered to a larger number of patients by a larger number of clinical investigators. Such trials usually take place at teaching hospitals or in large public institutions. Successful results achieved in this phase ordinarily lead to the licensing of the drug for general use.

In the clinical part of testing, careful procedures are followed to attempt to exclude bias in the results. Investigators want their tests to be successful and patients want to get well, and either or both of these factors may influence test results. Investigators may perceive a patient as "improved" just because they want or expect him to be. What is more, all medications produce a "placebo effect." That is, when patients are given inactive substances (placebos), they nevertheless often show improvement.

To rule out these kinds of influences, a common procedure followed in drug testing is the "double-blind" test design. In this design, a certain number of patients are given the drug being tested, and the remainder of the test group are given placebos. (In some cases, an established drug may be used instead of or in addition to placebos.) Neither the investigators nor the patients are allowed to know who is receiving the drug and who is not— both are kept "blind." Sometimes a test group is divided so that part receives placebos all of the time, part only some of the time, and part receives genuine medication all of the time.

Often placebos are no more than just sugar pills. Yet, frequently, substances are prepared to produce side effects like those of the drug being tested. If, for example, the drug causes drowsiness, a placebo will be used that produces drowsiness. In this way, investigators will not be able to learn which patients are being given placebos on the basis of irrelevant observations.

The double-blind test design is employed in many kinds of clinical investigation, not just in drug testing. Thus, the testing of new vaccines and therapies often follows the same form. A major variation is the "single-blind" design, in which those who must evaluate the results of some treatment are kept in ignorance of which patients have received it.

THE "INFORMED" PART OF INFORMED CONSENT

At first sight, consent is no more than agreement. A person consents when he or she says "yes" when asked to be a research subject. But legitimate or valid consent cannot be merely saying yes. If people are to be treated as autonomous agents, they must have the opportunity to *decide* whether they wish to become participants in research. Deciding, whatever else it may be, is a process in which we reason about an issue at hand. We consider such matters as the risks to our participation, its possible advantages to ourselves and others, the risks and advantages of other alternatives that are offered to us, and our own values. In short, valid consent requires that we deliberate before we decide.

But genuine deliberation requires both information and understanding. These two requirements are the source of difficulties and controversies. After all, medical research and treatment are highly technical enterprises. They are based on complicated scientific theories that are expressed in a special vocabulary and involve unfamiliar concepts.

For this reason, some physicians and investigators have argued that it is virtually useless to provide patients with relevant scientific information about research and treatment. Patients without the proper scientific background, they argue, simply don't know what to make of the information. Not only do patients find it puzzling, but they find it frightening. Thus, some have suggested, informed consent is at worst a pointless charade and at best a polite fiction. The patient's interest is best served by allowing a physician to make the decision.

This obviously paternalistic point of view (see Chapter 5) implies, in effect, that all patients are incompetent to decide their best interest and that physicians must assume the responsibility of acting for them. An obvious objection to this view is its assumption that, because patients lack a medical background, they cannot be given information in a form they can understand that is at least adequate to allow them to decide how they are to be treated. Thus, it can be argued, proponents of this view confuse the difficulty of communication with the impossibility of communication. It is true that it is often hard to explain technical medical matters to a layperson, but this hardly makes it legitimate to conclude that people should turn over their right to determine what is done to them to physicians. Rather, it imposes on physicians and researchers the obligation to find a way to explain medical matters to their patients.

The information provided to patients must be usable. That is, they must understand enough about the proposed research and treatment in order to deliberate and reach a decision. From the standpoint of the researcher, the problem here is to determine when the patient has an adequate understanding to make informed consent valid. Patients, being people, do not like to appear stupid and say they do not understand an explanation. Also, they may believe they understand an explanation when, as a matter of fact, they do not.

Until recently, very little effort was made to deal with the problem of determining when a patient understands the information provided and is competent to assess it. In the last few years, researchers have investigated situations in which individuals have been asked to consent to become experimental subjects. Drawing upon these data, some writers have attempted to formulate criteria for assessing competency for giving informed consent. The problem is not one that even now admits to an ideal solution, but, with additional empirical investigation and philosophical analysis, the situation may improve even more.

THE "CONSENT" PART OF INFORMED CONSENT

We have talked so far as though the issue of gaining the legitimate agreement of someone to be a research subject involved only providing information to an ordinary person in ordinary circumstances and then allowing the person to decide. But the matter is more complicated than this because often either the person or the circumstances possess special features. These features can call into question the very possibility of valid consent.

It is generally agreed that, in order to be valid, consent must be voluntary. The person must of his or her "own free will" agree to become a research subject. This means that the person must be capable of acting voluntarily. That is, the person must be _competent_.

This is an obvious and sensible requirement that is accepted by virtually everyone. But the difficulty lies in specifying just what it means to be competent. One answer is that a person is competent if he or she is capable of acting rationally. Since we have some idea of what it is to act rationally, this is a movement in the direction of an answer. The problem with it, however, is that people sometimes decide to act for the sake of moral (or religious) principles in ways that may not seem reasonable. For example, someone may volunteer to be a subject in a potentially hazardous experiment because she believes the experiment holds out the promise of helping countless others. In terms of self-interest alone, such an action would not be reasonable.

At present we do not have adequate criteria that can specify who is competent and who is not. Quite apart from this general theoretical problem is the issue of how children, the mentally retarded, and those suffering from psychiatric illnesses are to be considered with respect to consent. Should no person in any of these groups be considered capable of giving consent? If so, then is it ever legitimate to secure the consent from some third party—from a parent or guardian? One possibility is simply to rule out all research that involves such people as subjects. But this has the undesirable consequence of severely hampering efforts to gain the knowledge that might be of use either to the people themselves or to others with similar medical problems.

The questions we have raised here are still matters very much under dispute. Later we will consider some of the special problems that arise with children and other special groups as research subjects.

The circumstances in which research is done can also call into question the voluntariness of consent. This is particularly so with prisons, nursing homes, and mental hospitals. These are all what the sociologist Erving Goffman calls "total institutions," for within them all aspects of a person's life are connected with the social structure. People have a definite place in the structure and particular social roles. Moreover, there are social forces at work that both pressure and encourage an inmate to do what is expected of him or her.

We will discuss below some of the special problems that arise in research with prisoners. Here we need only to point out that the matter of gaining voluntary consent from inmates in institutions may not be possible at all. If it is possible, then it is necessary to specify the kinds of safeguards that must be followed in order to free them from the pressures that result from the very fact that they are inmates. Those who suffer from psychiatric illnesses may be considered just as capable intellectually of giving consent, but here too safeguards to protect them from the pressures of the institution need to be specified.

To avoid a misimpression, it is also worth pointing out that ordinary patients in hospitals may also be subject to pressures that call into question the voluntariness of the consent that they give. Patients are psychologically predisposed to act in ways that please physicians. Not only do physicians possess a social role that makes them figures of authority, but an ill person feels very dependent on those who may possess the power to make him well. Thus, he will be inclined to go along with any suggestion or recommendation made by a physician. The ordinary patient, like the inmate in an institution, needs protection from the social and psychological pressures that are exerted by circumstances. Otherwise, the voluntariness of consent will be compromised, and the patient cannot act as a free and autonomous agent.

MEDICAL RESEARCH AND MEDICAL THERAPY

Medical therapy aims at relieving the suffering of people and restoring them to health. It attempts to cure diseases, correct disorders, and bring about normal bodily functioning. Its focus is on the individual patient, and his or her welfare is its primary concern.

Medical research, by contrast, is a scientific enterprise. Its aim is to acquire a better understanding of the chemical and physiological processes that are involved in human functioning. It is concerned with the effectiveness of therapies in ending disease processes and restoring functioning. But this concern is not for the patient as an individual. Rather it is directed toward establishing theories. The hope, of course, is that this theoretical understanding can be used as a basis for treating individuals. But helping a particular patient get well is not a goal of medical research.

The related but distinct aims of medical research and medical therapy are a source of conflict in human experimentation. It is not unusual for a physician to be acting both as a researcher and as a therapist. This means that although she must be concerned with the welfare of her patient, her aims must also include acquiring data that are important to her research project. It is possible, then, that she may quite unconsciously encourage her patients to volunteer to be research subjects, provide them with inadequate information on which to base their decisions, or minimize the risks they are likely to be subject to.

The patient, for his part, may be reluctant to question his physician to acquire more information or to help him understand his role and risks in research. Also, as mentioned above, the patient may feel pressured into volunteering for research, just because he wants to do what his physician expects of him.

Medical research is a large-scale operation in this country and affects a great many people. It has been estimated that 400,000–800,000 people a year are patients in research programs investigating the effectiveness of drugs and other therapies. Since 1980, the number of clinical studies has increased about 30%, from about 3,400 to 4,400. Informed consent is more than an abstract moral issue.

The aims of therapy and the aims of research may also cause moral difficulties for the physician that go beyond the question of consent. This is particularly so in certain kinds of research. Let's look at some of the ethical issues more specifically.

Placebos and Research

As we saw earlier in the description of a typical drug experiment, placebos are considered to be essential in order to determine the true effectiveness of the drug being tested. In practice, this means that during all or some of the time they are being "treated," patients who are also subjects in a research program will not be receiving genuine medication. They are not, then, receiving the best available treatment for their specific condition.

This is one of the risks that a patient needs to know about before consenting to become a research subject. After all, most people become patients in order to be cured, if possible, of their ailments, not to further science or anything of the kind.

The physician-as-therapist will continue to provide medical care to a patient, for under double-blind conditions the physician does not know who is being given placebos and who is not. But the physician-as-researcher will know that a certain number of people will be receiving medication that cannot be expected to help their condition. Thus, the aims of the physician who is also a researcher come into conflict.

This conflict is particularly severe in cases in which it is reasonable to believe (on the basis of animal experimentation, in vitro research,

and so on) that an effective disease preventative exists, yet, to satisfy scientific rigor, tests of its effectiveness involve the giving of placebos. This was the case with the development of a polio vaccine by Thomas Weller, John F. Enders, and Frederick C. Robbins in 1960. The initial phase of the clinical testing involved injecting 30,000 children with a substance known to be useless in the prevention of polio—a placebo injection. It was realized, statistically, that some of those children would get the disease and die from it.

Since Weller, Enders, and Robbins believed that they had an effective vaccine, they can hardly be regarded as acting in the best interest of these children. As physicians they were not acting to protect the interest and well-being of the children. They did, of course, succeed in proving the safety and effectiveness of the polio vaccine. The moral question is whether they were justified in failing to provide 30,000 children with a vaccine they believed to be effective, even though it had not been tested on a wide scale with humans. That is, did they correctly resolve the conflict between their role as researchers and their role as physicians?

Placebos also present physician-researchers with another conflict. As we noticed in the earlier discussion, placebos are not always just "sugar pills." They often contain active ingredients that produce in patients effects that resemble those caused by the medication being tested—nervousness, vomiting, loss of appetite, and so on. This means that a patient receiving a placebo is sometimes not only failing to receive any medication for his illness, but also receiving a medication that may do him some harm. Thus, the physician committed to care for the patient and to relieve his suffering is at odds with the researcher who may be harming the patient. Do the aims of scientific research and its potential benefits to others justify treating patients in this fashion? Here is another moral question that the physician must face in particular and we must face in general.

We should not leave the topic of the use of placebos without mentioning that it is possible to make use of an experimental design in research that does not require giving placebos to a control group. An investigator can compare the results of two treatment forms: a standard treatment whose effectiveness is known and a new treatment with a possible but not proven effectiveness. This is not as satisfactory scientifically as the other approach because the researcher must do without a control group that has received no genuine treatment. But it does provide a way out of the dilemma of both providing medical care and conducting research.

Therapeutic and Nontherapeutic Research

We have mentioned the conflict that faces the physician who is also an investigator. But the patient who has to decide whether or not to consent to become a research subject is faced with a similar conflict.

Some research holds out the possibility of a direct and immediate advantage to those patients who agree to become subjects. For example, a new drug may, on the basis of limited trials, promise to be more effective in treating an illness than those drugs in standard use. Or a new surgical procedure may turn out to give better results than one that would ordinarily be used. By agreeing to participate in research involving such a drug or procedure, a patient may then have a chance of gaining something more beneficial than he or she would gain otherwise.

Yet the majority of medical research projects do not offer any direct therapeutic advantages to patients who consent to be subjects. The research may eventually benefit many patients, but seldom does it bring direct therapeutic benefits to research participants. Ordinarily, the most that participants can expect to gain is advantages such as having the attention of physicians who are more familiar with their illness than most physicians and receiving close observation and supervision in a research ward.

These are matters that ought to be presented to the patient as information relevant to the decision the patient must make. The patient must then decide whether he or she is willing to become a subject even if there are no special therapeutic advantages to be gained. It is in making this decision that one's moral beliefs can play a role. Some people volunteer to become research subjects without hope of reward because they believe that their action may eventually be of help to others.

Let us now turn to examining some of the problems posed by medical research in dealing with special groups. We will also consider some of the related issues that are involved in fetal research.

Research Involving Children

One of the most controversial areas of all medical experimentation has been that involving children as research subjects. The Willowbrook project discussed in the Case Presentation in this chapter is just one among many investigations that have drawn severe criticism and, quite often, court action.

The obvious question is: Why should children ever be made research subjects? Children clearly lack the physical, psychological, and intellectual maturity of adults. It does not seem that they are as capable as adults of giving informed consent because they can hardly be expected to grasp the nature of research and the possible risks to themselves. Furthermore, because they have not yet developed their capacities, it seems wrong to subject children to risks that might alter, for the worse, the course of their lives. They are in a position of relative dependency, relying upon adults to provide the conditions for their existence and development. It seems almost a betrayal of trust to allow children to be subjected to treatment that is of potential harm to them.

Such considerations help explain why we generally regard research involving children with deep suspicion. It is easy to imagine children being exploited and their lives heedlessly blighted by callous researchers. Some writers have been sufficiently concerned by the possibility of dangers and abuses that they have advocated an end to all research with children as subjects.

But there is another side to the coin. Biologically, children are not just small adults. Their bodies are developing, growing systems. Not only are there anatomical differences; there are also differences in metabolism and biochemistry. For example, some drugs are absorbed and metabolized more quickly in children than in adults, whereas other drugs continue to be active for a longer time. Often some drugs produce different effects when administered to children. Furthermore, just because the bodies of children are still developing, their nutritional needs are different. Findings based on adult subjects cannot simply be extrapolated to children, any more than results based on animal studies can be extrapolated to human beings.

Also, children are prone to certain kinds of diseases (measles, for example) that are either less common in adults or occur in different forms. It is important to know the kinds of therapies that are most successful in the treatment of children afflicted with them. Finally, even familiar surgical procedures cannot be employed in a straightforward way with children. Their developing organ systems are sufficiently different that special pediatric techniques must often be devised.

For many medical purposes, children must be thought of almost as if they were wholly different organisms. Their special biological features set them apart and mark them as subjects requiring special study. To gain the kind of knowledge and understanding required for effective medical treatment of children, it is often impossible to limit research solely to adults.

Failing to conduct research on children raises its own set of ethical issues. If children are excluded from investigations, then the development of pediatric medicine will be severely hindered. In general, this would mean that children would receive medical therapies that are less effective than might be possible. Also, since it is known that children differ significantly from adults in drug reactions, it seems wrong to subject children to the risks of drugs and drug dosages that have been tested only on adults.

Research involving children also seems necessary to avoid causing long-term harm to numerous people. The use of pure oxygen in the environments of prematurely born babies in the early 1940s resulted in blindness and impaired vision in a great number of cases. It was not until a controlled study was done that such damage was traced to the effects of the oxygen. Had the research not been allowed, the chances are very good that the practice would have continued and thousands more infants would have been blinded.

Yet, even if we agree that not all research involving children should be forbidden, we still have to face up to the issues that such research generates. Without attempting to be complete, we can mention the following three issues as among the more prominent.

First, who is to be considered a child? For infants and children in elementary school, this question is not a difficult one. But what about people in their teens? Then the line becomes hard to draw. Indeed, perhaps it is not possible to draw a line at all without being arbitrary. The concern behind the question is with the acquisition of autonomy, of self-direction and responsibility. It is obvious on the basis of ordinary experience that people develop at different rates, and some people at sixteen are more capable of taking charge of their own lives than others are at twenty. Some teenagers are more capable of understanding the nature and hazards of a research project than are many people who are much older.

This suggests that many people who are legally children may be quite capable of giving their informed consent. Of course, many others probably are not, so that decisions about capability would have to rest on an assessment of the individual. Where medical procedures that have a purely therapeutic aim are concerned, an individual who is capable of deciding whether it is in his or her best interest should probably be the one to decide. The issue may be somewhat different when the aim is not therapy. In such cases, a better policy might be to set a lower limit on the age at which consent can be given, and those below that limit should not be permitted to consent to participate in research. The problem is, of course, what should that limit be?

Second, can anyone else consent on behalf of a child? Parents or guardians have a duty to act for the sake of the welfare of a child under their care. In effect, they have a duty to substitute their judgment for that of the child. We generally agree to this because most often we consider the judgment of an adult more mature and informed than a child's. And because the responsibility for care rests with the adult, we customarily recognize that the adult has a right to decide. It is almost as though the adult's autonomy is being shared with the child—almost as though the child were an extension of the adult.

Society and its courts have recognized limits on the power of adults to decide for children. When it seems that the adult is acting in an irresponsible or unreasonable manner, then society steps in to act as a protector of the child's right to be cared for. Thus, courts have ordered that lifesaving procedures or blood transfusions be performed on children even when their parents or guardians have decided against it.

What sort of limits should govern a parent's or guardian's decision to allow a child to become a research subject? Can one person really give informed consent for another? Is it reasonable to believe that, if a parent would allow herself to be the subject of an experiment, then it is also right for her to consent to her child's becoming a subject? Or should something more be required before consent for a child's participation can be considered legitimate?

Third, should children be allowed to be subjects of research that does not offer them a chance of direct therapeutic benefits? Perhaps the "something more" that parents or guardians ought to require before consenting on behalf of a child is the genuine possibility that the research will bring the child direct benefits. This would be in accordance with a parent's duty to seek the welfare of the child. It is also a way of recognizing that the parent's autonomy is not identical with that of the child: one may have the right to take a risk oneself without having the right to impose the risk on someone else.

This seems like a reasonable limitation, and it has been advocated by some writers. (See the Freedman selection in this chapter, for example.) Yet there are difficulties with the position. Some research virtually free from risk (coordination tests, for example) might be stopped because of its lack of a "direct therapeutic value." More important, however, much research promising immense long-term benefits would have to be halted. Research frequently involves the withholding of accepted therapies without any guarantee that what is used in their place will be as effective. Sometimes the withholding of accepted treatment is beneficial. Thus, as it turned out, in the research on the incidence of blindness in premature infants in the 1940s, premature infants who were not kept in a pure oxygen environment were better off than those who received ordinary treatment. But no one could know this in advance, and such research as this is, at best, ambiguous as to the promise of direct therapy. Sheer ignorance imposes restrictions. Yet if the experiment had not been done, the standard treatment would have continued with its ordinary course of (statistically) disastrous results.

Here, at least, there was the possibility of better results from the experimental treatment. But in research that involves the substitution of placebos for medications or vaccines known to be effective, it is known in advance that some children will not receive medical care considered to be the best. A child who is a subject in such research is then put in a situation in which he or she is subjected to a definite hazard. The limitation on consent that we are considering would rule out such research. But the consequence of doing this would be to restrict the development of new and potentially more effective medications and treatment techniques. That is, future generations of children would be deprived of at least some possible medical advances.

These, then, are some of the issues that we have to face in arriving at a view of the role of children in research. Perhaps the greatest threat to children, however, has to do with social organization. Children, like prisoners, are often grouped together in institutions (schools, orphanages, detention centers, and so on) and are attractive targets for clinical investigators because they inhabit a limited and relatively controlled environment, can be made to follow orders, and do not ask too many questions that have to be answered. It is a misimpression to see researchers in such situations as "victimizing" children, but at the same time it is clear that careful controls are needed to see that research involving children is legitimate and carried out in a morally satisfactory way.

In response to some of these difficulties, in 1983 the Department of Health and Human Services issued guidelines specifically designed to protect children as research subjects. For children to become subjects, permission must be obtained from parents or guardians, and children must give their "assent." An Institutional Review Board is assigned the responsibility of considering the "ages, maturity, and psychological states" of the children and determining whether they are capable of assenting. (A failure to object cannot be construed as assent.) Children who are wards of the state or of an institution can become sub-

jects only if the research relates to their status as wards or takes place in circumstances in which the majority of subjects are not wards. Each child must also be supplied with an "advocate" to represent her or his interest.

Research Involving Prisoners

Prisoners are in some respects social outcasts. They have been found guilty of breaking the laws of society and, as a consequence, are removed from it. Stigmatized and isolated, prisoners in the relatively recent past were sometimes thought of as less than human. It seemed only reasonable that such depraved and corrupt creatures should be used as the subjects of experiments that might bring benefits to the members of the society that they wronged. Indeed, it seemed not only reasonable but fitting.

Accordingly, in the early part of this century, tropical medicine expert Richard P. Strong obtained permission from the Governor of the Philippines to inoculate a number of condemned criminals with plague bacillus. The prisoners were not asked for their consent, but they were rewarded by being provided with cigarettes and cigars.

Episodes of this sort were relatively common during the late nineteenth and early twentieth centuries. But as theories about the nature of crime and criminals changed, it became standard practice to use only volunteers and to secure the consent of the prisoners themselves. In the 1940s, for example, the University of Chicago infected over 400 prisoners with malaria in an attempt to discover new drugs to treat and prevent the disease. A committee set up by the Governor of Illinois recommended that potential volunteers be informed of the risks, be permitted to refuse without fear of such reprisals as withdrawal of privileges, and be protected from unnecessary suffering. The committee suggested also that volunteering to be a subject in a medical experiment is a form of good conduct that should be taken into account in deciding whether a prisoner should be paroled or have his sentence reduced.

But the committee also called attention to a problem of great moral significance. They pointed out that, if a prisoner's motive for volunteering is the wish to contribute to human welfare, then a reduction in his sentence would be a reward. But if his motive is to obtain a reduction in sentence, then the possibility of obtaining one is really a form of duress. In this case, the prisoner cannot be regarded as making a free decision.

The issue of duress or "undue influence," as it is called in law, is central to the question of deciding whether, and under what conditions, valid informed consent can be obtained for research involving prisoners. Some ethicists have argued that, to avoid undue influence, prisoners should never be promised any substantial advantages for volunteering to be research subjects. If they volunteer, they should do so for primarily moral or humane reasons.

Others have claimed that becoming research subjects offers prisoners personal advantages that they should not be denied. For example, participation in a research project frees them from the boredom of prison life, gives them an opportunity to increase their feelings of self-worth, and allows them to exercise their autonomy as moral agents. It has been argued, in fact, that prisoners have a *right* to participate in research if the opportunity is offered to them and they wish to do so. To forbid the use of prisoners as research subjects is thus to deny to them, without adequate grounds, a right that all human beings possess. As a denial of their basic autonomy, of their right to take risks and control their own bodies, *not* allowing them to be subjects might constitute a form of cruel and unusual punishment.

By contrast, it can also be argued that prisoners do not deserve to be allowed to exercise such autonomy. Because they have been sentenced for crimes, they should be deprived of the right to volunteer to be research subjects:

that right belongs to free citizens. Being deprived of the right to act autonomously is part of their punishment. This is basically the position taken in 1952 by the House of Delegates of the American Medical Association. The Delegates passed a resolution expressing disapproval of the use as research subjects of people convicted of "murder, rape, arson, kidnapping, treason, and other heinous crimes."

A more worrisome consideration is the question of whether prisoners can be sufficiently free of undue influence or duress to make their consent legitimate. As we mentioned earlier, prisons are total institutions, and the very institutional framework puts pressures on people to do what is desired or expected of them. There need not be, then, promises of rewards (such as reduced sentences) or overt threats (such as withdrawal of ordinary privileges) for coercion to be present. That people may volunteer to relieve boredom is itself an indication that they may be acting under duress. That "good conduct" is a factor in deciding whether to grant parole may function as another source of pressure.

The problem presented by prisoners is fundamentally the same as that presented by inmates in other institutions, such as nursing homes and mental hospitals. In these cases, once it has been determined that potential subjects are mentally competent to give consent, then it must also be decided whether the institutional arrangements allow the consent to be "free and voluntary."

Research Involving the Poor

In the eighteenth century, Princess Caroline of England requested the use of six "charity children" as subjects in the smallpox vaccination experiments she was directing. Then, and until quite recently, charity cases, like prisoners, were regarded by some medical researchers as prime research subjects.

A recent and horrible example of medical research involving the poor is the Tuskegee Syphilis Study that was conducted under the auspices of the U.S. Department of Public Health. From 1932 to 1970, a large but undetermined number of black males suffering from the later stages of syphilis were examined at regular intervals to determine the course their disease was taking. The men in the study were poor and uneducated and believed that they were receiving proper medical care from the state and local public health clinics. As a matter of fact, they were given either no treatment or inadequate treatment, and at least forty of them died as a result of factors connected with their disease. Their consent was never obtained, and the nature of the study, its risks, and the alternatives open to them were never explained. It was known when the study began that those with untreated syphilis have a higher death rate than those whose condition is treated, and although the study was started before the advent of penicillin (which is highly effective against syphilis), other drugs were available but were not used in ways to produce the best results. When penicillin became generally available, it still was not used.

The Tuskegee Study clearly violated the Nuremberg Code, but it was not stopped even after the War Crimes trials. It was reviewed in 1969 by a USPH ad hoc committee, and it was decided that the study should be phased out in 1970. The reasons for ending the study were not moral ones. It was simply believed that there was nothing of much scientific value to be gained by continuing the work. In 1973, a USPH Ad Hoc Advisory Panel, which had been established as a result of public and congressional pressure to review the Tuskegee Study, presented its final report. It condemned the study both on moral grounds and because of its lack of worth and rigor.

No one today argues seriously that disadvantaged people ought to be made subjects of research simply as a result of their social or economic status. The "back wards" in hospitals whose poor patients once served as a source of research subjects have mostly disappeared as a result of such programs as Medicare and Medicaid. Each person is now entitled to his or her own physician and is not merely under the care of the state or of a private charity.

Yet many research projects continue to be based in large public or municipal hospitals. And such hospitals have a higher percentage of disadvantaged people as patients than do private institutions. For this reason, such people are still more likely to become research subjects than are the educated and wealthy. If society continues to accept this state of affairs, special precautions must be taken to see to it that those who volunteer to become research subjects are genuinely informed and free in their decisions.

Research Involving Fetuses

In 1975 legal charges were brought against several physicians in Boston. They had injected antibiotics into living fetuses that were scheduled to be aborted. The aim of the research was to determine by autopsy, after the death of the fetuses, how much of the drug got into the fetal tissues.

Such information is considered to be of prime importance because it increases our knowledge of how to provide medical treatment for a fetus still developing in its mother's womb. It also helps to determine ways in which drugs taken by a pregnant woman may affect a fetus and so points the way toward improved prenatal care.

Other kinds of research involving the fetus also promise to provide important knowledge. Effective vaccines for preventing viral diseases, techniques for treating children with defective immune-system reactions, and hormonal measurements that indicate the status of the developing fetus are just some of the potential advances that are partially dependent on fetal research.

But a number of moral questions arise in connection with such research. Even assuming that a pregnant woman consents to allow the fetus she is carrying to be injected with drugs prior to abortion, is such research ethical? Does the fact that the fetus is going to be aborted alter in any way the moral situation? For example, prior to abortion should the fetus be treated with the same respect and concern for its well-being as a fetus that is not scheduled for abortion?

After the fetus is aborted, if it is viable—if it can live separated from the mother—then we seem to be under an obligation to protect its life. But what if a prenatal experiment threatens its viability? The expectation in abortion is that the fetus will not be viable, but this is not in fact always the case. Does this mean that it is wrong to do anything before abortion to threaten the life of the fetus or reduce its chance for life, even though we do not expect it to live?

These are very difficult questions to answer without first settling the question of whether the fetus is to be considered a person. (See the discussion of this issue in the introduction and selections in Chapter 1.) If the fetus is a person, then it is entitled to the same moral considerations that we extend to other persons. If we decide to take its life, if abortion is considered to be at least sometimes legitimate, then we must be prepared to offer justification. Similarly, if we are to perform experiments on a fetus, even one expected to die, then we must also be prepared to offer justification. Whether the importance of the research is adequate justification is a matter that currently remains to be settled.

If the fetus is not a person, then the question of fetal experimentation becomes less important morally. Since, however, the fetus may be regarded as a potential person, we may still believe it is necessary to treat it with consideration and respect. The burden of justification may be somewhat less weighty, but it may still be there.

Let us assume that the fetus is aborted and is apparently not viable. Typically, before such a fetus dies, its heart beats and its lungs function. Is it morally permissible to conduct research on the fetus before its death? The knowledge that can be gained, particularly of lung functions, can be used to help save the lives of premature infants, and the fetus is virtually certain of dying, whether or not it is made a subject of research.

After the death of a fetus that is either deliberately or spontaneously aborted, are there any moral restraints on what is done with the remains? It is possible to culture fetal tissues and use them for research purposes. These tissues might, in fact, be commercially grown and distributed by biological supply companies in the way that a variety of animal tissues are now dealt with. Exactly when a fetus can be considered to be dead so that its tissues and organs are available for experimentation, even assuming that one approves of their use in this manner, is itself an unanswered question.

Scientists have been concerned about proposed federal guidelines and state laws regulating fetal research. Most investigators fear that they will be forced to operate under such rigid restrictions that research will be slowed or even prohibited. Nearly everyone agrees, however, that some important moral and social decisions must be made about fetal research. (See Chapter 9.)

Fetal research has to be considered a part of human experimentation. Not only are many fetuses born alive even when deliberately aborted, but they all possess certain human characteristics and potentialities. But who shall give approval to what is done with the fetus? Who is responsible for consent?

It seems peculiar to say that a woman who has decided to have an abortion is also the one who should consent to research involving the aborted fetus. It can be argued that in deciding to have an abortion she has renounced all interest and responsibility with respect to the fetus. Yet, if the fetus does live, we would consider her, at least in part, legally and morally responsible for seeing to its continued well-being.

But if the woman (or the parents) is the one who must give consent for fetal experimentation, are there limits to what she can consent to on behalf of the fetus? With this question we are back where we began. It is obvious that fetal research raises both moral and social issues. We need to decide, then, what is right as a matter of personal conduct and what is right as a matter of social policy. At the moment, issues in each of these areas remain unsettled.

Research Involving Animals

The seventeenth-century philosopher René Descartes doubted whether animals experience pain. They may act *as if* they are in pain, but perhaps they are only complicated pieces of clockwork designed to act that way. Humans feel pain, but then, unlike animals, humans have a "soul" that gives them the capacity to reason, be self-conscious, and experience emotions. The bodies of humans are pieces of machinery, but the mental states that occur within the bodies are not.

If the view of animals represented by Descartes and others in the mechanistic tradition he initiated is correct, we need have no moral concern about the use of animals in research. Animals of whatever species have the status of any other piece of delicate and often expensive lab equipment. They may be used in any way for any purpose.

Here are some of the ways in which animals are used in biomedical research:

- A standard test for determining the toxicity of drugs or chemicals is the "lethal dose-50" (LD-50) test. This is the amount of a substance that, when administered to a group of experimental animals, will kill 50% of them.

- The Draize test, once widely used in the cosmetics industry, involves dripping a chemical substance into the lidless eyes of rabbits to determine its potential to cause eye damage.

- The effects of cigarette smoking were investigated by a series of experiments using beagles with tubes inserted into holes cut into their tracheas so that, when breathing, they were forced to inhale cigarette smoke. The dogs were then "sacrificed" and autopsied to look for significant changes in cells and tissues.

- Surgical procedures are both developed and acquired by using animals as experimental subjects. Surgical residents spend much time in "dog labs" learning to perform standard surgical procedures on live dogs. Limbs may be deliberately broken and organs damaged or destroyed to test the usefulness of surgical repair techniques.

- A traditional medical-school demonstration consisted in exsanguinating (bleeding to death) a dog to illustrate the circulation of the blood. High school and college biology courses sometimes require that students destroy the brains of frogs with long needles (pithing) and then dissect the frogs to learn about physiological processes.

- Chimpanzees and other primates have served as experimental subjects for the study of the induction and treatment of infectious diseases. Perfectly healthy chimps and monkeys have been inoculated with viruses resembling the AIDS virus; then the course of the resulting diseases is studied.

A list of the ways in which animals are used would include virtually all basic biomedical research. The discovery of an "animal model" of a disease typically signals a significant advancement in research. It means that the disease can be studied in ways it cannot be in humans. The assumption is that animals can be subjected to experimental conditions and treatments that humans cannot be subjected to without violating basic moral principles.

Is the assumption that we have no moral obligation toward animals warranted? Certainly the crude "animal machine" view of Descartes has been rejected, and no one is prepared to argue that no nonhuman animal can experience pain.

Exactly what animals have the capacity for suffering is a matter of dispute. Mammals undoubtedly do, and vertebrates in general seem to experience pain, but what about insects, worms, lobsters, and clams? Is the identification of endorphins, naturally occurring substances associated with pain relief in humans, adequate grounds for saying that an organism that produces endorphins must experience pain?

Once it is acknowledged that at least some animals can suffer, most philosophers agree that we have some moral responsibility with respect to them. At the least, some (like Ross) say that, since we have a prima facie duty not to cause unnecessary suffering, we should not inflict needless pain on animals.

This does not necessarily mean that biomedical research should discontinue the use of animals. Strictly construed, it means only that the animals should be treated in a *humane* way. For example, surgical techniques should be practiced only on dogs that have been anesthetized. Understood in this way, the principle raises no objection to humanely conducted animal research, even if its purpose is relatively trivial.

Philosophers like Kant and most of those in the natural law tradition would deny that we have any duties to animals at all. The only proper objects of duty are rational agents; unless we are prepared to argue that animals are rational, we have to refuse them the status of moral persons. We might treat animals humanely because we are magnanimous, but they are not in a position to lay claims against us. Animals have no rights.

Some contemporary philosophers (Tom Regan in particular) have argued that, although animals are not rational agents, they have preferences. This gives them an autonomy that makes them "moral patients." Like humans, animals possess the right to respectful treatment, and this entails that they not be treated only as a means to some other end.

They are ends in themselves, and this intrinsic worth makes it wrong to use them as subjects in research, even when alternatives to animal research are not available.

Contrary to Regan, a number of writers have taken a utilitarian approach to the issue of animal experimentation. Some (like Peter Singer) have argued that, although animals cannot be said to have rights, they have interests. If we recognize that the interests of humans are deserving of equal consideration, then so too are the interests of nonhuman animals. Hence, we can recognize that animals have inherent worth without assigning them rights, but this does not mean that we must treat them exactly as we treat humans.

Most people, whether utilitarians or not, argue that at least some forms of animal experimentation can be justified by the benefits produced. After all, they point out, the understanding of biological processes we have acquired since the time of Aristotle has been heavily dependent on animal experimentation. This understanding has given us insights into the causes and processes of diseases, and, most important, it has put us in a position to invent and test new therapies and modes of prevention.

Without animal experimentation, the identification of the role played by insulin, the development of the polio vaccine, and the perfection of hundreds of major surgical techniques surely would not have been possible. The list could be extended to include virtually every accomplishment of medicine and surgery. Countless millions of human lives have been saved by using the knowledge and understanding gained from animal studies.

Animals, too, have benefited from the theoretical and practical knowledge of research. An understanding of nutritional needs has led to healthier domestic animals, and an understanding of environmental needs has produced a movement to protect and preserve many kinds of wild animals. At the conceptual and scientific levels, veterinary medicine is not really distinct from human medicine. The same sorts of surgical procedures, medicines, and vaccines that benefit the human population also benefit many other species.

However, even from a broadly utilitarian perspective, accepting the general principle that the results justify the practice does not mean that every experiment with animals is warranted. Some experiments might be trivial, unnecessary, or poorly designed. Others might hold no promise of yielding the kind or amount of knowledge sufficient to justify causing the animal subjects to suffer pain and death.

Furthermore, the utilitarian approach supports (as does a rights view like Regan's) looking for an alternative to animal experimentation. If good results can be obtained, for example, by conducting experiments with cell cultures (in vitro), rather than with whole organisms (in vivo), then in vitro experiments are to be preferred. However, if alternatives to animal testing are not available and if the benefits secured promise to outweigh the cost, animal testing may be morally legitimate.

The utilitarian justification faces what some writers see as a major difficulty. It is one posed by the fact that animals like chimpanzees and even dogs and pigs can be shown to possess mental abilities superior to those of humans suffering from severe brain damage and retardation. If experiments on mammals are justifiable by appealing to the benefits, then why aren't experiments on humans with serious mental impairments equally justified? Indeed, shouldn't we experiment on a human in a chronic vegetative state, rather than on a healthy and alert dog?

The use made of animals in biomedical research is a significant issue, but it is no more than one aspect of the general philosophical question about the status of animals. Do animals have rights? If so, what grounds can be offered for them? Do animals have a right to coexist with humans? Do animals have a right to be free? Is it wrong to eat animals or use products made from their remains? These

questions and many others like them are now being given the most careful scrutiny they have received since the last century. How they are answered will do much to shape the character both of medical research and of our society.

Women and Medical Research

Critics have recently charged that medical research has typically failed to include women as experimental subjects, even when women might also stand to benefit from the results. Most strikingly, a study showing the effectiveness of small doses of aspirin in reducing the risk of heart attack included 2,201 subjects—all male. The relevance of the study to women is in doubt, for, although more men than women die of heart disease, after women reach menopause the difference between genders becomes much smaller.

Studies of the therapeutic effectiveness of drugs ordinarily include only males. Although the effects of many drugs are the same for women as for men, this is not always true. Hormonal differences may alter drug reactions, so conclusions based on the reactions of men may be misleading when applied to women.

In the view of critics, the traditionally male-dominated research establishment has been responsible for the current state of affairs. To change the situation so that both women and men are included in studies would add to their costs. It would introduce gender as a variable, and the study would have to include more subjects in order to get the degree of statistical reliability that could be achieved with fewer subjects of the same gender. However, such studies would have the additional value of yielding results known to be applicable to women.

That this issue is a matter of social fairness is obvious, but its connection with informed consent is less direct. As we mentioned in connection with prisoners, not allowing someone to consent may be viewed as treating that person as having less worth than someone who is allowed to consent. From this perspective, then, women have been denied the opportunity to be full persons in the moral sense. They have not been able to exercise their autonomy in ways permitted to men. Of course, they have also not been permitted to gain benefits that might be associated with the research projects from which they have been excluded.

Summary

There are other areas of medical experimentation that present special forms of moral problems. We have not discussed, for example, research involving military personnel, college and university students, or dying patients. Moreover, we mentioned only a few of the special difficulties presented by the mentally retarded, psychiatric patients, and old people confined to institutions.

We have, however, raised such a multiplicity of questions about consent and human experimentation that it is perhaps worthwhile to attempt to restate some of the basic issues in a general form. Three issues are particularly noteworthy:

1. Who is competent to consent? (Are children? Are mental patients? If a person is not competent, who—if anyone—should have the power to consent for him or her?) Given that animals have no power to consent, is research involving them legitimate?

2. When is consent voluntary? (Is any institutionalized person in a position to offer free consent? How can even hospitalized patients be made free of pressures to consent?)

3. When are information and understanding adequate for genuine decision making? (Can complicated medical information ever be adequately explained to laypeople? Should we attempt to devise tests for understanding?)

Although we have concentrated on the matter of consent in research, there are other morally relevant matters connected with the character of research that we have not discussed. These often relate to research standards. Among them are the following:

1. Is the research of sufficient scientific and medical worth to justify the human risk involved? Research that involves trivial aims or that is unnecessary (when, for example, it merely serves to confirm what is already well established) cannot be used to justify causing any threat to human well-being.

2. Can the knowledge sought be obtained without human experimentation? Can it be obtained without animal experimentation?

3. Have animal (and other) studies been done to minimize as far as is possible the risk to human subjects? A great deal can be learned about the effects of drugs, for example, by using "animal models," and the knowledge gained can be used to minimize the hazards in human trials. (Ethical issues involving animals in research may also be called into question.)

4. Does the design of the research meet accepted scientific standards? Sloppy research that is scientifically worthless means that people have been subjected to risks for no legitimate purpose and that animals have been harmed or sacrificed needlessly.

5. Do the investigators have the proper medical or scientific background to conduct the research effectively?

6. Is the research designed to minimize the risks and suffering of the participants? As we noted earlier, it is sometimes possible to test new drugs without using placebos. Thus, people in need of medication are not forced to be without treatment for their condition.

7. Have the aims and the design of the research and the qualifications of the investigators been reviewed by a group or committee competent to judge them? Such "peer review" is intended to assure that only research that is worthwhile and that meets accepted scientific standards is conducted. And although such review groups can fail to do their job properly, as they apparently did in the Tuskegee Syphilis Study, they are still necessary instruments of control.

Most writers on experimentation would agree that these are among the questions that must be answered satisfactorily before research involving human subjects is morally acceptable. Obviously, however, a patient who is asked to give his or her consent is in no position to judge whether the research project meets the standards implied by these questions. For this reason, it is important that there be social policies and practices governing research. Everyone should be confident that a research project is, in general, a legitimate one before having to decide whether to volunteer to become a participant.

Special problems are involved in seeing to it that these questions are properly answered. It is enough for our purposes, however, merely to notice that the character of the research and the manner in which it is to be performed are factors that are relevant to determining the moral legitimacy of experimentation involving human subjects.

ETHICAL THEORIES: MEDICAL RESEARCH AND INFORMED CONSENT

We have clearly raised too many issues in too many areas of experimentation to discuss how each of several ethical theories might apply to them all. We must limit ourselves to considering a few suggestions about the general issues of human experimentation and informed consent.

Utilitarianism's principle of utility tells us, in effect, to choose those actions that will produce the greatest amount of benefit. Utilitarianism must approve human experimentation in general, since there are cases in which the sacrifices of a few bring great benefits to many. We might, for example, design our social policies to make it worthwhile for people to volunteer for experiments with the view that, if people are paid to take risks and are compensated for their suffering or for any damage done to them during the course of a research project, then the society as a whole might benefit.

The principle of utility also tells us to design experiments to minimize suffering and the chance of harm. Also, it forbids us to do research of an unnecessary or trivial kind—research that is not worth its cost in either human or economic resources.

As far as informed consent is concerned, utilitarianism does not seem to require it. If more social good is to be gained by making people research subjects without securing their agreement, then this is morally legitimate. (It is not, of course, necessarily the best procedure to follow. A system of rewards to induce volunteers might be more likely to lead to an increase in general happiness.) Furthermore, the principle of utility suggests that the best research subjects would be "less valuable" members of the society, such as the mentally retarded, the habitual criminal, or the dying. This, again, is not a necessary consequence of utilitarianism, although it is a possible one. If the recognition of rights and dignity would produce a better society in general, then a utilitarian would also say that they must be taken into account in experimentation with human beings.

For utilitarianism, that individual is competent to give consent who is able to balance benefits and risks and then decide what course of action is best for him or her. Thus, if informed consent is taken to be a requirement supported by the principle of utility, those who are mentally ill or retarded or senile have to be excluded from the class of potential experimental subjects. Furthermore, investigators must provide enough relevant information to allow competent people to make a meaningful decision about what is likely to serve their own interests the most.

For Kant, an individual capable of giving consent is one who is rational and autonomous. Kant's principles would thus also rule out as experimental subjects people who are not able to understand experimental procedures, aims, risks, and benefits. People may volunteer for experiments if they expect them to be of therapeutic benefit to themselves, or they may act out of duty and volunteer, thus discharging their imperfect obligation to advance knowledge or to improve human life.

Yet, for Kant, there are limits to the risks that one should take. We have a duty to preserve our lives, so no one should agree to become a subject in an experiment in which the likelihood of death is great. Additionally, no one should subject himself to research in which there is considerable risk that his capacity for rational thought and autonomy will be destroyed. Indeed, Kant's principles appear to require us to regard as morally illegitimate those experiments that seriously threaten the lives or rationality of their subjects. Not only should we not subject ourselves to them, but we should not subject others to them.

Kant's principles also rule out as potential experimental subjects those who are not in a position to act voluntarily, those who cannot exercise their autonomy. This makes it important to determine, from a Kantian point of view, whether children and institutionalized people (including prisoners) can be regarded as free agents capable of moral choice. Also, as in the case of abortion, the status of the fetus must be determined. If the fetus is not a person, then fetal experimentation presents no particular moral problems. But if the fetus is a person, then we must accord it a moral status and act for its sake and not for the sake of knowledge or for others.

Kant's view of people as autonomous rational beings requires that informed consent be obtained for both medical treatment and research. We cannot be forced to accept treatment for "our own good," nor can we be turned into experimental subjects for "the good of others." We must always be treated as ends and never as means only. To be treated in this way requires that others never deliberately deceive us, no matter how good their intentions. In short, we have a right to be told what we are getting into so that we can decide whether we want to go through with it or not.

Ross's theory imposes on researchers prima facie duties to patients that are similar to Kant's requirements. The nature of people as autonomous moral agents requires that their informed consent be obtained. Researchers ought not deceive their subjects, and experiments should be designed in ways in which suffering and the risk of injury or death are minimized.

These are all prima facie duties, of course, and it is possible to imagine situations in which other duties might take precedence over them. In general, however, Ross, like Kant, tells us that human research cannot be based on what is useful; it must be based on what is right. Ross's principles, like Kant's, do not tell us, however, how we are to deal with such special problems as research involving children or prisoners.

As we saw in the introductory chapter, the principle of double effect and the principle of totality, which are based on the natural law theory of morality, have specific applications to experimentation. Because we hold our bodies in trust, we are responsible for assessing the degree of risk to which we might be put if we agree to become research subjects. Thus, others have an obligation to supply us with the information that we need in order to make our decision. If we decide to give our consent, it must be given freely and not be the consequence of deception or coercion.

If available evidence shows that a sick person may gain benefits from participating in an experiment, then the experiment is justified. But if the evidence shows that the benefits may be slight or if the chance of serious injury or death is relatively great, then the experiment is not justified. In general, the likelihood of a person's benefiting from an experiment must exceed the danger of the person's suffering greater losses. The four requirements that govern the application of the principle of double effect determine what is and what is not an allowable experiment. (See the introductory chapter for a discussion of these.)

People can volunteer for experiments from which they expect no direct benefits. The good they seek in doing so is not their own good but the good of others. But there are limits to what they can subject themselves to. A dying patient, for example, cannot be made the subject of a useless or trivial experiment. The probable value of the knowledge to be gained must balance the risk and suffering the patient is subjected to, and there must be no likelihood that the experiment will seriously injure or kill the patient.

These same restrictions also apply to experiments involving healthy people. The principle of totality forbids a healthy person to submit to an experiment that involves the probability of serious injury, impaired health, mutilation, or death.

The status of the fetus is clear in the Roman Catholic version of the natural law theory: the fetus is a person. As such, the fetus is entitled to the same dignity and respect we accord to other persons. Experiments that involve doing it injury or lessening its chances of life are morally prohibited. But not all fetal research is ruled out. That which may be of therapeutic benefit or which does not directly threaten the fetus's well-being is allowable. Furthermore, research involving fetal tissue or remains is permissible, if it is done for a serious and valuable purpose.

From Rawls's point of view, the difficulty with utilitarianism with respect to human experimentation is that the principle of utility would permit the exploitation of some groups (the dying, prisoners, the retarded) for the sake of others. By contrast, Rawls's principles of justice would forbid all experiments that involve violating a liberty to which a person is entitled by virtue of being a member of society. As a result, all experiments that make use of coercion or deception are ruled out. And since a person has a right to decide what risks she is willing to subject herself to, voluntary informed consent is required of all subjects. Society might, as in utilitarianism, decide to reward those who volunteer to become research subjects. As long as this is a possibility open to all, it is not objectionable.

It would never be right, according to Rawls, to take advantage of those in the society who are least well off to benefit those who are better off. In general, inequalities must be arranged so that they bring benefits (ideally) to everyone or at least to those who are most disadvantaged. Research involving direct therapeutic benefits is clearly acceptable (assuming that there is informed consent), but research that takes advantage of the sick, the poor, the retarded, or the institutionalized and does not benefit them is clearly unacceptable. The status of the fetus—whether or not it is a person in the moral sense—is an issue that has to be resolved before we know how to apply Rawls's principles to fetal research.

We have been able to provide only the briefest sketch here of some of the ways in which our moral theories might apply to the issues in human experimentation. The remarks are not meant to be anything more than suggestive. Clearly, a satisfactory moral theory of human experimentation requires working out the application of principles to problems in detail, as well as resolving such issues as the status of children and fetuses and the capability of institutionalized people to act freely.

Some Ethical Problems in Clinical Investigation

Louis Lasagna

Louis Lasagna discusses some of the issues that face the physician who is in the role of both therapist and researcher. But perhaps the most important aspect of his article is the review of the arguments against informed consent. Lasagna points out that sometimes researchers themselves do not know the risks that may be involved in research, that there are experiments in which information provided to potential subjects can alter the outcome, and that often patients themselves do not wish to be put into a position in which they must make a decision on the basis of information that they are not really competent to evaluate. Taking a basically utilitarian stance, Lasagna suggests that the "greater interest" of society must sometimes be given precedence over the rights of individuals.

One potentially important source of tension in clinical investigation is the fundamental discrepancy in outlook between the clinical investigator and the physician. The two positions are rarely identical. One reads that medical experimentation takes place continually in every doctor's office and that the therapy of disease is an experimental aspect of medicine, but in point of fact, the practice of medicine and the pursuit of a scientific problem are not equivalent.

The physician is primarily concerned with the patient *qua* patient, with getting him well as quickly as possible and with a minimum of discomfort, inconvenience, risk, and cost to the patient. In the practice of his art the doctor has to use any and every measure he considers justified, and he is concerned with what measure (if any) works, not with what contribution (if any) he makes to the body of scientific data.

For the investigator, the primary emphasis is on the research question. This does not mean that he need be callous or lacking in caution; indeed, patients who are in an experiment are likely to be more carefully observed and cared for than if they were not research subjects. (In fact, carefully designed experiments result more often in improved patient care than in exciting new scientific information.) There are good reasons for the preferred status of patients in an experiment. Physicians in a research ward or research institution have usually had the advantage of intensive training, experience, and the intellectual discipline of an academic atmosphere. Further, the patient is, paradoxically, often better served by the restraint observed in the therapeutic approach of the critical experimentalist. The uncritical use of many therapeutic measures can be less desirable than the wise use of a few well-chosen ones; in medicine two and two sometimes add up to minus four, as the patient finds his medications working at cross purposes and yielding iatrogenic illness to boot. Often in controlled trials, for example, the placebo-treated patients turn out to be the lucky ones, as the new "remedy" proves to be toxic or therapeutically ineffective.

Notwithstanding the admirable qualities of many research-oriented physicians, however, there still remain important differences in orientation between the physician and the investigator which may affect the individual patient to a significant degree and which deserve discussion. Take, for example, the patient with metastatic cancer. Here is a serious disease for which we lack good treatment. There would seem to be no ethical problem in giving a desperately ill patient a new compound which may do some good. Yet the situation is only superficially simple.

The first cancer patients to receive an investigational drug often fail to obtain significant therapeu-

Reprinted by permission of the publishers from Human Aspects of Biomedical Innovation, *by Everett Mendelsohn, Judith P. Swazey, and Irene Taviss, eds., Cambridge, Mass.: Harvard University Press, Copyright © 1971 by the President and Fellows of Harvard College.*

tic benefit, and the dose exploration and tolerability studies involved in such early pharmacologic trials are likely to entail a certain amount of serious risk because of the powerful drugs generally required to treat malignant disease. In such a situation, therefore, the physician might well say "No" to the earliest trial of a new drug in cases where the investigator might say "Yes." If one then moves to a problem such as the treatment of pain or of insomnia, where we have remedies which, while not perfect, are for most purposes excellent and reasonably safe, what is the physician to say? Statistically, there is no doubt that the patient has a better chance of adequate relief if given a standard and accepted drug rather than an untried one, no matter how impressive a case for research can be made from the standpoint of society's long-term needs.

Another difficulty stems from the use of both patients and volunteer subjects in medical research. This practice tends to blur the fundamental distinction between these two kinds of subjects. The volunteer (or the patient who is being studied in a way unrelated to his disease) is truly an experimental subject and usually stands to gain little or nothing medically—at least in the near future—from the experience of being exposed to an investigational compound. He may run considerable risk. It seems to me that such a volunteer must be handled quite differently from the patient who is also contributing to research goals but who may derive considerable benefit in the immediate future. To the degree that this distinction is blurred, ethical difficulties will be compounded.

It may be useful to consider the currently controversial issue of obtaining "informed consent" from subjects participating in drug investigation. The new Food and Drug Administration (FDA) regulations governing experimentation on human subjects make it clear that except in rare instances informed written consent must be obtained from anyone who is being given an investigational drug.[1] The FDA has spelled out in great detail the kinds of information that must be supplied to subjects of such experiments. It is interesting to contrast this approach with the usual practice of medicine, in which drug administration also plays an important role, and where patients almost certainly suffer more harm (some avoidable, much of it not) from the use of old drugs than experimental subjects suffer from the prescribing of new drugs by experienced investigators. In ordinary practice, consent is usually not informed, and it is almost never written, except for surgical procedures.

In favor of obtaining informed consent in clinical investigation is the reasonable (and generally held) belief that a person should know what is being done to him and what the risks of participation in an experiment may be. Of course, there are also important legal implications in procedures which—in the absence of consent—may be construed as civil or criminal assault on a person's body. There is a strong common law tradition in this regard which goes back at least as far as Justice Cardozo. In addition, unless a physician or committee other than the investigator is making the final decisions, the patient's informed consent represents a check on the motives of the investigator, motives which may be generally admirable but specifically undesirable, or at least questionable, for the individual patient.

What are the arguments *against* informed consent? To begin with, there are instances in which it would seem clearly not in the patient's best interest to discuss matters with full candor. A person dying of terminal cancer who has been given the few weakly effective available drugs, and whose condition is deteriorating, may gain little from an excessively detailed and frank discussion of the situation when a new drug is available which might possibly provide some benefit. Investigational drug use in psychiatric patients poses similar psychic hazards, including the special risk, if the use of drugs is made to look too much like an experiment, of permanently damaging or destroying the patient-doctor relationship.

One may also argue that obtaining informed consent involves the assumption that the investigator knows the risks of giving the drug, of withholding it, and the alternative risks from the use of other, older agents that might be used instead. The language of the FDA regulations does, it seems to me, imply all this. In fact, this information is available only in small measure.[2] One also assumes that the investigator is capable of the exposition required to present this information to the patient and that the patient is capable of grasping the information. One would also like to think that the patient is capable of making a decision in keeping with his own best interests after hearing the information, although a competent adult should, I suppose, have the freedom to make the wrong decision in the hospital or doctor's office no less than in the voting booth. All of these considerations are not, to be sure, so much arguments against informed consent as examples of the difference between the wish and the achievement.

Some important arguments against consent revolve around the possibility of impeding scientific progress if such consent is routinely obtained. (One could, for "scientific progress," substitute "providing benefit to others, including future generations.") There are some trials that will be impossible if a truly candid explanation has to be provided. One prominent investigator has evinced his skepticism about convincing people to participate in a trial that will last for years and in which some individuals are given drugs to lower their blood pressure and others receive placebos. Since it is not clear that all patients with hypertension should receive drugs, it would seem unethical *not* to perform the trial, but there is disagreement as to whether it is ethical to inform the patients of the nature of the trial while they are participating in it. With postpartum patients, we found in one experiment that if women were approached while they are actually having pain and asked to sign a consent form to participate in an experiment in which they might also receive inert preparations, some 80 to 85 percent refused to participate. (In work conducted on patients of this sort without written consent over a decade or so, we have never seen any evidence of serious harm or discontent; indeed, it is reasonably certain that these patients have received closer attention and better medical care than they would otherwise have received.) This would result in such an idiosyncratic selection of the population that we refused to conduct the trial, not only because of the time that would be required to complete it but because of the very real possibility that the results in such a minority of the population might not provide legitimate basis for predicting effects in the majority.

There is also the chance—even if patients consent to participate—that one may destroy the validity of a trial by inducing introspection of various kinds, producing a sort of Heisenberg effect. Some patients, when they know they are in a trial, will try to outwit the investigator by guessing which medications they are receiving. Other patients will be troubled by the nontherapeutic aspects of the experience, so that one may have difficulty in relating the responses to the usual clinical situation. Although investigators quite rightly tend to emphasize the difference between clinical practice and rigorous clinical investigation, it is nevertheless true that those studying new drugs experimentally wish very

much to collect data applicable to the use of the drugs in patients treated by "ordinary" doctors in "routine" medical practice.

Finally, there are some experiments which lose their entire point if all the cards are laid on the table. Take, for example, the investigation of the impact of a placebo. Although some patients report benefits from placebos even when they are told they are receiving "sugar pills," the full power of suggestibility and the patient-doctor relationship would almost certainly be affected by a discussion of the experiment with the subjects. This would be the medical equivalent of "bugging" a jury room to study the jurors' deliberations and then showing the jury the hidden microphones.[3]

Are there alternatives to "double-blind" placebo trials? (It is assumed that the obtaining of consent will be more feasible if patients do not have to agree to receive placebos.) One possibility, in drug investigation, is to demonstrate differences between a new drug and a standard drug. If the new one is significantly better, there is no problem. But what if it is significantly worse? This could mean that the drug is ineffective or merely that it is a *less* effective one—an important distinction. Another possibility is the use of dose-response relationships. If such relationships can be shown for new and old drugs in the same experiment, potency estimates can be made which are in no way dependent on the use of placebos. This is quite possible in a situation such as alleviation of postoperative pain, where the challenge is severe, the response to powerful analgesics is reasonably predictable, and placebos are thus rarely needed or used. In postpartum pain, however, dose-response relationships are rather difficult to elaborate, and the same may be true in studies of hypnotic drugs. This phenomenon has important implications for the admission of new drugs to the marketplace. If placebo studies are abandoned, will the FDA accept clinical comparisons where no dose-response relationships are evident? Not to do so may keep an effective drug off the market, but accepting at face value experiments where no difference is demonstrated between doses or drugs will surely result in the occasional admission of ineffective agents to the market.

Is some less formidable and stylized consent approach acceptable? It is apparently not, in regard to investigational drugs, unless one is willing to flaunt the FDA regulations. On the other hand, it may be possible to modify these regulations so as to make the consent provisions more flexible. If one eliminates the *written* aspects of the present informed consent regulations and substitutes verbal discussion (perhaps even placed on tape for the record) it may be possible to avoid some of the threats to experimentation discussed above while at the same time insuring that a certain amount of discussion with the patient has occurred.[4] I believe that the degree of candor utilized in obtaining consent should be related not only to the specific psychological and clinical problems but also to the expected risks of the experiment.

There is also the possibility of monitoring experimentation by use of peer committees or lay-scientific review boards which go over protocols, checking them carefully for flaws of various kinds, including ethical ones. No investigator should be engaged in research that he would be ashamed to have judged by his scientific colleagues or by a responsible group of laymen and scientists. There is at least theoretical advantage to sharing problems of conscience and morality with individuals not directly involved in the research, and of course ample precedent exists in society for delegation of important decision-making powers to others, although I doubt the legal acceptability of such review as an *alternative* to informed patient consent. It should be remembered, however, that a peer review mechanism may safeguard a subject more efficiently than informed consent; some people will agree to undergo risks that an expert committee would veto on their behalf.

It has been suggested that one way of discouraging unethical research is for editors to prevent the publication of data obtained in unsavory experiments by refusing to accept such manuscripts. Although this is an attractive notion at first glance, one wonders whether in fact important data unethically obtained could or should really be buried in this way. If an unscrupulous investigator were to discover a cure for cancer, would it be ethical to keep this knowledge from being used by others for the benefit of cancer patients, in compulsive adherence to "principle"? Although it is often affirmed that the ends do not justify the means, our society often functions as if they do.

One way of improving the present situation would be to acquaint the public, the regulatory agencies, the governmental granting agencies, and hospital committees with the needs and problems of experimentation. The present FDA regulations on informed consent, for example, quite clearly are the result of a particular climate of opinion. The law is susceptible to change. I heard one distinguished Baltimore judge say recently that the purpose of the law is to harmonize progress with stability. Years ago a property owner possessed the land underneath his feet as far as it went and all of the air directly above his property. With the coming of the airplane, this concept has changed. Similarly, educational facilities once considered "separate but equal" are no longer considered "equal." The law reflects the needs and desires of society as society sees these needs and desires, and it is entirely consistent with history to expect an appropriate legal response from society if it becomes educated to the needs of science and the social benefits of research.[5]

One wonders how many of medicine's greatest advances might have been delayed or prevented by the rigid application of some currently proposed principles to research at large. Even physicians were in a sense intellectually and emotionally unprepared for the earliest triumphs of cardiac surgery. What, then, would have been the layman's reaction to a full exposition of the problems involved in the original Blalock-Taussig shunts? And what of cardiac catheterization? The benefits of this technique have, quite appropriately, won Nobel Prizes for three of the physicians who pioneered in its use, but is it difficult to imagine lay journalists dubbing the early experimentation of these men barbaric and Nazi-like? ("and then, dear readers, these monsters have the temerity to thrust a tube down the length of one's arm into the very chambers of the human heart! The mind of anyone not completely brutalized by prolonged immersion in the bloody charnel houses of Science boggles at the thought"). I doubt, on the other hand, that the public would back—provided they had the facts—legislation like that originally proposed by Senator Thaler in New York State, which would have prohibited pediatric research *of all kinds* in the absence of court orders. Others have already pointed out that such legislation would have rendered impossible the development of the poliomyelitis and other vaccines.

If society is to be educated, there are many items that might be put on the agenda for discussion. The desire to involve the patient in the decision-making process in regard to details of medical care implies that there should be fuller and franker discussion about the use of everything from drugs to surgical techniques. Whether the public wants this is a matter for debate; I personally doubt it. In my own experience as a physician and investigator, not only are patients usually incapable of making the decisions in question (which is not surprising) but they are usually not desirous of making such decisions. In considerable anxiety a lay friend once called me to say that his physician had disclosed to him the controversy over the long-term use of anticoagulants in the management of patients who had recovered from a cardiac infarct. My friend protested that he was in no position to judge whether his wife should receive anticoagulants and that he really would have preferred his physician to make this judgment. In many complex decision-making situations in medicine, the patient is really more in the position of being on an airplane that has defective landing gear, is running out of gas, and whose pilot has to make some sort of landing in one of several alternate places than in the position of a passenger who is asked whether he wishes to board a plane whose pilot indicates that he is about to fly for the first time with his eyes closed and "no hands."

How much should be told to a patient by a surgeon who is requesting permission to perform an established operation, but one he personally is attempting for the first time? How much should be told to a patient about the hazards of a debilitating series of diagnostic abdominal X-rays, which may subject him to days of restricted food and fluid intake, as well as repeated cathartics? How much should be told to individuals exposed to radiation of any kind, for diagnosis or therapy, in view of the evidence in both insects and mammals that *no* amount of radiation is innocent in regard to genetic damage?

There are many other points that require consideration. What special safeguards are required for the study of prisoners? Of children? Of the psychiatrically ill? Of the mentally retarded? Of the dying patient? If an experimental live virus vaccine is to be given to subjects, should consent also be obtained from neighbors or schoolmates who may pick up the virus from the volunteers and come down with the disease? Should the patients in the adjoining beds be asked for permission when a new antibiotic is given to a patient, in view of the ability of antibiotics to disturb the ecology of the normal bacteria resident in the body and cause the development of resistant strains which can' then spread to these patients?

Should individuals be recompensed for damage suffered in the course of research, without any attempt to establish blame? The patient or volunteer who is injured by an experimental drug and loses his earning power thereby is entitled to compensation. The children of a patient who dies as the result of unanticipated mischief from a new diagnostic technique under investigation perhaps ought to expect financial remuneration. This implies not that the investigator must shoulder this burden alone but that the burden must be borne somehow. Who, then, shall pay the bill? In seeking an answer to this question, we should perhaps ask, "Who reaps the benefits of research?" While it is true that the investigator will gain when research is successful, and that with new drugs the pharmaceutical industry will profit, in the final analysis the beneficiary is really society as a whole. It would therefore seem incumbent on society to seek means of walking safely the narrow ledge between the twin abysses of hampered research and uncompensated patient injury. Scientists must not be reckless in their research; neither can they operate in an atmosphere of perpetual fear of disabling economic loss (or destroyed reputations) if unavoidable harm is the result of a well-planned experiment. Patients must not seek court settlements capriciously; neither must they silently suffer pain, injury, or death in the course of research. The problem is both subtle and complex and deserves an honest and equitable solution.

What should be society's attitude toward harm to the individual in return for benefits to the population as a whole? Mass chest X-ray surveys to detect treatable tuberculosis or other pulmonary diseases may cause leukemia in a few. Is the benefit worth the risk? Who shall decide? What means should be taken to safeguard the rights and health of individuals approached to participate in such a survey? Should a simple majority decide whether an entire community's water supply should be fluoridated? We have become reconciled to the ability of a governmental agency to expropriate our land or homes in order to build a new school or a new bridge, but it is not traditional to force anyone to participate in research. Yet society frequently tramples on the rights of individuals in the "greater interest." One can object, but can we deny the existence of the phenomenon? Should we have different guidelines for individual sacrifice when health or life is at stake, rather than property?

Finally, a word about the effective implantation of an ethical conscience in the minds of physicians and clinical investigators. The doctor becomes increasingly accustomed to a life which does not allow for leisurely contemplation. He is by trade a non-agnostic. Even when he makes a decision not to treat, for example, he is not suspending judgment but expressing the belief that "no treatment" is better than treatment. He must continually choose between remedies even when he has poor basis for making a choice. The doctor is likely to be propelled increasingly in the direction of quick decisions which at times resemble reflex responses. In this pragmatic, frenetic existence he may quickly absorb the moral atmosphere around him without questioning it. It is my conviction, therefore, that ethical problems must be integrated into the doctor's life at the earliest possible moment. I do not believe that it will be effective to bring up such matters relatively late in the medical career, although the doctor will certainly require constant reinforcement throughout his professional life. The medical student must be made, from the beginning, to consider the ethical aspects of medicine, in regard to *both* practice and research. Many a liver biopsy or laboratory test is now performed in the name of science, with little benefit to the patient. A medical student made emotionally immune to the casual performance of risky procedures by the tacit acceptance of such procedures by his mentors is unlikely to be excessively concerned as a physician or investigator with the subtleties of ethical and moral issues. Some way must be found to incorporate these matters so firmly into his moral fabric that he cannot avoid the ethical implications of his acts. I submit that the successful development of such an ethical conscience, combined with professional skill, will protect the patent or experimental subject much more effectively than any laws or regulations.

I have previously said that for the ethical, experienced investigator no laws are needed and for the unscrupulous incompetent no laws will help, except to allow the injured subjects to obtain compensation or to punish the offending scientists. Between these extremes there still remain many investigators who will unquestionably be constrained in some way by legislation. But it is unlikely that subjects will be *optimally* protected from harm without additional safeguards imposed by the scientific community itself. These safeguards will range all the way from exercise of wisdom and judgment to the invoking of statistical monitoring techniques to halt experiments that were ethical at the outset but cannot ethically be continued.

Some are fond of quoting Claude Bernard when he said, in *An Introduction to the Study of Experimental Medicine*, "The principle of medical and surgical morality, therefore, consists in never performing on man an experiment which might be harmful to him in any extent, even though the result might be highly advantageous to science, i.e., to the health of others."[6] This statement is irrelevant to much of clinical investigation, where patients usually are involved in procedures that may be of considerable benefit to them, although they necessarily involve some risk (like almost everything else in the world). One might point out that Claude Bernard also said, "So, among the experiments that may be tried on man, those that can only harm are forbidden, those that are innocent are permissible, and those that may do good are obligatory."[7] The investigator is responsible not only to the patients currently under his care but also to the many that will never be seen by him. Is this responsibility to mankind less noble than that of the physician concerned with the care of the individual patient?

Bernard's statement is—like my own remarks—full of ambivalence. As J. Bronowski has put it, one of society's major tasks is to reconcile the welfare of man with the welfare of men.[8] In clinical investigation, as in other societal activities, the good of the individual and the good of society are often not identical and sometimes mutually exclusive. I believe it is inevitable that the many will continue to benefit on occasion from the contributions—sometimes involuntary—of the few. The problem is to know when to say "Halt!" There are some societal "gains" that may only be available at an excessively high price. We cannot afford to have the cancer of moral decay that comes from frequent and flagrant disregard of human rights gnawing away at the body of science. We should, therefore, in a very real sense welcome the present and continuing debate on ethics in clinical investigation. That harm has come from exaggerated stories is unquestioned, as is the possibility that additional harm to patients may occur, but I believe that in the long run both the public and science will benefit from a searching analysis of the roots of our ethical conduct.

Notes

1. While the FDA rules apply only to investigational drugs, the issue of consent is relevant to all clinical

investigation because of both legal implications and current National Institutes of Health policies on human experimentation which affect the conduct of grantees.

2. It is surrealistic to read, in an editorial in a leading American medical journal, the statement: "How much more important it is to have informed consent, when the potential risk is unknown!"

3. Dinnerstein et al., in an interesting paper, have reviewed some of the literature on the differential effects of drugs in different experimental settings. Their desire to study the effects of drugs "in a completely concealed form, with the subject not even knowing when he has been drugged" and under situations with different "cover stories" would be out of the question if rigid application of this principle of "total disclosure" were made. Albert J. Dinnerstein, Milton Lowenthal, and Bernard Blitz, "The Interaction of Drugs with Placebos in the Control of Pain and Anxiety," *Perspectives in Biology and Medicine*, 10 (1966), 103–117.

4. It is important to remember that there is no *necessary* relation between a consent procedure that satisfies the law and one that safeguards the patient.

5. John Dewey once warned that part of the public protest against experimentation is related to old misunderstandings and dreads about science. He was talking about animal experimentation, but it may be useful to remember his warning to be "on the alert against every revival of the spirit of animosity to discovery and to the application of the fruits of discovery." One does not need to accuse everyone who is concerned about the ethics of clinical investigation of being antiscientific to believe that at least some of the hue and cry can be traced to antiscientism.

6. Claude Bernard, *An Introduction to the Study of Experimental Medicine* (New York: Dover Publications, 1957), p. 101.

7. Ibid., p. 102.

8. J. Bronowski, *Science and Human Values* (London: Hutchinson & Co., 1961), p. 78.

Philosophical Reflections on Experimenting with Human Subjects

Hans Jonas

Hans Jonas argues that, if we justify experiments by considering them a right of society, then we are exposing individuals to dangers for the general good. This, for Jonas, is inherently wrong, and no individual should be forced to surrender himself or herself to a social goal.

Any risk that is taken must be voluntary, but obtaining informed consent, Jonas claims, is not sufficient to justify the experimental use of human beings. Two other conditions must be met: first, subjects must be recruited from those who are most knowledgeable about the circumstances of research and who are intellectually most capable of grasping its purposes and procedures; second, the experiment must be undertaken for an adequate cause. Jonas cautions us that the progress that may come from research is not necessarily worth our efforts or approval, and he reminds us that there are moral values that we ought not to lose in the pursuit of science.

Experimenting with human subjects is going on in many fields of scientific and technological progress.

It is designed to replace the overall instruction by natural, occasional experience with the selective in-

Reprinted by permission of Daedalus, *Journal of the American Academy of Arts and Sciences, Spring 1969, Boston, Mass. This essay is included, on pp. 105–131, in a 1980 reedition of Jonas's* Philosophical Essays: From Current Creed to Technological Man, *published by the University of Chicago Press.*

formation from artificial, systematic experiment which physical science has found so effective in dealing with inanimate nature. Of the new experimentation with man, medical is surely the most legitimate; psychological, the most dubious; biological (still to come), the most dangerous. I have chosen here to deal with the first only, where the case *for* it is strongest and the task of adjudicating conflicting claims hardest. . . .

The Peculiarity of Human Experimentation

Experimentation was originally sanctioned by natural science. There it is performed on inanimate objects, and this raises no moral problems. But as soon as animate, feeling beings become the subjects of experiment, as they do in the life sciences and especially in medical research, this innocence of the search for knowledge is lost and questions of conscience arise. The depth to which moral and religious sensibilities can become aroused over these questions is shown by the vivisection issue. Human experimentation must sharpen the issue as it involves ultimate questions of personal dignity and sacrosanctity. One profound difference between the human experiment and the physical (besides that between animate and inanimate, feeling and unfeeling nature) is this: The physical experiment employs small-scale, artificially devised substitutes for that about which knowledge is to be obtained, and the experimenter extrapolates from these models and simulated conditions to nature at large. Something deputizes for the "real thing"—balls rolling down an inclined plane for sun and planets, electric discharges from a condenser for real lightning, and so on. For the most part, no such substitution is possible in the biological sphere. We must operate on the original itself, the real thing in the fullest sense, and perhaps affect it irreversibly. No simulacrum can take its place. Especially in the human sphere, experimentation loses entirely the advantage of the clear division between vicarious model and true object. Up to a point, animals may fulfill the proxy role of the classical physical experiment. But in the end man himself must furnish knowledge about himself, and the comfortable separation of noncommittal experiment and definitive action vanishes. An experiment in education affects the lives of its subjects, perhaps a whole generation of schoolchildren. Human experimentation for

whatever purpose is always *also* a responsible, nonexperimental, definitive dealing with the subject himself. And not even the noblest purpose abrogates the obligations this involves.

This is the root of the problem with which we are faced: Can both that purpose and this obligation be satisfied? If not, what would be a just compromise? Which side should give way to the other? The question is inherently philosophical as it concerns not merely pragmatic difficulties and their arbitration, but a genuine conflict of values involving principles of a high order. May I put conflict in these terms. On principle, it is felt, human beings *ought* not to be dealt with in that way (the "guinea pig" protest); on the other hand, such dealings are increasingly urged on us by considerations, in turn appealing to principle, that claim to override those objections. Such a claim must be carefully assessed, especially when it is swept along by a mighty tide. Putting the matter thus, we have already made one important assumption rooted in our "Western" cultural tradition: The prohibitive rule is, to that way of thinking, the primary and axiomatic one; the permissive counter-rule, as qualifying the first, is secondary and stands in need of justification. We must justify the infringement of a primary inviolability, which needs no justification itself; and the justification of its infringement must be by values and needs of a dignity commensurate with those to be sacrificed.

Health as a Public Good

The cause invoked [for medical experimentation] is health and, in its more critical aspect, life itself—clearly superlative goods that the physician serves directly by curing and the researcher indirectly by the knowledge gained through his experiments. There is no question about the good served or about the evil fought—disease and premature death. But a good to whom and an evil to whom? Here the issue tends to become somewhat clouded. In the attempt to give experimentation the proper dignity (on the problematic view that a value becomes greater by being "social" instead of merely individual), the health in question or the disease in question is somehow predicated on the social whole, as if it were society that, in the persons of its members enjoyed the one and suffered the other. For the purposes of our problem, public interest can then be pitted against private interest, the common good against the individual good. Indeed, I have found health called a national resource, which of course it is, but surely not in the first place.

In trying to resolve some of the complexities and ambiguities lurking in these conceptualizations, I have pondered a particular statement, made in the form of a question, which I found in the *Proceedings* of the earlier *Daedalus* conference: "Can society afford to discard the tissues and organs of the hopelessly unconscious patient when they could be used to restore the otherwise hopelessly ill, but still salvageable individual?" And somewhat later: "A strong case can be made that society can ill afford to discard the tissues and organs of the hopelessly unconscious patient; they are greatly needed for study and experimental trial to help those who can be salvaged."[1] I hasten to add that any suspicion of callousness that the "commodity" language of these statements may suggest is immediately dispelled by the name of the speaker, Dr. Henry K. Beecher, for whose humanity and moral sensibility there can be nothing but admiration. But the use, in all innocence, of this language gives food for thought. Let me, for a moment, take the question literally. "Discarding" implies proprietary rights—nobody can discard what does not belong to him in the first place. Does society then own my body? "Salvaging" implies the same and, moreover, a use-value to the owner. Is the life-extension of certain individuals then a public interest—that is, of the loss or gain involved. And "society" itself—what is it? When does a need, an aim, an obligation become social? Let us reflect on some of these terms.

What Society Can Afford

"Can Society afford . . .?" Afford what? To let people die intact, thereby withholding something from other people who desperately need it, who in consequence will have to die too? These other, unfortunate people indeed cannot afford not to have a kidney, heart, or other organ of the dying patient, on which they depend for an extension of their lease on life; but does that give them a right to it? And does it oblige society to procure it for them? What is it that *society* can or cannot afford—leaving aside for the moment the question of what it has a *right* to? It surely can afford to lose members through death; more than that, it is built on the balance of death and birth decreed by the order of life. This is too general, of course, for our question, but perhaps it is well to

remember. The specific question seems to be whether society can afford to let some people die whose death might be deferred by particular means if these were authorized by society. Again, if it is merely a question of what society can or cannot afford, rather than of what it ought or ought not to do, the answer must be: Of course, it can. If cancer, heart disease, and other organic, noncontagious ills, especially those tending to strike the old more than the young, continue to exact their toll at the normal rate of incidence (including the toll of private anguish and misery), society can go on flourishing in every way.

Here, by contrast, are some examples of what, in sober truth, society cannot afford. It cannot afford to let an epidemic rage unchecked; a persistent excess of deaths over births, but neither—we must add—too great an excess of births over deaths; too low an average life expectancy even if demographically balanced by fertility, but neither too great a longevity with the necessitated correlative dearth of youth in the social body; a debilitating state of general heath; and things of this kind. These are plain cases where the whole condition of society is critically affected, and the public interest can make its imperative claims. The Black Death of the Middle Ages was a *public* calamity of the acute kind; the life-sapping ravages of endemic malaria or sleeping sickness in certain areas are a public calamity of the chronic kind. Such situations a society as a whole can truly not "afford," and they may call for extraordinary remedies, including, perhaps, the invasion of private sacrosanctities.

This is not entirely a matter of numbers and numerical ratios. Society, in a subtler sense, cannot "afford" a single miscarriage of justice, a single inequity in the dispensation of its laws, the violation of the rights of even the tiniest minority, because these undermine the moral basis on which society's existence rests. Nor can it, for a similar reason, afford the absence or atrophy in its midst of compassion and of the effort to alleviate suffering—be it widespread or rare—one form of which is the effort to conquer disease of any kind, whether "socially" significant (by reasons of number) or not. And in short, society cannot afford the absence among its members of *virtue*, with its readiness for sacrifice beyond defined duty. Since its presence—that is to say, that of personal idealism—is a matter of grace and not of decree, we have the paradox that society depends for its existence on intangibles of nothing less than a religious order, for which it can hope, but which it cannot enforce. All the more must it protect this most precious capital from abuse.

For what objectives connected with the medico-biological sphere should this reserve be drawn upon—for example, in the form of accepting, soliciting, perhaps even imposing the submission of human subjects to experimentation? We postulate that this must be not just a worthy cause, as any promotion of the health of anybody doubtlessly is, but a cause qualifying for transcendent social sanction. Here one thinks first of those cases critically affecting the whole condition, present and future, of the community we have illustrated. Something equivalent to what in the political sphere is called "clear and present danger" may be invoked and a state of emergency proclaimed, thereby suspending certain otherwise inviolable prohibitions and taboos. We may observe that averting a disaster always carries greater weight than promoting a good. Extraordinary danger excuses extraordinary means. This covers human experimentation, which we would like to count, as far as possible, among the extraordinary rather than the ordinary means of serving the common good under public auspices. Naturally, since foresight and responsibility for the future are of the essence of institutional society, averting disaster extends into long-term prevention, although the lesser urgency will warrant less sweeping licenses.

Society and the Cause of Progress

Much weaker is the case where it is a matter not of saving but of improving society. Much of medical research falls into this category. As stated before, a permanent death rate from heart failure or cancer does not threaten society. So long as certain statistical ratios are maintained, the incidence of disease and of disease-induced mortality is not (in the strict sense) a "social" misfortune. I hasten to add that it is not therefore less of a human misfortune, and the call for relief issuing with silent eloquence from each victim and all potential victims is of no lesser dignity. But it is misleading to equate the fundamentally human response to it with what is owed to society: it is owed by man to man—and it is thereby owed by society to the individuals as soon as the adequate ministering to these concerns outgrows (as it progressively does) the scope of private spontaneity and is made a public mandate. It is thus that

society assumes responsibility for medical care, research, old age, and innumerable other things not originally of the public realm (in the original "social contract"), and they become duties toward "society" (rather than directly toward one's fellow man) by the fact that they are socially operated.

Indeed, we expect from organized society no longer mere protection against harm and the securing of the conditions of our preservation, but active and constant improvement in all the domains of life: the waging of the battle against nature, the enhancement of the human estate—in short, the promotion of progress. This is an expansive goal, one far surpassing the disaster norm of our previous reflections. It lacks the urgency of the latter, but has the nobility of the free, forward thrust. It surely is worth sacrifices. It is not at all a question of what society can afford, but of what it is committed to, beyond all necessity, by our mandate. Its trusteeship has become an established, ongoing, institutionalized business of the body politic. As eager beneficiaries of its gains, we now owe to "society," as its chief agent, our individual contributions toward its *continued pursuit*. I emphasize "continued pursuit." Maintaining the existing level requires no more than the orthodox means of taxation and enforcement of professional standards that raise no problems. The more optional goal of pushing forward is also more exacting. We have this syndrome: Progress is by our choosing an acknowledged interest of society, in which we have a stake in various degrees; science is a necessary instrument of progress; research is a necessary instrument of science; and in medical science experimentation on human subjects is a necessary instrument of research. Therefore, human experimentation has come to be a societal interest.

The destination of research is essentially melioristic. It does not serve the preservation of the existing good from which I profit myself and to which I am obligated. Unless the present state is intolerable, the melioristic goal is in a sense gratuitous, and this not only from the vantage point of the present. Our descendants have a right to be left an unplundered planet; they do not have a right to new miracle cures. We have sinned against them, if by our doing we have destroyed their inheritance—which we are doing at full blast; we have not sinned against them if by the time they come around arthritis has not yet been conquered (unless by sheer neglect). And generally, in the matter of progress, as humanity had no claim on a Newton, a Michelangelo, or a St.

Francis to appear, and no right to the blessings of their unscheduled deeds, so progress, with all our methodical labor for it, cannot be budgeted in advance and its fruits received as a due. Its coming-about at all and its turning out for good (of which we can never be sure) must rather be regarded as something akin to grace.

The Melioristic Goal, Medical Research, and Individual Duty

Nowhere is the melioristic goal more inherent than in medicine. To the physician, it is not gratuitous. He is committed to curing and thus to improving the power to cure. Gratuitous we called it (outside disaster conditions) as a *social* goal, but noble at the same time. Both the nobility and the gratuitousness must influence the manner in which self-sacrifice for it is elicited, and even its free offer accepted. Freedom is certainly the first condition to be observed here. The surrender of one's body to medical experimentation is entirely outside the enforceable "social contract."

Or can it be construed to fall within its terms—namely, as repayment for benefits from past experimentation that I have enjoyed myself? But I am indebted for these benefits not to society, but to the past "martyrs," to whom society is indebted itself, and society has no right to call in my personal debt by way of adding new to its own. Moreover, gratitude is not an enforceable social obligation; it anyway does not mean that I must emulate the deed. Most of all, if it was wrong to exact such sacrifice in the first place, it does not become right to exact it again with the plea of the profit it has brought me. If, however, it was not exacted, but entirely free, as it ought to have been, then it should remain so, and its precedence must not be used as a social pressure on others for doing the same under the sign of duty. . . .

The "Conscription" of Consent

The mere issuing of the appeal, the calling for volunteers, with the moral and social pressures it inevitably generates, amounts even under the most meticulous rules of consent to a sort of *conscripting*. And some soliciting is necessarily involved. . . . And this is why "consent," surely a nonnegotiable minimum requirement, is not the full answer to the problem. Granting then that soliciting and therefore some degree of conscripting are part of the situation, who may conscript and who may be conscripted? Or less harshly expressed: Who should issue appeals and to whom?

The naturally qualified issuer of the appeal is the research scientist himself, collectively the main carrier of the impulse and the only one with the technical competence to judge. But his being very much an interested party (with vested interests, indeed, not purely in the public good, but in the scientific enterprise as such, in "his" project, and even in his career) makes him also suspect. The ineradicable dialectic of this situation—a delicate incompatibility problem—calls for particular controls by the research community and by public authority that we need not discuss. They can mitigate, but not eliminate the problem. We have to live with the ambiguity, the treacherous impurity of everything human.

Self-Recruitment of the Community

To whom should the appeal be addressed? The natural issuer of the call is also the first natural addressee: the physician-researcher himself and the scientific confraternity at large. With such a coincidence—indeed, the noble tradition with which the whole business of human experimentation started—almost all of the associated legal, ethical, and metaphysical problems vanish. If it is full, autonomous identification of the subject with the purpose that is required for the dignifying of his serving as a subject—here it is; if strongest motivation—here it is; if fullest understanding—here it is; if freest decision—here it is; if greatest integration with the person's total, chosen pursuit—here it is. With the fact of self-solicitation the issue of consent in all its insoluble equivocality is bypassed per se. Not even the condition that the particular purpose be truly important and the project reasonably promising, which must hold in any solicitation of others, need be satisfied here. By himself, the scientist is free to obey his obsession, to play his hunch, to wager on chance, to follow the lure of ambition. It is all part of the "divine madness" that somehow animates the ceaseless pressing against frontiers. For the rest of society, which has a deep-seated disposition to look with reverence and awe upon the guardians of the mysteries of life, the profession assumes with this proof of its devotion the role of a self-chosen, consecrated fraternity, not unlike the monastic orders of the past, and this would come nearest to the actual, religious origins of the art of healing. . . .

"Identification" as the Principle of Recruitment in General

If the properties we adduced as the particular qualifications of the members of the scientific fraternity itself are taken as general criteria of selection, then one should look for additional subjects where a maximum of identification, understanding, and spontaneity can be expected—that is, among the most highly motivated, the most highly educated, and the least "captive" members of the community. From this naturally scarce resource, a descending order of permissibility leads to greater abundance and ease of supply, whose use should become proportionately more hesitant as the exculpating criteria are relaxed. An inversion of normal "market" behavior is demanded here—namely, to accept the lowest quotation last (and excused only by the greatest pressure of need); to pay the highest price first.

The ruling principle in our considerations is that the "wrong" of reification can only be made "right" by such authentic identification with the cause that it is the subject's as well as the researcher's cause—whereby his role in its service is not just permitted by him, but *willed*. That sovereign will of his which embraces the end as his own restores his personhood to the otherwise depersonalizing context. To be valid it must be autonomous and informed. The latter condition can, outside the research community, only be fulfilled by degrees; but the higher the degree of understanding regarding the purpose and the technique, the more valid becomes the endorsement of the will. A margin of mere trust inevitably remains. Ultimately, the appeal for volunteers should seek this free and generous endorsement, the appropriation of the research purpose into the person's own scheme of ends. Thus, the appeal is in truth addressed to the one, mysterious, and sacred source of any such generosity of the will—"devotion," whose forms and objects of commitment are various and may invest different motivations in different individuals. The following, for instance, may be responsive to the "call" we are discussing: compassion with human suffering, zeal for humanity, reverence for the Golden Rule, enthusiasm for progress, homage to the cause of knowledge, even longing for sacrificial

justification (do not call that "masochism," please). On all these, I say, it is defensible and right to draw when the research objective is worthy enough; and it is a prime duty of the research community (especially in view of what we called the "margin of trust") to see that this sacred source is never abused for frivolous ends. For a less than adequate cause, not even the freest, unsolicited offer should be accepted.

The Rule of the "Descending Order" and its Counterutility Sense

We have laid down what must seem to be a forbidding rule to the number-hungry research industry. Having faith in the transcendent potential of man, I do not fear that the "source" will ever fail a society that does not destroy it—and only such a one is worthy of the blessings of progress. But "elitistic" the rule is (as is the enterprise of progress itself), and elites are by nature small. The combined attribute of motivation and information, plus the absence of external pressures, tends to be socially so circumscribed that strict adherence to the rule might numerically starve the research process. This is why I spoke of a descending order of permissibility, which is itself permissive, but where the realization that it is a *descending* order is not without pragmatic import. Departing from the august norm, the appeal must needs shift from idealism to docility, from high-mindedness to compliance, from judgment to trust. Consent spreads over the whole spectrum. I will not go into the casuistics of this penumbral area. I merely indicate the principle of the order of preference: The poorer in knowledge, motivation, and freedom of decision (and that, alas, means the more readily available in terms of numbers and possible manipulation), the more sparingly and indeed reluctantly should the reservoir be used, and the more compelling must therefore become the countervailing justification.

Let us note that this is the opposite of a social utility standard, the reverse of the order by "availability and expendability": The most valuable and scarcest, the least expendable elements of the social organism, are to be the first candidates for risk and sacrifice. It is the standard of *noblesse oblige*; and with all its counterutility and seeming "wastefulness," we feel a rightness about it and perhaps even a higher "utility," for the soul of the community lives by this spirit.[2] It is also the opposite of what the day-to-day interests of research clamor for, and for the scientific community to honor it will mean that it will have to fight a strong temptation to go by routine to the readiest sources of supply—the suggestible, the ignorant, the dependent, the "captive" in various senses.[3] I do not believe that heightened resistance here must cripple research, which cannot be permitted; but it may indeed slow it down by the smaller numbers fed into experimentation in consequence. This price—a possibly slower rate of progress—may have to be paid for the preservation of the most precious capital of higher communal life.

Experimentation on Patients

So far we have been speaking on the tacit assumption that the subjects of experimentation are recruited from among the healthy. To the question "Who is conscriptable?" the spontaneous answer is: Least and last of all the sick—the most available of all as they are under treatment and observation anyway. That the afflicted should not be called upon to bear additional burden and risk, that they are society's special trust and the physician's trust in particular—these are elementary responses of our moral sense. Yet the very destination of medical research, the conquest of disease, requires at the crucial stage trial and verification on precisely the sufferers from the disease, and their total exemption would defeat the purpose itself. In acknowledging this inescapable necessity, we enter the most sensitive area of the whole complex, the one most keenly felt and most searchingly discussed by the practitioners themselves. No wonder, it touches the heart of the doctor-patient relation, putting its most solemn obligations to the test. There is nothing new in what I have to say about the ethics of the doctor-patient relation, but for the purpose of confronting it with the issue of experimentation some of the oldest verities must be recalled.

The Fundamental Privilege of the Sick

In the course of treatment, the physician is obligated to the patient and to no one else. He is not the agent of society, nor of the interests of medical science, nor of the patient's family, nor of his co-sufferers, nor of future sufferers from the same disease. The patient alone counts when he is under the physician's care. By the simple law of bilateral contract (analogous, for example, to the relation of lawyer to client and its "conflict of interest" rule), the physician is bound not to let any other interest interfere with that of the patient in being cured. But manifestly more sublime norms than contractual ones are involved. We may speak of a sacred trust; strictly by its terms, the doctor is, as it were, alone with his patient and God.

There is one normal exception to this—that is, to the doctor's not being the agent of society vis-à-vis the patient, but the trustee of his interests alone: the quarantining of the contagious sick. This is plainly not for the patient's interest, but for that of others threatened by him. (In vaccination, we have a combination of both: protection of the individual and others.) But preventing the patient from causing harm to others is not the same as exploiting him for the advantage of others. And there is, of course, the abnormal exception of collective catastrophe, the analogue to a state of war. The physician who desperately battles a raging epidemic is under a unique dispensation that suspends in a nonspecifiable way some of the structures of normal practice, including possibly those against experimental liberties with his patients. No rules can be devised for the waiving of rules in extremities. And as with the famous shipwreck examples of ethical theory, the less said about it the better. But what is allowable there and may later be passed over in forgiving silence cannot serve as a precedent. We are concerned with non-extreme, non-emergency conditions where the voice of principle can be heard and claims can be adjudicated free from duress. We have conceded that there are such claims, and that if there is to be medical advance at all, not even the superlative privilege of the suffering and the sick can be kept wholly intact from the intrusion of its needs. About this least palatable, most disquieting part of our subject, I have to offer only groping, inconclusive remarks.

The Principle of "Identification" Applied to Patients

On the whole, the same principles would seem to hold here as are found to hold with "normal subjects": motivation, identification, understanding on the part of the subject. But it is clear that these conditions are peculiarly difficult to satisfy with regard to a patient. His physical state, psychic preoccupation, dependent relation to the doctor, the submissive attitude induced by treatment—everything connected with his condition and situation makes the sick person inherently less of a sovereign person than the healthy one. Spontaneity of self-offering was almost to be ruled out; consent is marred by lower resistance or captive circumstance, and so on. In fact, all the factors that make the patient, as a category, particularly accessible and welcome for experimentation at the same time compromise the quality of the responding affirmation that must morally redeem the making use of them. This, in addition to the primacy of the physician's duty, puts a heightened onus on the physician-researcher to limit his undue power to the most important and defensible research objectives and, of course, to keep persuasion at a minimum.

Still, with all the disabilities noted, there is scope among patients for observing the rule of the "descending order of permissibility" that we have laid down for normal subjects, in vexing inversion of the utility order of quantitative abundance and qualitative "expendability." By the principle of this order, those patients who most identify with and are cognizant of the cause of research—members of the medical profession (who after all are sometimes patients themselves)—come first; the highly motivated and educated, also least dependent, among the lay patients come next; and so on down the line. An added consideration here is seriousness of condition, which again operates in inverse proportion. Here the profession must fight the tempting sophistry that the hopeless case is expendable (because in prospect already expended) and therefore especially usable; and generally the attitude that the poorer the chances of the patient, the more justifiable his recruitment for experimentation (other than for his own benefit). The opposite is true.

Nondisclosure as a Borderline Case

Then there is the case where ignorance of the subject, sometimes even of the experimenter, is of the essence of the experiment (the "double blind"-control group-placebo syndrome). It is said to be a necessary element of the scientific process. Whatever may be said about its ethics in regard to normal subjects, especially volunteers, it is an outright betrayal of trust in regard to the patient who believes that he is receiving treatment. Only supreme impor-

tance of the objective can exonerate it, without making it less of a transgression. The patient is definitely wronged even when not harmed. And ethics apart, the practice of such deception holds the danger of undermining the faith in the *bona fides* of treatment, the beneficial intent of the physician—the very basis of the doctor-patient relationship. In every respect it follows that concealed experiment on patients—that is, experiment under the guise of treatment—should be the rarest exception, at best, if it cannot be wholly avoided.

This has still the merit of a borderline problem. The same is not true of the other case of necessary ignorance of the subject—that of the unconscious patient. Drafting him for nontherapeutic experiments is simply and unqualifiedly impermissible; progress or not, he must never be used, on the inflexible principle that utter helplessness demands utter protection.

When preparing this paper, I filled pages with a casuistics of this harrowing field, but then scrapped most of it, realizing my dilettante status. The shadings are endless, and only the physician-researcher can discern them properly as the cases arise. Into his lap the decision is thrown. The philosophical rule, once it has admitted into itself the idea of a sliding scale, cannot really specify its own application. It can only impress on the practitioner a general maxim or attitude for the exercise of his judgment and conscience in the concrete occasions of his work. In our case, I am afraid, it means making life more difficult for him.

It will also be noted that, somewhat at variance with the emphasis in the literature, I have not dwelt on the element of "risk" and very little on that of "consent." Discussion of the first is beyond the layman's competence; the emphasis on the second has been lessened because of its equivocal character. It is a truism to say that one should strive to minimize the risk and to maximize the consent. The more demanding concept of "identification," which I have used, includes "consent" in its maximal or authentic form, and the assumption of risk is its privilege.

No Experiments on Patients Unrelated to Their Own Disease

Although my ponderings have, on the whole, yielded points of view rather than definite prescriptions, premises rather than conclusions, they have led me to a few unequivocal yeses and nos. The first is the emphatic rule that patients should be experimented upon, if at all, *only* with reference to *their disease*. Never should there be added to the gratuitousness of the experiment as such the gratuitousness of service to an unrelated cause. This follows simply from what we have found to be the only excuse for infracting the special exemption of the sick at all—namely, that the scientific war on disease cannot accomplish its goal without drawing the sufferers from disease into the investigative process. If under this excuse they become subjects of experiment, they do so *because*, and only because, of *their* disease.

This is the fundamental and self-sufficient consideration. That the patient cannot possibly benefit from the unrelated experiment therapeutically, while he might from experiment related to his condition, is also true, but lies beyond the problem area of pure experiment. I am in any case discussing nontherapeutic experimentation only, where *ex hypothesi* the patient does not benefit. Experiment as part of therapy—that is, directed toward helping the subject himself—is a different matter altogether and raises its own problems but hardly philosophical ones. As long as a doctor can say, even if only in his own thought: "There is no known cure for your condition (or: You have responded to none); but there is promise in a new treatment still under investigation, not quite tested yet as to effectiveness and safety; you will be taking a chance, but all things considered, I judge it in your best interest to let me try it on you"—as long as he can speak thus, he speaks as the patient's physician and may err, but does not transform the patient into a subject of experimentation. Introduction of an untried therapy into the treatment where the tried ones have failed is not "experimentation on the patient."

Generally, and almost needless to say, with all the rules of the book, there is something "experimental" (because tentative) about every individual treatment, beginning with the diagnosis itself; and he would be a poor doctor who would not learn from every case for the benefit of future cases, and a poor member of the profession who would not make any new insights gained from his treatments available to the profession at large. Thus, knowledge may be advanced in the treatment of any patient, and the interest of the medical art and all sufferers from the same affliction as well as the patient himself may be served if something happens to be learned from his case. But his gain to knowledge and future therapy is incidental to the *bona fide* service to the present patient. He has the right to expect that the doctor does nothing to him just in order to learn.

In that case, the doctor's imaginary speech would run, for instance, like this: "There is nothing more I can do for you. But you can do something for me. Speaking no longer as your physician but on behalf of medical science, we could learn a great deal about future cases of this kind if you would permit me to perform certain experiments on you. It is understood that you yourself would not benefit from any knowledge we might gain; but future patients would." This statement would express the purely experimental situation, assumedly here with the subject's concurrence and with all cards on the table. In Alexander Bicker's words: "It is a different situation when the doctor is no longer trying to make [the patient] well, but is trying to find out how to make others well in the future."[4]

But even in the second case, that of the nontherapeutic experiment where the patient does not benefit, at least the patient's own disease is enlisted in the cause of fighting that disease, even if only in others. It is yet another thing to say or think: "Since you are here—in the hospital with its facilities—anyway, under our care and observation anyway, away from your job (or, perhaps, doomed) anyway, we wish to profit from your being available for some other research of great interest we are presently engaged in." From the standpoint of merely medical ethics, which has only to consider risk, consent, and the worth of the objective, there may be no cardinal difference between this case and the last one. I hope that the medical reader will not think I am making too fine a point when I say that from the standpoint of the subject and his dignity there is a cardinal difference that crosses the line between the permissible and the impermissible, and this by the same principle of "Identification" I have been invoking all along. Whatever the rights and wrongs of any experimentation on any patient—in the one case, at least that residue of identification is left him that it is his own affliction by which he can contribute to the conquest of that affliction, his own kind of suffering which he helps to alleviate in others; and so in a sense it is his own cause. It is totally indefensible to rob the unfortunate of this intimacy with the purpose and make his misfortune a convenience for the furtherance of alien concerns.

Conclusion

. . . I wish only to say in conclusion that if some of the practical implications of my reasonings are felt to work out toward a slower rate of progress, this should not cause too great dismay. Let us not forget that progress is an optional goal, not an unconditional commitment, and that its tempo in particular, compulsive as it may become, has nothing sacred about it. Let us also remember that a slower progress in the conquest of disease would not threaten society, grievous as it is to those who have to deplore that their particular disease be not yet conquered, but that society would indeed be threatened by the erosion of those moral values whose loss, possibly caused by too ruthless a pursuit of scientific progress, would make its most dazzling triumphs not worth having. Let us finally remember that it cannot be the aim of progress to abolish the lot of mortality. Of some ill or other, each of us will die. Our mortal condition is upon us with its harshness but also its wisdom—because without it there would not be the eternally renewed promise of the freshness, immediacy, and eagerness of youth; nor would there be for any of us the incentive to number our days and make them count. With all our striving to wrest from our mortality what we can, we should bear its burden with patience and dignity.

Notes

1. *Proceedings of the Conference on the Ethical Aspects of Experimentation on Human Subjects,* November 3–4, 1967 (Boston, Mass.; hereafter called *Proceedings*), pp. 50–51.

2. Socially, everyone is expendable relatively—that is, in different degrees; religiously, no one is expendable absolutely: The "image of God" is in all. If it can be enhanced, then it is not by anyone being expended, but by someone expending himself.

3. This refers to captives of circumstance, not of justice. Prison inmates are, with respect to our problem, in a special class. If we hold to some idea of guilt, and to the supposition that our judicial system is not entirely at fault, they may be held to stand in a special debt to society, and their offer to serve—from whatever motive—may be accepted with a minimum of qualms as a means of reparation.

4. *Proceedings,* p. 33.

Informed (But Uneducated) Consent _____

F. J. Ingelfinger

F. J. Ingelfinger claims that efforts to secure informed consent from potential patients or subjects are mostly doomed to failure. "The chances are remote," Ingelfinger says, "that the subject really understands what he has consented to—in the sense that the responsible medical investigator understands the goals, nature, and hazards of his study." Nor can the subject be given information that is in any genuine sense complete. In fact, it might even be unethical to present a person with all the contingencies that may be involved in an experiment.

The current procedure, Ingelfinger asserts, is better than ones followed in the past, for then people were not even told that they were going to be research subjects. But, beyond this, the process of obtaining informed consent "is no more than an elaborate ritual that, when the patient is uneducated and uncomprehending, confers no more than the semblance of propriety on human experimentation." The subject's only real protection depends on the person directing the research.

The trouble with informed consent is that it is not educated consent. Let us assume that the experimental subject, whether a patient, a volunteer, or otherwise enlisted, is exposed to a completely hon-

Reprinted by permission from the New England Journal of Medicine 287, *9 (August 31, 1972):*
465–466. Editor's Note: The notes in this essay have been renumbered.

est array of factual detail. He is told of the medical uncertainty that exists and that must be resolved by research endeavors, of the time and discomfort involved, and of the tiny percentage risk of some serious consequences of the test procedure. He is also reassured of his rights and given a formal, quasi-legal statement to read. No exculpatory language is used. With his written signature, the subject then caps the transaction, and whether he sees himself as a heroic martyr for the sake of mankind, or as a reluctant guinea pig dragooned for the benefit of science, or whether, perhaps, he is merely bewildered, he obviously has given his "informed consent." Because established routines have been scrupulously observed, the doctor, the lawyer, and the ethicist are content.

But the chances are remote that the subject really understands what he has consented to—in the sense that the responsible medical investigator understands the goals, nature, and hazards of his study. How can the layman comprehend the importance of his perhaps not receiving, as determined by luck of the draw, the highly touted new treatment that his roommate will get? How can he appreciate the sensation of living for days with a multi-lumen intestinal tube passing through his mouth and pharynx? How can he interpret the information that an intravascular catheter and radiopaque dye injection have an 0.01 per cent probability of leading to a dangerous thrombosis or cardiac arrhythmia? It is moreover quite unlikely that any patient-subject can see himself accurately within the broad context of the situation, to weigh the inconveniences and hazards that he will have to undergo against the improvements that the research project may bring to the management of his disease in general and to his own case in particular. The difficulty that the public has in understanding information that is both medical and stressful is exemplified by [a report that] only half the families given genetic counseling grasped its impact.[1]

Nor can the information given to the experimental subject be in any sense totally complete. It would be impractical and probably unethical for the investigator to present the nearly endless list of all possible contingencies; in fact, he may not himself be aware of every untoward thing that might happen. Extensive detail, moreover, usually enhances the subject's confusion. Epstein and Lasagna showed that comprehension of medical information given to untutored subjects is inversely correlated with the elaborateness of the material presented.[2] The inconsiderate investigator, indeed, conceivably could exploit his authority and knowledge and extract "informed consent" by overwhelming the candidate-subject with information.

Ideally, the subject should give his consent freely, under no duress whatsoever. The facts are that some element of coercion is instrumental in any investigator-subject transaction. Volunteers for experiments will usually be influenced by hopes of obtaining better grades, earlier parole, more substantial egos, or just mundane cash. These pressures, however, are but fractional shadows of those enclosing the patient-subject. Incapacitated and hospitalized because of illness, frightened by strange and impersonal routines, and fearful for his health and perhaps life, he is far from exercising a free power of choice when the person to whom he anchors all his hopes asks, "Say, you wouldn't mind, would you, if you joined some of the other patients on this floor and helped us to carry out some very important research we are doing?" When "informed consent" is obtained, it is not the student, the destitute bum, or the prisoner to whom, by virtue of his condition, the thumb screws of coercion are most relentlessly applied; it is the most used and useful of all experimental subjects, the patient with disease.

When a man or woman agrees to act as an experimental subject, therefore, his or her consent is marked by neither adequate understanding nor total freedom of choice. The conditions of the agreement are a far cry from those visualized as ideal. Jonas would have the subject identify with the investigative endeavor so that he and the researcher would be seeking a common cause: "Ultimately, the appeal for volunteers should seek . . . free and generous endorsement, the appropriation of the research purpose into the person's [i.e., the subject's] own scheme of ends."[3] For Ramsey, "informed consent" should represent a "covenantal bond between consenting man and consenting man [that] makes them . . . joint adventurers in medical care and progress."[4] Clearly, to achieve motivations and attitudes of this lofty type, an educated and understanding, rather than merely informed, consent is necessary.

Although it is unlikely that the goals of Jonas and of Ramsey will ever be achieved, and that human research subjects will spontaneously volunteer rather than be "conscripted,"[3] efforts to promote educated consent are in order. In view of the current emphasis on involving "the community" in such activities as regional planning, operation of clinics, and assignment of priorities, the general public and its political leaders are showing an increased awareness and understanding of medical affairs. But the orientation of this public interest in medicine is chiefly socioeconomic. Little has been done to give the public a basic understanding of medical research and its requirements not only for the people's money but also for their participation. The public, to be sure, is being subjected to a bombardment of sensation-mongering news stories and books that feature "breakthroughs," or that reveal real or alleged exploitations—horror stories of Nazi-type experimentation on abused human minds and bodies. Muckraking is essential to expose malpractices, but unless accompanied by efforts to promote a broader appreciation of medical research and its methods, it merely compounds the difficulties for both the investigator and the subject when "informed consent" is solicited.

The procedure currently approved in the United States for enlisting human experimental subjects has one great virtue: patient-subjects are put on notice that their management is in part at least an experiment. The deceptions of the past are no longer tolerated. Beyond this accomplishment, however, the process of obtaining "informed consent," with all its regulations and conditions, is no more than an elaborate ritual, a device that, when the subject is uneducated and uncomprehending, confers no more than the semblance of propriety on human experimentation. The subject's only real protection, the public as well as the medical profession must recognize, depends on the conscience and compassion of the investigator and his peers.

Notes

1. Leonard, Claire O., et al. Genetic counseling: a consumer's view. N Engl J Med 287:433–449, 1972.

2. Epstein, L. C., Lasagna, L. Obtaining informed consent: form or substance. Arch Intern Med 123:682–688, 1969.

3. Jonas, H. Philosophical reflections on experimenting with human subjects. Daedalus 98:219–247, Spring, 1969.

4. Ramsey, P. The ethics of a cottage industry in an age of community and research medicine. N Engl J Med 294:700–706, 1971.

A Moral Theory of Consent

Benjamin Freedman

Benjamin Freedman claims that an account of what it is to be "free," "informed," and "competent" will allow us to decide when a person is mature enough to give consent and when prisoners are free to consent to participating in experiments. According to Freedman, there is a "right to consent" that arises from our status as persons. To deny someone a right to consent is to deprive him of personhood and autonomy. Also it is often to deprive him of such advantages as direct therapeutic benefits. For these reasons, we should recognize the possibility that prisoners can give valid consent.

Those who claim that full information can never be given to patients or subjects miss the point, Freedman says. The amount and kind of information are relative to the purpose at hand—namely, to permit the patient to make a meaningful decision. Informed consent, then, is possible. Consent must also be responsible, but the only way to decide this is by considering the character of the patient. Finally, consent must be voluntary, and this condition is met when the "reward" for participating does something more than merely raise a person to the ordinary level of rights and freedoms.

In discussing consent and the incompetent, Freedman rejects as invalid proxy consent for research on children. Children, in his view, have a right to "custody, not liberty." They have a right to be cared for, so consent in adults and proxy consent for children are very different.

Most medical codes of ethics, and most physicians, agree that the physician ought to obtain the "free and informed consent" of his subject or patient before attempting any serious medical procedures, experimental or therapeutic in nature. They agree, moreover, that a proxy consent ought to be obtained on behalf of the incompetent subject. And informed consent is seen as not merely a legal requirement, and not merely a formality: it is a substantial requirement of morality.

Acceptance of this doctrine, however, requires the solution of a number of problems. How much information need be imparted? At what age is a person mature enough to consent on his own behalf? Can prisoners give a "free and informed consent" to be experimented upon? Lurking behind these and similar questions there are more fundamental difficulties. What are the functions of consent for the competent and the incompetent? What is the sense in which the patient/subject must be "free," "informed," and "competent"? It is by way of an approach to these latter questions that I shall attempt to respond to the more specific questions.[1]

I. Consent and the Competent

The negative aspects of the doctrine of informed consent have ordinarily been the focus of attention; difficulties in obtaining the informed consent of the subject/patient render the ethics of experimentation and therapeutic measures questionable. Our common view of informed consent is that, when at all relevant, it represents a minimum condition which ethics imposes upon the physician. It is seen as a necessary condition for medical manipulation, but hardly as a sufficient condition.

The reasons why this is so—why it is not sufficient that an experimenter, for instance, have received informed consent from his subject before proceeding—are quite obvious. The scarcity of medical resources (which includes a scarcity of qualified physician-investigators) forbids us from wasting time upon poorly-designed experiments, or upon experiments which merely replicate well-established conclusions. There seems to be, as well, a limit to the dangers which we (ordinarily) allow subjects to face. We do not, as a matter of policy, think it wise to allow would-be suicides to accomplish their end with the aid of a scientific investigator. Many other reasons could be given for the proposition that a person does not have a right to be experimented upon, even when he has given valid consent to the procedure.

The Right to Consent

But there does seem to exist a positive right of informed consent, which exists in both therapeutic and experimental settings. A person who has the capacity to give valid consent, and who has in fact consented to the procedure in question, has a right to have that fact recognized by us. We all have a duty to recognize a valid consent when confronted with it.

From whence derives this right? It arises from the right which each of us possesses to be treated as a person, and in the duty which all of us have, to have respect for persons, to treat a person as such, and not as an object. For this entails that our capacities for personhood ought to be recognized by all—these capacities including the capacity for rational decision, and for action consequent upon rational decision. Perhaps the worst which we may do to a man is to deny him his humanity, for example, by classifying him as mentally incompetent when he is, in fact, sane. It is a terrible thing to be hated or persecuted; it is far worse to be ignored, to be notified that you "don't count."

If an individual is capable of and has given valid consent, I would argue that he has a right, as against the world but more particularly as against his physician, to have it recognized that valid consent has been given. (The same applies, of course, with still

Reprinted by permission of the author and publisher from the Hastings Center Report, 5 *(August 1975).*
© *Institute of Society, Ethics and Life Sciences.*

greater force, with regard to *refusals* to consent to medical procedures.) The limited force of this claim must be emphasized: it does not entail a right to be treated, or to be experimented upon. It is a most innocuous right, one which most of us would have little hesitation about granting.

It is, therefore, curious that the literature on informed consent has failed to recognize this right—has, in fact, tacitly denied this right, at least as regards experimentation. In writings on informed consent it seems to have been assumed that if, under certain conditions, it is *doubtful* that valid consent to an experiment has been granted, it is best to "play it safe" ethically. In cases of doubt, we prefer not to take chances: in this case, we will not take a chance upon violating the canons of ethics by experimenting without being certain that the subject has validly consented to the experiment. Since we do not at present know whether a prisoner can give a valid consent, let us not take chances: we call for a moratorium on prison experimentation. Since we do not know at what age a person has the capacity to give a valid consent, we avoid the problem by setting the age of majority at a point where it is beyond doubt that maturity has been attained. If we must err, we shall ensure that we err in being overly ethical.

The establishment of the innocuous right to have valid consent recognized as such eliminates this expedient. Other writers have conceptualized the conflict as one between a right and, at best, a mere liberty. From the patient's point of view, he has a right to have his health protected by the physician, and a mere liberty to be experimented upon. From the physician-investigator's point of view, he has a duty to protect the subject's health, and a mere liberty to experiment upon the subject (contingent, of course, upon obtaining the subject's consent). A recognition of the claims of personhood and autonomy, however, reveals this to be a conflict between rights and duties. The physician-investigator has a duty to recognize consent when validly offered. When the consent is of doubtful validity, therefore, the physician experiences a conflict between two duties. He will not be ethically well-protected by choosing not to experiment, for there exists the possibility—which, as cases are multiplied, becomes a probability—that he is violating a duty in so choosing. Problems in informed consent present us with a dilemma. It is no longer the case that the burden of proof devolves upon the would-be exper-

imenter. The would-be abstainer-from-experiments may have to prove his case as well.

These considerations give us a new point of departure in investigating problems of informed consent. They show us that there is no "fail-safe" procedure which we can fall back upon in cases of doubt. Rather, what is required is an exhaustive examination of each case and issue, to see whether or not a valid consent has in fact been obtained.

When we fail to recognize a valid consent, of course, more is involved than a denial of personhood. Other benefits may be denied as well. Dr. Vernon Mark, for example, maintains that psychosurgery should not be done on prisoners with epilepsy because of the problem in obtaining a voluntary consent from prisoners.[2] But a resolution of this problem has not been shown to be impossible. Surely, the proper thing to do here would be to see whether prisoners can or cannot give valid consent to such a procedure. To remain satisfied with doubts, to fail to investigate this question, complex though it be, results in a denial of medical treatment for the prisoner, as well as representing a negation of the prisoner's human capacities. In depriving prisoners of the opportunity to serve as subjects in medical experiments, there are losses other than those of human respect.[3] Not the least of these is the loss of an opportunity to be of altruistic service to mankind.[4] Even a child feels at times a need to be useful; in promoting a moratorium on prison experimentation we deny prisoners the satisfaction of this psychic need. We should not need a reminder from John Stuart Mill that there are "higher" as well as "lower" pleasures and needs.

The right to have valid consent recognized as such does not indicate that we must experiment on prisoners. What it does indicate is that we have a moral responsibility to investigate in detail the question of whether prisoners can, under certain conditions, validly consent to experimentation. It also requires that we not prevent a researcher from experimenting on the basis of over-scrupulousness. If prisoners can give valid consent, we wrong not only the researcher but the prisoner as well by forbidding prison experimentation.

The Requirement of Information

The most common locution for the requirement which I am discussing is "informed consent"—we require "informed consent" to protect a doctor from legal liability resultant from his therapeutic endeavors, or to ensure the "ethicacy" of an experiment. But I believe "informed consent" to be a serious misnomer for what we do, in fact, want medical practice to conform to.

No lengthy rehearsal of the absurdities consequent upon taking the term "informed consent" at face value is necessary. The claim has been made, and repeated with approval, that "fully informed consent" is a goal which we call never achieve, but toward which we must strive. In order to ensure that fully informed consent has been given, it has seriously been suggested that only medical students or graduate students in the life sciences ought to be accepted as subjects for experimentation. *Reductio ad absurdum* examples of "fully informed consent" have been elaborated, in forms which list all the minutiae of the proposed medical procedure, together with all of its conceivable sequelae. With such a view of "informed consent" and its requirements, it is not surprising to find doctors who claim that since they cannot fully inform patients, they will tell them nothing, but instead will personally assume the responsibility for assuring the subject's safety.

In truth, a *reductio ad absurdum* of this view of "informed consent" need not be constructed; it serves as its own *reductio ad absurdum*. For there is no end to "fully informing" patients. When the doctor wishes to insert a catheter, must he commend to the subject's attention a textbook of anatomy? Although this, of course, would not suffice: he must ensure that the patient understand the text as well. Must he tell the patient the story of Dr. X, that bogey of first-year medical students, who, in a state of inebriation, inserted ("by mistake") his pen-refill instead of the catheter? With, of course, the assurance that *this* physician never gets drunk ("Well, rarely, anyway"). Must the patient be informed of the chemical formula of the catheter? Its melting point?

The basic mistake which is committed by those who harp upon the difficulties in obtaining informed consent (and by critics of the doctrine) is in believing that we can talk about information in the abstract, without reference to any human purpose. It is very likely impossible to talk about "information" in this way; but impossible or not, when we do in fact talk about, or request, information, we do not mean "information in the abstract." If I ask someone to "tell me about those clouds" he will, ordinarily, know what I mean; and he will

answer me, in the spirit in which he was asked, by virtue of his professional expertise as an artist, meteorologist, astronomer, soothsayer, or what-have-you. The meteorologist will not object that he cannot tell you the optical refraction index of the clouds, and therefore that he cannot "fully answer" your question. He knows that you are asking him with a given end in mind, and that much information about the cloud is irrelevant *relative to that purpose*.

That this "abstract information" requirement is not in question in obtaining valid consent is hardly an original point, but it is worth repeating. One of the leading court opinions on human experimentation puts it like this: " . . . the patient's interest in information does not extend to a lengthy polysyllabic discourse on all possible complications. A mini-course in medical science is not required. . . ."[5]

The proper question to ask, then, is not "What information must be given?" That would be premature: we must first know for what purpose information is needed. *Why* must the patient be informed? Put that way, the answer is immediately forthcoming. The patient must be informed so that he will know what he is getting into, what he may expect from the procedure, what his likely alternatives are—in short, what the procedure (and forbearance from it) will mean, so that a responsible decision on the matter may be made. This is the legal stance, as well as, I think, a "common sensical" stance; as Alexander Capron writes, the information component in valid consent derives in law from the recognition that information is "necessary to make meaningful the power to decide."[6] The proper test of whether a given piece of information needs to be given is, then, whether the physician, knowing what he does about the patient/subject, feels that that patient/subject would want to know this before making up his mind. Outré, improbable consequences would not ordinarily, therefore, be relevant information. Exceptionally, they will be: for example, when there is a small risk of impotence consequent upon the procedure which the physician proposes to perform upon a man with a great stake in his sexual prowess. This is only sensible.

Our main conclusion, then, is that valid consent entails only the imparting of that information which the patient/subject requires in order to make a responsible decision. This entails, I think, the possibility of a valid yet ignorant consent.

Consider, first, the therapeutic context. It is, I believe, not unusual for a patient to give his doctor *carte blanche* to perform any medical procedure which the physician deems proper in order to effect a cure. He is telling the doctor to act as his agent in choosing which procedure to follow. This decision is neither unwise nor (in any serious sense) an abdication of responsibility and an unwarranted burden upon the physician. We each of us choose to delegate our power of choice in this way in dealing with our auto mechanic or stockbroker.

It may be harder to accept an ignorant consent as valid in the purely experimental context. I think, however, that much of this difficulty is due to our paucity of imagination, our failure to imagine circumstances in which a person might choose to proceed in this way. We might approach such a case, for example, by imagining a Quaker who chooses to serve society by acting as a research subject, but who has a morbid fear of knives and pointed instruments. The Quaker might say to the physician-investigator that he wants to serve science but is afraid that his phobia would overcome his better judgment. He might consequently request that any experiment which would involve use of scalpels, hypodermic needles, and such, be performed without informing him: while, say, he is asleep or unconscious. He might further ask the doctor not to proceed should the experiment involve considerable risk. In such a case, or one similar, we would find an instance of a valid yet ignorant consent to experimentation.

The ostensible differences between the therapeutic and experimental contexts may be resolved into two components: in the therapeutic context it is supposed that the physician knows what the sequelae to treatment will be, which information, by definition, is not available in the experimental situation; and in the therapeutic context the doctor may be said to be seeking his patient's good, in contrast to the experimental context where some other good is being sought. On the basis of these differences it may be claimed that a valid yet ignorant consent is enough permission for therapy, but not for experimentation.

Closer examination, however, reveals that these differences do not necessarily obtain. First, because I believe it would be granted that a valid yet ignorant consent can be given in the "therapeutic-experimental" situation, where a new drug or procedure is being attempted to aid the patient (in the absence of any traditional available therapy). In the therapeutic-experimental situation, as in the purely experimental situation, the sequelae are not known (although of course in both cases some definite result is expected or anticipated). If a valid yet ignorant consent is acceptable in the one, therefore, it must be acceptable in the other.

Secondly, because it is patently not the case that we can expect there to be no good accruing to the subject of an experiment by reason of his participation. There are, commonly, financial and other "tangible" benefits forthcoming (laboratory training, and so on). And it must once again be said that the pleasures of altruism are not negligible. The proposed differences between experimentation and therapy do not stand up, and so we must say that if a valid yet ignorant consent is acceptable in the one it must be acceptable in the other. It must be remembered that this statement only concerns itself with one part of the consent doctrine, which is, itself, only one of the requirements which the ethical experiment must satisfy.

To mention—without claiming totally to resolve—two problems which may be raised at this point: First, it is said that a doctor often does not know what will happen as a consequence of a recommended procedure, and so cannot tell the patient what the patient wants to know. The obvious response to this seems to be right: the physician should, in that case, tell the patient/subject that he does not know what will happen (which does not exclude an explanation of what the doctor expects to happen, and on what he bases this expectation).

Second, it will be objected that the adoption of a requirement such as I propose would forbid the use of placebos and blind experiments. I am not sure that this is so; sometimes it must be the case that the subjects in an experiment may be asked (without introducing artifacts into the results) to consent to an experiment knowing that some will, and some will not, be receiving placebos. Another alternative would be to inform the subjects that the experiment may or may not involve some subjects receiving placebos.[7] I am aware, however, that these remarks are less than adequate responses to these problems.

Our conclusion, then, is that the informing of the patient/subject is not a fundamental requirement of valid consent. It is, rather, derivative from the requirement that the consent be the expression of a responsible choice. The two requirements which I do see as fundamental in this doctrine are that the choice be responsible and that it be voluntary.

The Requirement of Responsibility

What is meant by saying that the choice must be "responsible"? Does this entail that the physician may at any time override a patient's judgment on the basis that, in the physician's view, the patient has not chosen responsibly? Surely not; to adopt such a criterion would defeat the purpose embodied in the doctrine of consent. It would mean that a person's exercise of autonomy is always subject to review.

Still, some such requirement would appear to be necessary. A small child can certainly make choices.[8] Small children can also be intelligent enough to understand the necessary information. Yet surely we would not want to say that a small child can give valid consent to a serious medical procedure.[9] The reason for this is that the child cannot choose *responsibly*.

We are faced with a dilemma. On the one hand, it appears that we must require that the choice be responsible. To require only that the choice be free would yield counter-intuitive results. On the other hand, if we do require that the choice made be a responsible one, we seem to presuppose some body which shall judge the reasonableness of choices; this represents a paternalism which is antithetical to the doctrine of consent. An elderly patient chooses to forgo further life-saving measures. How are we to judge whether or not this choice is a responsible one?

The path between the horns of this dilemma involves saying that the "responsibility" which we require is to be predicated not on the nature of the particular choice, but on the nature of the patient/subject. What we need to know is whether *he* is a responsible man ("in general," so to speak), not whether the choice which has been made is responsible. In this way, we avoid the danger of upholding as "responsible" only those choices which we ourselves feel are good choices. We can and do admit into the community of responsible persons individuals who make choices with which we do not agree.

In this sense, responsibility is a dispositional characteristic. To say that someone is a responsible individual means that he makes choices, typically on the basis of reasons, arguments, or beliefs—and that he remains open to the claims of reason, so that further rational argument might lead him to change

his mind. It is to say that a person is capable of making and carrying through a life-plan—that he is prepared to act on the basis of his choices. It is to say that a person is capable of living with his life-plan; he can live with the consequences of his choices, he *takes responsibility* for his choices.[10] Of course, none of these are absolutes: all responsible people are at times pigheaded, at times shortsighted, at times flighty. That is to say, all responsible men at times act irresponsibly. Should the lack of responsibility persist, of course, to an extreme degree, we may say that the person has left the community of responsible folk.

Voluntarism and Reward

The other requirement of valid consent is that it be given voluntarily. The choice which the consent expresses must be freely made.

We all know some conditions which, if satisfied, make us say that a consent has been given involuntarily. The case which immediately springs to mind occurs when an individual succumbs under a threat: we call this duress or coercion. But the threat need not be overt; and perhaps there need not be a threat at all to render consent involuntary.

Hence, the major problem currently engendered by the requirement of voluntariness. It is typified by the prisoner who "volunteers" for an experiment in the hope or expectation of a reward: significantly higher wages, an opportunity for job training, better health care while involved in the experiment, a favorable report to his parole board. Is the consent which the prisoner offers a voluntary consent? The problem may be stated more generally thus: At what point does reward render consent involuntary?

The problem of reward is particularly difficult, since it involves questions of degree. Is a prisoner's consent involuntary if the reward for his participation in the experiment is a three-month reduction of sentence? Is it relevant here that the prisoner is serving a twenty-year sentence, rather than a one-to-five-year sentence? Does a possible increase in wages from twenty-five cents per hour to one dollar per hour constitute duress? Should we consider the percentage increase, or the increase in absolute value, or the increase in actual value which the seventy-five cent disparity represents in the prison environment?

To some, of course, questions like these have little meaning. They have little meaning to those who are indifferent to the demands of justice and autonomy which the consent doctrine represents, to those who are willing to buy guinea pigs, rather than to reward human beings. And they have little meaning for those who are convinced that prisoners are inherently unfree, and who thus would call for a total cessation of prison experimentation. Each of these positions denies, in an *a priori* fashion, freedom to prisoners; each must be rejected. A recognition of the fact that decisions about consent may be over- as well as under-protective forces us to deal with this sort of question, complex though it may be.

As is so often the case, posing the question in a different way may facilitate response. We have been considering the question of how much reward nullifies the validity of consent, how much reward renders the subject unfree. But is it in fact the case that *reward* is the disruptive factor here?

This problem may be clarified by the following examples. Imagine an upper-middle-class individual, who can provide for his family all of their needs and most of the amenities of civilized life. Let us say that this person is offered one hundred dollars to cross the street—if you like, make it one thousand or ten thousand dollars? He chooses to cross the street. Is his choice *involuntary*? Despite the substantial reward, I think most of us would agree that the consent was freely offered (and would that we should have such problems!).

Consider a person who deeply wants to be an astronaut. He is told that as part of the program he must participate in experiments to determine resistance to high-G conditions. Is his consent to this invalid, involuntary? I think not. We would say, this is part of his job; he should have expected it; and if he can't stand the heat, he should get out of the kitchen. In this vein, consider Evel Knievel, a financially prosperous man, who is offered millions of dollars to perform daredevil stunts. His choice may be bizarre, even crazy; but has his reward rendered it unfree?

Finally, consider a man who is informed by his doctor that he will most likely die unless he has open-heart surgery. His "reward" for consenting is his life; the penalty for not consenting is death. Does this mean this man cannot give the doctor valid consent—morally valid consent—to proceed?

There are two distinctions which, I think, go a long way towards dispelling these problems. First, I think it must be granted that natural contingencies

("acts of God," things which come to pass naturally, those contingencies which we cannot hold anyone responsible for) do not render a person unfree, nor do they render unfree the choices which a person makes in light of those contingencies.[11]

That natural contingencies do not render a man unfree is a point which is apt to be forgotten in the present context. I am not—in the morally relevant sense—lacking in freedom because I cannot, unaided, fly through the air, or live on grass. Nor am I unfree because my heart is about to give out. Nor am I unfree when, recognizing that my heart may give out, I choose to undergo surgery. I may, of course, be so crazed by knowing that I am near death's door that I am in a state of general impotence, and hence must have the choice made for me; but general incompetence is not in question here. The distinction between choices forced by man, and choices forced by nature, is, then, of importance.

The second distinction is between those pressures which are, and those which are not, in Daube's words, "consonant with the dignity and responsibility of free life."[12] I would explain this as follows: there are certain basic freedoms and rights which we possess which *entitle* us (morally) to certain things (or states of affairs). We would all, no doubt, draw up different lists of these rights and freedoms; but included in them would be safety of person, freedom of conscience and religion, a right to a certain level of education, and, for some of us, a right to some level of health care. When the "reward" is such as only to give us the necessary conditions of these rights and freedoms—when all that the reward does is to bring us up to a level of living to which we are entitled, and of which we have been deprived by man—then the "reward," I think, constitutes duress. A reward which accrues to one who has achieved this level, or who can easily achieve it (other than by taking the reward-option), and which hence serves only to grant us "luxury" items, does not constitute duress, and hence does not render choice unfree, no matter how great this reward may be.

The rewards above the moral subsistence level are true rewards. In contrast, we may say (with some touch of metaphor) that the "rewards" which only bring us up to the level to which we were in any event entitled are properly viewed as functioning as *threats*: "Do this, or stay where you are"—when you should not have been "where you are" in the first place.

The astronaut, Evel Knievel, and the upper-middle-class street-crosser are being granted "luxury" items, and hence are capable of giving free consent. But consider a man who will not be admitted to the hospital for treatment unless he agrees to be a subject in an experiment (unrelated to his treatment). Those who feel, as I do, that we are, here and now, morally entitled to medical treatment would agree, I trust, that this illegitimate option coerces the man into agreeing. Or consider a man who has religious scruples against donating blood, who takes his daughter to a hospital for treatment. He is told that the doctors will not treat her unless the family donates a certain amount of blood. His freedom has been nullified: his "consent" to donating blood is morally invalid. Similarly, the college student whose grade is contingent upon his participation in the instructor's psychological experiments is not validly consenting to serve. He is entitled to have his grade based upon his classroom work.

It yet remains to apply this distinction to our original problem, prison experimentation. The application will not be attempted here, for we would first need to be clear in our minds what rights and freedoms a prisoner is entitled to. I would not hesitate to say, though, that when a situation is created whereby a prisoner can only receive decent health care by participating in an experiment, he is being coerced into that experiment. I would have little hesitation in claiming that if subjecting himself to experimentation is the only way in which a prisoner could learn a trade which may be used "outside," then that prisoner is being coerced, his consent is not free. When we take into account the condition of our society, these would seem to be reasonable entitlements for the prisoner. Other rewards—for example, higher pay—may or may not constitute rewards above the moral subsistence level; if they are, then consent in light of these rewards could be freely offered. Perhaps too much has been said already; judgments like these must be made in an individualized fashion, one which is sensitive to the realities of prison life.

II. Consent and the Incompetent

In this section will be discussed, first, the question of how the age of majority and minority with reference to valid consent ought to be set; and secondly, the problems associated with the concept of proxy consent.

The Age of Consent

It has been argued that the requirements for obtaining valid consent are that the patient/subject must have consented freely and that he must be a responsible individual. The requirement of voluntariness does not raise any novel problems when applied to minors. Rather, what we usually have in mind when restricting the power of the minor to consent is that he is not, in the sense required, a responsible individual.

I have claimed that to be a responsible individual one must be capable of rationally adopting, following through, and accepting the consequences of a life-plan. The age, therefore, at which society indicates a presumption that individuals can satisfy these conditions can be said to be the age at which society ought to grant the right to give valid consent to serious medical procedures. The examples which spring to mind are the age of conscription and the age of marriageability. At these ages society has indicated that one is capable of acting, in a complex society, as an individual.

This is not an argument like that which says "If you are old enough to fight, then you are old enough to vote." The requirements necessary for being a soldier may be wholly unrelated to the requirements necessary before the franchise may be properly exercised. In contrast, the responsibility which we assume to be possessed by those capable of soldiering and contracting marriage is the same responsibility which is required to make consent valid: the ability to work through and with a life-plan.

The first thing which needs to be said, then, is that the age of consent should be lowered from 21 to 18 in those jurisdictions which have not yet done so. This should not entail merely that an 18-year-old may consent in the absence of parental disapproval; it should be a full power to consent, irrespective of what others might say.

But the setting of an age of consent indicates only a presumption and nothing more. The fact that someone has passed the age of consent is not conclusive proof that he is responsible (in the sense required); the fact that someone is below the age of consent is not conclusive proof of irresponsibility. The presumption may be defeated in either direction.

It is clear, for example, that an adult is not, *ipso facto*, responsible. The adult may be insane.

It is equally clear that a minor need not be irresponsible. People mature at different rates. If evidence of responsibility may be supplied on behalf of one below the age of consent, the presumption of irresponsibility should be defeated. The sort of evidence which would be necessary is that which indicates that the person can work through a life-plan. It may be said that this notion is being approached by the law in the special provisions sometimes made for the "emancipated minor." Marriage or economic self-sufficiency are among the common requirements for being considered an emancipated minor. One of the special prerogatives of the emancipated minor is that he may consent on his own behalf to medical care. I would argue that this should be extended to cover participation in experimentation as well.

Proxy Consent

Proxy consent is consent given on behalf of an individual who is himself incapable of granting consent. The major category of those who require proxy consent are minors, but proxy consent may need to be obtained for the insane or the unconscious as well. My comments will nevertheless be restricted to the case of minors, leaving the other cases to be dealt with by implication. In minors, proxy consent is ordinarily granted by the child's parent or guardian; exceptionally, it may be given by another close relative or by an individual appointed by the court for the specific purpose of granting consent to some procedure.

I have argued that the function of informed consent is to respect the autonomy and dignity of the individual. This cannot be the function of proxy consent. The minor patient/subject cannot fully express autonomy and dignity through choices. It may be said that the function of proxy consent is to protect the right of the parents to raise their child as they see fit, to do with the child as they like. But the child is not the property of the parents; parents do not have an absolute right of disposal over the child. In law we recognize constraints upon the parental power, and common morality affirms the justice in this. What then is the function of proxy consent?

I think it would be best to turn this question on its head. By virtue of what right which the child possesses do we require the granting of proxy consent before a medical procedure may be initiated? What *could* be the source of such an obligation? We ordinarily recognize that there is only one funda-

mental right possessed by minors, a right to be protected and aided in development. " . . . A child, unlike an adult, has a right 'not to liberty but to custody.' "[13] All other rights which a child possesses, all other duties which we have towards children, are derivative from this single right, and are void when inconsistent with it. Broadly speaking, in consequence of this right, we must do what we may to promote the welfare of the child; we must abstain from doing what will injure the child, physically or otherwise; and, as far as this right goes, we are at liberty to deal with the child in ways which neither help nor hurt.

That proxy consent is ordinarily to be obtained from the parent or guardian of the child is understandable. We feel that the parent has the best interests of the child at heart, and knows how best to seek the child's welfare. It also follows from this right, however, that, when the parent does not have the best interests of the child in mind, the power of proxy consent should be transferred to another. It is on such a basis that society feels justified in removing a child from his parent's custody, and in appointing another to act *in parens patriae*. If this system is to be effective, society must, by and large, act on the basis of shared common views about what the welfare of the child consists of. We cannot allow anything which a parent considers to be a benefit to the child—being boiled in oil to save his eternal soul—to count as action in the child's best interests. This does not preclude a certain amount of leeway in a liberal society as to permitted views of welfare: if most feel that it is better, when the money is available, to send the child to a private school, we yet will not fault an affluent parent who decides to send his child to a public school.

The consequences of these propositions for cases when proxy consent is being sought for the purpose of giving therapy to a child accord well with the way the law handles this subject. The problem situation which arises concerns parents who, because of religious scruples, refuse to consent to needed medical treatment for their child. Jehovah's Witnesses, for example, who believe that blood transfusions are forbidden by the law of God, will not consent on behalf of their child to blood transfusions. Society feels that the benefit of the child is to be found in allowing the procedure. Because of this, the hospital will often turn to a judge, who appoints someone to act *in parens patriae* for the purpose of consenting to the specific procedure. I suggest that if it were clearly the view of society that it is to the mongoloid infant's benefit to survive, should a parent refuse to consent to a life-saving procedure for that infant, a similar course would be followed: the consent of a court-appointed guardian would be substituted.

Proxy consent to experimentation on children is a more complicated matter. In law, there are two kinds of intervention in the person of another which are actionable in the absence of consent: those interventions where harm does, and where harm does not, result. The latter are termed "wrongful" or "harmful touchings" (though no harm has occurred). In other words, the mere *doing* of something to a person without his consent is, in itself, an actionable wrong.

We may say that, corresponding to this division, there are two sorts of experiments: those which do, and those which do not, injure the subject appreciably. Beecher has noted, for example, that "Many thousands of psychomotor tests and sociological studies have been carried out in children during the child's development and have revealed much information of value. . . . Sound nutritional studies without risk have been carried out. So have certain blood studies."[14] It must be added that many studies of value cannot, due to metabolic and other differences, be carried out in adults with results which will be valid for children.

It is clear, on the basis of the principle of benefit, that proxy consent to dangerous or harmful experiments on children cannot be valid. What about those experiments which carry no appreciable risk—the "wrongful touchings" sort? In an adult, it would seem, the right to autonomy, the right "to be let alone," is sufficient basis for the action of wrongful touching. But the child does not have a right to autonomy, except insofar as some measure of autonomy is necessary to promote the child's development and well-being.

Harmless experiments on children, therefore, which satisfy the other canons of medical ethics—good design, well-trained experimenters, and so forth—could be performed. Parents would not be derelict in their duty should they consent, on behalf of their child, to experiments of this sort. Participation in these experiments does not infringe the child's right to welfare, unless they would result in a *harmful* (and not just any) restriction of autonomy.

As I see it, the fundamental problem with those who would forbid *all* experimentation upon children[15] is that they confuse consent in adults with proxy consent for children. These two are fundamentally different requirements. Children are not small adults; our relations with children must not be made to approach as nearly as possible to our relations with adults. There are things which you ought to grant to children which need not be granted to adults: if a child is thirsty you provide him with drink. And there are things which may licitly be done to children which could not be done with adults: if my parents annoy me I may not send them to their room. A child is (morally) a different sort of thing than is an adult; we must adjust our relations with them according to their claims upon us.

Conclusion

This paper represents an attempt to formulate what I call a "moral theory" of the requirement of consent to serious medical procedures. The method used involves an interplay between cases and principles, such that each influences the other. Well-established moral intuitions about cases suggested some principles and called for the rejection of others. These principles in turn, once established, enabled the clarification of a proper approach to other, borderline cases.

Under the influence of situation ethics, much of the work on medical ethics has stressed the respects in which cases differ. This has resulted in the development of an *ad hoc* literature on cases which pose difficulty for the doctrine of informed consent. As the cases accumulated, the doctrine began to seem more and more amorphous.

In contrast, this paper has sought to unify the doctrine of consent. Principles which are developed through considering the problems raised by prison experimentation in turn suggested solutions to other situations; rather than stressing the differences between the experimental and the therapeutic contexts, their similarities were emphasized. There is, I think, a need for such efforts at unification, as there is a need for a literature which is committed to the unique aspects of different cases.

Notes

The research for this paper was begun during an internship at the Institute of Society, Ethics and the Life Sciences in the month of June, 1973. I gratefully acknowledge the help of Drs. Daniel Callahan, Marc Lappé, Peter Steinfels, and Robert Veatch, of the Institute, who helped make my internship profitable and enjoyable. My wife Barbara read the manuscript and suggested a number of needed changes.

1. For examples of a similar method applied to different problems, see Thomas I. Emerson, *Toward a General Theory of the First Amendment* (New York: Vintage Books, 1967).

2. "Brain Surgery in Aggressive Epileptics," in *Hastings Center Report*, February 1973.

3. See the insert to Alexander M. Capron's call for a moratorium on prison experimentation, "Medical Research in Prisons," *Hastings Center Report*, June 1973. The insert is a report from the *New York Times*, April 15, 1973, and reads in part: "Ninety-six of the 175 inmates at Lancaster County prison have written to a newspaper here protesting a recent decision by the state to halt all medical experiments on state prisoners. In their letter to the *Lancaster New Era*, they urged that state to allow the research [which] did not harm them and enabled them to pay off their fines and court costs."

4. See Henry K. Beecher, *Research and the Individual: Human Studies* (Boston: Little, Brown, 1970), p. 56. Professor Beecher notes a study of prison inmates, who, for participation in an experiment involving malaria, received pay but no reduction of sentence. Half of the volunteers cited "altruism" rather than money as their motive for volunteering. Those inmates who did not volunteer "expressed or implied respect for those who did volunteer."

5. *Cobbs* v. *Grant*, 502 P. 2d 1, 11.

6. Alexander M. Capron, "Legal Rights and Moral Rights," in Hilton, *et al.*, eds., *Ethical Issues in Human Genetics* (Plenum Press, 1973), 228.

7. If this sort of explanation were given as a matter of course in *all* experiments, this might still further reduce the problem of artifacts. The remarks, it should be noted, are directed towards medical experiments. By and large, they are inapplicable to, say, experiments in social psychology.

8. The counter-suggestion may be made that children cannot *really* make choices. This would, I think, put too great a weight upon the requirement of voluntarism. We would be recruiting the concepts of choice and volition to do a job which they have not been designed for.

9. I am speaking of course in the moral, not the legal, context. It may be that in an emergency a child may, in the absence of his parents, give legally valid consent.

10. This gives us the link between "responsible" in the dispositional sense explained here, and "responsible" in the blame-sense of the word ("I'll hold you responsible for that").

11. The *caveat* must be added: natural contingencies do not have, as their *sole* result, the rendering of a person unfree, in the sense which vitiates consent: a man's brain tumor can make the man an idiot, schizophrenia can make a man insane, but these do not so much affect a person's volition as they do disturb his entire psychic structure.

12. David Daube, quoted in Beecher, p. 146.

13. *In re Gault*, 387 U.S. 1 (1967).

14. Beecher, p. 67.

15. See, for example, Paul Ramsey, "Consent as a Canon of Loyalty with Special Reference to Children in Medical Investigations," in *The Patient as Person* (New Haven: Yale University Press, 1970).

The Willowbrook Letters: Criticism and Defense

Stephen Goldby, Saul Krugman, M. H. Pappworth, and Geoffrey Edsall

"The Willowbrook Letters", by Stephen Goldby, Saul Krugman, M. H. Pappworth, and Geoffrey Edsall, concern the moral legitimacy of the study of viral hepatitis that was conducted at the Willowbrook School by Krugman and his associates. (See the Case Presentation for more detail.) Goldby charges that the study was "quite unjustifiable" because it was morally wrong to infect children when no benefit to them could result. Krugman defends himself by claiming that his results demonstrated a "therapeutic effect" for the children involved, as well as for others. He presents four reasons for holding that the infecting of the children was justified.

Pappworth claims that Krugman's defense is presented only after the fact, whereas an experiment is ethical or not in its inception. Moreover, he asserts, consent was obtained through the use of coercion. Parents who wished to put their children in the institution were told there was room only in the "hepatitis unit."

In the final letter, Edsall defends the Krugman study. The experiments, he asserts, involved no greater risk to the children involved than they would have run in any case. What is more, the results obtained were of general benefit.

Sɪʀ.—You have referred to the work of Krugman and his colleagues at the Willowbrook State School in three editorials. In the first article the work was cited as a notable study of hepatitis and a model for this type of investigation. No comment was made on the rightness of attempting to infect mentally retarded children with hepatitis for experimental purposes, in an institution where the disease was already endemic.

The second editorial again did not remark on the ethics of the study, but the third sounded a note of doubt as to the justification for extending these experiments. The reason given was that some children might have been made more susceptible to serious hepatitis as the result of the administration of previously heated icterogenic material.

I believe that not only this last experiment, but the whole of Krugman's study, is quite unjustifiable, whatever the aims, and however academically or therapeutically important are the results. I am amazed that the work was published and that it has been actively supported editorially by the *Journal of the American Medical Association* and by Ingelfinger in the 1967–68 *Year Book of Medicine*. To my knowledge only the *British Journal of Hospital Medicine* has clearly stated the ethical position on these experiments and shown that it was indefensible to give potentially dangerous infected material to children, particularly those who were mentally retarded, with or without parental consent, when no benefit to the child could conceivably result.

Krugman and Giles have continued to publish the results of their study, and in a recent paper go to some length to describe their method of obtaining parental consent and list a number of influential medical boards and committees that have approved the study. They point out again that, in their opin-ion, their work conforms to the World Medical Association Draft Code of Ethics on Human Experimentation. They also say that hepatitis is still highly endemic in the school.

This attempted defence is irrelevant to the central issue. Is it right to perform an experiment on a normal or mentally retarded child when no benefit can result to that individual? I think that the answer is no, and that the question of parental consent is irrelevant. In my view the studies of Krugman serve only to show that there is a serious loophole in the Draft Code, which under General Principles and Definitions puts the onus of consent for experimentation on children on the parent or guardian. It is this section that is quoted by Krugman. I would class his work as "experiments conducted solely for the acquisition of knowledge," under which heading the code states that "persons retained in mental hospital or hospitals for mental defectives should not be used for human experiment." Krugman may believe that his experiments were for the benefit of his patients, meaning the individual patients used in the study. If this is his belief he has a difficult case to defend. The duty of a pediatrician in a situation such as exists at Willowbrook State School is to attempt to improve that situation, not to turn it to his advantage for experimental purposes, however lofty the aims.

Every new reference to the work of Krugman and Giles adds to its apparent ethical respectability, and in my view such references should stop, or at least be heavily qualified. The editorial attitude of *The Lancet* to the work should be reviewed and openly stated. The issue is too important to be ignored.

If Krugman and Giles are keen to continue their experiments I suggest that they invite the parents of

Reprinted by permission of the authors and publisher from The Lancet, *April 10, May 8, June 5, and July 10, 1971.*

the children involved to participate. I wonder what the response would be.

Stephen Goldby

SIR.—Dr. Stephen Goldby's critical comments about our Willowbrook studies and our motives for conducting them were published without extending us the courtesy of replying in the same issue of *The Lancet.* Your acceptance of his criticisms without benefit of our response implies a blackout of all comment related to our studies. This decision is unfortunate because our recent studies on active and passive immunisation for the prevention of viral hepatitis, type B, have clearly demonstrated a "therapeutic effect" for the children involved. These studies have provided us with the first indication and hope that it may be possible to control hepatitis in this institution. If this aim can be achieved, it will benefit not only the children, but also their families and the employees who care for them in the school. It is unnecessary to point out the additional benefit to the worldwide populations which have been plagued by an insoluble hepatitis problem for many generations.

Dr. Joan Giles and I have been actively engaged in studies aimed to solve two infectious-disease problems in the Willowbrook State School—measles and viral hepatitis. These studies were investigated in this institution because they represented major health problems for the 5000 or more mentally retarded children who were residents. Uninformed critics have assumed or implied that we came to Willowbrook to "conduct experiments on mentally retarded children."

The results of our Willowbrook studies with the experimental live attenuated measles vaccine developed by Enders and his colleagues are well documented in the medical literature. As early as 1960 we demonstrated the protective effect of this vaccine during the course of an epidemic. Prior to licensure of the vaccine in 1963 epidemics occurred at two-year intervals in this institution. During the 1960 epidemic there were more than 600 cases of measles and 60 deaths. In the wake of our ongoing measles vaccine programme, measles has been eradicated as a disease in the Willowbrook State School. We have not had a single case of measles since 1963. In this regard the children at the Willowbrook State School have been more fortunate than unimmunised children in Oxford, England, other areas in Great Britain, as well as certain groups of children in the United States and other parts of the world.

The background of our hepatitis studies at Willowbrook has been described in detail in various publications. Viral hepatitis is so prevalent that newly admitted susceptible children become infected within 6 to 12 months after entry in the institution. These children are a source of infection for the personnel who care for them and for their families if they visit with them. We were convinced that the solution of the hepatitis problem in this institution was dependent on the acquisition of new knowledge leading to the development of an effective immunising agent. The achievements with smallpox, diphtheria, poliomyelitis, and more recently measles represent dramatic illustrations of this approach.

It is well known that viral hepatitis in children is milder and more benign than the same disease in adults. Experience has revealed that hepatitis in institutionalised, mentally retarded children is also mild, in contrast with measles, which is a more severe disease when it occurs in institutional epidemics involving the mentally retarded. Our proposal to expose a small number of newly admitted children to the Willowbrook strains of hepatitis virus was justified in our opinion for the following reasons: (1) they were bound to be exposed to the same strains under the natural conditions existing in the institution; (2) they would be admitted to a special, well-equipped, and well-staffed unit where they would be isolated from exposure to other infectious diseases which were prevalent in the institution—namely, shigellosis, parasitic infections, and respiratory infections—thus, their exposure in the hepatitis unit would be associated with less risk than the type of institutional exposure where multiple infections could occur; (3) they were likely to have a subclinical infection followed by immunity to the particular hepatitis virus; and (4) only children with parents who gave informed consent would be included.

The statement by Dr. Goldby accusing us of conducting experiments exclusively for the acquisition of knowledge with no benefit for the children cannot be supported by the true facts.

Saul Krugman

SIR.—The experiments at Willowbrook raise two important issues: What constitutes valid consent, and do ends justify means? English law definitely forbids experimentation on children, even if both parents consent, unless done specifically in the interests of each individual child. Perhaps in the U.S.A. the law is not so clear-cut. According to Beecher, the parents of the children at Willowbrook were informed that, because of overcrowding, the institution was to be closed; but only a week or two later they were told that there would be vacancies in the "hepatitis unit" for children whose parents allowed them to form part of the hepatitis research study. Such consent, ethically if not legally, is invalid because of its element of coercion, some parents being desperately anxious to institutionalise their mentally defective children. Moreover, obtaining consent after talking to parents in groups, as described by Krugman, is extremely unsatisfactory because even a single enthusiast can sway the diffident who do not wish to appear churlish in front of their fellow citizens.

Do ends justify the means? Krugman maintains that any newly admitted children would inevitably have contracted infective hepatitis, which was rife in the hospital. But this ignores the statement by the head of the State Department of Mental Hygiene that, during the major part of the 15 years these experiments have been conducted, a gamma-globulin inoculation programme had already resulted in over an 80 percent reduction of that disease in that hospital. Krugman and Pasamanick claim that subsequent therapeutic effects justify these experiments. This attitude is frequently adopted by experimenters and enthusiastic medical writers who wish us to forget completely how results are obtained but instead enjoy any benefits that may accrue. Immunisation was not the purpose of these Willowbrook experiments but merely a by-product that incidentally proved beneficial to the victims. Any experiment is ethical or not at its inception, and does not become so because it achieved some measure of success in extending the frontiers of medicine. I particularly object strongly to the views of Willey, " . . . risk being assumed by the subjects of the experimentation balanced against the potential benefit to the subjects *and* [Willey's italics] to society in general." I believe that experimental physicians never have the right to select martyrs for society. Every human being has the right to be treated with decency, and that right must always supersede every consideration of what may benefit mankind, what may advance medical science, what may contribute to public welfare. No doctor is ever justified in placing society or science first and his obligation to patents second. Any claim to act for the good of society should be regarded with distaste because it may be merely a highflown expression to cloak outrageous acts.

M. H. Pappworth

SIR.—I am astonished at the unquestioning way in which *The Lancet* has accepted the intemperate position taken by Dr. Stephen Goldby concerning the experimental studies of Krugman and Giles on hepatitis at the Willowbrook State School. These investigators have repeatedly explained for over a decade that natural hepatitis infection occurs sooner or later in virtually 100% of the patients admitted to Willowbrook, and that it is better for the patient to have a known, timed, controlled infection than an untimed, uncontrolled one. Moreover, the wisdom and human justification of these studies have been repeatedly and carefully examined and verified by a number of very distinguished, able individuals who are respected leaders in the making of such decisions.

The real issue is: Is it not proper and ethical to carry out experiments in children, which would apparently incur no greater risk than the children were likely to run by nature, in which the children generally receive better medical care when artificially infected than if they had been naturally infected, and in which the parents as well as the physician feel that a significant contribution to the future well-being of similar children is likely to result from the studies? It is true, to be sure, that the W.M.A. code says, "Children in institutions and not under the care of relatives should not be the subjects of human experiments." But this unqualified *obiter dictum* may represent merely the well-known inability of committees to think a problem through. However, it has been thought through by Sir Austin Bradford Hill, who has pointed out the unfortunate effects for these very children that would have resulted, were such a code to have been applied over the years.

Geoffrey Edsall

Judgment on Willowbrook

Paul Ramsey

Paul Ramsey reviews the justifications offered for the Willowbrook experiments presented by Krugman. Ramsey observes that there is nothing about hepatitis that requires that research be conducted on children, that no justification except the needs of the experiment is given for withholding gamma globulin from the subjects, and that nothing is said about attempting to control the low-grade epidemic by other means. Furthermore, Ramsey questions the morality of consent secured from the parents of the children. His basic recommendation is that the use of captive populations of children ought to be made legally impossible.

In 1958 and 1959 the *New England Journal of Medicine* reported a series of experiments performed upon patients and new admittees to the Willowbrook State School, a home for retarded children in Staten Island, New York.[1] These experiments were described as "an attempt to control the high prevalence of infectious hepatitis in an institution for mentally defective patients." The experiments were said to be justified because, under conditions of an existing controlled outbreak of hepatitis in the institution, "knowledge obtained from a series of suitable studies could well lead to its control." In actuality, the experiments were designed to duplicate and confirm the efficacy of gamma globulin in immunization against hepatitis, to develop and improve or improve upon that inoculum, and to learn more about infectious hepatitis in general.

The experiments were justified—doubtless, after a great deal of soul searching—for the following reasons: there was a smoldering epidemic throughout the institution and "it was apparent that most of the patients at Willowbrook were naturally exposed to hepatitis virus"; infectious hepatitis is a much milder disease in children; the strain at Willowbrook was especially mild; only the strain or strains of the virus already disseminated at Willowbrook were used; and only those small and incompetent patients whose parents gave consent were used.

The patient population at Willowbrook was 4478, growing at a rate of one patient a day over a three-year span, or from 10 to 15 new admissions per week. In the first trial the existing population was divided into two groups: one group served as uninoculated controls, and the other group was inoculated with 0.01 ml. of gamma globulin per pound of body weight. Then for a second trial new admittees and those left uninoculated before were again divided: one group served as uninoculated controls and the other was inoculated with 0.06 ml. of gamma globulin per pound of body weight. This proved that Stokes et al. had correctly demonstrated that the larger amount would give significant immunity for up to seven or eight months.[2]

Serious ethical questions may be raised about the trials so far described. No mention is made of any attempt to enlist the adult personnel of the institution, numbering nearly 1,000 including nearly 600 attendants on ward duty, and new additions to the staff, in these studies whose excusing reason was that almost everyone was "naturally" exposed to the Willowbrook virus. Nothing requires that major research into the natural history of hepatitis be first undertaken in children. Experiments have been carried out in the military and with prisoners as subjects. There have been fatalities from the experiments; but surely in all these cases the consent of the volunteers was as valid or better than the proxy consent of these children's "representatives." There would have been no question of the understanding consent that might have been given by the adult personnel at Willowbrook, if significant benefits were expected from studying that virus.

Second, nothing is said that would warrant withholding an inoculation of some degree of known efficacy from part of the population, or for withholding in the first trial less than the full amount of gamma globulin that had served to immunize in previous tests, except the need to test, confirm, and improve the inoculum. That, of course, was a desirable goal; but it does not seem possible to warrant withholding gamma globulin for the reason that is often said to justify controlled trials, namely, that one procedure is *as likely* to succeed as the other.

Third, nothing is said about attempts to control or defeat the low-grade epidemic at Willowbrook by more ordinary, if more costly and less experimental, procedures. Nor is anything said about admitting no more patients until this goal had been accomplished. This was not a massive urban hospital whose teeming population would have to be turned out into the streets, with resulting dangers to themselves and to public health, in order to sanitize the place. Instead, between 200 and 250 patients were housed in each of 18 buildings over approximately 400 acres in a semirural setting of fields, woods, and well-kept, spacious lawns. Clearly it would have been possible to secure other accommodation for new admissions away from the infection, while eradicating the infection at Willowbrook building by building. This might have cost money, and it would certainly have required astute detective work to discover the source of the infection. The doctors determined that the new patients likely were not carrying the infection upon admission, and that it did not arise from the procedures and routine inoculations given them at the time of admission. Why not go further in the search for the source of the epidemic? If this had been an orphanage for normal children or a floor of private patients, instead of a school for mentally defective children, one wonders whether the doctors would so readily have accepted the hepatitis as a "natural" occurrence and even as an opportunity for study.

The next step was to attempt to induce "passive-active immunity" by feeding the virus to patients already protected by gamma globulin. In this attempt to improve the inoculum, permission was obtained from the parents of children from 5 to 10 years of age newly admitted to Willowbrook, who were then isolated from contact with the rest of the institution. All were inoculated with gamma globulin and then divided into two groups: one served as controls while the other group of new patients were fed the Willowbrook virus, obtained from feces, in doses having 50 percent infectivity, i.e., in concentrations estimated to produce hepatitis with jaundice in half the subjects tested. Then twice the 50 percent infectivity was tried. This proved, among other things, that hepatitis has an "alimentary-tract phase" in which it can be transmitted from one person to another while still "inapparent" in the first person. This, doubtless, is exceedingly important information in learning how to control epidemics of infectious hepatitis. The second of the two articles mentioned above describes studies of the incubation period of the virus and of whether pooled serum remained infectious when aged and frozen. Still the small, mentally defective patients who were deliberately fed infectious hepatitis are described as having suffered mildly in most cases: "The liver became enlarged in the majority, occasionally a week or two before the onset of jaundice. Vomiting and anorexia usually lasted only a few days. Most of the children gained weight during the course of hepatitis."

That mild description of what happened to the children who were fed hepatitis (and who continued to be introduced into the unaltered environment of Willowbrook) is itself alarming, since it is now definitely known that cirrhosis of the liver results from infectious hepatitis more frequently than from excessive consumption of alcohol! Now, or in 1958 and 1959, no one knows what may be other serious consequences of contracting infectious hepatitis. Understanding human volunteers were then and are now needed in the study of this disease, although a South American monkey has now successfully been given a form of hepatitis, and can henceforth serve as our ally in its conquest. But not children who cannot consent knowingly. If Peace Corps workers are regularly given gamma globulin before going abroad as a guard against their contracting hepatitis, and are inoculated at intervals thereafter, it seems that this is the least we should do for mentally defective children before they "go abroad" to Willowbrook or other institutions set up for their care.

Discussions pro and con of the Willowbrook experiments that have come to my attention serve only to reinforce the ethical objections that can be raised against what was done simply from a careful analysis of the original articles reporting the research design and findings. In an address at the 1968

Ross Conference on Pediatric Research, Dr. Saul Krugman raised the question, Should vaccine trials be carried out in adult volunteers before subjecting children to similar tests?[3] He answered this question in the negative. The reason adduced was simply that "a vaccine virus trial may be a more hazardous procedure for adults than for children." Medical researchers, of course, are required to minimize the hazards, but not by moving from consenting to unconsenting subjects. This apology clearly shows that adults and children have become interchangeable in face of the overriding importance of obtaining the research goal. This means that the special moral claims of children for care and protection are forgotten, and especially the claims of children who are most weak and vulnerable. (Krugman's reference to the measles vaccine trials is not to the point.)

The *Medical Tribune* explains that the 16-bed isolation unit set up at Willowbrook served "to protect the study subjects from Willowbrook's other endemic diseases—such as shigellosis, measles, rubella and respiratory and parasitic infections—while exposing them to hepatitis."[4] This presumably compensated for the infection they were given. It is not convincingly shown that the children could by no means, however costly, have been protected from the epidemic of hepatitis. The statement that Willowbrook "had endemic infectious hepatitis and a sufficiently open population so that the disease could never be quieted by exhausting the supply of susceptibles" is at best enigmatic.

Oddly, physicians defending the propriety of the Willowbrook hepatitis project soon begin talking like poorly instructed "natural lawyers"! Dr. Louis Lasagna and Dr. Geoffrey Edsall, for example, find these experiments unobjectionable—both, for the reason stated by Edsall: "the children would apparently incur no greater risk than they were likely to run by nature." In any case, Edsall's examples of parents consenting with a son 17 years of age for him to go to war, and society's agreements with minors that they can drive cars and hurt themselves were entirely beside the point. Dr. David D. Rutstein adheres to a stricter standard in regard to research on infectious hepatitis: "It is not ethical to use human subjects for the growth of a virus for any purpose."[5]

The latter sweeping verdict may depend on knowledge of the effects of viruses on chromosomal difficulties, mongolism, etc., that was not available to the Willowbrook group when their researches were begun thirteen years ago. If so, this is a telling point against appeal to "no discernible risks" as the sole standard applicable to the use of children in medical experimentation. That would lend support to the proposition that we always know that there are unknown and undiscerned risks in the case of an invasion of the fortress of the body—which then can be consented to by an adult in behalf of a child only if it is in the child's behalf medically.

When asked what she told the parents of the subject-children at Willowbrook, Dr. Joan Giles replied, "I explain that there is no vaccine against infectious hepatitis. . . . I also tell them that we can modify the disease with gamma globulin but we can't provide lasting immunity without letting them get the disease."[6] Obviously vaccines giving "lasting immunity" are not the only kinds of vaccine to be used in caring for patients.

Doubtless the studies at Willowbrook resulted in improvement in the vaccine, to the benefit of present and future patients. In September 1966, "a routine program of GG [gamma globulin] administration to every new patient at Willowbrook" was begun. This cut the incidence of icteric hepatitis 80 to 85 percent. Then follows a significant statement in the *Medical Tribune* article: "A similar reduction in the icteric form of the disease has been accomplished among the employees, who began getting routine GG earlier in the study."[7] Not only did the research team (so far as these reports show) fail to consider and adopt the alternative that new admittees to the staff be asked to become volunteers for an investigation that might improve the vaccine against the strain of infectious hepatitis to which they as well as the children were exposed. Instead, the staff was routinely protected earlier than the inmates were! And, as we have seen, there was evidence from the beginning that gamma globulin provided at least some protection. A "modification" of the disease was still an inoculum, even if this provided no lasting immunization and had to be repeated. It is axiomatic to medical ethics that a known remedy or protection—even if not perfect or even if the best exact administration of it has not been proved—should not be withheld from individual patients. It seems to a layman that from the beginning various trials at immunization of all new admittees might have been made, and controlled observation made of their different degrees of effectiveness against "nature" at Willowbrook. This would doubtless have been a longer way round, namely, the "anecdotal" method of investigative treatment that comes off second best in comparison with controlled trials. Yet this seems to be the alternative dictated by our received medical ethics, and the only one expressive of minimal care of the primary patients themselves.

Finally, except for one episode, the obtaining of parental consent (on the premise that this is ethically valid) seems to have been very well handled. Wards of the state were not used, though by law the administrator at Willowbrook could have signed consent for them. Only new admittees whose parents were available were entered by proxy consent into the project. Explanation was made to groups of these parents, and they were given time to think about it and consult with their own family physicians. Then late in 1964 Willowbrook was closed to all new admissions because of overcrowding. What then happened can most impartially be described in the words of an article defending the Willowbrook project on medical and ethical grounds:

> Parents who applied for their children to get in were sent a form letter over Dr. Hammond's signature saying that there was no space for new admissions and that their name was being put on a waiting list.
>
> But the hepatitis program, occupying its own space in the institution, continued to admit new patients as each new study group began. "Where do you find new admissions except by canvassing the people who have applied for admission?" Dr. Hammond asked.
>
> So a new batch of form letters went out, saying that there were a few vacancies in the hepatitis research unit if the parents cared to consider volunteering their child for that. In some instances the second form letter apparently was received as closely as a week after the first letter arrived.[8]

Granting—as I do not—the validity of parental consent to research upon children not in their behalf medically, what sort of consent was that? Surely, the duress upon these parents with children so defective as to require institutionalization was far greater than the duress on prisoners given tobacco or paid or promised parole for their cooperation! I grant that the timing of these events was inadvertent. Since, however, ethics is a matter of criticizing institutions and not only of exculpating or making culprits of individual men, the inadvertence does not matter. This is the strongest possible argument for saying that even if parents have the right to

consent to submit the children who are directly and continuously in their care to nonbeneficial medical experimentation, this should not be the rule of practice governing institutions set up for their care.

Such use of captive populations of children for purely experimental purposes ought to be made legally impossible. My view is that this should be stopped by legal acknowledgement of the moral invalidity of parental or legal proxy consent for the child to procedures having no relation to a child's own diagnosis or treatment. If this is not done, canons of loyalty require that the rule of practice (by law, or otherwise) be that children in institutions and not directly under the care of parents or relatives should *never* be used in medical investigations having present pain or discomfort and unknown present and future risks to them, and promising future possible benefits only for others.

Notes

1. Robert Ward, Saul Krugman, Joan P. Giles, A. Milton Jacobs, and Oscar Bodansky, "Infectious Hepatitis: Studies of Its Natural History and Prevention," *New England Journal of Medicine* 258, no. 9 (February 27, 1958): 407–16; Saul Krugman, Robert Ward, Joan P. Giles, Oscar Bodansky, and A. Milton Jacobs, "Infectious Hepatitis: Detection of the Virus during the Incubation Period and in Clinically Inapparent Infection," *New England Journal of Medicine* 261, no. 15 (October 8, 1959): 729–34. The following account and unannotated quotations are taken from these articles.

2. J. Stokes, Jr., et al., "Infectious Hepatitis: Length of Protection by Immune Serum Globulin (Gamma Globulin) during Epidemics," *Journal of the American Medical Association* 147 (1951): 714–19. Since the half-life of gamma globulin is three weeks, no one knows exactly why it immunizes for so long a period. The "highly significant protection against hepatitis obtained by the use of gamma globulin," however, had been confirmed as early as 1945 (see Edward B. Grossman, Sloan G. Stewart, and Joseph Stokes, "Post-Transfusion Hepatitis in Battle Casualties," *Journal of the American Medical Association* 129, no. 15 [December 8, 1945]: 991–94). The inoculation *withheld* in the Willowbrook experiments had, therefore, proved valuable.

3. Saul Krugman, "Reflections on Pediatric Clinical Investigations," in *Problems of Drug Evaluation in Infants and Children,* Report of the Fifty-eighth Ross Conference on Pediatric Research, Dorado Beach, Puerto Rico, May 5–7, 1968 (Columbus: Ross Laboratories), pp. 41–42.

4. "Studies with Children Backed on Medical, Ethical Grounds," *Medical Tribune and Medical News* 8, no. 19 (February 20, 1967): 1, 23.

5. *Daedalus*, Spring 1969, pp. 471–72, 529. See also pp. 458, 470–72. Since it is the proper business of an ethicist to uphold the proposition that only retrogression in civility can result from bad moral reasoning and the use of inept examples, however innocent, it is fair to point out the startling comparison between Edsall's "argument" and the statement of Dr. Karl Brandt, plenipotentiary in charge of all medical activities in the Nazi Reich: "Do you think that one can obtain any worthwhile, fundamental results without a definite toll of lives? The same goes for technological development. You cannot build a great bridge, a gigantic building—you cannot establish a speed record without deaths!" (quoted by Leo Alexander, "War Crimes: Their Social-Psychological Aspects," *American Journal of Psychiatry* 105, no. 3 [September 1948]: 172). Casualties to progress, or injuries accepted in setting speed limits, are morally quite different from death or maiming or even only risks, or unknown risks, directly and deliberately imposed upon an unconsenting human being.

6. *Medical Tribune*, February 20, 1967, p. 23.

7. *Medical Tribune*, February 20, 1967, p. 23.

8. *Medical Tribune*, February 20, 1967, p. 23.

Competency to Give an Informed Consent: A Model for Making Clinical Assessments

James F. Drane

James Drane claims that respect for patients requires securing their informed consent in decisions about their welfare. However, we must not take patients' competence to consent for granted or we may fail in our duty to promote their well-being. We need a standard of competence, but no single standard is workable.

Drane proposes a sliding-scale model consisting of three standards: (1) if a treatment is not dangerous and is in the patient's best interest, the patient need only be *aware* of the general situation and *assent* to it; (2) if a disease is chronic, a diagnosis uncertain, a treatment dangerous, results uncertain, or alternative therapies available, the patient must be able to *understand* the options and *choose* among them (leaving the choice to one's physician is also a possibility); (3) when diagnosis is clear, treatment effective, and death likely to result from refusing treatment, the patient must have "a capacity to appreciate the nature and consequence of the decision." To meet this last standard, a patient must be able to give intelligible reasons for the decision, even if it varies from what most rational people would decide. Drane sees his position as balancing rationality, maximum autonomy, and maximum patient benefit.

In January 1980, as one more indication of the growing importance of medical ethics, a presidential commission was formed and began work on the moral questions posed by the practice of contemporary medicine. After three years of intense work, the commission published a separate volume on 11 dif-

This investigation was supported in part by grant ED 0652-78 from the National Endowment for the Humanities.

Reprinted from JAMA: Journal of the American Medical Association, *August 17, 1984, Vol. 252, No. 7, pp. 925–927. Copyright 1984, American Medical Association.*

ferent ethical problems in the hope of stimulating thoughtful discussion. Some broad principles were uncovered that apply to any and every bioethical issue, such as the principle of patient respect and its concrete application in the right of informed consent. But there were also recurring perplexities, one of which was competency or, in the language preferred by the commission, the patient's capacity to choose.[1]

Respect for patients means ensuring their participation in decisions affecting their lives. Such participation is a basic form of freedom and stands at the core of Western values. But freedom, participation, and self-determination suppose a capacity for such acts. No one, for example, assumes that an infant has such a capacity and, time and again, doubts arise about the capacity of some older patients. Not to respect a patient's freedom is undoubtedly wrong. But to respect what may be an expression of freedom only in appearance would be a violation of another basic principle of ethical medicine: promotion of the patient's well-being.

Although the commission's report referred many times to competency or capacity to choose, commissioners and staff members privately expressed frustration and disappointment about their conclusions. The commission reports spelled out what are considered to be the components of competency: the possession of a set of values and goals, the ability to communicate and understand information, and the ability to reason and deliberate. In addition, the commission criticized some standards for determining competency that either were too lenient and did not protect a patient sufficiently or were too strict and in effect transferred decision making to the physician. But the commission did not come up with its own standard and left unsettled the question of how to decide whether a particular patient's decision should be respected or overridden because of incompetency. Incompetency is not the only reason for overriding a patient's refusal or setting aside a consent, but it is the most common reason for doing so. Defining incompetency or establishing standards of competency is a complex problem because it involves law, ethics, and psychiatry.

Competency Assessment

Competency assessments focus on the patient's mental capacities, specifically, the mental capacities to make an informed medical decision. Does the patient understand what is being proposed? Can the patient come to a decision about treatment based on an adequate understanding? How much understanding and rational decision-making capacity are sufficient for this particular patient to be considered competent? Conversely, how deficient must this patient's decision-making capacity be before he is declared incompetent? A properly performed competency assessment should eliminate two types of error: (1) preventing a competent person from participating in treatment decisions and (2) failing to protect an incompetent person from the harmful effects of a bad decision.

Model for Making the Assessment

The President's commission did not recommend a single standard for determining competency because any one standard is inappropriate for the many different types of medical decisions that people face. What is proposed here is a sliding standard, i.e., the more dangerous the medical decision, the more stringent the standards of competency. The basic idea, following a suggestion of Mark Siegler,[2, 3] is to connect determination of competency to different medical situations (acute or chronic, critical or noncritical), and next to take this idea a step further by specifying three different standards or definitions of what it means to be competent. These standards are then correlated with three different medical situations, each more dangerous than the other. Finally, the sliding standards and different medical situations are correlated with the types of psychiatric abnormalities that ordinarily undermine competency. The interrelationship of all these entities creates a model that can aid the physician faced with a question about a patient's capacity to choose. This model brings together disparate academic disciplines, but its goal is thoroughly pragmatic: to provide a workable guide for clinical decision making.

Standard 1

The first and least stringent standard of competency to give a valid consent applies to those medical decisions that are not dangerous and objectively are in the patient's best interest. If the patient is critically ill because of an acute illness that is life threatening, if there is an effective treatment available that is low in risk, and if few or no alternatives are available, then consent to the treatment is prima facie rational. Even though patients are seriously ill and thereby impaired in both cognitive and conative functioning, they are usually competent to consent to a needed treatment.

The act of consent to such a treatment is considered to be an informed consent as long as the patient is aware of what is going on. *Awareness* in the sense of orientation or being conscious of the general situation satisfies the cognitive requirement of informed consent. *Assent* alone to what is the rational expectation in this medical context satisfies the decisional component. When adult patients go along with needed medical treatment, then a legal presumption of competency holds even though the patients are obviously impaired. To insist on higher standards for capacity to give a valid consent in such a medical setting would amount to requiring surplus mental capacities for a simple task and would result in millions of acutely ill patients being considered incompetent. Such an absurd requirement would produce absurd consequences. Altogether rational and appropriate decisions would be set aside as invalid, and surrogate decision makers would have to be selected to make the same decision. For what purpose? To accomplish what objective? To protect what value? None of the values and objectives meant to be safeguarded by the competency requirement is disregarded or set aside by a lenient standard for this type of decision.

Considering as competent seriously ill patients, even the mentally ill, who are aware and assent to treatment, eliminates the ambiguity and confusion associated with terms such as *virtually competent, marginally competent,* and *competent for practical purposes* that are used to excuse the commonsense practice of respecting the decisions of patients who would be judged incompetent by a more demanding single standard of decision-making capacity. Refusal by a patient dying of a chronic illness of treatments that are useless and only prolong the dying requires the same modest standard of competency.

Infants, unconscious persons, and the severely retarded would obviously fall short even of this least demanding standard. These persons, and patients who use psychotic defenses that severely compromise reality testing, are the only ones who fail to meet this first definition of decision-making capacity. Children who have reached the age of reason (6

years or older), on the other hand, as well as the senile, the mildly retarded, and the intoxicated, are considered competent.

The law considers 21 and sometimes 18 years to be the age below which persons are presumed incompetent to make binding contracts, including health care decisions. The President's commission, however, endorses a lower age of competency, and so do many authors who write about children and mental retardation. In this model, we are discussing ethical standards, but the physician cannot ignore the law and must obtain consent from the child's legal guardian.

Standard 2

If the illness is chronic rather than acute, or if the treatment is more dangerous or of less definite benefit (or if there are real alternatives to one or another course of action, e.g., death rather than lingering illness), then the risk-benefit balance is tipped differently than in the situation described in the previous section. Consequently, a different standard of competency to consent is required. The patient must be able to *understand* the risks and outcomes of the different options and then be able to *choose* a decision based on this understanding. At this point, competency means capacity to understand the real options and to make an understanding decision, a higher standard than that required for the first type of treatment choice.

Ability to understand is not the same as being able to articulate conceptual or verbal understanding. Some ethicists assume a rationalist epistemology and reduce all understanding to a conceptual or verbal type. Many, in fact, require that patients literally remember what they have been told as a proof of competence. Understanding, however, may be more affective than conceptual. Following an explanation, a patient may grasp what is best for him with strong feelings and convictions, and yet be hard pressed to articulate his understanding/conviction in words.

Competency as capacity for an understanding choice is also reconcilable with a decision to let a trusted physician decide what is the best treatment. Such a choice (waiver) may be made for good reasons and represent a decision in favor of one set of values (safety or anxiety reduction) over another (independence and personal initiative). As such, it can be considered as informed consent and creates no suspicion of incompetency.

Ignorance or inability to understand, however, undermines competency. The same is true of a severe mood disorder or severe shock, which may either impair thought processes or undermine capacity to make an understanding choice. Short-term memory loss, delusion, dementia, and delirium would also render a patient incompetent. On the other hand, mature adolescents, the mildly retarded, and persons with some personality disorders would be competent to make this type of decision.

Standard 3

The most stringent and demanding standard of competency is reserved for those decisions that are very dangerous and fly in the face of both professional and public rationality. When diagnostic uncertainty is minimal, the available treatment is effective, and death is likely to result from treatment refusal, a presumption is established against refusal of consent to treatment. The medical decision now is not a balancing of what are widely recognized as reasonable alternatives. Any decision other than the one to be treated seems to violate basic reasonableness. A decision to refuse treatment, then, is apparently irrational, besides being harmful. Yet, according to this model, such decisions can be respected as long as the patients satisfy the most demanding standard of competency.

Competency in this context requires a capacity to appreciate the nature and consequences of the decision being made. *Appreciation* is a term used to refer to the highest degree of understanding, one that grasps more than just the medical details of the illness and treatment. To be competent to make apparently irrational and very dangerous choices, the patient must be able to come to a decision based on the medical information and to appreciate the implications of this decision for his life. Competency of this type requires a capacity that is both technical and personal, both cognitive and affective.

Since the patient's decision flies in the face of objective standards of rationality, it must at least be subjectively critical and *rational*. A patient need not conform to what most rational people do to be considered competent, but the competent patient must be able to give reasons for his decision. The patient must be able to show that he has thought through the medical issues and related this information to his personal value system. The patient's personal reasons need not be medically or publicly accepted, but neither can they be purely private, idiosyncratic, or incoherent. Their intelligibility may derive from a set of religious beliefs or from a philosophical view that is shared by only a small minority. This toughest standard of competency does, however, demand a more rationalistic type understanding: one that includes verbalization, argumentation, and consistency.

The higher-level mental capacities required for competency to make this type of decision are impaired by less severe psychiatric abnormality. In fact, much less serious mental affliction suffices to create an assumption of incompetency to refuse a needed and effective treatment. On the other hand, however, not any mental or emotional disturbance would constitute an impairment of decisional capacity. A certain amount of anxiety, for example, goes with any serious decision and cannot make a patient incompetent. Some mild pain would not impair decisional capacity, but severe pain might do so. Even a slight reactive depression may not render a patient incompetent for this type of decision. But intense anxiety associated with mild or severe shock, and/or a mild endogenous depression, would be considered incapacitating. In fact, any mental or emotional disorder that compromises appreciation and rational decision making would make a patient incompetent. For example, persons who are incapable of making the effort required to control destructive behavior (substance abusers and sociopaths), as well as neurotic persons, hysterical persons, and persons who are ambivalent about their choice, would all be incompetent to refuse life-saving treatment. The same standard applies to consent to experiments not related to one's own illness.

Conclusion

Radical advocates of patient rights and doctrinaire libertarians will worry that this model shifts power back toward physicians who make competency determinations and away from patients whose choices ought to be respected. But only in situation 3 does the physician's power increase, and then only for the patient's welfare. Moreover, this loss in the patients' power never reaches the point where patients' self-determination is set aside. Patients can insist on their decision to refuse a treatment even when the physician knows that the outcome will be certain death, as long as every precaution is taken to ensure that such a decision is not the product of a pathological state.

A balancing of values is the cornerstone of a good competency assessment. Rationality is given its place throughout this model. Maximum autonomy is guaranteed for patients because they can choose to do what is not at all beneficial (a nontherapeutic experiment) or refuse to do what is most beneficial. Maximum benefit is also guaranteed because patients are protected against harmful choices that are more the product of abnormality than of their self-determination. All the values, in fact, on which competency requirements were originally based are guaranteed in this model.

No one proposal will settle the question of which standard or standards of competency are appropriate for medical decisions. More empirical research is required on the issue, and more physicians who have valuable practical experience with complex cases need to be heard from. After much more study and discussion, perhaps the medical profession itself, through its ethics committees, will take a stand on the issue. In the meantime, this proposal is meant to be a contribution to the discussion.

References

1. President's Commission for the Study of Ethical Problems in Medicine and Biomedical and Behavioral Research; *Deciding to Forego Life-Sustaining Treatment*. Washington, D.C., U.S. Government Printing Office, 1983.

2. Siegler, M., Goldblatt, A. D.: Clinical intuition: A procedure for balancing the rights of patients and the responsibilities of physicians, in Spicker, S. F., Healey, J. M., Engelhardt, H. T. (eds.): *The Law-Medicine Relation: A Philosophical Exploration*. Dordrecht, The Netherlands, D. Reidel Publishing Co., 1981, pp. 5–29.

3. Jonsen, A. R., Siegler, M., Winslade, W. J.: *Clinical Ethics*. New York, Macmillan Publishing Co., Inc., 1982, pp. 56–85.

When Well-Meaning Science Goes Too Far

Alexander Morgan Capron

Alexander Capron raises the question of whether Baby Fae was "hero, victim, or patient." (See the Baby Fae Case Presentation for additional information.) In his view, when a child is a patient and research is involved, then physicians have an obligation never to advance their research "at the expense of the child by foregoing an alternative treatment that offers a better chance." It is possible, Capron suggests, that Baby Fae was indeed "a victim of well-meaning science."

Baby Fae has joined such figures as Barney Clark and Karen Ann Quinlan in the vocabulary of popular bioethics. Her transformation from tiny baby to larger-than-life symbol is not without problems, however, partly because of the way in which it occurred and partly because of ambiguities about the role she played in the whole drama.

There was a time when the public learned of biomedical developments after they had been reviewed by, and generally reported to, the researchers' scientific and medical peers. This method not only preserved the dignity of all involved—from scientists to patients—but also meant that the public learned about genuine "advances" rather than merely being titillated by bizarre cases of as-yet unproven import.

Today, it seems that *People* magazine has replaced *The New England Journal of Medicine* as the preferred forum for reporting events on the medical frontiers. This occurs not only in instances where a court (and, hence, usually public records, as in the *Quinlan* case) is involved, but also when the hospital

From The Hastings Center Report, *February 1985, Vol. 15, no. 1, pp. 8–9. Reproduced by permission.*
© *The Hastings Center.*

actively courts the media or lamely asserts its inability to prevent media coverage. (Would we accept as readily a hospital's inability to prevent the spread of an infection into the community?)

As a result, the public receives a distorted view about the process by which scientific knowledge and useful technology actually unfold. Moreover, it may be misled about the usefulness of techniques like the baboon-heart transplant technique used on Baby Fae. Even when the press is able to obtain opinions on such an experimental procedure from members of the biomedical community, the latter are typically unable to offer the sorts of careful, well-informed evaluations that require the full data from a completed experiment (usually including matched or randomized controls or at least a series of cases).

And the research process itself may be distorted by the drive for publicity. As Ellen Goodman asked recently in questioning the way Humana Hospital was handling the William Schroeder artificial-heart implant, "Must every research project now come complete with a press kit and an attractive, articulate patient available perhaps for talk shows and certainly evening-news programs?" How can research in epidemiology or preventive care possibly compete?

One final concern about the manner in which Baby Fae was transformed into a familiar though fleeting part of our lives: this episode illustrates the unseemly way that traditional medical privacy is now frequently invaded by media spotlights merely because a patient is participating in unusual research. Some people may regard this concern as pure paternalism. After all, it might be argued, if a patient consents to the publicity (perhaps out of a desire for fame or to reward a researcher to whom the patient feels indebted), who am I to complain that his hematocrit level or urinary output is reported on the evening news?

But it is precisely here that the Baby Fae case becomes so sticky. Whatever difficulties attend the process of negotiation between a researcher and his or her subject—fraught as it is with barriers to understanding, with transferences and countertransferences, as Jay Katz has recently reminded us in *The Silent World of Doctor and Patient*—they are insignificant compared to those that arise when someone else (such as a parent) must consent on behalf of the patient-subject. Reading over the documents in the Barney Clark case, I have my doubts about the "informed consent" he gave to many aspects of what occurred, but at least some possibility of genuine communication and choice existed. Obviously, for Baby Fae, it was impossible.

This leads to the second, and more important, set of issues, which grow out of the role little Fae played in the drama that brought all that attention to Loma Linda University Medical Center. What was she: hero, victim, or patient?

The ancient dictum *primum non nocere* is simply inadequate guidance for those who treat very sick and dying patients. For them, the greatest kindness may not always to be avoid doing any harm, if they wish to risk harm for a chance at improvement. Indeed, some patients decide to join with physician-investigators in path-breaking research—almost as collaborators, as Renée Fox observed in *Experiment Perilous*. On such medical frontiers, they are rightly regarded as heroes.

A child who is "volunteered" for research is not in the same position, however. For this reason, some ethicists have opposed research involving children. Others have suggested that allowing children into experiments (on their parents' consent, for example) serves to teach a moral lesson, that people in a community owe it to one another to behave altruistically, as by contributing to the discovery of new, useful knowledge.

Such arguments may be persuasive for low-risk studies, but certainly not for innovative therapy of the baboon-heart transplant sort. Here the choice to use a child must rest on the firmest scientific and ethical grounds. Regarding the first, I argued some years ago for a "model of successive approximations," by which one would try to get down to the least vulnerable child-subjects for procedures designed and tested to involve the least possible risk (for example, only those that had first been proven on older subjects).

When a procedure cannot be tested first on other subjects because it is intended especially for infants (as is said to be the case for babies with Fae's heart problems), there should be no ambiguity about the obligations of all involved toward the child as patient. For the physicians this means never advancing their research at the expense of the child by foregoing an alternative treatment that offers a better chance. Did Dr. Leonard Bailey and his colleagues seek a human heart for Baby Fae? Apparently not. Was one available? So a transplant expert in Los Angeles has said.

Hence the concern that Baby Fae may have ended up—like the children in the Willowbrook hepatitis research—as a victim of well-meaning science. And like them, doubts linger not only about the adequacy of the information supplied to Baby Fae's parents but about whether their personal difficulties made it possible for them to choose freely, and whether the realization that their child was dying may have left them with the erroneous conclusion that consenting to the transplant was the only "right" thing to do.

More will have to be known about this case before these doubts can be answered. Until then, Baby Fae's short life will remain with us as a reminder that certain good things—like biomedical research—sometimes go too far, and that others—like the publicity that so often now attends such experiments-in-process—need a very critical reexamination.

Animal Rights and Experimentation

Tom Regan

In Tom Regan's view, animals (at least nonhuman, developed mammals) have a moral status. They are capable of acting on their preferences and thus have "preference autonomy." However, because they are unable to rise above preferences and objectively consider their duty, they lack "Kantian autonomy." Hence, although animals are not moral agents, their autonomy makes them moral patients.

Moral agents and patients, according to Regan, possess basic rights that are independent, universally shared, and universally equal. The basic right is "to respectful treatment," and this means treating moral beings as having equal inherent value. Thus, animals cannot be treated merely as a means to value; like all other moral entities, animals have "a prima facie basic moral right not to be harmed." Regan identifies two principles (the "miniride" and the "worse-off") that may justify overriding the prima facie right not to be harmed.

Regan asserts explicitly that scientific research on animals violates their rights and ought to cease. This is so, he claims, even if no alternatives can be found, for to act otherwise is to ignore the intrinsic value of animals. The moral challenge is to develop nonhuman, nonanimal testing procedures. In the final section, Regan explains why he rejects the utilitarian view in favor of his own "rights view."

Animal Rights

The principal conclusion reached in the present chapter is that all moral agents and patients have certain basic moral rights. To say that these individuals possess basic (or unacquired) moral rights means that (1) they possess certain rights independently of anyone's voluntary acts, either their own or those of others, and independently of the position they happen to occupy in any given institutional arrangement; (2) these rights are universal—that is, they are possessed by all relevantly similar individuals, independently of those considerations mentioned in (1); and (3) all who possess these rights possess them equally. Basic moral rights thus differ *both* from acquired moral rights (e.g., the right of the promisee against the promisor) because one acquires these rights as a result of someone's voluntary acts or one's place in an institutional arrangement *and* from legal rights (e.g., the

Reprinted with permission of the University of California Press, from Tom Regan, The Case for Animal Rights, *pp. 327–329, 382–388, 392–393. © 1983, The Regents of the University of California .*

right to vote) since legal rights, unlike basic moral rights, are not equal or universal.

Moral rights, whether basic or acquired, were analyzed as valid claims. To make a claim is to affirm that certain treatment is owed or is due, either to oneself or to another (or others). A claim is valid if and only if (a) it is a valid claim-against assignable individuals and (b) it is a valid claim-to treatment owed by these individuals, the validity of any claim-to resting ultimately on the validity of principles of direct duty. Because the primary concern of the present chapter was the question of basic moral rights, major emphasis was placed on validating rights of this kind.

The principal basic moral right possessed by all moral agents and patients is the right to respectful treatment. . . . All moral agents and patients are intelligibly and nonarbitrarily viewed as having a distinctive kind of value (inherent value) and as having this value equally. All moral agents and patients must always be treated in ways that are consistent with the recognition of their equal possession of value of this kind. These individuals have a basic moral right to respectful treatment because the claim made to it is (a) a valid claim-against assignable individuals (namely, all moral agents) and (b) a valid claim-to, the validity of the claim-to resting on appeal to the respect principle, the case for that principle's validity having been made in an earlier context. The basic moral right to respectful treatment prohibits treating moral agents or patients as if they were mere receptacles of intrinsic values (e.g., pleasure), lacking any value of their own, since such a view of these individuals would allow harming some (e.g., by making them suffer) on the grounds that the aggregate consequences for all those other "receptacles" affected by the outcome would be "the best." It was also argued that all moral agents and patients have a prima facie basic moral right not to be harmed.

To say that this latter right is a prima facie right means that (1) there are circumstances in which it is permissible to override it but (2) anyone who would override it must justify doing so by appeal to valid moral principles that can be shown to override this right in a given case. Two challenges to regarding this right as prima facie—first, the view that we ought never to use harmful violence (the pacifist principle) and, second, the view that we ought never to harm the innocent (the innocence princi-

ple)—were considered and shown to be deficient, and two moral principles (the miniride and the worse-off principles) were identified as valid principles, derivable from the respect principle, that can justify overriding the right of the innocent not to be harmed. The miniride principle implies that, special considerations aside, numbers count. When we are faced with choosing between harming the few who are innocent or harming the many, and when all those who will be harmed face prima facie comparable harm, then we ought to choose to override the rights of the few. The worse-off principle implies that, special considerations aside, numbers don't count. Special considerations aside, when we are faced with choosing to harm the many or the few who are innocent, and when the harm faced by the few would make them worse-off than any of the many, then we ought to override the rights of the many rather than the few. (The worse-off principle also applies to cases where only two individuals are involved. . . .)

Both the miniride and worse-off principles are logically distinct from and should not be confused with the minimize harm principle, the principle that we are to act so as to minimize the aggregate amount of harm done to all those affected by the outcome, including all the side effects. The rights view rejects such an aggregative principle as a basis for overriding individual rights, since all such principles assume that moral agents and patients are mere receptacles of value. For similar reasons, therefore, the rights view rejects, and at the same time provides an option to, utilitarian approaches to deciding when and, if so, why the innocent may be justifiably harmed. . . .

Thus has the case for animal rights been offered. If it is sound, then, like us, animals have certain basic moral rights, including in particular the fundamental right to be treated with the respect that, as possessors of inherent value, they are due as a matter of strict justice. Like us, therefore—assuming the soundness of the arguments that have gone before—they must never be treated as mere receptacles of intrinsic values (e.g., pleasure, or preference-satisfaction), and any harm that is done to them must be consistent with the recognition of their equal inherent value and their equal prima facie right not to be harmed. It remains to be asked whether our institutions or practices give animals the justice they are due. . . .

Scientific Research

To deny science use of animals in research is, it might be said, to bring scientific and allied medical progress to a halt, and that is reason enough to oppose it. The claim that progress would be "brought to a halt" is an exaggeration certainly. It is not an exaggeration to claim that, given its present dominant tendency, the rights view requires massive redirection of scientific research. The dominant tendency involves routinely harming animals. It should come as no surprise that the rights view has principled objections to its continuation.

A recent statement of the case for unrestricted use of animals in neurobiological research contrasts sharply with the rights view and will serve as an introduction to the critical assessment of using animals in basic research. The situation, as characterized by C. R. Gallistel, a psychologist at the University of Pennsylvania, is as follows:[1] "Behavioral neurobiology tries to establish the manner in which the nervous system mediates behavioral phenomena. It does so by studying the behavioral consequences of one or more of the following procedures: (a) destruction of a part of the nervous system, (b) stimulation of a part, (c) administration of drugs that alter neural functioning. These three techniques are as old as the discipline. A recent addition is (d) the recording of electrical activity. All four cause the animal at least temporary distress. In the past they have frequently caused intense pain, and they occasionally do so now. Also, they often impair an animal's proper functioning, sometimes transiently, sometimes permanently."[2] The animals subjected to these procedures are, in a word, harmed. When it comes to advancing our knowledge in neurobiology, however, "there is no way to establish the relation between the nervous system and behavior without some experimental surgery," where by "experimental surgery" Gallistel evidently means to include the four procedures just outlined. The issue, then, in Gallistel's mind, is not whether to allow such surgery or not; it is whether any restrictions should be placed on the use made of animals. Gallistel thinks not.

In defense of unrestricted use of animals in research, Gallistel claims that "most experiments conducted by neurobiologists, *like scientific experiments generally,* may be seen in retrospect to have been a waste of time, in the sense that they did not prove or yield any new insight." But, claims Gallistel, "there is no way of discriminating in advance the waste-of-time experiments from the illuminating ones with anything approaching certainty."[3] The logical upshot, so Gallistel believes, is that "restricting research on living animals is certain to restrict the progress in our understanding of the nervous system and behavior. Therefore," he concludes, "one should advocate such restrictions only if one believes that the moral value of this scientific knowledge and of the many human and humane benefits that flow from it cannot outweigh the suffering of a rat," something that, writing autobiographically, Gallistel finds "an affront to my ethical sensibility."[4]

Even those unpersuaded by the rights view ought to challenge Gallistel's argument at every point. Is it true, as he claims, "that there is *no* way to establish the relation between the nervous system and behavior without some experimental surgery"? Can we learn nothing whatever about this connection from, say, clinical observation of those who have been injured? Again, is it true that *we can never say in advance* that a given proposal has been drawn up by an incompetent researcher who doesn't know what he is looking for and wouldn't recognize it if he found it? What could be the grounds for peer review of research proposals if Gallistel's views were accepted? Why not draw straws instead? Those stirrings in the scientific community, away from unrestricted use of animals toward the refinement of one's protocol (thereby eliminating so-called unnecessary experiments) and reduction in the number of animals used, will find no support from the no-holds-barred approach Gallistel advocates. Since there is, in his view, no way to separate the scientific wheat from the chaff in advance of experimenting, why worry about refinement? Why worry about reduction?

These matters aside, the rights view rejects Gallistel's approach at a more fundamental level. On the rights view, we cannot justify harming a single rat *merely* by aggregating "the many human and humane benefits" that flow from doing it, since, as stated, this is to assume that the rat has value only as a receptacle, which, on the rights view, is not true. Moreover, the benefits argument that Gallistel deploys is deficient. Not even a single rat is to be treated as if that animal's value were reducible to his *possible utility* relative to the interests of others, which is what we would be doing if we intentionally harmed the rat on the grounds that this *just might* "prove" something, *just might* "yield" a "new insight," *just might* produce "benefits" for others.

It bears emphasizing that the rights view's critique of the use of animals in research is unlike some that find favor in the literature on this matter. Some object on methodological grounds, arguing that the results of such research offer very little hope of benefits for humanity because of the by-now well-established difficulty of extrapolating results from animal tests to the species *Homo sapiens;* others challenge the necessity of a variety of experiments, cases where animals have been cut, blinded, deformed, mutilated, shocked into "learned helplessness," and so on, all in the name of research. Neither of these critical approaches, though each has clear validity as far as it goes, gets to the moral heart of the matter. It is not that the methodology is suspect (though it is), nor that a great deal of research is, Gallistel's opinion to the contrary notwithstanding, known to be a waste of time before it is undertaken. The point to note is that both these challenges *invite the continuation of research on animals,* the latter because it would rule out only that research known to be a waste of time before it is conducted, and the former because it gives researchers a blank check to continue animal experiments in the hope of overcoming the deficiencies in the present methodology. If we are seriously to challenge the use of animals in research, we must challenge the *practice* itself, not only individual instances of it or merely the liabilities in its present methodology.

The rights view issues such a challenge. Routine use of animals in research assumes that their value is reducible to their possible utility relative to the interests of others. The rights view rejects this view of animals and their value, as it rejects the justice of institutions that treat them as renewable resources. They, like us, have a value of their own, logically independently of their utility for others and of their being the object of anyone else's interests. To treat them in ways that respect their value, therefore, requires that we *not* sanction practices that institutionalize treating them as if their value was reducible to their possible utility relative to our interests. Scientific research, when it involves routinely harming animals in the name of possible "human and humane benefits," violates this requirement of respectful treatment. Animals are not

to be treated as mere receptacles or as renewable resources. Thus does the practice of scientific research on animals violate their rights. Thus ought it to cease, according to the rights view. It is not enough first conscientiously to look for nonanimal alternatives and then, having failed to find any, to resort to using animals.[5] Though that approach is laudable as far as it goes, and though taking it would mark significant progress, it does not go far enough. It assumes that it is all right to allow practices that use animals as if their value were reducible to their possible utility relative to the interests of others, provided that we have done our best not to do so. The rights view's position would have us go further in terms of "doing our best." *The best we can do in terms of not using animals is not to use them.* Their inherent value does not disappear just because we have failed to find a way to avoid harming them in pursuit of our chosen goals. Their value is independent of these goals and their possible utility in achieving them.

Let us suppose [in a variant of an earlier case] that the lifeboat contains four normal adults and a dog. Provisions are plentiful this time, and there is more than enough room. Only now suppose the humans have a degenerative brain disease, while the dog is healthy. Also on board, so it happens, is a new medicine that just might be the long-awaited cure of the disease the humans have. The medicine has not been tested. However, it is known to contain some potentially fatal compounds. The means exist to give the degenerative disease to the dog. In these dire circumstances, would it be all right to do this and then to administer the medicine to the animal to assess its curative properties?

Quite possibly most people would give an affirmative reply, at least initially—but not those who subscribe to the rights view. Animals are not to be treated as if their value were reducible *merely* to their possible utility relative to human interests, which is what the survivors would be doing if they made the healthy animal (who, after all, stands to gain nothing and lose everything) run their risks in their stead.

Some might seize upon this verdict of the rights view as a basis for urging what they regard as a fatal objection: since most people think it would be all right to give the medicine to the dog, since the rights view allows appeals to what most people think as a basis for testing alternative moral principles and theories, and since what most people think in this case conflicts with the verdict of the rights view, it follows, some may think, that the practice of using animals in harmful research is justifiable.

Three replies must suffice. First, just because most people think the dog should be treated as described, assuming that most do so, it does not follow that most people think well in this case. Our prereflective intuitions . . . must be tested reflectively to determine how well they stand up under the conscientious attempt to reach an ideal moral judgment. Without making this attempt, those who are content to appeal to "what most people think" have no rational basis to assume that what most people think in any given case is not based on their shared ignorance, their shared prejudices, or their shared irrationality. *Merely* to appeal to "what most people think," in other words, is not decisive in this, or in any other, moral context.

Second, even in those cases where a given belief continues to be held by most people *after* they have made a conscientious effort to remove the insidious effects of ignorance, prejudice, and the like, the possibility still remains that the belief in question stands in need of revision or abandonment. For if a given belief cannot be squared with moral principles that themselves pass the relevant tests for assessing their validity (namely, scope, precision, consistency, and conformity with a host of other intuitions that stand up on reflection), one must come to doubt the rational grounds of that belief and others like it in the relevant respects. Again, then, *merely* to announce that, after having given the matter one's conscientious attention, one still thinks that the dog should be treated as described in the lifeboat case, is not to mount a serious challenge to the rights view or its verdict in this case. A serious challenge can be raised only if, in addition to citing one's belief in this case, one also adduces the general principles that would support it and shows that these principles are equal or superior to the rights view when these principles are themselves subjected to the tests of scope, precision, and the like.

But third . . . the justice of policies or practices are not guaranteed by generalizing on one's judgment in exceptional cases; and lifeboat cases, as was mentioned earlier, are exceptional cases. To make the danger of generalizing on such cases clearer, imagine that the lifeboard contains four exceptional and one average human. Suppose the four are preeminent scientists, each on the verge of making discoveries that portend enormous health benefits for humanity. The fifth man delivers Twinkies to retail stores in Brooklyn. The four scientists have the degenerative brain disease. The Twinkies deliveryman does not. Would it be permissible to give the disease to him and then test for the drug's efficacy by administering it to him first? No doubt many people would be inclined to reply affirmatively (though not, again, those who subscribe to the rights view). Even among those who think the deliveryman should serve as the proverbial guinea pig in these exceptional circumstances, however, none with the slightest egalitarian tendencies would be willing to generalize on the basis of this unusual case and favor a policy or practice of doing research on average humans so that humans who are very bright or who make large social contributions might benefit. Such a practice leaves the bad taste of perfectionism in our mouths. The rights view categorically rejects perfectionism as a basis for assessing the justice of practices involving humans, whether in science or elsewhere. And so should we all. But just as perfectionism is not an equitable basis for assessing the justice of practices involving humans, so it is an unacceptable basis for assessing the justice of practices involving animals. And it is implicit allegiance to perfectionism that would tempt one to sanction the harmful use of animals in research, their "lesser" value being "sacrificed" for the "greater" value of humanity. Grounded in the recognition of the equal inherent value of all those who have inherent value, the rights view denies that a distinction between lesser and greater should be made where the perfectionist defense of the use of animals in research requires it. Thus does it deplore the continuation of this practice.

The rights view does not oppose using what is teamed from conscientious efforts to treat a sick animal (or human) to facilitate and improve the treatment tendered other animals (or humans). In *this* respect, the rights view raises no objection to the "many human and humane benefits" that flow from medical science and the research with which it is allied. What the rights view opposes are practices that cause intentional harm to laboratory animals (for example, by means of burns, shock, amputation, poisoning, surgery, starvation, and sensory deprivation) preparatory to "looking for something that just might yield some human or humane bene-fit." Whatever benefits happen to accrue from such a practice are irrelevant to assessing its tragic injustice. Lab animals are not our tasters; we are not their kings.

The tired charge of being antiscientific is likely to fill the air once more. It is a moral smokescreen. The rights view is not against research on animals, if this research does not harm these animals or put them at risk of harm. It is apt to remark, however, that this objective will not be accomplished merely by ensuring that test animals are anaesthetized, or given postoperative drugs to ease their suffering, or kept in clean cages with ample food and water, and so forth. For it is not only the pain and suffering that matters—though they certainly matter—but it is the *harm* done to the animals, including the diminished welfare opportunities they endure as a result of the deprivations caused by the surgery, *and* their untimely death. It is unclear whether a *benign* use of animals in research is possible or, if possible, whether scientists could be persuaded to practice it. That being so, and given the serious risks run by relying on a steady supply of human volunteers, research should take the direction away from the use of any moral agent or patient. If nonanimal alternatives are available, they should be used; if they are not available, they should be sought. That is the moral challenge to research, given the rights view, and it is those scientists who protest that this "can't be done," in advance of the scientific commitment to try—not those who call for the exploration—who exhibit a lack of commitment to, and belief in, the scientific enterprise—who are, that is, antiscientific at the deepest level. Like Galileo's contemporaries, who would not look through the telescope because they had already convinced themselves of what they would see and thus saw no need to look, those scientists who have convinced themselves that there can't be viable scientific alternatives to the use of whole animals in research (or toxicity tests, etc.) are captives of mental habits that true science abhors. . . .

Animals in Science, Utilitarianism, and Animal Rights

The fundamental differences between utilitarianism and the rights view are never more apparent than in the case of the use of animals in science. For the utilitarian, whether the harm done to animals in pursuit of scientific ends is justified depends on the balance of the aggregated consequences for all those affected by the outcome. If the consequences that result from harming animals would produce the best aggregate balance of good over evil, then harmful experimentation is obligatory. If the resulting consequences would be at least as good as what are otherwise obtainable, then harmful experimentation is permissible. Only if harmful experimentation would produce less than the best consequences would it be wrong. For a utilitarian to oppose or support harmful experimentation on animals, therefore, requires that he have the relevant facts—who will be benefited or harmed, how much, and so on. *Everyone's* interests, including the interests of those who do the tests or conduct the research, their employers, the dependents of these persons, the retailers and wholesalers of cages, animal breeders, and others, must be taken into account and counted equitably. For utilitarians, such *side effects count*. The animals used in the test have no privileged moral status. Their interests must be taken into account, to be sure, but not any more than anybody else's interests.

As is "almost always" the case, utilitarians simply fail to give us what is needed—the relevant facts, facts that we must have, given their theory, to determine whether use of animals in science is or is not justified. Moreover, for a utilitarian to claim or imply that there must be something wrong with a given experiment, if the experimenter would not be willing to use a less intelligent, less aware human being but would be willing to use a more intelligent, more aware animal, simply lacks a utilitarian basis. For all we know, and for all the utilitarian has thus far told us, the consequences of using such an animal, all considered, might be better than those that would result from using the human being. It is not *who* is used, given utilitarian theory, that matters; it is *the consequences* that do.

The rights view takes a very different stand. No one, whether human or animal, is ever to be treated as if she were a mere receptacle, or as if her value were reducible to her possible utility for others. We are, that is, never to harm the individual merely on the grounds that this will or just might produce "the best" aggregate consequences. To do so is to violate the rights of the individual. That is why the harm done to animals in pursuit of scientific purposes is wrong. The benefits derived are real enough; but some gains are ill-gotten, and all gains are ill-gotten when secured unjustly.

So it is that the rights view issues its challenge to those who do science: advance knowledge, work for the general welfare, but not by allowing practices that violate the rights of the individual. These are, one might say, the terms of the new contract between science and society, a contract that, however belatedly, now contains the signature of those who speak for the rights of animals. *Those who accept the rights view, and who sign for animals, will not be satisfied with anything less than the total abolition of the harmful use of animals in science—in education, in toxicity testing, in basic research.* But the rights view plays no favorites. No scientific practice that violates human rights, whether the humans be moral agents or moral patients, is acceptable. . . .

Notes

1. C. R. Gallistel, "Bell, Magendie, and the Proposal to Restrict the Use of Animals in Neurobehavioral Research," *American Psychologist* (April 1981), pp. 357–360.

2. Ibid., p. 357.

3. Ibid., p. 358.

4. Ibid., p. 360.

5. This is the view recommended in Dale Jamieson and Tom Regan, "On the Ethics of the Use of Animals in Science" [in *And Justice for All*, ed. Tom Regan and Donald Van De Veer (Totowa, N.J.: Rowman and Littlefield, 1982), 169–196]. In disassociating myself from this earlier view, I speak only for myself. I am in no position to speak for Professor Jamieson.

The Moral Case for Experimentation on Animals

H. J. McCloskey

McCloskey argues that animal experimentation, for the sake of animals and for the sake of humans, is morally justifiable. He bases his claims on two principles: the "prima facie duty to maximize the balance of good over evil" and the "duty to respect persons." Morally justifiable experiments on animals for the good of animals include as requirements the conditions that: the knowledge produced cannot be obtained in a "morally less costly" way, pain must be minimized, and tests that are useless must be avoided. Because the results of an experiment are often uncertain and their worth difficult to judge, McCloskey considers that it is experimentation in general (as distinct from particular cases) that is justified by the principle of maximizing the balance of good over evil.

In McCloskey's view, experimenting on animals for the sake of persons (or persons and animals) can be justified by appealing both to our duty to maximize good and to our duty to respect persons. To permit avoidable suffering by not developing drugs and vaccines is to show a serious lack of respect for persons. Without past and continuing animal experimentation, suffering and death would be much greater than they are.

McCloskey reviews four possible alternatives to the use of animals in the testing of toxicity. He finds each of them lacking in merit. (In the part of the essay not included here, McCloskey criticizes Tom Regan's attempt to assign rights to animals.)

The moral case for experimentation on animals rests both on the goods to be realized, the evils to be avoided thereby, and on the duty to respect persons and to secure them in the enjoyment of their natural moral rights. Some experimentation on animals presents no problems of justification as it involves no harm at all to the animals which are the subject of experiments and is such as to seek to achieve an advance in knowledge. Experiments on non-sentient animals, like those on plant life, may harm the subjects but in ways that in themselves need raise no morally significant issues. Moral issues may arise if the subjects of experiments are members of an endangered species and for like reasons but not simply on account of the harm caused by the experiment to the subjects. Other experimentation on animals is to be justified solely in terms of its benefit to animals, even though it involves harm to the animals upon which experiments are performed. There are many poisons and diseases to which animals and not human beings are exposed which give rise to the need for experiments to determine effective therapies, treatments, or other remedies. Examples include annual rye grass toxicity, foot-and-mouth disease, the many fowl diseases, and so on. Human beings commonly have an interest in successfully experimenting to find effective remedies, either a financial interest as with farm animals, race horses and the like, amusement interest as with pets, or a concern not to have a species or variety become extinct. The moral case for such experiments may be strengthened by reference to such interests if they in turn have a moral basis, but generally it does not depend for its validity on this. Other experimentation that harms the animals involved is to be justified in terms of the benefits to be realized and evils lessened for persons by the knowledge and the use of the knowledge gained, where the knowledge is used to secure the enjoyment of their moral rights by persons. Much experimentation benefits both persons, contributing to the securing of their enjoyment of their moral rights, and animals which do not possess moral rights, and is to be morally justified on both counts. Obviously a great amount of experimentation occurs today which does not admit of justification along any of these lines, and hence, is such that it must be condemned as being morally wrong.

The experimentation that is to be considered in this paper relates to determining the toxicity of materials that may be harmful to animals and/or man, and the testing of possible antidotes and remedies, and to the investigation of substances, drugs, vaccines, therapies, treatments that may also be beneficial or harmful to animals and/or man.

The ethical basic of the view developed here is that there is prima facie duty to maximize the balance of good over evil, where pleasure and pain are among the important goods and evils and that among the other basic prima facie duties that hold of persons is the duty to respect persons, to treat persons as persons, as beings to be respected, and not simply as means to ends. (Other humanly orientated duties are those of honesty and justice, these holding of persons in respect of persons.) Persons as morally autonomous beings possess moral rights by virtue of their nature as persons, that is, as morally autonomous, rational, sentient, affective beings, the rights including the rights to life, health, bodily integrity, respect as a person and all that that implies, moral autonomy and integrity, self-development and education as dictated by that and other rights, and knowledge and true belief. There are obvious difficulties in the way of providing a justification of such an ethic. The principle of maximizing the balance of good over evil is exposed to the problem that it involves a rejection of the distinction between acts of supererogation and duties proper. However, for the purposes of this paper, it is not essential that this problem be met as it is the causing of avoidable suffering without good cause that is of central importance here. There is a general acknowledgement and acceptance of the duty not unnecessarily to cause or allow to continue unnecessary suffering. Objections may be urged against the claims that persons ought to be respected, and that, as persons with the nature they possess, they possess as rights of recipience the rights noted above. Here, as also with the principle relating to maximizing the balance of good over evil, appeal must ultimately be made to the self-evidence of the principles and of the possession of these rights by persons.[1]

It is important now to examine the nature of the moral justification of those experiments on animals for the good of animals that are justified. The experiments must be such that the knowledge sought from them cannot be obtained by means that are morally less costly. They must so be planned and structured as to minimize such pain and loss of pleasure as will occur, such scientifically and morally indefensible overtesting as by LD50 tests being avoided, and the pain being lessened where possible by the use of anaesthesia and/or analgesia, and terminated as soon as possible in terms of the completion of the experiment. Such suffering and distress as may be caused by confinement before and after the experiment, and by the confinement and transporting of animals is to be minimized by care in ensuring satisfactory accommodation and conditions of transportation. Experiments so-called which cause hurt or harm to the animals and which merely duplicate past experiments and this not by way of seeking necessary confirmation of past results are such as not to admit of moral justification.

It is not possible to lay down in detail necessary and sufficient conditions for eithically justifiable experiments. This is due in part to the great differences between animals in respect of their capacity to experience pain. All that can be done here is to indicate general guidelines and what practices can have no moral basis. Experiments must be constructed so as to minimize suffering and not use scientifically unnecessary over-testing, overkill methods. More important, animals that may experience pain should be used only when the relevant information sought can be obtained only through them or human beings and not by experiments on non-sentient animals. Further, it is essential, when well-thought-out ethical codes of conduct of animal experiments are laid down, it be ensured that experimentation conform with the required standards. Experimenters, whether they be experimenters on humans or on animals, notoriously fail to conform with the ethical standards laid down for experimentation in the absence of effective controls and supervision.

It is possible to ground a justification of experimentation on animals for the good of animals which conforms with sound ethical criteria of the kind indicated here when it is *experimentation in general* as a scientific tool used to gain knowledge about drugs, toxins, antidotes, and the like, that it is sought to justify, as the use of such a tool overall may be seen to lead to the greatest balance of good over evil. However there are problems in justifying specific, ethically and scientifically well-planned experiments which involve great suffering which it is hoped will produce results beneficial to animals, and which produce no useful outcome, no useful knowledge, and whose value seem to lie simply in the intrinsic value of this knowledge. Yet, in advance of the experiment, it is impossible to know which experiments will provide useful knowledge and useful outcomes. Even after an experiment, the knowledge that is gained may at that time appear to be of no value, and only much later come to be seen to be of great value. This suggests that it is experimentation as a whole activity, ethically and scientifically well-planned experimentation, not individual experiments as such, that admits of ethical justification by reference to the principle of maximizing the balance of good over evil.

The general justification of experimentation on animals for the sake of persons alone or of persons and animals together is to be set out by reference to the principle of maximizing the balance of good over evil and that of respecting persons. Clearly not to lessen unnecessary, avoidable pain and suffering, vast amounts of pain and suffering of very many persons as by producing and testing drugs, vaccines (these being produced using animals and animal experimentation), therapies to combat diseases such as smallpox, cholera, malaria, poliomyelitis, tuberculosis, and the like, is to act immorally both because it is thereby to fail to lessen preventable suffering of persons, and to show serious lack of respect for persons as persons. To respect the moral rights of persons is to seek to prevent suffering, disablement, degeneration of their bodies, and death that such diseases can bring. Consider the evils that would now be besetting mankind had animal experimentation never occurred in respect of antibiotics, vaccines, and such like, and the evils that would befall mankind if such experimentation were to be stopped today. Without animal experimentation in the past we should still be afflicted by such diseases on a vast scale, we should still be incapable of checking the ravages of septicaemia, gangrene, diabetes and a host of other diseases. Without continued experimentation we shall be exposed to the new strains and new diseases that continue to emerge, golden staphylococcal infection, Legionaire's disease, AIDS, and the very many other diseases that are emerging.

What distinguishes attempts to justify animal experimentation by reference to respect for persons and for human rights by contrast with maximizing the balance of good over evil is that lack of success in any specific experiment constitutes no problem, as respect for persons dictates not necessarily successful endeavour but endeavour that is rationally based. Much is made by critics of animal experimentation of the difficulty of extrapolating the results of animal experiments as they apply to human beings. There are of course problems here, but they lessen as the animals experimented upon are closer to man. Hence the use of mammals in so many important, productive experiments, experiments beneficial to man.

Those who are morally critical of animal experimentation argue that a vast amount of animal experimentation is unnecessary because it relates to inessentials that could be dispensed with, without loss, cosmetics in particular getting a very bad press on many counts, not least because of the scientifically unnecessary, morally indefensible use of overtesting as in the use of LD50 tests. Clearly a great deal of experimentation relating to substances such as cosmetics is unnecessary because we already have the relevant knowledge. Nonetheless, that cosmetics are inessentials is not in itself a reason for not testing them although it may be a reason for seeking to ban the production and sale of any new, untested cosmetics. However, as long as we have cosmetics in use, testing of their toxicity and their other effects in respect of causing diseases, will continue to be morally important and necessary. Cosmetics as inessentials do not constitute the very special kind of case it is suggested they do. There are many other essentials such tobacco, cannabis, the various hallucinatory drugs, addictive drugs such as alcohol, cocaine, and heroin, for example, which need not be used by persons but which are so used, even when their use is prohibited by states, the effects of which it is important to determine. In so far as animal experimentation can help to reveal their effects, and help in the search for counter-measures, antidotes, and the like, to that extent at least animal experimentation has a moral justification provided of course the experiments conform with the kinds of ethical criteria noted above. Not to seek to extend our knowledge of the effects of such substances and of ways of counteracting them, given the difficulty of checking their use, is to show serious disrespect for persons.

It is useful now to consider possible alternatives to the testing of substances, drugs, therapies, treatments that may harmfully affect or benefit mankind by the use of experimentation on animals.

(i) It has been suggested that we could opt immediately to stop animal experimentation, to develop no new substance, drugs, materials by and in industry, treatments, therapies, and to use only those substances we now use and which have been tested up to the present time. So to act would be both foolish and immoral. We do not know all the properties, all the effects, harmful or otherwise, of substances, drugs, therapies used today. It has taken a very long time to gain the very limited knowledge we now have. Consider how long it has taken to learn of many of the important, harmful effects of smoking tobacco, using asbestos, the carcinogenetic and other harmful effects of substances and drugs so long unsuspected of having any adverse effects. Very many new substances, pesticides, fertilizers, complex compounds, preservatives, food dyes, sweeteners, thickeners, drugs, antibiotics, have come into use since World War II, such that we know little about their effects today. Our knowledge of the effects of such familiar substances as alcohol, cannabis, heroin, cocaine is very limited; much knowledge remains to be gained, and this in part at least by and through animal experimentation. New poisons are becoming important in our ecosystems because of new interactions, through industrial waste, pollution, the spread of plants to new areas with new climates, and so on. Consider the serious problems that annual rye grass toxicity, industrial waste seeping into river and bay ecosystems, and atmospheric pollution are causing in Australia. It is therefore essential that we extend our kowledge using animal experimentation. Further, bacteria and their hosts, and the hosts of viruses, are continually developing resistance to antibiotics, pesticides, such that new antibiotics and pesticides are continually needed if we are not to be ravaged by new strains of old diseases and old diseases carried by resistant hosts. Golden stapholococcal infection, the spread of malaria after the near conquest of malaria, and like phenomena, bring out the nature of the problem. These new strains create the need for new tests for new drugs and pesticides. Further, new diseases such as AIDS and genital herpes are developing or moving into new populations in such a way as to call for further research using animals where possible, and this, perhaps, in order to develop vaccines as our knowledge increases. It is quite unrealistic to speak as if it is overall possible and desirable to opt to use only those substances now in use. The growing world population, the increased use of resources that must come if the standard of living of those in the Third World is to improve, necessitate the use of new substances and the finding of new uses for substances already in use, with new problems arising, many of which cannot satisfactorily be tackled or solved without resort to experimentation on animals.

There is a school of ethical thought, one which I reject, to the effect that it is immoral to make use of knowledge gained by seriously immoral means, and hence that it is immoral to use such knowledge as that gained by the Nazis in their experiments on inmates of concentration camps. If that reasoning were to be accepted by those opposed to animal experimentation, they would need to put aside all that we know of substances, drugs, therapies, by means of animal experimentation. They would in addition need to abandon the production and use of vaccines produced using animals whether or not such vaccines were discovered via animal experimentation. So to act would be to opt for vast epidemics, for a vast increase in human suffering, and untimely deaths for untold numbers of persons. So to act would be to opt for a course of blatant immorality.

(ii) Alternatively or complementary to the course advocated in (i), it is suggested that knowledge be sought and that it can be gained using avenues other than experimentation on animals. This suggestion is little short of irresponsible. Our knowledge of physics, chemistry, bio-sciences, is much too limited for us to be able to determine by reference to them what substances in what quantities will be toxic to animals and humans, what will be safe antidotes, which will cause chromosome damage, impairments, which cancer, and the like, and which drugs and treatments will be beneficial. Some of the alternatives to animal experimentation which could if morally available have a limited use are experiments on aborted live human foetuses, human embryos, 'brain dead' human beings—more could be done by way of experiments on such organisms if human body banks where the bodies were kept functioning on support machines were to be instituted—themselves raise significant moral issues which need to be resolved. It is morally vital that those methods of gaining knowledge that involve the least moral cost be used if other things are equal. However it is extremely misleading to suggest that more than an almost insignificant amount of relevant knowlege that is now gained using experiments on animals could at present be obtained by means of morally acceptable methods of other kinds.

(iii) Another approach might be that of relying on observations of effects of substances on humans and animals by way of post-mortems as well as in life, where the substances are those that are encountered or used by some in the course of their lives, for example, in respect of pollutants such as leaded petrol, DDT and other pesticides, addictive drugs used by addicts, and in respect of other materials and drugs, using also observations of the reactions of persons who volunteer to be subjects of experiments where they give free and informed consent to the experiments. Alternatively, it might be suggested that some persons, criminals, incompetents, or the like, be conscripted to be subjects of such experiments. Most accounts of the ethics of human experimentation insist, rightly, that experiments on human beings are morally desirable only if embarked upon after all the relevant preliminary animal experiments have been carried out. To forbid experimentation on animals but to permit experimentation on human conscripts and/or human volunteers who are made necessary because animal experimentation is outlawed, is morally outrageous.

(iv) It might be urged that new drugs, vaccines, therapies, treatments, food dyes, fertilizers, materials used in industry, be used without any testing at all by means of animal experimentation. This is distinct from position (i). There the suggestion is that we opt not to use new substances and processes. Here the proposal is that we use new substances and processes and in effect engage in inefficient testing by observing their effects on humans and animals. Since such haphazard testing would be even more costly in terms of human welfare and human life, and human and animal suffering than would be controlled experiments on a limited number of human beings—conscripts and/or volunteers—and since it would amount to having involuntary subjects of the experiments, it is morally completely unacceptable as an alternative to animal experimentation. . . .

Principles of the Nuremberg Code _____

1. The voluntary consent of the human subject is absolutely essential.

2. The experiment should be such as to yield fruitful results for the good of society, unprocurable by other methods or means of study, and not random and unnecessary in nature.

3. The experiment should be so designed and based on the results of animal experimentation and a knowledge of the natural history of the disease or other problem under study that the anticipated results will justify the performance of the experiment.

4. The experiment should be so conducted as to avoid all unnecessary physical and mental suffering and injury.

5. No experiment should be conducted where there is an a priori reason to believe that death or disabling injury will occur; except, perhaps, in those experiments where the experimental physicians also serve as subjects.

6. The degree of risk to be taken should never exceed that determined by the humanitarian importance of the problem to be solved by the experiment.

7. Proper preparations should be made and adequate facilities provided to protect the experimental subject against even remote possibilities of injury, disability, or death.

8. The experiment should be conducted only by scientifically qualified persons. The highest degree of skill and care should be required through all stages of the experiment of those who conduct or engage in the experiment.

9. During the course of the experiment the human subject should be at liberty to bring the experiment to an end if he has reached the physical or mental state where continuation of the experiment seems to him to be impossible.

10. During the course of the experiment the scientist in charge must be prepared to terminate the experiment at any stage, if he has probable cause to believe, in the exercise of good faith, superior skill and careful judgment required of him that a continuation of the experiment is likely to result in injury, disability, or death to the experimental subject.

Principles of the Declaration of Helsinki _____

World Medical Association

I. Basic Principles

1. Biomedical research involving human subjects must conform to generally accepted scientific principles and should be based on adequately performed laboratory and animal experimentation and on a thorough knowledge of the scientific literature.

2. The design and performance of each experimental procedure involving human subjects should be clearly formulated in an experimental protocol which should be transmitted to a specially appointed independent committee for consideration, comment, and guidance.

3. Biomedical research involving human subjects should be conducted only by scientifically qualified persons and under the supervision of a clinically competent medical person. The responsibility for the human subject must always rest with a medically qualified person and never rest on the subject of research, even though the subject has given his or her consent.

4. Biomedical research involving human subjects cannot legitimately be carried out unless the importance of the objective is in proportion to the inherent risk to the subject.

From Trials of War Criminals before the Nuremberg Military Tribunals under Control Council Law No. 10, *vol. 2, pp. 181–182. Washington, D.C.: United States Government Printing Office, 1949.*

Adopted by the 18th World Medical Assembly, Helsinki, Finland, 1964, and revised by the 29th World Medical Assembly, Tokyo, Japan, October 1975. Reprinted with permission of the World Medical Association, Inc., from the "Declaration of Helsinki," revised edition.

5. Every biomedical research project involving human subjects should be preceded by careful assessment of predictable risks in comparison with foreseeable benefits to the subject or to others. Concern for the interests of the subject must always prevail over the interests of science and society.

6. The right of the research subject to safeguard his or her integrity must always be respected. Every precaution should be taken to respect the privacy of the subject and to minimize the impact of the study on the subject's physical and mental integrity and on the personality of the subject.

7. Doctors should abstain from engaging in research projects involving human subjects unless they are satisfied that the hazards involved are believed to be predictable. Doctors should cease any investigation if the hazards are found to outweigh the potential benefits.

8. In publication of the results of his or her research, the doctor is obliged to preserve the accuracy of the results. Reports of experimentation not in accordance with the principles laid down in this Declaration should not be accepted for publication.

9. In any research on human beings, each potential subject must be adequately informed of the aims, methods, anticipated benefits and potential hazards of the study and the discomfort it may entail. He or she should be informed that he or she is at liberty to abstain from participation in the study and that he or she is free to withdraw his or her consent to participation at any time. The doctor should then obtain the subject's freely given informed consent, preferably in writing.

10. When obtaining informed consent for the research project the doctor should be particularly cautious if the subject is in a dependent relationship to him or her or may consent under duress. In that case the informed consent should be obtained by a doctor who is not engaged in the investigation and who is completely independent of this official relationship.

11. In case of legal incompetence, informed consent should be obtained from the legal guardian in accordance with national legislation. Where physical or mental incapacity makes it impossible to obtain informed consent, or when the subject is a minor, permission from the responsible relative replaces that of the subject in accordance with national legislation.

12. The research protocol should always contain a statement of the ethical consideration involved and should indicate that the principles enunciated in the present Declaration are complied with.

II. Medical Research Combined with Professional Care (Clinical Research)

1. In the treatment of the sick person, the doctor must be free to use a new diagnostic and therapeutic measure, if in his or her judgment it offers hope of saving life, reestablishing health or alleviating suffering.

2. The potential benefits, hazards and discomfort of a new method should be weighed against the advantages of the best current diagnostic and therapeutic methods.

3. In any medical study, every patient—including those of a control group, if any—should be assured of the best proven diagnostic and therapeutic method.

4. The refusal of the patient to participate in a study must never interfere with the doctor-patient relationship.

5. If the doctor considers it essential not to obtain informed consent, the specific reasons for this proposal should be stated in the experimental protocol for transmission to the independent committee (I, 2).

6. The doctor can combine medical research with professional care, the objective being the acquisition of new medical knowledge, only to the extent that medical research is justified by its potential diagnostic or therapeutic value for the patient.

III. Non-therapeutic Biomedical Research Involving Human Subjects (Non-clinical Biomedical Research)

1. In any purely scientific application of medical research carried out on a human being, it is the duty of the doctor to remain the protector of the life and health of that person on whom biomedical research is being carried out.

2. The subjects should be volunteers—either healthy persons or patients for whom the experimental design is not related to the patient's illness.

3. The investigator or the investigating team should discontinue the research if in his/her or their judgment it may, if continued, be harmful to the individual.

4. In research on man, the interest of science and society should never take precedence over considerations related to the well-being of the subject.

Decision Scenario 1 ....

You are an agent of the Ethics Committee of the National Association of Physicians. You have been sent to Laural, Mississippi, to look into the experimental work of Dr. Joseph Camwell at the Laural State Hospital.

"Our basic concern," Dr. Camwell tells you, "was to test the effectiveness of a hormone-based substance in controlling conception by the regulation of ovulation."

"A birth-control pill."

"Exactly," says Dr. Camwell. "We ran a double-blind test with HB-4, the test substance, and a sucrose-based compound flavored and shaped to be phenomenologically indistinguishable from the tablets of HB-4."

"So that neither the experimenter nor the subjects knew who was getting HB-4 and who was getting the sugar pills. But who were your test subjects?"

"Patients who presented themselves at our state-sponsored outpatient clinic and requested contraceptive medication formed our candidate population. We drew from them subjects with a good medical history, and no present major illnesses, who seemed reliable enough to take their medications on schedule."

"What were the racial percentages?"

"We didn't consider that to be a relevant factor in the experiment. It just happened that about 90% of our subjects were black, although race was not a criterion for selection."

"Did you secure from these women their informed consent to be subjects in this experiment?"

"Of course," Dr. Camwell says. "I personally explained to each of them that they were going to

participate in an experiment but that it wouldn't hurt them any. I told them they would be given birth-control pills that we were testing for effectiveness. 'You might get pregnant while you're taking these pills,' I said."

"But you didn't tell them that at least half of them would be receiving sugar pills that would do absolutely nothing to prevent pregnancy?"

"I think that I warned them sufficiently," says Dr. Camwell. "I told them they might get pregnant. None of these women is able to understand medical sophistications. If I tried to tell them about the experiment, they wouldn't understand me. They knew they might get pregnant, and I figured that was enough."

"Did they all agree to participate?"

"Every last person we approached agreed to participate," Dr. Camwell says. "People always want to help out doctors, and they'll do it if you just put it to them in the right way. I never have any trouble getting subjects for my work."

1. *Would you recommend to the Ethics Committee that Dr. Camwell's consent procedures be condemned? If so, on what grounds?*

2. *Camwell apparently endorses Ingelfinger's view that informed consent is impossible. Evaluate this claim.*

3. *What sort of information would have to be provided to the potential subjects to satisfy the principles of informed consent argued for by Freedman?*

4. *How does Drane's "sliding-scale" model of consent apply to such cases?*

Decision Scenario 2 ....

"In effect," said Dr. Sanchez, "the drug is a powerful tranquilizer. We are not sure how it works, but we know that it has a great calming effect on people diagnosed as schizophrenics. It's much like thorazine, which you may have heard of."

"Does it have any side effects?" Monica Jones asked.

"If taken over a period of a couple of weeks, it produces a palsied condition—muscular tremors, difficulty in walking and in controlling the face muscles, and so on. These don't seem to be permanent."

"That's in schizophrenics," Monica said.

"That's right. We don't know the likely effects in other people. Perhaps you will notice no change whatsoever, and perhaps you will never develop the muscular tremors. But perhaps you'll develop them sooner or more severely. That's part of what we need to find out."

"I'm not in danger of death, then?"

"Not to any great extent. That is, all medication has associated with it some risk. But we don't believe the risk here to be great. There is some possibility of long-term nerve or brain damage. We simply don't know the risks here."

"And you need so-called normal people like me to act as subjects so that you can compare the effects of the drug on us with its effects on schizophrenics?"

"Exactly right," said Dr. Sanchez. "But I should tell you that you may not get the drug. None of us involved in the experiment as patients or experimenters will know who is getting the tranquilizer and who is getting a placebo."

"So maybe I'm not running any risk at all," said Monica.

"Maybe not. But your participation is still important. This drug may do much to relieve the symptoms of a great number of schizophrenics."

"Now, if I understand correctly," said Monica Jones, "I will be paid for my participation."

"That's right. You will be paid a flat fee for participation—half at the beginning of the study and the rest at the end. I want you to be clear on one thing, however. You must waive your right to claim compensation due to any injury or ill effects you may suffer as a result of the medication."

"I understand that. I've got to take a risk. I'm not too happy about that, but I can't get a job and I need the money so I can go back to school next semester."

"Fine," said Dr. Sanchez. "I have the consent forms right here."

1. *Is a society in which risking one's health for financial gain one compatible with Rawls's principles of justice?*

2. *Do Kant's principles allow one to take such a risk?*

3. *Does the natural law doctrine of Catholicism?*

4. *Would the view of human experimentation advocated by Jonas regard such an experiment as legitimate? Would the view of Lasagna? Would Freedman's theory allow such a financial transaction?*

5. *Do you think it is possible for Sanchez to give Jones good reasons for participating that do not involve some form of pressure or duress?*

Decision Scenario 3 . . . .

The drug DES—diethylstilbestrol—was once believed to be effective in preventing miscarriages. But in 1971 sufficient evidence was available to establish a link between DES and vaginal cancer and cervical cell abnormalities in the daughters of women given the drug. About one million women were given DES in the first trimester of pregnancy, and over 120 daughters of these women have been shown to have cancer. Sons, apparently, do not develop cancer, but the group shows a higher-than-average proportion of genital abnormalities and sterility.

In late 1951 and early 1952, women receiving prenatal care at the University of Chicago's Lying-In Hospital were given unmarked tablets of DES as part of a study conducted by Dr. William Dieckmann. One of those receiving the tablets was Ms. Patsy T. Mink, who later became an Assistant Secretary of State.

"I remember quite clearly the doctor giving me those pills and telling me they were vitamins," Ms. Mink says.

Ms. Mink's daughter Gwendolyn was born in the hospital in 1952. Ms. Mink was not notified that she had been given DES until twenty-four years later. She rushed her daughter to a medical examination, and it was discovered that Gwendolyn had abnormal cell changes in the cervix—a condition known as adenosis and thought to be a precursor of cancer.

Ms. Mink is outraged by the experiment in which she was an unwitting subject. She feels that she was not given the drug for a legitimate medical reason and that she was deceived by her doctor. "There's no way we could know," she says. "If they had given me a choice, if they had said, 'We think you are a risk case and this drug may help you,' that's different. That's the choice we should have been presented with. But I wasn't a risk case, and I wasn't told anything."

1. *Did those who gave her DES act immorally? After all, at the time she was given the drug there was no reason to believe that it might have harmful effects.*

2. *If Ms. Mink's informed consent had been obtained, the outcome would have been exactly the same because she could not have been warned of dangers that no one knew existed. Doesn't this show that the whole notion of informed consent is pointless and that one simply must trust in the integrity and best judgment of a physician, as Ingelfinger suggests?*

Decision Scenario 4 •

"You realize," Dr. Thorne said, "that you may not be in the group that receives medication? You may be in the placebo group for at least part of the time."

"Right," Ms. Ross said. "You're just going to give me some medicine."

"And do you understand the aims of the experiment?"

"You want to help me get better," Ms. Ross suggested hesitantly.

"We hope you get better, of course. But that's not what we're trying to accomplish here. We're trying to find out if this particular medication will help other people in your condition if we can treat them earlier than we were able to treat you."

"You want to help people," Ms. Ross said.

"That's right. Now, do you understand that we may not be helping you in this experiment?"

"But you're going to try?"

"Not exactly. I mean, we aren't going to try to harm you. But we aren't necessarily going to be giving you the preferred treatment for your complaint either. Do you know the difference between research and therapy?"

"Research is when you're trying to find something out. You're searching around."

"That's right. And we're asking you to be part of a research effort. As I told you, there are some risks. Besides the possibility of not getting treatment that you need, the drug may produce some limited hepatic portal damage. We're not sure how much."

"I think I understand," Ms. Ross said.

"I hope so," said Dr. Thorne. "Now I understand that you are freely volunteering to participate in this research."

"Yes, sir. Mrs. Woolerd, she told me if I volunteered I'd get a letter put in my file and I could get early release."

"Mrs. Woolerd told you the Review Board would take your volunteering into account when they considered whether you should be put on work-release."

"Yes, sir. And I'm awfully anxious to get out of here. I've got two children staying with my aunt, and I need to get out of this place as quick as I can."

"I understand. We can't promise you release, of course. But your participation will look good on your record. Now I have some papers here I want you to sign."

1. *Discuss some of the difficulties involved in explaining research procedures to nonexperts and determining whether they are aware of the nature and risks of their participation.*

2. *What reasons are there for believing that Ms. Ross does not understand what she is volunteering for?*

3. *Also discuss the problems involved in securing free and voluntary consent from a person involuntarily confined to an institution (a prisoner, for example).*

4. *Is there a reason to believe that Ms. Ross is not giving free consent?*

5. *What conditions does Freedman require to be satisfied before a prisoner's consent can be regarded as legitimate?*

6. *Which, if any, of Drane's three standards seems relevant in this case?*

Decision Scenario 5 •

The ad in the newspapers was simple and uninformative:

Subjects (male and female) wanted to participate in scientific study. Must be 21 or over. $2.00 per hour.

Karen Barty wrote down the address. She could use the money, and in 1962 $2.00 an hour wasn't bad pay for what was sure to be very little work. Besides, the hours were probably flexible, and she could fit the time into her class schedule.

The next Tuesday morning at ten o'clock, Karen and nine other people reported to Room 711 of the Basic Sciences Building in the Western Medical Center. A man who introduced himself as Dr. Carlo Raphael explained what would be required of them as research subjects.

"First of all, you must all sign consent forms," he said. "These state that you are voluntary participants in this study and that for your assistance you will receive a financial reward. If you are not willing to sign the forms, then we cannot accept you as a subject."

He interrupted himself to pass out badly mimeographed sheets of paper that had "Voluntary Consent of Research Subjects" printed at the top. Karen signed hers at once, without bothering to read it. The others in her group, she noticed, did the same thing.

"Very good," Dr. Raphael said, after collecting the forms. "We are going to ask that you provide us with the answers to a series of questions. Some of you may think of these as 'tests,' but I want to assure you that they are not tests in the way you ordinarily think of them. You can neither pass nor fail. Just give us your immediate and truthful responses."

With the help of two assistants, Dr. Raphael distributed test booklets with coded answer sheets tucked inside. Everyone was then supplied with a black IBM pencil with soft, black lead.

Karen listened, half bored, as Dr. Raphael explained how the answer sheets were to be filled in. She had heard the same kind of explanation a dozen times before, but she guessed that the same thing always had to be said as part of the test procedure. Despite herself, she felt a twinge of anxiety. It was all well and good to say these weren't tests they were taking, but they were enough like every other test she had taken to make her adrenalin flow.

At noon, they handed in their test booklets and took a break for lunch. When they reported back, it was to another room in the same building. It was not a classroom this time but a lounge. Steel-framed chairs and sofas covered in gray and orange plastic were set about the room, and the floor was covered with beige carpet, its industrial finish looking flat and somewhat dirty.

A long table at the front was draped with white crepe paper, and pitchers of water surrounded by glasses were set at one end. At the opposite end, a red cafeteria tray with small paper cups was watched over by a woman Karen hadn't seen before.

The cups looked like the sort that are usually filled with nuts or hard candies. When Karen got close enough, she saw that each cup contained only what looked like a single cube of sugar.

That's what it tasted like when Karen got hers. Dr. Raphael lined up the ten subjects, and as each one reached the table, the woman handed over one of the cups.

"Let the cube dissolve in your mouth," Dr. Raphael told them. "Then have some water, if you like, but don't eat or drink anything else. Then you may just sit around in this room and talk to each other."

It was pretty disgusting, just eating plain sugar. But within twenty minutes, Karen knew that it wasn't just plain sugar. She was sitting on one of the sofas talking to another woman about an English group called the Beatles. The woman had never heard of them, and Karen spelled the name for her.

But as she started to spell it, she suddenly found it very hard to concentrate. She knew where she was and what she was doing, but the woman in front of her began to look strange. She seemed to be surrounded by a halo of brightly colored light. The features of her face lost their outlines and became twisted and distorted.

In a few minutes, Karen gave up trying to talk. Somewhere at the back of her mind, she felt fear and confusion. But what was happening to her wasn't unpleasant. It was interesting, really, and she surrendered herself to the fantastic images that seemed to take over her mind without her being able to control them.

Somewhere in that time, Karen fell asleep or at least she thought she did. She vaguely remembered one of Dr. Raphael's assistants holding her by the arm and leading her back to the classroom. She tried to talk to him, but she wasn't sure what she said. When she was handed another test booklet, she was surprised to find how easy it was to fill out the answer sheet. This time there was no anxiety at all.

By five o'clock that afternoon, Karen was herself again. It was not until seventeen years later that she realized she had been an unwitting participant in a research project sponsored by the Army to determine psychological effects of LSD.

1. *What kind of information would Karen Barty have had to be given to satisfy Freedman's principles of informed consent?*

2. *On what grounds would Jonas disapprove of the way in which Karen was employed as a subject?*

3. *This was clearly a case of nontherapeutic research. Can a case be made for it on utilitarian grounds?*

4. *Does Karen have any grounds for claiming compensation if in years after the research she suffers from*

effects that may reasonably be attributed to her participation as a subject?

5. *Suppose that Dr. Raphael had fully informed the group about the nature and aims of the research and warned them about potential dangers. Given that very little was known in 1962 about the possible effects of LSD, would any person be justified in risking life or health by participating in the experiment?*

Decision Scenario 6 . . . .

"That is truly absurd," Dr. Kuhmwar Raita said. "The mother wanted to get rid of the fetus. That's why she elected to have the abortion in the first place. The fetus has no status. It's just a lump of tissue."

Dr. Allan Smith shook his head in disagreement. "It is not, Kuhmwar. That's just the point. The fetus is not viable, but it's out of the uterus and alive at this very instant."

"Well, it will be dead in a short while. Then it will be of no use to me. If I'm going to find out anything about cerebral glucose uptake, I've got to have a functioning system."

"But we can't just kill this child."

"The child, as you call it, is as good as dead. And if we can ever gain an understanding of the fundamental processes involved here, we may

actually be able to save the lives of countless babies."

"I can't believe you would resort to such a crude argument."

"Call it whatever you want to, but I think it's right."

1. *Is it possible to construct a utilitarian argument to support the position taken by Dr. Raita?*

2. *In what way is the status of the fetus relevant to this issue of fetal experimentation?*

3. *Are the issues of fetal experimentation exactly analogous to the arguments about abortion? Or are they more closely analogous to the arguments about human experimentation?*

4. *What view might a Kantian take on this question?*

Decision Scenario 7 . . . .

In April of 1979, a suit was filed in Illinois by the Cook County Public Guardian against the Illinois Department of Mental Health. The suit alleged that during the 1950s and 1960s between 25 and 100 patients underwent "unauthorized and secret" surgery at a state mental health center.

The suit charged that the patients, without their consent, were subjected to experimental surgery to remove their adrenal glands. A memo from a psychiatrist was cited that described the health center as "virtually a human dog lab."

A spokesman for the mental health department publicly denied the charges in the suit. He claimed that an internal investigation showed that consent from the patients had been obtained and each had

been informed of the possible risks and of the short- and long-term effects.

Moreover, the surgery was said to have a therapeutic aim, as well as an experimental one. A theory at the time suggested that the removal of the adrenal gland might correct a hormonal imbalance that some research psychiatrists believed to be a cause of schizophrenia. Furthermore, it was claimed that only four schizophrenic patients were involved.

As a matter of fact, the surgery did not lead to improvement in any of the patients, and the theory suggesting that it might is no longer held. Those who had their adrenal glands removed required injections of cortisone for the rest of their lives to compensate for the loss of natural secretions from the gland.

1. *Suppose that the charge made by the Public Guardian is correct. What utilitarian argument might be offered to support the use of mental patients as subjects in the experimental surgery?*

2. *Clearly the only proper candidates for an experimental procedure aimed at treating schizophrenia are people who are schizophrenics. Is it reasonable to believe that people who suffer from psychosis are capable of giving informed consent?*

3. *On Freedman's view, would proxy consent obtained for such people be legitimate?*

4. *Is it possible to argue that the principle of autonomy requires that patients diagnosed as psychotic ought to be allowed to consent to any procedure that may help their condition? If not, why not?*

5. *How relevant to the moral issue of consent is the nonmoral question of the degree of confirmation of a theory that is the basis of an experimental procedure with a therapeutic aim?*

Decision Scenario 8 ·

At six A.M. on Wednesday, March 6, 1985, Dr. Kevin Cheng of Phoenix got a call from cardiac surgeon Dr. Cecil Vaughn. "Is your heart ready to be implanted?" Dr. Vaughn asked.

Dr. Cheng thought the question was about implanting the artificial heart he had invented into a calf, an experiment he and Dr. Vaughn had done once before and were planning to do again. When he learned that the intended recipient was a human, he hesitated. "Wait a minute," Dr. Cheng said. "It's designed for a calf and not ready for a human yet."

"Think about it, decide, and I'll call back in ten minutes," Dr. Vaughn told him.

The heart was needed because Thomas Creighton, a thirty-three-year-old automobile mechanic and divorced father of two, had rejected the heart he had received from an accident victim. Dr. Jack Copeland and the transplant team at University Medical Center in Tucson immediately began a search for another donor heart, and Mr. Creighton was placed on the heart–lung machine. Dr. Copeland had also called Utah and requested that the Jarvik-7 heart be flown in.

"I knelt and prayed," Dr. Cheng recalled later. When Dr. Vaughn called him back, he said "The pump is sterile and ready to go."

Around noon of the same day, Dr. Vaughn implanted the device in Mr. Creighton. Mr. Creighton's physicians had decided that it would be dangerous to leave him on the heart–lung machine any longer, and the Jarvik-7 heart had not yet arrived. The Phoenix heart maintained Mr. Creighton's circulation until a donor heart was located.

At eleven that night, the device was turned off, and Mr. Creighton was put back on the heart–lung machine. At three A.M. on Thursday, Dr. Copeland transplanted the second donor heart. However, despite all efforts, Mr. Creighton died the following day. The Phoenix heart had had nothing to do with causing his death.

However, in deciding to use the Phoenix heart, Dr. Vaughn and Dr. Copeland had apparently violated FDA regulations by employing a device that had not been approved for experimental use in humans. They and their defenders justified their action by claiming that their use of the device was an emergency measure. They were not performing an experiment with Mr. Creighton, but attempting to save his life. The only other option was just to let him die. "We had nothing to lose" by using the heart, Dr. Copeland said.

1. *Would the line of reasoning taken by Dr. Copeland lead to the conclusion that anything at all can be done to a patient, if it can be justified as an effort to save the patient's life?*

2. *What response can be given to the charge that Mr. Creighton's condition was not a true medical emergency, because transplant rejection is one of the anticipated risks of that kind of surgery?*

3. *Although Mr. Creighton gave consent to the original surgery, he was in no condition to give consent to the use of the artificial heart. (Consent was given by his mother and sister.) Because of the risks known to be associated with artificial hearts (strokes and consequent brain damage, for example), the fact that he*

consented to a heart transplant does not mean that he would have consented to even the temporary use of an artificial heart. As far as he knew, the matter would never arise. Does this mean that Mr. Creighton was illegitimately denied the opportunity to decide what sort of risks he was willing to take?

Decision Scenario 9 •

The first human heart was transplanted in 1967 in South Africa by Dr. Christiaan Barnard. However, this was not the first heart transplant on a human being. In January of 1964, Dr. James D. Hardy of the University of Mississippi transplanted a chimpanzee heart into Boyd Rush.

Boyd Rush was a deaf-mute who was brought to the University of Mississippi Medical Center unconscious and on the verge of dying. A stepsister, the only relative who could be located, signed a consent form permitting, if necessary, "the insertion of a suitable heart transplant." The form made no reference to the sort of heart that might be employed. Mr. Rush lived for two hours after the transplant.

Dr. Hardy justified his use of the chimpanzee heart on the ground that it was impossible to obtain a human heart. Also, he was encouraged to think the transplant might be successful because of the limited success obtained by Dr. Keith Reemtsma in transplanting chimpanzee kidneys into a man dying of glomerulonephritis. The kidney recipient lived for two months.

Dr. Leonard Bailey, the surgeon who trans-

planted the baboon heart into the child known as Baby Fae, expressed his view of Dr. Hardy in an interview: "He's an idol of mine because he followed through and did what he should have done . . . he took a gamble to try to save a human life."

1. Evaluate the quality of the consent that was secured for transplant surgery in this case.

2. Suppose that Mr. Rush's stepsister did know that it was possible that a chimpanzee heart might be used. Should anyone be permitted to give consent to such a transplant on behalf of someone else?

3. If the only way to save the life of Mr. Rush was to transplant a chimpanzee heart, was the surgery justified?

4. If the transplant could have been expected to postpone Mr. Rush's death for only a relatively short time, was the surgery justifiable?

5. Evaluate the criticism that Dr. Hardy was doing no more than performing a medical experiment in which Mr. Rush was the unknowing and unconsenting subject.

Decision Scenario 10 •

In 1988 cardiologist William O'Neill decided he would have to go to Germany to do a clinical test on a device to clean out clogged arteries. Several years previously, researchers at the Centers for Disease Control planned to test the effectiveness of giving vitamin supplements to pregnant women to prevent spina bifida in their children. The National Institute for Child Health and Development objected to the plan to withhold vitamins from the control group. The researchers found Chinese collaborators who arranged for the clinical studies to be done.

Some clinical researchers are of the opinion that such cases are widespread and increasing in number. In general, they claim, more and more often

researchers and drug companies are choosing to test medical devices, therapies, and drugs in foreign countries. As a result, some researchers fear that the American reputation for innovative, cutting-edge clinical research is being eroded. If the process continues, the United States will eventually lose its well-established and respected tradition of clinical research, and the trained researchers the tradition produces will disappear. Furthermore, Americans will no longer be able to count on being among the first to receive the most effective medical treatments.

Two reasons are frequently mentioned as causing this switch in testing to foreign countries. First, the Federal Drug Administration and other federal agencies require so many levels of approval and so much paperwork that efforts to mount clinical trials are discouraged. Second, overzealous advocates of patients' rights have both complicated the approval process and made it difficult to recruit test subjects. Speaking of informed-consent forms to test a new clot-dissolving drug used during a heart attack, one British researcher said "The American documents were three pages of legalistic junk. That's not the sort of thing you want to push under someone's nose as he's having a heart attack, terrified with chest pain, on morphine. You want to tell him about the trial, but you want to be humane." Furthermore, critics of testing have made people so suspicious of medical experimentation that they refuse to participate when asked. By contrast, patients in other countries are more trusting and give their consent more readily.

The situation has been encouraged by an FDA decision to accept data from some foreign trials. The aim of the policy change was to make effective drugs more quickly available in the United States, but a consequence has been to encourage researchers to avoid problems at home by going abroad.

1. *Do we have an obligation to make sure that clinical trials in other countries involve the free and informed consent of participants? How might a Kantian answer this question? Do we have a prima facie duty to protect research subjects everywhere?*

2. *Suppose that in a scientifically well-designed trial a drug to prevent strokes was found to be amazingly effective, but we learn that the trial was conducted in a Third-World country and that none of the patients in the study were aware of their status as experimental subjects. Should we refuse to use the drug until the same studies were repeated with subjects who were informed and consenting participants?*

3. *Is there a possibility that the FDA policy of accepting data from foreign studies will encourage the exploitation of people in countries with practices offering less protection to patients than those in the United States? If so, then should the FDA policy be reversed in order to discourage such exploitation?*

4. *Might a utilitarian find the reasons mentioned for shifting testing to foreign countries relevant grounds for weakening current laws designed to protect research subjects?*

Decision Scenario 11 •

During the two years he had worked for the Bioplus Foundation, Dennis Quade had been in many labs. Before he could renew the funding of a grant, he was required to make an on-site inspection of the facilities and review the work of the investigators. Now he was sitting in a small, chilly conference room about to watch a videotape of a phase of the work done at Carolyn Sing's lab.

Sing herself was sitting at the table with him, and she leaned forward and pushed the play button. "The experimental subjects we used are baboons," she told him. "We think they possess facial and cranial similarities sufficiently similar to humans to make them the best animal models."

Dennis nodded, then watched the monitor in complete silence. He was appalled by what he saw. An adult animal, apparently limp from anesthesia, was strapped to a stainless-steel table. Its head was fitted into a viselike device and several clamps tightened to hold it immobile. The upper-left side of the baboon's head had been shaved and the area painted with a faintly purple antiseptic solution. A

dark circle had been drawn in the center of the painted area.

The white-coated arms of an assistant appeared in the tight focus of the picture. The assistant was holding a device that looked like an oversized electric drill. A long, transparent plastic sleeve stuck out from the chuck-end of the device, and through it Dennis could see a round, stainless-steel plate. A calibrated dial was visible on the side of the device, but Dennis couldn't read the marks.

"That's an impact hammer," Dr. Sing said. "We thought at first we were going to be able to use one off the shelf, but we had to modify one. That's an item we didn't anticipate in our initial budget."

The assistant centered the plastic tube over the spot marked on the baboon's head and pulled the trigger of the impact hammer. The motion of the steel plate was too swift for Dennis to see, but he saw the results. The animal's body jerked in spasm, and a froth of blood, brain tissue, and bone fragments welled up from the purple spot.

Dennis Quade turned away from the monitor, unable to stand the images any longer.

"Through induced head trauma studies, we have been able to learn an enormous amount," Carolyn Sing said. "Not only do we know more about what happens to brain tissue during the first few minutes after trauma, but we've used that knowledge to develop some new management techniques that may save literally tens of thousands of people from permanent brain damage."

Dennis Quade nodded.

1. *Why would Tom Regan oppose such experiments? Suppose it is true that brain damage from head trauma may be reduced or eliminated in thousands of people. Would this make a difference to Regan's view?*

2. *If you knew that the information gained from the study described would prevent your child from suffering from brain damage, should this count in your decision about whether such an experiment is justifiable?*

3. *Is there any reason to suppose that a human life (of any sort) is worth more than an animal life (of any sort)? On what moral grounds, if any, might one object to using patients in a chronic vegetative state as experimental subjects in the study?*

4. *Would McCloskey find the experiment described morally justified? What features does the experiment have that might lead him to approve it? What principles does he ask that we consider in assessing the moral worth of the testing? What, in particular, does the duty to respect persons have to do with animal experiments?*

PART III

CONTROLS

CHAPTER 7

GENETICS:

INTERVENTION, CONTROL,

AND RESEARCH

CASE PRESENTATION
Huntington's Disease: The Search for a Marker

Huntington's disease (HD) is a particularly cruel and frightening genetic disorder. Those diagnosed as having the disease soon become aware of the facts that the disease is invariably fatal and that there is no effective treatment for it. What is more, each of their children has a 50% chance of developing the disease.

The disease typically makes its appearance between the ages of thirty-five and forty-five in men and women who have shown no previous symptoms. The signs of its onset may be quite subtle—a certain clumsiness in performing small tasks, a slight slurring of speech, a few facial twitches. But the disease is progressive. Eventually the small, subtle signs develop into massive physical and mental changes. Walking becomes jerky and unsteady, the face contorts into wild grimaces, the hands repeatedly clench and relax, and the whole body writhes with involuntary muscle spasms. The victim eventually loses the power of speech, becomes disoriented, and gives way to irrational emotional outbursts. Before mental deterioration becomes too advanced, HD victims often kill themselves out of sheer hopelessness and despair. Death may occur naturally from fifteen to twenty years after the beginning of the symptoms. Usually it results from

massive infection and malnutrition, for, as the disease progresses, the victim loses the ability to swallow normally.

In the United States, at any given time, some 20,000 people are diagnosed as having the disease. It has been estimated that as many as 100,000 more may have the gene responsible for the disease. The incidence of the disease is only 1 in 10,000, but for the child of a victim of the disease the chances are 1 out of 2.

The disease is transmitted from generation to generation in a hereditary pattern that indicates that it is caused by a single gene. However, since the disease makes its appearance relatively late in life, an unsuspecting victim may already have passed on the gene to a child before he or she shows any sign of the disease. In the absence of a genetic test to detect the presence of the gene, there is no way for an individual to know whether he or she is a carrier of the gene.

In 1983 a major step toward the development of a genetic test for determining the presence of the HD gene was announced by Dr. James F. Gusella and his group at Massachusetts General Hospital. The team did not locate the gene itself, but a "genetic marker" that appears to indicate that it is present.

403

The group began by studying the DNA taken from members of a large American family with a history of Huntington's disease. They then employed recombinant-DNA techniques to attempt to locate a genetic marker for the HD gene. The techniques involve using a group of proteins known as restriction enzymes. A particular enzyme, when mixed with a single strand of DNA, cuts the strand at specific locations known as recognition sites. After the DNA strand has been cut up by restriction enzymes, short sections of radioactive, single-stranded DNA are added to serve as probes. The probes bind to particular segments of the DNA. Because the probes are radioactive, the segments of DNA to which they are attached can be identified on photographic film.

The number and location of recognition sites vary among individuals and appear to be inherited. The various fragments of DNA produced by the restriction enzymes and identified by probes form a pattern that is typical of individuals. A mutation of a normal gene may change the point at which an enzyme makes a cut. This produces a DNA fragment that is not the usual length and alters the pattern of that person. Thus, if the pattern of someone who does not have the disease is compared with the pattern of a family member who does, the fragments that include the faulty gene can be identified, even though the gene itself is unknown. The abnormal pattern serves as a *marker* for the presence of the gene.

Dr. Gusella's group faced the problem of attempting to find a marker that was consistently inherited by those with Huntington's disease but not inherited by those free of the disease. This meant identifying perhaps as many as 800 markers and determining whether one could serve as the marker for the HD gene. Fortunately, after only eleven attempts the team identified a good candidate. It was a marker found in all members of the family they were studying. All those with the disease had the same form of the marker, and those free of the disease had some other form.

In collaboration with the Hereditary Disease Foundation, plans were made to test this finding in a larger population. It was known that a large family with a high incidence of HD lived along the shores of Lake Maracaibo in Venezuela. Nancy Wexler led a team to this remote location to collect the family history and to obtain blood and skin samples for analysis. The lake-dwelling family included some 100 people with the disease and 1,100 children with the risk of developing it.

Analysis of the samples showed that those with the disease also carried the same form of the marker as their American counterparts. Gusella estimated that the odds are 100 million to 1 that the marker is linked to the HD gene. Subsequent work by Susan Naylor located the marker on chromosome number four. The gene itself still has not been identified, and it is still not known whether the gene is located on chromosome four of all who carry the HD gene. Also, the mechanisms through which the gene acts to cause the disease are not yet known.

A standard genetic test for the presence of the HD marker has yet to be developed. It is reasonably certain that one will be soon. The current test is elaborate and expensive and can be used only with those who have large enough families to detect a linkage with the marker. The identification of the gene should permit a blood test and the use of a DNA probe to search for the presence of the gene.

A study conducted in Wales in the 1970s revealed that more than half of those whose parents or relatives were victims of Huntington's disease would not want to have a test that would tell them whether they had the HD gene, even if such a test were available. Considering that the disease is virtually untreatable and invariably fatal, this is perhaps not a surprising finding. It is difficult to imagine the dread and horror that would be suffered by someone who knows that eventually the disease will announce itself and who must wait for that moment.

But what about obligations to others? If a test is available, is it fair to a potential marriage partner to marry without finding out whether one is a carrier of the HD gene and informing the potential partner of the result? Perhaps he or she may be willing to take the chance that the offspring of an HD victim will not have the disease. Yet, because of the tremendous burden the disease places on the other spouse, the possibility of being tested for the presence of the gene deserves serious consideration.

The decision about whether to have children might also be affected by the knowledge that, because one partner is a carrier of the HD gene, there is a 50% chance any child will also inherit the gene and develop the disease. Should a potential carrier of the gene impose the risk of having a child who will inherit the disease on the other partner? Should such a risk be imposed on a potential child? A genetic test could determine whether there is any risk at all. If the risk is present, then the couple could at least make a decision with a knowledge of the relevant facts.

The present test can also be used in conjunction with amniocentesis to determine whether a developing fetus has the marker for the HD gene, and any subsequent test will also have this capability. Possessing such information adds a particular difficulty to making an abortion decision, for those who do not oppose abortion in principle. A child born with the HD gene will inevitably develop the disease but may not do so for three, four, or even five or more decades. Is the fact that the child will eventually succumb to the disease reason enough to make an abortion morally obligatory?

The development of a standard, inexpensive test for the HD gene is sure to raise other moral and social issues as well. For example, it is possible that insurance companies may refuse to provide life or health insurance to those from families with Huntington's disease, unless they prove that they are not carriers of the gene. Employers may refuse to provide health benefits to family members unless they are tested and found to lack the gene.

Informing someone that he or she carries the marker or the gene also has problems associated with it. Such news can be devastating, both to the person and to the person's family. About 10–12% of HD victims kill themselves, and 30% of those at risk say that this is what they will do if they learn they have the disease. Thus, the mere act of conveying the information that someone will later develop the signs of a fatal disease can itself constitute a threat to life.

In the best of all worlds, an effective means of avoiding or treating the disease would be available. Then the moral and social issues associated with a genetic test for it would disappear without having to be resolved. Regrettably, that world still lies in the future.

CASE PRESENTATION
Gene Therapy

In 1980 Dr. Martin J. Cline of UCLA treated two patients suffering from an incurable blood disorder called beta-zero thalassemia with an entirely new therapeutic technique. The disease is one in which the gene for beta globulin, one of the constituents of the hemoglobin in red blood cells, is either missing or unexpressed. Those with the disease usually die very early, and frequently they suffer from anemia, cirrhosis of the liver, and serious heart problems because of the inability of their blood to transport sufficient oxygen to their tissues.

The aim of Dr. Cline's treatment was to provide the patients with the gene required to produce normal hemoglobin. The technique he employed, called *transformation*, is one that had been developed through research with animals. The basic idea behind the technique is simple.

Copies of a normal gene are inserted into the cells of a patient who lacks the gene or who possesses it only in a malfunctioning form. The DNA of the cells is induced to incorporate the new gene so that, when the cells reproduce themselves, copies of the new gene are made along with copies of the other genes encoded by the cellular DNA. In this way, the patient acquires a population of normal cells. The problem that was caused by the missing or defective gene is thus corrected. The technique as applied by Cline in this particular situation depended on the chemical properties of DNA and on the fact that cells take in calcium from their environment. Under proper conditions, the cells will take up DNA fragments, which include new genes, along with the calcium. Cells in the bone marrow (stem cells) are among those responsible for the production of red blood cells. Accordingly, Cline and his associates took bone marrow from the patients and added the appropriate DNA segments to a cell culture of that material. The hope was that the DNA would be incorporated into the genetic code of the cells—that the cells would be transformed. Afterward, the treated cells would then multiply, and their copies would include the new genes. The patients would thus be supplied with the cells necessary to produce beta globulin.

The plan was not successful. Transformation is a very ineffective process, and very few cells in a culture actually incorporate the foreign DNA. Perhaps the material injected into the patients did not contain enough transformed cells to make a difference. Or perhaps the transformed cells did not multiply sufficiently or otherwise perform as expected. In any case, the patients were not helped by the attempt at therapy, although there was no indication they were harmed, either.

Cline was reprimanded by the National Institutes of Health for engaging in medical experiments without securing the approval of the appropriate UCLA committees. In his own view, the experiments were both scientifically and morally justifiable.

The techniques developed in recombinant-DNA research are crucial to the procedures of gene therapy. It must be possible to identify the defective gene and manipulate the cell's DNA so that a new DNA segment containing a functioning gene is included in it. What is more, these tasks must be accomplished without damaging the cell or destroying its ability to reproduce normally. Although Cline made use of transformation as a technique, the more common technique in animal research is to employ a genetically engineered retrovirus to introduce the new gene into the cellular DNA. Unmodified retroviruses frequently cause diseases in humans, such as AIDS and certain forms of cancer. Consequently, one of the aims of recent gene-therapy research has been to modify retroviruses so that they will insert a desired gene into the DNA of a human cell but will not cause a dangerous infection. (See the Introduction for more information about recombinant DNA.)

In June 1990, W. French Anderson and R. Michael Blaese received approval from the National Institutes of Health Institutional Biosafety Committee to employ recombinant-DNA methods to treat children suffering from a deficiency of the enzyme adenosine deaminase (ADA).

The lack of the ADA enzyme leads to a destruction of special white blood cells known as T-cells and B-cells in the immune system. As a consequence, those with the disease die of massive infections early in life. The disease is rare, affecting only about twenty people at any time. (The "Bubble Boy" who lived for years in a sealed sterile environment in Houston had the disease. He died when a bone marrow transplant failed to help his dysfunctional immune system.)

On September 14, 1990, Anderson and his colleagues performed the first authorized therapeutic procedure employing genetically altered human cells—the first gene therapy. The patient was a four-year-old girl suffering from ADA.

The treatment involved taking blood from the patient, isolating the T-cells, then growing a massive number of them. These cells were then infected with a weakened retrovirus into which a copy of the human gene for ADA had been spliced. The cells were then injected into the patient in a blood transfusion.

If everything works, the ADA gene will migrate to the cellular DNA, switch on, and begin producing ADA. If the cells can produce enough of the enzyme, the child's immune system will not be destroyed. Because most T-cells live for only weeks or months, the process will have to be repeated at regular intervals. The hope is eventually to identify T-cells that will last for years.

The promise that gene therapy holds for those who suffer from a variety of genetic disorders is enormous. In the view of most researchers, the first diseases to receive attention should be those like ADA that both are life threatening and hold out the possibility of successful treatment. Prime candidates meeting these criteria are deficiency diseases in which a crucial enzyme is missing because of a single defective gene. Like ADA, most of these diseases are invariably fatal and caused by the lack of a single effective gene. Replacing the gene in a patient's cells would allow the cells to produce the missing enzyme. In principle, people suffering from such diseases could be completely cured by genetic modification.

In the future, it may be possible to treat such relatively common diseases as cystic fibrosis, hemophilia, phenylketonuria, and sickle-cell anemia by gene therapy. Current strategy is to concentrate on diseases with causes that are comparatively simple. Initial success seems certain to spur research to make it possible to treat more complicated diseases, including genetic disorders that are the result of more than one malfunctioning gene.

Paralleling the development of gene therapy are other treatment strategies also based on the technology of recombinant DNA. One of the most promising is the use of drugs to alter the function of genes that are not behaving normally. The drugs in effect "turn on" a malfunctioning gene so that it plays the role it is supposed to. Some promising results in the treatment of thalassemia and sickle-cell anemia have been reported.

Another technique involves transplanting cells into the brain, and it has been used experimentally in the treatment of Parkinson's disease. (See Chapter 8 for a fuller discussion.) The disease appears to result from the destruction of brain cells in the substantia nigra and the consequent reduction in dopamine production. Dopamine is a neurotransmitter involved in the movement of voluntary muscles. Its absence results in loss of control and shaky, involuntary movements. Researchers in Sweden in 1990 reported success in transplanting cells from fetal tissue into the substantia nigra of the brain. Other recent work also supports the idea that transplant therapy for diseases such as Parkinson's and Alzheimer's will be effective in the not-too-distant future.

The gene therapy in humans that is currently under development is somatic-cell therapy. That is, the modifications are in the body cells of patients, not in the sex cells. This means that, even if the therapy can eliminate the disease produced in an individual who has inherited a defective gene, the therapy will do nothing to alter the probability that a child of that person will inherit the same defective gene. To change this circumstance, so-called germ-line cells would have to be altered. That is, the defective gene in an ovum or sperm cell would have to be replaced.

If this were possible, then certain genetic diseases could be eliminated from families. Germ-line therapy would make it unnecessary to perform somatic-cell therapy for each generation of affected individuals. As appealing as this prospect is, at the present germ-line therapy has many more technical difficulties associated with it than does somatic-cell therapy. Uniformly encouraging results have not so far been produced in animal research, and somatic-cell therapy in humans remains a distant prospect.

Most of the moral issues discussed in connection with gene therapy have centered around germ-line therapy. It holds out the prospect of genetically engineering sex cells to produce offspring with virtually any set of characteristics desired. This possibility has led many critics to warn that "genetic surgery" may be leading us into a sort of Brave New World in which we practice eugenics and manufacture our children to order. (See the Introduction for a fuller discussion.) However, any dangers posed by germ-line therapy are far from immediate.

Somatic-cell therapy in humans is likely to become an established form of treatment within the next two to five years. It will for some time remain an experimental treatment, and as such it raises the same sorts of moral questions typical of any experimental procedure—ones of informed consent, benefit, and risk.

INTRODUCTION

The two great triumphs of nineteenth-century biology were Darwin's formulation of the theory of organic evolution and Mendel's statement of the laws of transmission genetics. One of the twentieth century's outstanding accomplishments has been the development of an understanding of the molecular structures and processes that are involved in genetic inheritance. All three great achievements give rise to moral and social issues of considerable complexity. The theories are abstract, but the problems they generate are concrete and immediate.

Major problems are associated with our increased knowledge of inheritance and genetic change. One class of problems concerns the use we make of the knowledge we possess in dealing with individuals. We know a great deal about the ways in which genetic diseases are transmitted and about the sorts of errors that can occur in human development. We have the means to make reliable predictions about the chances of the occurrence of a disease in a particular case, and we have the medical technology to detect some disorders before birth.

To what extent should we employ this knowledge? One possibility is that we might use it to detect, treat, or prevent genetic disorders. Thus, we might require that everyone submit to screening and counseling before having children. Or we might require that children be tested either prenatally or immediately after birth. We might recommend or require selective abortions. In this way, it might be possible to bring many genetic diseases under control in much the same way that we have brought contagious diseases under control.

Requiring screening and testing suggests another possibility, one that involves taking a broader view of human genetics. Eliminating genetic disease might simply become part of a much more ambitious plan for deliberately improving the entire species. Shall we attempt to control human evolution by formulating policies and practices designed to alter the genetic composition of the human population? Shall we make use of "gene surgery" and recombinant-DNA technology to shape physical and mental attributes of our species? That is, shall we practice some form of eugenics?

Another class of problems has to do with the wider social and environmental consequences of genetic research and technology. Research in molecular genetics that is concerned with recombinant DNA has already revealed to us ways in which the machinery of cells can be altered in beneficial ways. We are able to make bacteria synthesize such important biological products as human insulin, and we are able to alter bacteria to serve as vaccines against some diseases. In effect, recombinant-DNA technology produces life forms that have never existed before. Should biotech industries be allowed to patent such forms, in exactly the same way as new inventions are patented? Or do organisms belong to us all?

Also, what are we to say about the deliberate release of genetically altered organisms into the environment? Is the threat that such organisms pose greater than the benefits they are likely to produce? We have already witnessed the great damage that can be done by pesticides and chemical pollution. Is there any way that we can avoid the potential damage that might be caused by genetically engineered organisms?

In the following three sections, we shall focus attention on the issues that are raised by the actual and potential use of genetic information. Our topics are these: genetic intervention (screening, counseling, and prenatal diagnosis), eugenics, and genetic research (therapy, technology, and biohazards).

GENETIC INTERVENTION: SCREENING, COUNSELING, AND DIAGNOSIS

Our genes play a major role in making us what we are. Biological programs of genetic information work amazingly well to produce normal, healthy individuals. But sometimes things can go wrong, and when they do, the results can be tragic.

Almost 2,000 human diseases have been identified as involving genetic factors. Some of the diseases are quite rare, whereas others are relatively common. Some are invariably fatal, whereas others are comparatively minor. Some respond well to treatment, whereas others do not.

The use of genetic information in predicting and diagnosing diseases has significantly increased during the last two decades. New scientific information, new medical techniques, and new social programs have all contributed to this increase.

Three approaches in particular have been adopted by the medical community as means of acquiring and employing genetic information related to diseases: genetic screening, genetic counseling, and prenatal genetic diagnosis. Each approach has been the source of significant ethical and social issues, but before examining the approaches and the problems they present, we need to consider what is usually meant in talking about genetic disease.

Genetic Disease

The concept of a "genetic" disease is far from being clear. Generally speaking, a genetic disease is one in which genes or the ways in which they are expressed are causally responsible for particular biochemical, cellular, or physiological defects. Rather than rely upon such a general definition, it is more useful for the purpose of understanding genetic diagnosis to consider some of the ways in which genes may play a role in producing diseases.

Gene Defects.   The program of information that is coded into DNA (the genetic material) may in some way be abnormal because of the occurrence of a mutation at some time or other. (That is, a particular gene may have been lost or damaged, or a new gene added.) Consequently, when the DNA blueprint is "read" and its instructions followed, the child that develops will have defects.

For example, a number of diseases (such as PKU and Tauri's disease) are the result of so-called "inborn errors of metabolism." The diseases are produced by the lack of a particular enzyme necessary for ordinary metabolic functioning. In each case, the genetic information required in coding for the production of the enzyme is simply not present. The gene for the enzyme is missing.

A missing or defective gene may be due to a new mutation, but more often the condition has been inherited. It has been transmitted to the offspring through the genetic material contributed by its parents. Because defective genes can be passed on in this way, the diseases that they produce are themselves described as heritable. (Thus, PKU is a genetically transmissible disease.) The diseases follow regular patterns through generations, and tracing out those patterns has been one of the great accomplishments of modern biology and medicine.

Developmental Defects.   The biological development of a human being from a fertilized egg to a newborn child is an immensely complicated process. It involves an interplay between both genetic and environmental factors, and the possibility of the occurrence of errors is quite real.

Mistakes that result as part of the developmental process are ordinarily called "congenital." Such defects are not in the original blueprint (genes) but result either from genetic damage or from the reading of the blueprint. When either happens, the manufacture and assembly of materials required for normal fetal development are affected.

Radiation, drugs, chemicals, and nutritional deficiencies can all cause changes in an otherwise normal process. Also, biological disease agents, such as certain viruses, may intervene in development. They may alter the machinery of the cells, interfere with the formation of tissues, and defeat the carefully programmed processes that lead to a normal child.

Finally, factors internal to fetal development may also alter the process and lead to defects. The most common form of Down's syndrome, for example, is known to be caused by a failure of chromosomes to separate normally. (However, the cause of this failure is at present unknown.) The result is a child that has failed to develop properly and displays physical anomalies and some degree of mental retardation.

Defects that occur during the developmental process are not themselves the results of inheritance, and they cannot be passed on to the next generation.

Genetic Carriers.   Some diseases are produced only when an individual inherits both genes (alleles) for the disease from his or her parents. The parents themselves possess only one gene for the disease and generally show none of its symptoms. However, sometimes a parent may have symptoms of the same kind as are associated with the disease, although to a much lesser degree of severity.

In the metabolic disease PKU, for example, individuals who have inherited only one of the genes (that is, the offspring are heterozygous, rather than homozygous) may show a greater-than-normal level of phenylalanine in their blood. Such people are somewhat deficient in the enzyme required to metabolize this substance. The level of the substance may not be high enough to have caused any damage to them. Yet they are the carriers of a gene that, when passed on with the same gene from the other parent, can cause the disease PKU in their offspring. (As we will see later, the same is also true for those who are carriers of sickle-cell trait.) The individual who receives both genes for PKU obviously has the disease, but what about the parents? Clearly, the point at which a condition becomes a disease is often a matter of degree.

Genetic Predisposition.   It has been suggested that virtually every disease involves a genetic component in some way or other. Whether or not this is true, there is good evidence that hypertension, heart disease, various forms of cancer, and differential responses to environmental agents (such as sunlight, molds, or chemical pollutants) run in families, and it has been established in a number of cases that the genetic makeup of particular individuals may predispose them to specific diseases.

At present, it is not generally possible to say just what genetic factor might be partly responsible for a particular disease, just what role it plays, or through what mechanism it expresses itself. It is important to keep in mind that predispositions are not themselves diseases. At best, they can be regarded only as causal conditions that, in conjunction with other conditions, can produce disease.

The action of genes in disease processes is much more complicated than we have been able to discuss here. Nevertheless, our general categories are adequate to allow us to talk about the use made of information in genetic diagnosis.

Genetic Screening

In 1962 Dr. Robert Guthrie of the State University of New York developed an automated procedure for testing the blood of newborn children for the disease PKU. Although a diagnostic test for PKU had been available since 1934, it was time consuming and labor intensive. The Guthrie test made it practical to diagnose a large number of infants at a relatively low price.

PKU (phenylketonuria) is a serious metabolic disorder. Infants affected are deficient in the enzyme phenylalanine hydroxylase. Since the enzyme is necessary to convert the amino acid phenylalanine into tyrosine, as part of the normal metabolic process, a deficiency of the enzyme leads to a high concentration of phenylalanine in the infant's blood. The almost invariable result is severe mental retardation.

However, if the high level of phenylalanine in an infant's blood is detected very early, the infant can be put on a diet that is very low in that particular amino acid. Keeping children on the diet until they are around the age of six significantly reduces the severity of the retardation that is otherwise inescapable.

The availability of the Guthrie test and the prospects of saving newborn children from irreparable damage encouraged state legislatures to pass mandatory screening laws. Massachusetts passed the first such law in 1963, and by 1967 similar legislation had been adopted by forty-one states.

The term "genetic screening" is sometimes used to refer to any activity having to do with locating or advising people with genetically connected diseases. In our discussion, we will restrict the term's application and use it to refer only to public health programs that survey or test target populations with the aim of detecting individuals who are at risk of disease for genetic reasons.

The Massachusetts PKU law pointed the way for the development of public screening programs. PKU was the first disease tested for, but before long others were added to the list. For example, New York state law requires that an infant be tested for seven diseases. A number of public health programs now screen particular populations for such conditions as sickle-cell anemia, sickle-cell trait, metabolic disorders, hypothyroidism, and chromosome anomalies.

Although genetic screening is relatively new as a social program, the concept is historically connected with public health measures for the detection of communicable diseases like tuberculosis and syphilis. If an individual with such a disease is identified, then he or she can receive treatment. Furthermore, the diseased individual can be prevented from spreading the disease to other members of the population.

Similarly, it is possible to think of diseases with a genetic basis as resembling contagious diseases. Individuals are affected, and they can pass on the disease. But with genetic diseases the potential spread is not horizontal through the population, but vertical through the generations.

In terms of this model, public health measures similar to the ones that continue to be so effective in the control of contagious diseases might be used to help bring genetic diseases under control. When screening locates an individual with a genetic disorder, then steps can be taken to ensure that he or she receives appropriate therapy. Furthermore, when carriers of genes that produce diseases are identified, then they can be warned about their chances of having children that are genetically defective. Thus, at least a limited amount of control over the spread of genetic disease can be exercised, and the suffering of at least some individuals can be reduced or eliminated.

The justification of laws mandating screening programs can be sought in the power and responsibility of government to see to the welfare of its citizens. Here again, the public health measures employed to control contagion might be looked to as a model. We do not permit the parents of a child to decide on their own whether the child should be vaccinated against smallpox. We believe that the society, operating through its government, has a duty to protect the child. Similarly, it can be argued that the society owes it to the child with PKU to see to it that the condition is discovered as quickly as possible so that appropriate treatment can be instituted.

Critics of screening programs have not been convinced that the contagious-disease model is at all appropriate in dealing with genetic diseases. Because the way in which genetic diseases are spread is so different, only a very small part of the population can be said to suffer any risk at all. By contrast, an epidemic of smallpox may threaten millions of people. Furthermore, some genetic screening programs do not have follow-up or counseling services attached to them, so often nothing is done that benefits participants. By being told that they are the carriers of a genetic disease, people may be more harmed than helped by the programs.

In general, there are serious questions about whether the benefits of screening programs are sufficient to outweigh the liabilities. In particular, are screening programs so worthwhile that they justify the denial of individual choice entailed by required participation?

These issues and others related to them are easier to appreciate when they are considered in the context of particular kinds of screening programs. We will discuss briefly two programs that have been both important and controversial.

PKU Screening.   As we pointed out earlier, screening for PKU was the first mass testing program to be mandated by state laws. It is generally agreed that it has also been the most successful program.

PKU is a relatively rare disease. It accounts for only about 0.8% of mentally retarded people who are institutionalized, and among the infants screened during a year in a state like Massachusetts, only about three or four cases of PKU may be discovered. (The incidence is 5.4 per 100,000 infants.) Given this relatively low incidence of the disease, some critics have argued that the abrogation of the freedom of choice required by a mandatory program does not make the results worthwhile.

This is particularly true, they suggest, because of the difficulties with the testing procedure itself. The level of phenylalanine in the blood may fluctuate so that not all infants with a higher-than-normal level at the time of the test actually have PKU. If they are put on the restricted diet, then they may suffer consequences from the diet that are harmful to their health. Thus, in attempting to protect the health of some infants, a mandatory program may unintentionally injure the health of other infants.

Tests more refined than the Guthrie one are possible. However, their use increases considerably the cost of the screening program, even if they are employed only when the Guthrie test is positive for PKU. In social terms, then, the financial cost of preventing a few cases of PKU may be much greater than allowing the cases to remain undetected and untreated.

Furthermore, there are additional hidden social costs. Female infants who are successfully treated for PKU may grow into adults and have children of their own. Their children run a very high risk of being born with brain damage. The reason for this is not genetic but developmental. The uterine environment of PKU mothers is one high in phenylalanine, and in high concentrations it causes damage to the infant. Thus, one generation may be saved from mental retardation by screening only to cause mental retardation in the next.

Sickle-Cell.   Sickle-cell disease is a disorder of the hemoglobin in red blood cells. The cells assume a characteristic sickle shape and do not transport oxygen as well as normal red cells. They are also fragile and break apart more frequently. The result is anemia and, often, the blocking of blood vessels by fragments of ruptured cells.

The disease occurs only in those who have inherited both genes for the disease from their parents. (That is, the gene for the disease is recessive, and those who are homozygous for the gene are the ones who develop the disease.) Those with only one gene for the disease (that is, are heterozygous) are said to have sickle-cell trait.

Sickle-cell disease may develop at infancy, or it may manifest itself later in life in painful and debilitating symptoms. Those with sickle-cell trait rarely show any of the clinical symptoms.

In the United States, the disease is most common among African Americans and those of Mediterranean ancestry. The trait is carried by about 7-9% of the African American population, and the disease occurs in about 0.3% of the general population. Many people with the disease are not severely affected and can live relatively normal lives. However, the disease may also be fatal, and at present there is no adequate therapy for it. There is no cure, although there is now a means of diagnosing the disease prenatally.

In 1970 a relatively inexpensive and accurate test for sickle-cell hemoglobin was developed, making it possible to identify the carriers of sickle-cell trait. This technological development, combined with political pressures generated by rising consciousness in the African American population, was to lead to the passage of state laws mandating sickle-cell screening. During 1971 and 1972, twelve states enacted sickle-cell legislation.

The results were socially disastrous. Some laws required African Americans who applied for a marriage license to undergo screening. Since the only way to reduce the incidence of the disease is for two carriers to avoid having children, many African Americans charged that the mandatory screening laws were a manifestation of a plan for genocide.

Medical reports that carriers of sickle-cell trait sometimes suffered from the pain and disability of sickling crises came to serve as a new basis of discrimination. Some employers and insurance companies began to require tests of African American employees, and as a result some job possibilities were closed off to African Americans with sickle-cell trait.

In 1972, Congress passed the National Sickle-Cell Anemia Control Act. In order to qualify for federal grants under the act, states were required to make sickle-cell screening voluntary, provide genetic counseling, and take steps to protect the confidentiality of participants. The most significant impact of the act was to force states to modify their laws to bring them into conformity with the act's requirements. In response, the seventeen states with sickle-cell screening laws now require only voluntary programs.

The National Genetic Diseases Act, passed in 1976 and funded annually since then, provides testing and counseling for the diagnosis and treatment of a number of genetic diseases. The act further strengthens the commitment to voluntary participation and to guarantees of confidentiality.

The lesson learned from the public controversy over the first sickle-cell screening programs is that genetic information can be used in ways that are harmful to the interests of individuals. Furthermore, the information can be used as a basis for systematic discrimination.

Cystic Fibrosis

Cystic fibrosis is a disease affecting the lungs, pancreas, and sweat glands. Until recently, most individuals with the disease died as children. With intensive antibiotic therapy and proper care, many now live into their early twenties. It is the most common genetic disease in the United States. Affecting Caucasians almost exclusively, it occurs in 1 of every 2,500 births.

In 1989 Francis Collins and Lap-Chee Tsui, using the techniques of reverse genetics, succeeded in identifying the mutated gene responsible for cystic fibrosis. In reverse genetics, a gene is isolated and the protein it makes identified. Afterward, research is directed at discovering the role of the protein and whether it is involved in a disease process. The protein in cystic fibrosis appears to be involved in the movement of chloride and sodium across cell membranes in the pancreas and lungs. Cells that are faulty absorb an abnormal amount of water from their surroundings. This dries out

mucous secretions. In the pancreas, the dried mucus inhibits enzyme secretions and is responsible for digestive problems. In the lungs, the dried mucus makes the person more prone to bacterial infections. Repeated infections destroy the lung tissue.

One in every twenty-five white Americans is a carrier of the cystic fibrosis gene. Accordingly, there is a one-in-four chance that a child will have the disease. A recent test analyzing the DNA in a blood sample for the missing sequence responsible for the disease has been successful in identifying 76% of those who are carriers. (Researchers estimate that as many as half a dozen other mutated forms of the gene may also be responsible for the disease, and work is underway to try to identify them.)

The availability of a carrier test for cystic fibrosis opens the possibility of screening for the disease. A couple who are both carriers would have several options. If they wish to have their own biological child, they might have the fetus tested. Should the results show the presence of the disease, they would then have to decide about abortion. (To choose not to have an abortion would, of course, mean choosing to have a child, despite knowing that the child will have a serious disease.) They might choose artificial insemination with sperm from a donor who is not a carrier.

Cystic fibrosis is also seen as a disease that is potentially treatable by gene therapy. By using a viral carrier to transport normal copies of the gene for the missing protein to lung tissue, the gene might become incorporated into the proper chromosome. If the gene that then became activated produced normal protein in sufficient quantity, the respiratory symptoms of the disease might be brought under control.

Genetic Counseling

Much is known about the ways in which a number of genetic diseases are inherited. Ones like PKU, sickle-cell, and Tay-Sachs follow the laws of Mendelian transmission genetics. Accordingly, given the appropriate information, it is often possible to determine how likely it is that a particular couple will have a child with a certain disease.

Suppose, for example, that an African American couple is concerned about the possibility of having a child with sickle-cell disease. They will be tested to discover whether either or both of them are carriers of sickle-cell trait.

Sickle-cell disease occurs only when two recessive genes are both present—one inherited from the mother, one from the father. If only one of the parents is a carrier of the trait (is heterozygous), then no child will have the disease. However, if both parents are carriers of the trait, then the chances are one out of four that their child will have the disease. (This is determined simply by considering which combinations of the two genes belonging to each parent will produce a combination that is a homozygous recessive. The combination of Ss and Ss will produce ss in only 25% of the possible cases.)

Such information can be used to explain to potential parents the risks they might run in having children. But, as the case of sickle-cell disease illustrates quite well, it is often very difficult for individuals to know what to do with such information.

Is a 25% risk of having a child with sickle-cell disease sufficiently high that a couple ought to decide to have no children at all? Since the prenatal test for the disease is not easily available to everyone, this question is one that is best considered in advance of a pregnancy. If the couple is opposed to abortion, the question becomes especially crucial. Answering it is made more difficult by the fact that sickle-cell disease varies greatly in severity. A child with the disease may be virtually normal, or doomed to a short life filled with suffering. No one can say in advance of its birth which possibility is more likely.

It is generally agreed that the question of whether to have a child when a serious risk is involved is a decision that must be made by the couple. The counselor may provide informa-tion about the risk, and—just as important—the counselor may provide information about medical therapies that are available for a child born with a hereditary disease.

In diseases in which prenatal diagnosis is possible, the option of abortion may be open to potential parents. Here, too, the object of counseling is to see to it that the couple is educated in ways relevant to their needs.

Prenatal Genetic Diagnosis

A variety of new technological developments now make it possible to secure a great amount of information about the developing fetus while it is still in the uterus. Ultrasound, radiography, and fiber optics allow examination of soft-tissue and skeletal development. Anatomical abnormalities can be detected early enough to permit an abortion to be safely performed, if that is the decision of the woman carrying the fetus.

Yet the most common methods of prenatal diagnosis are amniocentesis and chorionic villus sampling (CVS), which involve direct cell studies. In amniocentesis, the amnion (the membrane surrounding the fetus) is punctured with a needle and some of the amniotic fluid removed for study. The procedure cannot be usefully performed until fourteen to sixteen weeks into the pregnancy. Until that time, there is an inadequate amount of fluid. The risk to the woman and to the fetus from the procedure is relatively small, usually less than 1%.

Chorionic villus sampling employs cells taken directly from the developing fetus. The advantage of the test is that it can be employed eight to ten weeks after conception, and a major study published in 1988 showed it to be virtually as safe as amniocentesis. A variant of CVS developed by J. D. Schulman involves using a vaginally inserted ultrasound probe. The probe is guided through the cervix and into the uterus. A needle on the end makes it possible to retrieve a tissue sample. Because the procedure can be performed as early as the sixth week of pregnancy, it is considered to offer a genuine advantage.

Amniocentesis came into wide use only in the early 1960s. At first, it was mostly restricted to testing fetuses in cases in which there was a risk of Rh incompatibility. When the mother lacks a group of blood proteins called the Rh (or Rhesus) factor, and the fetus has it, then the immune system of the mother may produce antibodies against the fetus. The result for the fetus may be anemia, brain damage, and even death.

It was soon realized that additional information about the fetus could be gained from further analysis of the amniotic fluid and the fetal cells in it. The fluid can be chemically assayed, and the cells can be grown in cultures for study. An examination of the chromosomes from the cells will show whether there are any known abnormalities that are likely to cause serious physical or mental defects. The presence or absence of the Y chromosome will also show the sex of the fetus. (Only males have a Y chromosome, so it is impossible to examine the chromosomes without discovering the sex of the fetus.)

A new test for Down's syndrome under development by Nicholas J. Wald in London employs a blood sample taken from the pregnant woman. The sample is examined for the presence of three fetal proteins. About sixteen to eighteen weeks after gestation, fetuses with the syndrome are known to produce abnormally small quantities of estriol and alpha fetoprotein and abnormally large amounts of chorionic gonadotropin. The levels of the proteins, plus such factors as the woman's age, can be used to determine the statistical probability of the syndrome.

Amniocentesis and CVS do have some hazard attached to them. Accordingly, neither is regarded as a routine procedure to be performed in every pregnancy. There must be some indication that the fetus is at risk from a genetic or developmental disorder.

One indication is the age of the mother. Down's syndrome is much more likely to occur in fetuses conceived in women over the age of thirty-five. Since the syndrome is produced by a chromosome abnormality, an examination of the chromosomes in the cells of the fetus can reveal the defect. (See the introduction to Chapter 2 for a fuller discussion.)

Genetic screening can also provide an indication of a need to perform amniocentesis. For example, Tay-Sachs disease is a metabolic disorder that occurs ten times as often among Jews originating in central and eastern Europe (the Ashkenazy) as in the general population. (The disease is invariably fatal and follows a sad course. An apparently normal child progressively develops blindness and brain damage, then dies at an early age.) Carriers of the Tay-Sachs gene can be identified by a blood test, and couples who are both carriers of the trait run a 25% risk of having a child with the disease. In such a case, there would be a good reason to perform amniocentesis.

Selective Abortion

In most cases in which prenatal diagnosis indicates that the fetus suffers from a genetic disorder or developmental defect, the only means of avoiding the birth of an impaired child is abortion.

Because those who go through the tests required to determine the condition of the fetus are concerned with having a child, abortion performed under such circumstances is called *selective*. That is, the woman decides to have an abortion to avoid producing a child with birth defects, not just to avoid having a child.

Those who oppose abortion in principle (see Chapter 1) also oppose selective abortion. In the view of some, the fact that a child will be born impaired is in no way a justification for terminating the life of the fetus.

Those who are prepared to endorse abortion at all typically approve of selective abortion as an acceptable way of avoiding suffering. In their view, it is better that the potential person that is the fetus not become an actual person, full of pain, disease, and disability.

At this time, there is some hope that the painful decision between having an abortion and giving birth to an impaired child may someday be avoided. For example, C. Thomas Caskey has been working on a procedure for screening ova to determine whether a woman heterozygous for a disease has produced an ovum that contains the abnormal allele. The technique involves examining the first polar body, a group of cells containing half the genetic material that is dropped off the ovum during cell division.

Repairs to the heart, the insertion of shunts to drain off excess brain fluids, and the placement of tubes to inflate collapsed lungs are some of the intrauterine surgical procedures now being performed. It is believed that it may be possible to expose the fetus within the uterus, perform surgery, then close up the amnion again. This would make possible more extensive surgery for a greater variety of conditions.

The present hope is that, as new surgical techniques for the treatment of fetuses are perfected and expanded, the need to rely on abortion to avoid the birth of defective children will significantly decline. Of course, surgery cannot, even in principle, provide a remedy for a large number of hereditary disorders. Surgery can do nothing for a child with Tay-Sachs disease or PKU.

Helplessness in this regard is matched by another hope. Perhaps in future years pharmaceutical and biochemical therapies will be available for cases involving missing enzymes. Or perhaps "gene surgery" will make it possible to insert the proper gene for manufacturing a needed biochemical into the DNA of the cells of a fetus.

Hopeful though we may be, the painful present reality is that, for most children born with genetic diseases or defects, very little can be done. Selective abortion continues to be the primary means to avoid the birth of a child known to be genetically impaired.

Difficulties with Genetic Intervention

Genetic screening, counseling, and prenatal diagnosis present bright possibilities for those who believe in the importance of exercising control through rational planning and decision making. The prospect of avoiding the birth of children with crippling impairments is seen by them as one of the triumphs of contemporary medicine.

Furthermore, the additional prospect of wholly eliminating some genetic diseases by counseling and control holds the promise of an even better future. For example, if people who are carriers of diseases caused by a dominant gene (such as Huntington's) produced no children with the disease, the disease would soon disappear entirely. The gene causing the disease would simply not be passed on to the next generation.

A vision of a world without the misery caused by genetic defects is a motivating factor among those who are strong advocates of programs of genetic intervention. (See the section on eugenics in this chapter for more details.) The vision must have its appeal to all who are moved by compassion in the face of suffering. Yet whether or not one shares this vision and is prepared to use it as a basis for social action, there are serious ethical questions about genetic intervention that must be faced.

We have already mentioned some of the issues in connection with particular programs and procedures. We can now add some more general questions to that list, but it should be kept in mind that our discussion cannot be complete. The moral and social issues connected with genetic intervention are woven into a complicated fabric of personal and social considerations. We can merely sketch the main outline of the pattern.

1. Is there a right to have children who are likely to be impaired? Suppose that a woman is informed, after an alphafetoprotein (AFP) test and amniocentesis, that the child she is carrying will be born with a neural tube defect.

Does she have the right to refuse an abortion and have the child anyway?

Those who are opposed to all abortion on the grounds of natural law would favor the woman's having the child. By contrast, a utilitarian might well argue that the decision would be wrong. The amount of suffering the potential child might be expected to undergo outweighs any parental loss. For different reasons, a Kantian might endorse this same point of view. Even if we assume the fetus is a person, a Kantian might argue that we are obliged to prevent its suffering. (For more details of these and similar arguments, see Chapters 1 and 2.)

Suppose we decide that a woman does have a right to have a child that is almost certain to be impaired. If so, then is the society obligated to bear the expense of caring for such a child? On the natural law view, the answer is almost certainly yes. The child, impaired or not, is a human person and, as such, is entitled to the support and protection of the society. If we agree that the impaired child is a person, then he or she is also a disadvantaged person. Thus, an argument based on Rawls's principles of justice would support the view that the child is entitled to social support. (Again, see Chapter 2 for more detail.)

2. Is society justified in requiring that people submit to genetic screening, counseling, and prenatal diagnosis? Children born with genetic diseases and defects require the expenditure of large amounts of public funds. Mandatory diagnosis need not be coupled with mandatory abortion or abstention from bearing children. (A related question is whether society ought to make available genetic testing to all who wish it, regardless of their ability to pay.)

On utilitarian grounds, it might be argued that society has a legitimate interest in seeing to it that, no matter what people ultimately decide, they should at least have the information about the likelihood that they will produce an impaired child.

If this view is adopted, then a number of specific medically related questions become relevant. For example, who should be screened? It is impractical and unnecessary to screen everyone. Why should we screen schoolchildren or prisoners, those who are sterile, or those past the age of childbearing?

This is closely connected with a second question: What should people be screened for? Should everyone be screened for Tay-Sachs disease, even though it is the Jewish population that is most at risk? Should everyone be screened for sickle-cell trait, even though it is primarily the African American population that is at risk?

Those who accept the contagious-disease model of genetic screening frequently defend it on the utilitarian grounds that screening promotes the general social welfare. However, one might argue that screening can also be justified on deontological grounds. It could be claimed that we owe it to developing fetuses, regarded as persons, to see to it that they receive the opportunity for the most effective treatment. For example, it might be said that we have an obligation to provide a PKU child with the immediate therapy required to save him or her from severe mental retardation. The restriction of the autonomy of individuals by requiring screening might be regarded as justified by this obligation. If screening is voluntary, then the welfare of the child is made to depend on ignorance and accidental opportunity.

3. Do physicians have an obligation to inform their patients who are prospective parents about the kinds of genetic tests that are available? A study of one population of women screened for Tay-Sachs disease showed that none had sought testing on the recommendation of her physician.

If the autonomy of the individual is to be preserved, then it seems clear that it is the duty of a physician to inform patients about genetic testing. A physician who disapproves of abortion might be reluctant to inform patients about tests that might encourage them to seek an abortion. Nevertheless, to the extent that abortion is a moral decision, it is a decision properly made by the individual, not by someone acting paternalistically in her behalf.

The duty of a physician to inform patients about the possibility of genetic tests seems quite straightforward. Yet the issue becomes more complicated in light of the next question about truth telling.

4. Do patients have a right to be informed of all of the results of a genetic test? Ethical theories that are based on respect for the autonomy of the individual (such as Kant's and Ross's) suggest that patients are entitled to know what has been learned from the tests.

But what if the test reveals that the fetus has only a quite minor genetically transmissible disease? Should the physician run the risk of the patient's deciding to have an abortion merely because she is committed to the ideal of a "perfect" baby? Is such a decision really one for the physician to make?

Furthermore, what about the matter of sex determination? Screening tests that involve chromosome examination also reveal the sex of the fetus. Are prospective parents entitled to know this information? When abortion is elective, it is quite possible for the woman to decide to have an abortion to avoid giving birth to a child of a particular sex.

It might be argued on both utilitarian and deontological grounds that the sex of the fetus is information that is not relevant to the health of the fetus. Accordingly, the physician is under no obligation to reveal the sex of the fetus. Indeed, the physician may be under an obligation *not* to reveal the sex of the fetus in order to avoid the possibility of its destruction for a basically trivial reason. But, again, is this really a decision for the physician?

5. Should public funds be used to pay for genetic tests when an individual is unable to pay? This is a question that holders of various ethical theories may not be prepared to answer in a simple yes-or-no fashion. Those who oppose abortion on natural law grounds might advocate providing funds only for genetic screening and counseling. That is, they might

favor providing prospective parents with information that they might then use to decide whether to refrain from having children. Yet opponents of abortion might be against spending public money on tests that might encourage the use of abortion to prevent the birth of a defective child.

The views of Rawls and of utilitarianism might well support the use of public funds for genetic testing as part of a more general program of providing for health-care needs. Whether genetic testing programs are funded and what the level of funding might be would then depend on judgments about their expected value in comparison with other health-care programs.

A present ethical and social difficulty is caused by the fact that federal funds may be employed to pay for genetic screening and testing, yet federal money cannot legally be used to pay for abortions. Consequently, it is possible for a woman to discover that she is carrying a fetus with a serious genetic disease, wish to have an abortion, yet lack the financial means to pay for it.

Issues about the confidentiality of test results, informed consent, the use of genetic testing to gather epidemiological information, and a variety of other matters might be mentioned here in connection with genetic intervention. Those that have been discussed are sufficient to indicate that the difficulties presented by genetic intervention are at least as numerous as the benefits it promises.

EUGENICS

Like other organisms, we are the products of millions of years of evolutionary development. This process has taken place through the operation of natural selection on randomly produced genetic mutations. Individual organisms are successful in an evolutionary sense when they contribute a number of genes to the gene pool of their species proportionately greater than the number contributed by others. Most often, this means that the evolutionarily successful individuals are those with the largest number of offspring. These are the individuals favored by natural selection. That is, they possess the genes for certain properties that are favored by existing environmental factors. (This favoring of properties is natural selection.) The genes of "favored" individuals will occur with greater frequency than the genes of others in the next generation. If the same environmental factors continue to operate, these genes will spread through the entire population.

Thanks to Darwin and the evolutionary biologists who have come after him, we now have a sound understanding of the evolutionary process and the mechanisms by which it operates. This understanding puts us in a position to intervene in the process. That is, we no longer have to consider ourselves subject to the blind working of natural selection. If we choose to do so, we can modify the course of human evolution. As the evolutionary biologist Theodosius Dobzhansky expressed the point: "Evolution need no longer be a destiny imposed from without; it may conceivably be controlled by man, in accordance with his wisdom and values."

Those who advocate eugenics accept just this point of view. They favor social policies and practices that, over time, offer the possibility of increasing the number of genes in the human population responsible for producing or improving traits (for example, intelligence) that we value.

The aim of increasing the number of favorable genes in the human population is called *positive eugenics*. By contrast, *negative eugenics* aims at decreasing the number of undesirable or harmful genes. Those who advocate negative eugenics are generally most interested in eliminating or reducing the number of those genes that are responsible for various kinds of birth defects and genetic diseases.

Both positive and negative eugenics require instituting some sort of control over human reproduction. Several kinds of policies and procedures have been advocated, and we will discuss a few of the possibilities.

Genetic Intervention

The discussion in the preceding section of genetic screening, counseling, and prenatal genetic diagnosis makes it unnecessary to repeat here information about the possibilities and procedures we currently possess for predicting and diagnosing genetic diseases. It is enough to recall that, given information about the genetic makeup and background of potential parents, a number of genetic diseases can be predicted with a certain degree of probability as likely to occur in a child of such parents. This is true of such diseases as PKU, sickle-cell anemia, hemophilia, Huntington's disease, and Tay-Sachs disease.

When genetic information is not adequate to serve as a basis for a reliable prediction, then information about the developing fetus can often be obtained by employing one of several procedures of prenatal diagnosis. Even when genetic information is adequate for a statistical prediction, whether the fetus has a certain disease can be determined by prenatal testing. Thus, in addition to the disorders named above, prenatal tests can be performed for such other defects as neural tube anomalies and Down's syndrome.

A proponent of negative eugenics might advocate that a screening process for all or some currently detectable genetic diseases be required by law. When the probability of the occurrence of a disease is high (whatever figure that might be taken to be), then the potential parents might be encouraged to have no children. Indeed, the law might *require* that such a couple abstain from having children and prescribe a penalty for going against the decision of the screening board. If those carrying the genes for some genetic diseases could be prevented from having children, then over time the incidence of the diseases in the population would decrease. In some cases when the disease is the result of a dominant gene (as it is in Huntington's disease), the disease would eventually disappear.

When the disease is a kind that can be detected only after a child is conceived, then if the results of a prenatal diagnosis show that the developing fetus has a heritable disease, an abortion might be encouraged. Short of a law requiring abortion, a variety of social policies might be adopted to make abortion an attractive option. (For example, the cost of an abortion might be paid for by government funds, or women choosing abortion might be financially rewarded.) The aborting of a fetus found to have a transmissible genetic disease would not only prevent the birth of an impaired infant, but it would also eliminate a potential carrier of the genes responsible for the disease.

Similarly, the sterilization of people identified as having genes that are responsible for certain kinds of physical or mental impairments would prevent them from passing on these defective genes. (See Chapter 8 for a discussion of sterilization.) In this way, the number of such genes in the population would be proportionately reduced.

Currently, there are no state or federal laws that make it a crime for couples who are genetically a bad risk to have children. Yet a tendency toward more genetic regulation may be developing. As we mentioned earlier, several states now require the screening of newborn infants in order to detect the presence of certain genetic diseases that respond well to early treatment. Also, genetic screening programs are frequently offered in communities to encourage people to seek information about particular diseases.

At present, genetic screening (for adults) and genetic counseling are voluntary. They aim at providing information and then leave reproductive decisions up to the individuals concerned. Most often, they are directed to-

ward the immediate goal of decreasing the number of children suffering from birth defects and genetic diseases. Yet genetic screening and counseling might also be viewed as a part of negative eugenics. To the extent that they discourage the birth of children carrying deleterious genes, they also discourage the spread of those genes in the human population.

Obviously, screening programs and genetic counseling might also be used to promote *positive* eugenics. Individuals possessing genes for traits that society values might be encouraged to have large numbers of children. In this way, genes for traits that are considered worthwhile would increase in relative frequency within the population.

There are no programs of positive eugenics. Yet it is easy to imagine a variety of social and economic incentives (for example, government bonuses) that might be introduced as part of a plan to promote the spread of certain genes by rewarding favored groups of people for having children.

Use of Desirable Germ Cells

Artificial insemination by the use of stored sperm is already a reality. The implantation of a donor ovum in the wall of the uterus is also possible, and we have developed a biotechnology that permits the long-term storage of ova. Thus, a man or woman might choose to have a child by selecting stored germ cells contributed by individuals possessing traits that they admire. Sperm banks and ova banks would then provide a way for the human population to improve itself—that is, to increase the number of genes for desirable traits in the population. (See Chapter 8.)

Difficulties with Eugenics

Critics have been quick to point out that the proposals we have discussed suffer from serious drawbacks. First, negative eugenics is not likely to make much of a change in the species as a whole. Most hereditary diseases are genetically recessive and so occur only when both parents possess the same defective gene. Even though a particular couple might be counseled (or required) not to have children, the gene will still be widespread in the population among people we would consider wholly normal. For a similar reason, sterilization would have few long-range effects. Also, there is the uncomfortable fact that geneticists have estimated that, on the average, everyone carries recessive genes for five genetic defects or diseases. Genetic counseling may help individuals, but negative eugenics does not promise much for the population as a whole.

Positive eugenics can promise little more. It is difficult to imagine that we would all agree on what traits we would like to see increased in the human species. But even if we could, it is not clear that we would be able to increase them in any simple way. For one thing, we have little understanding of the genetic basis of traits such as "intelligence," "honesty," "musical ability," and so on. It is clear, however, that there is not just a single gene for them, and the chances are that they are the result of a complicated interplay between genetic endowment and social and environmental factors. Consequently, the task of increasing their frequency is quite different from that of, say, increasing the frequency of short-horned cattle. Furthermore, the desirable traits may well be accompanied by less desirable traits, and we may not be able to increase the first without also increasing the second.

Quite apart from biological objections, eugenics also raises questions of a moral kind. Have we indeed become the "business manager of evolution," as Julian Huxley once claimed? If so, then do we have a responsibility to future generations to improve the human race? Would this responsibility justify our requiring genetic screening? Would it justify our establishing a program of positive eugenics? Affirmative answers to these questions may generate conflicts with notions of individual dignity and self-determination.

Of the ethical theories we have discussed, it seems likely that only utilitarianism might be construed as favoring a program of positive eugenics. The possibility of increasing the frequency of desirable traits in the human species might, in terms of the principle of utility, justify present restrictions on reproduction. It is not clear that this is so, however. The goal of an improved society or human race might well be regarded as too distant and uncertain to warrant the imposition of restrictions that would increase current human unhappiness.

As far as negative eugenics is concerned, the principle of utility could certainly be appealed to in order to justify social policies that would discourage or prohibit parents who are serious genetic risks from having children. The aim here need not be the remote one of improving the human population but the more immediate one of preventing the increase in sorrows and pains that would be caused by an impaired child.

Natural law doctrines of Roman Catholicism forbid abortion (see the introduction to Chapter 1 and the introductory chapter) and sterilization. Thus, these means of practicing negative eugenics are ruled out. Also, the natural law view that reproduction is a natural function of sexual intercourse seems, at least prima facie, to rule out negative eugenics as a deliberate policy altogether. It could be argued, however, that voluntary abstinence from sexual intercourse or some other acceptable form of birth control would be a legitimate means of practicing negative eugenics.

Ross's prima facie duty of causing no harm might be invoked to justify negative eugenics. If there is good reason to believe that a child is going to suffer from a genetic disease, then we may have a duty to prevent the child from being born. Similarly, Rawls's theory might permit a policy that would require the practice of some form of negative eugenics for the benefit of its immediate effects of preventing suffering and sparing all the cost of supporting those with genetic diseases.

It is difficult to determine what sort of answer to the question of negative eugenics might be offered in terms of Kant's ethical principles. Laws regulating conception or forced abortion or sterilization might well be considered to violate the dignity and autonomy of individuals. Yet moral agents as rational decision makers require information on which to base their decisions. Thus, programs of genetic screening and counseling might be considered to be legitimate.

GENETIC RESEARCH, THERAPY, AND TECHNOLOGY

By replacing natural selection with artificial selection that is directly under our control, we can, over time, alter the genetic composition of populations of organisms. This has been done for thousands of years by animal and plant breeders, and our improved understanding of genetics allows us to do it today with more effectiveness and certainty of results. Yet such alterations require long periods of time. Molecular genetics holds out the possibility of immediate changes. Bacteria continue to be the major organisms of research, but genetic technology is already being applied to plants and animals. The same technology is now on the verge of being applied to humans.

Recombinant DNA

The information required for genetic inheritance is coded in the two intertwined strands of DNA (deoxyribonucleic acid) found in plant and animal cells—the double helix. The strands are made up of four kinds of chemical units called nucleotides, and the genetic message is determined by the particular sequence of nucleotides. Three nucleotides in sequence form a triplet codon. Each codon directs the synthesis of a particular amino acid and determines the place that it will occupy in

making up a protein molecule. Since virtually all properties of organisms (enzymes, organs, eye color, and so on) depend on proteins, the processes directed by DNA are fundamental.

Alterations in the nucleotide sequence in DNA occur naturally as mutations—random changes introduced as "copying errors" when DNA replicates (reproduces) itself. These alterations result in changes in the properties of organisms since the properties are under the control of DNA. Much research in current molecular genetics is directed toward bringing about desired changes by deliberately manipulating the nucleotide sequences in DNA. The major steps toward this goal have involved the development of techniques for recombining DNA from different sources.

The recombinant process begins by taking proteins known as restriction enzymes from bacteria and mixing them with DNA that has been removed from cells. These enzymes cut open the DNA strands at particular nucleotide locations. DNA nucleotide sequences from another source can then be added, and certain of these will attach to the cut ends. Thus, DNA from distinct sources can be recombined to form a single molecule.

This recombinant DNA can then be made to enter a host cell. The organism almost universally employed as a host is the one-celled bacterium E. coli that inhabits the human intestine by the billions. In addition to the DNA that makes up the chromosome of the cell, E. coli also possesses small circular strands of DNA known as plasmids. The DNA of a plasmid can be recombined with the DNA of a foreign source and returned to the cell. There the plasmid will start replicating again. It will make copies of the original nucleotides *plus* copies of the added segments. Thus, a strain of bacteria can be produced that will make limitless numbers of copies of the foreign DNA.

The obvious question is, what benefits might this recombinant technique produce? It might lead to the understanding and control of the molecular processes involved in such diseases as cancer, diabetes, and hemophilia. It might provide more effective treatment for metabolic diseases like PKU and Tay-Sachs.

From the more commercial standpoint, recombinant-DNA technology might lead to the development of new breeds of plants that are able to utilize nitrogen from the air and thus require no fertilizer. Specially engineered bacteria might be used to clean up the environment by breaking down currently nonbiodegradable compounds like DDT and Agent Orange. Other bacteria might be used to convert petroleum into other useful chemical compounds, including plastics.

The most immediate benefits of recombinant DNA are likely to be the use of modified bacteria as chemical factories to produce biological materials of medical importance. In addition, the transplanting of human genes into nonhuman embryos promises to lead to an understanding of the ways in which genes can be made to reproduce themselves and be passed on to succeeding generations.

Just a glance at a few of the many recent research developments is enough to gain an appreciation of the powerful potential of genetic technology:

- Hypopituitary dwarfism is a condition caused by a deficiency in growth hormone. The hormone itself consists of molecules that are too large and structurally complex to synthesize in the laboratory. In 1979 researchers in California employed recombinant-DNA technology to induce bacteria to produce the hormone. It is now available in quantities large enough to be used in medical therapy.

- In 1982 Dr. John D. Baxter and his associates developed a bacterial strain capable of producing endorphin. Because endorphin is a natural opiate, the hope is that it can be used as an effective substitute for such addictive drugs as morphine.

- Modified bacteria now produce human insulin in quantities large enough to meet the need of diabetics who are allergic to swine or bovine insulin.

- Genetically engineered bacteria have also been used to produce a vaccine against hepatitis B and against a strain of genital herpes. The clotting factor employed in the treatment of hemophilia has been similarly produced.

- In 1985 the Cetus Corporation was awarded the first patent for an altered form of the protein interleukin-2. Il-2 activates the immune system and shows promise in the treatment of some forms of cancer. It occurs naturally but in very small amounts; thus, it was not possible to test its effectiveness until it was produced in quantity by genetically altered bacteria.

- Researchers have inserted human genes into plants and induced the plants to produce large quantities of medically significant proteins. Antibodies, serum albumin, enkephalins, hormones, and growth factors are among those currently produced.

- Substances occurring in the human body in minute amounts that can be important as drugs when available are now being produced in large quantities by genetic engineering. For example, tissue plasminogen activator, which is produced in blood vessels, dissolves blood clots and is a useful drug in the treatment of heart attacks. Also, blood factor-8, a clotting agent, may improve the lives and health of hemophiliacs by reducing their chances of viral infection from donated blood.

Gene Therapy

The rapid advancement in genetic knowledge during the last few years makes it seem likely to most experts that the use of recombinant-DNA techniques as part of a program of medical therapy is now virtually at hand. Therapy in which a needed gene is inserted has already been employed in an experimental way. (See the Case Presentation for more details.)

The ability to alter the basic machinery of life to correct its malfunctioning is surely the most powerful form of therapy imaginable. The immediate prospects for gene therapy are most likely to involve the relatively modest, but very dramatic, task of splicing into the DNA of body cells a gene that controls the production of a specific substance. Diseases such as PKU that are caused by the absence of a particular enzyme might then be corrected by inducing the patient's cells to manufacture that enzyme. Some genetic diseases involve dozens or even hundreds of genes, and often the mechanism by which the genes produce the disease is not understood. Consequently, it is likely to be a long while before most genetic diseases can be treated by gene therapy. However, the treatment of single-gene disorders is a most promising possibility.

Few special moral or social issues are raised by the use of gene therapy as long as the cells modified are somatic (body) cells. However, the issues change significantly with the prospect of modifying human germ-line (sex) cells. Somatic-cell changes cannot be inherited, but germ-line cell changes can be. This possibility holds out the benign prospect of eliminating forever a number of sex-linked diseases. However, it also points toward the more frightening outcome of "engineering" human beings to produce people who meet our predetermined specifications. We will discuss this possibility further below. Here it is relevant only to note that the technology that would be required to alter the sex cells of human beings does not exist at present.

The Human Genome Project

The 46 human chromosomes contain an estimated 100,000 genes. This complete set of genes is known as the human genome. Metaphorically, the genome is the blueprint for assembling a human being that is stored in the nuclius of each cell. At present, only about 1,400 genes have been located or "mapped" on the DNA strands, and only about 600 genes have been sequenced—that is, the precise order of their base pairs determined.

In 1985 Robert Sinsheimer began promoting the idea that the entire human genome should be mapped and its genes sequenced. Since the genome is believed to consist of some 3 billion base pairs, the genome project would be on a scale unprecedented in the biological sciences. It would compare with efforts of physical scientists to develop the atomic bomb during World War II and with the launching of the manned space project in the 1960s.

The size of the genome project made many bioscientists skeptical about supporting it. Many believed it would drain money away from smaller projects of immediate value in favor of one with only distant and uncertain value. Also, some feared the genome project would turn out to be too much like the space project and emphasize the solution to engineering problems more than the advancement of basic science.

Attitudes changed in 1988, when the National Research Council endorsed the genome project and outlined a gradual approach of coordinated research that would protect the interest of the basic sciences. When James Watson agreed to be director of the project, most critics dropped their opposition, and many became enthusiastic participants.

Mapping and sequencing the human genome is expected to take fifteen to twenty years and cost around $3-5 billion. In 1989 Congress approved $31 million to initiate the program. Eventually hundreds of scientists and scores of university, federal, and institute laboratories will be participating in the research and contributing to the final product.

The payoff of the genome project is considered to be of inestimable worth by its supporters. They claim that the information should provide us with a better understanding of the patterns and processes of human evolution and clarify our degree of genetic relatedness with other organisms. Further, the connections between genes and human behavior should become clearer. Most important, the detailed genetic information the project will supply may allow us to understand the relationships between certain genes and particular diseases. This information in turn may permit us to develop gene therapy to such a degree that genetic diseases can be wholly eliminated or their results effectively controlled.

Such technology is not yet available, any more than a complete map of the genome is available. Meanwhile, some thinkers worry that newly acquired understanding of parts of the human genome will permit genetic discrimination based on a new form of genetic screening.

Genetic Discrimination

The enzyme AHH (amyl hydrocarbon hydroxylase) acts to break down hydrocarbons in smoke and other industrial pollutants. About 10% of the population possesses variant forms of the genes that produce the enzyme, and their bodies produce it in an excessive amount. The excess enzyme reacts with hydrocarbons and turns them into carcinogenic substances. People with the variant genes are thus some twenty-six times more likely than others to get lung cancer from breathing air polluted with hydrocarbons.

This is just one example of the way in which genetic factors may predispose individuals to certain kinds of diseases. Researchers are well on the way to identifying an entire catalogue of such factors and their associated diseases. Such information offers the opportunity for individuals who are screened and found to be particularly susceptible to a certain environmental pollutant or manufacturing substance to avoid contact with that agent. For example, people who are prone to develop an acute form of anemia after exposure to naphthalene should avoid jobs in which that chemical is employed.

In principle, susceptible workers could be assigned to jobs that would allow them to avoid being exposed to the chemicals particularly harmful to them. With such an end in view, in 1982 some 59% of large companies surveyed indicated that they either had a genetic screening program or intended to institute one. Their motivation was partly based on economic self-interest, for the costs of damage suits and insurance premiums could be lowered by keeping susceptible workers out of danger.

By 1986 most plans to screen workers had been abandoned by corporations that had initially favored them. This was mostly in response to criticisms from civil-rights groups, women's organizations, and labor unions. The critics pointed out that the results of the genetic screening could be used to discriminate against the hiring of entire classes of workers. Because African Americans are more susceptible to environmentally induced anemia, they would be effectively shut out of jobs in which the risk to them is greater than to other workers. Similarly, because fetuses are likely to be affected by a number of chemicals used in manufacturing, pregnant women would not be hired for a wide variety of jobs. Indeed, the possibility that a woman might be or might become pregnant might result in the exclusion of women as a group.

As Morton Hunt points out, the possibility of genetic screening in connection with employment presents us with a number of dilemmas of a moral and social kind. We wish to promote equal opportunity for workers, yet we also wish to protect their health and safety. If those genetically predisposed to certain diseases are allowed to compete for jobs that place them at risk, then we are not seeing to their health and safety. Yet, if we see to their health, we are not allowing them equal opportunity. Similarly, we wish to promote individual freedom in the society, but at what point do we decide that an individual is taking an unacceptable risk? If we allow someone to risk her health, are we willing to bear the social cost associated with her falling ill?

A worker found to be susceptible to a common manufacturing chemical would be at a clear disadvantage in attempting to get a job and might claim that an employer who required him to take a screening test as a condition of employment was violating his right to privacy. Yet should employers be allowed no protection from the added costs of damage suits and higher insurance premiums caused by a higher rate of illness among susceptible workers?

Quite apart from the issues of employment, individuals who are screened for whatever reason and found to be at risk for the development of some genetically predisposed disease may find they can get only very expensive health insurance, if they can get it at all. Insurance companies, for their part, may decide to make genetic screening for probabilities of known disorders a condition of insurability. Are individuals entitled to keep such information about themselves private? Are insurers entitled to know what risk they are taking before insuring an applicant?

These are some of the difficulties that are raised by the new possibilities of screening for genetic predisposition to diseases. The promise of being able to prevent the occurrence of disease in many individuals is a genuine one, but we have yet to make an adequate effort to resolve the social and moral issues that fulfilling the promise presents. Until we resolve them, a powerful technology will remain unutilized.

Biohazards

The issues connected with gene therapy and screening may be overshadowed in significance by questions concerning dangers inherent in the development of genetic technology and in the release of its products into the natural environment.

The question of whether recombinant-DNA research ought to be halted is no longer a serious social issue. However, this has not always been so. In 1974 a group of scientists active in such research issued a report recommending that scientists be asked to suspend work voluntarily on recombinant experiments involving tumor viruses, increased drug resistance in harmful bacteria, and increased toxicity in bacteria. The discussion that ensued resulted in the formulation of guidelines by the National Institutes of Health to regulate research.

The major concern initially was that recombinant techniques might be employed to produce essentially new organisms that would threaten human health. Suppose that the nucleotide sequence for manufacturing a lethal toxin were combined with the DNA of *E. coli*. This currently harmless inhabitant of the intestine might be transformed into a deadly organism that would threaten the existence of the entire human population. Or perhaps a nucleotide sequence that transforms normal cells into cancerous ones might trigger an epidemic of cancer. Without a thorough knowledge of the molecular mechanisms involved, little could be done to halt the outbreak. Indeed it is not even clear what would happen if an insulin-producing strain of bacteria spread through the human population.

These and similar dangers prompted some critics to call for an end to all genetic-engineering research. However, almost two decades of recombinant-DNA research have passed without the occurrence of any biological catastrophes. Most observers regard this as sufficient proof of the essential safety of the research. Yet, in the view of others, the fact that no catastrophes have yet occurred must not be allowed to give us a false sense of security. Almost no one advocates that the research be abandoned, but several molecular geneticists have argued that the very fact that we still do not know enough to estimate the risks involved with a high degree of certainty is a good reason for continuing to control it severely.

The release of genetically altered organisms into the environment still remains a focus of concern, more so than does research itself. In 1988 health officials in Argentina concluded that several farm workers had became infected with a genetically altered vaccinia virus containing a gene from the rabies virus. The modified virus was experimentally injected into cattle to stimulate the production of antibodies against rabies.

Although American experts expressed skepticism about the possibility of the altered virus affecting humans, critics pointed out that the incident indicates the ways in which researchers are beginning to turn to overseas trials to escape having to comply with protective regulation. Also, a number of other incidents show how easy it is to skirt the complex regulatory process that is supposed to provide protection from the products of genetically altered organisms.

The concern of critics is based on the possibility that such organisms may multiply, mutate, and cause unforeseeable damage. Most animal viruses do not infect people, but an altered virus may. Also, it almost certainly could spread to other animals, both domestic and wild. The virus might act in ways that would cause disease in other animals or make them more susceptible to numerous diseases.

In response to a variety of incidents, the Environmental Protection Agency has tightened standards governing environmental testing of genetically altered organisms. Very few critics are calling for abandoning the use of such organisms, for they hold too much promise as vaccines, growth enhancers, and pesticides. However, within the scientific community there is a widespread attitude of caution and a demand for rigorous testing.

Quite apart from the possible hazards associated with genetic engineering, many people continue to be uneasy about the direction of research. A number of biotechnological possibilities are on the horizon, some of which might have far-reaching consequences. As we noticed earlier, gene surgery offers more possibilities than just medical therapy. If undesirable DNA segments can be sliced out of the genetic code and replaced by others, then this would permit the "engineering" of human beings to an extent and to a degree of precision never before imagined. The eugenic dream of producing people to match an ideal model would be a reality. What would happen then to such traditional and moral values as autonomy, diversity, and the inherent worth of the individual?

The same techniques employed to manufacture the ideal person might also be used to design others to fit special needs. It is not difficult to imagine using genetic surgery to engineer a subhuman race to serve as a slave class for the society. The scenarios of cautionary science fiction might be acted out in our own future.

In addition, the biological technique of asexual reproduction known as cloning might be employed to produce individuals that are exact genetic copies of the DNA donor. These "Xeroxed" organisms—including human beings—are within the scope of technological imagination.

To mention just one last possibility, virtually new organisms might be produced by splicing together DNA from two or more sources. Thus, the world might be faced with creatures of an unknown and unpredictable nature that are not the product of the natural processes of evolution.

It is little wonder that molecular biologists have become concerned about the nature and direction of their research. As Robert Sinsheimer of the California Institute of Technology says, "Biologists have become, without wanting it, custodians of great and terrible power." Such power in the hands of a tyrannical government could be used with irresistible effectiveness to control its subjects. Societies might create a race of semihuman slaves or armies of genetically engineered soldiers. The possibilities are both fantastic and unlimited.

Difficulties with Genetic Research, Therapy, and Technology

The risks involved in gene therapy are not unique ones. In most respects, they exactly parallel those involved in any new medical treatment. Accordingly, it seems reasonable to believe that the same standards of safety and the same consideration for the welfare of the patient that are relevant to the use of other forms of therapy should be regarded as relevant to gene therapy.

The principles of Kant and Ross would suggest that the autonomy of the individual be respected and preserved. In particular, the individual ought not be viewed as an experimental case for testing out a procedure that may later prove helpful. If the person is well enough to be adequately informed and to give consent, and if there is no alternative therapy likely to be effective, it would be morally legitimate for the patient to be given the opportunity to benefit from the therapy. However, if the hazards are great or if they are completely unknown, then it is doubtful whether the patient would be justified in risking his or her life.

By contrast, on utilitarian principles, if the outcome of gene therapy can be reasonably expected to produce more benefit than harm, then the use of the therapy might be considered justifiable. If we assume that a person is likely to die anyway, then that in itself might be enough to warrant the use of the therapy. In addition, since each case treated is likely to contribute to increased understanding and to benefit others, this tends to support the use of gene therapy, even in cases in which it is of doubtful help to the individual. (See Chapter 6 for a fuller discussion.)

Genetic research and its associated technology present issues that are much greater in scope than those raised by gene therapy. They are issues that require us to decide what sort of society we want to live in.

Very few responsible people currently believe that we should call a halt to research in molecular genetics and forgo the increase in power and understanding that it is likely to bring. However, the possibilities of genetic engineering include ones that are frightening and threatening, ones that could wholly alter our society and destroy some of our most cherished values. These are the possibilities that require that we make decisions about whether or to what extent we want to see them realized.

The natural law view of ethics would not, in general, support any policy of restricting scientific inquiry in the area of molecular genetics. For on this view there is a natural inclination (and hence a natural duty) to seek knowledge. Yet certain types of experiments and gene engineering would be ruled out. Those that aim at altering human beings or creating new species from mixed DNA are most likely to be considered to violate the natural order. On the Roman Catholic view, such a violation of nature would run counter to God's plan and purpose and so be immoral.

The principle of utility might be invoked to justify limiting, directing, or even ending research in molecular genetics. If research or its results are more likely to bring about more harm than benefit, then regulation would be called for. Yet if the promise of relieving misery or increasing well-being is great, then some risk that we might also acquire dangerous knowledge in the process might be acceptable. On the utilitarian view, knowledge may be recognized as a good, but it is only one good among others. Possessing the knowledge to alter human beings in accordance with a eugenic ideal or to create new species means that we have to make a decision about whether doing so would result in an overall benefit. That judgment will then be reflected in our social policies and practices. Such an analysis also seems to be consistent with Rawls's principles. There is not, for Rawls, an absolute right to seek knowledge, nor is there any obligation to employ knowledge that is available. Restriction might well be imposed on scientific research and on the technological possibilities it presents if the good of society seems to demand it.

Genetic Diseases: Can Having Children Be Immoral?

L. M. Purdy

L. M. Purdy claims that it is wrong to reproduce when we know there is a high risk of transmitting a serious genetic disease to an offspring. In support of this claim, Purdy presents three interconnected arguments: (1) we have a duty to provide every child with a normal opportunity for a good life; (2) we do not harm possible children by preventing them from existing; (3) the duty to provide a normal opportunity for a good life takes precedence over a potential parent's right to reproduce.

Purdy uses Huntington's disease (chorea) as an example in her argument. The recent identification of a genetic marker (see the Case Presentation) has opened up new possibilities for early detection of the disease in some cases. However, this fact does not substantially affect Purdy's argument. Also, the line of reasoning she develops is applicable to a wide variety of genetic diseases, such as thallasemia and cystic fibrosis, and is not uniquely tied to Huntington's disease.

I. Introduction

Suppose you know that there is a fifty percent chance you have Huntington's chorea, even though you are still free of symptoms, and that if you do have it, each of your children has a fifty percent chance of having it also.

Should you now have children?

There is always some possibility that a pregnancy will result in a diseased or handicapped child. But certain persons run a higher than average risk of producing such a child. Genetic counselors are increasingly able to calculate the probability that certain problems will occur; this means that more people can find out whether they are in danger of creating unhealthy offspring before the birth of a child.

Since this kind of knowledge is available, we ought to use it wisely. I want in this paper to defend the thesis that it is wrong to reproduce when we know there is a high risk of transmitting a serious disease or defect. My argument for this claim is in three parts. The first is that we should try to provide every child with a normal opportunity for health; the second is that in the course of doing this it is not wrong to prevent possible children from existing. The third is that this duty may require us to refrain from childbearing.[1]

One methodological point must be made. I am investigating a problem in biomedical ethics: this is a philosophical enterprise. But the conclusion has practical importance since individuals do face the choice I examine. This raises a question: what relation ought the outcome of this inquiry bear to social policy?[2] It may be held that a person's reproductive life should not be interfered with. Perhaps this is a reasonable position, but it does not follow from it that it is never wrong for an individual to have

Reprinted with permission of the author.

children or that we should not try to determine when this is the case. All that does follow is that we may not coerce persons with regard to childbearing. Evaluation of this last claim is a separate issue which cannot be handled here.

I want to deal with this issue concretely. The reason for this is that, otherwise, discussion is apt to be vague and inconclusive. An additional reason is that it will serve to make us appreciate the magnitude of the difficulties faced by diseased or handicapped individuals. Thus it will be helpful to consider a specific disease. For this purpose I have chosen Huntington's chorea.[3]

II. Huntington's Chorea: Course and Risk

Let us now look at Huntington's chorea. First we will consider the course of the disease, then its inheritance pattern.

The symptoms of Huntington's chorea usually begin between the ages of thirty and fifty, but young children can also be affected. It happens this way:

> Onset is insidious. Personality changes (obstinacy, moodiness, lack of initiative) frequently antedate or accompany the involuntary choreic movements. These usually appear first in the face, neck, and arms, and are jerky, irregular, and stretching in character. Contractions of the facial muscles result in grimaces; those of the respiratory muscles, lips, and tongue lead to hesitating, explosive speech. Irregular movements of the trunk are present; the gait is shuffling and dancing. Tendon reflexes are increased . . .
> Some patients display a fatuous euphoria; others are spite- ful, irascible, destructive, and violent. Paranoid reactions are common. Poverty of thought and impairment of attention, memory, and judgment occur. As the disease progresses, walking becomes impossible, swallowing difficult, and dementia profound. Suicide is not uncommon.[4]

The illness lasts about fifteen years, terminating in death.

Who gets Huntington's chorea? It is an autosomal dominant disease; this means it is caused by a single mutant gene located on a non-sex chromosome. It is passed from one generation to the next via affected individuals. When one has the disease, whether one has symptoms and thus knows one has

it or not, there is a fifty percent chance that each child will have it also. If one has escaped it then there is no risk to one's children.[5]

How serious is this risk? For geneticists, a ten percent risk is high.[6] But not every high risk is unacceptable: this depends on what is at stake.

There are two separate evaluations in any judgment about a given risk. The first measures the gravity of the worst possible result; the second perceives a given risk as great or small. As for the first, in medicine as elsewhere, people may regard the same result differently:

> . . . The subjective attitude to the disease or lesion itself may be quite at variance with what informed medical opinion may regard as a realistic appraisal. Relatively minor limb defects with cosmetic overtones are examples here. On the other hand, some patients regard with equanimity genetic lesions which are of major medical importance.[7]

For devastating diseases like Huntington's chorea, this part of the judgment should be unproblematic: no one could want a loved one to suffer so.

There may be considerable disagreement, however, about whether a given probability is big or little. Individuals vary a good deal in their attitude toward this aspect of risk.[8] This suggests that it would be difficult to define the "right" attitude to a particular risk in many circumstances. Nevertheless, there are good grounds for arguing in favor of a conservative approach here. For it is reasonable to take special precautions to avoid very bad consequences, even if the risk is small. But the possible consequences here *are* very bad: a child who may inherit Huntington's chorea is a child with a much larger than average chance of being subjected to severe and prolonged suffering. Even if the child does not have the disease, it may anticipate and fear it, and anticipating an evil, as we all know, may be worse than experiencing it. In addition, if a parent loses the gamble, his child will suffer the consequences. But it is one thing to take a high risk for oneself; to submit someone else to it without his consent is another.

I think that these points indicate that the morality of procreation in situations like this demands further study. I propose to do this by looking first at the position of the possible child, then at that of the potential parent.[9]

III. Reproduction: The Possible Child's Position

The first task in treating the problem from the child's point of view is to find a way of referring to possible future offspring without seeming to confer some sort of morally significant existence upon them. I will call children who might be born in the future but who are not now conceived "possible" children, offspring, individuals, or persons. I stipulate that this term implies nothing about their moral standing.

The second task is to decide what claims about children or possible children are relevant to the morality of childbearing in the circumstances being considered. There are, I think, two such claims. One is that we ought to provide every child with at least a normal opportunity for a good life. The other is that we do not harm possible children if we prevent them from existing. Let us consider both these matters in turn.

A. Opportunity for a Good Life

Accepting the claim that we ought to try to provide for every child a normal opportunity for a good life involves two basic problems: justification and practical application.

Justification of the claim could be derived fairly straightforwardly from either utilitarian or contractarian theories of justice, I think, although a proper discussion would be too lengthy to include here. Of prime importance in any such discussion would be the judgment that to neglect this duty would be to create unnecessary unhappiness or unfair disadvantage for some persons.

The attempt to apply the claim that we should try to provide a normal opportunity for a good life leads to a couple of difficulties. One is knowing what it requires of us. Another is defining "normal opportunity." Let us tackle the latter problem first.

Conceptions of "normal opportunity" vary among societies and also within them: *de rigueur* in some circles are private music lessons and trips to Europe, while in others providing eight years of schooling is a major sacrifice. But there is no need to consider this complication since we are here concerned only with health as a prerequisite for normal opportunity. Thus we can retreat to the more limited claim that every parent should try to ensure normal health for his child. It might be thought that even this moderate claim is unsatisfactory since in some places debilitating conditions are the norm. One could circumvent this objection by saying that parents ought to try to provide for their children health normal for that culture, even though it may be inadequate if measured by some outside standard. This conservative position would still justify efforts to avoid the birth of children at risk for Huntington's chorea and other serious genetic diseases.

But then what does this stand require of us: is sacrifice entailed by the duty to try to provide normal health for our children? The most plausible answer seems to be that as the danger of serious disability increases, the greater the sacrifice demanded of the potential parent. This means it would be more justifiable to recommend that an individual refrain from childbearing if he risks passing on spina bifida than if he risks passing on webbed feet. Working out all the details of such a schema would clearly be a difficult matter: I do not think it would be impossible to set up workable guidelines, though.

Assuming a rough theoretical framework of this sort, the next question we must ask is whether Huntington's chorea substantially impairs an individual's opportunity for a good life.

People appear to have different opinions about the plight of such persons. Optimists argue that a child born into a family afflicted with Huntington's chorea has a reasonable chance of living a satisfactory life. After all, there is a fifty percent chance it will escape the disease even if a parent has already manifested it, and a still greater chance if this is not so. Even if it does have the illness, it will probably enjoy thirty years of healthy life before symptoms appear; and, perhaps, it may not find the disease destructive. Optimists can list diseased or handicapped persons who have lived fruitful lives. They can also find individuals who seem genuinely glad to be alive. One is Rick Donahue, a sufferer from the Joseph family disease: "You know, if my mom hadn't had me, I wouldn't be here for the life I have had. So there is a good possibility I will have children."[10] Optimists therefore conclude that it would be a shame if these persons had not lived.

Pessimists concede these truths, but they take a less sanguine view of them. They think a fifty percent risk of serious disease like Huntington's chorea appallingly high. They suspect that a child born into an afflicted family is liable to spend its youth in dreadful anticipation and fear of the disease. They expect that the disease, if it appears, will be perceived as a tragic and painful end to a blighted life. They point out that Rick Donahue is still young and has not yet experienced the full horror of his sickness.

Empirical research is clearly needed to resolve this dispute: we need much more information about the psychology and life history of sufferers and potential sufferers. Until we have it we cannot know whether the optimist or the pessimist has a better case: definitive judgment must therefore be suspended. In the meantime, however, common sense suggests that the pessimist has the edge.

If some diseased persons do turn out to have a worse than average life there appears to be a case against further childbearing in afflicted families. To support this claim two more judgments are necessary, however. The first is that it is not wrong to refrain from childbearing. The second is that asking individuals to so refrain is less of a sacrifice than might be thought.[11] I will examine each of these judgments.

B. The Morality of Preventing the Birth of Possible Persons

Before going on to look at reasons why it would not be wrong to prevent the birth of possible persons, let me try to clarify the picture a bit. To understand the claim it must be kept in mind that we are considering a prospective situation here, not a retrospective one: we are trying to rank the desirability of various alternative future states of affairs. One possible future state is this: a world where nobody is at risk for Huntington's chorea except as a result of random mutation. This state has been achieved by sons and daughters of persons afflicted with Huntington's chorea ceasing to reproduce. This means that an indeterminate number of children who might have been born were not born. These possible children can be divided into two categories: those who would have been miserable and those who would have lived good lives. To prevent the existence of members of the first category it was necessary to prevent the existence of all. Whether or not this is a good state of affairs depends on the morality of the means and the end. The end, preventing the existence of miserable beings, is surely

good; I will argue that preventing the birth of possible persons is not intrinsically wrong. Hence this state of affairs is a morally good one.

Why then is it not in itself wrong to prevent the birth of possible persons? It is not wrong because there seems to be no reason to believe that possible individuals are either deprived or injured if they do not exist. They are not deprived because to be deprived in a morally significant sense one must be able to have experiences. But possible persons do not exist. Since they do not exist, they cannot have experiences. Another way to make this point is to say that each of us might not have been born, although most of us are glad we were. But this does not mean that it makes sense to say that we would have been deprived of something had we not been born. For if we had not been born, we would not exist, and there would be nobody to be deprived of anything. To assert the contrary is to imagine that we are looking at a world in which we do not exist. But this is not the way it would be: there would be nobody to look.

The contention that it is wrong to prevent possible persons from existing because they have a right to exist appears to be equally baseless. The most fundamental objection to this view is that there is no reason to ascribe rights to entities which do not exist. It is one thing to say that as-yet-nonexistent persons will have certain rights if and when they exist: this claim is plausible if made with an eye toward preserving social and environmental goods.[12] But what justification could there be for the claim that nonexistent beings have a right to exist?

Even if one conceded that there was a presumption in favor of letting some nonexistent beings exist, stronger claims could surely override it.[13] For one thing, it would be unfair not to recognize the prior claim of already existing children who are not being properly cared for. One might also argue that it is simply wrong to prevent persons who might have existed from doing so. But this implies that contraception and population control are also wrong.

It is therefore reasonable to maintain that because possible persons have no right to exist, they are not injured if not created. Even if they had that right, it could rather easily be overridden by counterclaims. Hence, since possible persons are neither deprived nor injured if not conceived, it is not wrong to prevent their existence.

C. Conclusion to Part III

At the beginning of Part III I said that two claims are relevant to the morality of childbearing in the circumstances being considered. The first is that we ought to provide every child with at least a normal opportunity for a good life. The second is that we do not deprive or injure possible persons if we prevent their existence.

I suggested that the first claim could be derived from currently accepted theories of justice: a healthy body is generally necessary for happiness and it is also a prerequisite for a fair chance at a good life in our competitive world. Thus it is right to try to ensure that each child is healthy.

I argued, with regard to the second claim, that we do not deprive or injure possible persons if we fail to create them. They cannot be deprived of anything because they do not exist and hence cannot have experiences. They cannot be injured because only an entity with a right to exist could be injured if prevented from existing: but there are no good grounds for believing that they are such entities.

From the conjunction of these two claims I conclude that it is right to try to ensure that a child is healthy even if by doing so we preclude the existence of certain possible persons. Thus it is right for individuals to prevent the birth of children at risk for Huntington's chorea by avoiding parenthood. The next question is whether it is seriously wrong *not* to avoid parenthood.

IV. Reproduction: The Potential Parent's Situation

I have so far argued that if choreics live substantially worse lives than average, then it is right for afflicted families to cease reproduction. But this conflicts with the generally recognized freedom to procreate and so it does not automatically follow that family members ought not to have children. How can we decide whether the duty to try to provide normal health for one's child should take precedence over the right to reproduce?

This is essentially the same question I asked earlier: how much must one sacrifice to try to ensure that one's offspring is healthy? In answer to this I suggested that the greater the danger of serious disability, the more justifiable considerable sacrifice is.

Now asking someone who wants a child to refrain from procreation seems to be asking for a large sacrifice. It may, in fact, appear to be too large to demand of anyone. Yet I think it can be shown that it is not as great as it initially seems.

Why do people want children? There are probably many reasons, but I suspect that the following include some of the most common. One set of reasons has to do with the gratification to be derived from a happy family life—love, companionship, watching a child grow, helping mold it into a good person, sharing its pains and triumphs. Another set of reasons centers about the parents as individuals—validation of their place within a genetically continuous family line, the conception of children as a source of immortality, being surrounded by replicas of themselves.

Are there alternative ways of satisfying these desires? Adoption or technological means provide ways to satisfy most of the desires pertaining to family life without passing on specific genetic defects. Artificial insemination by donor is already available; implantation of donor ova is likely within a few years. Still another option will exist if cloning becomes a reality. In the meantime, we might permit women to conceive and bear babies for those who do not want to do so themselves.[14] But the desire to extend the genetic line, the desire for immortality, and the desire for children that physically resemble one cannot be met by these methods.

Many individuals probably feel these latter desires strongly. This creates a genuine conflict for persons at risk for transmitting serious genetic diseases like Huntington's chorea. The situation seems especially unfair because, unlike normal people, through no fault of their own, doing something they badly want to do may greatly harm others.

But if my common sense assumption that they are in grave danger of harming others is true, then it is imperative to scrutinize their options carefully. On the one hand, they can have children: they satisfy their desires but risk eventual crippling illness and death for their offspring. On the other, they can remain childless or seek nonstandard ways of creating a family: they have some unfulfilled desires, but they avoid risking harm to their children.

I think it is clear which of these two alternatives is best. For the desires which must remain unsatisfied if they forgo normal procreation are less than admirable. To see the genetic line continued entails a sinister legacy of illness and death; the desire for immortality cannot really be satisfied by reproduction anyway; and the desire for children that physically resemble one is narcissistic and its fulfillment cannot be guaranteed even by normal reproduction. Hence the only defence of these desires is that people do in fact feel them.

Now, I am inclined to accept William James' dictum regarding desires: "Take any demand, however slight, which any creature, however weak, may make. Ought it not, for its own sole sake be satisfied? If not, prove why not."[15] Thus I judge a world where more desires are satisfied to be better than one in which fewer are. But not all desires should be regarded as legitimate, since, as James suggests, there may be good reasons why these ought to be disregarded. The fact that their fulfillment will seriously harm others is surely such a reason. And I believe that the circumstances I have described are a clear example of the sort of case where a desire must be judged illegitimate, at least until it can be shown that sufferers from serious genetic diseases like Huntington's chorea do not live considerably worse than average lives. Therefore, I think it is wrong for individuals in this predicament to reproduce.

V. Conclusion

Let me recapitulate. At the beginning of this paper I asked whether it is wrong for those who risk transmitting severe genetic disease like Huntington's chorea to have "blood" children. Some despair of reaching an answer to this question.[16] But I think such pessimism is not wholly warranted, and that if generally accepted would lead to much unnecessary harm. It is true that in many cases it is difficult to know what ought to be done. But this does not mean that we should throw up our hands and espouse a completely laissez-faire approach: philosophers can help by probing the central issues and trying to find guidelines for action.

Naturally there is no way to derive an answer to this kind of problem by deductive argument from self-evident premises, for it must depend on a complicated interplay of facts and moral judgments. My preliminary exploration of Huntington's chorea is of this nature. In the course of discussion I suggested that, if it is true that sufferers live substantially worse lives than do normal persons, those who might transmit it should not have children. This conclusion is supported by the judgments that we

ought to try to provide for every child a normal opportunity for a good life, that possible individuals are not harmed if not conceived, and that it is sometimes less justifiable for persons to exercise their right to procreate than one might think.

I want to stress, in conclusion, that my argument is incomplete. To investigate fully even a single disease, like Huntington's chorea, empirical research on the lives of members of afflicted families is necessary. Then, after developing further the themes touched upon here, evaluation of the probable consequences of different policies on society and on future generations is needed. Until the results of a complete study are available, my argument could serve best as a reason for persons at risk for transmitting Huntington's chorea and similar diseases to put off having children. Perhaps this paper will stimulate such inquiry.

Notes

1. There are a series of cases ranging from low risk of mild disease or handicap to high risk of serious disease or handicap. It would be difficult to decide where the duty to refrain from procreation becomes compelling. My point here is that there are some clear cases.

   I'd like to thank Lawrence Davis and Sidney Siskin for their helpful comments on an earlier version of this paper.

2. This issue is one which must be faced most urgently by genetic counselors. The proper role of the genetic counselor with regard to such decisions has been the subject of much debate. The dominant view seems to be that espoused by Lytt Gardner who maintains that it is unethical for a counselor to make ethical judgments about what his clients ought to do. ("Counseling in Genetics." *Early Diagnosis of Human Genetic Defects: Scientific & Ethical Considerations*, ed. Maureen Harris [H.E.W. Publication No. (NIH), 72–25; Fogarty Center Proceedings No. 6], p. 192.) Typically this view is unsupported by an argument. For other views see Bentley Glass, "Human Heredity and Ethical Problems," *Perspectives in Biology & Medicine*, Vol. 15 (winter '72), 237–53, esp. 242–52; Marc Lappé, "The Genetic Counselor Responsible to Whom?" *Hastings Center Report*, Vol. 1, No. 2 (Sept. '71), 6–8; E. C. Fraser, "Genetic Counseling," *Am J. of Human Genetics* 26: 636–659, 1974.

3. I have chosen Huntington's chorea because it seems to me to be one of the clearest cases of high risk serious genetic disease known to the public, despite the fact that it does not usually manifest itself until the prime of life. The latter entails two

further facts. First an individual of reproductive age may not know whether he has the disease; he therefore does not know the risk of passing on the disease. Secondly, an affected person may have a substantial number of years of healthy life before it shows itself. I do not think that this factor materially changes my case, however. Even if an individual does not in fact risk passing the disease to his children, *he cannot know that this is true*. And even thirty years of healthy life may well be seriously shadowed by anticipation and fear of the disease. Thus the fact that the disease develops late does not diminish its horror. If it could be shown that these factors could be adequately circumvented, my claim that there is a *class* of genetic disease of such severity that it would be wrong to risk passing them on would not be undermined.

It might also be thought that Huntington's chorea is insufficiently common to merit such attention. But, depending on reproductive patterns, the disease could become a good deal more widespread. Consider the fact that in 1916 nine hundred and sixty-two cases could be traced from six seventeenth-century arrivals in America. (Gordon Rattray Taylor, *The Biological Time Bomb*, [New York, 1968], p. 176.) But more importantly, even if the disease did not spread, it would still be seriously wrong. I think, to inflict it unnecessarily on *any* members of new generations. Finally, it should be kept in mind that I am using Huntington's chorea as an example of the sort of disease we should try to eradicate. Thus the arguments presented here would be relevant to a wide range of genetic diseases.

4. *The Merck Manual* (Rahway, N.J.: Merck, 1972), p. 1346.

5. Hymie Gordon, "Genetic Counseling," JAMA, Vol. 217, No. 9 (August 30, 1971), 1217.

6. Charles Smith, Susan Holloway, and Alan E. H. Emery, "Individuals at Risk in Families—Genetic Disease," *J. of Medical Genetics*, 8 (1971), 453. See also Townes in *Genetic Counseling*, ed. Daniel Bergsma, *Birth Defects Original Article Series*, Vol. VL, No. I (May 1970).

7. J. H. Pearn, "Patients' Subjective Interpretation of Risks offered in Genetic Counseling," *Journal of Medical Genetics*, 10 (1973) 131.

8. Pearn, p. 132.

9. There are many important and interesting points that might be raised with respect to future generations and present society. There is no space to deal with them here, although I strongly suspect that conclusions regarding them would support my judgment that it is wrong for those who risk transmitting certain diseases to reproduce—for some discussion of future generations, see Gerald Leach, *The Biocrats* (Middlesex, England: Penguin Books, 1972), p. 150; M. P. Golding, "Obligations to Future Generations," *Monist* 56 (Jan. 1972), 84–99; Gordon Rattray Taylor, *The Biological Time Bomb* (New York, 1968), esp. p. 176. For some discussions of society, see Daniel Callahan, "The Meaning and Significance of Genetic Disease: Philosophical Perspectives," *Ethical Issues in Human Genetics*, ed. Bruce Hilton et al., (New York, 1973), p. 87ff.; John Fletcher, "The Brink: The Parent-Child Bond in the Genetic Revolution," *Theological Studies* 33 (Sept. '72), 457–486; Glass (supra 2ª); Marc Lappé, "Human Genetics," Annals of the *New York Academy of Sciences*, Vol. 26 (May 18, 1973), 152–59; Marc Lappé, "Moral Obligations and the Fallacies of Genetic Control," *Theological Studies*, Vol. 33, No. 3 (Sept. '72), 411–427; Martin P. Golding, "Ethical Issues in Biological Engineering," *UCLA Law Review*, Vol. 15: 267 (1968), 443–479; L. C. Dunn, *Heredity and Evolution in Human Populations* (Cambridge, Mass., 1959), p. 145; Robert S. Morison in *Ethical Issues in Human Genetics*, ed. Bruce Hilton et al. (New York, 1973), p. 208.

10. *The New York Times*, September 30, 1975, p. 1, col. 6. The Joseph family disease is similar to Huntington's chorea except that symptoms start appearing in the twenties. Rick Donahue is in his early twenties.

11. There may be a price for the individuals who refrain from having children. We will be looking at the situation from their point of view shortly.

12. This is in fact the basis for certain parental duties. An example is the maternal duty to obtain proper nutrition before and during pregnancy, for this is necessary if the child is to have normal health when it is born.

13. One might argue that as many persons as possible should exist so that they may enjoy life.

14. Some thinkers have qualms about the use of some or all of these methods. They have so far failed to show why they are immoral, although, naturally, much careful study will be required before they could be unqualifiedly recommended. See, for example, Richard Hull, "Genetic Engineering: Comment on Headings," *The Humanist*, Vol. 32 (Sept./Oct. 1972), 13.

15. *Essays in Pragmatism*, ed. A. Castell (New York, 1948), p. 73.

16. For example, see Leach, p. 138. One of the ways the dilemma described by Leach could be lessened would be if society emphasized those aspects of family life not dependent on "blood" relationships and downplayed those that are.

Implications of Prenatal Diagnosis for the Human Right to Life

Leon R. Kass

Leon R. Kass expresses concern that the practice of "genetic abortion" will strongly affect our attitudes toward all who are "defective" or abnormal. Those who escape the net of selective abortion might receive less care and might even come to think of themselves as second-class specimens. Furthermore, on Kass's view, genetic abortion might encourage us to accept the general principle that defectives of any kind ought not be born. This, in turn, would threaten our commitment to the basic moral principle that each person, despite any physical or mental handicap, is the inherent equal of every other person.

Kass presents six criteria that he suggests ought to be satisfied to justify the abortion of a fetus for genetic reasons. In the remainder of his paper, he focuses on the question raised by the last criterion: According to what standards should we judge a fetus with genetic abnormalities unfit to live? As candidates for such standards, Kass examines the concepts of social good, family good, and the "healthy and sound" fetus. He finds difficulty with all, and in the end he professes himself unable to provide a satisfactory justification for genetic abortion. Kass's difficulty with the "healthy and sound" fetus as a standard puts his general position in conflict with that taken by Purdy. What Purdy regards as a relatively clear-cut criterion, Kass views as a relatively vague and arbitrary social standard.

Any discussion of the ethical issues of genetic counseling and prenatal diagnosis is unavoidably haunted by a ghost called the morality of abortion. This ghost I shall not vex. More precisely, I shall not vex the reader by telling ghost stories. However, I would be neither surprised nor disappointed if my discussion of an admittedly related matter, the ethics of aborting the genetically defective, summons that hovering spirit to the reader's mind. For the morality of abortion is a matter not easily laid to rest, recent efforts to do so notwithstanding. . . .

Yet before leaving the general question of abortion, let me pause to drop some anchors for the discussion that follows. Despite great differences of opinion both as to what to think and how to reason about abortion, nearly everyone agrees that abortion is a moral issue.[1] What does this mean? Formally, it means that a woman seeking or refusing an abortion can expect to be asked to justify her action. And we can expect that she should be able to give reasons for her choice other than "I like it" or "I don't like it." Substantively, it means that, in the absence of good reasons for intervention, there is some presumption in favor of allowing the pregnancy to continue once it has begun. A common way of expressing this presumption is to say that "the fetus has a right to continued life."[2] In this context, disagreement concerning the moral permissibility of abortion concerns what rights (or interests or needs), and whose, override (take precedence over, or outweigh) this fetal "right." Even most of the "opponents" of abortion agree that the

Reprinted from Ethical Issues in Human Genetics: Genetic counseling and the Use of Genetic Knowledge, *edited by Bruce Hilton, Daniel Callahan, Maureen Harris, Peter Condliffe, and Burton Berkeley (New York: Plenum Press, 1973), pp. 185–199. A revised version of this essay ("Perfect Babies: Prenatal Diagnosis and the Equal Right to Life") appears in Dr. Kass's book,* Toward a More Natural Science: Biology and Human Affairs *(New York: The Free Press, 1985).*

mother's right to live takes precedence, and that abortion to save her life is permissible, perhaps obligatory. Some believe that a woman's right to determine the number and spacing of her children takes precedence, while yet others argue that the need to curb population growth is, at least at this time, overriding.

Hopefully, this brief analysis of what it means to say that abortion is a moral issue is sufficient to establish two points. First, that the fetus is a living thing with some moral claim on us not to do it violence, and therefore, second, that justification must be given for destroying it.

Turning now from the general questions of the ethics of abortion, I wish to focus on the special ethical issues raised by the abortion of "defective" fetuses (so-called "abortion for fetal indications"). I shall consider only the cleanest cases, those cases where well-characterized genetic diseases are diagnosed with a high degree of certainty by means of amniocentesis, in order to sidestep the added moral dilemmas posed when the diagnosis is suspected or possible, but unconfirmed. However, many of the questions I shall discuss could also be raised about cases where genetic analysis gives only a statistical prediction about the genotype of the fetus, and also about cases where the defect has an infectious or chemical rather than a genetic cause (e.g., rubella, thalidomide).

My first and possibly most difficult task is to show that there is anything left to discuss once we have agreed not to discuss the morality of abortion in general. There is a sense in which abortion for genetic defect is, after abortion to save the life of the mother, perhaps the most defensible kind of abortion. Certainly, it is a serious and not a frivolous reason for abortion, defended by its proponents in sober and rational speech—unlike justifications based upon the false notion that a fetus is a mere part of a woman's body, to be used and abused at her pleasure. Standing behind genetic abortion are serious and well-intentioned people, with reasonable ends in view: the prevention of genetic diseases, the elimination of suffering in families, the preservation of precious financial and medical resources, the protection of our genetic heritage. No profiteers, no sex-ploiters, no racists. No arguments about the connection of abortion with promiscuity and licentiousness, no perjured testimony about the mental health of the mother, no arguments about the seriousness of the population problem. In short, clear objective data, a worthy cause, decent men and women. If abortion, what better reason for it?

Yet if genetic abortion is but a happily wagging tail on the dog of abortion, it is simultaneously the nose of a camel protruding under a rather different tent. Precisely because the quality of the fetus is central to the decision to abort, the practice of genetic abortion has implications which go beyond those raised by abortion in general. What may be at stake here is the belief in the radical moral equality of all human beings, the belief that all human beings possess equally and independent of merit certain fundamental rights, one among which is, of course, the right to life.

To be sure, the belief that fundamental human rights belong equally to all human beings has been but an ideal, never realized, often ignored, sometimes shamelessly. Yet it has been perhaps the most powerful moral idea at work in the world for at least two centuries. It is this idea and ideal that animates most of the current political and social criticism around the globe. It is ironic that we should acquire the power to detect and eliminate the genetically unequal at a time when we have finally succeeded in removing much of the stigma and disgrace previously attached to victims of congenital illness, in providing them with improved care and support, and in preventing, by means of education, feelings of guilt on the part of their parents. One might even wonder whether the development of amniocentesis and prenatal diagnosis may represent a backlash against these same humanitarian and egalitarian tendencies in the practice of medicine, which, by helping to sustain to the age of reproduction persons with genetic disease has itself contributed to the increasing incidence of genetic disease, and with it, to increased pressures for genetic screening, genetic counseling, and genetic abortion.

No doubt our humanitarian and egalitarian principles and practices have caused us some new difficulties, but if we mean to weaken or turn our backs on them, we should do so consciously and thoughtfully. If, as I believe, the idea and practice of genetic abortion points in that direction, we should make ourselves aware of it. And if, as I believe, the way in which genetic abortion is described, discussed, and justified is perhaps of even greater consequence than its practice for our notions of human rights and of their equal possession by all human beings, we should pay special attention to questions of language and in particular, to the question of justification. . . .

Genetic Abortion and the Living Defective

The practice of abortion of the genetically defective will no doubt affect our view of and our behavior toward those abnormals who escape the net of detection and abortion. A child with Down's syndrome or with hemophilia or with muscular dystrophy born at a time when most of his (potential) fellow sufferers were destroyed prenatally is liable to be looked upon by the community as one unfit to be alive, as a second-class (or even lower) human type. He may be seen as a person who need not have been, and who would not have been, if only someone had gotten to him in time.

The parents of such children are also likely to treat them differently, especially if the mother would have wished but failed to get an amniocentesis because of ignorance, poverty, or distance from the testing station, or if the prenatal diagnosis was in error. In such cases, parents are especially likely to resent the child. They may be disinclined to give it the kind of care they might have before the advent of amniocentesis and genetic abortion, rationalizing that a second-class specimen is not entitled to first-class treatment. If pressed to do so, say by physicians, the parents might refuse, and the courts may become involved. This has already begun to happen.

In Maryland, parents of a child with Down's syndrome refused permission to have the child operated on for an intestinal obstruction present at birth. The physicians and the hospital sought an injunction to require the parents to allow surgery. The judge ruled in favor of the parents, despite what I understand to be the weight of precedent to the contrary, on the grounds that the child was Mongoloid, that is, had the child been "normal," the decision would have gone the other way. Although the decision was not appealed to and hence not affirmed by a higher court, we can see through the prism of this case the possibility that the new powers of human genetics will strip the blindfold from the lady of justice and will make official the dangerous doctrine that some men are more equal than others.

The abnormal child may also feel resentful. A child with Down's syndrome or Tay-Sachs disease

will probably never know or care, but what about a child with hemophilia or with Turner's syndrome? In the past decade, with medical knowledge and power over the prenatal child increasing and with parental authority over the postnatal child decreasing, we have seen the appearance of a new type of legal action, suits for wrongful life. Children have brought suit against their parents (and others) seeking to recover damages for physical and social handicaps inextricably tied to their birth (e.g., congenital deformities, congenital syphilis, illegitimacy). In some of the American cases, the courts have recognized the justice of the child's claim (that he was injured due to parental negligence), although they have so far refused to award damages, due to policy considerations. In other countries, e.g., in Germany, judgments with compensation have gone for the plaintiffs. With the spread of amniocentesis and genetic abortion, we can only expect such cases to increase. And here it will be the soft-hearted rather than the hard-hearted judges who will establish the doctrine of second-class human beings, out of compassion for the mutants who escaped the traps set out for them.

It may be argued that I am dealing with a problem which, even if it is real, will affect very few people. It may be suggested that very few will escape the traps once we have set them properly and widely, once people are informed about amniocentesis, once the power to detect prenatally grows to its full capacity, and once our "superstitious" opposition to abortion dies out or is extirpated. But in order even to come close to this vision of success, amniocentesis will have to become part of every pregnancy—either by making it mandatory, like the test for syphilis, or by making it "routine medical practice," like the Pap smear. Leaving aside the other problems with universal amniocentesis, we could expect that the problem for the few who escape is likely to be even worse precisely because they will be few.

The point, however, should be generalized. How will we come to view and act toward the many "abnormals" that will remain among us—the retarded, the crippled, the senile, the deformed, and the true mutants—once we embark on a program to root out genetic abnormality? For it must be remembered that we shall always have abnormals some who escape detection or whose disease is undetectable *in utero*, others as a result of new mutations, birth injuries, accidents, maltreatment, or disease—

who will require our care and protection. The existence of "defectives" cannot be fully prevented, not even by totalitarian breeding and weeding programs. Is it not likely that our principle with respect to these people will change from "We try harder" to "Why accept second best?" The idea of "the unwanted because abnormal child" may become a self-fulfilling prophecy, whose consequences may be worse than those of the abnormality itself.

Genetic and Other Defectives

The mention of other abnormals points to a second danger of the practice of genetic abortion. Genetic abortion may come to be seen not so much as the prevention of genetic disease, but as the prevention of birth of defective or abnormal children—and, in a way, understandably so. For in the case of what other diseases does preventive medicine consist in the elimination of the patient-at-risk? Moreover, the very language used to discuss genetic disease leads us to the easy but wrong conclusion that the afflicted fetus or person is rather than has a disease. True, one is partly defined by his genotype, but only partly. A person is more than his disease. And yet we slide easily from the language of possession to the language of identity, from "He has hemophilia" to "He is a hemophiliac," from "She has diabetes" through "She is diabetic" to "She is a diabetic," from "The fetus has Down's syndrome" to "The fetus is a Down's." This way of speaking supports the belief that it is defective persons (or potential persons) that are being eliminated, rather than diseases.

If this is so, then it becomes simply accidental that the defect has a genetic cause. Surely, it is only because of the high regard for medicine and science, and for the accuracy of genetic diagnosis, that genotypic defectives are likely to be the first to go. But once the principle, "Defectives should not be born," is established, grounds other than cytological and biochemical may very well be sought. Even ignoring racialists and others equally misguided—of course, they cannot be ignored—we should know that there are social scientists, for example, who believe that one can predict with a high degree of accuracy how a child will turn out from a careful, systematic study of the socioeconomic and psychodynamic environment into which he is born and in which he grows up. They might press for the prevention of sociopsychological disease, even of

"criminality," by means of prenatal environmental diagnosis and abortion. I have heard rumor that a crude, unscientific form of eliminating potential "phenotypic defectives" is already being practiced in some cities, in that submission to abortion is allegedly being made a condition for the receipt of welfare payments. "Defectives should not be born" is a principle without limits. We can ill-afford to have it established.

Up to this point, I have been discussing the possible implications of the practice of genetic abortion for our belief in and adherence to the idea that, at least in fundamental human matters such as life and liberty, all men are to be considered as equals, that for these matters we should ignore as irrelevant the real qualitative differences amongst men, however important these differences may be for other purposes. Those who are concerned about abortion fear that the permissible time of eliminating the unwanted will be moved forward along the time continuum, against newborns, infants, and children. Similarly, I suggest that we should be concerned lest the attack on gross genetic inequality in fetuses be advanced along the continuum of quality and into the later stages of life.

I am not engaged in predicting the future; I am not saying that amniocentesis and genetic abortion will lead down the road to Nazi Germany. Rather, I am suggesting that the principles underlying genetic abortion simultaneously justify many further steps down that road. The point was very well made by Abraham Lincoln (1854):

> If A can prove, however conclusively, that he may, of right, enslave B—Why may not B snatch the same argument and prove equally, that he may enslave A?
>
> You say A is white, and B is black. It is color, then; the lighter having the right to enslave the darker? Take care. By this rule, you are to be slave to the first man you meet with a fairer skin than your own.
>
> You do not mean color exactly? You mean the whites are intellectually the superiors of the blacks, and, therefore have the right to enslave them? Take care again. By this rule, you are to be slave to the first man you meet with an intellect superior to your own.
>
> But, say you, it is a question of interest, and, if you can make it your interest, you have the right to enslave another. Very well. And if he can make it his interest, he has the right to enslave you.

Perhaps I have exaggerated the dangers; perhaps we will not abandon our inexplicable preference for generous humanitarianism over consistency. But we should indeed be cautious and move slowly as we give serious consideration to the question "What price the perfect baby?"[3]

Standards for Justifying Genetic Abortion

The rest of this paper deals with the problem of justification. What would constitute an adequate justification of the decision to abort a genetically defective fetus? Let me suggest the following formal characteristics, each of which still begs many questions. (1) The reasons given should be logically consistent, and should lead to relatively unambiguous guidelines—note that I do not say "rules"—for action in most cases. (2) The justification should make evident to a reasonable person that the interest or need or right being served by abortion is sufficient to override the otherwise presumptive claim on us to protect and preserve the life of the fetus. (3) Hopefully, the justification would be such as to help provide intellectual support for drawing distinctions between acceptable and unacceptable kinds of genetic abortion and between genetic abortion itself and the further practices we would all find abhorrent. (4) The justification ought to be capable of generalization to all persons in identical circumstances. (5) The justification should not lead to different actions from month to month or from year to year. (6) The justification should be grounded on standards that can, both in principle and in fact, sustain and support our actions in the case of genetic abortion and our notions of human rights in general.

Though I would ask the reader to consider all these criteria, I shall focus primarily on the last. According to what standards can and should we judge a fetus with genetic abnormalities unfit to live, i.e., abortable? It seems to me that there are at least three dominant standards to which we are likely to repair.

The first is societal good. The needs and interests of society are often invoked to justify the practices of prenatal diagnosis and abortion of the genetically abnormal. The argument, full blown, runs something like this. Society has an interest in the genetic fitness of its members. It is foolish for society to squander its precious resources ministering to and caring for the unfit, especially for those who will never become "productive , or who will never in any way "benefit" society. Therefore, the interests of society are best served by the elimination of the genetically defective prior to their birth.

The societal standard is all-too-often reduced to its lowest common denominator: money. Thus one physician, claiming that he has "made a cost-benefit analysis of Tay-Sachs disease," notes that "the total cost of carrier detection, prenatal diagnosis and termination of at-risk pregnancies for all Jewish individuals in the United States under 30 who will marry is $5,730,281. If the program is set up to screen only one married partner, the cost is $3,122,695. The hospital costs for the 990 cases of Tay-Sachs disease these individuals would produce over a thirty-year period in the United States is $34,650,000."[4] Another physician, apparently less interested or able to make such a precise audit has written: "Cost-benefit analyses have been made for the total prospective detection and monitoring of Tay-Sachs disease, cystic fibrosis (when prenatal detection becomes available for cystic fibrosis) and other disorders, and in most cases, the expenditures for hospitalization and medical care far exceed the cost of prenatal detection in properly selected risk populations, followed by selective abortion." Yet a third physician has calculated that the costs to the state of caring for children with Down's syndrome is more than three times that of detecting and aborting them. (These authors all acknowledge the additional nonsocietal "costs" of personal suffering, but insofar as they consider society, the costs are purely economic.)

There are many questions that can be raised about this approach. First, there are the questions about the accuracy of the calculations. Not all the costs have been reckoned. The aborted defective child will be "replaced" by a "normal" child. In keeping the ledger, the "costs" to society of his care and maintenance cannot be ignored—costs of educating him, or removing his wastes and pollutions, not to mention the "costs" in nonreplaceable natural resources that he consumes. Who is a greater drain on society's precious resources, the average inmate of a home for the retarded or the average graduate of Harvard College? I am not sure we know or can even find out. Then there are the costs of training the physician, and genetic counselors, equipping their laboratories, supporting their research, and sending them and us to conferences to worry about what they are doing. An accurate economic analysis seems to me to be impossible, even in principle. And even if it were possible, one could fall back on the words of the ordinary language philosopher, Andy Capp, who, when his wife said that she was getting really worried about the cost of living, replied: "Sweet'eart, name me one person who wants t'stop livin' on account of the cost."

A second defect of the economic analysis is that there are matters of social importance that are not reducible to financial costs, and others that may not be quantifiable at all. How does one quantitate the costs of real and potential social conflict, either between children and parents, or between the community and the "deviants" who refuse amniocentesis and continue to bear abnormal children? Can one measure the effect on racial tensions of attempting to screen for and prevent the birth of children homozygous (or heterozygous) for sickle-cell anemia? What numbers does one attach to any decreased willingness or ability to take care of the less fortunate, or to cope with difficult problems? And what about the "costs" of rising expectations? Will we become increasingly dissatisfied with anything short of the "optimum baby"? How does one quantify anxiety? Humiliation? Guilt? Finally, might not the medical profession pay an unmeasurable price if genetic abortion and other revolutionary activities bring about changes in medical ethics and medical practice that lead to the further erosion of trust in the physician?

An appeal to social worthiness or usefulness is a less vulgar form of the standard of societal good. It is true that great social contributions are unlikely to be forthcoming from persons who suffer from most serious genetic diseases, especially since many of them die in childhood. Yet consider the following remarks of Pearl Buck (1968) on the subject of being a mother of a child retarded from phenylketonuria:

> My child's life has not been meaningless. She has indeed brought comfort and practical help to many people who are parents of retarded children or are themselves handicapped. True, she has done it through me, yet without her I would not have had the means of learning how to accept the inevitable sorrow, and how to make that acceptance useful to others. Would I be so heartless as to say that it has been worthwhile for my child to be born retarded? Certainly not, but I am saying that even though gravely retarded it has been worthwile for her to have lived.

It can be summed up, perhaps, by saying that in this world, where cruelty prevails in so many aspects of our life, I would not add the weight of choice to kill rather than to let live. A retarded child, a handicapped person, brings its own gift to life, even to the life of normal human beings. That gift is comprehended in the lessons of patience, understanding, and mercy, lessons which we all need to receive and to practice with one another, whatever we are.

The standard of potential social worthiness is little better in deciding about abortion in particular cases than is the standard of economic cost. To drive the point home, each of us might consider retrospectively whether he would have been willing to stand trial for his life while a fetus, pleading only his worth to society as he now can evaluate it. How many of us are not socially "defective" and with none of the excuses possible for a child with phenylketonuria? If there is to be human life at all, potential social worthiness cannot be its entitlement.

Finally, we should take note of the ambiguities in the very notion of societal good. Some use the term "society" to mean their own particular political community, others to mean the whole human race, and still others speak as if they mean both simultaneously, following that all-too-human belief that what is good for me and mine is good for mankind. Who knows what is genetically best for mankind, even with respect to Down's syndrome? I would submit that the genetic heritage of the human species is largely in the care of persons who do not live along the amniocentesis frontier. If we in the industrialized West wish to be really serious about the genetic future of the species, we would concentrate our attack on mutagenesis, and especially on our large contribution to the pool of environmental mutagens.

But even the more narrow use of society is ambiguous. Do we mean our "society" as it is today? Or do we mean our "society" as it ought to be? If the former, our standards will be ephemeral, for ours is a faddish "society." (By far the most worrisome feature of the changing attitudes on abortion is the suddenness with which they changed.) Any such socially determined standards are likely to provide too precarious a foundation for decisions about genetic abortion, let alone for our notions of human rights. If we mean the latter, then we have transcended the societal standard, since the "good society" is not to be found in "society" itself, nor is it likely to be discovered by taking a vote. In sum, societal good as a standard for justifying genetic abortion seems to be unsatisfactory. It is hard to define in general, difficult to apply clearly to particular cases, susceptible to overreaching and abuse (hence, very dangerous), and not sufficient unto itself if considerations of the good community are held to be automatically implied.

A second major alternative is the standard of parental or familial good. Here the argument of justification might run as follows. Parents have a right to determine, according to their own wishes and based upon their own notions of what is good for them, the qualitative as well as the quantitative character of their families. If they believe that the birth of a seriously deformed child will be the cause of great sorrow and suffering to themselves and to their other children and a drain on their time and resources, then they may ethically decide to prevent the birth of such a child, even by abortion.

This argument I would expect to be more attractive to most people than the argument appealing to the good of society. For one thing, we are more likely to trust a person's conception of what is good for him than his notion of what is good for society. Also, the number of persons involved is small, making it seem less impossible to weigh all the relevant factors in determining the good of the family. Most powerfully, one can see and appreciate the possible harm done to healthy children if the parents are obliged to devote most of their energies to caring for the afflicted child.

Yet there are ambiguities and difficulties perhaps as great as with the standard of societal good. In the first place, it is not entirely clear what would be good for the other children. In a strong family, the experience with a suffering and dying child might help the healthy siblings learn to face and cope with adversity. Some have even speculated that the lack of experience with death and serious illness in our affluent young people is an important element in their difficulty in trying to find a way of life and in responding patiently yet steadily to the serious problems of our society (Cassell, 1969). I suspect that one cannot generalize. In some children and in some families, experience with suffering may be strengthening, and in others, disabling. My point here is that the matter is uncertain, and that parents deciding on this basis are as likely as not to be mistaken.

The family or parental standard, like the societal standard, is unavoidably elastic because "suffering" does not come in discontinuous units, and because parental wishes and desires know no limits. Both are utterly subjective, relative, and notoriously subject to change. Some parents claim that they could not tolerate having to raise a child of the undesired sex; I know of one case where the woman in the delivery room, on being informed that her child was a son, told the physician that she did not even wish to see it and that he should get rid of it. We may judge her attitude to be pathological, but even pathological suffering is suffering. Would such suffering justify aborting her normal male fetus?

Or take the converse case of two parents, who for their own very peculiar reasons, wish to have an abnormal child, say, a child who will suffer from the same disease as grandfather or a child whose arrested development would preclude the threat of adolescent rebellion and separation. Are these acceptable grounds for the abortion of "normals"?

Granted, such cases will be rare. But they serve to show the dangers inherent in talking about the parental right to determine, according to their wishes, the quality of their children. Indeed, the whole idea of parental rights with respect to children strikes me as problematic. It suggests that children are like property, that they exist for the parents. One need only look around to see some of the results of this notion of parenthood. The language of duties to children would be more in keeping with the heavy responsibility we bear in affirming the continuity of life with life and in trying to transmit what wisdom we have acquired to the next generation. Our children are not our children. Hopefully, reflection on these matters could lead to a greater appreciation of why it is people do and should have children. No better consequence can be hoped for from the advent of amniocentesis and other technologies for controlling human reproduction.

If one speaks of familial good in terms of parental duty, one could argue that parents have an obligation to do what they can to insure that their children are born healthy and sound. But this formulation transcends the limitation of parental wishes and desires. As in the case of the good society, the idea of "healthy and sound" requires an objective standard, a standard in reality. Hard as it may be to uncover it, this is what we are seeking. Nature as a standard is the third alternative.

The justification according to the natural standard might run like this. As a result of our knowledge of genetic diseases, we know that persons afflicted with certain diseases will never be capable of living the full life of a human being. Just as a no-necked giraffe could never live a giraffe's life, or a needleless porcupine would not attain true "porcupine-hood," so a child or fetus with Tay-Sachs disease or Down's syndrome, for example, will never be truly human. They will never be able to care for themselves, nor have they even the potential for developing the distinctively human capacities for thought or self-consciousness. Nature herself has aborted many similar cases, and has provided for the early death of many who happen to get born. There is no reason to keep them alive; instead, we should prevent their birth by contraception or sterilization if possible, and abortion if necessary.

The advantages of this approach are clear. The standards are objective and in the fetus itself, thus avoiding the relativity and ambiguity in societal and parental good. The standard can be easily generalized to cover all such cases and will be resistant to the shifting sands of public opinion.

This standard, I would suggest, is the one which most physicians and genetic counselors appeal to in their heart of hearts, no matter what they say or do about letting the parents choose. Why else would they have developed genetic counseling and amniocentesis? Indeed, the notions of disease, of abnormal, of defective, make no sense at all in the absence of a natural norm of health. This norm is the foundation of the art of the physician and of the inquiry of the health scientist. Yet, as Motulsky and others in this volume have pointed out, the standard is elusive. Ironically, we are gaining increasing power to manipulate and control our own nature at a time in which we are increasingly confused about what is normal, healthy, and fit.

Although possibly acceptable in principle, the natural standard runs into problems in application when attempts are made to fix the boundary between potentially human and potentially not human. Professor Lejeune (1970) has clearly demonstrated the difficulty, if not the impossibility, of setting clear molecular, cytological, or developmental signposts for this boundary. Attempts to induce signposts by considering the phenotypes of the worst cases is equally difficult. Which features would we take to be the most relevant in, say, Tay-Sachs disease, Lesch-Nyhan syndrome, Cri du chat, Down's syndrome? Certainly, severe mental retardation. But how "severe" is "severe"? As Abraham Lincoln and I argued earlier, mental retardation admits of degree. It too is relative. Moreover, it is not clear that certain other defects and deformities might not equally foreclose the possibility of a truly or fully human life. What about blindness or deafness? Quadriplegia? Aphasia? Several of these in combination? Not only does each kind of defect admit of a continuous scale of severity, but it also merges with other defects on a continuous scale of defectiveness. Where on this scale is the line to be drawn: after mental retardation? blindness? muscular dystrophy? cystic fibrosis? hemophilia? diabetes? galactosemia? Turner's syndrome? XYY? club foot? Moreover, the identical two continuous scales—kind and severity—are found also among the living. In fact, it is the natural standard which may be the most dangerous one in that it leads most directly to the idea that there are second-class human beings and subhuman human beings.

But the story is not complete. The very idea of nature is ambiguous. According to one view, the one I have been using, nature points to or implies a peak, a perfection. According to this view, human rights depend upon attaining the status of humanness. The fetus is only potential; it has no rights, according to this view. But all kinds of people fall short of the norm: children, idiots, some adults. This understanding of nature has been used to justify not only abortion and infanticide, but also slavery.

There is another notion of nature, less splendid, more humane and, though less able to sustain a notion of health, more acceptable to the findings of modern science. Animal nature is characterized by impulses of self-preservation and by the capacity to feel pleasure and to suffer pain. Man and other animals are alike on this understanding of nature. And the right to life is ascribed to all such self-preserving and suffering creatures. Yet on this understanding of nature, the fetus—even a defective fetus—is not potential, but actual. The right to life belongs to him. But for this reason, this understanding of nature does not provide and may even deny what it is we are seeking, namely a justification for genetic abortion, adequate unto itself, which does not simultaneously justify infanticide, homicide, and enslavement of the genetically abnormal.

There is a third understanding of nature, akin to the second, nature as sacrosanct, nature as created by a Creator. Indeed, to speak about this reminds us that there is a fourth possible standard for judgments about genetic abortion: the religious standard. I shall leave the discussion of this standard to those who are able to speak of it in better faith.

Now that I am at the end, the reader can better share my sense of frustration. I have failed to provide myself with a satisfactory intellectual and moral justification for the practice of genetic abortion. Perhaps others more able than I can supply one. Perhaps the pragmatists can persuade me that we should abandon the search for principled justification, that if we just trust people's situational decisions or their gut reactions, everything will turn out fine. Maybe they are right. But we should not forget the sage observation of Bertrand Russell: "Pragmatism is like a warm bath that heats up so imperceptibly that you don't know when to scream." I would add that before we submerge ourselves irrevocably in amniotic fluid, we take note of the connection to our own baths, into which we have started the hot water running.

Notes

1. This strikes me as by far the most important inference to be drawn from the fact that men in different times and cultures have answered the abortion question differently. Seen in this light, the differing and changing answers themselves suggest that it is a question not easily put under, at least not for very long.

2. Other ways include: one should not do violence to living or growing things; life is sacred; respect nature; fetal life has value; refrain from taking innocent life; protect and preserve life. As some have pointed out, the terms chosen are of different weight, and would require reasons of different weight to tip the balance in favor of abortion. My choice of the "rights" terminology is not meant to beg the questions of whether such rights really exist, or of where they come from. However, the notion of a "fetal right to life" presents only a little more difficulty in this regard than does the notion of a "human right to life," since the former does not depend on a claim that the human fetus is already "human." In my sense of the terms "right" and "life," we might even say that a dog or a fetal dog has a "right to life," and that it would be cruel and immoral for a man to go around performing abortions even on dogs for no good reason.

3. For a discussion of the possible biological rather than moral price of attempts to prevent the birth of defective children, see Neel (1970) and Motulsky, Fraser, and Felsenstein (1971).

4. I assume this calculation ignores the possibilities of inflation, devaluation, and revolution.

References

Buck, P. S. (1968). Foreword to *The Terrible Choice: The Abortion Dilemma*. New York: Bantam Books, pp. ix–xi.

Cassell, E. (1969). "Death and the Physician," Commentary (June), pp. 73–79.

Lejeune J. (1970). *American Journal of Human Genetics*, 22, p. 121.

Lincoln, A. (1854). In *The Collected Works of Abraham Lincoln*, R. P. Basler, editor. New Brunswick, N.J.: Rutgers University Press, Vol. II, p. 222.

Motulsky, A. G., G. R. Fraser, and J. Felsenstein (1971). In Symposium on Intrauterine Diagnosis, D. Bergsma, editor. *Birth Defects: Original Article Series*, Vol. 7, No. 5.

Neel, J. (1972). In *Early Diagnosis of Human Genetic Defects: Scientific and Ethical Considerations*, M. Harris, editor. Washington, D.C.: U.S. Government Printing Office, pp. 366–380.

Moral Issues in Human Genetics: Counseling or Control?

Ruth Macklin

Critics of genetic screening and selective abortion have often charged that it is only a small social step from such programs to the practice of eugenics. Ruth Macklin reviews four arguments against any proposal to establish a eugenics program. Macklin holds that, if we accept these arguments as sound, then there is no justification for restricting individual decision making in matters of reproduction for eugenic considerations. Eugenics programs are likely to be misguided or dangerous, and decisions about genetic screening, selective abortion, and the like are best left to the individuals concerned.

The notion of genetic engineering appears to have a narrower and a broader definition. The narrow conception refers to approaches involving laboratory manipulation of genes or cells: somatic cell alteration and germ cell alteration.[1] When this meaning is assigned to genetic engineering, the term 'eugenics' is used to refer to selection of parents or of their germ cells.[2] But sometimes the term 'genetic engineering' is used in a fully general sense, to refer to any manipulation of the reproductive acts or capacities of persons or their parts. It is this latter sense that will be used in the remainder of this account.

At least the idea behind eugenics—if not the practice itself in some form—is ancient. Positive eugenics was promoted in Plato's *Republic*, long before the science of genetics provided the theoretical basis and systematic data that today's proponents of genetic engineering have to work with. The lack of personal freedoms allowed the citizens in the *Republic* is well known to those familiar with Plato's work, and is evident in the following passage discussing regulation of unions between the sexes:

> It is for you, then, as their lawgiver, who have already selected the men, to select for association with them women who are so far as possible of the same natural capacity. . . . [A]nything like unregulated unions would be a profanation in a state whose citizens lead the good life. The Rulers will not allow such a thing. . . . [I]f we are to keep our flock at the highest pitch of excellence, there should be as many unions of the best of both sexes, and as few of the inferior, as possible, and . . . only the offspring of the better unions should be kept. . . . Moreover, young men who acquit themselves well in war and other duties, should be given, among other rewards and privileges, more liberal opportunities to sleep with a wife, for the further purpose that, with good excuse,

as many as possible of the children may be begotten of such fathers.[3]

But lest we conclude that a eugenics movement can only be promoted or gain adherents in a rigidly controlled society like Plato's *Republic* or a totalitarian regime such as Nazi Germany, let us consider the view of a 20th century Nobel Prize winning geneticist. The late Hermann Muller was an arch proponent of positive eugenics, based on his belief that the human gene pool is deteriorating. Muller argued for voluntary programmes of positive eugenics, rejecting any form of state-imposed regulations. He claimed that "democratic control . . . implies an upgrading of the people in general in both their intellectual and social faculties, together with a maintenance or, preferably, an improvement in their bodily condition."[4] Muller was one of a number of contemporary geneticists who have made gloomy prophecies about the increasing load of mutations in the human gene pool. The particular brand of positive eugenics that he advocated was a voluntary artificial insemination programme using donor semen (AID). He envisaged preserving the semen of outstanding men for future use in artificial insemination, choosing such greats as Einstein, Pasteur, Descartes, Leonardo and Lincoln as men whose child no woman would refuse to bear.[5]

Muller's method of freezing the semen of intellectual and creative men is only one of several proposals favouring some form of *positive* eugenics—a programme for improving the species, breeding a better race, or trying to prevent further deterioration by taking active countermeasures. Greater attention has been directed to the question of whether *negative* eugenics should be practiced on carriers or those afflicted with heritable diseases, in the form of enforced or encouraged abortions, sterilization, or less repressive but nonetheless coercive measures. The

Reprinted by permission from Dialogue, *Vol. XVI, no. 3 (1977), pp. 386–396.* [Editor's note. *In the first part of this article, which is omitted here, Macklin discusses genetic counseling and argues that individuals "should have final decision-making authority" in matters of reproduction when "the reasons for these decisions refer to genetic factors."*]

dilemma of choosing between preserving the individual freedom to marry and procreate as one chooses, and preventing further pollution of the gene pool would, indeed, pose an agonizing moral choice if the facts were as clear-cut as the eugenicists take them to be. There seems, however, to be enough uncertainty about the possible and probable outcomes of any attempts at eugenics to warrant extreme caution in mounting such grandiose schemes for genetic improvement. Many scientists agree that trying to reduce the load of mutations in the human gene pool through negative eugenics would be ineffective, at best. And the arguments against positive eugenics point to a number of potentially infelicitous outcomes. There are at least five separate arguments against the feasibility or desirability of any large-scale attempt at genetic engineering for eugenic purposes—arguments which, if taken together, give strong support to my conclusion that genetic engineering with this aim is misguided or dangerous or both. A sixth argument is the religious one that creating or modifying the human species is a task not for man, but for God.[6] For those to whom this sort of argument is compelling, it may lend added strength to the other five. I shall confine my discussion to four of the five considerations that do not require belief in a supernatural deity. Each of the following arguments against a systematic effort to mount any sort of eugenics programme will be discussed in turn below:

1. We're too ignorant to do it right;

2. In any case, we are likely to alter the gene pool for ill;

3. Negative eugenics can't possibly work unless carriers are eliminated, but this would soon eliminate the entire species;

4. Some methods of genetic engineering carry grave moral risks of mishap.

The fifth argument is essentially that most—if not all—methods of genetic engineering are dehumanizing in basic ways.[7] While I think this attack contains some interesting points and raises questions of the value that generally deserve important consideration, it is a gratuitous argument in this context. If the first four arguments are sound, they obviate the necessity for the fifth, since the scientific and practical objections to eugenic programmes would rule them out before the value issues need be brought into consideration. So I shall treat only the first four arguments in what follows.

(1) The claim that we are too ignorant to do the job right has several variants, each with significant implications. The first consideration points to our general ignorance about the value of a gene to a given race to the species. As one prominent geneticist notes:

> We know only about its value to the individual carrying it and then only in instances where the effect is severe. In the light of such ignorance, it seems to me that the best procedure is to avoid all changes in the environment which are likely to change the mutation rate. . . . The quality of a gene or genotype may be determined only by the reaction of the associated phenotype in the environment in which it exists. A phenotype may be disadvantageous in some environments, essentially neutral in others, and advantageous in others. In the face of a rapidly changing and entirely new environment (new in an evolutionary sense), I do not believe that we can determine the value of specific genotypes to the species.[8]

This brand of ignorance constitutes our lack of knowledge of what to select for—a form of ignorance that some may argue is confined to the present state of development of the science of genetics. But a second variant of the "we're too ignorant" argument notes that "if we alter the gene pool, independent of environment, we are acting on the basis of present environmental criteria to select a gene pool for the future. Since the environment is changing a thousandfold times faster than our gene pool, it would be a disastrous approach.[9] But the difficulty here is not simply one of our inability to predict accurately what the future will be like. Questions of value enter in—questions that invariably resurrect the memory of attempts at positive eugenics among the Nazis. One writer asks:

> Who will be the judges and where will be the separation between good and bad? The most difficult decisions will come in defining the borderline cases. Will we breed against tallness because space requirements become more critical? Will we breed against nearsightedness because people with glasses may not make good astronauts? Will we forbid intellectually inferior individuals from procreating despite their proved ability to produce a number of superior individuals?[10]

The last variant on the "we're too ignorant" theme that we shall consider here requires us to recall Hermann Muller's proposal for positive eugenics. Muller would not be alone in including Abraham Lincoln on a list of men whose child no woman would refuse to bear. Yet there is now considerable evidence that Lincoln was afflicted with Marfan's syndrome, a heritable disease of the connective tissue that is transmitted by a dominant gene. The evidence is based on a number of factors. Lincoln's bodily characteristics and facial features—the very qualities we term "Lincolnesque"—are typical features of bone deformities common to Marfan's syndrome. The disease was first named in 1896, some thirty years after Lincoln's death. It was believed for some time that Lincoln had Marfan's disease, on the basis of physical defects he was known to have had, as well as the early death of one of his children. One sign of the disease was Lincoln's abnormally long limbs. Also, casts made of Lincoln's body in the year of his inauguration reveal that his left hand was much longer than his right hand, and his left middle finger was elongated. He is also known to have suffered from severe farsightedness, in addition to having difficulty with his eyesight that stemmed from distortions in his facial bone structure. These bodily asymmetries are common to Marfan's syndrome, as is cardiac disease. It is believed that Lincoln inherited the disease from his father's side. His father was blind in one eye, his son Robert had difficulties with his eyes, and his son Tad had a speech defect and died at the age of eighteen, probably from cardiac trouble. The likelihood that Lincoln himself suffered from Marfan's syndrome was further confirmed in 1959, when a California physician named Harold Schwartz recognized the disease in a boy of seven who was known to share an ancestor with Lincoln.[11] Since the gene for Marfan's disease is dominant, those who have it and reach child-bearing age stand a fifty percent chance of having an afflicted child.

Now consider the consequences for the gene pool if Lincoln's frozen sperm were to be disseminated widely in the population. At least until the facts became evident, the result would be exactly the opposite of what Muller intended by his proposal. And if the mistake went beyond the case of Lincoln and Marfan's syndrome, including other individuals who, despite their outstanding achievements might be afflicted with or be carriers of other little known or as yet undiagnosed genetic diseases, the results would be dysgenic in the extreme. This last consideration leads directly to the second argument against eugenics programmes to which we turn next.

(2) This argument holds that in any event, we are likely to alter the gene pool for ill. Leaving aside the less likely incidence of this occurrence as exemplified just now in the Abraham Lincoln story, we may look at another prominent consideration noted by some geneticists.

This consideration is often referred to as "heterozygote advantage." One geneticist explains as follows:

> There is . . . good evidence that individuals who carry two different forms of the same gene, that is, are heterozygous, appear to have an advantage. This is true even if that gene in double dose, that is, in the homozygous state, produces a severe disease. For example, individuals homozygous for the gene coding for sickle-cell hemoglobin invariably develop sickle-cell anemia which is generally fatal before the reproductive years. Heterozygotes for the gene are, however, protected more than normals from the effects of the most malignant form of malaria. It has been shown that women who carry the gene in single dose have a higher fertility in malarial areas than do normals.[12]

Here again, it is not only in the cases where there is known heterozygote advantage that the likelihood exists of altering the gene pool for ill by trying to eliminate genes for heritable diseases. There are, in addition, all of the cases where heterozygote advantage may exist but is at present unknown. If one uses risk-benefit ratios or something like a utilitarian schema for deciding moral issues in biomedical contexts, the evidence seems clearly to indicate a greater risk of dysgenic consequences than a possibility of beneficial results from attempts to alter the human gene pool by means of negative eugenics. A successful effort to eliminate carriers for heritable diseases would result at the same time in eliminating heterozygote advantage, which is believed to be beneficial to the species or to sub-populations within the species. While little is known at the present stage of inquiry in genetics about all of the particular advantages that exist, it is an inference made by many experts in the field on the basis of present data and well-confirmed genetic theory. One biologist asks us to:

Consider the gene leading to cystic fibrosis (C.F.). Until quite recently homozygotes for this gene died in infancy. Yet the gene causing C.F. is very common among all Caucasoid populations thus far studied. . . . It is too widespread in the race to be accounted for by genetic drift. The gene is also too frequent for it to be likely to be maintained by mutation pressure. Hence, we are driven to assume heterozygote advantage.[13]

It would seem, then, that what is gained by the elimination of homozygotes may well be lost by the elimination of heterozygotes, resulting in no clear benefits and possibly some significant disadvantages in populations that suffer from genetic diseases. But the argument just given assumes that it would in fact be possible to eliminate genes for heritable diseases by preventing carriers from reproducing and thereby passing on such genes to future generations. The next argument against genetic engineering questions such a possibility.

(3) This argument maintains, in sum, that negative eugenics can't possibly work unless carriers are eliminated as well as diseased individuals; but a successful attempt to prevent all carriers of potentially lethal genes from reproducing would effectively eliminate the entire species. The effects of negative eugenics on the general population are assessed by one geneticist as follows:

With a few exceptions, dominant diseases are rare and interfere severely with reproductive ability. They are generally maintained in the population by new mutations. Therefore, there is either no need or essentially no need for discouraging these individuals from reproduction . . . The story is quite different for recessive conditions. . . . [A]ny attempt to decrease the gene frequency of these common genetic disorders in the population by prevention of fertility of all carriers would be doomed to failure. First, we all carry between three and eight of these genes in a single dose. Secondly, for many of these conditions, the frequency of carriers in the population is about 1 in 50 or even greater. Prevention of fertility for even one of these disorders would stop a sizable proportion of the population from reproducing. . . .[14]

If this assessment is sound, it has significant implications for the prospects of favorably altering the human gene pool by negative eugenics. Such an argument is persuasive if the purpose of negative eugenics is viewed as that of improving the human gene pool for the sake of future generations. But if the purpose of negative eugenics is seen as improving the quality of life for those in the present and next generation, then the argument just given is beside the point. We should recall the dual purpose for which proposals for genetic engineering are put forth. The one we have been discussing here is the proposed improvement or prevention of deterioration of the gene pool for the sake of future generations of humans. The other purpose, tied to voluntary genetic screening programmes and the activity of genetic counseling, is to present options to individuals or couples that will help them avoid the birth of a defective child whose quality of life will be poor and who will most likely be a burden on both parents and society. For this latter purpose, the practice of negative eugenics through voluntary screening and sensitive genetic counseling can serve to improve the quality of life of persons in this and the next generation. But when transformed into a programme designed to control the reproductive acts or capacities of people for the sake of future generations, then the practice of negative eugenics seems to be scientifically and practically misguided. Indeed, taking this argument and the previous one together, the conclusion may be put succinctly in the words of one writer:

Neither positive nor negative eugenics can ever significantly improve the gene pool of the population and simultaneously allow for adequate evolutionary improvement of the human race. The only useful aspect of negative eugenics is in individual counseling of specific families in order to prevent some of the births of abnormal individuals.[15]

(4) The fourth argument against genetic engineering focuses specifically on those practices involving manipulation of genetic material itself. This argument raises questions about the grave risks involved in any such manipulation, especially since mishaps that may arise are likely to be far worse than what happens when nature takes its course. One geneticist sees the prospects as follows:

The problem of altering an individual's genes by direct chemical change of his DNA presents technically an enormously difficult task. Even if it became possible to do this, the chance of error would be high. Such an error, of course, would have the diametrically opposite effect to that desired and would be irreversible; in other words, the individual would become even more abnormal.[16]

Some observers fear the creation of hapless monsters as a result of various manipulations on genetic material. Whether or not the laboratory techniques are sufficiently refined at present to enable researchers to develop procedures for widespread use, it is likely that these techniques will be available soon enough to deserve careful reflection now. We need to ask, once again, whether the purpose served by laboratory methods of genetic engineering is helping those who are at risk for bearing defective children to prevent such occurrences, or instead, breeding a genetically improved species for the future. If such techniques are perfected and become available for use in spite of the attendant risks of mishap, they would then be offered to couples on a voluntary basis in the same way that current methods of genetic intervention are employed. Where a practice is aimed at the genetic improvement of a couple's own progeny, there are no grounds for methods that involve coercion. What is needed in such cases is counseling and education, not coercion and control.

At the outset, I said I would argue for two separate but related theses. First, the individual or couple should have final decision-making authority in matters of his or her own reproductive acts and capacities, as well as continuation or termination of pregnancy where the reasons for these decisions refer to genetic factors. Second, attempts at government-based or scientist-directed eugenic programmes are bound to be misguided or dangerous or both. The four arguments at the end were offered in support of the second thesis. If those arguments are sound, they demonstrate that there is no warrant for those in power to take final decision-making authority away from the individual where the reasons for such actions refer to eugenic considerations. Recall also our earlier conclusion that final decision-making should be left to the individual or couple in the context of genetic counseling, except in cases where the decision requires medical expertise that a patient is unlikely to have. Now if genetic screening should be practiced on a voluntary basis; and if decisions arising out of counseling should be left to the individual; and if in addition, positive and negative eugenics aimed at future generations is basically misguided; then there seems to be only one consideration remaining that might argue in favour of limiting individual rights for the sake of social benefits. That consideration points to the burden placed on society for treating and maintaining defective infants and others who might have been aborted or never even conceived by dint of state policy. Time does not permit an examination of this last issue, but is worth making a final observation in closing. If the notion of social benefit is understood largely in terms of increased financial resources that would otherwise be allocated to caring for those afflicted with heritable diseases, then something crucial is being left out of the balance between individual rights and social benefits. What is socially beneficial must be viewed not only in terms of increases in financial and other tangible resources, but also in terms of a range of freedom and autonomy that members of a society can reasonably expect to enjoy. It is important to preserve that freedom and autonomy through insuring the individual's right to decide about his or her own reproductive acts and capacities. With increased availability of voluntary genetic screening programmes and widespread education of the public, it is hard to imagine that most people will choose to burden themselves and society with defective children when other options are open to them. Even if there are some who refuse screening or abortion, society as a whole would be better off to accommodate their freely chosen reproductive acts than to impose compulsory genetic screening, abortion, or sterilization on its members.

Notes

1. Bernard D. Davis, "Threat and Promise in Genetic Engineering," ed. by Preston Williams in *Ethical Issues in Biology and Medicine* (Cambridge, Mass.: Schenkman Publishing Company, 1973), pp. 17–24.

2. *Ibid.*

3. Francis MacDonald Cornford (tr.), *The Republic of Plato* (New York: Oxford University Press), pp. 157–60.

4. Hermann J. Muller, "Genetic Progress by Voluntarily Conducted Germinal Choice," ed. by Gordon Wolstenholme, in *Man and His Future* (Boston: Little, Brown and Co., 1963), p. 256.

5. Theodosius Dobzhansky, *Mankind Evolving* (New Haven: Yale University Press, 1962), p. 328.

6. Such arguments are offered by Paul Ramsey in *Fabricated Man* (New Haven: Yale University Press, 1970).

7. This argument is given by Ramsey, *op. cit.*, and also by Leon R. Kass, "Making Babies—The New Biology and the 'Old' Morality," *The Public Interest*, Vol. 26, Winter, 1972.

8. Arthur Steinberg, "The Genetic Pool. Its Evolution and Significance—'Desirable' and 'Undesirable'

Genetic Traits," in C.I.O.M.S. *Recent Progress in Biology and Medicine*, pp. 83–93.

9. Kurt Hirschhorn, "Symposium: Ethics of Genetic Counseling," *Contemporary OB/GYN*," Vol. 2, no. 4, p. 128.

10. Kurt Hirschhorn, "Practical and Ethical Problems in Human Genetics," *Birth Defects*, Vol. VIII, July, 1972, p. 28.

11. *Ibid.* p. 23.

12. Steinberg, *op. cit.*

13. Rene Dubos and Maya Pines, *Health and Disease* (New York: Time, Inc., 1965), pp. 123–24.

14. Kurt Hirschhorn, "Practical and Ethical Problems in Human Genetics," pp. 22–23.

15. *Ibid*, p. 25.

16. *Ibid*, p. 27.

Genetics and Human Malleability

W. French Anderson

Anderson argues that gene transplants should be used only for the treatment of serious diseases and should never be performed for the purpose of "improving" human beings. Somatic cell therapy can be supported by the principle of beneficence, but any change that would detract from "the dignity of man" would be wrong. Anderson admits that it might be difficult to draw the line between serious diseases and conditions that we might want to treat, but he emphasizes that we should reject all forms of "enhancement engineering." (Anderson was a member of the team that performed the first authorized gene transfer in September 1990.)

Just how much can and should we change human nature . . . by genetic engineering? Our response to that hinges on the answers to three further questions: (1) What *can* we do now? Or more precisely, what *are* we doing now in the area of human genetic engineering? (2) What *will* we be able to do? In other words, what technical advances are we likely to achieve over the next five to ten years? (3) What *should* we do? I will argue that a line can be drawn and should be drawn to use gene transfer only for the treatment of serious disease, and not for any other purpose. Gene transfer should never be undertaken in an attempt to enhance or "improve" human beings.

What Can We Do?

In 1980 John Fletcher and I published a paper in the *New England Journal of Medicine* in which we delineated what would be necessary before it would be ethical to carry out human gene therapy.[1] As with any other new therapeutic procedure, the fundamental principle is that it should be determined in advance that the probable benefits outweigh the probable risks. We analyzed the risk/benefit determination for somatic cell gene therapy and proposed three questions that need to have been answered from prior animal experimentation: Can the new gene be inserted stably into the correct target cells? Will the new gene be expressed (that is, function) in the cells at an appropriate level? Will the new gene harm the cell or the animal? These criteria are very similar to those required before use of any new therapeutic procedure, surgical operation, or drug. They simply require that the new treatment should get to the area of disease, correct it, and do more good than harm.

A great deal of scientific progress has occurred in the nine years since that paper was published. The technology does now exist for inserting genes into some types of target cells.[2] The procedure being used is called "retroviral-mediated gene transfer."

From The Hastings Center Report, *January/February 1990, pp. 21–24. Reprinted by permission of the author.*

In brief, a disabled murine retrovirus serves as a delivery vehicle for transporting a gene into a population of cells that have been removed from a patient. The gene-engineered cells are then returned to the patient.

The first clinical application of this procedure was approved by the National Institutes of Health and the Food and Drug Administration on January 19, 1989.[3] Our protocol received the most thorough prior review of any clinical protocol in history: It was approved only after being reviewed fifteen times by seven different regulatory bodies. In the end it received unanimous approval from every one of those committees. But the simple fact that the NIH and FDA, as well as the public, felt that the protocol needed such extensive review demonstrates that the concept of gene therapy raises serious concerns.

We can answer our initial question, "What can we do now in the area of human genetic engineering?," by examining this approved clinical protocol. Gene transfer is used to mark cancer-fighting cells in the body as a way of better understanding a new form of cancer therapy. The cancer-fighting cells are called TIL (tumor-infiltrating-lymphocytes), and are isolated from a patient's own tumor, grown up to a large number, and then given back to the patient along with one of the body's immune growth factors, a molecule called interleuken 2 (IL-2). The procedure, developed by Steven Rosenberg of the NIH, is known to help about half the patients treated.[4]

The difficulty is that there is at present no way to study the TIL once they are returned to the patient to determine why they work when they do work (that is, kill cancer cells), and why they do not work when they do not work. The goal of the gene transfer protocol was to put a label on the infused TIL, that is, to mark these cells so that they could be studied in blood and tumor specimens from the patient over time.

The TIL were marked with a vector (called N2) containing a bacterial gene that could be easily identified through recombinant DNA techniques. Our protocol was called, therefore, the N2-TIL Human Gene Transfer Clinical Protocol. The first patient received gene-marked TIL on May 22, 1989. Five patients have now received marked cells. No side effects or problems have thus far arisen from the gene transfer portion of the therapy. Useful data on the fate of the gene-marked TIL are being obtained.

But what was done that was new? Simply, a single gene was inserted into a population of cells that had been obtained from a patient's body. There are an estimated 100,000 genes in every human cell. Therefore the actual addition of material was extremely minute, nothing to correspond to the fears expressed by some that human beings would be "re-engineered." Nonetheless, a functioning piece of genetic material was successfully inserted into human cells and the gene-engineered cells did survive in human patients.

What Will We Be Able to Do?

Although only one clinical protocol is presently being conducted, it is clear that there are several applications for gene transfer that probably will be carried out over the next five to ten years. Many genetic diseases that are caused by a defect in a single gene should be treatable, such as ADA deficiency (a severe immune deficiency disease of children), sickle cell anemia, hemophilia, and Gaucher disease. Some types of cancer, viral diseases such as AIDS, and some forms of cardiovascular disease are targets for treatment by gene therapy. In addition, germline gene therapy, that is, the insertion of a gene into the reproductive cells of a patient, will probably be technically possible in the foreseeable future. My position on the ethics of germline gene therapy is published elsewhere.[5]

But successful somatic cell gene therapy also opens the door for enhancement genetic engineering, that is, for supplying a specific characteristic that individuals might want for themselves (somatic cell engineering) or their children (germline engineering) which would not involve the treatment of a disease. The most obvious example at the moment would be the insertion of a growth hormone gene into a normal child in the hope that this would make the child grow larger. Should parents be allowed to choose (if the science should ever make it possible) whatever useful characteristics they wish for their children?

What Should We Do?

A line can and should be drawn between somatic cell gene therapy and enhancement genetic engineering.[6] Our society has repeatedly demonstrated that it can draw a line in biomedical research when necessary. The Belmont Report illustrates how guidelines were formulated to delineate ethical from unethical clinical research and to distinguish clinical research from clinical practice. Our responsibility is to determine how and where to draw lines with respect to genetic engineering.

Somatic cell gene therapy for the treatment of severe disease is considered ethical because it can be supported by the fundamental moral principle of beneficence: It would relieve human suffering. Gene therapy would be, therefore, a moral good. Under what circumstances would human genetic engineering not be a moral good? In the broadest sense, when it detracts from, rather than contributes to, the dignity of man. Whether viewed from a theological perspective or a secular humanist one, the justification for drawing a line is founded on the argument that, beyond the line, human values that our society considers important for the dignity of man would be significantly threatened.

Somatic cell enhancement engineering would threaten important human values in two ways: It could be medically hazardous, in that the risks could exceed the potential benefits and the procedure therefore cause harm. And it would be morally precarious, in that it would require moral decisions our society is not now prepared to make, and it could lead to an increase in inequality and discriminatory practices.

Medicine is a very inexact science. We understand roughly how a simple gene works and that there are many thousands of housekeeping genes, that is, genes that do the job of running a cell. We predict that there are genes which make regulatory messages that are involved in the overall control and regulation of the many housekeeping genes. Yet we have only limited understanding of how a body organ develops into the size and shape it does. We know many things about how the central nervous system works—for example, we are beginning to comprehend how molecules are involved in electric circuits, in memory storage, in transmission of signals. But we are a long way from understanding thought and consciousness. And we are even further from understanding the spiritual side of our existence.

Even though we do not understand how a thinking, loving, interacting organism can be derived from its molecules, we are approaching the time when we can change some of those molecules. Might there be genes that influence the brain's or-

ganization or structure or metabolism or circuitry in some way so as to allow abstract thinking, contemplation of good and evil, fear of death, awe of a "God"? What if in our innocent attempts to improve our genetic make-up we alter one or more of those genes? Could we test for the alteration? Certainly not at present. If we caused a problem that would affect the individual or his or her offspring, could we repair the damage? Certainly not at present. Every parent who has several children knows that some babies accept and give more affection than others, in the same environment. Do genes control this? What if these genes were accidentally altered? How would we even know if such a gene were altered?

My concern is that, at this point in the development of our culture's scientific expertise, we might be like the young boy who loves to take things apart. He is bright enough to disassemble a watch, and maybe even bright enough to get it back together again so that it works. But what if he tries to "improve" it? Maybe put on bigger hands so that the time can be read more easily. But if the hands are too heavy for the mechanism, the watch will run slowly, erratically, or not at all. The boy can understand what is visible, but he cannot comprehend the precise engineering calculations that determined exactly how strong each spring should be, why the gears interact in the ways that they do, etc. Attempts on his part to improve the watch will probably only harm it. We are now able to provide a new gene so that a property involved in a human life would be changed, for example, a growth hormone gene. If we were to do so simply because we could, I fear we would be like that young boy who changed the watch's hands. We, too, do not really understand what makes the object we are tinkering with tick.

In summary, it could be harmful to insert a gene into humans. In somatic cell gene therapy for an already existing disease the potential benefits could outweigh the risks. In enhancement engineering, however, the risks would be greater while the benefits would be considerably less clear.

Yet even aside from the medical risks, somatic cell enhancement engineering should not be performed because it would be morally precarious. Let us assume that there were no medical risks at all from somatic cell enhancement engineering. There would still be reasons for objecting to this procedure. To illustrate, let us consider some examples. What if a human gene were cloned that could produce a brain chemical resulting in markedly increased memory capacity in monkeys after gene transfer? Should a person be allowed to receive such a gene on request? Should a pubescent adolescent whose parents are both five feet tall be provided with a growth hormone gene on request? Should a worker who is continually exposed to an industrial toxin receive a gene to give him resistance on his, or his employer's request?

These scenarios suggest three problems that would be difficult to resolve: What genes should be provided; who should receive a gene; and, how to prevent discrimination against individuals who do or do not receive a gene.

We allow that it would be ethically appropriate to use somatic cell gene therapy for treatment of serious disease. But what distinguishes a serious disease from a "minor" disease from cultural "discomfort"? What is suffering? What is significant suffering? Does the absence of growth hormone that results in a growth limitation to two feet in height represent a genetic disease? What about a limitation to a height of four feet, to five feet? Each observer might draw the lines between serious disease, minor disease, and genetic variation differently. But all can agree that there are extreme cases that produce significant suffering and premature death. Here then is where an initial line should be drawn for determining what genes should be provided: treatment of serious disease.

If the position is established that only patients suffering from serious diseases are candidates for gene insertion, then the issues of patient selection are no different than in other medical situations: the determination is based on medical need within a supply and demand framework. But if the use of gene transfer extends to allow a normal individual to acquire, for example, a memory-enhancing gene, profound problems would result. On what basis is the decision made to allow one individual to receive the gene but not another: Should it go to those best able to benefit society (the smartest already?)? To those most in need (those with low intelligence? But how low? Will enhancing memory help a mentally retarded child?)? To those chosen by a lottery? To those who can afford to pay? As long as our society lacks a significant consensus about these answers, the best way to make equitable decisions in this case

should be to base them on the seriousness of the objective medical need, rather than on the personal wishes or resources of an individual.

Discrimination can occur in many forms. If individuals are carriers of a disease (for example, sickle cell anemia), would they be pressured to be treated? Would they have difficulty in obtaining health insurance unless they agreed to be treated? These are ethical issues raised also by genetic screening and by the Human Genome project. But the concerns would become even more troublesome if there were the possibility for "correction" by the use of human genetic engineering.

Finally, we must face the issue of eugenics, the attempt to make hereditary "improvements." The abuse of power that societies have historically demonstrated in the pursuit of eugenic goals is well documented.[7] Might we slide into a new age of eugenic thinking by starting with small "improvements"? It would be difficult, if not impossible, to determine where to draw a line once enhancement engineering had begun. Therefore, gene transfer should be used only for the treatment of serious disease and not for putative improvements.

Our society is comfortable with the use of genetic engineering to treat individuals with serious disease. On medical and ethical grounds we should draw a line excluding any form of enhancement engineering. We should not step over the line that delineates treatment from enhancement.

References

1. W. French Anderson and John C. Fletcher, "Gene Therapy in Human Beings: When Is It Ethical to Begin?," *New England Journal of Medicine* 303:22 (1980), 1293–97.

2. See also W. French Anderson, "Prospects for Human Gene Therapy," *Science*, 26 October 1984, 401–409; T. Friedman, "Progress towards Human Gene Therapy," *Science*, 16 June 1989, 1275–81.

3. J. Wyngaarden, "Human Gene Transfer Protocol," *Federal Register* (1989), vol. 54, no. 47, pp. 10508–10510.

4. Steven A. Rosenberg *et al.*, "Use of Tumor-Infiltrating Lymphocytes and Interleukin-2 in the Immunotherapy of Patients with Metastatic Melanoma," *New England Journal of Medicine* 319:25 (1988), 1676–80.

5. W. French Anderson, "Human Gene Therapy: Scientific and Ethical Considerations," *Journal of Medicine and Philosophy* 10 (1985): 275–91.

6. W. French Anderson, "Human Gene Therapy: Why Draw a Line?," *Journal of Medicine and Philosophy* 14 (1989), 681–93.

7. See, for example, Kenneth M. Ludmerer, *Genetics and American Society* (Baltimore: The Johns Hopkins University Press, 1972), and Daniel J. Kevles, *In the Name of Eugenics* (New York: Alfred A. Knopf, 1985).

Decision Scenario 1 . . . .

"My mother was fifty when she died," Lauri Ross said. "From the time the first symptoms of Huntington's appeared until the time she died was about twelve years. It was terribly sad to watch. I would hate to think that I was going to put a child through the ordeal my sister and I suffered."

"Do you ever worry about yourself?" Dr. Haskins asked.

"About whether I'm going to develop Huntington's? Yes, I do. I know that there is a fifty-fifty chance that I will. I'm twenty-five now, and I can't keep from thinking about what the next ten or fifteen years may bring." Lauri smiled and shrugged. "But life has been pretty good to me in a lot of ways. We all have to go some way so I guess I'm prepared for it."

"You don't seem to have let the possibility affect your life too much. You've gone to college, established yourself in a career, gotten married. You've done all the things others do, and I think that's a tribute to your courage."

"I haven't done quite everything," Lauri said. "Bob and I would like to have children. Quite frankly, I don't know whether we should. That's connected with what I wanted to ask you. Is there any prenatal test that can be used to determine whether a child is going to have Huntington's? Or is there any test I can take that will show whether I'm going to have it?"

"Without going into detail, the answer is: not yet. If we had a lot of family history and we had blood samples from you and a large number of family members, it would be possible to use a genetic probe technique to see whether you are carrying the gene. But all of that is still in the experimental stage, and for the moment it doesn't offer any practical solution."

"So Bob and I just have to decide for ourselves whether we're willing to take the risk."

"Fundamentally, that is correct."

Lauri nodded. "What bothers me most, I guess, is that we also have to decide the fate of the potential child. I don't know whether it's right to saddle a child with our decision."

Dr. Haskins shrugged. "If you decide not to have a child, then you're deciding not to let that potential child live at all. Maybe it's better to allow the child at least some years of a normal life, rather than no life at all."

1. According to Purdy, would it be wrong for Lauri and Bob to decide to have no children?

2. On what grounds can it be argued that we have an obligation to provide every child with at least a normal opportunity for a good life?

3. Is there a right to reproduce? If so, does it override the duty to provide a child with a normal life?

Decision Scenario 2 . . . .

Sara Straus was frightened. She sat in the counselor's office with her hands folded in her lap, trying to look calm.

"Mrs. Straus," the counselor said, "I have the results back on your AFP test. I'm sorry to tell you that the level of alpha protein in your blood is quite high."

"What does that mean?" Mrs. Straus asked.

"It means," said the counselor, "that your chances of having a baby with what we call neural tube defect are quite high. Your child might be born with an open spine or with part of its brain missing."

"Oh, my God. Is there anything I can do?"

The counselor shook her head. "If you mean can you do anything to make the baby normal, the answer is no. This test is about 90% accurate. The only reasonable course is to have an abortion and begin another child when you feel ready."

"But I don't believe in abortion," said Mrs. Straus.

"There's no way we can force you to have one. But, according to the law, if you have been informed of the chances of a defect and do not have an abortion, then you and your husband must accept full financial responsibility for the care of the impaired child."

"How much would that cost?"

"Probably around $50,000 a year. "

"We can't afford that," said Mrs. Straus. "Nobody could afford to pay money like that."

"I'm just telling you the law," said the counselor.

"What if we have the child and then can't pay?"

"The law requires that you and your husband declare yourselves bankrupt. The child will then be placed in a public institution, and a fixed percentage of your future earnings will go to pay for its upkeep. Even after its death you must continue to pay until the accumulated costs to the state have been repaid."

"That's unfair," said Mrs. Straus. "We're being forced to go against what we think is right."

1. At this time, there is no such law as that mentioned by the counselor. Should there be such a law? After all, don't we generally believe that people should accept responsibility for their actions and decisions?

2. Is it ever right for society to force people to act in ways they consider to be morally wrong?

3. Does involuntary prenatal or genetic screening necessarily involve a violation of the autonomy of individuals?

4. Should screening programs be voluntary and advisory, or should they be backed up by laws that aim to protect society by requiring that individuals act in certain ways as a result of the screening?

5. Following Purdy's line of argument, might one claim that, when there is a reason to believe that a child may suffer from a serious genetic disease, the parents have a duty to undergo genetic screening?

Decision Scenario 3

"I'm sorry I wasn't able to bring you better news," Dr. Valery Mendez said. "I hope our first consultation helped prepare you for it."

Timothy Schwartz shook his head. "We gambled and lost," he said. "We can't say we didn't know what we were doing."

"That doesn't make it much easier," Judith Schwartz said. "When you said we were both Tay-Sachs carriers, I thought 'Well, it won't happen to us.' But I was wrong."

"The odds were in our favor," Mr. Schwartz said. "I still think we did the right thing."

"Maybe we shouldn't even have had ourselves tested," Mrs. Schwartz said. "Then we wouldn't even know we've got a problem."

"But we'd have one anyway," her husband said. "Ignorance is bliss only when it's folly to be wise. Now we at least know what we're up against."

"What about this new test?" Mrs. Schwartz asked. "Can we really trust the results?"

"I'm afraid so," said Dr. Mendez. "The fetal cells taken during amniocentesis were cultured, and

the chromosome study showed that the child you're carrying will have Tay-Sachs."

"What do you recommend?" Mr. Schwartz asked.

"It's not for me to recommend. I can give you some information—tell you the options—but you've got to make your own decision."

"Is abortion the only solution?" Mrs. Schwartz asked.

"If you call it a solution," Mr. Schwartz said.

"The disease is almost invariably fatal," Dr. Mendez said. "And there is really no effective treatment for it. A lot of people think there may be in the future, but that doesn't help right now."

"So what does it involve?" Mr. Schwartz asked.

"At first your child will seem quite normal, but that's only because it takes time for a particular chemical to build up in the brain. After the first year or so, the child will start to show signs of deterioration. He'll start losing his sight. Then, as brain damage progresses, he'll lose control over his muscles, and eventually he will die."

"And we just have to stand by and watch that happen?" Mrs. Schwartz asked.

"Nothing can be done to stop it," Dr. Mendez said. "It's a terrible and sad disease."

"We certainly do want to have a child," Mr. Schwartz said. "But we don't want to have one that is going to suffer all his life. I don't think I could stand that."

1.   How persuasive is Kass's argument that genetic abortion constitutes a threat to the principle that all persons are of equal worth?

2.   Can Purdy's argument that every child deserves a normal opportunity for a good life be used to justify requiring abortion in a case such as this?

3.   Kass contends that none of the three standards he examines can allow us to justify selective abortion. State and evaluate his arguments.

4.   How unfavorable must the odds be against having a normal child before (according to Purdy) parents have a duty not to reproduce? In what way is the seriousness of the disease at issue relevant to the odds?

Decision Scenario 4 . . . .

"The concept behind the bill is very simple, Senator," said Mrs. Laude. "We want to improve the human race, and we know exactly how to do it. The principles of genetics can be used to guide changes in the population."

"You mean," said the Senator, "you can make people smarter?"

"Not as individuals. But we can increase the level of intelligence in society. We can do this by seeing to it that intelligent people have more children than the less intelligent. Over time, the statistical balance will shift toward intelligence."

"And does your draft of the bill make that possible?"

"By a system of financial incentives and disincentives," said Mrs. Laude. "Those above a certain level of intelligence will be offered a yearly stipend to pay part of the expenses for each of their children. Those below that level will receive nothing, and, having to bear the full cost themselves, they are likely to limit the number of children they have. We will also make use of genetic counseling programs to encourage or discourage children, whatever is appropriate in each case."

"These genetic counseling programs will be government run and supported?" the Senator asked.

"That's right. The law will require that everyone be screened and classified before his or her fifteenth birthday."

"Is intelligence all that you'll screen for?"

"It's the only positive trait we will try to increase. We will also screen against genetic diseases, like Tay-Sachs and sickle-cell anemia."

"This will be very controversial, you know," said the Senator.

"We know," Mrs. Laude said. "It will take a person of courage to introduce such a bill into the Senate. But we think it's the most important piece of legislation imaginable. The improvement of our society and of the whole human race will be the end result."

1.   What problems and dangers are inherent in Mrs. Laude's proposal for a program of positive and negative eugenics?

2.   What can be said in defense of such a program?

3.   Would a utilitarian be likely to favor such a program?

4.   Could such a program be defended as compatible with Rawls's principles of justice?

5.   What arguments against any such program does Macklin present?

Decision Scenario 5 . . . .

"I don't know what your problem is," Harold Lucas said. "We have the opportunity to eliminate sickle-cell forever. This is a disease that has caused suffer-

ing and death to untold generations of human beings, yet you seem to want to keep it around. What possible reasons could you have?"

"I'm not sure you'll understand," Amy Lamont said. "I'm not in favor of sickle-cell. It's a horrible disease, and I have nothing but sympathy for those who have the disease or carry the trait."

"So, let's slice out the defective gene that produces the abnormal hemoglobin and splice in one that does the job right," Lucas said. "We can use somatic-cell therapy to treat those who have the disease now, but let's look to the future. Let's use cell-line therapy to modify the sex cell of the carriers and just get rid of the disease."

Amy Lamont shook her head. "It sounds humane, but it's not so easy as that," she said. "To do that means modifying human beings, and if we start doing that, I don't know when we would stop. We might do anything at all with them."

"You're afraid of some kind of wild eugenics scheme?"

"That's one problem I have," Amy Lamont said. "It's something deeper than that, though. I just don't like the idea of tampering with human life and human destiny. To change ourselves deliberately is, I think, to make us something less than human."

"If I understand you correctly, I couldn't disagree with you more," Harold Lucas said.

1. *Rephrase Amy Lamont's arguments so they are in an explicit form.*

2. *Possessing sickle-cell trait has been found to offer protection from a particular form of malaria. Is this an adequate reason for not eliminating the gene from the human gene pool, if we were able to do so?*

3. *Does Anderson share Lamont's point of view so far as eugenic enhancement is concerned?*

4. *Does Anderson endorse Lamont's objection that germ-line therapy would be wrong just because it alters the human genome?*

Decision Scenario 6 . . . .

"The screening program is for the *benefit* of our employees," Carl Larski said. "Amchem production involves radiologic agents and potentially harmful chemical substances. It is absolute madness not to monitor people for overexposure to radiation. I'm sure you agree with that. And it's ridiculous to expose women who are pregnant to a radiation hazard, because that could cause serious impairments in the child. Of course, sometimes women are pregnant for a while before they realize it, so it makes sense to keep all women of childbearing age away from radiation."

Susan Spencer shook her head to show that she disagreed. "You're using company policy to make decisions that people ought to make for themselves," she said. "If a woman wants to take a risk, she should be allowed to. After all, radiation can make men sterile, as well as causing them direct harm. Amchem's practices are inherently discriminatory. And they don't stop with radiation, and they don't stop with women. The company excludes African Americans from jobs that put them into contact with naphthalene."

"That's correct," Larski said. "That's because they are much more likely to develop a serious form of anemia than most other workers. And we also keep women away from most of the chemicals we work with. We're concerned about them, of course, but no more so than we are concerned about the men who work with them. We are, once again, worried about the effects on their children."

"Mostly you are worried about insurance claims and lawsuits."

"That's a factor," Larski admitted. "If some people are more prone to develop serious illnesses than others and we can detect it in advance, then we have a corporate duty to keep them out of harm's way. It's true that we help control our insurance cost by doing that, but we also help people avoid getting ill."

"We are impressed with Amchem's humane concerns," Spencer said. "But the Committee Against Screening is much more interested in protecting the individual's right to seek employment of her or his choice. Also, CAS believes that the data used to exclude people from jobs may also be used to exclude them from other benefits. For example, insurance companies are likely to refuse health insurance to someone who runs a greater than average risk of developing a serious disease. The result is that people are penalized because of their genetic makeup, and that's an accident of birth. Our society has a duty to protect individuals from just that sort of discrimination, and CAS intends to do all it can to make sure that society lives up to that duty."

"That's very eloquent," Larski said. "But you're trying to force equality where none exists. People are different, and the society can't alter that fact."

1. Is it a legitimate function of society to protect individuals from hazards in the workplace? Is there a limit to steps that can be taken to provide protection?

2. If certain jobs present greater hazards to women and African Americans than to others, then excluding these minorities is discriminatory. Are all forms of discrimination that are not directly related to job performance unjustifiable?

3. "We value individual autonomy, and it may seem enough to warn people of the hazards they may face in accepting a particular job. However, the need to earn a living may force some to accept jobs that put them at a greater-than-average risk. Consequently, it is misleading to think that we are preserving autonomy by allowing individuals to decide for themselves whether they wish to accept a job that is more than normally hazardous to them. Economic necessity makes a mockery out of the notion that people are free to choose." Evaluate this argument.

Decision Scenario 7 . . . .

"The trick," said Martin Anders, "is to make use of the virus as part of our production system."

"How's that?" Hilda Presti asked.

"The DNA of the virus contains a segment of DNA that we introduced into it. When the virus attacks a bacterial cell, it injects the DNA into it. The viral DNA then takes over the cell machinery enough to get the cell to make copies of the DNA and get it to synthesize the proteins coded for by the DNA segment we spliced in."

"That means that, if the proteins are something that are useful—like a hormone—then you've got a chemical factory working to produce it."

"That's the idea," Anders said. "We can harness the power of literally billions of bacteria to make what we want."

"Isn't that dangerous, though?" Presti asked. "Isn't it at least possible that the viruses might contain some DNA segments that would make the bacteria resistant to antibiotics?"

"That's the sort of Andromeda Strain scenario people used to worry about in the seventies, but we realize today that that's just not something that's going to happen."

"Can you really be sure of that?" Presti asked.

"Reasonably certain," Anders said. "Nothing serious has happened so far. Besides, we've taken a lot of steps to avoid the danger. Even when genetically altered bacteria are released directly into the environment or when altered viruses have been used as vaccines, everything reasonable has been done to make them safe. The bacteria are harmless ones, and the viruses are always weakened strains."

"Probably you're right," Presti said. "But the risks seem to me genuine. Why can't we do without genetically altered organisms? What is there to be gained?"

"The most immediate gain is that we can exploit an entirely new form of technology. We can grow better crops, manufacture better and more effective drugs. There is really no end to what we might be able to do in the future."

"If there is one," Presti said.

1. What are the potential dangers of genetically altered organisms? What are the potential benefits?

2. Why do some scientists believe that the so-called Andromeda Strain scenario is not one that we need to take seriously?

3. What considerations suggest that we ought to proceed with caution in exploiting the promises of genetic engineering?

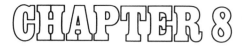

CHAPTER 8

REPRODUCTIVE CONTROL: IN VITRO FERTILIZATION, ARTIFICIAL INSEMINATION, AND SURROGATE PREGNANCY

CASE PRESENTATION
Louise Brown: The First "Test-Tube Baby"

Under other circumstances, the birth announcement might have been perfectly ordinary, the sort that appears in newspapers every day: *Born to John and Lesley Brown: a baby girl, Louise, 5 lbs. 12 ozs., 11:47 P.M., July 25, 1978, Oldham General Hospital (Oldham, England).*

But the birth of Louise Brown was far from being an ordinary event, and the announcement of its occurrence appeared in headlines throughout the world. For the first time in history, a child was born who was conceived outside the mother's body under controlled laboratory conditions.

Louise Brown was the world's first "test-tube baby."

For John and Lesley Brown, the birth of Louise was a truly marvelous event. "She's so small, so beautiful, so perfect," her mother told a reporter. "It was like a dream. I couldn't believe it," her father said.

The joy of the Browns was understandable, for, from the time of their marriage in 1969, they had both very much wanted to have a child. Then they discovered that Mrs. Brown was unable to conceive because of blocked Fallopian tubes—the ova would not descend so fertilization could not occur. In 1970, she underwent an operation in an attempt to correct the condition, but the procedure was unsuccessful.

The Browns decided they would adopt a child, since they couldn't have one of their own. After two years on a waiting list, they gave up that plan. But the idea of having their own child was rekindled when a nurse familiar with the work of embryologist Robert Edwards and gynecologist Patrick Steptoe referred the Browns to them.

For the previous twelve years, Steptoe and Edwards had been working on the medical and biochemical techniques required for embryo transfer. Steptoe developed techniques for removing a ripened ovum from a woman's ovaries, then reimplanting it in the uterus after it has been fertilized. Edwards improved the chemical solutions needed to keep ova functioning and healthy outside the body and perfected a method of external fertilization with sperm.

Using their techniques, Steptoe and Edwards had successfully produced a pregnancy in one of their patients in 1975, but it had resulted in a miscarriage. They continued to refine their procedures and were confident that their techniques could produce a normal pregnancy that would result in a healthy baby.

They considered Lesley Brown an excellent candidate for an embryo transfer. She was in excellent general health, at thirty-one she was not too old for pregnancy, and she was highly fertile. In 1976, Steptoe did an exploratory operation and found that Mrs. Brown's Fallopian tubes were not functional and could not be surgically repaired. He removed them so that he would have clear access to the ovaries.

In November of 1977, Mrs. Brown was given injections of a hormone to increase the maturation rate of her egg cells. Then, in a small private hospital in Oldham, Dr. Steptoe performed a minor surgical procedure. Using a laparoscope to guide him—a tube with a built-in eyepiece and light source that is inserted through a tiny slit in the abdomen—he extracted an ovum with a suction needle from a ripened follicle.

The ovum was then placed in a small glass vessel containing biochemical nutrients and sperm that had been secured from John Brown. Once the egg was fertilized, it was transferred to another nutrient solution. More than fifty hours later, the ovum had reached the eight-cell stage of division. Guided by their previous experience and research, Steptoe and Edwards had decided that it was at this stage that an ovum should be returned to the womb. Although in normal human development the ovum has divided to produce sixty-four or more cells before it completes its descent down the Fallopian tube and becomes attached to the uterine wall, they had learned that attachment is possible at an earlier stage. The stupendous difficulties in creating and maintaining the proper biochemical environment for a multiplying cell made it reasonable to reduce the time outside the body as much as possible.

Mrs. Brown had been given another series of hormone injections to prepare her uterus. Two and a half days after the ovum was removed, the fertilized egg—an embryo—was reimplanted. Using a laparoscope and a hollow plastic tube (a cannula), Dr. Steptoe introduced the small sphere of cells into Mrs. Brown's uterus. It successfully attached itself to the uterine wall.

Mrs. Brown's pregnancy proceeded normally. But, because of the special nature of her case, seven weeks before the baby was due she entered the Oldham Hospital maternity ward so that she could be continuously monitored. About a week before the birth was expected, the baby was delivered by Caesarean section. Mrs. Brown had developed toxemia, a condition associated with high blood pressure that can lead to stillbirth.

The baby was normal, and all concerned were jubilant. "The last time I saw the baby it was just eight cells in a test tube," Dr. Edwards said. "It was beautiful then, and it's still beautiful now." After the delivery, Dr. Steptoe said "She came out crying her head off, a beautiful normal baby."

Mr. Brown almost missed the great event, because no one on the hospital staff had bothered to tell him that his wife was scheduled for the operation. Only when he had been gone for about two hours and called back to talk to his wife did he find out what was about to happen.

He rushed back and waited anxiously until a nurse came out and told him "You're the father of a wonderful little girl." As he later told a reporter, "Almost before I knew it, there I was holding our daughter in my arms."

Like many ordinary fathers, he ran down the halls of the hospital telling people he passed "It's a girl! I've got a baby daughter."

To calm down, he went outside and stood in the rain. It was there that a reporter from a London newspaper captured Mr. Brown's view of the event. "The man who deserves all the praise is Mr. Steptoe," he said. "What a man to be able to do such a wonderful thing."

CASE PRESENTATION

The Orphaned Embryos of Mario and Elsa Rios

In 1983 Mario and Elsa Rios died in a plane crash. Their deaths left others to face some unique moral and legal issues.

The Los Angeles couple had been trying to have a child. Ova from Mrs. Rios and sperm from an anonymous donor were combined, and the embryos that developed were frozen and stored at the Queen Victoria Medical Center in Melbourne, Australia. The aim of freezing the embryos was to allow other attempts at pregnancy without subjecting Mrs. Rios to additional surgery.

A scholarly committee that was asked to study the question of what should be done with the embryos recommended that they be destroyed. However, the Parliament of the State of Victoria rejected the recommendation and passed a bill with an amendment that required the embryos to be put up for adoption and implanted in surrogate mothers. (The amendment was intended to cover only the Rioses' embryos, not to establish a general policy. In the future, couples participating in in vitro fertilization programs will be required to indicate what should be done with frozen embryos in the event of death or separation.)

The Rios estate was valued at about one million dollars, and what claim, if any, the embryos might have on it is a complicating factor. According to Victoria law, the embryo implants would be considered the children only of their surrogate/adoptive parents. California courts have disqualified such children from making any claims on the Rios estate on the basis of a state law requiring that a beneficiary be born or in utero at the time of parental death.

Almost a decade after the embryos were frozen, they remain submerged in a tank of liquid nitrogen, unimplanted and controversial. Their chance of survival if thawed is estimated by researchers to be less than 5%.

CASE PRESENTATION
Embryos in Court: The Davis Case

The subject of the dispute between Mary Sue Davis and her estranged husband, Junior Davis, was seven embryos lying frozen in liquid nitrogen in the Fertility Center of East Tennessee.

Junior Davis did not want Mary Sue Davis to use the embryos to bear their child after their divorce. Mary Sue Davis wished to be free to do just that. In her view, the embryos were already living children, while for Junior Davis they were not alive in any significant way. For him, the only issue was the legal one of settling a joint property dispute, and he had no wish to be forced into fatherhood against his wishes. That was why he sued his estranged wife to gain recognition of what he considered to be his right to exercise a veto power over the use of the embryos.

The Davises had met when both were in the army and stationed in Germany. They married in 1979 and, after their military discharge, moved to Maryville, Tennessee. Mrs. Davis got a job as a service representative for a boat dealer, and Mr. Davis found work as a refrigeration technician. They tried to start a family, but luck was not with them. Mrs. Davis suffered through five ectopic pregnancies. The last resulted in the rupturing and scarring of one Fallopian tube and the tying off of the other for medical reasons.

Convinced that normal conception was impossible, in October of 1988 the couple entered an in vitro fertilization program in Knoxville. Originally nine ova were retrieved and fertilized with Mr. Davis's sperm. An attempt was made to implant two of the embryos, but it was unsuccessful. The plan was to try again at a more propitious time in Mrs. Davis's reproductive cycle, and the remaining seven embryos were frozen. Unfortunately, for reasons the Davises have not made public, their marriage began to break down, and on February 24, 1989, Junior Davis filed for divorce.

Junior Davis also filed suit to exercise joint control over the frozen embryos. During the trial, Mary Sue Davis took the position that the embryos were the product of her years of suffering through surgery, tests, and injections and represented her best chance to have a child. "I consider [the embryos] life," Mrs. Davis said. "To me it would be killing them if you destroyed them." In her view, the case involved the issues of custody of children and a woman's right to decide whether to bring a pregnancy to term. Her lawyer argued that the frozen embryos should be regarded as "preborn children."

In contrast with Mary Sue Davis's position, Junior Davis testified that he would feel "raped of my reproductive rights" if his wife were allowed to use the embryos to produce a child. He also opposed their donation for use by someone else. He insisted that he did not wish to be a father and that he had the right to make that decision. His attorney argued that the embryos were "mere tissue" and that they should be kept frozen indefinitely.

Testimony by fertility experts put Mary Sue Davis's chances of bearing a child with the implanted embryos at about 10%. Testimony also supported the view that the embryos would probably cease to be viable after two years.

Circuit Judge W. Dale Young rendered his decision on September 21, 1989. He ruled that "The temporary custody of the seven human embryos is vested in Mrs. Davis for the purpose of implantation." Furthermore, "Human embryos are not property. Human life begins at conception. Mr. and Mrs. Davis have produced human beings, in vitro, to be known as their child or children."

The judge's decision was explicitly based on the notion that the embryos already have the status of children. According to the decision, "It is in the manifest interest of the child or children that they be available for implantation. It serves the best interest of the child or children for their mother, Mrs. Davis, to be permitted the opportunity to bring them to term through implantation." Furthermore, Judge Young held, "To allow the seven human embryos to remain so preserved for a period exceeding two years is tantamount to the destruction of these human beings."

Judge Young declared that, if Mrs. Davis had a baby after implantation of the embryos, he would then decide the issues of child custody, support, and visitation rights.

Mr. Davis announced that he would appeal the ruling, and Mary Sue Davis said she would make no attempt to implant the ova until the appeal was heard. Soon afterward she married again, and in May 1990, without explaining her reasons, she said she didn't want to use the embryos. However, she wanted to be free to donate them to some childless couple who might be able to benefit from them. Junior Davis said he was totally against this. In September 1990 the Appeals Court granted joint custody of the embryos to Junior Davis and Mary Sue Davis Stowe.

CASE PRESENTATION

Baby M: Surrogate Pregnancy in Court

On March 30, 1986, Dr. Elizabeth Stern, a professor of pediatrics, and her husband, William, accepted from Mary Beth Whitehead a baby who had been born four days earlier. The child's biological mother was Mrs. Whitehead, but she had been engaged by the Sterns as a surrogate mother. Even so, it was not until almost exactly a year later that the Sterns were able to claim legal custody of the child.

The Sterns, working through the Infertility Center of New York, had first met with Mrs. Whitehead and her husband, Richard, in January of 1985. Mrs. Whitehead, who already had a son and a daughter, had indicated her willingness to become a surrogate mother by signing up at the Infertility Center. "What brought her there was empathy with childless couples who were infertile," her attorney later stated. Her own sister had been unable to conceive.

According to court testimony, the Sterns considered Mrs. Whitehead a "perfect person" to bear a child for them. Mr. Stern said that it was "compelling" for him to have children, for he had no relatives "anywhere in the world." He and his wife planned to have children, but they put off attempts to conceive until his wife completed her medical residency in 1981. However, in 1979 she was diagnosed as having an eye condition indicating that she probably had multiple sclerosis. When she learned that the symptoms of the disease might be worsened by pregnancy and that she might become temporarily or even permanently paralyzed, the Sterns "decided the risk wasn't worth it." It was this decision that led them to the Infertility Center and to Mary Beth Whitehead.

The Sterns agreed to pay Mrs. Whitehead $10,000 to be artificially inseminated with Mr. Stern's sperm and to bear a child. Mrs. Whitehead would then turn the child over to the Sterns, and Dr. Stern would be allowed to adopt the child legally. The agreement was drawn up by a lawyer specializing in surrogacy arrangements. Mr. Stern later testified that Mrs. Whitehead seemed perfectly pleased with the agreement and expressed no interest in keeping the baby she was to bear. "She said she would not come to our doorstep," he said. "All she wanted from us was a photograph each year and a little letter on what transpired that year."

The baby was born on March 27, 1986. According to Dr. Stern, the first indication that Mrs. Whitehead might not keep the agreement was her statement to the Sterns in the hospital two days after the baby's birth. "She said she didn't know if 'I can go through with it,' " Dr. Stern testified. Although Mrs. Whitehead did turn the baby over to the Sterns on March 30, she called a few hours later. "She said she didn't know if she could live any more," Dr. Stern said. She called again the next morning and asked to see the baby, and she and her sister arrived at the Sterns' house before noon.

According to Dr. Stern, Mrs. Whitehead told her that she "woke up screaming in the middle of the night" because the baby was gone, that her husband was threatening to leave her, and that she had "considered taking a bottle of Valium." Dr. Stern quoted Mrs. Whitehead as saying, "I just want her for a week, and I'll be out of your lives forever." The Sterns allowed Mrs. Whitehead to take the baby home with her.

Mrs. Whitehead then refused to return the baby voluntarily and took the infant with her to the home of her parents in Florida. The Sterns obtained a court order, and on July 31 the child was seized from Mrs. Whitehead. The Sterns were granted temporary custody. Then Mr. Stern, as the father of the child, and Mrs. Whitehead, as the mother, each sought permanent custody from the Superior Court of the State of New Jersey.

The seven-week trial attracted considerable attention, for the legal issues were virtually without precedent. Mrs. Whitehead was the first to challenge the legal legitimacy of a surrogate agreement in a U.S. court. She argued that the agreement was "against public policy" and violated New Jersey prohibitions against selling babies. In contrast, Mr. Stern was the first to seek a legal decision to uphold the "specific performance" of the terms of a surrogate contract. In particular, he argued that Mrs. Whitehead should be ordered to uphold her agreement and to surrender her parental rights and permit his wife to become the baby's legal mother. In addition to the contractual issues, the judge had to deal with the "best interest" of the child as required by New Jersey child-custody law. In addition to being a vague concept, the "best interest" standard had never been applied in a surrogacy case.

On March 31, 1987, Judge Harvey R. Sorkow announced his decision. He upheld the legality of the surrogate-mother agreement between the Sterns and Mrs. Whitehead and dismissed all argu-

ments that the contract violated public policy or prohibitions against selling babies. Immediately after he read his decision, Judge Sorkow summoned Elizabeth Stern into his chambers and allowed her to sign documents permitting her to adopt the baby she and her husband called Melissa. The court decision effectively stripped Mary Beth Whitehead of all parental rights concerning this same baby, the one she called Sara.

The Baby M story did not stop with Judge Sorkow's decision. Mrs. Whitehead's attorney appealed the ruling to the New Jersey Supreme Court, and on February 3, 1988, the seven members of the court, in a unanimous decision, reversed Judge Sorkow's ruling on the surrogacy agreement. The court held that the agreement violated the state's adoption laws, because it involved a payment for a child. "This is the sale of a child, or at the very least, the sale of a mother's right to her child," Chief Justice Wilentz wrote. The agreement "guarantees the separation of a child from its mother . . .; it takes the child from the mother regardless of her wishes and her maternal fitness . . .; and it accomplishes all of its goals through the use of money." The court held that surrogacy agreements might be acceptable if they involved no payment and if a surrogate mother voluntarily surrendered her parental rights. In the present case, though, the court regarded paying for surrogacy "illegal, perhaps criminal, and potentially degrading to women."

The court let stand the award of custody to the Sterns, because "Their household and their personalities promise a much more likely foundation for Melissa to grow and thrive." Mary Beth Whitehead, having divorced her husband three months earlier, was romantically involved with a man named Dean Gould and was pregnant at the time of the court decision.

Despite awarding custody to the Sterns, the court set aside the adoption agreement signed by Elizabeth Stern. Mary Beth Whitehead remained a legal parent of Baby M, and the court ordered a lower court hearing to consider visitation rights for the mother.

The immediate future of the child known to the court and to the public as Baby M was settled. Neither the Sterns nor Mary Beth Whitehead had won exactly what they had sought, but neither had they lost all.

CASE PRESENTATION
The Unclaimed Infant

In January 1983, Judy Stiver of Lansing, Michigan, gave birth to a child nine months after she was artificially inseminated with sperm from Alexander Malahoff of Queens, New York. Mr. Malahoff had agreed to pay Mrs. Stiver $10,000 for her services as a surrogate mother.

Mrs. Stiver had a long and difficult labor, and trouble started as soon as the child was born. The child, a boy, was microcephalic and suffered from a severe infection. Mr. Malahoff, as the presumed father, refused to authorize the treatment necessary to sustain the life of the infant. However, the hospital obtained a court order, and the infant was successfully treated.

Before Mrs. Stiver and her husband could cash the check given to her by Mr. Malahoff, Mr. Malahoff informed them that there was a problem. The baby's blood type was O-positive, while Mr. Malahoff's was AB-positive. Thus, the child could not be his, and he refused to accept responsibility for it. Before that time, according to Mr. Stiver, Mr. Malahoff had accepted the baby's impairment, had the child baptized, and planned to place him in an institution.

"We don't feel the baby is ours," Mr. Stiver said. "We feel no maternal or paternal relationship. We feel sorry for it, but we don't want it." Mrs. Stiver reported that she felt "some affection" for the baby but "there is no bond."

Mrs. Stiver said that she had a thorough medical examination to guarantee that she was not pregnant before she was inseminated with Mr. Malahoff's sperm. She and her husband then avoided sexual intercourse for thirty days. Mr. Malahoff, who had separated from his wife, sued the Stivers for $30,000, alleging that they violated the terms of the contract by having intercourse during the insemination period. The Stivers sued the physician who performed the insemination, and several suits and countersuits are still in litigation.

The child, who was named Christopher, is a patient at the Beekman Center for Therapy. According to Mrs. Stiver, "They say he has the capabilities of a two- to four-month old, and he probably won't get much beyond that."

The case of Christopher Stiver prompted the introduction of legislation in Michigan to protect the interests of children born through various fertility techniques, including surrogate pregnancy, and to establish legal rights and responsibilities of contractual parents. New Jersey and Washington, two states in which legislation directly addresses the issues of surrogacy, require that the contractual father be recognized as the legal father.

CASE PRESENTATION
The Calvert Case: Gestational Surrogacy

Disease forced Crispina Calvert of Orange County, California, to have a hysterectomy, but only her uterus was removed by surgery, not her ovaries. She and her husband, Mark, wanted a child of their own, but without a uterus Crispina would not be able to bear it. For a fee of $10,000 they arranged with Anna Johnson to act as a surrogate.

Unlike the more common form of surrogate pregnancy, Johnson would have no genetic investment in the child. The ovum that would be fertilized would not be hers. Mary Beth Whitehead, the surrogate in the controversial Baby M case, had received artificial insemination. Thus, she made as much genetic contribution to the child as did the biological father.

Johnson, however, would be the gestational surrogate. In a standard in vitro fertilization process, ova were extracted from Crispina Calvert and mixed with sperm from Mark. A fertilized ovum was implanted in Anna Johnson's uterus, and a fetus began to develop.

Johnson's pregnancy proceeded along a normal course, but in her seventh month she announced that she had changed her mind about giving up the child. She filed suit against the Calverts to seek custody of the unborn child. "Just because you donate a sperm and an egg doesn't make you a parent," said Johnson's attorney. "Anna is not a machine, an incubator."

"That child is biologically Chris and Mark's," said the Calverts' lawyer. "That contract is valid."

Johnson was not the first woman to serve as a gestational surrogate. No official records are kept, but the Center for Surrogate Parenting in Beverly Hills estimates that about 80 such births have occurred since 1987. This compares to some 2,000 surrogate pregnancies during the same period. According to the Center's figures, probably around 4,000 surrogate births have occurred since the late 1970s.

Critics of genetic surrogate pregnancy are equally critical of gestational surrogate pregnancy. Both methods, some claim, exploit women, particularly poor women. Further, in gestational pregnancy the surrogate is the one who must run the risks and suffer the discomforts and dangers of pregnancy. She has a certain biological claim to be the mother, because it was her body that produced the child according to the genetic information.

Defenders of surrogate pregnancy respond to the first criticism by denying that surrogates are exploited. They enter freely into a contract to serve as a surrogate for pay, just as anyone might agree to perform any other form of service for pay. Pregnancy has hazards and leaves its marks on the body, but so do many other paid occupations. As far as gestational surrogacy is concerned, defenders say, since the surrogate makes no genetic contribution to the developing child, in no reasonable way can she be regarded as the child's parent.

The Ethics Committee of the American Fertility Society has endorsed a policy opposing surrogate pregnancy "for non-medical reasons." The apparent aim of the policy is to permit the use of gestational surrogate pregnancy in cases like that of Mrs. Calvert, while condemning it when its motivation is mere convenience or an unwillingness to be pregnant. When a woman is fertile but, because of diabetes, uncontrollable hypertension, or some other life-threatening disorder, is unable to bear the burden of pregnancy, then gestational surrogacy would be a legitimate medical option.

The child carried by Anna Johnson, a boy, was born on September 19, and for a while, under a court order, Johnson and the Calverts shared visitation rights. Then, in October, 1990, a California Superior Court denied to Anna Johnson the parental rights she had sought. Justice R. N. Parslow awarded complete custody of the child to the Calverts and terminated Johnson's visitation rights.

"I decline to split the child emotionally between two mothers," the judge said. He said Johnson had nurtured and fed the fetus in the way a foster parent might take care of a child, but she was still a "genetic stranger" to the boy and could not claim parenthood because of surrogacy.

Justice Parslow found the contract between the Calverts and Johnson to be valid, and he expressed doubt about Johnson's contention that she had "bonded" with the fetus she was carrying. "There is substantial evidence in the record that Anna Johnson never bonded with the child till she filed her lawsuit, if then," he said. While the trial was in progress, Johnson had been accused of planning to sue the Calverts from the beginning to attempt to make the case famous so she could make money from book and movie rights.

Justice Parslow also urged the California Legislature to establish legal guidelines to deal with surrogacy cases. He suggested a process in which all parties undergo psychological evaluation and agree at the beginning that the surrogate mother will have no custody rights. He also suggested that a surrogate be required to have had previous successful experience with childbirth and that surrogacy be used only in cases in which the genetic mother is unable to give birth.

"I see no problem with someone getting paid for her pain and suffering," he said. "There is nothing wrong with getting paid for nine months of what I understand is a lot of misery and a lot of bad days. They are not selling a baby; they are selling pain and suffering."

The Calverts were overjoyed by the decision.

INTRODUCTION

"Oh, brave new world that has such people in it!" exclaims Miranda in Shakespeare's *The Tempest*.

It is a phrase from this line that provided Aldous Huxley with the title for his dystopian novel *Brave New World*. A dystopia is the opposite of a utopia, and the future society depicted by Huxley is one that we are invited to view with shock and disapproval.

In this society, "pregnancy" is a dirty word, sex is purely recreational, and children are produced according to explicit genetic standards in the artificial wombs of state "hatcheries." Furthermore, an individual's genetic endowment determines the social position and obligations that he or she has within the society. Of course, everyone is conditioned to believe that the role he finds himself in is the best one to have.

In significant ways, that future is now. The new and still-developing medical technologies of human reproduction have now reached a stage in which the technical innovations imagined by Huxley in 1932 to make such a society possible are well within the limits of feasibility.

We have no state hatcheries and no artificial uteruses. But we do have sperm banks and surrogate mothers. We have it within our power to remove an ovum from a woman's body, fertilize it, then return it so that it may develop into a child. By relatively simple surgical procedures, we can end forever the reproductive potentialities of otherwise fertile men or women.

The new technology associated with human reproduction is so powerful that it differs only in degree from that of Huxley's dystopian world. What we have yet to do is to employ the technology as part of a deliberate social policy to restructure our world along the lines imagined by Huxley.

Yet the potentiality is there. Perhaps more than anything else, it is the bleak vision of such a mechanistic and dehumanized future that has motivated much of the criticism of current reproductive technology. The "brave new world" of Huxley is one in which traditional values associated with reproduction and family life, values based on individual autonomy, have been replaced by values of a purely social kind. In such a society, it is the good of the society or of the species, not the good of

individuals, that is the touchstone of justification.

The possible loss of personal values is a legitimate and serious concern. The technologies of human reproduction are sometimes viewed as machines that may be employed to pave the road leading to a world of bleakness and loss. Yet it is important to remember that those same technologies also promise to enhance the lives of those presently living and to prevent potential suffering and despair.

Some women who are unable to bear children may now find it possible to do so through the use of in vitro fertilization techniques. Artificial insemination offers a means of impregnation when biological dysfunction makes the normal means impossible. Further, those women who would be at risk from becoming pregnant may now be protected by choosing surgical sterilization.

These are all potentialities that have become actualities; in vitro fertilization, artificial insemination, and sterilization are all procedures currently being performed. In the view of some, these procedures merely mark a beginning, and the possibilities inherent in reproductive technology still remain relatively unrealized. If we wish, we can employ the technology to change the very fabric and pattern of our society.

Should we do that? Or will the use of the technology necessarily promote the development of a dystopia? One way of thinking about these general questions is to turn once more to Huxley.

It is frequently overlooked that in 1962 Huxley published a utopian novel entitled *Island*. Like the society in *Brave New World*, Huxley's ideal society also relies upon the principles of science, but in the ideal society they are used to promote autonomy and personal development.

Island portrays a society on the island of Pala that for over a hundred years has developed itself in accordance with the principles of reason and science. Living is communal, sexual repression is nonexistent, children are cared for by both their biological parents and other adults, drugs are used to enhance perceptual awareness, and social obligations are assigned on the basis of personal interest and ability.

More to the present point, the society makes use of reproductive technology to achieve its ends. It practices contraception, eugenics, and artificial insemination. Negative eugenics to eliminate genetic diseases is considered only rational. But more than this, by the use of "DF" and "AI" (Deep Freeze and Artificial Insemination), sperm from donors with superior genetic endowments is available for the use of couples who wish to improve their chances of having a child with special talents or with higher-than-usual intelligence.

Huxley's ideal society is not above criticism, even from those who are sympathetic toward the values he endorses. Yet *Brave New World* is such a powerful cautionary tale of what might happen if science were pressed into the service of repressive political goals that it makes it difficult to imagine other possible futures in which some of the same technology plays a more benign role. Since *Island* is an attempt to present such an alternative future, in thinking about the possibilities inherent in reproductive technology, fairness demands that we also consider Palinese society and not restrict our attention to the world of soma and state hatcheries.

IN VITRO FERTILIZATION

The birth of Louise Brown in 1978 (see the Case Presentation) was treated as a major media event. Photographs, television coverage, interviews, and news stories presented the world with minute details of the lives of the people involved and with close accounts of the technical procedures that had led to Louise's conception.

Despite the unprecedented character of the event, few people seemed surprised by it. The idea of a "test-tube baby" was one already familiar from fiction and folklore. The medi-eval alchemist was thought capable of generating life within his retorts, and hundreds of science fiction stories depicted a future in which the creation of life within the laboratory was an ordinary occurrence. In some ways, then, the birth of Louise Brown was seen as merely a matter of science and medicine catching up with imagination. (Indeed, they didn't quite catch up, for the "test tube" contained sperm and an egg, not just a mixture of chemicals.)

Although it is doubtful whether the public appreciated the magnitude of the achievement that resulted in the birth of Louise Brown, it was one of considerable significance. The first embryo transfer was performed in rabbits in 1890, but it was not until the role of hormones in reproduction, the nutritional requirements of developing cells, and the reproductive process itself were better understood that it became possible to consider seriously the idea of fertilizing an egg outside the mother's body and then returning it for ordinary development.

"In vitro" is a Latin phrase that means "in glass," and in embryology it is used in contrast with "in utero" or "in the uterus." Ordinary human fertilization takes place in utero (strictly speaking, in the Fallopian tubes) when a sperm cell unites with an ovum. In vitro fertilization, then, is fertilization that is artificially performed outside the woman's body—in a test tube, so to speak.

The ovum that produced Louise Brown was fertilized in vitro. But the entire process involved *embryo transfer*. That is, an ovum had to be taken from her mother's body. Then, after it was fertilized and had become an embryo, it was returned for in utero development.

Robert Edwards and Patrick Steptoe were the individuals responsible for developing and performing the techniques of in vitro fertilization and embryo transfer that led to the birth of Louise Brown. Basically, they followed a four-step process that has now become almost standard.

1.   The patient is given a reproductive hormone in order to cause ova to ripen. A

few hours before ovulation can be expected to occur, a small incision is made in the abdomen just below the navel. A laparoscope is inserted through the incision, and the ovaries are examined directly. When mature eggs are found that are about to break free from the thin walls of the ovarian follicle, the walls are punctured and the contents are removed by a vacuum aspirator (a hollow suction needle). Several eggs may be removed.

2. The eggs are transferred to a nutrient solution that is biochemically similar to that found in the Fallopian tubes. Sperm is then added to the solution. As soon as a single sperm cell penetrates the ovum, the ovum is fertilized.

3. The fertilized egg is transferred to another nutrient solution where, after about a day, it begins to undergo cell division. When the ovum reaches the eight-cell stage, it is ready to be returned to the uterus. The patient is given injections of hormones to prepare her uterus to receive the fertilized egg.

4. The small ball of cells is placed in the uterus through the cervix (the opening that leads to the vagina) by means of a hollow plastic tube called a cannula. The fertilized egg continues to divide, and, somewhere between the thirty-two- and sixty-four-cell stage, it attaches itself to the uterine wall.

If the attachment is successful, from this point on development should proceed as though fertilization had taken place in the ordinary fashion.

On December 28, 1981, Elizabeth Jordan Carr was born at Norfolk General Hospital, Norfolk, Virginia. She has the distinction of being the first baby conceived in vitro born in the United States. Like Louise Brown, she also weighed five pounds, twelve ounces, was born ahead of schedule, and was perfectly healthy.

As of 1989, over 15,000 births have resulted from using in vitro techniques, and in the United States alone more than 100 clinics performing the procedure have been opened since the Norfolk program was initiated. (Some estimates place the number of programs worldwide at over 200.) Success rates vary, but in the best programs the chance of a woman's becoming pregnant is about 23–25%, roughly the same odds as those of a normal, healthy couple attempting conception during the woman's regular monthly cycle. Each fertilization and transplantation attempt costs around $5,000, and in most cases such expenses are not covered by insurance.

The technical procedures are still fundamentally the same as those pioneered by Steptoe and Edwards. However, modifications and extensions have been introduced. One of the more important ones is the development of a nonsurgical procedure for securing ova. After hormones are used to stimulate the ovarian follicles, ultrasound is employed to locate the follicles, and a hollow needle is inserted through the vaginal wall and into a follicle. Fluid is withdrawn, and egg cells are identified under the microscope. The egg cells are then fertilized with the sperm, cultured, and reimplanted.

An additional modification is to attempt to implant two, three, or even more fertilized ova at a time. This increases the chances that at least one of them will attach to the uterine wall and develop normally. Of course, the procedure also increases the chances of multiple births, and clinics that use this technique have patients that produce a higher-than-average percentage of twins and triplets.

A variation of standard in vitro techniques is gamete intrafallopian transfer, or GIFT. The procedure was developed in 1984 by Ricardo Asch and involves inserting both ova and sperm into the Fallopian tubes. If fertilization takes place, it does so inside the woman's body. This feature has seemed to some as being in some sense more "natural" than in vitro fertilization.

Intravaginal culture (IVC) is another attempt at naturalness. Ova are placed in a tube to which sperm cells are added, and the tube is then inserted into the vagina and kept next to the cervix by a diaphragm. Normal sexual intercourse can occur with the tube in place. Two days later the tube is removed, the contents decanted, and fertilized ova transferred into the uterus.

Another important development is the perfection of techniques for freezing embryos. Evidence to date indicates that embryos can be stored in a frozen condition and then unfrozen and implanted without any damage to the chromosomes. The advantage of the procedure is that it eliminates the need for a woman to undergo the surgery and the lengthy and uncomfortable process required to secure additional ova. If a woman fails to become pregnant at a first attempt, an embryo saved from the initial fertilization can be employed in another effort. Furthermore, the technique makes it possible to delay an embryo transplant until the potential mother has reached the most favorable time in her menstrual cycle.

By virtue of being first, Louise Brown continues to be a symbol of what it is possible to achieve by means of the techniques developed by Steptoe and Edwards. But in the future it is likely she will quietly take her place among the ranks of the literally thousands of others whose conception occurred in a glass bottle.

Benefits

Obviously, the processes involved in in vitro fertilization and embryo transfer are complicated and require a great amount of skill and knowledge. An obvious question to ask about the whole procedure is, what is to be gained by it? That is, what are the benefits of such a technically difficult and expensive medical procedure?

The most direct and perhaps the most persuasive answer is that in vitro fertilization makes it possible for many couples to conceive children who would not otherwise be able to do so. At a time when problems with fertility seem to be on the increase, this is a particularly important consideration. Research shows that 10% of married couples in the United States are infertile—that they have attempted to conceive a child for a year or longer without success. During the period 1981–1982, physicians reported a record 2 million visits for infertility problems, twice as many as for comparable two-year periods. Also, infertility among younger women seems to be on the increase. In 1965 infertility in women aged 20 to 26 was estimated to be 4%; in 1982 the figure was 11%.

In vitro fertilization is obviously not a solution to all problems of fertility. However, it is the only solution possible in a large number of cases. Figures show that as much as 45% of all cases of female infertility are caused by abnormal or obstructed Fallopian tubes. In such cases, although normal ova are produced, they cannot move down the tubes to be fertilized. In some cases, tissue blocking the tubes may be removed, or the tubes reconstructed. In other cases, however, the tubes may be impossible to repair or may be entirely absent. (Only 40–50% of infertile women can be helped through surgery.) This means that the only way in which the woman can expect to have a child of her own is by means of in vitro fertilization. Thus, the procedure offers a realistic possibility of becoming parents to many people who once had no hope at all of having a child.

Despite some early doubts, the public acceptance of in vitro fertilization has been overwhelmingly positive. A public-opinion poll conducted in 1978 showed that by a margin of more than two to one Americans favored making in vitro fertilization an option available to childless couples. Furthermore, there can be little doubt that the great majority of eligible couples who want a child are in favor of the procedure. The Norfolk clinic is reported to have a waiting list of some 8,000 names—a backlog of sixteen years.

A second, and quite ironic, benefit of research into improving in vitro fertilization and embryo transfer is that it may lead to better and more effective contraceptives. This almost paradoxical result is due to the fact that the sort of knowledge required to make fertilization and reimplantation of the embryo successful is also knowledge that can be employed to prevent pregnancy. For example, a knowledge of the biochemical mechanism by which a sperm penetrates an ovum and renders the ovum impenetrable to all other sperm cells can be turned in the direction either of promoting fertilization or of preventing it. Similarly, understanding how the embryo attaches itself to the wall of the uterus may lead to methods for either decreasing or increasing the likelihood of an embryo's becoming attached.

Third, research with animals using the techniques of in vitro fertilization and embryo transfer can be employed to determine the ways in which various environmental toxins and drugs affect the developing fetus. At present, research groups are exposing fertilized monkey ova to chemicals, then reimplanting them. The aim is to discover the means by which specific chemicals alter development and result in defective offspring.

Such information is of obvious value. If we are to be successful in eliminating or reducing human birth defects that are caused by chemical agents, then we must know what the chemicals do. Only in such ways can safe levels of exposure be determined and steps taken to avoid or prevent the presence of environmental toxins and harmful ingredients in drugs.

These are just three of the more direct advantages associated with in vitro fertilization. Other possibilities inherent in the procedure might make up a substantial list. Here are merely two of them.

Gene Repair.   The way in which the genetic code contained in the DNA of a fertilized egg directs the development of the egg into a baby is far from being understood. Nonetheless, fragments of the total picture are now emerging. The technology of recombinant DNA (see the introduction to Chapter 7) has made it possible to isolate single genes and to identify their products. It is a long way from this stage to being able, for example, to outline all of the steps by which the heart develops. Yet such work is promising enough to fuel the hope that we shall eventually understand the way in which DNA controls the entire developmental process.

This kind of detailed knowledge might make it possible to locate defects in genes that, when uncorrected, lead to faulty development of the fetus. At present, to avoid the birth of a child with birth defects associated with damaged or missing genes, abortion is the only recourse.

Additional knowledge might allow faulty genes to be replaced or repaired. Thus, developmental failures like Down's syndrome and spinal bifida or heritable genetic defects like Tay-Sachs disease might be treated at the level of the genes. An entirely new chapter of fetal medicine would then be opened.

Gestational Surrogates.   This is perhaps the most dramatic possibility opened up by in vitro fertilization and embryo transfer. A woman whose uterus has been removed and who is not capable of a normal pregnancy can contribute an ovum that, after being fertilized in vitro, is implanted in the uterus of a second woman whose uterus has been prepared to receive it. The "host" or gestational surrogate mother then carries the baby to term.

Some observers think that since 1987 about eighty children have been born to gestational surrogates. Traditional surrogate mothers, those impregnated by artificial insemination, have given birth to around 4,000 children since the late 1970s.

Gestational surrogacy is relatively new, but it is only the extension of a practice that has already become established to a limited degree. At present, the wives of couples using the services of a surrogate are themselves unable to bear children. However, it is only a short step from being unable to bear children to being *unwilling* to bear children, though physically able.

Thus, it is easy to imagine that some women might choose to free themselves from the rigors of pregnancy by hiring a gestational surrogate mother. The employer would be the source of the ovum, which would then be fertilized in vitro and implanted as an embryo in the uterus of the surrogate. Women who could afford to do so could have their own natural children without ever having to be pregnant.

An additional possibility is what has been called "prenatal adoption." A woman unable to ovulate normally, but otherwise capable of pregnancy, might choose to "adopt" an embryo carried by another woman. The embryo would be transferred to the first woman's uterus (after she had been prepared by appropriate hormone injections), and there it would develop into a child. This procedure is not one that has been performed yet.

Although a few have advocated using "genetically superior" women as a source of ova and "less superior" women as gestational surrogates, it is highly unlikely that such a program will ever be endorsed by society. (See the introduction to Chapter 7 for the difficulties in determining genetic "superiority.") Nevertheless, the basic procedure is entirely possible.

The possibilities inherent in in vitro fertilization and embryo transfer mentioned here as sources of immediate or future benefits are all ones considered to be quite realistic by most researchers. By contrast, although it is possible to imagine such a thing, the development of "baby factories" or "hatcheries" similar to those described in *Brave New World* is technologically unlikely, judged in terms of current science and medicine. Machines would have to serve the function now served by the uterus, and designing such machines would require knowing enough about the needs of the developing fetus to reproduce that function. At present it is not possible even to state all the problems that would have to be solved.

Difficulties

This is not the place to discuss the ethical and social issues connected with the possibilities of in vitro fertilization mentioned above. There are aspects of the procedure itself and the current way in which it is being employed that some people find troublesome. Very briefly, we shall consider just five.

1. The ova that are removed for fertilization are not all used. Although they may all be mixed with sperm and several may be fertilized, no more than four fertilized ova are selected for implantation. The others are simply discarded.

For those who believe that human life begins at the moment of conception, the destruction of fertilized ova may be viewed as tantamount to abortion. Thus, for some people, the destruction may be regarded as destroying innocent human life.

Others, who are not prepared to ascribe the status of being a person to a fertilized ovum, may still be troubled by its pointless destruction. They may believe that its potentiality to develop, under certain conditions, into a human being at least requires that it be treated with concern and respect. Those who subscribe to such a view might well argue that the only legitimate form of in vitro fertilization is one in which the effort is made to fertilize only a single ovum. A failure in fertilization would then be similar to the failure that occurs naturally, and what would be eliminated would be the necessity of destroying fertilized eggs that cannot be implanted.

2. At present, when human in vitro fertilization is a relatively new procedure, it is impossible to assess the risks to the fetus and to the person it may become. A fetus conceived from an ovum that is removed to an alien environment and sustained by a nutrient solution that may not contain some necessary ingredients for development may well be at much greater risk than a fetus conceived in the ordinary way. Not only may the child be more likely to suffer defects evident at birth, but it

may suffer some defects that will not show up until years later. (Mrs. Brown is rumored to have signed an agreement stating that she would submit to an abortion if there were signs that the fetus she was carrying was not developing normally.)

Experience has rather much taken the teeth out of this objection. The rate of birth defects in children born of in vitro fertilization is about 3%, virtually the same as that of ordinary births. So far there is no evidence that children conceived in vitro differ in any way from other children.

3. In vitro fertilization may encourage the development of eugenic ideas about improving the species. Rather than having children of their own, would-be parents might be motivated to seek out ova (and sperm) from people who possess physical and intellectual characteristics that are particularly admired. Thus, even without an organized plan of social eugenics (see Chapter 7), individuals might be tempted to follow their own eugenic notions.

4. Similarly, would-be parents might be inclined to exercise the potential for control over the sex of their offspring. Only males contain both an X and a Y chromosome, and their presence is detectable in the cells of the developing embryo. Determination of the sex of the embryo would allow the potential parents to decide whether they wish to have a male or female child. Consequently, a potential human being (the developing fetus) might be destroyed for what is basically a trivial reason.

5. In vitro fertilization is likely to promote a social climate in which having children becomes severed from the family. The procedure places emphasis on the mechanics of fertilization and, in doing so, minimizes the significance of the shared love and commitments of the parents of a child conceived by normal intercourse. Furthermore, the procedure offers the opportunity for an unmarried woman to have a child without having anything at all to do with the biological father of the child.

Obviously, these difficulties are not ones likely to be considered equally serious by everyone. Those who do not believe that life begins at conception will hardly be troubled by the discarding of unimplanted embryos. Additional research and experience will no doubt reduce whatever risks there may be to a fetus conceived in vitro. Sex choice is possible now by the use of amniocentesis so is not a problem unique to in vitro fertilization, and the same is true of the implementation of eugenic ideas. Finally, whether in vitro procedures actually lead to a weakening of the values associated with the family is partly an empirical question that only additional use of the method will show. Even if childbearing does become severed from current family structure, it still must be shown that this is itself something of which we ought to disapprove. It is clearly not impossible that alternative social structures for childbearing and childrearing might be superior to ones currently dominant in Western culture.

Research on in vitro fertilization was effectively halted in the United States when Congress declared a temporary moratorium on fetal research in 1974. Technically, the moratorium ended a year later when the former Department of Health, Education, and Welfare declared that all proposals for research involving federal funding would have to be approved by an Ethics Advisory Board. Although such a board was established, it never approved a single proposal. Before it was dissolved in 1979, the board held hearings and solicited testimony from experts in a variety of fields. In its final report, the board held that research into in vitro fertilization and embryo transfer is ethically acceptable.

Despite the board's conclusion, no secretary of the department has seen fit to lift the de facto moratorium. As a result, most of the research done in the United States has involved little more than observation of patients. Some privately funded work has been done, but for the most part American researchers have been dependent on research conducted in England and Australia.

Understandably frustrated, some researchers worry that the lack of major research efforts will slow our understanding of basic biological processes that are involved in conception and development. In particular, the hope that we might detect and repair defective genes in vitro and generally increase our understanding of genetic diseases may suffer a long delay in being realized.

ARTIFICIAL INSEMINATION

In 1909, an unusual letter appeared in the professional journal *Medical World*. A. D. Hard, the author of the letter, claimed that when he was a student at Jefferson Medical College in Philadelphia, a wealthy businessman and his wife consulted a physician on the faculty about their inability to conceive a child.

A detailed examination of each of the spouses showed that the man was incapable of producing sperm. The case was presented for discussion in a class of which Hard was a member. According to Hard, the class suggested that semen should be taken from the "best-looking member of the class" and used to inseminate the wife.

The letter claimed that this was done while the woman was anesthetized and that neither the husband nor the wife was told about the process. The patient became pregnant and gave birth to a son. The husband was then told how the pregnancy was produced, and, although he was pleased with the result, he asked that his wife not be informed.

The event described by Hard took place in 1884, and there is reason to believe that Hard was "the best-looking member of the class."

The Philadelphia case is generally acknowledged to be the first recorded instance of artificial insemination of donor sperm in a human patient. However, the process of artificial insemination itself has a much longer history. Arab horsemen in the fourteenth century

apparently inseminated mares with semen-soaked sponges, and in the eighteenth century the Italian physiologist Spallansani documented experiments in which he fertilized dogs, reptiles, and frogs.

The first recorded case of the artificial insemination of a human being occurred in 1790, when the English physician John Hunter used semen obtained from a husband to inseminate his wife. Sporadic uses of the technique continued to occur in England, France, and the United States, and during the early part of the present century, they became more and more frequent. At present, probably more than 2,000 children a year are born in this country who were conceived by artificial insemination.

Artificial insemination has become generally recognized as a legitimate medical procedure. The process is employed by hospitals, fertility clinics, and physicians who specialize in problems involving conception. Before looking at some of the ethical and legal issues involved in artificial insemination, it is useful to consider some relevant factual information about the process.

The Artificial Insemination Procedure

Artificial insemination is a relatively simple procedure. It is initiated when the woman's body temperature indicates that ovulation is to take place in one or two days. It is then repeated one or two more times until her body temperature shows that ovulation is completed. Typically, three inseminations are performed during a monthly cycle.

In the insemination, the patient is usually placed in a position so that her hips are raised. A semen specimen, collected earlier through masturbation or taken from a sperm bank, is placed in a syringe attached to a narrow tube or catheter. The catheter is gently inserted into the cervical canal, and the semen is slowly injected into the uterus. The patient then stays in her position for fifteen or twenty minutes to increase the chances that the sperm will fertilize an ovum.

The overall success rate of artificial insemination is about 85%. Success on the first attempt is quite rare, and the highest rate occurs in the third month. In unusual cases, efforts may be made every month for as long as six months or a year. Such efforts are continued, however, only when a detailed examination shows that the woman is not suffering from some unrecognized problem preventing her from becoming pregnant.

When sperm taken from donors is used, the rate of congenital abnormalities is a little lower than that for the general population. There seems to be no evidence to support the fear that manipulating the sperm causes any harm. (Many physicians prefer to employ fresh, rather than frozen, sperm to minimize the amount of environmental change the sperm is subjected to. Other physicians claim that frozen sperm is to be preferred, for it provides a means of screening out defective cells or chromosome abnormalities.)

Reasons for Seeking Artificial Insemination

Artificial insemination may be sought for a variety of reasons. When a couple is involved, the reasons are almost always associated with physiological or physical factors that make it impossible for the couple to conceive a child in the usual sexual way.

About 10% of all married couples are infertile, and 40% of those cases are due to factors involving the male. In some instances, the male may be unable to produce any sperm at all (a condition called asospermia), or the number of sperm the male produces may be too low to make impregnation of the female likely (a condition called oligospermia). In other cases, adequate numbers of sperm cells may be produced, but they may not function normally. They may not be sufficiently motile to make their way past the vaginal canal and through the opening to the uterus. Hence, their chances of reaching and penetrating an ovum are slight. Finally, the male may suffer from a neurological condition that makes ejaculation impossible or from a disease (such as diabetes) that renders him impotent.

If the female cannot ovulate, or if her Fallopian tubes are blocked so that ova cannot descend, then artificial insemination can accomplish nothing. (See the section above on in vitro fertilization.) Yet there are factors affecting the female that artificial insemination can be helpful in overcoming. For example, if the female has a vaginal environment that is biochemically inhospitable to sperm, then artificial insemination may be successful. Because the sperm need not pass through the vagina, they have a better chance of surviving. Also, if the female has a small cervix (the opening to the uterus) or if her uterus is in an abnormal position, then artificial insemination may be used to deliver the sperm to an advantageous position for fertilization, a position they otherwise might not reach.

A couple might also seek artificial insemination for genetic reasons. Both may be carriers of a recessive gene for a genetic disorder (Tay-Sachs disease, for example) or the male may be the carrier of a dominant gene for a genetic disorder (Huntington's chorea, for example). In either case, the couple may not want to run the statistical risk of their child's being born with a genetic disease. To avoid the possibility, they may choose to make use of artificial insemination with sperm secured from a donor.

The traditional recipient of artificial insemination is a married woman who, in consultation with her husband, has decided to have a child. Some physiological or physical difficulty in conceiving leads them to turn to artificial insemination.

But the traditional recipient is no longer the only recipient. Those seeking to have the procedure performed now include single women who wish to have a child but do not wish to have it fathered in the usual fashion. Some estimates place the number of such women at 150 a year. The percentages of such inseminations may increase in the future if the notion of being a single parent continues to be met with acceptance or approval within our society. The increase may be quite rapid if the attitudes of physicians, in particular, change. At present, single women who wish to become mothers are likely to be discouraged, and some physicians will not accept them as candidates for artificial insemination.

Types of Artificial Insemination

Artificial insemination can be divided into types in accordance with the source of the sperm employed in the procedure.

Artificial insemination (homologous) uses sperm obtained from the male partner. The name of the process is usually abbreviated as AIH, and the H is frequently taken to stand for "husband." While it is true that the male of a couple is most frequently the woman's husband, legal marriage is not necessary for AIH. The male need only be, in some sense, the functional equivalent of a husband.

Artificial insemination (heterologous) uses sperm from a sperm donor. For this reason, the process is usually referred to by the abbreviation AID. The use of semen obtained from a donor is the most frequent of AI procedures, and it is the one that gives rise to most of the social and legal issues surrounding the practice.

Artificial insemination (confused) employs a mixture of sperm from the male partner and sperm obtained from a donor. CAI, as it is commonly called, has no particular biological advantage, but it does offer a couple a degree of psychological support. Because they cannot be sure that it was not sperm from the male partner that resulted in conception, they may be more inclined to accept the child as the product of their union. The role of the third-party sperm donor is thus psychologically minimized.

Sperm Donors

Sperm donors are typically selected from medical-student and hospital-staff volunteers. An effort is made to employ as donors people in excellent health with a high level of intellectual ability. Their family histories are reviewed to reduce the possibility of transmitting a genetic disorder, and their blood type is checked to determine its compatibility with that of the AID recipient.

Such general physical features of the donor as body type, hair and eye color, and complexion are matched in a rough way with those of the potential parents. To be a donor, an individual must also be known to be fertile. This means that he must already be a biological parent or that he must fall within the normal range in several semen analyses.

Donors are typically paid for their services. What is more, their identity is kept secret from the recipient and her husband. A coding system is ordinarily used both to preserve the anonymity of the donor and to ensure that the same donor is used in all inseminations.

Sperm contributed by a donor might be employed in an insemination within one to three hours after the semen is obtained. As mentioned earlier, some physicians prefer to use freshly obtained sperm in the procedure. But sperm may also be maintained in a frozen condition and, after being restored to the proper temperature, used in the same way as fresh sperm. Sperm banks are no more than freezers containing racks of coded plastic tubes holding donated sperm.

The semen stored in sperm banks is not necessarily that of anonymous donors. For a variety of reasons, individuals may wish to have their sperm preserved and pay a fee to a sperm-bank operator for this service. For example, a man planning a vasectomy (see the section on sterilization below) or one expecting to become sterile because of a progressive disease may store his sperm in the event that he may later want to father a child.

Issues in Artificial Insemination

Artificial insemination presents a great variety of moral, legal, and social issues. The truth is, most of those issues have not been addressed in a thorough fashion. Legal scholars have explored some of the consequences that AI has for traditional legal doctrines of paternity, legitimacy, and inheritance. They have also made recommendations for formulating new laws (or reformulating old ones) to take into account the reality of the practice of AI.

Others who have written about AI have mostly focused on its potential for altering the relationship between husbands and wives and for producing undesirable social changes. Many of the objections to in vitro fertilization have also been offered to artificial insemination. For example, it has been argued that AI will take the love out of sexual procreation and make it a purely mechanical process, that AI will promote the practice of eugenics and so denigrate the worth of babies that fall short of some ideal, and that AI is just another step down the road toward the society of *Brave New World*.

While such issues are of great importance, they have usually been discussed in such a general fashion that specific ethical questions about the use of artificial insemination as a medical procedure have rarely been raised. As a result, those questions have not been subjected to the dialectical process of argument and criticism that is important in helping us arrive at reasoned opinions.

Some of the issues that need close attention from philosophers concern individual rights and responsibilities. For example, does a man who has served as a sperm donor have any special moral responsibilities? He certainly must have some responsibilities. For example, it would be wrong for him to lie about any genetic diseases in his family history. But does he have any responsibilities to the child that is produced by AI employing his sperm? If donating sperm is no different from donating blood, then perhaps he does not. But is such a comparison apt?

Can a child born as a result of AI legitimately demand to know the name of his biological father? We need not assume that mere curiosity might motivate such a request. Someone might need to know his family background in order to determine how likely it is that a potential child might have a genetic disorder. After all, it is unreasonable to assume that a donor is fully informed about his own biological background. Perhaps the current practice of maintaining the anonymity of sperm donors is not one that can stand critical scrutiny.

Should a woman be allowed to order sperm donated by someone who approximates her concept of an ideal person? Should she be able to request a donor from a certain ethnic group, with particular eye and hair color, certain minimum or maximum height, physical attractiveness, with evidence of intelligence, and so on? At present, the physician who performs the procedure also makes the choice of the donor. But why should the physician be granted the right to make the selection? One might argue that allowing the physician to exercise such a power violates the autonomy of the AI recipient.

A number of other ethical questions are easily raised about AI: Does any woman (married or single, of any age) have the right to demand AI? Should a physician make AID available to a married woman even if her husband is opposed?

Other questions concerning the proper procedures to follow in the practice of AI are also of considerable significance. For example, how thoroughly must sperm donors be screened for genetic defects? What standards of quality must sperm as a biological material be required to satisfy? What physical, educational, or general social traits (if any) should individual donors possess? Should records be maintained and shared through an established network to prevent the marriage or mating of individuals born from AID with the same biological father?

At present, these questions have been answered only by individual physicians or clinics, if at all. There are no general medical or legal policies that govern the practice of AI. Even if present practices are adequate, most people would agree that there is a need to develop uniform policies to regulate AI.

Obviously, we have touched upon only a few of the ethical and social issues that the practice of artificial insemination generates. Indeed, at the moment, it is not wholly clear even what the more significant issues may be. In this area of medical ethics, in particular, philosophers still have a great deal of work to do.

SURROGATE PREGNANCY

We have already mentioned surrogate mothers in connection with in vitro fertilization. In that connection, a surrogate mother is one who supplies an ovum that may be fertilized and implanted into a host mother or one who serves as the host mother (a gestational surrogate) and receives an embryo from the biological parents.

Surrogate mothers in the more usual sense are women who agree to become pregnant by means of artificial insemination with sperm from the male of a married couple. The surrogate mother carries the baby to term, then turns the baby over to the couple for adoption. Surrogate mothers are typically sought by couples who wish to have a child with whom they have some genetic link and who have been unsuccessful in conceiving one themselves.

Various legal complications surround surrogate pregnancy. Although it is not prohibited by state laws, it is not acknowledged as legitimate, either. A number of bills have been introduced into state legislatures either to regulate the arrangements or to forbid them, but none has been passed into law.

A major problem has been finding a legal way to pay women who undertake to be surrogate mothers. Adoption laws forbid the selling of children or even the payment of money to one of the parents in connection with adoption. A Michigan appellate court decision, which the Supreme Court refused to review, held that a couple had the right to the services of a surrogate mother but did not have the right to compensate her for acting in that capacity.

Since a child born to a surrogate mother is legally her child, the child must be adopted by the couple securing her services. How, then, can the surrogate mother be paid? Some women have simply volunteered to be surrogate mothers so that the issue of payment would not arise. In general the difficulty has been resolved by paying the mother to compensate her for the loss of her time and for her inconvenience. Technically, then, the surrogate mother is not being paid for conceiving and bearing a child, nor is she being paid for the child who is handed over for adoption.

The typical fee paid a surrogate mother is about $10,000. If the arrangements are made by an attorney or by an organization like the Infertility Center of New York, additional fees must be paid. The couple seeking the service must also pay the medical and hospital-delivery expenses of the surrogate mother. Total costs range from $20,000 to $25,000.

Some of the same reasons that can be offered to justify in vitro fertilization and embryo transfer can also be offered for surrogate pregnancy. Fundamentally, those couples who wish to have a child of their own but are unable to do so because of some uncorrectable medical difficulty experienced by the woman view surrogate pregnancy as the only hope remaining to them. Some rule out adoption because of the relative shortage of available infants, and some simply want there to be some genetic connection between them and the child. Some people are simply quite desperate to have a child of their own.

Some critics have charged that surrogate pregnancy is no more than a specialized form of prostitution. A woman, in effect, rents out her body for a period of time and is paid for doing so. Such a criticism rests on the assumption that prostitution is morally wrong, and this is a claim that at least some would deny is correct. Furthermore, the criticism fails to take into account the differences in aims. Some surrogate mothers have volunteered their services with no expectation of monetary reward, and some women have agreed to be surrogate mothers at the request of their sisters. Even those who are paid mention that part of their motivation is to help those couples who so desperately want a child. Far from condemning surrogate mothers as acting immorally, it is perhaps possible to view at least some of them as acting in a morally heroic way by contributing to the good of others through their actions.

Perhaps the most serious objection to surrogate mothers is that they are likely to be recruited from the ranks of those most in need of money. Women of the upper and middle income groups are not likely to serve as surrogate mothers. Women with low-paying jobs or no jobs at all are obviously the prime candidates for recruiters. It might be charged, then, that women who become surrogate mothers are being exploited by those who have money enough to pay for their services.

However, merely paying someone in need of money to do something does not constitute exploitation. To make such a charge stick, it would be necessary to show that women who become surrogate mothers are under a great deal of social and economic pressure and have no other realistic options. Furthermore, it could be argued that, within limits, individuals have a right to do with their bodies as they choose. If a woman freely decides to earn money by serving as a surrogate mother, then we have no more reason to object to her decision than we would have to object to a man's decision to earn money by working as a construction laborer.

There is good reason to believe that the practice of employing surrogate mothers is likely to increase in the near future. The ethical and social issues are far from being resolved to the general satisfaction of our society. Al-though surrogate mothers have been featured numerous times in newspapers and magazines, the whole issue of surrogate parenthood has received much less attention than it deserves from philosophers and other ethical theorists.

ETHICAL THEORIES AND REPRODUCTIVE CONTROL

One of the themes of Mary Shelley's famous novel *Frankenstein* is that it is both wrong and dangerous to tamper with the natural forces of life. It is wrong because it disturbs the natural order of things, and it is dangerous because it unleashes forces beyond human control. The "monster" that is animated by Dr. Victor Frankenstein stands as a warning and reproach to all who seek to impose their will on the world through the powers of scientific technology.

The fundamental ethical question about the technology of human reproductive control is whether it ought to be employed at all. Is it simply wrong for us to use our knowledge of human biology to exercise power over the processes of human reproduction?

The natural law view, as represented by currently accepted doctrines of the Roman Catholic Church, suggests that all the techniques for controlling human reproduction that we have discussed here are fundamentally wrong.

Children may ordinarily be expected as a result of sexual union within marriage. However, if no measures are wrongfully taken to frustrate the possibility of their birth (contraception, for example), then a married couple has no obligation to attempt to conceive children by means such as artificial insemination or in vitro fertilization.

Indeed, those processes themselves are inherently objectionable. Artificial insemination requires male masturbation, which is prima facie wrong, since it is an act that can be considered to be unnatural, given the natural end of sex. Furthermore, AI, even when semen from the husband is used, tends to destroy the values inherent in the married state. It makes conception a mechanical act.

In vitro fertilization is open to the same objections. In addition, the process itself involves the destruction of fertilized ova. On the view that human conception takes place at the moment of fertilization, this means that the discarding of unimplanted embryos amounts to the destruction of human life.

On the utilitarian view, no reproductive technology is in itself objectionable. The question that has to be answered is whether the use of any particular procedure, in general or in a certain case, is likely to lead to more good than not. In general, it is reasonable to believe that a utilitarian would be likely to approve of the three sorts of procedures we have discussed here.

However, it is worth mentioning that a rule utilitarian might well oppose any or all of the procedures. If there is strong evidence to support the view that the use of reproductive technology will lead to a society in which the welfare of its members will not be served, then a rule utilitarian would be on firm ground in arguing that reproductive technology ought to be abandoned.

According to Ross's ethical theory, we have prima facie duties of beneficence. That is,

we have an obligation to assist others in bettering their lives. This suggests that the use of reproductive technology may be justified as a means to promote the well-being of others. For example, if a couple desires to have a child but is unable to conceive one, then either in vitro fertilization procedures or artificial insemination might be employed to help them satisfy their shared desire.

Kantian principles do not seem to supply grounds for objecting either to in vitro fertilization or to artificial insemination as inherently wrong. However, the maxim involved in each action must always be one that satisfies the categorical imperative. Consequently, some instances of in vitro fertilization and artificial insemination would no doubt be morally wrong.

The technology of reproduction is a reality of ordinary life. So far it has made our society into neither a dystopia nor a utopia. It is just one set of tools among the many others that science and medicine have forged.

Yet the tools are powerful ones, and we should beware of allowing familiarity to produce indifference. The moral and social issues raised by reproductive technology are just as real as the technology. So far we have not treated some of them with the seriousness that they deserve.

Instruction on Respect for Human Life in Its Origin and on the Dignity of Procreation: Replies to Certain Questions of the Day

Congregation for the Doctrine of the Faith

This "Instruction" was issued on February 22, 1987. It was approved and ordered published by Pope John Paul II and thus may be taken as representing the official position of the Roman Catholic Church on the issues addressed.

The document takes the position that a number of current or potential practices connected with reproductive technology are morally illegitimate. Included are the following:

- Prenatal diagnosis by amniocentesis or ultrasound for the purpose of identifying impaired fetuses so that abortion can be performed;

- Therapeutic intervention that may cause a risk to a fetus disproportionate to a potential benefit;

- Experimentation on a living embryo that is not directly therapeutic;

- Keeping alive human embryos for experimental or commercial purposes;

- Destroying human embryos produced by in vitro techniques for the purpose of either research or procreation;

- Cross-species fertilization involving human and animal gametes;

- The gestation of a human embryo in an animal uterus or an artificial uterus;

- The use of human genetic material in procedures like cloning, parthenogenesis, and twin fission (the splitting of gametes);

- Attempts to manipulate genetic material for the purpose of sex selection or to promote desirable characteristics;

- Artificial insemination involving unmarried individuals or the artificial insemination of an unmarried woman or a widow, even if the sperm is that of her deceased husband;

- Acquiring sperm by means of masturbation;

- Surrogate motherhood.

Some techniques and practices, according to the document, are morally legitimate. Included are the following:

- Medical intervention to remove the causes of infertility;

- The prescription of drugs to promote fertility;

- Prenatal diagnosis with the aim of promoting the welfare of the fetus;

- Prenatal therapeutic intervention (including genetic manipulation) with the aim of healing the developing embryo or fetus;

- Prenatal research that is limited to monitoring or observing the embryo.

The document also makes a number of specific recommendations to governments to establish laws and policies governing reproductive technologies. It asks that civil laws be passed to prohibit the donation of sperm or ova between unmarried people. Laws should "expressly forbid" the use of living embryos for experimentation and protect them from mutilation and destruction. Further, legislation should prohibit "embryo banks, postmortem insemination and 'surrogate motherhood.' "

Some Roman Catholic theologians disagreed sharply with parts of the document. "The document argues that a child can be born only from a sexual act," Richard A. McCormick pointed out. "The most that can be argued is that a child should be born within a marriage from a loving act. Sexual intercourse is not the only loving act." Some suggested that individuals would make up their own minds on the issues, quite apart from the Vatican position. The significance of the document to non-Catholics is that the positions taken and the arguments for them are likely to affect the character of the discussion about reproductive technology and have an impact on legislation that will place restraints on research and practices many currently consider legitimate.

Notes and references are omitted in this excerpt.

Part 1: Respect for Human Embryos

Careful reflection on this teaching of the Magisterium and on the evidence of reason . . . enables us to respond to the numerous moral problems posed by technical interventions upon the human being in the first phases of his life and upon the processes of his conception.

1. What Respect Is Due to the Human Embryo, Taking into Account His Nature and Identity?

The human being must be respected—as a person— from the very first instant of his existence.

The implementation of procedures of artificial fertilization has made possible various interventions upon embryos and human fetuses. The aims pursued are of various kinds: diagnostic and therapeutic, scientific and commercial. From all of this, serious problems arise. Can one speak of a right to experimentation upon human embryos for the purpose of scientific research? What norms or laws should be worked out with regard to this matter? The response to these problems presupposes a detailed reflection on the nature and specific identity— the word "status" is used—of the human embryo itself. . . .

This Congregation is aware of the current debates concerning the beginning of human life, concerning the individuality of the human being and concerning the identity of the human person. The Congregation recalls the teachings found in the Declaration on Procured Abortion: "From the time that the ovum is fertilized, a new life is begun which is neither that of the father nor of the mother: it is rather the life of a new human being with his own growth. It would never be made human if it were not human already. To this perpetual evidence . . . modern genetic science brings valuable confirmation. It has demonstrated that, from the first instant, the programme is fixed as to what this living being will be: a man, this individual-man with his characteristic aspects already well determined. Right from fertilization is begun the adventure of a human life, and each of its great capacities requires time . . . to find its place and to be in a position to act." This teaching remains valid and is further confirmed, if confirmation were needed, by recent findings of human biological science which recognize that in the zygote* resulting from fertilization the biological identity of a new human individual is already constituted. . . .

Thus the fruit of human generation, from the first moment of its existence, that is to say from the moment the zygote has formed, demands the unconditional respect that is morally due to the human being in his bodily and spiritual totality. The human being is to be respected and treated as a person from the moment of conception; and therefore from that same moment his rights as a person must be recognized, among which in the first place is the inviolable right of every innocent human being to life.

The doctrinal reminder provides the fundamental criterion for the solution of the various problems posed by the development of the biomedical sciences in this field: since the embryo must be treated as a person, it must also be defended in its integrity, tended and cared for, to the extent possible, in the same way as any other human being as far as medical assistance is concerned.

2. Is Prenatal Diagnosis Morally Licit?

If prenatal diagnosis respects the life and integrity of the embryo and the human fetus and is directed towards its safeguarding or healing as an individual, then the answer is affirmative.

For prenatal diagnosis makes it possible to know the condition of the embryo and of the fetus when still in the mother's womb. It permits, or makes it possible to anticipate earlier and more ef-

---

*The zygote is the cell produced when the nuclei of the two gametes have fused.

fectively, certain therapeutic, medical or surgical procedures.

Such diagnosis is permissible, with the consent of the parents after they have been adequately informed, if the methods employed safeguard the life and integrity of the embryo and the mother, without subjecting them to disproportionate risks. But this diagnosis is gravely opposed to the moral law when it is done with the thought of possibly inducing an abortion depending upon the results: a diagnosis which shows the existence of a malformation or a hereditary illness must not be the equivalent of a death-sentence. Thus a woman would be committing a gravely illicit act if she were to request such a diagnosis with the deliberate intention of having an abortion should the results confirm the existence of a malformation or abnormality. The spouse or relatives or anyone else would similarly be acting in a manner contrary to the moral law if they were to counsel or impose such a diagnostic procedure on the expectant mother with the same intention of possibly proceeding to an abortion. So too the specialist would be guilty of illicit collaboration if, in conducting the diagnosis and in communicating its results, he were deliberately to contribute to establishing or favoring a link between prenatal diagnosis and abortion.

In conclusion, any directive or program of the civil and health authorities or of scientific organizations which in any way were to favor a link between prenatal diagnosis and abortion, or which were to go as far as directly to induce expectant mothers to submit to prenatal diagnosis planned for the purpose of eliminating fetuses which are affected by malformations or which are carriers of hereditary illness, is to be condemned as a violation of the unborn child's right to life and as an abuse of the prior rights and duties of the spouses.

3. Are Therapeutic Procedures Carried Out on the Human Embryo Licit?

As with all medical interventions on patients, *one must uphold as licit procedures carried out on the human embryo which respect the life and integrity of the embryo and do not involve disproportionate risks for it but are directed towards its healing, the improvement of its condition of health, or its individual survival.*

Whatever the type of medical, surgical or other therapy, the free and informed consent of the parents is required, according to the deontological rules followed in the case of children. The application of this moral principle may call for delicate and particular precautions in the case of embryonic or fetal life. . . .

4. How Is One to Evaluate Morally Research and Experimentation on Human Embryos and Fetuses?

Medical research must refrain from operations on live embryos, unless there is a moral certainty of not causing harm to the life or integrity of the unborn child and the mother, and on condition that the parents have given their free and informed consent to the procedure. It follows that all research, even when limited to the simple observation of the embryo, would become illicit were it to involve risk to the embryo's physical integrity or life by reason of the methods used or the effects induced.

As regards experimentation, and presupposing the general distinction between experimentation for purposes which are not directly therapeutic and experimentation which is clearly therapeutic for the subject himself, in the case in point one must also distinguish between experimentation carried out on embryos which are still alive and experimentation carried out on embryos which are dead. *If the embryos are living, whether viable or not, they must be respected just like any other human person; experimentation on embryos which is not directly therapeutic is illicit.*

No objective, even though noble in itself, such as a foreseeable advantage to science, to other human beings or to society, can in any way justify experimentation on living human embryos or fetuses, whether viable or not, either inside or outside the mother's womb. The informed consent ordinarily required for clinical experimentation on adults cannot be granted by the parents, who may not freely dispose of the physical integrity or life of the unborn child. Moreover, experimentation on embryos and fetuses always involves risk, and indeed in most cases it involves the certain expectation of harm to their physical integrity or even their death. . . .

In the case of experimentation that is clearly therapeutic, namely, when it is a matter of experimental forms of therapy used for the benefit of the embryo itself in a final attempt to save its life, and in the absence of other reliable forms of therapy, recourse to drugs or procedures not yet fully tested can be licit. . . .

5. How Is One to Evaluate Morally the Use for Research Purposes of Embryos Obtained by Fertilization "In Vitro"?

Human embryos obtained in vitro are human beings and subjects with rights: their dignity and right to life must be respected from the first moment of their existence. *It is immoral to produce human embryos destined to be exploited as disposable "biological material."*

In the usual practice of in vitro fertilization, not all of the embryos are transferred to the woman's body; some are destroyed. Just as the Church condemns induced abortion, so she also forbids acts against the life of these human beings. *It is a duty to condemn the particular gravity of the voluntary destruction of human embryos obtained "in vitro" for the sole purpose of research, either by means of artificial insemination or by means of "twin fission."* By acting in this way the researcher usurps the place of God; and, even though he may be unaware of this, he sets himself up as the master of the destiny of others inasmuch as he arbitrarily chooses whom he will allow to live and whom he will send to death and kills defenseless human beings.

Methods of observation or experimentation which damage or impose grave and disproportionate risks upon embryos obtained in vitro are morally illicit for the same reasons. Every human being is to be respected for himself, and cannot be reduced in worth to a pure and simple instrument for the advantage of others. *It is therefore not in conformity with the moral law deliberately to expose to death human embryos obtained "in vitro."* In consequence of the fact that they have been produced in vitro, those embryos which are not transferred into the body of the mother and are called "spare" are exposed to an absurd fate, with no possibility of their being offered safe means of survival which can be licitly pursued.

6. What Judgment Should Be Made on Other Procedures of Manipulating Embryos Connected with the "Techniques of Human Reproduction"?

Techniques of fertilization in vitro can open the way to other forms of biological and genetic manipulation of human embryos, such as attempts or plans for fertilization between human and animal gametes and the gestation of human embryos in the uterus of animals, or the hypothesis or project of constructing artificial uteruses for the human em-

bryos. *These procedures are contrary to the human dignity proper to the embryo, and at the same time they are contrary to the right of every person to be conceived and to be born within marriage and from marriage. Also, attempts or hypotheses for obtaining a human being without any connection with sexuality through "twin fission," cloning or parthenogenesis are to be considered contrary to the moral law, since they are in opposition to the dignity both of human procreation and of the conjugal union.*

The *freezing of embryos*, even when carried out in order to preserve the life of an embryo— cryopreservation—*constitutes an offense against the respect due to human beings* by exposing them to grave risks of death or harm to their physical integrity and depriving them, at least temporarily, of maternal shelter and gestation, thus placing them in a situation in which further offenses and manipulation are possible.

Certain attempts to influence chromosomic or genetic inheritance are not therapeutic but are aimed at producing human beings selected according to sex or other predetermined qualities. These manipulations are contrary to the personal dignity of the human being and his or her integrity and identity. Therefore in no way can they be justified on the grounds of possible beneficial consequences for future humanity. Every person must be respected for himself: in this consists the dignity and right of every human being from his or her beginning.

Part II: Interventions upon Human Procreation

By "artificial procreation" or "artificial fertilization" are understood here the different technical procedures directed towards obtaining a human conception in a manner other than the sexual union of man and woman. This Instruction deals with fertilization of an ovum in a test-tube (in vitro fertilization) and artificial insemination through transfer into the woman's genital tracts of previously collected sperm.

A preliminary point for the moral evaluation of such technical procedures is constituted by the consideration of the circumstances and consequences which those procedures involve in relation to the respect due the human embryo. Development of the practice of in vitro fertilization has required innumerable fertilizations and destructions of human embryos. Even today, the usual practice presupposes a hyper-ovulation on the part of the woman: a number of ova are withdrawn, fertilized and then cultivated in vitro for some days. Usually not all are transferred into the genital tracts of the woman; some embryos, generally called "spare," are destroyed or frozen. On occasion, some of the implanted embryos are sacrificed for various eugenic, economic or psychological reasons. Such deliberate destruction of human beings or their utilization for different purposes to the detriment of their integrity and life is contrary to the doctrine on procured abortion already recalled.

The connection between in vitro fertilization and the voluntary destruction of human embryos occurs too often. This is significant: through these procedures, with apparently contrary purposes, life and death are subjected to the decision of man, who thus sets himself up as the giver of life and death by decree. This dynamic of violence and domination may remain unnoticed by those very individuals who, in wishing to utilize this procedure, become subject to it themselves. The facts recorded and the cold logic which links them must be taken into consideration for a moral judgment on IVF and ET (in vitro fertilization and embryo transfer): the abortion-mentality which has made this procedure possible thus leads, whether one wants it or not, to man's domination over the life and death of his fellow human beings and can lead to a system of radical eugenics.

Nevertheless, such abuses do not exempt one from a further and thorough ethical study of the techniques of artificial procreation considered in themselves, abstracting as far as possible from the destruction of embryos produced in vitro.

The present Instruction will therefore take into consideration in the first place the problems posed by heterologous artificial fertilization (II, 1–3),* and

subsequently those linked with homologous artificial fertilization (II, 4–6).†

Before formulating an ethical judgment on each of these procedures, the principles and values which determine the moral evaluation of each of them will be considered.

A. Heterologous Artificial Fertilization

1. Why Must Human Procreation Take Place in Marriage? *Every human being is always to be accepted as a gift and blessing of God. However, from the moral point of view a truly responsible procreation vis-a-vis the unborn child must be the fruit of marriage.*

For human procreation has specific characteristics by virtue of the personal dignity of the parents and of the children: the procreation of a new person, whereby the man and the woman collaborate with the power of the Creator, must be the fruit and the sign of the mutual self-giving of the spouses, of their love and of their fidelity. *The fidelity of the spouses in the unity of marriage involves reciprocal respect of their right to become a father and a mother only through each other.*

The child has the right to be conceived, carried in the womb, brought into the world and brought up within marriage: it is through the secure and recognized relationship to his own parents that the child can discover his own identity and achieve his own proper human development.

The parents find in their child a confirmation and completion of their reciprocal self-giving: the child is the living image of their love, the permanent sign of their conjugal union, the living and indissoluble concrete expression of their paternity and maternity.

By reason of the vocation and social responsibilities of the person, the good of the children and of the parents contributes to the good of civil society;

---

*By the term heterologous artificial fertilization or procreation, the Instruction means techniques used to obtain a human conception artificially by the use of gametes coming from at least one donor other than the spouses who are joined in marriage. Such techniques can be of two types:

a. Heterologous IVF and ET: the technique used to obtain a human conception through the meeting in vitro of gametes taken from at least one donor other than the two spouses joined in marriage.

b. Heterologous artificial insemination: the technique used to obtain a human conception through the transfer into the genital tracts of the woman of the sperm previously collected from a donor other than the husband.

---

†By artificial homologous fertilization or procreation, the Instruction means the technique used to obtain a human conception using the gametes of the two spouses joined in marriage. Homologous artificial fertilization can be carried out by two different methods:

a. Homologous IVF and ET: the technique used to obtain a human conception through the meeting in vitro of the gametes of the spouses joined in marriage.

b. Homologous artificial insemination: the technique used to obtain a human conception through the transfer into the genital tracts of a married woman of the sperm previously collected from her husband.

the vitality and stability of society require that children come into the world within a family and that the family be firmly based on marriage.

The tradition of the Church and anthropological reflection recognize in marriage and in its indissoluble unity the only setting worthy of truly responsible procreation.

2. Does Heterologous Artificial Fertilization Conform to the Dignity of the Couple and to the Truth of Marriage?

Through IVF and ET and heterologous artificial insemination, human conception is achieved through the fusion of gametes of at least one donor other than the spouses who are united in marriage. *Heterologous artificial fertilization is contrary to the unity of marriage, to the dignity of the spouses, to the vocation proper to parents, and to the child's right to be conceived and brought into the world in marriage and from marriage. . . .*

These reasons lead to a negative moral judgment concerning heterologous artificial fertilization: consequently fertilization of a married woman with the sperm of a donor different from her husband and fertilization with the husband's sperm of an ovum not coming from his wife are morally illicit. Furthermore, the artificial fertilization of a woman who is unmarried or a widow, whoever the donor may be, cannot be morally justified.

The desire to have a child and the love between spouses who long to obviate a sterility which cannot be overcome in any other way constitute understandable motivations; but subjectively good intentions do not render heterologous artificial fertilization conformable to the objective and inalienable properties of marriage or respectful of the rights of the child and of the spouses.

3. Is "Surrogate"* Motherhood Morally Licit?

No, for the same reasons which lead one to reject heterol-

*By "surrogate mother" the Instruction means:

a. the woman who carries in pregnancy an embryo implanted in her uterus and who is genetically a stranger to the embryo because it has been obtained through the union of the gametes of "donors." She carries the pregnancy with a pledge to surrender the baby once it is born to the party who commissioned or made the agreement for the pregnancy.

b. the woman who carries in pregnancy an embryo to whose procreation she has contributed the donation of her own ovum, fertilized through insemination with the sperm of a man other than her husband. She carries the pregnancy with a pledge to surrender the child once it is born to the party who commissioned or made the agreement for the pregnancy.

ogous artificial fertilization: for it is contrary to the unity of marriage and to the dignity of the procreation of the human person.

Surrogate motherhood represents an objective failure to meet the obligations of maternal love, of conjugal fidelity and of responsible motherhood; it offends the dignity and the right of the child to be conceived, carried in the womb, brought into the world and brought up by his own parents; it sets up, to the detriment of families, a division between the physical, psychological and moral elements which constitute those families.

B. Homologous Artificial Fertilization

Since heterologous artificial fertilization has been declared unacceptable, the question arises of how to evaluate morally the process of homologous artificial fertilization: IVF and ET and artificial insemination between husband and wife. First a question of principle must be clarified.

4. What Connection Is Required from the Moral Point of View between Procreation and the Conjugal Act?

. . . In reality, the origin of a human person is the result of an act of giving. The one conceived must be the fruit of his parents' love. He cannot be desired or conceived as the product of an intervention of medical or biological techniques; that would be equivalent to reducing him to an object of scientific technology. No one may subject the coming of a child into the world to conditions of technical efficiency which are to be evaluated according to standards of control and dominion.

The moral relevance of the link between the meanings of the conjugal act and between the goods of marriage, as well as the unity of the human being and the dignity of his origin, demand that the procreation of a human person be brought about as the fruit of the conjugal act specific to the love between spouses. The link between procreation and the conjugal act is thus shown to be of great importance on the anthropological and moral planes, and it throws light on the positions of the Magisterium with regard to homologous artificial fertilization.

5. Is Homologous "In Vitro" Fertilization Morally Licit?

The answer to this question is strictly dependent on the principles just mentioned. Certainly one cannot ignore the legitimate aspirations of sterile couples. For some, recourse to homologous IVF and ET appears to be the only way of fulfilling their sincere desire for a child. The question is asked whether the totality of conjugal life in such situations is not sufficient to insure the dignity proper to human procreation. It is acknowledged that IVF and ET certainly cannot supply for the absence of sexual relations and cannot be preferred to the specific acts of conjugal union, given the risks involved for the child and the difficulties of the procedure. But it is asked whether, when there is no other way of overcoming the sterility which is a source of suffering, homologous in vitro fertilization may not constitute an aid, if not a form of therapy, whereby its moral licitness could be admitted.

The desire for a child—or at the very least an openness to the transmission of life—is a necessary prerequisite from the moral point of view for responsible human procreation. But this good intention is not sufficient for making a positive moral evaluation of in vitro fertilization between spouses. The process of IVF and ET must be judged in itself and cannot borrow its definitive moral quality from the totality of conjugal life of which it becomes part nor from the conjugal acts which may precede or follow it.

It has already been recalled that, in the circumstances in which it is regularly practiced, IVF and ET involves the destruction of human beings, which is something contrary to the doctrine on the illicitness of abortion previously mentioned. But even in a situation in which every precaution were taken to avoid the death of human embryos, homologous IVF and ET dissociates from the conjugal act the actions which are directed to human fertilization. For this reason the very nature of homologous IVF and ET also must be taken into account, even abstracting from the link with procured abortion.

Homologous IVF and ET is brought about outside the bodies of the couple through actions of third parties whose competence and technical activity determine the success of the procedure. Such fertilization entrusts the life and identity of the embryo into the power of doctors and biologists and establishes the domination of technology over the origin and destiny of the human person. Such a relationship of domination is in itself contrary to the dignity and equality that must be common to parents and children.

Conception in vitro is the result of the technical action which presides over fertilization. *Such fertilization is neither in fact achieved or positively willed as the expression and fruit of specific acts of the conjugal union. In homologous IVF and ET, therefore, even if it is considered in the context of "de facto" existing sexual relations, the generation of the human person is objectively deprived of its proper perfection: namely, that of being the result and fruit of a conjugal act* in which the spouses can become "cooperators with God for giving life to a new person." . . .

Certainly, homologous IVF and ET fertilization is not marked by all that ethical negativity found in extra-conjugal procreation; the family and marriage continue to constitute the setting for the birth and upbringing of the children. Nevertheless, in conformity with the traditional doctrine relating to the goods of marriage and the dignity of the person, *the Church remain opposed from the moral point of view to homologous "in vitro" fertilization. Such fertilization is in itself illicit and in opposition to the dignity of procreation and of the conjugal union, even when everything is done to avoid the death of the human embryo.*

Although the manner in which human conception is achieved with IVF and ET cannot be approved, every child which comes into the world must in any case be accepted as a living gift of the divine Goodness and must be brought up with love.

6. How Is Homologous Artificial Insemination to Be Evaluated from the Moral Point of View?

Homologous artificial insemination within marriage cannot be admitted except for those cases in which the technical means is not a substitute for the conjugal act but serves to facilitate and to help so that the act attains its natural purpose.

The teaching of the Magisterium on this point has already been stated. This teaching is not just an expression of particular historical circumstances but is based on the Church's doctrine concerning the connection between the conjugal union and procreation and on a consideration of the personal nature of the conjugal act and of a human procreation. "In its natural structure, the conjugal act is a personal action, a simultaneous and immediate cooperation on the part of the husband and wife, which by the very nature of the agents and the proper nature of the act is the expression of the mutual gift which, according to the words of Scripture, brings about union 'in one flesh.' " Thus moral conscience "does not necessarily proscribe the use of certain artificial means destined solely either to the facilitating of the natural act or to insuring that the natural act normally performed achieves its proper end." If the technical means facilitates the conjugal act or helps it to reach its natural objectives, it can be morally acceptable. If, on the other hand, the procedure were to replace the conjugal act, it is morally illicit.

Artificial insemination as a substitute for the conjugal act is prohibited by reason of the voluntarily achieved dissociation of the two meanings of the conjugal act. Masturbation, through which the sperm is normally obtained, is another sign of this dissociation: even when it is done for the purpose of procreation, the act remains deprived of its unitive meaning: "It lacks the sexual relationship called for by the moral order, namely the relationship which realizes 'the full sense of mutual self-giving and human procreation in the context of true love.' " . . .

8. The Suffering Caused by Infertility in Marriage. *The suffering of spouses who cannot have children or who are afraid of bringing a handicapped child into the world is a suffering that everyone must understand and properly evaluate.*

On the part of the spouses, the desire for a child is natural: it expresses the vocation to fatherhood and motherhood inscribed in conjugal love. This desire can be even stronger if the couple is affected by sterility which appears incurable. Nevertheless, marriage does not confer upon the spouses the right to have a child, but only the right to perform those natural acts which are per se ordered to procreation.

A true and proper right to a child would be contrary to the child's dignity and nature. The child is not an object to which one has a right, nor can he be considered as an object of ownership: rather, a child is a gift, "the supreme gift" and the most gratuitous gift of marriage, and is a living testimony of the mutual giving of his parents. For this reason, the child has the right, as already mentioned, to be the fruit of the specific act of the conjugal love of his parents; and he also has the right to be respected as a person from the moment of his conception.

Nevertheless, whatever its cause or prognosis, sterility is certainly a difficult trial. The community of believers is called to shed light upon and support the suffering of those who are unable to fulfill their legitimate aspiration to motherhood and fatherhood. Spouses who find themselves in this sad situation are called to find in it an opportunity for sharing in a particular way in the Lord's Cross, the source of spiritual fruitfulness. Sterile couples must not forget that "even when procreation is not possible, conjugal life does not for this reason lose its value. Physical sterility in fact can be for spouses the occasion for other important services to the life of the human person, for example, adoption, various forms of educational work, and assistance to other families and to poor or handicapped children."

Many researchers are engaged in the fight against sterility. While fully safeguarding the dignity of human procreation, some have achieved results which previously seemed unattainable. Scientists therefore are to be encouraged to continue their research with the aim of preventing the causes of sterility and of being able to remedy them so that sterile couples will be able to procreate in full respect for their own personal dignity and that of the child to be born. . . .

Creating Embryos _____

Peter Singer

_____

Peter Singer begins by showing that the "standard argument" used to support ascribing a right to life to an embryo fails to be convincing. The premise "Every human being has a right to life" is acceptable only if we appeal to specific mental qualities; yet doing so raises questions about the premise "A human embryo is a human being," for the embryo lacks just these qualities. The standard argument employs "human" equivocally, and Singer finds attempts to rescue the argument unpersuasive.

In his "positive approach," Singer argues that the minimum characteristic that gives an embryo claim to consideration is "the capacity to feel pain or pleasure." At this stage, like many nonhuman animals, the embryo is "conscious but not self-conscious," and we must rigorously control research. Before then, with parental consent, there is no moral objection to discarding early embryos.

The Moral Status of the Embryo

The Standard Argument

The standard argument in favor of attributing a right to life to the embryo goes like this:

> Every human being has a right to life.
> A human embryo is a human being.
> Therefore the embryo has a right to life.

To avoid questions about capital punishment, or killing in self-defense, it can be stipulated that the term "innocent" is assumed whenever we are talking of human beings and their rights.

The standard argument has a standard response. The standard response is to accept the first premise, that all human beings have a right to life, but to deny the second premise, that the human embryo is a human being. This standard response, however, runs into difficulties, because the embryo is clearly a being of some sort, and it can't possibly be of any other species than *Homo sapiens*. So it seems to follow that it must be a human being. Attempts to say that it only becomes a human being at viability, or at birth, are not entirely convincing. Viability is so closely tied to the state of development of neonatal intensive care that it is hardly the kind of thing that can determine when a being gets a right to live. As for birth, those who draw the line there must explain why an infant born premature at 26 weeks should have a right to life, whereas a fetus of 32 weeks, more developed in every respect, should not. Can location relative to the cervix really make so much difference to one's right to life?

Questioning the First Premise

So the standard argument for attributing a right to life to the embryo can withstand the standard response. It is not easy to mount a direct challenge to the claim that the embryo is a human being. What the standard argument cannot withstand, however, is a more critical examination of its first premise: the premise that every human being has a right to life. At first glance, this seems the stronger premise. Do we really want to deny that every (innocent) human being has a right to life? Are we about to condone murder? No wonder it is at the second premise that most of the fire has been directed. But the first premise is surprisingly vulnerable. Its vulnerability becomes apparent as soon as we cease to take "Every human being has a right to life" as some kind of unquestionable moral axiom, and instead inquire into the moral basis for our particular objection to killing human beings.

By "our particular objection to killing human beings" I mean the objection we have to killing human beings, over and above any objections we may have to killing other living beings, such as pigs and cows and dogs and cats, and even trees and lettuces. Why is it that we think killing human beings is so much more serious than killing these other beings?

The obvious answer is that human beings are different from other animals, and the greater seriousness of killing them is a result of these differences. But which of the many differences between humans and other animals justify such a distinction? Again, the obvious response is that the morally relevant differences are those based on our superior mental powers—our self-awareness, our rationality, our moral sense, our autonomy, or some combination of these. They are the kinds of thing, we are inclined to say, which make us "truly human." To be more precise, they are the kinds of thing which make us *persons*.

That the particular objection to killing human beings rests on such qualities is very plausible. To take the most extreme of the differences between living things, consider a person who is enjoying life, is part of a network of relationships with other people, is looking forward to what tomorrow may bring, and freely choosing the course her or his life will take for the years to come. Now think about a lettuce, which, we can safely assume, knows and feels nothing at all. One would have to be quite mad, or morally blind, or warped, not to see that killing the person is far more serious than killing the lettuce.

We shall postpone, for the present, asking just which of the mental qualities make the difference in the moral seriousness between the killing of a person and the killing of a lettuce. For our immediate purposes, all we need to note is that the plausibility of the assertion that human beings have a right to life depends on the fact that human beings generally possess mental qualities which other living beings do not possess. So should we accept the premise that every human being has a right to life? We may do so, but *only* if we bear in mind that by "human being" here we refer to those beings who have the mental qualities that generally distinguish members of our species from members of other species.

Two Senses of "Human"

If this is the sense in which we can accept the first premise, however, what of the second premise? It is immediately clear that in the sense of the term "human being" which is required to make the first premise acceptable, the second premise is false. The embryo, especially the early embryo, is obviously not a being with the mental qualities which generally distinguish members of our species from members of other species. The early embryo has no brain, no nervous system. It is reasonable to assume that, so far as its mental life goes, it has no more awareness than a lettuce.

It is still true that the human embryo is a member of the species *Homo sapiens*. That is, as we saw, why it is difficult to deny that the human embryo is a human being. But we can now see that this is not the sense of "human being" we need to make the standard argument work. A valid argument cannot equivocate on the meanings of the central terms it uses. If the first premise is true when "human" means "a being with certain mental qualities" and the second premise is true when "human" means "member of the species *Homo sapiens*," the argument is based on a slide between the two meanings and is invalid.

Speciesism

Can the argument be rescued? It obviously cannot be rescued by claiming that the embryo is a being with the requisite mental qualities. That *might* be arguable for some later stage of the development of the embryo or fetus, but it is impossible to make out the claim for the early embryo. If the second premise cannot be reconciled with the first in this way, can the first perhaps be defended in a form which makes it compatible with the second? Can it be argued that human beings have a right to life, not because of any moral qualities they may possess, but because they—and not pigs, cows, dogs, or lettuces—are members of the species *Homo sapiens*?

This is a desperate move. Those who make it find themselves having to defend the claim that species membership is *in itself* morally relevant to the wrongness of killing a being. But why should species membership in itself be morally crucial? If we are considering whether it is wrong to destroy something, surely we must look at its actual characteristics, not just the species to which it belongs. If ET and similar visitors from other planets turn out to be sensitive, thinking, planning beings, who get homesick just like we do, would it be acceptable to kill them simply because they are not members of our species? Should you be in any doubt, ask yourself the same kind of question, but with "race" substituted for "species." If we reject the claim that membership of a particular race is *in itself* morally relevant to the wrongness of killing a being, it is not easy to see how we could accept the same claim when based on species membership. Remember that the fact that other races, like our own, can feel, think, and plan for the future is not relevant to this question, for we are considering the simple fact of membership of the particular group—whether race or species—as the *sole* basis for distinguishing between the wrongness of killing those who belong to *our* group, and those who are of some *other* group. As long as we keep this in mind, I am sure that we will conclude that neither race nor species can, *in itself*, provide any justifiable basis for such a distinction.

So the standard argument fails. It fails not because of the standard response that the embryo is not a human being, but because the sense in which the embryo is a human being is not the sense in which we should accept that every human being has a right to life.

The Argument from Potential

At this point in the discussion, those who wish to defend the embryo's right to life often switch ground. We should not, they say, base our views of the status of the embryo on the mental qualities it *actually has while an embryo*; we must, rather, consider what it has the potential to *become*.

Indeed, we do need to consider the moral relevance of the embryo's potential. But this argument is not as easy to grasp as it may appear. If we attempt to set it out in an argument of standard form, as we did with the previous argument, we get

> Every potential human being has a right to life.
> The embryo is a potential human being.
> Therefore the embryo has a right to life.

There is no equivocation in this argument, and its second premise is undoubtedly true. The problem is with the first premise. The claim that every potential human being has a right to life is by no means self-evidently true. We would need to be given good grounds for accepting it. What grounds could there be?

One might try to argue that since full-fledged human beings (those with at least some of the mental qualities I have been discussing) have a right to life, anything with the potential to become a full-fledged human being must also have a right to life. But there is no general rule that a potential X has the rights of an X. If there were, Prince Charles, who is a potential King of England, would now have the rights of a King of England. But he does not.

Another possible argument might go like this: there is nothing of greater moral significance than a thinking, choosing rational being. We value such beings above almost everything else. Therefore anything which can give rise to such a being has value because of what it can become.

What is this argument asserting? It suggests that the destruction of an embryo is wrong because it means that a person who might have existed will now not exist; and since we value people, the destruction of the embryo has caused us to lose something of value. But this proves too much. For destroying an embryo is not the only way of ensuring that a person who might have existed will not exist. If a couple decide, after their second, or third, or fourth child, that their family is complete, it is also the case that a person who might have existed—in fact, several people who might have existed—will not exist. Since some people who oppose abortion also oppose the use of contraceptives, it is worth pointing out that this is true whether the couple use contraceptives, or simply abstain from sexual intercourse during the woman's fertile periods (though admittedly the latter method gives the possible people a greater chance of existence). Yet those who condemn the destruction of embryos do not condemn with equal weight the use of contraceptives, and they generally do not condemn at all the use of

sexual abstinence to limit the size of one's family. So it seems that the basis for their objection to the destruction of the embryo cannot be that a person who might have existed will now not exist.

Another example, more relevant to the question of embryo research, suggests the same conclusion. Suppose that a scientist has obtained two ripe eggs from two women, let us call them Jan and Maria. They are hoping to have their eggs fertilized with their husbands' sperm and transferred to their wombs. Jan had her laparoscopy first, her egg was put into a petri dish, and her husband's sperm added to it some hours ago. On checking it, the scientist finds that fertilization has taken place. In the case of Maria's egg the sperm has only just been added to the dish, so fertilization cannot yet have taken place, but the laboratory has a 90 percent success rate for achieving fertilization in these circumstances, and the scientist is reasonably confident that fertilization will take place within the next few hours. Some would say that to destroy Jan's embryo would be gravely wrong, but to destroy the egg and sperm from Maria and her husband would not be wrong at all, or would be much less seriously wrong. In terms of preventing a possible person from existing, however, the difference is only that there is a slightly higher probability of a person resulting from what is in Jan's petri dish than there is of a person resulting from what is in Maria's petri dish. If the difference in the wrongness of disposing of the contents of the two dishes is greater than this slightly higher probability would justify, it cannot be preventing the existence of a possible future person that makes such disposal wrong. To borrow a phrase from the Oxford philosopher Jonathan Glover, if it is cake we are after, it doesn't make much difference whether we throw away the ingredients separately, or ofter they are mixed together (7).

Uniqueness

At this point some will say that it is wrong to destroy an embryo because the embryo already contains the unique genetic basis for a particular person. When a couple abstain from intercourse, or the scientist washes out the petri dish before fertilization has taken place, the genetic constitution of the person who might have existed has yet to be determined. This is true, of course, but does it matter? *All* human beings are genetically determinate, and all, except identical siblings, are genetically unique.

Imagine that instead of just dropping lots of sperm into a petri dish containing a ripe egg, we carried out a program of artificial reproduction by singling out just *one* sperm and placing it with the egg. Then, once the sperm had been singled out and placed with the egg, the genetic constitution of the person who could develop from the egg-and-sperm would also have been uniquely determined. Suppose now that after the egg and sperm have been placed together, but before fertilization has taken place, the woman is found to have a medical condition which makes pregnancy inadvisable. Freezing is not available, and there are no patients interested in a donated embryo. Would it be wrong to throw out the egg and sperm at this stage? If you do not think that it would be wrong to dispose of the egg and the sperm in *this* situation (and worse than it would be if the usual procedure, involving millions of sperm, had been used) then you cannot be attributing much moral significance to the existence of a genetically unique entity.

I have pursued the will-o'-wisp of potential for a long time—not just today, but over the past five years in which I have been working on this topic. I can understand the view that fertilization is one step in the development of a person and that if potentiality is a matter of degree, the embryo is a degree closer to being a person than a collection of egg and sperm in a petri dish before fertilization has taken place. What I still cannot find is any basis for the view that this difference of degree makes an enormous difference in the moral status of what we have before us.

A Positive Approach

We have now seen the inadequacy of attempts to argue that the early embryo has a right to life. It remains only to say something positive about when in its development the embryo may acquire rights.

The answer must depend on the actual characteristics of the embryo. The minimal characteristic which is needed to give the embryo a claim to consideration is sentience, or the capacity to feel pain or pleasure. Until the embryo reaches that point, there is nothing we can do to the embryo which causes harm to *it*. We can, of course, damage it in such a way as to cause harm to the person it will become, if it lives, but if it never becomes a person, the embryo has not been harmed, because its total lack of awareness means that it can have no interest in becoming a person.

Once an embryo may be capable of feeling pain, there is a clear case for very strict controls over the experimentation which can be done with it. At this point the embryo ranks, morally, with other creatures who are conscious but not self-conscious. Many nonhuman animals come into this category, and in my view they have often been unjustifiably made to suffer in scientific research. We should have stringent controls over research to ensure that this cannot happen to embryos, just as we should have stringent controls to ensure that it cannot happen to animals.

Practical Implications of the Moral Status of Embryos

The conclusion to draw from this is that as long as the parents give their consent, there is no ethical objection to discarding a very early embryo. If the early embryo can be used for significant research, so much the better. What is crucial is that the embryo not be kept beyond the point at which it has formed a brain and a nervous system, and might be capable of suffering. Two government committees—the Warnock Committee in Britain (8) and the Waller Committee in Victoria, Australia (9)—have recently recommended that research on embryos should be allowed, but only up to 14 days after fertilization. This is the period at which the so-called "primitive streak," the first indication of the development of a nervous system, begins to form, and up to this stage there is certainly no possibility of the embryo feeling anything at all. In fact, the 14-day limit is unnecessarily conservative. A limit of, say, 28 days would still be very much on the safe side of the best estimates of when the embryo may be able to feel pain; but such a limit would, in contrast to the 14-day limit, allow research on embryos at the stage at which some of the more specialized cells have begun to form. As we saw earlier, this research would, according to Robert Edwards, have the potential to cure such terrible diseases as sickle cell anemia and leukemia (2).

As for freezing the embryo with a view to later implantation, the question here is essentially one of risk. If freezing carries no special risk of abnormality, there seems to be nothing objectionable about it. With embryo freezing, this appears to be the case. The ethical objections some people have to freezing embryos has led to the suggestions that it would be better to freeze eggs (8); for this and other reasons there has been a considerable research effort di-

rected at freezing eggs. Human eggs are more difficult to freeze than human embryos, and until recently it had not proved possible to freeze them in
a manner which allowed fertilization after thawing.
In December 1985, however, an IVF team at Flinders
University, in Adelaide, South Australia, announced that it had succeeded in obtaining a pregnancy from an egg which had been frozen and
thawed before being fertilized (10). The technique
used involved stripping away a protective outer
layer from the egg, so that it would take up a chemical which would protect it during the freezing process. This technique does overcome the ethical
problems some find in freezing embryos, but it does
so at the cost of introducing a new potential cause
of risk to the offspring, the risk that the chemicals
absorbed by the egg may have some harmful effect
(11). Whether or not this risk proves to be a real one,
from the point of view of ethics, one may doubt
whether the risk is worth running, if the primary
reason for running it is to avoid objections, which
we have now seen to be ill-founded, to the freezing
of embryos. . . .

References

1. Singer P., Wells D. Making babies. New York: Scribner's, 1985.

2. Edwards RG. Paper presented at the Fourth World Congress on IVF. Melbourne, Australia, Nov 22, 1985.

3. Abstract. Proceedings of the Fifth Scientific Meeting of the Fertility Society of Australia, Adelaide, Dec. 2-6, 1986.

4. Rowland R. Reproductive technologies: the final solution to the woman question? In: Arditti R, Klein RD, Minden S, eds, Test-tube women: what future for motherhood? London: Pandora, 1984.

5. Firestone S. The dialectic of sex. New York: Bantam, 1971.

6. Breeze N. Who is going to rock the petri dish? In: Arditti R, Klein RD, Minden S, eds, Test-tube women: what future for motherhood? London: Pandora, 1984.

7. Glover J. Causing death and saving lives. Harmondsworth, England: Penguin, 1977.

8. Warnock M (Chairperson). Report on the Committee of Inquiry into Human Fertilisation and Embryology. London: Her Majesty's Stationery Office, 1984, p 66.

9. Waller L (Chairman). Victorian Government Committee to Consider the Social, Ethical and Legal Issues Arising from In Vitro Fertilization. Report on the disposition of embryos produced by in vitro fertilization. Melbourne: Victorian Government Printer, 1984, p 47.

10. The Australian, Dec 19, 1985.

11. Trounson A. Paper presented at the Fourth World Congress on IVF, Melbourne, Australia, Nov 22, 1985.

Surrogate Motherhood as Prenatal Adoption ————————

Bonnie Steinbock

Bonnie Steinbock reviews the Baby M case and maintains that the court decision was inconsistent in considering the best interest of the child. The aim of legislation, she claims, should be to minimize potential harms and prevent cases like that of Baby M from happening again. This can be so only if surrogacy is not intrinsically wrong.

This leads Steinbock to examine three lines of argument and attempt to show that neither paternalism of the sort outlined by Gerald Dworkin (see Chapter 5) nor such considerations as threats of exploitation, loss of dignity, or harm to the child are adequate to show that surrogacy is inherently objectionable. In Steinbock's view, regulating surrogacy—and protecting liberty—is preferable to prohibiting it.

The recent case of "Baby M" has brought surrogate motherhood to the forefront of American attention. Ultimately, whether we permit or prohibit surrogacy depends on what we take to be good reasons for preventing people from acting as they wish. A growing number of people want to be, or hire, surrogates; are there legitimate reasons to prevent them? Apart from its intrinsic interest, the issue of surrogate motherhood provides us with an opportunity to examine different justifications for limiting individual freedom.

In the first section, I examine the Baby M case, and the lessons it offers. In the second section, I examine claims that surrogacy is ethically unacceptable because exploitive, inconsistent with human dignity, or harmful to the children born of such arrangements. I conclude that these reasons justify restrictions on surrogate contracts, rather than an outright ban.

I. Baby M

Mary Beth Whitehead, a married mother of two, agreed to be inseminated with the sperm of William Stern, and to give up the child to him for a fee of $10,000. The baby (whom Mrs. Whitehead named Sara, and the Sterns named Melissa) was born on March 27, 1986. Three days later, Mrs. Whitehead took her home from the hospital, and turned her over to the Sterns.

Then Mrs. Whitehead changed her mind. She went to the Sterns' home, distraught, and pleaded to have the baby temporarily. Afraid that she would kill herself, the Sterns agreed. The next week, Mrs. Whitehead informed the Sterns that she had decided to keep the child, and threatened to leave the country if court action was taken.

At that point, the situation deteriorated into a cross between the Keystone Kops and Nazi storm troopers. Accompanied by five policemen, the Sterns went to the Whitehead residence armed with a court order giving them temporary custody of the child. Mrs. Whitehead managed to slip the baby out of a window to her husband, and the following morning the Whiteheads fled with the child to Florida, where Mrs. Whitehead's parents lived. During the next three months, the Whiteheads lived in roughly twenty different hotels, motels, and homes to avoid apprehension. From time to time, Mrs. Whitehead telephoned Mr. Stern to discuss the matter: He taped these conversations on advice of counsel. Mrs. Whitehead threatened to kill herself, to kill the child, and falsely to accuse Mr. Stern of sexually molesting her older daughter.

At the end of July 1986, while Mrs. Whitehead was hospitalized with a kidney infection, Florida police raided her mother's home, knocking her down, and seized the child. Baby M was placed in the custody of Mr. Stern, and the Whiteheads returned to New Jersey, where they attempted to regain custody. After a long and emotional court battle, Judge Harvey R. Sorkow ruled on March 31, 1987, that the surrogacy contract was valid, and that specific performance was justified in the best interests of the child. Immediately after reading his decision, he called the Sterns into his chambers so that Mr. Stern's wife, Dr. Elizabeth Stern, could legally adopt the child.

This outcome was unexpected and unprecedented. Most commentators had thought that a court would be unlikely to order a reluctant surrogate to give up an infant merely on the basis of a contract. Indeed, if Mrs. Whitehead had never surrendered the child to the Sterns, but had simply taken her home and kept her there, the outcome undoubtedly would have been different. It is also likely that Mrs. Whitehead's failure to obey the initial custody order angered Judge Sorkow, and affected his decision.

The decision was appealed to the New Jersey Supreme Court, which issued its decision on February 3, 1988. Writing for a unanimous court, Chief Justice Wilentz reversed the lower court's ruling that the surrogacy contract was valid. The court held that a surrogacy contract which provides money for the surrogate mother, and which includes her irrevocable agreement to surrender her child at birth, is invalid and unenforceable. Since the contract was invalid, Mrs. Whitehead did not relinquish, nor were there any other grounds for terminating, her parental rights. Therefore, the adoption of Baby M by Mrs. Stern was improperly granted, and Mrs. Whitehead remains the child's legal mother.

The Court further held that the issue of custody is determined solely by the child's best interests,

From "Surrogate Motherhood as Prenatal Adoption," by Bonnie Steinbock, Law, Medicine and Health Care, Vol. 16, No. 1 (Spring/Summer 1988), 44–50.

and it agreed with the lower court that it was in Melissa's best interests to remain with the Sterns. However, Mrs. Whitehead, as Baby M's legal as well as natural mother, is entitled to have her own interest in visitation considered. The determination of what kind of visitation rights should be granted to her, and under what conditions, was remanded to the trial court.

The distressing details of this case have led many people to reject surrogacy altogether. Do we really want police officers wrenching infants from their mothers' arms, and prolonged custody battles when surrogates find they are unable to surrender their children, as agreed? Advocates of surrogacy say that to reject the practice wholesale, because of one unfortunate instance, is an example of a "hard case" making bad policy. Opponents reply that it is entirely reasonable to focus on the worst potential outcomes when deciding public policy. Everyone can agree on at least one thing: This particular case seems to have been mismanaged from start to finish, and could serve as a manual of how not to arrange a surrogate birth.

First, it is now clear that Mary Beth Whitehead was not a suitable candidate for surrogate motherhood. Her ambivalence about giving up the child was recognized early on, although this information was not passed on to the Sterns.[1] Second, she had contact with the baby after birth, which is usually avoided in "successful" cases. Typically, the adoptive mother is actively involved in the pregnancy, often serving as the pregnant woman's coach in labor. At birth, the baby is given to the adoptive, not the biological, mother. The joy of the adoptive parents in holding their child serves both to promote their bonding, and to lessen the pain of separation of the biological mother.

At Mrs. Whitehead's request, no one at the hospital was aware of the surrogacy arrangement. She and her husband appeared as the proud parents of "Sara Elizabeth Whitehead," the name on her birth certificate. Mrs. Whitehead held her baby, nursed her, and took her home from the hospital—just as she would have done in a normal pregnancy and birth. Not surprisingly, she thought of Sara as her child, and she fought with every weapon at her disposal, honorable and dishonorable, to prevent her being taken away. She can hardly be blamed for doing so.[2]

Why did Dr. Stern, who supposedly had a very good relation with Mrs. Whitehead before the birth,

not act as her labor coach? One possibility is that Mrs. Whitehead, ambivalent about giving up her baby, did not want Dr. Stern involved. At her request, the Sterns' visits to the hospital to see the newborn baby were unobtrusive. It is also possible that Dr. Stern was ambivalent about having a child. The original idea of hiring a surrogate was not hers, but her husband's. It was Mr. Stern who felt a "compelling" need to have a child related to him by blood, having lost all his relatives to the Nazis.

Furthermore, Dr. Stern was not infertile, as was stated in the surrogacy agreement. Rather, in 1979 she was diagnosed by two eye specialists as suffering from optic neuritis, which meant that she "probably" had multiple sclerosis. (This was confirmed by all four experts who testified.) Normal conception was ruled out by the Sterns in late 1982, when a medical colleague told Dr. Stern that his wife, a victim of multiple sclerosis, had suffered a temporary paralysis during pregnancy. "We decided the risk wasn't worth it," Mr. Stern said.[3]

Mrs. Whitehead's lawyer, Harold J. Cassidy, dismissed the suggestion that Dr. Stern's "mildest case" of multiple sclerosis determined their decision to seek a surrogate. He noted that she was not even treated for multiple sclerosis until after the Baby M dispute had started. "It's almost as though it's an afterthought," he said.[4]

Judge Sorkow deemed the decision to avoid conception "medically reasonable and understandable." The Supreme Court did not go so far, noting that "her anxiety appears to have exceeded the actual risk, which current medical authorities assess as minimal."[5] Nonetheless the court acknowledged that her anxiety, including fears that pregnancy might precipitate blindness and paraplegia, was "quite real." Certainly, even a woman who wants a child very much, may reasonably wish to avoid becoming blind and paralyzed as a result of pregnancy. Yet is it believable that a woman who really wanted a child would decide against pregnancy *solely* on the basis of *someone else's* medical experience? Would she not consult at least one specialist on her *own* medical condition before deciding it wasn't worth the risk? The conclusion that she was at best ambivalent about bearing a child seems irresistible.

This possibility conjures up many people's worst fears about surrogacy: That prosperous women, who do not want to interrupt their careers, will use poor and educationally disadvantaged women to bear their children. I will return shortly to the question of whether this is exploitive. The issue here is psychological: What kind of mother is Dr. Stern likely to be? If she is unwilling to undergo pregnancy, with its discomforts, inconveniences, and risks, will she be willing to make the considerable sacrifices which good parenting requires? Mrs. Whitehead's ability to be a good mother was repeatedly questioned during the trial. She was portrayed as immature, untruthful, hysterical, overly identified with her children, and prone to smothering their independence. Even if all this is true—and I think that Mrs. Whitehead's inadequacies were exaggerated—Dr. Stern may not be such a prize either. The choice for Baby M may have been between a highly strung, emotional, over-involved mother, and a remote, detached, even cold one.

The assessment of Mrs. Whitehead's ability to be a good mother was biased by the middle-class prejudices of the judge and mental health officials who testified. Mrs. Whitehead left school at 15, and is not conversant with the latest theories on child rearing: She made the egregious error of giving Sara teddy bears to play with, instead of the more "age-appropriate," expert-approved pans and spoons. She proved to be a total failure at patty-cake. If this is evidence of parental inadequacy, we're all in danger of losing our children.

The Supreme Court felt that Mrs. Whitehead was "rather harshly judged" and acknowledged the possibility that the trial court was wrong in its initial award of custody. Nevertheless, it affirmed Judge Sorkow's decision to allow the Sterns to retain custody, as being in Melissa's best interests. George Annas disagrees with the "best interests" approach. He points out that Judge Sorkow awarded temporary custody of Baby M to the Sterns in May 1986 without giving the Whiteheads notice or an opportunity to obtain legal representation. That was a serious wrong and injustice to the Whiteheads. To allow the Sterns to keep the child compounds the original unfairness: ". . . justice requires that reasonable consideration be given to returning Baby M to the permanent custody of the Whiteheads."[6]

But a child is not a possession, to be returned to the rightful owner. It is not fairness to all parties that should determine a child's fate, but what is best for her. As Chief Justice Wilentz rightly stated, "The child's interests come first: We will not punish it for judicial errors, assuming any were made."[7]

Subsequent events have substantiated the claim that giving custody to the Sterns was in Melissa's best interests. After losing custody, Mrs. Whitehead, whose husband had undergone a vasectomy, became pregnant by another man. She divorced her husband and married Dean R. Gould last November. These developments indicate that the Whiteheads were not able to offer a stable home, although the argument can be made that their marriage might have survived, but for the strains introduced by the court battle, and the loss of Baby M. But even if Judge Sorkow had no reason to prefer the Sterns to the Whiteheads back in May 1986, he was still right to give the Sterns custody in March 1987. To take her away then, at nearly eighteen months of age, from the only parents she had ever known, would have been disruptive, cruel, and unfair to her.

Annas' preference for a just solution is premised partly on his belief that there is no "best interest" solution to this "tragic custody case." I take it that he means that however custody is resolved, Baby M is the loser. Either way, she will be deprived of one parent. However, a best interests solution is not a perfect solution. It is simply the solution which is on balance best for the child, given the realities of the situation. Applying this standard, Judge Sorkow was right to give the Sterns custody, and the Supreme Court was right to uphold the decision.

The best interests argument is based on the assumption that Mr. Stern has at least a *prima facie* claim to Baby M. We certainly would not consider allowing a stranger who kidnapped a baby, and managed to elude the police for a year, to retain custody on the grounds that he was providing a good home to a child who had known no other parent. However, the Baby M case is not analogous. First, Mr. Stern is Baby M's biological father and, as such, has at least some claim to raise her, which no non-parental kidnapper has. Second, Mary Beth Whitehead agreed to give him their baby. Unlike the miller's daughter in *Rumpelstiltskin*, the fairy tale to which the Baby M case is sometimes compared, she was not forced into the agreement. Because both Mary Beth Whitehead and Mr. Stern have *prima facie* claims to Baby M, the decision as to who should raise her should be based on her present best interests. Therefore we must, regretfully, tolerate the injustice to Mrs. Whitehead, and try to avoid such problems in the future.

It is unfortunate that the Court did not decide the issue of visitation on the same basis as custody. By declaring Mrs. Whitehead Gould the legal mother, and maintaining that she is entitled to visitation, the Court has prolonged the fight over Baby M. It is hard to see how this can be in her best interests. This is no ordinary divorce case, where the child has a relation with both parents which it is desirable to maintain. As Mr. Stern said at the start of the court hearing to determine visitation, "Melissa has a right to grow and be happy and not be torn between two parents."[8]

The court's decision was well-meaning but internally inconsistent. Out of concern for the best interests of the child, it granted the Sterns custody. At the same time, by holding Mrs. Whitehead Gould to be the legal mother, with visitation rights, it precluded precisely what is most in Melissa's interest, a resolution of the situation. Further, the decision leaves open the distressing possibility that a Baby M situation could happen again. Legislative efforts should be directed toward ensuring that this worst-case scenario never occurs.

II. Should Surrogacy Be Prohibited?

On June 27, 1988, Michigan became the first state to outlaw commercial contracts for women to bear children for others. Yet making a practice illegal does not necessarily make it go away: Witness black market adoption. The legitimate concerns which support a ban on surrogacy might be better served by careful regulation. However, some practices, such as slavery, are ethically unacceptable, regardless of how carefully regulated they are. Let us consider the arguments that surrogacy is intrinsically unacceptable.

A. Paternalistic Arguments

These arguments against surrogacy take the form of protecting a potential surrogate from a choice she may later regret. As an argument for banning surrogacy, as opposed to providing safeguards to ensure that contracts are freely and knowledgeably undertaken, this is a form of paternalism.

At one time, the characterization of a prohibition as paternalistic was a sufficient reason to reject it. The pendulum has swung back, and many people are willing to accept at least some paternalistic restrictions on freedom. Gerald Dworkin points out that even Mill made one exception to his otherwise absolute rejection of paternalism: He thought that no one should be allowed to sell himself into slavery, because to do so would be to destroy his future autonomy.

This provides a narrow principle to justify some paternalistic interventions. To preserve freedom in the long run, we give up the freedom to make certain choices, those which have results which are "far-reaching, potentially dangerous and irreversible."[9] An example would be a ban on the sale of crack. Virtually everyone who uses crack becomes addicted and, once addicted, a slave to its use. We reasonably and willingly give up our freedom to buy the drug, to protect our ability to make free decisions in the future.

Can a Dworkinian argument be made to rule out surrogacy agreements? Admittedly, the decision to give up a child is permanent, and may have disastrous effects on the surrogate mother. However, many decisions may have long-term, disastrous effects (e.g., postponing childbirth for a career, having an abortion, giving a child up for adoption). Clearly we do not want the state to make decisions for us in all these matters. Dworkin's argument is rightly restricted to paternalistic interferences which protect the individual's autonomy or ability to make decisions in the future. Surrogacy does not involve giving up one's autonomy, which distinguishes it from both the crack and selling-oneself-into-slavery examples. Respect for individual freedom requires us to permit people to make choices which they may later regret.

B. Moral Objections

Four main moral objections to surrogacy were outlined in the Warnock Report.[10]

1. It is inconsistent with human dignity that a woman should use her uterus for financial profit.

2. To deliberately become pregnant with the intention of giving up the child distorts the relationship between mother and child.

3. Surrogacy is degrading because it amounts to child-selling.

4. Since there are some risks attached to pregnancy, no woman ought to be asked to undertake pregnancy for another in order to earn money.

We must all agree that a practice which exploits people or violates human dignity is immoral. However, it is not clear that surrogacy is guilty on either count.

1. Exploitation.   The mere fact that pregnancy is *risky* does not make surrogate agreements exploitive, and therefore morally wrong. People often do risky things for money; why should the line be drawn at undergoing pregnancy? The usual response is to compare surrogacy and kidney-selling. The selling of organs is prohibited because of the potential for coercion and exploitation. But why should kidney-selling be viewed as intrinsically coercive? A possible explanation is that no one would do it, unless driven by poverty. The choice is both forced and dangerous, and hence coercive.

The situation is quite different in the case of the race car driver or stuntman. We do not think that they are *forced* to perform risky activities for money: They freely choose to do so. Unlike selling one's kidneys, these are activities which we can understand (intellectually, anyway) someone choosing to do. Movie stuntmen, for example, often enjoy their work, and derive satisfaction from doing it well. Of course they "do it for the money," in the sense that they would not do it without compensation; few people are willing to work "for free." The element of coercion is missing, however, because they enjoy the job, despite the risks, and could do something else if they chose.

The same is apparently true of most surrogates. "They choose the surrogate role primarily because the fee provides a better economic opportunity than alternative occupations, but also because they enjoy being pregnant and the respect and attention that it draws."[11] Some may derive a feeling of self-worth from an act they regard as highly altruistic: Providing a couple with a child they could not otherwise have. If these motives are present, it is far from clear that the surrogate is being exploited. Indeed, it seems objectionably paternalistic to insist that she is.

2. Human Dignity.   It may be argued that even if womb-leasing is not necessarily exploitive, it should still be rejected as inconsistent with human dignity. But why? As John Harris points out, hair, blood and other tissue is often donated or sold; what is so special about the uterus?[12]

Human dignity is more plausibly invoked in the strongest argument against surrogacy, namely,

that it is the sale of a child. Children are not property, nor can they be bought or sold. It could be argued that surrogacy is wrong because it is analogous to slavery, and so is inconsistent with human dignity.

However, there are important differences between slavery and a surrogate agreement. The child born of a surrogate is not treated cruelly or deprived of freedom or resold; none of the things which make slavery so awful are part of surrogacy. Still, it may be thought that simply putting a market value on a child is wrong. Human life has intrinsic value; it is literally priceless. Arrangements which ignore this violate our deepest notions of the value of human life. It is profoundly disturbing to hear the boyfriend of a surrogate say, quite candidly in a television documentary on surrogacy, "We're in it for the money."

Judge Sorkow accepted the premise that producing a child for money denigrates human dignity, but he denied that this happens in a surrogate agreement. Mrs. Whitehead was not paid for the surrender of the child to the father: She was paid for her willingness to be impregnated and carry Mr. Stern's child to term. The child, once born, is his biological child. "He cannot purchase what is already his."

This is misleading, and not merely because Baby M is as much Mrs. Whitehead's child as Mr. Stern's. It is misleading because it glosses over the fact that the surrender of the child was part—indeed, the whole point—of the agreement. If the surrogate were paid merely for being willing to be impregnated and carrying the child to term, then she would fulfill the contract upon giving birth. She could take the money *and* the child. Mr. Stern did not agree to pay Mrs. Whitehead merely to *have* his child, but to provide him with a child. The New Jersey Supreme Court held that this violated New Jersey's laws prohibiting the payment or acceptance of money in connection with adoption.

One way to remove the taint of baby-selling would be to limit payment to medical expenses associated with the birth or incurred by the surrogate during pregnancy (as is allowed in many jurisdictions, including New Jersey, in ordinary adoptions). Surrogacy could be seen, not as baby-selling, but as a form of adoption. Nowhere did the Supreme Court find any legal prohibition against surrogacy when there is no payment, and when the surrogate has the right to change her mind and keep the child. However, this solution effectively prohibits surrogacy, since few women would become surrogates solely for self-fulfillment or reasons of altruism.

The question, then, is whether we can reconcile paying the surrogate, beyond her medical expenses, with the idea of surrogacy as prenatal adoption. We can do this by separating the terms of the agreement, which include surrendering the infant at birth to the biological father, from the justification for payment. The payment should be seen as compensation for the risks, sacrifice, and discomfort the surrogate undergoes during pregnancy. This means that if, through no fault on the part of the surrogate, the baby is stillborn, she should still be paid in full, since she has kept her part of the bargain. (By contrast, in the Stern-Whitehead agreement, Mrs. Whitehead was to receive only $1,000 for a stillbirth.) If, on the other hand, the surrogate changes her mind and decides to keep the child, she would break the agreement, and would not be entitled to any fee, or compensation for expenses incurred during pregnancy.

C. The Right of Privacy

Most commentators who invoke the right of privacy do so in support of surrogacy. However, George Annas makes the novel argument that the right to rear a child you have borne is also a privacy right, which cannot be prospectively waived. He says:

> [Judge Sorkow] grudgingly concedes that [Mrs. Whitehead] could not prospectively give up her right to have an abortion during pregnancy. . . . This would be an intolerable restriction on her liberty and under *Roe* v. *Wade,* the state has no constitutional authority to enforce a contract that prohibits her from terminating her pregnancy.
>
> But why isn't the same logic applicable to the right to rear a child you have given birth to? Her constitutional rights to rear the child she has given birth to are even stronger since they involve even more intimately, and over a lifetime, her privacy rights to reproduce and rear a child in a family setting.[15]

Absent a compelling state interest (such as protecting a child from unfit parents), it certainly would be an intolerable invasion of privacy for the state to take children from their parents. But Baby M has two parents, both of whom now want her. It is not clear why only people who can give birth (i.e.,

women) should enjoy the right to rear their children.

Moreover, we do allow women to give their children up for adoption after birth. The state enforces those agreements, even if the natural mother, after the prescribed waiting period, changes her mind. Why should the right to rear a child be unwaivable before, but not after, birth? Why should the state have the constitutional authority to uphold postnatal, but not prenatal, adoption agreements? It is not clear why birth should affect the waivability of this right, or have the constitutional significance which Annas attributes to it.

Nevertheless, there are sound moral and policy, if not constitutional, reasons to provide a postnatal waiting period in surrogate agreements. As the Baby M case makes painfully clear, the surrogate may underestimate the bond created by gestation, and the emotional trauma caused by relinquishing the baby. Compassion requires that we acknowledge these feelings, and not deprive a woman of the baby she has carried because, before conception, she underestimated the strength of her feelings for it. Providing a waiting period, as in ordinary postnatal adoptions, will help protect women from making irrevocable mistakes, without banning the practice.

Some may object that this gives too little protection to the prospective adoptive parents. They cannot be sure that the baby is theirs until the waiting period is over. While this is hard on them, a similar burden is placed on other adoptive parents. If the absence of a guarantee serves to discourage people from entering surrogacy agreements, that is not necessarily a bad thing, given all the risks inherent in such contracts. In addition, this requirement would make stricter screening and counselling of surrogates essential, a desirable side effect.

D. Harm to Others

Paternalistic and moral objections to surrogacy do not seem to justify an outright ban. What about the effect on the offspring of such contracts? We do not yet have solid data on the effects of being a "surrogate child." Any claim that surrogacy creates psychological problems in the children is purely speculative. But what if we did discover that such children have deep feelings of worthlessness from learning that their natural mothers deliberately created them with the intention of giving them away? Might we ban surrogacy as posing an unacceptable risk of psychological harm to the resulting children?

Feelings of worthlessness are harmful. They can prevent people from living happy, fulfilling lives. However, a surrogate child, even one whose life is miserable because of these feelings, cannot claim to have been harmed by the surrogate agreement. Without the agreement, the child would never have existed. Unless she is willing to say that her life is not worth living because of these feelings, that she would be better off never having been born, she cannot claim to have been harmed by being born of a surrogate mother.

Children can be *wronged* by being brought into existence, even if they are not, strictly speaking, *harmed*. They are wronged if they are deprived of the minimally decent existence to which all citizens are entitled. We owe it to our children to see that they are not born with such serious impairments that their most basic interests will be doomed in advance. If being born to a surrogate is a handicap of this magnitude, comparable to being born blind or deaf or severely mentally retarded, then surrogacy can be seen as wronging the offspring. This would be a strong reason against permitting such contracts. However, it does not seem likely. Probably the problems arising from surrogacy will be like those faced by adopted children and children whose parents divorce. Such problems are not trivial, but neither are they so serious that the child's very existence can be seen as wrongful.

If surrogate children are neither harmed nor wronged by surrogacy, it may seem that the argument for banning surrogacy on grounds of its harmfulness to the offspring evaporates. After all, if the children themselves have no cause for complaint, how can anyone else claim to reject it on their behalf? Yet it seems extremely counter-intuitive to suggest that the risk of emotional damage to the children born of such arrangements is not even relevant to our deliberations. It seems quite reasonable and proper—even morally obligatory—for policymakers to think about the possible detrimental effects of new reproductive technologies, and to reject those likely to create physically or emotionally damaged people. The explanation for this must involve the idea that it is wrong to bring people into the world in a harmful condition, even if they are not, strictly speaking, harmed by having been brought into existence. Should evidence emerge that surrogacy produces children with serious psychological problems, that would be a strong reason for banning the practice.

There is some evidence on the effect of surrogacy on the other children of the surrogate mother. One woman reported that her daughter, now 17, who was 11 at the time of the surrogate birth, ". . . is still having problems with what I did, and as a result she is still angry with me." She explains, "Nobody told me that a child could bond with a baby while you're still pregnant. I didn't realize then that all the times she listened to his heartbeat and felt his legs kick that she was becoming attached to him."[14]

A less sentimental explanation is possible. It seems likely that her daughter, seeing one child given away, was fearful that the same might be done to her. We can expect anxiety and resentment on the part of children whose mothers give away a brother or sister. The psychological harm to these children is clearly relevant to a determination of whether surrogacy is contrary to public policy. At the same time, it should be remembered that many things, including divorce, remarriage, and even moving to a new neighborhood, create anxiety and resentment in children. We should not use the effect on children as an excuse for banning a practice we find bizarre or offensive.

Conclusion

There are many reasons to be extremely cautious of surrogacy. I cannot imagine becoming a surrogate, nor would I advise anyone else to enter into a contract so fraught with peril. But the fact that a practice is risky, foolish, or even morally distasteful is not sufficient reason to outlaw it. It would be better for the state to regulate the practice, and minimize the potential for harm, without infringing on the liberty of citizens.

Notes

1. Had the Sterns been informed of the psychologist's concerns as to Mrs. Whitehead's suitability to be a surrogate, they might have ended the arrangement, costing the Infertility Center its fee. As Chief Justice Wilentz said, "It is apparent that the profit motive got the better of the Infertility Center." In the matter of Baby M, Supreme Court of New Jersey, A-39, at 45.

2. "[W]e think it is expecting something well beyond normal human capabilities to suggest that this mother should have parted with her newly born infant without a struggle. . . . We . . . cannot conceive of any other case where a perfectly fit

mother was expected to surrender her newly born infant, perhaps forever, and was then told she was a bad mother because she did not." *Id.* at 79.

3. Father recalls surrogate was "perfect." *New York Times*, January 6, 1987, B2.

4. *Id.*

5. In the matter of Baby M, *supra* note 1 at 8.

6. Annas GJ: Baby M: babies (and justice) for sale. *Hastings Center Report* 17 (3): 15, 1987.

7. In the matter of Baby M, *supra* note 1, at 75.

8. Anger and Anguish at Baby M Visitation Hearing, *New York Times*, March 29, 1988, 17.

9. Dworkin G: Paternalism. In Wasserstrom RA, ed.: *Morality and the Law*. Belmont, Calif., Wadsworth,

1971; reprinted in Feinberg J, Gross H, eds., *Philosophy of Law*, 3rd ed. Wadsworth, 1986, p. 265.

10. Warnock M, chair: *Report of the committee of inquiry into human fertilisation and embryology*. London, Her Majesty's Stationery Office, 1984.

11. Robertson JA: Surrogate mothers: not so novel after all. *Hastings Center Report* 13 (5): 29, 1983. Citing Parker P: Surrogate mother's motivations: initial findings. *American Journal of Psychiatry* (140): 1, 1983.

12. Harris J: *The Value of Life*. London: Routledge & Kegan Paul, 1985, 144.

13. Annas, *supra* note 6.

14. Baby M case stirs feelings of surrogate mothers. *New York Times*, March 2, 1987, B1.

The Case against Surrogate Parenting

Herbert T. Krimmel

Herbert T. Krimmel argues that it is morally wrong for someone "to create a human life with the intention of giving it up." Thus, Krimmel disapproves both of the role of surrogate mother and of artificial insemination with donor sperm. In both cases, he argues, a child should be desired for its own sake, not as a means for attaining some other end.

If surrogate motherhood is permitted, Krimmel claims, there is a risk that we will come to view children as little more than commodities that we can exploit for our own ends. Further, the way is opened for the practice of eugenics. Finally, both surrogate pregnancies and artificial insemination with donor sperm exert pressures upon the family structure. The child of the surrogate mother is taken away from her, the sperm donor never knows his children, and both single females and males can become parents.

Is it ethical for someone to create a human life with the intention of giving it up? This seems to be the primary question for both surrogate mother arrangements and artificial insemination by donor (AID), since in both situations a person who is providing germinal material does so only upon the assurance that someone else will assume full responsibility for the child he or she helps to create.

The Ethical Issue

In analyzing the ethics of surrogate mother arrangements, it is helpful to begin by examining the roles the surrogate mother performs. First, she acts as a procreator in providing an ovum to be fertilized. Second, after her ovum has been fertilized by the sperm of the man who wishes to parent the child, she acts as host to the fetus, providing nurture and

From The Hastings Center Report, *October 1983, Vol. 13, no. 5, 35–39. Reproduced by permission.*
© *The Hastings Center.*

protection while the newly conceived individual develops.

I see no insurmountable moral objections to the functions the mother performs in this second role as host. Her actions are analogous to those of a foster mother or of a wet-nurse who cares for a child when the natural mother cannot or does not do so. Using a surrogate mother as a host for the fetus when the biological mother cannot bear the child is no more morally objectionable than employing others to help educate, train, or otherwise care for a child. Except in extremes, where the parent relinquishes or delegates responsibilities for a child for trivial reasons, the practice would not seem to raise a serious moral issue.

I would argue, however, that the first role that the surrogate mother performs—providing germinal material to be fertilized—does pose a major ethical problem. The surrogate mother provides her ovum, and enters into a surrogate mother arrangement, with the clear understanding that she is to avoid responsibility for the life she creates. Surrogate mother arrangements are designed to separate in the mind of the surrogate mother the decision to create a child from the decision to have and raise that child. The cause of this dissociation is some other benefit she will receive, most often money.[1] In other words, her desire to create a child is born of some motive other than the desire to be a parent. This separation of the decision to create a child from the decision to parent it is ethically suspect. The child is conceived not because he is wanted by his biological mother, but because he can be useful to someone else. He is conceived in order to be given away.

At their deepest level, surrogate mother arrangements involve a change in motive for creating children: from a desire to have them for their own sake, to a desire to have them because they can provide some other benefit. The surrogate mother creates a child with the intention to abdicate parental responsibilities. Can we view this as ethical? My answer is no. I will explain why by analyzing various situations in which surrogate mother arrangements might be used.

Why Motive Matters

Let's begin with the single parent. A single woman might use AID, or a single man might use a surrogate mother arrangement, if she or he wanted a child but did not want to be burdened with a spouse.[2] Either practice would intentionally deprive the child of a mother or a father. This, I assert, is fundamentally unfair to the child.

Those who disagree might point to divorce or to the death of a parent as situations in which a child is deprived of one parent and must rely solely or primarily upon the other. The comparison, however, is inapt. After divorce or the death of a parent, a child may find herself with a single parent due to circumstances that were unfortunate, unintended, and undesired. But when surrogate mother arrangements are used by a single parent, depriving the child of a second parent is one of the intended and desired effects. It is one thing to ask how to make the best of a bad situation when it is thrust upon a person. It is different altogether to ask whether one may intentionally set out to achieve the same result. The morality of identical results (for example, killings) will oftentimes differ depending upon whether the situation is invited by, or involuntarily thrust upon, the actor. Legal distinctions following and based upon this ethical distinction are abundant. The law of self-defense provides a notable example.[3]

Since a woman can get pregnant if she wishes whether or not she is married, and since there is little that society can do to prevent women from creating children even if their intention is to deprive the children of a father, why should we be so concerned about single men using surrogate mother arrangements if they too want a child but not a spouse? To say that women can intentionally plan to be unwed mothers is not to condone the practice. Besides, society will hold the father liable in a paternity action if he can be found and identified, which indicates some social concern that people should not be able to abdicate the responsibilities that they incur in generating children. Otherwise, why do we condemn the proverbial sailor with a pregnant girlfriend in every port?

In many surrogate mother arrangements, of course, the surrogate mother will not be transferring custody of the child to a single man, but to a couple: the child's biological and a stepmother, his wife. What are the ethics of surrogate mother arrangements when the child is taken into a two-parent family? Again, surrogate mother arrangements and AID pose similar ethical questions: The surrogate mother transfers her parental responsibilities to the wife of the biological father, while with AID the sperm donor relinquishes his interest in the child to the husband of the biological mother. In both cases the child is created with the intention of transferring the responsibility for its care to a new set of parents. The surrogate mother situation is more dramatic than AID since the transfer occurs after the child is born, while in the case of AID the transfer takes place at the time of the insemination. Nevertheless, the ethical point is the same: creating children for the purpose of transferring them. For a surrogate mother the question remains: Is it ethical to create a child for the purpose of transferring it to the wife of the biological father?

At first blush this looks to be little different from the typical adoption, for what is an adoption other than a transfer of responsibility from one set of parents to another? The analogy is misleading, however, for two reasons. First, it is difficult to imagine anyone conceiving children for the purpose of putting them up for adoption. And, if such a bizarre event were to occur, I doubt that we would look upon it with moral approval. Most adoptions arise either because an undesired conception is brought to term, or because the parents wanted to have the child, but find that they are unable to provide for it because of some unfortunate circumstances that develop after conception.

Second, even if surrogate mother arrangements were to be classified as a type of adoption, not all offerings of children for adoption are necessarily moral. For example, would it be moral for parents to offer their three-year-old for adoption because they are bored with the child? Would it be moral for a couple to offer for adoption their newborn female baby because they wanted a boy?

Therefore, even though surrogate mother arrangements may in some superficial ways be likened to adoption, one must still ask whether it is ethical to separate the decision to create children from the desire to have them. I would answer no. The procreator should desire for its own sake, and not as a means to attaining some other end. Even though one of the ends may be stated altruistically as an attempt to bring happiness to an infertile couple, the child is still being used by the surrogate. She creates it not because she desires it, but because she desires something from it.

To sanction the use and treatment of human beings as means to the achievement of other goals instead of as ends in themselves is to accept an ethic

with a tragic past, and to establish a precedent with a dangerous future. Already the press has reported the decision of one couple to conceive a child for the purpose of using it as a bone marrow donor for its sibling (*Los Angeles Times*, April 17, 1979, p. 1–2). And the bioethics literature contains articles seriously considering whether we should clone human beings to serve as an inventory of spare parts for organ transplants[4] and articles that foresee the use of comatose human beings as self-replenishing blood banks and manufacturing plants for human hormones.[5] How far our society is willing to proceed down this road is uncertain, but it is clear that the first step to all these practices is the acceptance of the same principle that the Nazis attempted to use to justify their medical experiments at the Nuremberg War Crimes Trials: that human beings may be used as means to the achievement of other goals, and need not be treated as ends in themselves.[6]

But why, it might be asked, is it so terrible if the surrogate mother does not desire the child for its own sake, when under the proposed surrogate mother arrangements there will be a couple eagerly desiring to have the child and to be its parents? That this argument may not be entirely accurate will be illustrated in the following section, but the basic reply is that creating a child without desiring it fundamentally changes the way we look at children—instead of viewing them as unique individual personalities to be desired in their own right, we may come to view them as commodities or items of manufacture to be desired because of their utility. A recent newspaper account describes the business of an agency that matches surrogate mothers with barren couples as follows:

> Its first product is due for delivery today. Twelve others are on the way and an additional 20 have been ordered. The "company" is Surrogate Mothering Ltd. and the "product" is babies.[7]

The dangers of this view are best illustrated by examining what might go wrong in a surrogate mother arrangement, and most important, by viewing how the various parties to the contract may react to the disappointment.

What Might Go Wrong

Ninety-nine percent of the surrogate mother arrangements may work out just fine; the child will be born normal, and the adopting parents (that is, the biological father and his wife) will want it. But, what happens when, unforeseeably, the child is born deformed? Since many defects cannot be discovered prenatally by amniocentesis or other means, the situation is bound to arise.[8] Similarly, consider what would happen if the biological father were to die before the birth of the child. Or if the "child" turns out to be twins or triplets. Each of these instances poses an inevitable situation where the adopting parents may be unhappy with the prospect of getting the child or children. Although legislation can mandate that the adopting parents take the child or children in whatever condition they come or whatever the situation, provided the surrogate mother has abided by all the contractual provisions of the surrogate mother arrangement, the important point for our discussion is the attitude that the surrogate mother or the adopting parent might have. Consider the example of the deformed child.

When I participated in the Surrogate Parent Foundation's inaugural symposium in November 1981, I was struck by the attitude of both the surrogate mothers and the adopting parents to these problems. The adopting parents worried, "Do we have to take such a child?" and the surrogate mothers said in response, "Well, we don't want to be stuck with it." Clearly, both groups were anxious not to be responsible for the "undesirable child" born of the surrogate mother arrangement. What does this portend?

It is human nature that when one pays money, one expects value. Things that one pays for have a way of being seen as commodities. Unavoidable in surrogate mother arrangements are questions such as: "Did I get a good one?" We see similar behavior with respect to the adoption of children: comparatively speaking, there is no shortage of black, Mexican-American, mentally retarded, or older children seeking homes; the shortage is in attractive, intelligent-looking Caucasian babies.[9] Similarly, surrogate mother arrangements involve more than just the desire to have a child. The desire is for a certain type of child.

But, it may be objected, don't all parents voice these same concerns in the normal course of having children? Not exactly. No one doubts or minimizes the pain and disappointment parents feel when they learn that their child is born with some genetic or congenital birth defect. But this is different from the surrogate mother situation, where neither the surrogate mother nor the adopting parents may feel responsible, and both sides may feel that they have a legitimate excuse not to assume responsibility for the child. The surrogate mother might blame the biological father for having "defective sperm," as the adopting parents might blame the surrogate mother for a "defective ovum" or for improper care of the fetus during pregnancy. The adopting parents desire a normal child, not *this* child in any condition, and the surrogate mother doesn't want it in any event. So both sides will feel threatened by the birth of an "undesirable child." Like bruised fruit in the produce bin of a supermarket, this child is likely to become an object of avoidance.

Certainly, in the natural course of having children a mother may doubt whether she wants a child if the father has died before its birth; parents may shy away from a defective infant, or be distressed at the thought of multiple births. Nevertheless, I believe they are more likely to accept these contingencies as a matter of fate. I do not think this is the case with surrogate mother arrangements. After all, in the surrogate mother arrangement the adopting parents can blame someone outside the marital relationship. The surrogate mother has been hosting this child all along, and she is delivering it. It certainly looks far more like a commodity than the child that arrives in the natural course within the family unit.

A Dangerous Agenda

Another social problem which arises out of the first, is the fear that surrogate mother arrangements will fall prey to eugenic concerns.[10] Surrogate mother contracts typically have clauses requiring genetic tests of the fetus and stating that the surrogate mother must have an abortion (or keep the child herself) if the child does not pass these tests.[11]

In the last decade we have witnessed a renaissance of interest in eugenics. This, coupled with advances in biomedical technology, has created a host of abuses and new moral problems. For example, genetic counseling clinics now face a dilemma: amniocentesis, the same procedure that identifies whether a fetus suffers from certain genetic defects, also discloses the sex of a fetus. Genetic counseling clinics have reported that even when the fetus is normal, a disproportionate number of mothers abort female children.[12] Aborting normal fetuses simply because the prospective parents desire children of a certain sex is one result of viewing children as commodities. The recent scandal at the Repository for Germinal Choice, the so-called "Nobel Sperm Bank," provides another chilling example. Their first "customer" was, unbeknownst to the staff, a woman who "had lost custody of two other children because they were abused in an effort to 'make them smart.' "[13] Of course, these and similar evils may occur whether or not surrogate mother arrangements are allowed by law. But to the extent that they promote the view of children as commodities, these arrangements contribute to these problems. There is nothing wrong with striving for betterment, as long as it does not result in intolerance to that which is not perfect. But I fear that the latter attitude will become prevalent.

Sanctioning surrogate mother arrangements can also exert pressures upon the family structure. First, as was noted earlier, there is nothing technically to prevent the use of surrogate mother arrangements by single males desiring to become parents. Indeed, single females can already do this with AID or even without it. But even if legislation were to limit the use of the surrogate mother arrangements to infertile couples, other pressures would occur: namely the intrusion of a third adult into the marital community.[14] I do not think that society is ready to accept either single parenting or quasi-adulterous arrangements as normal.

Another stress on the family structure arises within the family of the surrogate mother. When the child is surrendered to the adopting parents it is removed not only from the surrogate mother, but also from her family. They too have interests to be considered. Do not the siblings of that child have an interest in the fact that their little baby brother has been "given" away?[15] One woman, the mother of a medical student who had often donated sperm for artificial insemination, expressed her feelings to me eloquently. She asked, "I wonder how many grandchildren I have that I have never seen and never been able to hold or cuddle."

Intrafamily tensions can also be expected to result in the family of the adopting parents due to the asymmetry of relationship the adopting parents will have toward the child. The adopting mother has no biological relationship to the child, whereas the adopting father is also the child's biological father. Won't this unequal biological claim on the child be used as a wedge in child-rearing arguments? Can't we imagine the father saying, "Well, he is my son, not yours"? What if the couple eventually gets divorced? Should custody in a subsequent divorce between the adopting mother and the biological father be treated simply as a normal child custody dispute? Or should the biological relationship between father and child weigh more heavily? These questions do not arise in typical adoption situations since both parents are equally unrelated biologically to the child. Indeed, in adoption there is symmetry. The surrogate mother situation is more analogous to second marriages, where the children of one party by a prior marriage are adopted by the new spouse. Since asymmetry in second marriage situations causes problems, we can anticipate similar difficulties arising from surrogate mother arrangements.

There is also the worry that the offspring of a surrogate mother arrangement will be deprived of important information about his or her heritage. This also happens with adopted children or children conceived by AID,[16] who lack information about their biological parents, which could be important to them medically. Another less popularly recognized problem is the danger of half-sibling marriages,[17] where the child of the surrogate mother unwittingly falls in love with a half sister or brother. The only way to avoid these problems is to dispense with the confidentiality of parental records; however, the natural parents may not always want their identity disclosed.

The legalization of surrogate mother arrangements may also put undue pressure upon poor women to use their bodies in this way to support themselves and their families. Analogous problems have arisen in the past with the use of paid blood donors.[18] And occasionally the press reports someone desperate enough to offer to sell an eye or some other organ.[19] I believe that certain things should be viewed as too important to be sold as commodities, and I hope that we have advanced from the time when parents raised children for profitable labor, or found themselves forced to sell their children.

While many of the social dilemmas I have outlined here have their analogies in other present-day occurrences such as divorced families or in adoption, every addition is hurtful. Legalizing surrogate mother arrangements will increase the frequency of these problems and put more stress on our society's shared moral values.[20]

A Tale for Our Time

An infertile couple might prefer to raise a child with a biological relationship to the husband, rather than to raise an adopted child who has no biological relationship to either the husband or the wife. But does the marginal increase in joy that they might therefore experience outweigh the potential pain that they, or the child conceived in such arrangements, or others might suffer? Does their preference outweigh the social costs and problems that the legalization of surrogate mothering might well engender? I honestly do not know. I don't even know on what hypothetical scale such interests could be weighed and balanced. But even if we could weigh such interests, and even if personal preference outweighed the costs, I still would not be able to say that we could justify achieving those ends by these means; that ethically it would be permissible for a person to create a child, not because she desired it, but because it could be useful to her.

Edmond Cahn has termed this ignoring of means in the attainment of ends the "Pompey syndrome".[21]

> I have taken the name from young Sextus Pompey, who appears in Shakespeare's *Antony and Cleopatra* in an incident drawn directly from Plutarch. Pompey, whose navy has won control of the seas around Italy, comes to negotiate peace with the Roman triumvirs Mark Antony, Octavius Caesar, and Lepidus, and they meet in a roistering party on Pompey's ship. As they carouse, one of Pompey's lieutenants draws him aside and whispers that he can become lord of all the world if he will only grant the lieutenant leave to cut first the mooring cable and then the throats of the triumvirs. Pompey pauses, then replies in these words:
>
> Ah, this thou shouldst have done,
> And not have spoke on't!
> In me 'tis villainy:
> In thee't had been good service.
> Thou must know tis not my profit that does
>   lend mine honour;
> Mine honour, it. Repent that e'er thy tongue
> Hath so betrayed thine act; being done
>   unknown;
> I should have found it afterwards well done,
> But must condemn it now. Desist, and drink.

Here we have the most pervasive of moral syndromes, the one most characteristic of so-called re-spectable men in a civilized society. To possess the end and yet not be responsible for the means, to grasp the fruit while disavowing the tree, to escape being told the cost until someone else has paid it irrevocably; this is the Pompey syndrome and the chief hypocrisy of our time.

Notes

1. See Philip J. Parker, "Motivation of Surrogate Mothers: Initial Findings," *American Journal of Psychiatry* 140:1 (January 1983), 117–18; see also Doe v. Kelley, Circuit Court of Wayne County Michigan (1980) reported in 1980 Rep. on Human Reproduction and Law II-A-1.

2. See, e.g., C. M. v C. C., 152 N.J. Supp. 160, 377 A2d 821 (1977); "Why She Went to 'Nobel Sperm Bank' for Child," *Los Angeles Herald Examiner*, Aug. 6, 1982, p. A9; "Womb for Rent," *Los Angeles Herald Examiner*, Sept. 21, 1981, p. A3.

3. See also Richard McCormick, "Reproductive Technologies: Ethical Issues" in *Encyclopedia of Bioethics*, edited by Walter Reich, Vol. 4 (New York: The Free Press, 1978) pp. 1454, 1459; Robert Snowden and G. D. Mitchell, *The Artificial Family* (London: George Allen & Unwin, 1981), p. 71.

4. See, e.g., Alexander Peters, "The Brave New World: Can the Law Bring Order within Traditional Concepts of Due Process?" *Suffolk Law Review* 4 (1970), 894, 901–02; Roderie Gorney, "The New Biology and the Future of Man," UCLA Law Review 15 (1968), 273, 302; J. G. Castel, "Legal Implications of Biomedical Science and Technology in the Twenty-First Century," *Canadian Bar Review* 51 (1973), 119, 127.

5. See Harry Nelson, "Maintaining Dead to Serve as Blood Makers Proposed: Logical, Sociologist Says," *Los Angeles Times*, February 26, 1974 p. II-1; Hans Jonas, "Against the Stream: Comments on the Definition and Redefinition of Death," in *Philosophical Essays: From Ancient Creed to Technological Man* (Chicago: University of Chicago Press, 1974), pp. 132–140.

6. See Leo Alexander, "Medical Science under Dictatorship," *New England Journal of Medicine* 241:2 (1949), 39; United States v. Brandt, Trial of the Major War Criminals, International Military Tribunal: Nuremberg, 14 November 1945-1 October 1946.

7. Bob Dvorchak, "Surrogate Mothers: Pregnant Idea Now a Pregnant Business," *Los Angeles Herald Examiner*, December 27, 1983, p. Al.

8. "Surrogate's Baby Born with Deformities Rejected by All," *Los Angeles Times*, January 22, 1983, p. I-17;

"Man Who Hired Surrogate Did Not Father Ailing Baby," *Los Angeles Herald Examiner*, February 3, 1983, p. A-6.

9. See, e.g., Adoption in America, Hearing before the Subcommittee on Aging, Family and Human Services of the Senate Committee on Labor and Human Resources, 97th Congress, 1st Session (1981), p. 3 (comments of Senator Jeremiah Denton) and pp. 16–17 (statement of Warren Master, Acting Commissioner of Administration for Children, Youth and Families, HHS).

10. Cf. "Discussion: Moral, Social and Ethical Issues," in *Law and Ethics of A.I.D. and Embryo Transfer* (1973) (comments of Himmelweit), reprinted in Michael Shapiro and Roy Spece. *Bioethics and Law* (St. Paul: West Publishing Company, 1981), p. 548.

11. See, e.g., Lane (*Newsday*), "Womb for Rent," *Tucson Citizen* (Weekender), June 7, 1980, p. 3: Susan Lewis, "Baby Bartering? Surrogate Mothers Pose Issues for Lawyers, Courts," *The Los Angeles Daily Journal*, April 20, 1981; see also Elaine Markoutsas, "Women Who Have Babies for Other Women," *Good Housekeeping* 96 (April 1981), 104.

12. See Morton A. Stenchever, "An Abuse of Prenatal Diagnosis," *Journal of the American Medical Association* 221 (1972), 408, Charles Westoff and Ronald R. Rindfus, "Sex Preselection in the United States: Some Implications," *Science* 184 (1974), 633, 636; see also Phyllis Battelle, "Is It a Boy or a Girl"? *Los Angeles Herald Examiner*, Oct. 8, 1981, p. A17.

13. "2 Children Taken from Sperm Bank Mother," *Los Angeles Times*, July 14, 1982, p. I-3; "The Sperm-Bank Scandal," *Newsweek* 24 (July 26, 1982).

14. See Helmut Thielicke, *The Ethics of Sex*, John W. Doberstein, trans. (New York: Harper & Row, 1964).

15. According to one newspaper account, when a surrogate mother informed her nine-year-old daughter that the new baby would be given away, the daughter replied, "Oh, good. If it's a girl we can keep it and give Jeffrey [her two-year-old half brother] away," "Womb for Rent," *Los Angeles Herald Examiner*, Sept. 21, 1981, p. A3.

16. See, e.g., Lorraine Dusky, "Brave New Babies"? *Newsweek* 30 (December 6, 1982). Also testimony of Suzanne Rubin before the California Assembly Committee on Judiciary, Surrogate Parenting Contracts, Assembly Publication No. 962, pp. 72–75 (November 19, 1982).

17. This has posed an increasing problem for children conceived through AID. See, e.g., Martin Curie-Cohen, et al., "Current Practice of Artificial Insemination by Donor in the United States," *New England Journal of Medicine* 300 (1979), 585–89.

18. See, e.g., Richard M. Titmuss, *The Gift Relationship: From Human Blood to Social Policy* (New York: Random House, 1971).

19. See, e.g., "Man Desperate for Funds: Eye for Sale at $35,000," *Los Angeles Times*, February 1, 1975, p. II-1; "100 Answer Man's Ad for New Kidney," *Los Angeles Times*, September 12, 1974, p. I-4.

20. See generally Guido Calabresi, "Reflections on Medical Experimentation in Humans," *Daedalus* 98 (1969), 387–93; also see Michael Shapiro and Roy Spece, "On Being 'Unprincipled on Principle': The Limits of Decision Making 'On the Merits' " in *Bioethics and Law*, pp. 67–71.

21. Edmond Cahn, "Drug Experiments and the Public Conscience," in *Drugs in Our Society*, edited by Paul Talalay (Baltimore: The Johns Hopkins Press, 1964), pp. 255, 258–61.

The Right to Lesbian Parenthood

Gillian Hanscombe

Gillian Hanscombe sees the possibility of becoming a single parent a major advantage of reproductive technology. She argues that homosexual parents are entitled to the same treatment from physicians and institutions as heterosexual ones. The objection that lesbian women should not be allowed to reproduce by artificial insemination is not one that can be supported by relevant evidence, Hanscombe claims. No studies have demonstrated that lesbian mothering is any different than heterosexual mothering or that children of lesbian mothers "fall victim to negative psychosexual developmental influences." She mentions instances of what she considers to be groundless prejudice against lesbian women by the medical establishment.

Anyone daring to address the subject of human rights faces both an appalling responsibility and being accused of an unnatural arrogance of utterance. I accept these risks not because I think myself expert on the subject of human rights, but because my experience is that human rights in the domain of parenthood are so very often denied existence.

I refer to a large minority in our population, that of lesbian women and gay men. Even at the most conservative estimate—which is that at least 1 in 20 adult people are homosexual—a group comprising 5 per cent—we are dealing with a group larger than the 4 per cent ethnic minorities group which already receives, as indeed it deserves to do, special attention. Lesbian women and gay men have to date, in all matters of social policy, been traditionally regarded as a deviant group.

It is the case, nonetheless, that the pathologising of this group is increasingly questioned, not only by members of the gay community themselves, but also by the agencies of our institutional life: that is, by medical practitioners, by teachers and social workers, and by working parties of religious and/or political orientation.

I am the co-author of a book about lesbian mothers.[1] It is written for the general public, rather than for specialists, but is nevertheless the only book to date on the subject which I know of. It records the experiences of a selected group of lesbian mothers—selected to range over the varieties of social existence these parents and their children experience—from divorced women to single women who have deliberately chosen to conceive their children by artificial insemination by donor (AID).

The question asked by many heterosexual professionals who are charged with the theory or practice of social policy, is whether lesbian women, for example, should be (a) allowed, and (b) aided, to become mothers.

Objections to lesbian women being *allowed* to reproduce can only be social, since no physiological studies seeking to find physical differences between

lesbian and non-lesbian women have ever succeeded in demonstrating such a difference.

Social objections fall into two categories: (a) the extent to which the psychopathology of the lesbian mother is assumed or demonstrated to deviate negatively from the norm. No studies to date have demonstrated that lesbian mothering is either significantly different from heterosexual mothering or that the lesbian mother is psychologically inadequately equipped to mother;[2] (b) the extent to which the children of lesbian mothers are assumed to fall victim to negative psychosexual developmental influences. No study to date has succeeded in demonstrating such a phenomenon.[3]

There remain social objections issuing from prejudice, which in turn issues from ignorance. Since the medical profession forms a professional part of our social policy-making institutional life, it is required that medical practitioners do not form judgments based on ignorance. A mere assumption that because, historically, lesbian women have been pathologised this somehow proves that they are "not normal" (and that in a negative sense) is, of course, unacceptable.

A good way of thinking about this is to begin with what is known about female sexuality. In the first place, it is clear that women, unlike men, are able to separate their sexual practice from their reproductive practice. It is possible, that is, for a woman (a) to become sexually aroused and reach orgasm without any possibility that she will become pregnant and (b) for a woman to be inseminated—either naturally or artificially—and become pregnant whether or not, at the same time, she experiences any sexual pleasure. Whatever might be thought, therefore, about lesbian sexual practice, it is clear that lesbian women are able to conceive and bear children in the same way as non-lesbian women do.

Hence, attempting not to allow them to do so would be highly problematic, even apart from the massive dilemma—were such a decision taken—of not being able to enforce the sanction. Contrary to

Reprinted by permission of Journal of Medical Ethics, *1983, vol. 9, 133–135.*

popular prejudice, it is the case that lesbian women, like other women, are quite capable of engaging in sexual intercourse with a man and, like other women, often solely for the reason that they intend to become pregnant.

Prejudice is not only rife within what are called the "helping professions," it is rife, too, in the courts. Lesbian mothers in dispute with husbands almost all lose custody of their children solely on the grounds of their lesbianism.[4] Because of this, as well as for many other reasons, young women in the last decade have turned increasingly to the alternative of AID. They have found, by and large, that medical practitioners are not willing to provide AID for them, again solely on the grounds of their lesbianism. They have decided, increasingly, in response to this attitude, to conduct AID by themselves, with the assistance of sympathetic men. This is neither technically difficult nor is it illegal. Many AID daughters and sons of lesbian women are now in our nurseries and schools.

There are over two million lesbian mothers in the United States. Calculations for Britain are well-nigh impossible, owing to the professional non-recognition of the existence of the group, together with the mothers' reticence in the face of prejudice. They are rightly anxious to conceal their sexuality since, like nearly all mothers, they love their children and will not willingly give them up, either to the courts or to any other social agency.

We might consider one case in particular. A lesbian woman, of middle-class background and professional standing in her own right, decided that she wanted to become a mother. It was, for her, a natural fulfillment of her womanhood, just as it is for millions of other women.

She became pregnant, deliberately, but unfortunately suffered a miscarriage, accompanied by much distress and depression. The usual practice of the hospital treating her was that, following the customary D & C, the patient should report to her own general practitioner. This she did, some six weeks later, wanting very much to know whether there were any clinical reasons why she might suffer further miscarriages. She asked the GP whether the hospital had sent her report.

"Yes, why?" came the reply.

"I want to know whether there is anything wrong with me which explains why I lost the baby," the woman explained.

"Why do you want to know?" persisted the GP.

"Because if there isn't, I want to become pregnant again," said the woman. "It was so dreadful losing the baby that I wouldn't knowingly go through it again. But if I can have a normal, full-term pregnancy, I want to try."

"But you can't have a baby," replied the GP, appalled; "you're not married!"

"What's that got to do with it?" asked the woman. And so ensued an embarrassing session of moralistic instruction from the GP to the silent woman. Her question remained unanswered.

She asked a friend who was a GP in a different area to write to the hospital for the information. This was done. There was no clinical reason for the miscarriage and the woman was pronounced normal and healthy.

The woman became pregnant again. But instead of feeling she could be cared for by her GP, she felt forced to opt for ante-natal care in the impersonal atmosphere of the hospital, where hundreds of women attended the clinic and where the same practitioner hardly ever appeared twice. At each visit, she was seen by different staff, which was comfortless but which at least ensured minimal questioning.

When she was nearly three months pregnant, the sister-in-charge said she must see the social worker. It was "hospital policy." But only, of course, for the unmarried. The woman felt angry and hurt, but didn't want to be accused of "making trouble." The social worker was sympathetic. "Just for the record, do you want your baby?" she asked. "Just for the record," the woman replied, "I planned my baby."

After delivery, she and her baby were not placed in an ordinary ward, but in one where mothers with handicapped babies were placed, together with mothers who had not had normal deliveries. In addition, she was "strongly advised" to stay for the full period, rather than to go home after 48 hours. And yet both she and her baby were fit and healthy.

This mother keeps away from the "helping professions." She is not open with her present GP, her child's school or the para-medical services, either about the circumstances of her child's birth or about her own sexuality. When she is offered contraception during her cervical smear tests, she simply declines it, not daring to explain that she is one of thousands of lesbian women who don't need it.

This woman is a proud and independent mother.[5] And her story is only one among scores. There is the mother who was refused AID by her local medical services and who then answered an advertisement in a lonely hearts column in order to find a man who would make her pregnant. She charted her ovulation cycle, and when she was fertile, dated the man, who only and clearly wanted casual sex. Her "experiment" worked and she bore a healthy child. There is the mother who came home from work one day to find a weeping partner who had to tell her that both her children—a son aged nine and a daughter aged seven—had been taken into care, because someone had told the social worker that the two women were lesbians.[6]

Hardly any histories of lesbian mothers and their children are on the record. But they are amongst us and they deserve the same care from professional careers as do other mothers and their children.

There are, too, gay men who parent and there are lesbian women and gay men who, though not biological parents themselves, are necessarily involved in childcare by virtue of their partners' parenthood. And there are men who donate semen for the insemination of women who take on themselves the responsibility of conception in order to exercise their right to reproduce and to bring up children. None of the considered and intricate planning undertaken by all these people is mentioned in the vast literature about the family, either in professional or popular publications. Hardly any of this material finds its way into discussions and seminars about family policy, about education, about poverty and so on.

In addition, cruel and heartless lobbying from powerful religious and political quarters—aimed against the human rights of adult homosexual women and men—is ongoing, despite its lack of scientific objectivity. Such pressure is also richly funded. The onus is therefore on the rational, well-informed and compassionate professionals in our caring institutions to consider how they will respond to those of our number born to homosexual parents. Removing the right to reproduce is both immoral and impractical. Neglecting the need of parents for normal support is both discriminatory and cruel. Removing their children from the natural custody of their parents—merely on grounds of the parents' sexuality—is a monstrous interference, with consequences for the children which are no better than the fate of children who are unwanted by their natural mothers. What is needed is education, not legislation.

There are no data—scientific, psychological, or social—which could support the thesis that homosexual people should not have the right to reproduce and to bring up their children. There are only differing opinions and prejudices, which are not capable of sustaining the rigorous intellectual analysis upon which any given body of knowledge must rest. Hitler didn't like homosexuals. Or the handicapped. Or Jews. His answer was to attempt to exterminate them. Our cruelties are not so extreme. What we do is simply to ignore groups of people whose existence troubles us.

I submit, humbly but confidently, that using an argument to exclude adult people from parenthood which is based solely on the definition of an individual's sexual practice, is untenable and uncivilised. Adult people have in their gift the right to dispose of their own reproductive potential as they themselves think suitable. And the rest of us share, all of us, in the responsibility to care for all those committed to parenting and for the children for whom they care.

References and Notes

1. Hanscombe G E, Forster J. *Rocking the cradle*. London: Peter Owen, 1981 and Sheba Feminist Publishers, 1982.

2. Green R. Sexual identity of 37 children raised by homosexual or transexual parents. *American Journal of Psychiatry* 1978; 6: 692–697.

3. See project comparing the psychosexual development of lesbians' children with that of single non-lesbians' children, undertaken by Michael Rutter, Susan Golombok and Ann Spencer, of the Institute of Psychiatry in London. Not all the data is yet published—to my present knowledge—but see reference (1) 85–87.

4. In February of this year the Court of Appeal ruled in favour of a lesbian mother retaining custody of her two daughters. The case made newspaper headlines, not least because such rulings have been so rare.

5. Identity and details withheld.

6. Identities and details withheld.

Artificial Insemination and Donor Responsibility _____

Ronald Munson

Ronald Munson argues that there are no morally significant differences between the sperm donor and the blood donor. Prima facie it may seem that there should be, given the fact that sperm may lead to the production of a child. Sperm and blood donors both have some responsibilities by virtue of the fact that both supply a product. However, even though the sperm donor supplies a causal condition for pregnancy, he is not the causal agent of the pregnancy. Lacking causal responsibility, he also lacks moral responsibility for any resulting child.

When Onan cast his seed on the ground, according to the Biblical account, that was the end of the possibility that his sperm might generate offspring. Modern biomedical technology has substantially altered the situation. Sperm cast into a sterile plastic container may immediately be used in an attempt to fertilize an ovum of a woman who has requested the procedure. Or the sperm might be frozen and later used toward the same end.

Onan may have had responsibilities to his God, but neither he nor anyone else had any particular moral responsibilities concerning the use of his cast-off sperm. By contrast, artificial insemination (AI) presents a great variety of moral, legal, and social issues. Some of the questions concern individual rights and responsibilities: Can a child born from AI legitimately demand to know the name of her biological father? Should any woman be permitted to be inseminated "on demand"? Should self-described lesbians be acknowledged as having a right to have children by AI? Should a woman be allowed to order sperm donated by a man who approximates her ideal (ethnic group, hair and eye color, height, body type, intelligence, physical attractiveness, sexual orientation)?

Other questions concern the proper role and responsibilities of sperm banks as social institutions: How thoroughly must sperm donors be screened for genetic diseases? Should acknowledged homosexuals be permitted to be sperm donors? What physical, educational, or general social traits (if any) should individuals possess to qualify as donors? Should national records be maintained and shared to prevent the marriage or mating of individuals born from AI with the same biological father (that is, the same anonymous donor)?

My concern here clearly cannot be with all of the issues raised by AI. I wish to limit consideration to a single, although central, issue. The question can be formulated in this way: *Are there any special moral difficulties associated with the donation of sperm for use in AI?* In particular, does the sperm donor have any special responsibilities or rights? If the sperm donor is exactly similar to the blood donor or organ donor, then there will be no special moral difficulties associated with the role. The responsibilities of each sort of donor will be the same. Yet if there are morally relevant features that distinguish donating sperm from donating blood, it is possible that the sperm donor may have rights or responsibilities not shared by the blood donor.

Before addressing the question directly, it is worth considering the issues involved in two court cases concerning AI. The legal issues show that the moral issues are not purely speculative ones.

1. Two Court Cases

Since the turn of the century, a variety of legal issues have been discussed in connection with AI. Most of them have concerned inheritance and legitimacy, but two relatively recent court decisions raise issues that bear more directly on moral rights and responsibilities. One is the 1968 California Supreme Court decision in the case of *People* v. *Sorenson*.[1] The Sorensons, a married couple, agreed that Mrs.

Sorenson would be artificially inseminated by a physician employing the sperm of an anonymous donor. The procedure was carried out, Mrs. Sorenson became pregnant, and a child was born. Four years afterwards, the couple separated, and Mrs. Sorenson took custody of the child. She requested child-support payments, but Mr. Sorenson refused to pay on the grounds that he was not the father of the child.

The court rejected Mr. Sorenson's argument and held that he was liable for child support. According to the court, "the word 'father' is construed to include a husband who, unable to accomplish his objective of creating a child by using his own semen, purchases semen from a donor and uses it to inseminate his wife to achieve his purpose."[2] Furthermore, the court held that the donor could not be regarded as the father, for "he is no more responsible for the use made of his sperm than is the donor of blood or a kidney."[3] For the court, then, the "natural father" of the child was the husband who consented to his wife's being inseminated with donor sperm. The sperm donor was explicitly held to be no different from a blood donor or an organ donor.

A more unusual court case also focused on the question of identifying the "natural father" of a child conceived by AI. The case of *CM* v. *CC* in the New Jersey Juvenile and Domestic Relations Court involved a situation considered to be without legal precedent.[4] The woman in the case, CC, wished to have a child, but she neither wished to marry at the time nor to have intercourse before marriage. Her male friend, CM, whom she was dating exclusively, offered to provide the sperm to be used in AI. The physician at the sperm bank to which CC applied for assistance refused to perform the procedure, but CC acquired sufficient information to inseminate herself. This she did, with the cooperation of CM, and became pregnant by that means. Three months before the birth of the child, CC and CM severed their relationship.

After the child was born, CC refused to allow CM to visit, and CM turned to the court to claim visitation rights. The issue, as the court saw it, was whether CM should be recognized as the natural father of the child, given that his sperm had been "transferred to CC by other than natural conventional means." If so, then CM would have visitation rights, for courts have repeatedly held that the nat-ural fathers of illegitimate children have such a right.

In making its decision, the court reasoned that if a child is conceived by intercourse between two unmarried people, the fact that they are unmarried does not alter the fact that the man is the father. Similarly, if a child is conceived between two unmarried people by employing the sperm of the man, the fact that the sperm was delivered by artificial means does not alter the fact that the man is the father. CM was a willing participant in CC's becoming pregnant, and in the circumstances, the manner in which the sperm was "delivered" was irrelevant. The court accordingly granted CM visitation rights, but it also enjoined him with the parental obligation of providing "support and maintenance of the child and payment of any expenses incurred in his birth."[5]

2. Donors as Supplying a Product to Be Used by Others

In the Sorenson case, the court held that the sperm donor was no more responsible for the use made of his sperm than a blood donor is for the use made of his blood. In either case, the donor is only supplying a product that is to be used by others. Presumably, then, if there are relevant moral differences between blood transfusions and AI, the differences are ones connected with the actions. Consequently, only the agents who perform the actions or consent to them are the proper subjects of moral evaluation.

The court was concerned primarily with the question of legal paternity, and it would be wrong to read the decision as implying that blood donors have no moral responsibilities so neither do sperm donors. This view of the moral situation is obviously too simple.

A person who knowingly sells a quantity of rat poison to a reputed bluebeard is not guilty of any ensuing act of poisoning by his customer, but he is surely guilty of something. Similarly, someone who donates blood knowing that it is going to be used to lengthen the life of someone who is being tortured to death bears some degree of blame for contributing to the action. Likewise, a sperm donor who sells sperm that he suspects is going to be used to impregnate a woman against her will is surely blameworthy in some way and to some extent.

Such cases make it plain that a person who knowingly supplies the material conditions necessary for an immoral act does not escape all responsibility for the act merely because he does not perform it himself. Under appropriate conditions, supplying materials is one way of acquiring responsibility. In this respect, there is no morally relevant difference between being a blood donor and being a sperm donor. In either case, the donor has some responsibility for the use to which his contributed product is put. This also means that he has some responsibility for finding out how it will be used before he contributes (or sells) it.

Some have contended that AI is inherently immoral, for it requires masturbation, which violates the "natural end" of sex. On this view, the very act of donating sperm would be wrong. However, if AI is not in itself wrong and masturbation is not in itself wrong (views I accept but will not argue for), then whatever responsibilities a sperm donor may have, they do not stem from contributing to or performing an invariably wrong act.

3. Donors as Responsible for the Quality of the Product

So far in discussing blood and sperm donors we have focused on the material supplied for use in an action performed by another. Thus, potential wrongfulness in both instances is acquired only at secondhand, since it depends on the actions of those who make use of the materials. However, there is a way in which wrongfulness may attach directly to the action of a donor.

Suppose that a donor falsifies his genetic history or lies about being the carrier of a heritable genetic defect (such as Tay-Sachs disease). In such an instance, he is directly responsible for the birth of a child with the associated relevant genetic defect. The physician who performs the insemination has not acted wrongly. Rather, the blame attaches to the donor. The donor has knowingly provided a defective and potentially deadly product.

Here again there is no disanalogy between sperm donation and blood donation. Before the procedure for testing blood for the presence of AIDS antibodies was introduced, someone who had been diagnosed as having AIDS could have concealed that fact and quite knowingly put others at risk of dying from the disease communicated via his blood.

So far as blameworthiness is concerned, there seems to be no real difference between donating blood and donating sperm. In both instances, wrongfulness may be attributed directly to the action of a donor.

4. Sperm Donation and Sexual Intercourse

The comparison between donating blood and donating sperm has produced results that support the view that there are no special moral problems or responsibilities connected with sperm donation. But perhaps by focusing on the fact that both are donations of a product we have been led to overlook significant disanalogies between the two sorts of acts.

Certainly there are important differences between donating blood and "donating" sperm through intercourse. The most significant difference is connected with the potential outcome of the acts. While donating blood is at most a contribution toward someone's interest (health, well-being, treatment, etc.), "donating" sperm may lead to the conception and birth of another human being—a dependent child. The biological difference between blood and sperm makes the acts of giving quite different. Thus, in considering AI, it may be more reasonable to compare the results of sperm donation to the results of sexual intercourse, rather than to the results of blood donation.

The responsibility for a child normally falls to the biological parents. Exceptions to this are made in law only in special circumstances. For example, a child conceived by a woman as a result of an adulterous relationship may be considered the legal progeny of the woman's husband for certain purposes. However, except in such cases, responsibility is typically assigned to both biological parents, and whether or not they are married to one another is irrelevant. Thus, if we take seriously the fact that AI and intercourse may lead to the same outcome, should we not say that the sperm donor is responsible for the child conceived from his sperm?

This view seems both counterintuitive and simplistic. But why should this be? Are there really morally relevant differences between delivering sperm by intercourse and delivering it by AI? The question is one that merits an answer if we are to avoid an uncritical dogmatism that assumes that the answer is obvious and needs no argument to support it.

At least two differences between the two sorts of cases stand out, and prima facie they may seem to explain why we are unwilling to count the sperm donor as the, so to speak, moral father of a child, even though he may be the biological father. First, it might be argued that the sperm donor has no intention of impregnating the woman who might receive his sperm. She is, most likely, a total stranger, someone he has never met and probably never will meet. Thus, it is totally ridiculous to suggest that he could have the intention of making her pregnant or becoming a father. Most likely, the donor has only the intention of making money by being paid a fee for donating his sperm. Or, at best, the sperm donor, like the blood donor, has the intention of providing a material that may be of assistance to someone who has a specific need that he is in a position to satisfy.

The obvious flaw in this argument is that men who "deliver" sperm by having sex do not always have the intention of impregnating their partners. The news has been out for some time that men engage in intercourse for a variety of reasons, and impregnating the female is not invariably one of them. Consequently, the man who delivers sperm through intercourse may be just as lacking in intention as the sperm donor may be imagined to be. In neither case need pregnancy have anything to do with the aim of action, and intention cannot be the grounds for holding that the man who engages in intercourse is the biological father who must accept attendant responsibilities, while the man who donates his sperm is the biological father who has no such responsibilities.

Second, it might be held that the likelihood of producing a pregnancy marks the difference between intercourse-and-responsibility and sperm donation-and-no-responsibility. After all, in having sex there is always a real probability of the female partner's becoming pregnant. The probability might be lowered by birth-control procedures, including vasectomy, but some degree of probability always remains. If we assume that the male knows that there is at least some risk, no matter how small, of pregnancy resulting from intercourse, then it is reasonable to hold him responsible if it occurs. By contrast, a sperm donor has no way of knowing what is going to be done with his sperm. It might be used for research purposes, it might be discarded after its "shelf-life" has passed, it might be mixed with the husband's sperm, or it might be used as merely one of a series of inseminations in which the sperm of others is also employed.

Once again, however, such a contrast is more apparent than real. Ordinarily, the sperm donor can be assumed to know that there is at least some degree of probability that his sperm will be used in AI. In this respect, then, he is in exactly the same position as the man who engages in intercourse, and there is no morally relevant difference (based on likelihood of pregnancy) between the cases.

However, let us assume that the sperm donor is completely ignorant of the likelihood that his sperm will be used to produce a pregnancy. This ignorance does not alter the fact that there is a certain degree of probability that someone will become pregnant by means of his sperm. Notice, though, that it is also possible for a male engaging in intercourse to be ignorant of the fact that there is a probability that his partner will become pregnant. (He may simply be ignorant of the realities of sex or he may hold certain false beliefs. For example, he may think that it is impossible for a nursing mother to become pregnant, or he may believe that his vasectomy guarantees that he is incapable of insemination.)

It is difficult to imagine a situation in which we would hold that ignorance on the part of the male who engages in intercourse excuses him from the responsibilities that attach to being the biological father of a resulting child. But if ignorance in the intercourse case is not a reason for setting aside the responsibilities of the biological father, then there seems to be no reason why it should be in the sperm-donation case.

Are we thus forced to accept the counterintuitive conclusion that since the sperm donor is the biological father, then he must also be the moral father? We are not if we can show that being the biological father is not a sufficient condition for being the moral father.

Under ordinary conditions, we are inclined to identify the biological father with the moral father. The reason for this lies in the general principle that someone who causes something to happen is responsible for its happening. Indeed, the question "Who is responsible for this?" asked about the occurrence of an event is a request for the identity of a person or persons who can be considered candidates for praise or blame. We expect and require that people, as we say, accept the consequences of their actions.

If a woman becomes pregnant as a result of having sex with A, we hold A responsible (partially) for the child, just because A is the cause of the pregnancy. It is irrelevant that the woman also had sex with B and C. They might have been responsible for the pregnancy, but as a matter of fact they were not. A is not responsible because he has genetic characteristics that are different from B and C or anything of the kind. A is responsible, we hold, because he is causally responsible, because the pregnancy resulted from his actions. We then expect and require him to accept the consequences of his actions. We thus identify him as both the biological and the moral father of the child.

By contrast with the actions of A in our example, the sperm donor does nothing to impregnate the recipient of the sperm. He is *not responsible* for her becoming pregnant, even though it is his sperm that makes her pregnant. He is the biological father, just as is A, but he is not the moral father, for unlike A, he is not the causal agent. Not being the causal agent, the sperm donor is not appropriately placed to "accept the consequences of his actions," when this means accepting responsibility for the child produced by the use of his sperm. The donor's actions consist only in donating (selling) his sperm, and as we discussed earlier, some responsibilities attach to such actions, but the responsibility of being a moral father is not among them.

In saying that the donor is not the causal agent of the pregnancy, I do not mean to deny that he is part of the causal complex. If "the cause" of an event is the entire set of conditions sufficient for the occurrence of the event, then the donor provides what is usually called a contributory condition. In this respect, his role is no different from that of the person who supplied the pigments Michaelangelo used to paint the Sistine ceiling. Just as it would be absurd to identify the paint supplier as responsible for the paintings, it would be absurd to identify the sperm donor as responsible for the child. (It is tempting to say that the donor's sperm is a necessary condition for the occurrence of the pregnancy, but that is not correct. Sperm is a necessary condition, but not his sperm. At most, he supplies a necessary condition

relative to that particular set of conditions that is jointly sufficient.)

It is in causal agency that we can locate the relevant moral difference between being a sperm donor whose sperm is used in AI and someone who impregnates a woman through intercourse. However, this seems to require us to conclude that the physician who uses the sperm to perform AI is the moral father of the child. Since the physician causes the pregnancy, it would seem to follow that he or she is responsible for it.

This particular counterintuitive outcome indicates that the AI situation is more complicated than we have allowed for so far. We have assumed that an action that causes an outcome entails a responsibility for the outcome. This is true so far as causal responsibility is concerned; however, causal responsibility is, at most, a necessary condition for moral responsibility. If a terrorist has filled a hospital ward with methane gas and by unsuspectingly turning on the light I cause the gas to explode, I am causally responsible for the explosion. That is, I performed the action that completed the causal chain. However, moral responsibility lies with the terrorist who filled the room with explosive gas.

The physician who performs AI is causally responsible for a woman's becoming pregnant. It is his act that makes her pregnant. However, she does not become pregnant because, to use an apt phrase from the last century, he "has his way with her." She becomes pregnant because the physician is not merely acting with her consent, but acting as her agent. She is as morally responsible for her own pregnancy as the terrorist is morally responsible for the explosion.

It is true that the physician must agree to act as the agent and, in doing so, accepts certain responsibilities. The physician must be assured that the woman is in a state of health compatible with being pregnant, that she genuinely wants to be pregnant, that she is not having a baby merely to sell for profit, and so on. Additional responsibilities attach to how the physician performs the task—has a serious effort been made to choose a sperm donor free of genetic disease, is the procedure performed in accordance with professional standards, and has meaningful consent been secured? However, in acting as the woman's agent, the physician is in no way responsible for the child that is conceived. The real causal agent is the woman herself.

What about the circumstance in which a male marriage partner agrees to the AI of his wife, with her consent, by the use of donor sperm? Does the husband then have no responsibilities, since he has not acted as a causal agent? The reasoning of the court in *Sorenson* seems quite correct in such a case. The husband, as one of the parties to the initial agreement, explicitly assumes responsibility for the child. He acknowledges himself to be the moral father. If he later changes his mind, he is still responsible because of his original commitment. His wife becomes pregnant with his consent and he can no more cease to be the moral father than he could if he were also the biological father. If the wife acts as a result of the agreement with her husband, then to some degree he too is causally responsible for the birth of the child.

It is now easy to see why the courts in *Sorenson* and in *CM* v. *CC* adopted different views toward the sperm donors. In *Sorenson*, the husband was a causal agent in the sense described above, for his wife became pregnant with his consent. Accordingly, the anonymous sperm donor played no role at all as a causal agent. By contrast, in *CM* v. *CC*, CM cooperated with CC in her becoming pregnant, and each played the same sort of causal role they would have played had actual intercourse taken place. CM was a sperm "donor" only in a Pickwickian sense.

A general result that follows from the position we have argued for is the recognition that being a biological father is not sufficient condition for being a moral or social father. We must now acknowledge that the special circumstances of AI make the role of biological father irrelevant to assigning responsibilities for the care of a child after it is born. The biological father in AI also has no rights as moral or social father. Since he played no role as a causal agent in the conception of the child, he can make no claim on the child, nor can the child or the child's representatives make any claim on him.

The exception to this concerns the area in which the sperm donor does have responsibilities. If he has in ignorance or through deception been responsible for the birth of a child with a genetic disorder, then he is liable to be held at least morally accountable for his action of contributing sperm. If he acted in ignorance, the only claim on him might be to provide medical information that might be of help to the child. If he acted with the intent to deceive, then we might believe that he should be liable for

more than our moral condemnation. We might argue, for example, that he should be forced to pay an indemnity.

Conclusion

The question we began with was whether a sperm donor has any special responsibilities or rights. In particular, we asked, are there any morally relevant differences between the sperm donor and the blood donor? Prima facie it seemed that there might be, for donating blood does not lead to the same sort of potential outcome that donating sperm does, for sperm may result in the birth of a dependent child.

What we have found is that there is no reason to hold that a sperm donor is the moral father of the child conceived by this sperm. Being the biological father, we argued, is not sufficient condition for being the moral father. The sperm donor is not a *causal agent* in the conception of the child and so is not responsible for the child. Further, although the physician who inseminates plays a causal role, he or she is not responsible for the child either. Causal responsibility is only a necessary condition for moral responsibility, and the physician is acting as the agent of the woman who has requested AI. A husband who agrees that his wife will have a child by AI is also acting as a causal agent, and in his agreement he has committed himself to becoming the moral father of the child. His wife has become pregnant by his word, rather than by his sperm.

There are differences between the sperm donor and the blood donor, but the differences are not morally relevant ones. Both have responsibilities, but they are responsibilities that come from providing a product. The fact that sperm can be used to produce a child and blood cannot be is not morally significant.

References

1. The People v. Falmer J. Sorenson. Supreme Court of California, Cr. 11708 (Feb. 26, 1968). 437 P. 2d 495.

2. Op. cit., 500.

3. Op. cit., 498.

4. C. M. v. C. C. Juvenile and Domestic Relations Court, Cumberland County, N.J., 152 N.J. Super. 160 (July 19, 1977). 377A. 2d 821.

5. Op. cit., 825.

Decision Scenario 1 . . . .

"I'm sorry we can't help you," Patricia Spring said. "But what you want is simply against our policy."

Charles Blendon and Carla Neuman didn't try to hide their disappointment. The San Diego Reproductive Clinic had been their last hope. They very badly wanted to have a child, but Carla's Fallopian tubes had been surgically removed as part of a successful effort to treat precancerous growths.

"In fact," Patricia Spring said, "you don't meet at least two of our criteria."

"We can afford to pay," Charles Blendon said.

"That's not it. First of all, Carla is thirty-eight, and we set thirty-five as the upper limit. And second, you two are not married, and we require that the donor and the patient be husband and wife."

"Who makes those rules?" Carla Neuman asked. "It seems to me that if we want to have a child, then that's our business and nobody else's."

"The Clinic makes the rules," Patricia Spring said. "You see, there is some greater risk of birth defects in women who are over the age of thirty-five. There are sound medical reasons for our criteria."

"But what if we're willing to take the risk?" Charles Blendon asked.

"You can't take a risk that is likely to affect an unborn child."

"But I'm willing to have tests," Carla Neuman said. "And neither of us is against abortion. If there is something wrong with the fetus, then I'll have an abortion."

"And just what sort of medical basis is there for the marriage requirement?" Charles Blendon asked. "It seems to me that the Clinic is just imposing its own moral standards on Carla and me."

"Look," Patricia Spring said, "I know you're both upset and disappointed. I sympathize with you. But the Clinic operates in a community, and our criteria reflect both good medical judgment and the standards of the community."

"Does the Clinic receive any public money?" Carla Neuman asked.

"We have some research grants."

"Then it seems to me that we have grounds for a suit," Carla said. "The Clinic is discriminating against us because we aren't married, and it's denying us the right to take a risk we're willing to take."

"I can only tell you what our criteria are," Patricia Spring said. "I can't arrange for you to be accepted as a patient here, and there's nothing you or I can do about it."

"That remains to be seen," Charles Blendon said.

1. *Is the Clinic justified in setting an age limit on the women it will accept as patients? If so, why?*

2. *How might a rule utilitarian justify the Clinic's requirement that a couple be married in order for the woman to be accepted as a patient?*

3. *Does the fact that the Clinic receives public funds provide any reason to believe that its services should be open to everyone?*

4. *On what grounds might the Vatican "Instruction" and Krimmel object to the very existence of such a clinic? Is such a clinic consistent with Steinbock's views?*

Decision Scenario 2 . . . .

In January of 1985, the British High Court took custody of a five-day-old girl, the first child known to be born in Britain to a woman paid to be a surrogate mother.

An American couple, known only as "Mr. and Mrs. A," were reported to have paid about $7,500 to a twenty-eight-year-old woman who allowed herself to be artificially inseminated with sperm from Mr. A. The woman, Kim Cotton, was prevented from turning the child over to Mr. and Mrs. A by a court order issued because of the un-

certainty over the legal status of a surrogate mother.

The court permitted "interested parties, including the natural father" to apply for custody of the child. Mr. A applied, and judge Sir John Latey ruled that the couple could take the baby girl out of the country, because they could offer her the chance of "a very good upbringing."

1. *Are there any moral reasons that might have made the court hesitate before turning over the child to her*

biological father? For example, could it be persuasively argued that Kim Cotton was, in effect, selling her baby to Mr. and Mrs. A?

2. *Kim Cotton agreed to be a surrogate mother for the sake of the money. Is surrogate pregnancy a practice that tends to exploit the poor? Or is it a legitimate way to earn money by providing a needed service? How might Steinbock respond to these questions?*

3. *Is serving as a surrogate mother essentially the same as prostitution? If it is not, then what are the relevant differences?*

4. *On what grounds do the Vatican "Instruction" and Krimmel oppose the practice of surrogate pregnancy? How persuasive are the arguments?*

Decision Scenario 3 . . . .

Dr. Charles Davis quickly scanned the data sheet on his desk, then looked at the woman seated across from him. Her name was Nancy Callahan. She was twenty-five years old and worked as a print conservator at an art museum.

"I see that you aren't married," Dr. Davis said.

"That's right," Nancy Callahan said. "That's basically the reason I'm here." When Dr. Davis looked puzzled, she added, "I still want to have a child."

Dr. Davis nodded and thought for a moment. Nancy Callahan was the first unmarried person to come to the Bayside Fertility Clinic to request AID. As the legal owner and operator of the Clinic, as well as the Chief of Medical Services, Dr. Davis was the one ultimately responsible for the Clinic's policies.

"I hope you understand that I have to ask you some personal questions," Dr. Davis said. "Of course."

"You're not engaged or planning to get married?"

"No. At least not at the moment. I don't want to rule out the possibility that I will want to get married someday."

"Don't you know anybody you would want to have a child with in the ordinary sexual way?"

"I might be able to find someone," Nancy Callahan said. "But you see, I don't want to get involved with anybody right now. I'm ready to be a mother, but I'm not ready to get into the kind of situation that having a child in what you call 'the ordinary sexual way' would require."

"I see."

"I hope you do. This is something I really want to do. I think I'll be a good mother. I want a child very much, and I can afford to support one."

"It's just somewhat unusual," Dr. Davis said.

"But it's not illegal, is it?"

"No," Dr. Davis said. "It's not illegal."

"So what's the problem? I'm healthy. I'm financially sound and mentally stable, and I'm both able and eager to accept the responsibility of being a mother."

"It's just that at the moment the policy of our Clinic requires that patients be married and that both husbands and wives agree to the insemination procedure."

"But there's nothing magical about a policy," Nancy Callahan said. "It can be changed for good reasons, can't it?"

"Perhaps so," said Dr. Davis.

1. *Suppose that Ms. Callahan is a lesbian. Should this be a relevant consideration in deciding whether she should receive AID? Why, according to Hanscombe, should it not be?*

2. *What utilitarian argument can be advanced in favor of the Clinic's policy?*

3. *Does the Vatican's natural law view support such a policy?*

4. *How might it be argued that respect for Ms. Callahan's autonomy makes it wrong to deny her the service she requests, while providing it to a married woman? Is Steinbock's position consistent with the Clinic's policy?*

Decision Scenario 4 . . . .

"My husband and I have talked over the matter in great detail," Marge Gower said. "We don't care

about the sex of the child, but we know exactly the kinds of features we want to try for."

"Mrs. Gower," Dr. Louise Singh said. "You've got to understand that we're not running a mail-order-catalogue business for babies."

"I'm not trying to order a *baby*. I just want to tell you what I'm looking for in a sperm donor. I want somebody who is at least six feet tall, muscular—not fat—has light-colored hair and is very good looking. Also, I want some proof that he has a good sense of humor and is intelligent. He has to have at least a college degree. I'll leave all the rest to you. I mean, things about health."

"Thank you," said Dr. Singh. "But I really don't think I can go along with that."

"I don't see why not. If I were going to have a child in the usual way and I were deliberately going to get pregnant, I would certainly choose somebody like I described."

"But you aren't doing it in the usual way. You're going to be using donor semen."

"But who is going to choose the donor? You are, aren't you?"

"I plan to. I'll select somebody from our list of applicants who resembles you and your husband in a general way."

"I don't see why you should have that kind of power," Mrs. Gower said. "It's going to be my baby. I think I have the right to say what the father should be like."

"That's against Reproductive Medicine's policy."

"Well, that's too bad. Just tell me who to talk to to get the policy changed. I'm going to have a baby like my husband and I want. As long as I have to have artificial insemination, I want to get the most good out of it."

1. On what grounds might a utilitarian support the claim that Dr. Singh ought to be wholly responsible for choosing the sperm donor?

2. On what grounds might a utilitarian support the claim that Mrs. Gower and her husband ought to be able to select the features that a sperm donor should have?

3. Would it be better for the potential recipient of artificial insemination if the sperm donor were known personally to her and her husband? What are some of the problems caused by anonymity?

4. Might the choice of a sperm donor by the physician be regarded as an unacceptable form of paternalism? (See the discussion of paternalism in Chapter 5.)

5. Consider the issue involved here from the standpoint of the potential sperm donor. Should a sperm donor have some control over the use of his sperm in artificial insemination? Mrs. Gower argues that since the child will be hers, she should be the one who specifies what traits the donor should have. Since, biologically speaking, the child will equally be the offspring of the sperm donor, should he be able to specify the traits the sperm recipient should have?

Decision Scenario 5 ·

"I'm going to sell my sperm for the simple reason that I need the money," John Lolton said. "It's no big deal."

"I think it is," Mary Cooper said. "You seem to think it's like selling your blood, but it isn't. If somebody is transfused with your blood, that's an end to things. But if a woman is inseminated with your sperm, a child may result."

"I don't have any responsibilities for what people do with my sperm," Lolton replied. "It's just a product."

"Not so," Cooper said. "It's a product all right, but if it's used in artificial insemination, that means that you're the father of a child. And if you're the father of a child, that means you have to be willing to accept responsibility for that child. "

"That is absolute nonsense," Lolton said.

1. If sperm is just a product, is Lolton correct in saying that he has no responsibilities for its use?

2. State as explicitly as possible Cooper's argument that a sperm donor is responsible for any child resulting from AI using his donated sperm.

3. According to Munson, why is being the biological father of a child born as a result of AI not a sufficient condition for being the moral father of the child?

4. According to the Vatican "Instruction," are there instances in which AI is morally licit? What is the moral status of a child conceived by AI?

Decision Scenario 6 ·

"I'm curious," Lois Ramer said. "What happens to the eggs you take from me that get fertilized but not implanted?"

"We destroy them," Dr. Martha Herman said.

"Oh," Lois Ramer said, sounding surprised. "I guess I never really thought about it before, but maybe I shouldn't be doing this."

"Why is that?"

"Because I believe life begins at conception. And I guess that means I think that the fertilized eggs that you destroy are human beings with the same rights I have."

"If you genuinely believe that," Dr. Herman said, "then you really shouldn't be having this procedure."

1. *What position does the Vatican "Instruction" take on the question of the status of an egg that is fertilized for the purpose of implantation, but then not used?*

2. *If every egg fertilized was implanted, would this make the procedure of embryo transfer morally legitimate according to the Vatican "Instruction"?*

3. *Does the Vatican's position on these matters rely on what Singer calls the "standard argument"? State Singer's version of the argument, and explain why he considers it unpersuasive.*

4. *Why does Singer believe the destruction of early embryos is morally legitimate? When does he consider it morally wrong to destroy an embryo?*

PART IV

RESOURCES

CHAPTER 9

ACQUIRING AND ALLOCATING SCARCE MEDICAL RESOURCES

CASE PRESENTATION
The Ayalas' Solution: Having a Child to Save a Life

Anissa Ayala was fifteen years old in 1988 when she was diagnosed with chronic myelogenous leukemia. She received radiation and chemotherapy treatments to destroy diseased bone marrow and blood cells, but the usual outcome of such treatments is that the bone marrow is left unable to produce an adequate number of normal blood cells.

Anissa's parents, Mary and Andy Ayala, were informed that without a bone marrow transplant of stem cells her survival chances were virtually zero, while with a transplant she would have a 70–80% chance.

Tests showed that neither the Ayalas nor their nineteen-year-old son, Airon, had bone marrow that was sufficiently compatible for them to be donors for Anissa. They turned to a public registry to assist them and during the next two years searched for a donor. The odds of a match between two nonrelated people is only one in 20,000, and as time passed and no one was found, the Ayalas began to feel increasingly desperate. Anissa's health had stabilized, yet that condition couldn't be counted on to last forever.

The Ayalas decided that the only way they could do more to help save their daughter's life was to try to have another child. Anissa's physician tried to discourage them, pointing out that the odds were

only one in four that the child would have the right tissue type to be a stem-cell donor. Furthermore, the possibility that they could conceive another child was doubtful. Andy Ayala was 45 and had had a vasectomy performed sixteen years earlier. Mary Ayala was 42, well past the period of highest fertility. Nevertheless, the Ayalas decided to go ahead with their plan, and as the first step Andy Ayala had surgery to repair the vasectomy.

Against the odds, Mary Ayala became pregnant.

When it became known that the Ayalas planned to have a child because their daughter needed compatible bone marrow, they became the subjects of intense media attention and received much harsh criticism. Some said that they were treating the baby they expected to have as a means only and not as a person of unique worth. One commentator described their actions as "outrageous." Others said they were taking a step down the path that would lead to conceiving children merely as a source of tissue and organs.

A few opposed this outpouring of criticism by pointing out that people decide to have children for many and complex reasons and sometimes for no reason at all. No one observed that a reason for having a child need not determine how one regards the child. Also, those who condemned the Ayalas often emphasized the "child-as-an-organ bank" notion but never mentioned the relative safety of a bone marrow transplant.

The Ayalas themselves reported that they were hurt by the criticisms. Mary Ayala said she had wanted a third child for a number of years but had been unable to get her husband to agree. Andy Ayala admitted that he would not have wanted another child had Anissa not become ill, but he said he also had in mind the comfort a child would bring to the family should Anissa die. The whole family said they would want and love the child, whether or not its bone marrow was a good match.

In February 1990 the Ayalas found they had beat the odds once more. Tests of the developing fetus showed that the stem cells were nearly identical with Anissa's. During an interview after the results were known, Anissa Ayala said "A lot of people think 'How can you do this? How can you be having this baby for your daughter?' But she's my baby sister and we're going to love her for who she is, not for what she can give me."

Then, on April 6, in a suburban Los Angeles hospital, more than a week before the predicted date, Mary Ayala gave birth to a healthy six-pound baby girl. The Ayalas named her Marissa Eve.

Anissa's physician, pediatric oncologist Patricia Konrad, collected and froze blood from the baby's umbilical cord. Umbilical blood contains a high concentration of stem cells, and she wanted the blood available should Anissa need it before Marissa is old enough to be a donor.

When Marissa is about six months old and has an adequate weight, she will be given general anesthesia and marrow extracted from her hipbone. The marrow will be prepared and then injected into one of Anissa's veins. If the procedure is successful, the stem cells will migrate to Anissa's marrow and begin to multiply. The hope is that this will enable Anissa's bone marrow to produce normal blood cells.

SOCIAL CONTEXT: THE PROMISE OF FETAL CELL IMPLANTS

Parkinson's disease often begins with tremors and a mild stiffening of the limbs that is followed by a gradual but progressive loss of muscle control. Although remaining intellectually lucid, people with the disease are often unable to walk, use the toilet, wash, or even eat without assistance.

Their behavior also has a peculiar and disturbing off/on aspect. Someone may be walking or talking when, without the least warning, he freezes during the action. Some find this feature of the disease so disconcerting that they become recluses, fearful of freezing in mid-motion in public or in a dangerous place. Over 1.5 million people are estimated to suffer from the disease.

The disease is causally connected with the dying off of cells in a darkly pigmented part of the brain called the substantia nigra. These cells produce dopamine, a neurotransmitter essential in conveying impulses to brain cells that control muscle movements. A major therapeutic advance in the treatment of Parkinsonism occurred with the introduction of the drug L-dopa. L-dopa is a biochemical precursor of dopamine, and when the body converts the drug to dopamine, people often make an amazing recovery from the effects of the disease. Unfortunately, within a few years L-dopa ceases to be effective, and the old problems of rigidity, "freezing," and general loss of muscle control return. (The recent film *Awakenings* depicts the effects of L-dopa treatments on a number of Parkinson's sufferers.)

In 1987 Ignacio Madrazo in Mexico reported that he had successfully transplanted cells from the adrenal cortex of two Parkinson patients into the caudate nucleus area of their brains. The adrenal gland is known to produce dopamine, and Madrazo described his patients as making substantial functional recoveries that he expected to continue over the long term. (Five years previously, Swedish researchers performed a similar operation but reported that their patients made only slight and transitory improvements.) Madrazo's results were never reported in a scientific journal, and although efforts were made to repeat the work he reported, no one was successful. Thus early hopes for adrenal cell transplants as an effective treatment for Parkinsonism were disappointed.

Then in February 1990, matters began to look hopeful again. Olle Lindvall of University Hospital, Lund, Sweden, reported in *Science* that he and his research team had implanted fetal brain cells into the brain of a forty-nine-year-old man with severe Parkinson's disease. The cells were injected into the left putamen, an area known to be the site of numerous dopamine pathways.

The man's symptoms were significantly relieved. Previously, even with medication, he had spent more than half his time in a frozen "off" position, but within three months after the implant he had only one or two brief "off" periods a day. (The man's course was followed from eleven months before the surgery, and it was still being followed at the time of publication five months afterward.) Most important, brain imaging methods indicated that the fetal cells were continuing to function and to produce dopamine.

Lindvall's team had been working on the problem since 1979, and the team's reputation, experimental procedures, and data convinced most of the biomedical community that their results were reliable. Other researchers indicated that they had experiments underway that were likely to confirm Lindvall's results.

The Swedish procedure involved taking neural tissue from four fetuses eight to nine weeks old. Fetal brain tissue offers the possibility of a better biological match than cells even from an individual's own adrenal gland. Further, neural fetal tissue seems to be unlikely to provoke an autoimmune response and cause graft-host rejection. Treating Parkinsonism with fetal cell implants is an exciting therapeutic possibility that may benefit hundreds of thousands of sufferers. Furthermore, the treatment points the way toward the development of other therapies involving fetal tissues.

Fetal liver cells may be used to generate new bone marrow to treat those suffering from leukemia, sickle-cell anemia, thalassemia, aplastic anemia, or radiation sickness. (Robert Gale employed fetal liver cells to treat some victims of the Chernobyl disaster, although without success.) Alzheimer's disease, Huntington's disease, and spinal cord injuries may all yield to treatments involving fetal neural cells. Fetal heart tissue may be used to replace damaged heart muscle, and the bodies of the more than 2 million insulin-dependent (Type-I) diabetics may someday be able to produce their own insulin, if implants of islet cells from fetal pancreatic tissue should be successful.

The potential therapeutic marvels promised by fetal cells hold out the only hope for literally millions of people suffering from a wide range of diseases. However, fetal cell implants and their use in research and therapy have also produced serious moral and social issues we have yet to resolve.

The most vexed issue is that of induced abortion as the source of fetal tissue. Opponents of elective abortion argue that research and therapy using fetal tissue would both condone and encourage abortion. According to the president of the National Right to Life Committee, John C. Wilke, the medical use of fetal tissue will just "offer an additional rationalization to those who defend the killings."

Also, both opponents and advocates of elective abortion express concern over the possibility that some women might deliberately conceive a child and then have an abortion for the sole purpose of obtaining the fetal tissue. The tissue could then either be used to help some member of the woman's family or be sold as a commodity. Although a 1988 amendment to the National Organ Transplant Act prohibits the sale of fetal organs and tissue, the success of fetal cell therapy could lead to a repeal. Some have suggested that fetal tissue, like blood, bone marrow, and sperm, can be considered a renewable resource. The potential for a fetal tissue market exists, and some have speculated that the current law may only encourage the establishment of an offshore source of supply. People will seek out illegal sources of supplies of fetal tissue in much the same way they seek illegal sources of drugs they believe are crucial to their survival.

Kate Michaelman of the National Abortion Rights Action League sees "a potential for the abuse of women in this whole thing." The idea that women might be put under pressure by social expectations or by their friends, husbands, or families to have an abortion to provide fetal tissue needed to treat an ailing relative is not farfetched. Further, if there were a market in fetal tissue, women might be under similar pressure to produce a fetus to secure money needed to support themselves or their families. (It should be kept in mind, though, that, even in the absence of pressure, a woman might choose to sell or donate fetal tissue for a variety of reasons.)

While the Catholic Church condemns induced abortion, it condones the use of fetal tissue, particularly that secured by spontaneous abortion, within certain limits. The "fetal organ donor" must be treated with the same respect as any other organ donor, and it is necessary to be certain that the donor is dead. This requirement presents a difficulty, however, for the standards for fetal brain death are far from clear.

Almost 1.5 million abortions are performed each year, and most fetal tissue used in research is obtained from those performed during the first four months of pregnancy. Although the matter is in dispute, some researchers regard tissue from eight- to nine-week-old fetuses to be preferable, while some claim older tissue is better. In either case, social and economic pressure on a woman to delay an abortion may start to build, and the best interest of the woman may be compromised by the need for mature fetal tissue. Instead of using a drug like RU-486 (should one become available in the United States) to inhibit the implantation of a fertilized ovum or instead of having an early abortion, a woman might carry the fetus until a time dictated by needs other than her own health.

The possibility of using only spontaneously aborted fetuses is dimmed by the fact that up to 60% show chromosomal abnormalities or other defects that might affect the tissue recipient.

In 1987 the Department of Health and Human Services suspended the support of research projects using fetal tissue obtained through induced abortions. After two reviews of the issues, a special panel of the National Institutes of Health decided in 1988 that the use of fetal tissue for research and treatment can be morally legitimate. The panel separated the question of elective abortion from that of the use of fetal tissue and took no position on the moral status of abortion. The panel also recommended that women not be permitted to donate fetal tissue for the treatment of their friends or family.

In April 1989, NIH, following most of the recommendations of its panel, issued guidelines for the use of fetal tissue in research and experimental therapy. However, the ban on the use of such tissue initiated during the Reagan administration was continued by the Bush administration, and at present (1991) federal funds cannot be used for human fetal tissue implants. In addition, at least seven states have passed laws forbidding the use of fetal tissue obtained from induced abortions.

Many researchers object to these restrictions. Some have claimed that the restrictions themselves are immoral, because they will seriously impede the development of effective treatments for devastating diseases. Some scientists have suggested that they may ignore state prohibitions and use funds from private foundations to continue their research.

One possibility under development is to employ cells from a single fetus, grow them in cultures, then harvest them as needed. This would eliminate the need for a large number of mature fetuses and make the research and treatment more independent of abortion.

Another possibility is to use the techniques of molecular biology to clone cells taken from an individual patient. If the cells can be made to multiply in sufficient quantity, then the patient can be treated with his own cells.

The problem of an immune reaction would be eliminated, and cell therapy would be severed from abortion.

Because fetal cells are now available and are not dependent on technological development, people suffering from Parkinson's disease and other disorders that might be helped by fetal cell implants are understandably frustrated by seeing research in this area slowed by a lack of federal funding. For a great number, the development of a future technology that will disconnect cell therapy and abortion will come too late to help.

SOCIAL CONTEXT: DISTRIBUTING TRANSPLANT ORGANS

Organ transplantation is perhaps the most dramatic example of how the high technology of contemporary medicine can save the lives of thousands of people who would have died untimely deaths only a few years earlier. However, behind the wonder and drama of transplant surgery lies the troubling fact that allocation decisions must be made. Daily, physicians, surgeons, and committees are put in the position of making judgments that will supply hope for some while destroying the last vestige of hope for others.

Replacing damaged, diseased, or defective organs by surgically transplanting donor organs has become increasingly common during the last decade. Although transplanting kidneys began as early as the 1950s, the list of organs now transplanted with a significant degree of success has been expanded to include corneas, bone marrow, bone and skin grafts, livers, pancreases, and hearts.

Worldwide, over 85,000 kidney transplants have been performed, and over 90% of the organs are still functioning a year later. (Some recipients are still alive after thirty years.) Thomas Starzl and his team successfully transplanted the first liver in 1967, and

now some 3,000 transplants have been done. The success rate is put at 75%. Also in 1967, Christian Barnard transplanted a human heart, and since then about 4,000 more such surgeries have been performed. More than three-quarters of the procedures are considered successful. New techniques of management and the development of drugs to suppress part of the immune response promise to make possible even more transplants in the future. (See the introduction for more details.)

A major social and moral difficulty of transplant surgery is that it is extremely expensive. For example, a kidney transplant may cost around $40,000, a heart transplant about $120,000, and a liver transplant in the range of $200,000 to $300,000. Questions have been raised in recent years about what restrictions, if any, should be placed on access to transplants. Should society deny them to everyone, pay for all who need them but cannot afford them, or pay for only some who cannot pay? (For a discussion of some of these issues, see Chapter 10.)

The second major problem, after cost, is the availability of donor organs. The increase in the number of transplant operations performed during the last fifteen years has resulted in a condition of chronic scarcity for most organs. For example, in the five-year period 1981–1985, the demand for livers increased by a factor of thirty-five and the demand for hearts by a factor of twenty-two. Unlike corneas or bones, kidneys, hearts, and livers are always in short supply, for there is no way in which they can be preserved in usable condition for more than a few hours.

This chronic shortage means that at any given time, thousands of people in the United States are waiting for organ transplants. In 1988 some 30,000 people needed a kidney, but 11,800 were forced to wait until one became available for transplant. Hundreds are currently in need of livers, pancreases, and hearts, and many of these people are likely to die before appropriate organs become available. Those in need of a kidney or pancreas can rely on dialysis and insulin injections to treat their diseases, but those in need of a liver or heart have almost no alternative treatment. For them the lack of a suitable transplant organ spells almost certain death.

Given the currently limited supply of transplant organs, we face two key questions today: How can the supply of organs be increased? How are those who will actually receive organs to be selected from the pool of candidates?

The obvious answer to the first question is that the supply of organs can be increased by increasing donations. The overwhelming majority of organs that could be used for transplant are not salvaged from the recently dead. According to one estimate, only about 15% of available organs are retrieved. Most people are simply buried with all their organs. This is true even in states that print an organ donation card on the back of driver's licenses. Most often, physicians and hospital administrators are reluctant to intrude on a family's grief by asking that a deceased patient's organs be donated for use as transplants. (Even if a patient has signed an organ donation card, the permission of the immediate family is required, in most cases, before the organs can be removed.)

In an attempt to overcome this reluctance, a 1987 federal law requires that hospitals receiving Medicare or Medicaid payments (97% of the nation's 6,800 hospitals) identify those patients who could become organ donors at death. The law also requires that hospitals discuss organ donations with the families of such patients and inform them of their legal power to authorize donations. Before the law was enacted, only about 4,000 people a year donated their organs. If organs could be retrieved after brain death, this alone would increase the number of donors to 20,000. However, because of difficulties in administering the law and a lag in developing a coordination of organ-sharing networks, it is still too early to see how successful the law will be. The hope is that a national policy will reduce, if not eliminate, the chronic shortage of transplant organs.

Another possibility for increasing the organ supply is to permit organs to be offered for sale on the open market. Before death, an individual might arrange payment for the posthumous use of one or more of his organs. Or, after the individual's death, his survivors might sell his organs to those in need of them. In a variation of this proposal, donors or their families might receive certain forms of tax credits, or a donor might be legally guaranteed that, if a family member or friend required a transplant organ, then that person would be given priority in the distribution. Under either plan, there would be a strong incentive to make organs available for transplant.

The public reaction to any plan for marketing organs has been strongly negative. People generally regard the prospect of individuals in need of transplants bidding against one another in an "organ auction" as ghoulish and morally repugnant, and this attitude extends to all forms of the market approach. In 1984 the National Organ Transplantation Act made the sale of organs for transplant illegal in the United States. At least twenty other countries, including Canada, Britain, and most of Europe, have similar laws.

A third possibility would be to allow living individuals to sell their nonvital organs to those in need of transplants. Taking hearts and livers from living people would be illegal, for it would involve homicide by the surgeon who removed them. However, kidneys occur in pairs, and we already permit individuals to donate one of their kidneys to a family member—indeed, we celebrate those who do. It is only a short step from the heroic act of giving away a kidney to the commercial act of selling one.

Such a procedure would be in keeping with the generally acknowledged principle that people ought to be free to do what they wish with their own bodies. However, the decisive disadvantage to allowing such transactions as a matter of social policy is that it would be the poor who would be most likely to suffer from it.

It is all too easy to imagine a mother, wishing to improve the lives and opportunities of her children, deciding to sell a kidney to help make that possible. That the economically advantaged should thrive by literally exploiting the bodies of the poor is morally repulsive to most people. It is no answer to state that someone should be permitted to do as she wishes with her body in order to provide for the welfare of her family. If selling a kidney and putting her own life and health at risk constitute the only option open to someone with that aim, then this in itself constitutes a prima facie case for major social reform.

A final possibility that has been widely discussed as a means of increasing the number of organs available for transplant is the adoption of a policy of "presumed consent." That is, a state or federal law would allow hospitals to take it for granted that a recently deceased person has tacitly consented to having any needed organs removed, unless the person had indicated otherwise or unless the family objects. The burden of securing consent would be removed from physicians and hospitals, but the burden of denying consent would be imposed on individuals or their families. To withdraw consent would require a positive action.

A policy of presumed consent has been adopted by several European countries. Critics of the policy point out that this has not, in general, done much to reduce the shortage of transplant organs in those countries. Although legally empowered to remove organs without a family's permission, physicians continue to be reluctant to do so. It is doubtful that a policy of presumed consent would be any more successful in this country. Also, if families are to be given the opportunity to deny consent, they must be notified of the death of the patient, and in many cases this would involve not only complicated practical arrangements but also a considerable loss of time.

Thus, it is somewhat doubtful that presumed consent would do a great deal to increase the number of usable transplant organs.

In the view of many observers, the present system of organ procurement by voluntary donation is the best system. It appeals to the best in people, rather than to greed and self-interest; it avoids exploiting the poor; and it is efficient. Many believe that without any fundamental alterations in the system it is possible to increase the number of available organs. As one observer commented, there is no shortage of donors, just a shortage of askers. If so, then the current U.S. policy of requiring that the next of kin be asked to donate organs holds the promise of relieving the chronic shortage.

Whatever the future may promise, the fact remains that at present there is a limited supply of transplant organs, and the demand exceeds the supply. Thus, the key question today is "How are organs to be distributed when they become available?" There are currently no national policies or procedures for answering this question. Typically, such decisions are made in accordance with policies adopted by particular regional or hospital-based transplant programs.

In a characteristic instance, a member of a hospital staff notifies someone in a transplant program of a potential donor, often a patient recently declared brain-dead. Someone from the program then approaches the family to secure consent. If consent is granted, the organs are removed and arrangements made to transplant them as soon as possible. Patients who are judged to be most in need medically and who have a good (not necessarily perfect) tissue match with the donor organ are chosen as the recipients.

Medical need is not the only factor considered in all instances, however. Decisions are also based on the patient's general medical condition, how much he might be expected to benefit from the transplant, his age, his ability to pay for the operation, whether he has a family that will assist him during recovery, and whether he belongs to the constituency that the hospital is committed to serving. In addition, other factors, such as the individual's "social worth" (education, occupation, accomplishments), may be taken into account.

Some of these factors, particularly the patient's social worth and ability to pay, have been strongly criticized as morally irrelevant to deciding who is to receive a transplant organ. A good example of an effort to formulate acceptable guidelines for making such decisions about allocating transplant organs is the Massachusetts Task Force on Organ Transplantation. The group issued a unanimous report that included the following recommendations:

1. Transplant surgery should be provided "to those who can benefit most from it in terms of probability of living for a significant period of time with a reasonable prospect for rehabilitation."

2. Decisions should not be based on "social worth" criteria.

3. Age may be considered as a factor in the selection process, but only to the extent that age is relevant to life expectancy and prospects for rehabilitation. Age must not be the only factor considered.

4. If not enough organs are available for all those who might benefit from them, final selections should be made by some random process (e.g., a lottery or a first-come, first-served basis).

5. Transplants should be provided to residents of New England on the basis of need, regardless of their ability to pay, so long as this does not adversely affect health-care services with a higher priority. Those who are not residents of New England should be accepted as transplant candidates only after they have demonstrated their ability to pay for the procedure.

A Presidential Commission in 1986 proposed that a national network of organ procurement and matching be established, one that would include all private, nonprofit agencies that currently undertake this work. It also recommended that a transplant program be funded so that no American in need of a heart, liver, or kidney transplant would be kept from receiving one because of an inability to pay.

The Reagan administration did not endorse the recommendations. It expressed the view that it would be more appropriate for the private sector, rather than the federal government, to accept the responsibilities associated with organ transplantation. Recent efforts have been made to tie private agencies into a single national network. However, for many people the inability to pay for an organ transplant still remains an unbreachable barrier to receiving one.

CASE PRESENTATION
Policy Decision and the Neonatal Unit

Jake Hanna (as we will call him) stood by the admitting desk in the emergency room of Commerce County Hospital and couldn't believe what was happening. It was like being trapped in a nightmare.

Less than ten miles away, his wife Christine lay in a recovery room at Valley View Hospital. She had just given birth to their first child and was still groggy from the anesthesia.

Martha, as they had already decided to name their daughter before her birth, had been premature. She was almost six weeks early, and both Jake and Chris had been surprised when Chris began to experience labor pains. At first they didn't know what the pains were; then they decided that, to be safe, they had better get Chris to the hospital Chris's obstetrician had told them to go to. They were lucky to have gotten to Valley View in time, because the birth was a difficult one, and Chris had needed help and reassurance.

In another respect, they hadn't been so lucky. Valley View was a small private hospital with restricted facilities. It had an emergency room but no intensive-care or neonatal units.

And Martha needed help. She was small and underdeveloped. Her heart sounds were weak and slightly irregular, she was having difficulty breathing, and her blood chemistry was unbalanced and showed inadequate kidney function. If she was to have a good chance at living, she needed special treatment and continuous monitoring.

"You need to get her into a special facility," Dr. Birk told Jake. "We're doing all we can for her here, but that's not very much. We aren't even set up to do dialysis. We simply don't have the equipment or the personnel to provide her with the kind of care she needs."

"Where could she go?" Jake asked.

"Commerce County Hospital—it's the only place in the area with a neonatal setup."

"Can you make the arrangements?"

"I'm sorry, I can't. They won't take referrals anymore. Somebody on their staff has to do the admitting. I think they're trying to cut back on their program."

"Can I get her in?"

"I'm not sure," Dr. Birk said. "But she needs to be there. They may take her as a walk-in. So you're going to have to go in person and take the baby with you. Do you have a friend or family member here?"

"Chris's mother is with her. But isn't it dangerous to move the baby?"

"Not really. She's in a stable condition, and if you take her you'll save a lot of time. She needs help as fast as she can get it."

With Martha wrapped in a gray hospital blanket and held by Chris's mother, Jake drove the ten miles to Commerce County Hospital and double-parked at the emergency entrance. He literally ran through the wide doors.

He explained to the clerk at the admitting desk that Dr. Birk had said that the baby needed to be in a neonatal unit at once. The clerk said that he had no authority to make that kind of admission and told

Jake to sit down while he paged Dr. Donna Chavez, the director of the unit.

The wait seemed interminable to Jake, but in less than ten minutes Dr. Chavez appeared in the emergency room. Jake walked over to her, and while they stood by the admitting desk with a dozen people waiting for their names to be called, he explained the problem once again.

When Jake had finished, Dr. Chavez shook her head. "We can't admit the child," she said. "I'm sorry, but we just can't do it."

"Why not?" Jake asked. "Don't you have room or something?"

"That's not the problem. We actually have enough space."

"Then what is it?"

"This is going to be hard for you to understand," Dr. Chavez said. "But the hospital has adopted a new policy. At no time can we have more than twenty patients in the neonatal unit, and that's the number we have now. The problem is with costs."

"But I'm willing to pay, and I have insurance."

"It's not particular costs, Mr. Hanna. It's the cost of the whole unit, and Commerce has just decided to cut back on its size. That's why they've imposed a twenty-infant limit."

"But what about my child?" Jake asked. "She needs help, and she needs it right now."

"I'm very, very sorry," Dr. Chavez said. "If the decision were mine alone, I would admit her at once. But as things are, I simply have to follow the hospital's policy guidelines."

"So you refuse to take her?"

"I must. I don't have any real choice in the matter."

"What am I supposed to do? Just let her die?"

"I suggest you take the child back to Valley View. They will do everything they can, and with luck things will work out for her. I certainly hope so."

Jake thought he had never had a nightmare as bad as this. He had never before felt so helpless, so powerless. There was no way he could force them to admit Martha, and there was nothing he could do for her himself. It surprised him that he didn't feel particularly angry at Dr. Chavez or at the hospital. He was simply too numb to feel much of anything.

Jake said nothing more to Dr. Chavez. He went out to the car and drove back to Valley View. Mrs.

Williams cried all the way back, and Jake wished that he could.

Inside the emergency room at Valley View, a nurse took the baby from Mrs. Williams. They took Martha to a small treatment room and gave her oxygen to help her breathing.

Jake and Mrs. Williams sat in the waiting area. They agreed that there was no need to tell Chris anything yet. She was asleep and no purpose would be served by waking her.

Three hours later, a doctor Jake had never seen before came to tell him that Martha was dead.

CASE PRESENTATION
Selection Committee for Dialysis

In 1966 Brattle, Texas, proper had a population of about 10,000 people. In Brattle County there were 20,000 more people who lived on isolated farms deep within the pine forests, or in crossroads towns with a filling station, a feed store, one or two white frame churches, and maybe twenty or twenty-five houses.

Brattle was the marketing town and county seat, the place all the farmers, their wives, and children went to on Saturday afternoon. It was also the medical center because it had the only hospitals in the county. One of them, Conklin Clinic, was hardly more than a group of doctors' offices. But Crane Memorial Hospital was quite a different sort of place. Occupying a relatively new three-story brick building in downtown Brattle, the hospital offered new equipment, a well-trained staff, and high-quality medical care.

This was mostly due to the efforts of Dr. J. B. Crane, Jr. The hospital was dedicated to the memory of his father, a man who practiced medicine in Brattle County for almost fifty years. Before Crane became a memorial hospital, it was Crane Clinic. But J. B. Crane, Jr., after returning from The Johns Hopkins Medical School, was determined to expand the clinic and transform it into a modern hospital. The need was there, and private investors were easy to find. Only a year after his father's death, Dr. Crane was able to offer Brattle County a genuine hospital.

It was only natural that, when the County Commissioner decided that Brattle County should have a dialysis machine, he would turn to Dr. Crane's hospital. The machine was bought with county funds, but Crane Memorial Hospital would operate it under a contract agreement. The hospital was guaranteed against loss by the county, but the hospital was also not permitted to make a profit on dialysis. Furthermore, although access to the machine was not restricted to county residents, residents were to be given priority.

Dr. Crane was not pleased with this stipulation. "I don't like to have medical decisions influenced by political considerations," he told the Commissioner. "If a guy comes in and needs dialysis, I don't want to tell him that he can't have it because somebody else who doesn't need it as much is on the machine and that person is a county resident."

"I don't know what to tell you," the Commissioner said. "It was county tax money that paid for the machine, and the County Council decided that the people who supplied the money ought to get top priority."

"What about the kind of case that I mentioned?" Dr. Crane asked. "What about somebody who could wait for dialysis who is a resident as opposed to somebody who needs it immediately who's not a resident?"

"We'll just leave that sort of case to our discretion," the Commissioner said. "People around here have confidence in you and your doctors. If you say they can wait, then they can wait. I know you won't let them down. Of course, if somebody died while some outsider was on the machine . . . Well, that would be embarrassing for all of us, I guess."

Dr. Crane was pleased to have the dialysis machine in his hospital. Not only was it the only one in Brattle County, but none of the neighboring counties had even one. Only the big hospitals in places like Dallas, Houston, and San Antonio had the machines. It put Crane Memorial up in the top rank.

Dr. Crane was totally unprepared for the problem when it came. He hadn't known there were so many people with chronic renal disease in Brattle County. But when news spread that there was a kidney machine available at Crane Memorial Hospital, twenty-three people applied for the dialysis program. Some were Dr. Crane's own patients or patients of his associates on the hospital staff. But a number of them were ones referred to the hospital by other physicians in Brattle and surrounding towns. Two of them were from neighboring Lopez County.

Working at a maximum, the machine could accommodate fourteen patients. But the staff decided that maximum operation would be likely to lead to dangerous equipment malfunctions and breakdowns. They settled on ten as the number of patients that should be admitted to the program.

Dr. Crane and his staff interviewed each of the program's applicants, reviewed their medical history, and got a thorough medical workup on each. They persuaded two of the patients to continue to commute to Houston, where they were already in dialysis. In four cases, renal disease had already progressed to the point that the staff decided that the patients could not benefit sufficiently from the program to make them good medical risks. In one other case, a patient suffering intestinal cancer and in generally poor health was rejected as a candidate. Two people were not in genuine need of dialysis but could be best treated by a program of medication.

That left fourteen candidates for the ten positions. Thirteen were from Brattle County and one from Lopez County.

"This is not a medical problem," Dr. Crane told the Commissioner. "And I'm not going to take the responsibility of deciding which people to condemn to death and which to give an extra chance at life."

"What do you want me to do?" the Commissioner asked. "I wouldn't object if you made the decision. I mean, you wouldn't have to tell everybody about it. You could just decide."

"That's something I won't do," Dr. Crane said. "All of this has to be open and aboveboard. It's got to be fair. If I decide, then everybody will think I am favoring my own patients or just taking the people who can pay the most money."

"I see what you mean. If I appoint a selection committee, will you serve on it?"

"I will. As long as my vote is the same as everybody else's."

"That's what I'll do, then," the Commissioner said.

The Brattle County Renal Dialysis Selection Committee was appointed and operating within the week. In addition to Dr. Crane, it was made up of three people chosen by the Commissioner. Amy Langford, a Brattle housewife in her middle fifties whose husband owned the largest automobile and truck agency in Brattle County, was one member. Reverend David Johnson was another member. He was the only African American on the committee and the pastor of the largest predominantly African American church in Brattle. The last member was Jacob Sims, owner of a hardware store in the nearby town of Silsbee. He was the only member of the committee not from the town of Brattle.

"Now I'm inclined to favor this fellow," said Mr. Sims at the Selection Committee's first meeting. "He's twenty-four years old, he's married, and he has a child two years old."

"You're talking about James Nelson?" Mrs. Langford asked. "I had some trouble with him. I've heard that he used to drink a lot before he got sick, and from the looks of his record he's had a hard time keeping a job."

"That's hard to say," said Reverend Johnson. "He works as a pulp-wood hauler, and people who do that change jobs a lot. You just have to go where the work is."

"That's right," said Mr. Sims. "One thing, though. I can't find any indication of his church membership. He says he's a Methodist, but I don't see where he's told us what his church is."

"I don't either," said Mrs. Langford. "And he's not a member of the Masons or the Lions Club or any other sort of civic group. I wouldn't say he's made much of a contribution to this community."

"That's right," said Reverend Johnson. "But let's don't forget that he's got a wife and baby depending on him. That child is going to need a father."

"I think he is a good psychological candidate," said Dr. Crane. "That is, I think if he starts the program he'll stick to it. I've talked with his wife, and I know she'll encourage him."

"We should notice that he's a high school dropout," Mrs. Langford said. "I don't think we can ever expect him to make much of a contribution to this town or to the county."

"Do you want to vote on this case?" asked Mr. Sims, the chairman of the committee.

"Let's talk about all of them, then go back and vote," Reverend Johnson suggested.

Everyone around the table nodded in agreement. The files were arranged by date of application, and Mr. Sims picked up the next one from the stack in front of him.

"Alva Algers," he said. "He's a fifty-three-year-old lawyer with three grown children. His wife is still alive, and he's still married to her. He's Secretary of the Layman's Board of the Brattle Episcopal Church, a member of the Rotary Club and the Elks. He used to be a scoutmaster."

"From the practical point of view," said Dr. Crane, "he would be a good candidate. He's intelligent and educated and understands what's involved in dialysis."

"I think he's definitely the sort of person we want to help," said Mrs. Langford. "He's the kind of person that makes this a better town. I'm definitely in favor of him."

"I am too," said Reverend Johnson. "Even if he does go to the wrong church."

"I'm not so sure," said Mr. Sims. "I don't think fifty-three is old—I'd better not, because I'm fifty-two myself. Still, his children are grown; he's led a good life. I'm not sure I wouldn't give the edge to some younger fellow."

"How can you say that?" Mrs. Langford said. "He's got a lot of good years left. He's a person of good character who might still do a lot for other people. He's not like that Nelson, who's not going to do any good for anybody except himself."

"I guess I'm not convinced that lawyers and members of the Rotary Club do a lot more good for the community than drivers of pulp-wood trucks," Mr. Sims said.

"Perhaps we ought to go on to the next candidate," Reverend Johnson said.

"We have Mrs. Holly Holton, a forty-three-year-old housewife from Mineral Springs," Mr. Sims said.

"That's in Lopez County, isn't it?" Mrs. Langford asked. "I think we can just reject her right off. She didn't pay the taxes that bought the machine, and our county doesn't have any responsibility for her."

"That's right," said Reverend Johnson.

Mr. Sims agreed, and Dr. Crane raised no objection.

"Now," said Mr. Sims, "here's Alton Conway. I believe he's our only African American candidate."

"I know him well," said Reverend Johnson. "He owns a dry-cleaning business, and people in the black community think very highly of him."

"I'm in favor of him," Mrs. Langford said. "He's a married man and seems quite settled and respectable."

"I wouldn't want us to take him just because he's black," Reverend Johnson said. "But I think he's got a lot in his favor."

"Well," said Mr. Sims, "unless Dr. Crane wants to add anything, let's go on to Nora Bainridge. She's a thirty-year-old divorced woman whose eight-year-old boy lives with his father over in Louisiana. She's a waitress at the Pep Cafe."

"She is a very vital woman," said Dr. Crane. "She's had a lot of trouble in her life, but I think she's a real fighter."

"I don't believe she's much of a churchgoer," said Reverend Johnson. "At least she doesn't give us a pastor's name."

"That's right," said Mrs. Langford. "And I just wonder what kind of morals a woman like her has. I mean, being divorced and working as a waitress and all."

"I don't believe we're trying to award sainthood here," said Mr. Sims.

"But surely moral character is relevant," said Mrs. Langford.

"I don't know anything against her moral character," said Mr. Sims. "Do you?"

"I'm only guessing," said Mrs. Langford. "But I wouldn't say that a woman of her background and apparent character is somebody we ought to give top priority to."

"I don't want to be the one to cast the first stone," said Reverend Johnson. "But I wouldn't put her at the top of our list either."

"I think we had better be careful not to discriminate against people who are poor and uneducated," said Dr. Crane.

"I agree," said Mrs. Langford. "But surely we have to take account of a person's worth."

"Can you tell us how we can measure a person's worth?" asked Mr. Sims.

"I believe I can," Mrs. Langford said. "Does the person have a steady job? Is he or she somebody we would be proud to know? Is he a churchgoer? Does he or she do things for other people? We can see what kind of education the person has had, and consider whether he is somebody we would like to have around."

"I guess that's some of it, all right," said Mr. Sims. "But I don't like to rely on things like education, money, and public service. A lot of people just haven't had a decent chance in this world. Maybe they were born poor or have had a lot of bad luck. I'm beginning to think that we ought to make our choices just by drawing lots."

"I can't approve of that," said Reverend Johnson. "That seems like a form of gambling to me. We ought to choose the good over the wicked, reward those who have led a virtuous life."

"I agree," Mrs. Langford said. "Choosing by drawing straws or something like that would mean we are just too cowardly to make decisions. We would be shirking our responsibility. Clearly, some people are more deserving than others, and we ought to have the courage to say so."

"All right," said Mr. Sims. "I guess we'd better get on with it, then. Simon Gootz is a forty-eight-year-old baker. He's got a wife and four children. Owns his own bakery—probably all of us have been there. He's Jewish."

"I'm not sure he's the sort of person who can stick to the required diet and go through the dialysis program," Dr. Crane said.

"I'll bet his wife and children would be a good incentive," said Mrs. Langford.

"There's not a Jewish church in town," said Reverend Johnson. "So of course we can't expect him to be a regular churchgoer."

"He's an immigrant," said Mr. Sims. "I don't believe he has any education to speak of, but he did start that bakery and build it up from nothing. I think that says a lot about his character."

"I think we can agree he's a good candidate," said Mrs. Langford.

"Let's just take one more before we break for dinner," Mr. Sims said. "Rebecca Scarborough. She's a sixty-three-year-old widow. Her children are all grown and living somewhere else."

"She's my patient," Dr. Crane said. "She's a tough and resourceful old woman. I believe she can follow orders and stand up to the rigors of the program, and her health in general is good."

Reverend Johnson said, "I just wonder if we shouldn't put a lady like her pretty far down on our list. She's lived a long life already, and she hasn't got anybody depending on her."

"I'm against that," Mrs. Langford said. "Everybody knows Mrs. Scarborough. Her family has been in this town for ages. She's one of our most substan-tial citizens. People would be scandalized if we didn't select her."

"Of course, I'm not from Brattle," said Mr. Sims. "And maybe that's an advantage here, because I don't see that she's got much in her favor except being from an old family."

"I think that's worth something," said Mrs. Langford.

"I'm not sure it's enough, though," said Reverend Johnson.

After dinner at the Crane Memorial Hospital cafeteria, the Selection Committee met again to discuss the seven remaining candidates. It was past ten o'clock before their final decisions were made. James Nelson, the pulp-wood truck driver, Holly Holton, the housewife from Mineral Springs, and Nora Bainridge, the waitress, were all rejected as candidates. Mrs. Scarborough was rejected also. The lawyer, Alva Algers, the dry cleaner, Alton Conway, and the baker, Simon Gootz, were selected to participate in the dialysis program. Others selected were a retired secondary schoolteacher, an assembly-line worker at the Rigid Box Company, a Brattle County Sheriff's Department patrolman, and a twenty-seven-year-old woman file clerk in the office of the Texas Western Insurance Company.

Dr. Crane was glad that the choices were made so that the program could begin operation. But he was not pleased with the selection method and resolved to talk to his own staff and with the County Commissioner about devising some other kind of selection procedure.

Without giving any reasons, Mr. Sims sent a letter to the County Commissioner resigning from the Renal Dialysis Selection Committee.

Mrs. Langford and Reverend Johnson also sent letters to the Commissioner. They thanked him for appointing them to the committee and indicated their willingness to continue to serve.

INTRODUCTION

TRANSPLANTS, KIDNEYS, MACHINES

The story of Robin Cook's novel *Coma* takes place in a large Boston hospital at the present time. What sets the novel apart from dozens of others with similar settings and characters is the fact that the plot hinges on the operations of a large-scale black market in transplant organs. For enormous fees, the criminals running the operation will supply corneas, kidneys, or hearts to those who can pay.

Cook claims that the inspiration for his novel came from an advertisement in a California newspaper. The anonymous ad offered to sell for $5,000 any organ that a reader wanted to buy. Thus, Cook's novel seems to be a book rooted firmly in the world we know today and not just a leap into the speculative realms of science fiction.

Organ transplants have attracted a considerable amount of attention in the last few years. Not only are transplants dramatic, often offering last-minute salvation from an almost certain death, but the very possibility of organ transplants is bright with promise. We can easily imagine a future in which any injured or diseased organ can be replaced almost as easily as the parts on a car. The present state of biomedical technology makes this more than a distant dream, although not a current reality.

The basic problem with organ transplants is the phenomenon of tissue rejection by the immune system. Alien proteins trigger the body's defense mechanisms. In the past, the proteins in the transplanted tissues were matched as carefully as possible with those of the recipient; then powerful immunosuppressive drugs were used in an effort to allow the host body to accommodate itself to the foreign tissue. These drugs left the body open to infections that it could normally cope with without much difficulty.

Increased use of the drug cyclosporine has done a great deal to improve the success of organ transplants. Cyclosporine selectively inhibits only part of the immune system and leaves enough of the system sufficiently functional to fight off most of the infections that were once fatal to large numbers of transplant recipients. Also, although tissue matching is still important, particularly for kidneys, the matches do not have to be as close as before.

Now 90–96% of transplanted kidneys function after one year; in the 1970s only about 50% did. Since 1970, the one-year survival rate for children with liver transplants has increased from 38% to around 70%, and there is good reason to believe that, if children survive as long as one year, they have a genuine chance to live a normal life. About 85% of heart transplant recipients now live for at least one year, a major increase from the 20% of the 1970s.

Some recent reports have suggested that long-term use of cyclosporine can result in kidney damage. This has led some to question whether the reduction in the rejection rate of transplants is offset by the chronic kidney damage caused by the drug. It is clear that cyclosporine is, at its best, only part of the solution to the tissue-rejection problem.

Because of the relatively high rate of success in organ transplants, the need for organs (kidneys in particular) is always greater than the supply. (The black-market operation in Cook's novel may not be wholly unrealistic.) In such a situation, where scarcity and need conflict, it is frequently necessary to decide who among the candidates for a transplant will receive an available organ. Relatively objective considerations such as the "goodness" of tissue matching, the size of the organ, and the general medical condition of the candidates may rule out some individuals. But it does happen that choices have to be made.

Who should make such choices? Should they be made by a physician, following his or her own intuitions? Should they be made by a committee or board? If so, who should be on the committee? Should a patient have a representative to speak for his or her interest—someone to "make a case" for receiving the transplant organ?

Should the decision be made in accordance with a set of explicit criteria? If so, then what criteria are appropriate? Are matters such as age, race, sex, and place of residence irrelevant? Should the character and accomplishments of the candidates be given any weight? Should people be judged by their estimated "worth to the community"? Should the fact that someone is a parent be given any weight?

These are just some of the questions relevant to the general issue of deciding how to allocate medical goods in situations in which the available supply is surpassed by a present need. Transplant organs are an example of one type of goods. In the future, assuming an improvement in transplant technology, the allocation of organs will no doubt become an even more frequent problem than at present. It is, of course, already a morally serious problem.

It was not organ transplants that first called public attention to the issue of resource allocation. This occurred most dramatically in the early 1960s, when the Artificial Kidney Center in Seattle, Washington, initiated an effective large-scale treatment program for people with renal diseases. Normal kidneys filter waste products from the blood that have accumulated as a result of ordinary cellular metabolism—salt, urea, creatinine, potassium, uric acid, and other substances. These waste products are sent from the kidneys to the bladder, where they are then secreted as urine. Kidney failure, which can result from one of a number of diseases, allows waste products to build up in the blood. This can cause high blood pressure and even heart failure, tissue edema (swelling), and muscular seizure. If unremedied, the condition results in death.

When renal failure occurs, hemodialysis is a way of cleansing the blood of waste products by passing it through a cellophane-like tube immersed in a chemical bath. The impurities in the blood pass through the membrane and into the chemical bath by osmosis, and the purified blood is then returned to the patient's body.

At the beginning of the Seattle program, there were many more candidates for dialysis than there were units ("kidney machines") to accommodate them. As a response to this situation, the Kidney Center set up a committee to select patients who would receive treatment. (See the Case Presentation for an account of how such a committee might work.) In effect, the committee was offering to some

a better chance for life than they would have without access to dialysis equipment.

As other centers and hospitals established renal units, they faced the same painful decisions that Seattle did. Almost always there were many more patients needing hemodialysis than there was equipment available to treat them. It was partly in response to this situation that Section 299-1 of Public Law 92-603 was passed by Congress in 1972. Those who require hemodialysis or kidney transplants are now eligible for Medicare payments that cover as much as 80% of the costs involved.

More than 70,000 patients are now receiving dialysis supported by Medicare. Present costs are over $2 billion a year, and the patient load is expected to increase at a rate of some 20% a year.

Quite apart from the cost, which is much higher than originally expected, dialysis continues to present moral difficulties. Resources are still finite so that at a given time more patients may both need and want dialysis than can be accommodated. Hence the need to make choices among patients is still present. It brings with it all the problems that we mentioned above.

In addition, because more dialysis equipment is accessible and is financially available to virtually everyone, physicians face a serious difficulty. Even if a physician believes that a patient is not likely to gain benefits from dialysis sufficient to justify the expense, should she recommend the patient for dialysis anyway? Not to do so may mean almost certain death for the patient in the near future, yet the social cost (measured in terms of the cost of equipment and its operation, hospital facilities, and the time of physicians, nurses, and technicians) may be immense. It can be $100,000 or more a year for a single person. Typically, however, the government spends about $20,000 for each of the approximately 90,000 dialysis patients annually.

Nor does dialysis solve all problems for patients with terminal kidney diseases. Although time spent on the machine varies, some patients spend five hours, three days a week, attached to the machine. Medical and psychological problems are typical even when the process works at its most efficient. Prolonged dialysis can produce neurological disorders, severe headaches, gastrointestinal bleeding, and bone diseases. Psychological and physical stress is always present, and particularly before dialysis treatments, severe depression is common. A 1971 study showed that 5% of dialysis patients take their own lives, and a number of others simply drop out of treatment programs and allow themselves to die. For these reasons, strong motivation, psychological stability, age, and a generally sound physical condition are factors considered important in deciding whether to admit a person to dialysis.

The characteristics required to make someone a "successful" dialysis patient are to some extent "middle-class virtues." A patient must not only be motivated to save his life, but he must also understand the need for the dialysis, be capable of adhering to a strict diet, show up for scheduled dialysis sessions, and so on. As a consequence, where decisions about whether to admit a patient to dialysis are based on estimates of the likelihood of the patient's doing what is required, members of the white middle class have a definite edge over others. Selection criteria that are apparently objective may actually involve hidden class or racial bias.

Various ways of dealing with both the costs and the personal problems presented by dialysis are currently under discussion. In the view of some, increasing the number of kidney transplants would do the most to improve the lives of patients and to reduce the cost of the kidney program. (This would have the result of increasing even more the demand for transplant organs. See the Social Context section for a discussion of proposals for doing this.) Others have pressed for training more patients to perform home dialysis, which is substantially cheaper than dialysis performed in clinics or hospitals. However, those who are elderly, live alone, or lack adequate facilities are not likely to be able to use and maintain the complicated equipment involved. Other things being equal, should such people be given priority for transplants?

The problems of transplants and dialysis involve decisions that affect individuals in a direct and immediate way. For example, either a person is accepted into a dialysis program or he is not. As we will see in the next chapter, there are a number of broader social issues connected with providing and distributing medical resources. But our concern here is with the sort of decision making that involves the welfare of particular people in specific situations. The situations are ones in which there is not enough of what is needed to go around. The basic question, of course, is who shall get it and who shall go without?

Any commodity or service that can be in short supply relative to the need for it raises the issue of fair and justifiable distribution. Decisions that control the supply itself, that determine, for example, what proportion of the federal budget will be spent on medical care, are generally referred to as *macroallocation* decisions. These are the large-scale decisions that do not involve individuals in a direct way. Similarly, deciding what proportion of the money allocated to health care should be spent on dialysis is another example of a macroallocation decision.

By contrast, *microallocation* decisions are ones that directly impinge on individuals. Thus, when one donor heart is available and six people in need of a transplant make a claim on it, the decision as to who gets the heart is a microallocation decision. In Chapter 10, in discussing the claim to health care, we will focus more on macroallocation, but in this chapter we will be concerned mostly with microallocation. (The distinction between macroallocation and microallocation is often less clear than the explanation here suggests. After all, there are many levels of decision making in the distribution of resources, and the terms "macro" and "micro" are relative ones.)

Although the examples we have considered have been restricted to transplant organs and dialysis machines, the question of fair distribution can be raised just as appropriately about cardiac resuscitation teams, microsurgical teams, space in burn units or intensive-care wards, hospital beds, drugs and vaccines, medical-evacuation helicopters, operating rooms, physicians' time, and all other medical goods and services that are in limited supply with respect to the demand for them.

Earlier, in connection with transplants, we considered some of the more specific questions that have to be asked about distribution. The questions generally fall into two categories: Who shall decide? What criteria or standards should be employed in making the allocation decision? These are the questions that must be answered whenever there is scarcity relative to needs and wants.

ETHICAL THEORIES AND THE ALLOCATION OF MEDICAL RESOURCES

An analogy that is frequently used in the discussion of the distribution of limited medical resources compares such a situation to the plight of a group of people adrift in a lifeboat. If some of the group are sacrificed, then the others will have a much better chance of surviving. But who should be sacrificed?

One answer to this question is that no one should be. Simply by virtue of being human, each person in the lifeboat has an equal worth. An action that involved sacrificing anyone for the good of the others in the boat would not be morally defensible. This suggests that the only right course of action would be simply to do nothing.

This point of view is one that may be regarded as compatible with Kant's ethical principles. Because each individual may be considered to have inherent value, considerations such as talent, intelligence, age, social worth, and so on are morally irrelevant. Accordingly, there seem to be no grounds for

distinguishing those who are to be sacrificed from those who may be saved. In the medical context, this would mean that when there are not enough goods and services to go around, then no one should receive them.

This is not a result that is dictated by Kant's principles, however. One might also argue that the fact that every person is equal to every other in dignity and worth does not require the sacrifice of all. A random procedure—such as drawing straws—might be used to determine who is to have an increased chance of survival. In such a case, each person is being treated as having equal value, and the person who loses might be regarded as exercising autonomy by sacrificing himself or herself.

The maxim underlying the sacrifice would, apparently, be one that would meet the test of the categorical imperative. Any rational person might be expected to sacrifice himself in such a situation and under the conditions in which the decision was made. In the case of medical resources, a random procedure would seem to be a morally legitimate procedure.

The natural law view and Ross's would seem to support a similar line of argument. Although we all have a duty, on these views, to preserve our lives, this does not mean that we do not sometimes have to risk them. Just such a risk might be involved in agreeing to abide by the outcome of a random procedure to decide who will be sacrificed and who saved.

Utilitarianism does not dictate a specific answer to the question of who, if anyone, should be saved. It does differ radically in one respect, however, from those moral views that ascribe an intrinsic value to each human life. The principle of utility suggests that we ought to take into account the consequences of sacrificing some people rather than others. Who, for example, is more likely to make a contribution to the general welfare of the society, an accountant or a nurse? This approach opens the way to considering the "social worth" of people and makes morally relevant such characteristics as education, occupation, age, record of accomplishment, and so on.

To take this approach would require working out a set of criteria to assign value to various properties of people. Those to be sacrificed would be those whose point total put them at the low end of the ranking. Here, then, a typical "calculus of utilities" would be relied on to solve the decision problem. The decision problem about the allocation of medical resources would follow exactly the same pattern.

This approach is not one required by the principle of utility, however. Someone might argue that a policy formulated along those lines would have so many harmful social consequences that some other solution would be preferable. Thus, a utilitarian might argue that a better policy would be one based on some random process. In connection with medical goods and services, a "first-come, first-served" approach might be superior. (This is a possible option for rule utilitarianism. It could be argued that an act utilitarian would be forced to adopt the first approach.)

Rawls's principles of justice seem clearly to rule out distributing medical resources on the criterion of "social worth." Where special benefits are to be obtained, those benefits must be of value to all and open to all. It is compatible with Rawls's view, of course, that there should be no special medical resources. But if there are, and they must be distributed under conditions of scarcity, then some genuinely fair procedure, such as random selection, must be the procedure used.

No ethical theory that we have considered gives a straightforward answer to the question of who shall make the selection. Where a procedure is random or first-come, first-served, the decision-making process requires only establishing the right kind of social arrangements to implement the policy. Only when social worth must be judged and considered as a relevant factor in decision making does the procedure assume importance. (This is assuming that medical decisions about appropriateness—decisions that establish a class of candidates for the limited resources—have already been made.)

A utilitarian answer as to who shall make the allocation decision might be that the decision should be made by those who are in a good position to judge the likelihood of an individual's contributing to the welfare of society as a whole. Since physicians are not uniquely qualified to make such judgments, leaving decisions to an individual physician or a committee of physicians would not be the best approach. A better one would probably be to rely on a committee composed of a variety of people representative of the society.

There are many more questions of a moral kind connected with the allocation of scarce resources than we have mentioned here. We have not, for example, considered whether an individual should be allowed to make a case for receiving resources. Nor have we examined any of the problems with employing specific criteria for selection (such as requiring that a person be a resident of a certain community or state). We have, however, touched upon enough of the basic issues that it should be easy to see how other appropriate questions might be asked.

The Allocation of Exotic Medical Lifesaving Therapy

Nicholas Rescher

Nicholas Rescher makes a useful distinction between two kinds of criteria: criteria of inclusion (for the selection of candidates) and criteria of comparison (for selection of recipients). Rescher argues that three areas need to be considered in establishing a class of candidates: (1) constituency (Is the person a member of the community the institution is designed to serve?); (2) progress of science (Can new knowledge be gained from the case?); and (3) success (Is the treatment of the person likely to be effective?).

Five factors, Rescher claims, ought to be considered in deciding upon recipients of the goods or services: (1) the likelihood of successful treatment compared with others in the group; (2) the life expectancy of the person; (3) the person's family role, (4) the potential of the person in making future contributions; and (5) the person's record of services or contributions.

Rescher argues that it is necessary to have a rational selection system, but he admits that the exact manner in which a system takes into account relevant factors cannot be fixed and exact. In his view, which is basically a utilitarian one, an acceptable selection system might be one that makes use of point ratings of the factors mentioned above. This would establish a smaller group, but as a final step, he suggests, the best procedure might well be to make use of a chance factor (such as a lottery) to choose recipients.

I. The Problem

Technological progress has in recent years transformed the limits of the possible in medical therapy. However, the elevated state of sophistication of modern medical technology has brought the economists' classic problem of scarcity in its wake as an unfortunate side product. The enormously sophisticated and complex equipment and the highly trained teams of experts requisite for its utilization are scarce resources in relation to potential demand. The administrators of the great medical institutions that preside over these scarce resources thus come to be faced increasingly with the awesome choice: *Whose life to save?*

A (somewhat hypothetical) paradigm example of this problem may be sketched within the following set of definitive assumptions: We suppose that persons in some particular medically morbid condition are "mortally afflicted": It is virtually certain that they will die within a short time period (say ninety days). We assume that some very complex course of treatment (e.g., a heart transplant) represents a substantial probability of life prolongation for persons in this mortally afflicted condition. We assume that the facilities available in terms of

human resources, mechanical instrumentalities, and requisite materials (e.g., hearts in the case of a heart transplant) make it possible to give a certain treatment—this "exotic (medical) lifesaving therapy," or ELT for short—to a certain, relatively small number of people. And finally we assume that a substantially greater pool of people in the mortally afflicted condition is at hand. The problem then may be formulated as follows: How is one to select within the pool of afflicted patients the ones to be given the ELT treatment in question; how to select those "whose lives are to be saved"? Faced with many candidates for an ELT process that can be made available to only a few, doctors and medical administrators confront the decision of who is to be given a chance at survival and who is, in effect, to be condemned to die.

As has already been implied, the "heroic" variety of spare-part surgery can pretty well be assimilated to this paradigm. One can foresee the time when heart transplantation, for example, will have become pretty much a routine medical procedure, albeit on a very limited basis, since a cardiac surgeon with the technical competence to transplant hearts can operate at best a rather small number of times each week and the elaborate facilities for such oper-

Reprinted from Ethics 79 *(April 1969), by permission of The University of Chicago Press and the author.* © *The University of Chicago Press.*

ations will most probably exist on a modest scale. Moreover, in "spare-part" surgery there is always the problem of availability of the "spare parts" themselves. A report in one British newspaper gives the following picture: "Of the 150,000 who die of heart disease each year [in the U.K.], Mr. Donald Longmore, research surgeon at the National Heart Hospital [in London] estimated that 22,000 might be eligible for heart surgery. Another 30,000 would need heart and lung transplants. But there are probably only between 7,000 and 14,000 potential donors a year."[1] Envisaging this situation in which at the very most something like one in four heart-malfunction victims can be saved, we clearly confront a problem in ELT allocation.

A perhaps even more drastic case in point is afforded by long-term haemodialysis, an ongoing process by which a complex device—an "artificial kidney machine"—is used periodically in cases of chronic renal failure to substitute for a nonfunctional kidney in "cleaning" potential poisons from the blood. Only a few major institutions have chronic haemodialysis units, whose complex operation is an extremely expensive proposition. For the present and foreseeable future the situation is that "the number of places available for chronic haemodialysis is hopelessly inadequate."[2]

The traditional medical ethos has insulated the physician against facing the very existence of this problem. When swearing the Hippocratic Oath, he commits himself to work for the benefit of the sick in "whatsoever house I enter."[3] In taking this stance, the physician substantially renounces the explicit choice of saving certain lives rather than others. Of course, doctors have always in fact had to face such choices on the battlefield or in times of disaster, but there the issue had to be resolved hurriedly, under pressure, and in circumstances in which the very nature of the case effectively precluded calm deliberation by the decision maker as well as criticism by others. In sharp contrast, however, cases of the type we have postulated in the present discussion arise predictably, and represent choices to be made deliberately and "in cold blood."

It is, to begin with, appropriate to remark that this problem is not fundamentally a medical problem. For when there are sufficiently many afflicted candidates for ELT then—so we may assume—there will also be more than enough for whom the purely medical grounds for ELT allocation are decisively strong in any individual case, and just about equally strong throughout the group. But in this circumstance a selection of some afflicted patients over and against others cannot *ex hypothesi* be made on the basis of purely medical considerations.

The selection problem, as we have said, is in substantial measure not a medical one. It is a problem *for* medical men, which must somehow be solved by them, but that does not make it a medical issue—any more than the problem of hospital building is a medical issue. As a problem it belongs to the category of philosophical problems—specifically a problem of moral philosophy or ethics. Structurally, it bears a substantial kinship with those issues in this field that revolve about the notorious whom-to-save-on-the-lifeboat and whom-to-throw-to-the-wolves-pursuing-the-sled questions. But whereas questions of this just-indicated sort are artificial, hypothetical, and farfetched, the ELT issue poses a genuine policy question for the responsible administrators in medical institutions, indeed a question that threatens to become commonplace in the foreseeable future.

Now what the medical administrator needs to have, and what the philosopher is presumably *ex officio* in a position to help in providing, is a body of *rational guidelines* for making choices in these literally life-or-death situations. This is an issue in which many interested parties have a substantial stake, including the responsible decision maker who wants to satisfy his conscience that he is acting in a reasonable way. Moreover, the family and associates of the man who is turned away—to say nothing of the man himself—have the right to an acceptable explanation. And indeed even the general public wants to know that what is being done is fitting and proper. All of these interested parties are entitled to insist that a reasonable code of operating principles provides a defensible rationale for making the life-and-death choices involved in ELT.

II. The Two Types of Criteria

Two distinguishable types of criteria are bound up in the issue of making ELT choices. We shall call these *Criteria of Inclusion* and *Criteria of Comparison*, respectively. The distinction at issue here requires some explanation. We can think of the selection as being made by a two-stage process: (1) the selection from among all possible candidates (by a suitable screening process) of a group to be taken under serious consideration as candidates for therapy, and then (2) the actual singling out, within this group, of the particular individuals to whom therapy is to be given. Thus the first process narrows down the range of comparative choices by eliminating *en bloc* whole categories of potential candidates. The second process calls for a more refined case-by-case comparison of those candidates that remain. By means of the first set of criteria one forms a selection group; by means of the second set, an actual selection is made within this group.

Thus what we shall call a "selection system" for the choice of patients to receive therapy of the ELT type will consist of criteria of these two kinds. Such a system will be acceptable only when the reasonableness of its component criteria can be established.

III. Essential Features of an Acceptable ELT Selection System

To qualify as reasonable, an ELT selection must meet two important "regulative" requirements: it must be *simple* enough to be readily intelligible, and it must be *plausible*, that is, patently reasonable in a way that can be apprehended easily and without involving ramified subtleties. Those medical administrators responsible for ELT choices must follow a modus operandi that virtually all the people involved can readily understand to be acceptable (at a reasonable level of generality, at any rate). Appearances are critically important here. It is not enough that the choice be made in a *justifiable* way; it must be possible for people—*plain* people—to "see" (i.e., understand without elaborate teaching or indoctrination) that *it is justified*, insofar as any mode of procedure can be justified in cases of this sort.

One "constitutive" requirement is obviously an essential feature of a reasonable selection system: all of its component criteria—those of inclusion and those of comparison alike—must be reasonable in the sense of being *rationally defensible*. The ramifications of this requirement call for detailed consideration. But one of its aspects should be noted without further ado: it must be *fair*—it must treat relevantly like cases alike, leaving no room for "influence" or favoritism, etc.

IV. The Basic Screening Stage: Criteria of Inclusion (and Exclusion)

Three sorts of considerations are prominent among the plausible criteria of inclusion/exclusion at the basic screening stage: the constituency factor, the progress-of-science factor, and the prospect-of-success factor.

A. The Constituency Factor

It is a "fact of life" that ELT can be available only in the institutional setting of a hospital or medical institute or the like. Such institutions generally have normal clientele boundaries. A veterans' hospital will not concern itself primarily with treating non-veterans, a children's hospital cannot be expected to accommodate the "senior citizen," an army hospital can regard college professors as outside its sphere. Sometimes the boundaries are geographic—a state hospital may admit only residents of a certain state. (There are, of course, indefensible constituency principles—say race or religion, party membership, or ability to pay; and there are cases of borderline legitimacy, e.g., sex.[4]) A medical institution is justified in considering for ELT only persons within its own constituency, provided this constituency is constituted upon a defensible basis. Thus the haemodialysis selection committee in Seattle "agreed to consider only those applications who were residents of the state of Washington. They justified this stand on the grounds that since the basic research . . . had been done at . . . a state-supported institution—the people whose taxes had paid for the research should be its first beneficiaries."[5]

While thus insisting that constituency considerations represent a valid and legitimate factor in ELT selection, I do feel there is much to be said for minimizing their role in life-or-death cases. Indeed a refusal to recognize them at all is a significant part of medical tradition, going back to the very oath of Hippocrates. They represent a departure from the ideal arising with the institutionalization of medicine, moving it away from its original status as an art practiced by an individual practitioner.

B. The Progress-of-Science Factor

The needs of medical research can provide a second valid principle of inclusion. The research interests of the medical staff in relation to the specific nature of the cases at issue is a significant consideration. It may be important for the progress of medical science—and thus of potential benefit to many persons in the future—to determine how effective the ELT at issue is with diabetics or persons over sixty or with a negative RH factor. Considerations of this sort represent another type of legitimate factor in ELT selection. A very definitely *borderline* case under this head would revolve around the question of a patient's willingness to pay, not in monetary terms, but in offering himself as an experimental subject, say by contracting to return at designated times for a series of tests substantially unrelated to his own health, but yielding data of importance to medical knowledge in general.

C. The Prospect-of-Success Factor

It may be that while the ELT at issue is not without *some* effectiveness in general, it has been established to be highly effective only with patients in certain specific categories (e.g., females under forty of a specific blood type). This difference in effectiveness—in the absolute or in the probability of success—is (we assume) so marked as to constitute virtually a difference in kind rather than in degree. In this case, it would be perfectly legitimate to adopt the general rule of making the ELT at issue available only or primarily to persons in this substantial-promise-of-success category. (It is on grounds of this sort that young children and persons over fifty are generally ruled out as candidates for haemodialysis.)

We have maintained that the three factors of constituency, progress of science, and prospect of success represent legitimate criteria of inclusion for ELT selection. But it remains to examine the considerations which legitimate them. The legitimating factors are in the final analysis practical or pragmatic in nature. From the practical angle it is advantageous—indeed to some extent necessary that the arrangements governing medical institutions should embody certain constituency principles. It makes good pragmatic and utilitarian sense that progress-of-science considerations should be operative here. And, finally, the practical aspect is reinforced by a whole host of other considerations—including moral ones—in supporting the prospect-of-success

criterion. The workings of each of these factors are of course conditioned by the ever-present element of limited availability. They are operative only in this context, that is, prospect of success is a legitimate consideration at all only because we are dealing with a situation of scarcity.

V. The Final Selection Stage: Criteria of Selection

Five sorts of elements must, as we see it, figure primarily among the plausible criteria of selection that are to be brought to bear in further screening the group constituted after application of the criteria of inclusion: the relative-likelihood-of-success factor, the life-expectancy factor, the family role factor, the potential-contributions factor, and the services-rendered factor. The first two represent the *biomedical* aspect, the second three the *social* aspect.

A. The Relative-Likelihood-of-Success Factor

It is clear that the relative likelihood of success is a legitimate and appropriate factor in making a selection within the group of qualified patients that are to receive ELT. This is obviously one of the considerations that must count very significantly in a reasonable selection procedure.

The present criterion is of course closely related to item C of the preceding section. There we were concerned with prospect-of-success considerations categorically and *en bloc*. Here at present they come into play in a particularized case-by-case comparison among individuals. If the therapy at issue is not a once-and-for-all proposition and requires ongoing treatment, cognate considerations must be brought in. Thus, for example, in the case of a chronic ELT procedure such as haemodialysis it would clearly make sense to give priority to patients with a potentially reversible condition (who would thus need treatment for only a fraction of their remaining lives).

B. The Life-Expectancy Factor

Even if the ELT is "successful" in the patient's case he may, considering his age and/or other aspects of his general medical condition, look forward to only a very short probable future life. This is obviously another factor that must be taken into account.

C. The Family Role Factor

A person's life is a thing of importance not only to himself but to others—friends, associates, neighbors, colleagues, etc. But his (or her) relationship to his immediate family is a thing of unique intimacy and significance. The nature of his relationship to his wife, children, and parents, and the issue of their financial and psychological dependence upon him, are obviously matters that deserve to be given weight in the ELT selection process. Other things being anything like equal, the mother of minor children must take priority over the middle-aged bachelor.

D. The Potential Future-Contributions Factor (Prospective Service)

In "choosing to save" one life rather than another, "the society," through the mediation of the particular medical institution in question—which should certainly look upon itself as a trustee for the social interest—is clearly warranted in considering the likely pattern of future *services to be rendered* by the patient (adequate recovery assumed), considering his age, talent, training, and past record of performance. In its allocations of ELT, society "invests" a scarce resource in one person as against another and is thus entitled to look to the probable prospective "return" on its investment.

It may well be that a thoroughly egalitarian society is reluctant to put someone's social contribution into the scale in situations of the sort at issue. One popular article states that "the most difficult standard would be the candidate's value to society," and goes on to quote someone who said: "You can't just pick a brilliant painter over a laborer. The average citizen would be quickly eliminated."[6] But what if it were not a brilliant painter but a brilliant surgeon or medical researcher that was at issue? One wonders if the author of the *obiter dictum* that one "can't just pick" would still feel equally sure of his ground. In any case, the fact that the standard is difficult to apply is certainly no reason for not attempting to apply it. The problem of ELT selection is inevitably burdened with difficult standards.

Some might feel that in assessing a patient's value to society one should ask not only who if permitted to continue living can make the greatest contribution to society in some creative or constructive way, but also who by dying would leave behind the greatest burden on society in assuming the discharge of their residual responsibilities.[7] Certainly the philosophical utilitarian would give equal weight to both these considerations. Just here is where I would part ways with orthodox utilitarianism. For—though this is not the place to do so—I should be prepared to argue that a civilized society has an obligation to promote the furtherance of positive achievements in cultural and related areas even if this means the assumption of certain added burdens.[8]

E. The Past Services-Rendered Factor (Retrospective Service)

A person's services to another person or group have always been taken to constitute a valid basis for a claim upon this person or group—of course a moral and not necessarily a legal claim. Society's obligation for the recognition and reward of services rendered—an obligation whose discharge is also very possibly conducive to self-interest in the long run—is thus another factor to be taken into account. This should be viewed as a morally necessary correlative of the previously considered factor of *prospective* service. It would be morally indefensible of society in effect to say: "Never mind about services you rendered yesterday—it is only the services to be rendered tomorrow that will count with us today." We live in very future-oriented times, constantly preoccupied in a distinctly utilitarian way with future satisfactions. And this disinclines us to give much recognition to past services. But parity considerations of the sort just adduced indicate that such recognition should be given *on grounds of equity*. No doubt a justification for giving weight to services rendered can also be attempted along utilitarian lines. ("The reward of past services rendered spurs people on to greater future efforts and is thus socially advantageous in the long-run future.") In saying that past services should be counted "on grounds of equity"—rather than "on grounds of utility"—I take the view that even if this utilitarian defense could somehow be shown to be fallacious, I should still be prepared to maintain the propriety of taking services rendered into account. The position does not rest on a utilitarian basis and so would not collapse with the removal of such a basis.[9]

As we have said, these five factors fall into three groups: the biomedical factors *A* and *B*, the familial factor *C*, and the social factors *D* and *E*. With items

A and *B* the need for a detailed analysis of the medical considerations comes to the fore. The age of the patient, his medical history, his physical and psychological condition, his specific disease, etc., will all need to be taken into exact account. These biomedical factors represent technical issues: they call for the physicians' expert judgment and the medical statisticians' hard data. And they are ethically uncontroversial factors— their legitimacy and appropriateness are evident from the very nature of the case.

Greater problems arise with the familial aid social factors. They involve intangibles that are difficult to judge. How is one to develop subcriteria for weighing the relative social contributions of (say) an architect or a librarian or a mother of young children? And they involve highly problematic issues. (For example, should good moral character be rated a plus and bad a minus in judging services rendered?) And there is something strikingly unpleasant in grappling with issues of this sort for people brought up in times greatly inclined towards maxims of the type "Judge not!" and "Live and let live!" All the same, in the situation that concerns us here such distasteful problems must be faced, since a failure to choose to save some is tantamount to sentencing all. Unpleasant choices are intrinsic to the problem of ELT selection; they are of the very essence of the matter.[10]

But is reference to all these factors indeed inevitable? The justification for taking account of the medical factors is pretty obvious. But why should the social aspect of services rendered and to be rendered be taken into account at all? The answer is that they must be taken into account not from the *medical* but from the *ethical* point of view. Despite disagreement on many fundamental issues, moral philosophers of the present day are pretty well in consensus that the justification of human actions is to be sought largely and primarily—if not exclusively—in the principles of utility and of justice.[11] But utility requires reference of services to be rendered and justice calls for a recognition of services that have been rendered. Moral considerations would thus demand recognition of these two factors. (This, of course, still leaves open the question of whether the point of view provides a valid basis of action: Why base one's actions upon moral principles?—or, to put it bluntly—Why be moral? The present paper is, however, hardly the place to grapple with so fundamental an issue, which has been canvassed in the literature of philosophical ethics since Plato.)

VI. More than Medical Issues Are Involved

An active controversy has of late sprung up in medical circles over the question of whether non-physician laymen should be given a role in ELT selection (in the specific context of chronic haemodialysis). One physician writes: "I think that the assessment of the candidates should be made by a senior doctor on the [dialysis] unit, but I am sure that it would be helpful to him—both in sharing responsibility and in avoiding personal pressure if a small unnamed group of people [presumably including laymen] officially made the final decision. I visualize the doctor bringing the data to the group, explaining the points in relation to each case, and obtaining their approval of his order of priority."[12]

Essentially this procedure of a selection committee of laymen has for some years been in use in one of the most publicized chronic dialysis units, that of the Swedish Hospital of Seattle, Washington.[13] Many physicians are apparently reluctant to see the choice of allocation of medical therapy pass out of strictly medical hands. Thus in a recent symposium on the "Selection of Patients for Haemodialysis,"[14] Dr. Ralph Shakman writes: "Who is to implement the selection? In my opinion it must ultimately be the responsibility of the consultants in charge of the renal units . . . I can see no reason for delegating this responsibility to lay persons. Surely the latter would be better employed if they could be persuaded to devote their time and energy to raise more and more money for us to spend on our patients."[15] Other contributors to this symposium strike much the same note. Dr. F. M. Parsons writes: "In an attempt to overcome . . . difficulties in selection some have advocated introducing certain specified lay people into the discussions. Is it wise? I doubt whether a committee of this type can adjudicate as satisfactorily as two medical colleagues, particularly as successful therapy involves close cooperation between doctor and patient."[16] And Dr. M. A. Wilson writes in the same symposium: "The suggestion has been made that lay panels should select individuals for dialysis from among a group who are medically suitable. Though this would relieve the doctor-in-charge of a heavy load of responsibility, it would place the burden on those who have no personal knowledge and have to base their judgments on medical or social reports. I do not believe this would result in better decisions for the group or improve the doctor-patient relationship in individual cases."[17]

But no amount of flag waving about the doctor's facing up to his responsibility—or prostrations before the idol of the doctor-patient relationship and reluctance to admit laymen into the sacred precincts of the conference chambers of medical consultations—can obscure the essential fact that ELT selection is not a wholly medical problem. When there are more than enough places in an ELT program to accommodate all who need it, then it will clearly be a medical question to decide who does have the need and which among these would successfully respond. But when an admitted gross insufficiency of places exists, when there are ten or fifty or one hundred highly eligible candidates for each place in the program, then it is unrealistic to take the view that purely medical criteria can furnish a sufficient basis for selection. The question of ELT selection becomes serious as a phenomenon of scale—because, as more candidates present themselves, strictly medical factors are increasingly less adequate as a selection criterion precisely because by numerical category-crowding there will be more and more cases whose "status is much the same" so far as purely medical considerations go.

The ELT selection problem clearly poses issues that transcend the medical sphere because—in the nature of the case—many residual issues remain to be dealt with once *all* of the medical questions have been faced. Because of this there is good reason why laymen as well as physicians should be involved in the selection process. Once the medical considerations have been brought to bear, fundamental social issues remain to be resolved. The instrumentalities of ELT have been created through the social investment of scarce resources, and the interests of the society deserve to play a role in their utilization. As representatives of their social interests, lay opinions should function to complement and supplement medical views once the proper arena of medical considerations is left behind.[18] Those physicians who have urged the presence of lay members on selection panels can, from this point of view, be recognized as having seen the issue in proper perspective.

One physician has argued against lay representation on selection panels for haemodialysis as fol-

lows: "If the doctor advises dialysis and the lay panel refuses, the patient will regard this as a death sentence passed by an anonymous court from which he has no right of appeal."[19] But this drawback is not specific to the use of a lay panel. Rather, it is a feature inherent in every *selection* procedure, regardless of whether the selection is done by the head doctor of the unit, by a panel of physicians, etc. No matter who does the selecting among patients recommended for dialysis, the feelings of the patient who has been rejected (and knows it) can be expected to be much the same, provided that he recognizes the actual nature of the choice (and is not deceived by the possibly convenient but ultimately poisonous fiction that because the selection was made by physicians it was made entirely on medical grounds).

In summary, then, the question of ELT selection would appear to be one that is in its very nature heavily laden with issues of medical research, practice, and administration. But it will not be a question that can be resolved on solely medical grounds. Strictly social issues of justice and utility will invariably arise in this area—questions going outside the medical area in whose resolution medical laymen can and should play a substantial role.

VII. The Inherent Imperfection (Non-Optimality) of Any Selection System

Our discussion to this point of the design of a selection system for ELT has left a gap that is a very fundamental and serious omission. We have argued that five factors must be taken into substantial and explicit account:

A. *Relative likelihood of success.* Is the chance of the treatment's being "successful" to be rated as high, good, average, etc.?[20]

B. *Expectancy of future life.* Assuming the "success" of the treatment, how much longer does the patient stand a good chance (75 per cent or better) of living—considering his age and general condition?

C. *Family role.* To what extent does the patient have responsibilities to others in his immediate family?

D. *Social contributions to be rendered.* Are the patient's past services to his society outstanding, substantial, average, etc.?

E. *Social contributions to be rendered.* Considering his age, talents, training, and past record of performance, is there a substantial probability that the patient will—*adequate recovery being assured*— render in the future services to his society that can be characterized as outstanding, substantial, average, etc.?

This list is clearly insufficient for the construction of a reasonable selection system, since that would require not only *that these factors be taken into account* (somehow or other), but—going beyond this—would specify a *specific set of procedures for taking account of them.* The specific procedures that would constitute such a system would have to take account of the interrelationship of these factors (e.g., *B* and *E*), and to set out exact guidelines as to the relevant weight that is to be given to each of them. This is something our discussion has not as yet considered.

In fact, I should want to maintain that there is no such thing here as a single rationally superior selection system. The position of affairs seems to me to be something like this: (1) It is necessary (for reasons already canvassed) to have a system, and to have a system that is rationally defensible, and (2) to be rationally defensible, this system must take the factors *A–E* into substantial and explicit account. But (3) the exact manner in which a rationally defensible system takes account of these factors cannot be fixed in any one specific way on the basis of general considerations. Any of the variety of ways that give *A–E* "their due" will be acceptable and viable. One cannot hope to find within this range of workable systems some one that is optimal in relation to the alternatives. There is no one system that does "the (uniquely) best"—only a variety of systems that do "as well as one can expect to do" in cases of this sort.

The situation is structurally very much akin to that of rules of partition of an estate among the relations of a decedent. It is important *that there be* such rules. And it is reasonable that spouse, children, parents, siblings, etc., be taken account of in these rules. But the question of the exact method of division—say that when the decedent has neither living spouse nor living children then his estate is to be divided, dividing 60 per cent between parents, 40 per cent between siblings versus dividing 90 per cent between parents, 10 per cent between siblings—cannot be settled on the basis of any general

abstract considerations of reasonableness. Within broad limits, a *variety* of resolutions are all perfectly acceptable—so that no one procedure can justifiably be regarded as "the (uniquely) best" because it is superior to all others .[21]

VIII. A Possible Basis for a Reasonable Selection System

Having said that there is no such thing as *the optimal* selection system for ELT, I want now to sketch out the broad features of what I would regard as *one acceptable* system.

The basis for the system would be a point rating. The scoring here at issue would give roughly equal weight to the medical considerations (*A* and *B*) in comparison with the extramedical considerations (*C* = family role, *D* = services rendered, and *E* = services to be rendered), also giving roughly equal weight to the three items involved here (*C, D,* and *E*). The result of such a scoring procedure would provide the essential starting point of our ELT selection mechanism. I deliberately say "starting point" because it seems to me that one should not follow the results of this scoring in an *automatic* way. I would propose that the actual selection should only be guided but not actually be dictated by this scoring procedure, along lines now to be explained.

IX. The Desirability of Introducing an Element of Chance

The detailed procedure I would propose—not of course as optimal (for reasons we have seen), but as eminently acceptable—would combine the scoring procedure just discussed with an element of chance. The resulting selection system would function as follows:

1. First the criteria of inclusion of Section IV above would be applied to constitute a *first phase selection group*—which (we shall suppose) is substantially larger than the number *n* of persons who can actually be accommodated with ELT.

2. Next the criteria of selection of Section V are brought to bear via a scoring procedure of the type described in Section VIII. On this basis a *second phase selection group* is constituted which

is only *somewhat* larger—say by a third or a half—than the critical number *n* at issue.

3. If this second phase selection group is relatively homogeneous as regards rating by the scoring procedure—that is, if there are no really major disparities within this group (as would be likely if the initial group was significantly larger than *n*)—then the final selection is made by *random* selection of *n* persons from within this group.

This introduction of the element of chance—in what could be dramatized as a "lottery of life and death"—must be justified. The fact is that such a procedure would bring with it three substantial advantages.

First, as we have argued above (in Section VII), any acceptable selection system is inherently non-optimal. The introduction of the element of chance prevents the results that life-and-death choices are made by the automatic application of an admittedly imperfect selection method.

Second, a recourse to chance would doubtless make matters easier for the rejected patient and those who have a specific interest in him. It would surely be quite hard for them to accept his exclusion by relatively mechanical application of objective criteria in whose implementation subjective judgment is involved. But the circumstances of life have conditioned us to accept the workings of chance and to tolerate the element of luck (good or bad): human life is an inherently contingent process. Nobody, after all, has an absolute right to ELT—but most of us would feel that we have "every bit as much right" to it as anyone else in significantly similar circumstances. The introduction of the element of chance assures a like handling of like cases over the widest possible area that seems reasonable in the circumstances.

Third (and perhaps least), such a recourse to random selection does much to relieve the administrators of the selection system of the awesome burden of ultimate and absolute responsibility.

These three considerations would seem to build up a substantial case for introducing the element of chance into the mechanism of the system for ELT selection in a way limited and circumscribed by other weightier considerations, along some such lines as those set forth above.[22]

It should be recognized that this injection of *man-made* chance supplements the element of *natural* chance that is present inevitably and in any case

(apart from the role of chance in singling out certain persons as victims for the affliction at issue). As F. M. Parsons has observed: "any vacancies [in an ELT program—specifically haemodialysis] will be filled immediately by the first suitable patients, even though their claims for therapy may subsequently prove less than those of other patients refused later."[23] Life is a chancy business and even the most rational of human arrangements can cover this over to a very limited extent at best.

Notes

1. Christine Doyle, "Spare-Part Heart Surgeons Worried by Their Success," *Observer*, May 12, 1968.

2. J. D. N. Nabarro, "Selection of Patients for Haemodialysis," *British Medical Journal* (March 11, 1967), p. 623. Although several thousand patients die in the U.K. each year from renal failure—there are about thirty new cases per million of population—only 10 per cent of these can for the foreseeable future be accommodated with chronic haemodialysis. Kidney transplantation—itself a very tricky procedure—cannot make a more than minor contribution here. As this article goes to press, I learn that patients can be maintained in home dialysis at an operating cost about half that of maintaining them in a hospital dialysis unit (roughly an $8,000 minimum). In the United States, around 7,000 patients with terminal uremia who could benefit from haemodialysis evolve yearly. As of mid-1968, some 1,000 of these can be accommodated in existing hospital units. By June 1967, a world-wide total of some 120 patients were in treatment by home dialysis. (Data from a forthcoming paper, "Home Dialysis," by C. M. Conty and H. V. Murdaugh. See also R. A. Baillod *et al.*, "Overnight Haemodialysis in the Home," *Proceedings of the European Dialysis and Transplant Association*, VI [1965], 99 ff.)

3. For the Hippocratic Oath see *Hippocrates: Works* (Loeb ed.; London, 1959), I, p. 298.

4. Another example of borderline legitimacy is posed by an endowment "with strings attached," e.g., "In accepting this legacy the hospital agrees to admit and provide all needed treatment for any direct descendant of myself, its founder."

5. Shana Alexander, "They Decide Who Lives, Who Dies," *Life*, LIII (November 9, 1962), 102–25 (see p. 107).

6. Lawrence Lader, "Who Has the Right to Live?" *Good Housekeeping* (January 1968), p. 144.

7. This approach could thus be continued to embrace the previous factor, that of family role, the preceding item (C).

8. Moreover a doctrinaire utilitarian would presumably be willing to withdraw a continuing mode of ELT such as haemodialysis from a patient to make room for a more promising candidate who came to view at a later stage and who could not otherwise be accommodated. I should be unwilling to adopt this course, partly on grounds of utility (with a view to the demoralization of insecurity), partly on the non-utilitarian ground that a "moral commitment" has been made and must be honored.

9. Of course the difficult question remains of the relative weight that should be given to prospective and retrospective service in cases where these factors conflict. There is good reason to treat them on a par.

10. This in the symposium on "Selection of Patients for Haemodialysis," *British Medical Journal* (March 11, 1967), pp. 622–24. F. M. Parsons writes: "But other forms of selecting patients [distinct from first come, first served] are suspect in my view if they imply evaluation of man by man. What criteria could be used? Who could justify a claim that the life of a mayor would be more valuable than that of the humblest citizen of his borough? Whatever we may think as individuals none of us is indispensable." But having just set out this hard-line view he immediately backs away from it: "On the other hand, to assume that there was little to choose between Alexander Fleming and Adolf Hitler . . . would be nonsense, and we should be naive if we were to pretend that we could not be influenced by their achievements and characters if we had to choose between the two of them. Whether we like it or not we cannot escape the fact that this kind of selection for long-term haemodialysis will be required until very large sums of money become available for equipment and services [so that *everyone* who needs treatment can be accommodated]."

11. The relative fundamentality of these principles is, however, a substantially disputed issue.

12. J. D. N. Nabarro, *op. cit.*, p. 622.

13. See Shana Alexander, *op. cit.*

14. *British Medical Journal* (March 11, 1967), pp. 622–24.

15. *Ibid.*, p. 624. Another contributor writes in the same symposium, "The selection of the few [to receive haemodialysis] is proving very difficult—a true 'Doctor's Dilemma'—for almost everybody would agree that this must be a medical decision, preferably reached by consultation among colleagues" (Dr. F. M. Parsons, *ibid.*, p. 623).

16. "The Selection of Patients for Haemodialysis," *op. cit.* (n. 10 above), p. 623.

17. Dr. Wilson's article concludes with the perplexing suggestion—wildly beside the point given the structure of the situation at issue—that "the final decision will be made by the patient." But this contention is only marginally more ludicrous than Parsons's contention that in selecting patients for haemodialysis "gainful employment in a well chosen occupation is necessary to achieve the best results" since "only the minority wish to live on charity" (*ibid.*).

18. To say this is of course not to deny that such questions of applied medical ethics will invariably involve a host of medical considerations—it is only to insist that extra-medical considerations will also invariably be at issue.

19. M. A. Wilson, "Selection of Patients for Haemodialysis," *op. cit.*, p. 624.

20. In the case of all ongoing treatment involving complex procedure and dietary and other mode-of-life restrictions—and chronic haemodialysis definitely falls into this category—the patient's psychological makeup, his willpower to "stick with it" in the face of substantial discouragements—will obviously also be a substantial factor here. The man who gives up, takes not his life alone, but (figuratively speaking) also that of the person he replaced in the treatment schedule.

21. To say that acceptable solutions can range over broad limits is not to say that there are no limits at all. It is an obviously intriguing and fundamental problem to raise the question of the factors that set these limits. This complex issue cannot be dealt with adequately here. Suffice it to say that considerations regarding precedent and people's expectations, factor of social utility, and matters of fairness and sense of justice all come into play.

22. One writer has mooted the suggestion that: "Perhaps the right thing to do, difficult as it may be to accept, is to select [for haemodialysis] from among the medical and psychologically qualified patients on a strictly random basis" (S. Gorovitz, "Ethics and the Allocation of Medical Resources," *Medical Research Engineering*, V [1966], p. 7). Out-right random selection, would, however, seem indefensible because of its refusal to give weight to considerations which, under the circumstances, *deserve* to be given weight. The proposed procedure of superimposing a certain degree of randomness upon the rational-choice criteria would seem to combine the advantages of the two without importing the worst defects of either.

23. "Selection of Patients for Haemodialysis," *op. cit.*, p. 623. The question of whether a patient for

chronic treatment should ever be terminated from the program (say, if he contracts cancer) poses a variety of difficult ethical problems with which we need not at present concern ourselves. But it does seem plausible to take the (somewhat anti-utilitarian) view that a patient should not be terminated simply because a "better qualified" patient comes along later on. It would seem that a quasi-contractual relationship has been created through established expectations and reciprocal understandings, and that the situation is in this regard akin to that of the man who, having undertaken to sell his house to one buyer, cannot afterward unilaterally undo this arrangement to sell it to a higher bidder who "needs it worse" (thus maximizing the over-all utility).

24. I acknowledge with thanks the help of Miss Hazel Johnson, Reference Librarian at the University of Pittsburgh Library, in connection with the bibliography.

Bibliography [24]

S. Alexander. "They Decide Who Lives, Who Dies," *Life*, LIII (November 9, 1962), 102–25.

C. Doyle. "Spare-Part Surgeons Worried by Their Success," *Observer* (London), May 12, 1968.

J. Fletcher. *Morals and Medicine*. London, 1955.

S. Gorovitz. "Ethics and the Allocation of Medical Resources," *Medical Research Engineering*, V (1966), 5–7.

L. Lader. "Who Has the Right to Live?" *Good Housekeeping* (January, 1968), pp. 85 and 144–50.

J. D. N. Nabarro, F. M. Parsons, R. Shakman, and M. A. Wilson. "Selection of Patients for Haemodialysis," *British Medical Journal* (March 11, 1967), pp. 622–24.

H. M. Schmeck, Jr. "Panel Holds Life-or-Death Vote in Allotting of Artificial Kidney," *New York Times*, May 6, 1962, pp. 1, 83.

G. E. W. Wolstenholme and M. O'Connor (eds.). *Ethics in Medical Progress*. London, 1966.

The Prostitute, the Playboy, and the Poet: Rationing Schemes for Organ Transplantation

George J. Annas

George Annas takes a position on transplant selection that introduces a modification of the first-come, first-served principle. He reviews four approaches to rationing scarce medical resources—market, selection committee, lottery, and customary—and finds each has disadvantages so serious as to make them all unacceptable. An acceptable approach, he suggests, is one that combines efficiency, fairness, and a respect for the value of life. Because candidates should both want a transplant and be able to derive significant benefits from one, the first phase of selection should involve a screening process that is based exclusively on medical criteria that are objective and as free as possible of judgments about social worth.

Since selection might still have to be made from this pool of candidates, it might be done by social-worth criteria or by lottery. However, social-worth criteria seem arbitrary, and a lottery would be unfair to those who are in more immediate need of a transplant—ones who might die quickly without it. After reviewing the relevant considerations, a committee operating at this stage might allow those in immediate need of a transplant to be moved to the head of a waiting list. To those not in immediate need, organs would be distributed in a first-come, first-served fashion. Although absolute equality is not embodied in this process, the procedure is sufficiently flexible to recognize that some may have needs that are greater (more immediate) than others.

In the public debate about the availability of heart and liver transplants, the issue of rationing on a massive scale has been credibly raised for the first time in United States medical care. In an era of scarce resources, the eventual arrival of such a discussion was, of course, inevitable.[1] Unless we decide to ban heart and liver transplantation, or make them available to everyone, some rationing scheme must be used to choose among potential transplant candidates. The debate has existed throughout the history of medical ethics. Traditionally it has been stated as a choice between saving one of two patients, both of whom require the immediate assistance of the only available physician to survive.

National attention was focused on decisions regarding the rationing of kidney dialysis machines when they were first used on a limited basis in the late 1960s. As one commentator described the debate within the medical profession:

> "Shall machines or organs go to the sickest, or to the ones with most promise of recovery; on a first-come, first-served basis; to the most 'valuable' patient (based on wealth, education, position, what?); to the one with the most dependents; to women and children first; to those who can pay; to whom? Or should lots be cast, impersonally and uncritically?"[2]

In Seattle, Washington, an anonymous screening committee was set up to pick who among competing candidates would receive the life-saving technology. One lay member of the screening committee is quoted as saying:

> "The choices were hard . . . I remember voting against a young woman who was a known prostitute. I found I couldn't vote for her, rather than another candidate, a young wife and mother. I also voted against a young man who, until he learned he had renal failure, had been a ne'er do-well, a real playboy. He promised he would reform his character, go back to school, and so on, if only he were selected for treatment. But I felt I'd lived long enough to know that a person like that won't really do what he was promising at the time."[3]

When the biases and selection criteria of the committee were made public, there was a general negative reaction against this type of arbitrary device. Two experts reacted to the "numbing accounts of how close to the surface lie the prejudices and mindless cliches that pollute the committee's deliberations," by concluding that the committee was "measuring persons in accordance with its own middle-class values." The committee process, they noted, ruled out "creative nonconformists" and made the Pacific Northwest "no place for a Henry David Thoreau with bad kidneys."[4]

To avoid having to make such explicit, arbitrary, "social worth" determinations, the Congress, in 1972, enacted legislation that provided federal funds for virtually all kidney dialysis and kidney transplantation procedures in the United States.[5] This decision, however, simply served to postpone the time when identical decisions will have to be made about candidates for heart and liver transplantation in a society that does not provide sufficient financial and medical resources to provide all "suitable" candidates with the operation.

There are four major approaches to rationing scarce medical resources: the market approach; the selection committee approach; the lottery approach; and the "customary" approach.[1]

The Market Approach

The market approach would provide an organ to everyone who could pay for it with their own funds or private insurance. It puts a very high value on individual rights, and a very low value on equality and fairness. It has properly been criticized on a number of bases, including that the transplant technologies have been developed and are supported with public funds, that medical resources used for transplantation will not be available for higher priority care, and that financial success alone is an insufficient justification for demanding a medical procedure. Most telling is its complete lack of concern for fairness and equity.[6]

A "bake sale" or charity approach that requires the less financially fortunate to make public appeals for funding is demeaning to the individuals involved, and to society as a whole. Rationing by financial ability says we do not believe in equality, but believe that a price can and should be placed on human life and that it should be paid by the individ-

Reprinted by permission of the author and The American Journal of Public Health, Vol. 75, no. 2, 1985, pp. 187–189.

ual whose life is at stake. Neither belief is tolerable in a society in which income is inequitably distributed.

The Committee Selection Process

The Seattle Selection Committee is a model of the committee process. Ethics Committees set up in some hospitals to decide whether or not certain handicapped newborn infants should be given medical care may represent another.[7] These committees have developed because it was seen as unworkable or unwise to explicitly set forth the criteria on which selection decisions would be made. But only two results are possible, as Professor Guido Calabresi has pointed out: either a pattern of decision-making will develop or it will not. If a pattern does develop (e.g., in Seattle, the imposition of middle-class values), then it can be articulated and those decision "rules" codified and used directly, without resort to the committee. If a pattern does not develop, the committee is vulnerable to the charge that it is acting arbitrarily, or dishonestly, and therefore cannot be permitted to continue to make such important decisions.[1]

In the end, public designation of a committee to make selection decisions on vague criteria will fail because it too closely involves the state and all members of society in explicitly preferring specific individuals over others, and in devaluing the interests those others have in living. It thus directly undermines, as surely as the market system does, society's view of equality and the value of human life.

The Lottery Approach

The lottery approach is the ultimate equalizer which puts equality ahead of every other value. This makes it extremely attractive, since all comers have an equal chance at selection regardless of race, color, creed, or financial status. On the other hand, it offends our notions of efficiency and fairness since it makes *no* distinctions among such things as the strength of the desires of the candidates, their potential survival, and their quality of life. In this sense it is a mindless method of trying to solve society's dilemma which is caused by its unwillingness or inability to spend enough resources to make a lottery unnecessary. By making this macro spending decision evident to all, it also undermines society's view of the pricelessness of human life. A first-

come, first-served system is a type of natural lottery since referral to a transplant program is generally random in time. Nonetheless, higher income groups have quicker access to referral networks and thus have an inherent advantage over the poor in a strict first-come, first-served system.[8,9]

The Customary Approach

Society has traditionally attempted to avoid explicitly recognizing that we are making a choice not to save individual lives because it is too expensive to do so. As long as such decisions are not explicitly acknowledged, they can be tolerated by society. For example, until recently there was said to be a general understanding among general practitioners in Britain that individuals over age 55 suffering from end-stage kidney disease not be referred for dialysis or transplant. In 1984, however, this unwritten practice became highly publicized, with figures that showed a rate of new cases of end-stage kidney disease treated in Britain at 40 per million (versus the US figure of 80 per million) resulting in 1500–3000 "unnecessary deaths" annually.[10] This has, predictably, led to movements to enlarge the National Health Service budget to expand dialysis services to meet this need, a more socially acceptable solution than permitting the now publicly recognized situation to continue.

In the US, the customary approach permits individual physicians to select their patients on the basis of medical criteria or clinical suitability. This, however, contains much hidden social worth criteria. For example, one criterion, common in the transplant literature, requires an individual to have sufficient family support for successful aftercare. This discriminates against individuals without families and those who have become alienated from their families. The criterion may be relevant, but it is hardly medical.

Similar observations can be made about medical criteria that include IQ, mental illness, criminal records, employment, indigency, alcoholism, drug addiction, or geographical location. Age is perhaps more difficult, since it may be impressionistically related to outcome. But it is not medically logical to assume that an individual who is 49 years old is necessarily a better medical candidate for a transplant than one who is 50 years old. Unless specific examination of the characteristics of older persons that make them less desirable candidates is undertaken, such a cut off is arbitrary, and thus devalues the lives of older citizens. The same can be said of blanket exclusions of alcoholics and drug addicts.

In short, the customary approach has one great advantage for society and one great disadvantage: it gives us the illusion that we do not have to make choices; but the cost is mass deception, and when this deception is uncovered, we must deal with it either by universal entitlement or by choosing another method of patient selection.

A Combination of Approaches

A socially acceptable approach must be fair, efficient, and reflective of important social values. The most important values at stake in organ transplantation are fairness itself, equity in the sense of equality, and the value of life. To promote efficiency, it is important that no one receive a transplant unless they want one and are likely to obtain significant benefit from it in the sense of years of life at a reasonable level of functioning.

Accordingly, it is appropriate for there to be an initial screening process that is based *exclusively* on medical criteria designed to measure the probability of a successful transplant, i.e., one in which the patient survives for at least a number of years and is rehabilitated. There is room in medical criteria for social worth judgments, but there is probably no way to avoid this completely. For example, it has been noted that "in many respects social and medical criteria are inextricably intertwined" and that therefore medical criteria might "exclude the poor and disadvantaged because health and socioeconomic status are highly interdependent."[11] Roger Evans gives an example. In the End Stage Renal Disease Program, "those of lower socioeconomic status are likely to have multiple comorbid health conditions such as diabetes, hepatitis, and hypertension" making them both less desirable candidates and more expensive to treat.[11]

To prevent the gulf between the haves and have nots from widening, we must make every reasonable attempt to develop medical criteria that are objective and independent of social worth categories. One minimal way to approach this is to require that medical screening be reviewed and approved by an ethics committee with significant public representation, filed with a public agency, and made readily available to the public for comment. In the event that more than one hospital in a state or region is offering a particular transplant service, it would be most fair and efficient for the individual hospitals to perform the initial medical screening themselves (based on the uniform, objective criteria), but to have all subsequent nonmedical selection done by a method approved by a single selection committee composed of representatives of all hospitals engaged in a particular transplant procedure, as well as significant representation of the public at large.

As this implies, after the medical screening is performed, there may be more acceptable candidates in the "pool" than there are organs or surgical teams to go around. Selection among waiting candidates will then be necessary. This situation occurs now in kidney transplantation, but since the organ matching is much more sophisticated than in hearts and livers (permitting much more precise matching of organ and recipient), and since dialysis permits individuals to wait almost indefinitely for an organ without risking death, the situations are not close enough to permit use of the same matching criteria. On the other hand, to the extent that organs are specifically tissue- and size-matched and fairly distributed to the best matched candidate, the organ distribution system itself will resemble a natural lottery.

When a pool of acceptable candidates is developed, a decision about who gets the next available, suitable organ must be made. We must choose between using a conscious, value-laden, social worth selection criterion (including a committee to make the actual choice), or some type of random device. In view of the unacceptability and arbitrariness of social worth criteria being applied, implicitly or explicitly, by committee, this method is neither viable nor proper. On the other hand, strict adherence to a lottery might create a situation where an individual who has only a one-in-four chance of living five years with a transplant (but who could survive another six months without one) would get an organ before an individual who could survive as long or longer, but who will die within days or hours if he or she is not immediately transplanted. Accordingly, the most reasonable approach seems to be to allocate organs on a first-come, first-served basis to members of the pool but permit individuals to "jump" the queue if the second level selection committee believes they are in immediate danger of death (but still have a reasonable prospect for long-term survival with a transplant) and the person who would otherwise get the organ can survive long enough to be reasonably assured that he or she will be able to get another organ.

The first-come, first-served method of basic selection (after a medical screen) seems the preferred method because it most closely approximates the randomness of a straight lottery without the obviousness of making equity the only promoted value. Some unfairness is introduced by the fact that the more wealthy and medically astute will likely get into the pool first, and thus be ahead in line, but this advantage should decrease sharply as public awareness of the system grows. The possibility of unfairness is also inherent in permitting individuals to jump the queue, but some flexibility needs to be retained in the system to permit it to respond to reasonable contingencies.

We will have to face the fact that should the resources devoted to organ transplantation be limited (as they are now and are likely to be in the future), at some point it is likely that significant numbers of individuals will die in the pool waiting for a transplant. Three things can be done to avoid this: 1) medical criteria can be made stricter, perhaps by adding a more rigorous notion of "quality" of life to longevity and prospects for rehabilitation; 2) resources devoted to transplantation and organ procurement can be increased; or 3) individuals can be persuaded not to attempt to join the pool.

Of these three options, only the third has the promise of both conserving resources and promoting autonomy. While most persons medically eligible for a transplant would probably want one, some would not—at least if they understood all that was involved, including the need for a lifetime commitment to daily immunosuppression medications, and periodic medical monitoring for rejection symptoms. Accordingly, it makes public policy sense to publicize the risks and side effects of transplantation, and to require careful explanations of the procedure be given to prospective patients *before* they undergo medical screening. It is likely that by the time patients come to the transplant center they have made up their minds and would do almost anything to get the transplant. Nonetheless, if there are patients who, when confronted with all the facts, would voluntarily elect not to proceed, we enhance both their own freedom and the efficiency and cost-effectiveness of the transplantation system by screening them out as early as possible.

Conclusion

Choices among patients that seem to condemn some to death and give others an opportunity to survive will always be tragic. Society has developed a number of mechanisms to make such decisions more acceptable by camouflaging them. In an era of scarce resources and conscious cost containment, such mechanisms will become public, and they will be usable only if they are fair and efficient. If they are not so perceived, we will shift from one mechanism to another in an effort to continue the illusion that tragic choices really don't have to be made, and that we can simultaneously move toward equity of access, quality of services, and cost containment without any challenges to our values. Along with the prostitute, the playboy, and the poet, we all need to be involved in the development of an access model to extreme and expensive medical technologies with which we can live.

Notes

1. Calabresi G, Bobbitt P: *Tragic Choices.* New York: Norton, 1978.

2. Fletcher J: Our shameful waste of human tissue. In: Cutler DR (ed): *The Religious Situation.* Boston: Beacon Press, 1969; 223–252.

3. Quoted in Fox R, Swazey J: *The Courage to Fail.* Chicago: Univ of Chicago Press, 1974; 232.

4. Sanders & Dukeminier: Medical advance and legal lag: hemodialysis and kidney transplantation. UCLA L Rev 1968; 15:357.

5. Rettig RA: The policy debate on patient care financing for victims of end stage renal disease. Law & Contemporary Problems 1976; 40:196.

6. President's Commission for the Study of Ethical Problems in Medicine: *Securing Access to Health Care.* US Govt Printing Office, 1983; 25.

7. Annas GJ: Ethics committees on neonatal care: substantive protection or procedural diversion? Am J Public Health 1984; 74:843–845.

8. Bayer R: Justice and health care in an era of cost containment: allocating scarce medical resources. Soc Responsibility 1984; 9:37–52.

9. Annas GJ: Allocation of artificial hearts in the year 2002: *Minerva v National Health Agency.* Am J Law Med 1977; 3:59–76.

10. Commentary: UK's poor record in treatment of renal failure. Lancet, July 7, 1984; 53.

11. Evans R: Health care technology and the inevitability of resource allocation and rationing decisions, Part 11. JAMA 1983; 249:2208, 2217.

Allocation of Scarce Medical Resources

Michael D. Bayles

Michael Bayles argues that "individual patient benefit" should be the primary criterion for allocating scarce resources, although it may be supplemented by "randomization for ties and responsibility and social worth as side-constraints."

Reasonable people, Bayles says, require an allocation principle to meet the tests of being impartial, adequate, and workable. He then argues that social worth, responsibility for one's medical condition, and randomization each fails as a primary principle, while the criterion that "resources should be allocated to those individuals who will derive the most benefit from them" satisfies all the tests.

Bayles ends by illustrating how a scheme for selecting patients for in vitro fertilization based on his primary and secondary criteria might work. In giving priority to individual benefit, Bayles's scheme differs significantly from the ones endorsed by Rescher and Annas.

Some medical resources are occasionally scarce, such as drugs and hospital beds on a given day; others are chronically scarce, such as intensive care units and organs for transplant. The resources need not be life-saving ones. This article concerns the allocation of medical resources to persons when there are not enough for all potential recipients. It does not concern allocation of scarce resources between various programs, such as surgical and non-surgical treatment of heart disease, or whether certain resources should be made available at all, such as permanent artificial hearts. The topic is simply how, given limited resources that cannot be provided to everyone, an allocation should be made among individuals. This topic involves two broad issues. One concerns the appropriate substantive grounds for allocating resources to one person rather than another. The other issue pertains to procedures for making allocation decisions—who does so, with what information, and so on. The procedural issue is largely left for another occasion.

The present discussion will argue that the primary principle or criterion for allocating scarce medical resources should be individual patient benefit. Surprisingly, this common-sense principle has been largely neglected in the more prominent discussions of the issue.[1] The introductory section presents the method of argument and indicates the patient pool. The following section briefly reviews alternative criteria social worth, responsibility, and randomization. Sometimes the practically most important criterion is the ability of a recipient to pay for resources either personally, by private insurance, or by governmental benefits. That criterion is ignored here, because often there are more persons who can pay than for whom there are resources available.

Introduction

Method. The method used is to ask what allocative principles reasonable persons would accept for a society in which they expected to live.[2] Reasonable persons use logical reasoning and all available pertinent information. For present purposes, they do not know what their circumstances will be if they need the resources; they are to make an *ex ante* decision about principles. Thus, whether they are self-interested or benevolent is largely irrelevant. Most arguments are based on self-interest, but in one place limited benevolence is considered.

It is unlikely that only one allocative principle would be accepted. Instead, reasonable people would likely accept a primary principle that provides the basic ground for allocative decisions along with various supplementary principles. For exam-

Reprinted with permission from Public Affairs Quarterly, *Vol. 4, No. 1 (January 1990), pp. 1–16.*

ple, a principle of social worth is likely to be supplemented by randomization among persons of equal social worth. However, important differences in allocative systems depend on which principle is primary. The argument here is that individual benefit should be primary, supplemented by randomization for ties and responsibility and social worth as side-constraints.

Reasonable people would have several tests for acceptable allocative principles or sets of principles. First, they should be impartial. This involves both procedural and substantive concerns. Principles should be capable of being applied with little bias and few conflicts of interest. Substantively, they generally should not distinguish between recipients on the basis of race, sex, and so on or persons' conceptions of a personally good life. For an allocative scheme to work, it must be acceptable to many people. Reasonable people would realize that their goals and circumstances might change. In a pluralistic society, this requires openness to alternative conceptions of a good life. Exceptions can be made only if they would be acceptable to reasonable persons, for example, for persons whose conduct or conceptions of a good life are contrary to core moral principles such as those in the criminal law. Second, a primary principle should be adequate; that is, provide guidance for most situations. A principle that seldom provides concrete guidance because it is inapplicable or unclear is best used as a supplemental principle. Third, a principle or set of principles should be workable; for example, some might be too complex to be useful.

Patient Pool. Potential recipients are persons within a jurisdiction who might benefit from the resource and who want it for themselves, or if incompetent, whose representatives want it for them. First, any jurisdictional or constituency factor is met. Government funded medical resources might be limited to residents of the territory. For example, resources in a national health insurance system, as in Canada, might be restricted to residents. Even private hospitals might have a local community constituency. This factor can be quite controversial in a system for allocating organs.

Second, a medical criterion is relevant. There is some likelihood of success from providing resources to individuals. It is pointless to perform a heart transplant on a patient who will not survive the operation. This factor obviously admits of de-

grees, and higher or lower standards can be used for admission to the pool. Although most authors do not require a very high probability of success, any requirement recognizes a possibility of individual benefit as a prerequisite for admission to the patient pool.

The third factor is patient desire for the resource. Presumably, if patients are competent and fully informed and do not desire a resource, it is unethical to provide it. Thus, even if persons might medically benefit from a resource, if they do not want it, they are not in the pool. A system could be devised in which persons who do not want or will not benefit from a resource are in the pool. If a system allocates a resource to them, they then own the resource and can determine its use. This possibility is ignored, because it would normally decrease achievement of the goals of the original allocation criteria. (It would not defeat the goal of a fair allocation with individual freedom to dispose of shares.)

Alternative Criteria

Social Worth. The social worth criterion refers to a person's effects on others. It can be split into several subcriteria by dividing those affected into the immediate family and the rest of society and effects into past (desert) and future. This gives four possible principles: past and future effects on family and past and future effects on the rest of society. The usual concern with family has been either that the individual has dependents or that there is a family to provide support during and after treatment. The latter is not an effect on others, but others' effect on the patient and so is not properly part of a social worth criterion. It can affect probability of success in allocating some resources and is thus included in that criterion. The following discussion emphasizes effects on persons outside the patient's family.

Social worth criteria fail the tests of impartiality and workability. Early decisions to allocate scarce hemodialysis machines on their basis failed these requirements. The decisions produced were not generally acceptable. Almost any criterion can produce undesirable results if applied unthinkingly or by biased persons, yet the likelihood of such results is intrinsic to social worth criteria. First, social worth inherently violates impartiality. Because life plans have different effects on others, various morally permissible ones have different social values. Moreover, what effects on others are good or bad is controversial in a pluralistic society. Do political operatives or nuclear engineers contribute to the social good? Subcriteria are likely to be vague. Charity, kindness, and so forth are not precise concepts. Because many people can be affected one way or another, the analysis can be quite complex. Suppose a business person saves a failing firm by laying off twenty percent of the employees and selling parts of it to foreign corporations. Did the person contribute to the net social good? Given the controversial, vague, and complex elements of most social worth criteria, even the best willed persons will arrive at different conclusions. With busy, biased, and only partially informed decisionmakers, the potential for abuse and mistakes is great. Thus, reasonable people could not accept distinguishing on the basis of social worth generally or by categories of occupations.

Although social worth as a primary criterion is unacceptable, specific subcriteria as supplemental principles are less objectionable and can be accepted. Whether a patient has dependents and how many are objective matters. So is a patient's status as a veteran. Being a veteran is currently a basis for allocating financial resources to pay for at least some medical care and thus affects the allocation of scarce medical resources such as transplants other than kidneys. Moreover, some detrimental effects on others are clear. The past conduct, desert, of a convicted multiple murderer violated core moral principles. It would be unreasonable to deny a good and effective president a heart transplant so that one could provide one to the convict. Consequently, reasonable people can accept some social worth subcriteria as supplemental principles either for people's admission into the potential pool or as specific exceptions to an allocation scheme. Precisely what supplemental principles or exceptions would be accepted must be determined in the context of specific exemptions to particular programs.

Responsibility.   This principle takes persons' responsibility for their condition as a criterion for allocating resources. Persons not responsible for their medical conditions have priority over those who are. Responsibility for health has been significantly discussed in the context of policies to discourage health risky behavior;[3] it has not been as much discussed in the context of allocating scarce resources among specific persons. As a primary principle it fails the impartiality, workability, and adequacy tests.

Its defects are related to the mental and causal conditions of responsibility. Mental conditions of responsibility for one's medical condition can vary significantly, from weakness of will in controlling one's weight and exercising, through negligence in causing an accident and reckless disregard for one's health, to deliberately self-inflicted wounds. The causal relationship can also vary from a lack of exercise causing generally poor health to a direct, immediate causal relationship.

First, because of the variability of the mental and causal conditions of responsibility, there are many situations where the responsibility criterion does not apply clearly. For example, to what extent are cigarette smokers responsible for various diseases? Second, venereal diseases, AIDS, and cirrhosis of the liver indicate that the opportunities for abuse, bias, and other factors are perhaps as great with it as with the social worth criterion. Third, it often provides no guidance. No infants are responsible for their medical condition, and adults are not plausibly responsible for many of their diseases or conditions.

In clear cases a responsibility criterion can be used as a supplemental criterion to distinguish otherwise similar persons on a priority list of recipients. Suppose Mr. *A* has previously received a kidney transplant. Because he failed to stick to the proper diet and to take his medication regularly, his transplanted kidney is failing; he is a possible candidate for another transplant. A responsibility criterion would give priority to Mrs. *B*, a similar candidate who is not responsible for her condition.

Reasonable persons could accept a responsibility criterion for such use, because they have an opportunity to avoid the condition. If their health risking behavior was voluntary, then the lesser priority can be a known risk that they assumed. However, they must have a reasonable opportunity not to risk their health and it should be known that so doing affects priority for resources. To implement such a principle immediately can be unfair if, at the time of their conduct, persons had no reason to believe it would affect their eligibility for resources. A responsibility criterion for transplants could be quickly implemented by simply informing all transplant recipients that if they fail to follow medical advice, they will have lower priority for a replacement.

Randomization.   A principle of randomization provides equality of opportunity. Everyone in the patient pool has an equal chance of receiving scarce medical resources. Thus, such policies will generally be impartial, adequate, and workable. The issue of their acceptability, then, is whether these conditions are met at the cost of ignoring other relevant considerations, in particular, individual benefit.

There are two versions of randomization—a lottery and "first come, first served." A lottery is plausibly more objective and procedurally impartial than even "first come, first served." Anyone who in the United States has waited to be served at a counter without a queue recognizes the potential difficulties with the latter principle. With a lottery, potential abuse is likely to be restricted to admission to the patient pool, because choice of individuals can be public and abuse easily detected. The motivation for abuse is likely to be weaker than with first come, because entry to the pool does not determine one's order of receiving the resource. However, the more stringent the medical criterion for admission to the pool, the greater the likelihood of and motivation for abuse. There will be significant pressure to make the medical criterion for admission stringent. A lottery always permits persons with lesser prospects of success and subsequent life to receive resources over those with greater prospects of success and subsequent life, even if the former can survive without the resource and the latter cannot. A reasonable person who might be in either position has no reason to accept such a result if an acceptable method can be found to avoid it. In effect, a lottery ignores differences in the individual benefit of potential recipients. A more stringent medical criterion for membership in the pool decreases such disparities. Consequently, the less medically homogeneous the pool, the less acceptable a lottery.

As indicated, first come is more open to potential abuse than a lottery. For example, who is first could be determined by who first had the need (became ill), first presented to a physician, was first recommended for the pool, or first fully qualified. This is largely a question of drawing a bright line. Whatever line is drawn is generally acceptable provided one sticks to it. In practice, the line is usually who first fully qualifies. However, if there is a financial qualification, as for some transplants, people who must raise the money by personal means can end up significantly farther back on the list than similar persons who did not have to raise money.

Like a lottery, it can result in persons with lesser prospects receiving resources over those with greater ones, even if they can survive without them and the latter cannot. Again, to avoid this, it is reasonable to use a more stringent medical criterion for admission—to make the pool more homogeneous.

Even a more stringent medical criterion for admission to a pool leaves significant disparities. With a first come principle and life-saving resources, some people on the list will die before they reach the top. A common response is to move a critically ill person who is not likely to survive without the resource to the top. George Annas recommends jumping a person in immediate danger of death over a person with a significantly lower chance of five year survival and not in immediate need provided the person jumped has a reasonable chance of receiving the resource before dying.[4] Suppose C, D, E, and F got on the list in alphabetical order. If D has greater prospects than C and is in immediate danger of death, Annas would jump D ahead of C provided C would still receive the resource.

At first glance, Annas's proposal seems acceptable, because both C and D receive the resource. However, this condition changes the situation to one where everyone being considered can receive the benefit. Yet, the situation is changed merely by forgetting E and F. If D receives the resource and would not have without jumping because he or she would have died, someone behind D, for example E, does not. E might have a greater prospect than D. Not knowing which person one might be, one would prefer that the resource go to the person with greater prospects because one might benefit more. If one drops the requirement that the person jumped, C, is likely to receive the resource, then the principle gives priority to those with a greater chance to benefit and collapses into a version of the individual benefit criterion.

If one drops both the requirements that the person jumped also receive the resource and that the jumper have greater prospects, one simply jumps persons who are in immediate danger of dying. An acceptable rationale for such a decision is not evident. To modify the example, suppose that with the resource C, D, E, and F have equal prospects of five year survival. Further suppose F is in immediate danger of death and the others are not. If C receives the resource, F dies. If one jumps F to the top of the list, then as resources are not adequate to provide for all, someone else—D or E—dies before receiving the resource when he or she would not have, had F not jumped the line. The principle is not first come, first served, but first near death, first served. Not knowing where one might be in a queue, one has no reason to prefer life for one person over another and thus no reason to accept this principle.

One reason that might be offered to support the first near death principle is that it is wrong to allow a person to die when one could prevent it. One could prevent F's death. When D or E dies, no resource will be available to save him or her, so one could not have prevented the death. However, from D or E's perspective, his or her death could have been prevented; had one followed the original list, he or she would have lived.

Randomization in either of its forms is appropriate for choosing between equals—when there are no relevant grounds to distinguish between persons. To the extent that relevant substantive grounds exist, randomization is inappropriate. As we have already seen, some social worth and responsibility subcriteria are acceptable supplemental principles in specific contexts. More importantly, a reasonable person who might be any member of a pool of potential recipients has good self-interested reasons to consider the benefit to individual recipients. Thus, randomization is not ethically acceptable as the primary criterion. It remains only as a supplemental principle for use when, after applying the other relevant criteria, more potential recipients remain than can be provided resources.

Individual Benefit

General Reasons.   The individual benefit criterion is that resources should be allocated to those individuals who will derive the most benefit from them. In its weak negative form that resources should not be allocated to people who cannot benefit from them, it is almost always at least a supplemental principle. Reasonable self-interested persons who did not know which potential recipient they might be would accept individual benefit as the primary principle because it maximizes their expectable benefits. The usual objection to accepting benefit maximizing principles is that a person might have to sacrifice over a long-term for the well-being of others who might benefit more. However, as the need for scarce medical resources is usually episodic

rather than chronic, people are unlikely to fall into or constitute a permanent deprived class. Moreover, as discussed below, a proper concept of benefit is impartial among social groups. The only exception is the elderly, but the tendency of an individual benefit criterion to operate against the elderly is justifiable.

The individual benefit criterion can be supported by other ethical views, though perhaps only as a supplemental principle. It is an obvious implication of a principle of beneficence. Thus, any moral theory that supports a duty of beneficence supports a criterion of individual benefit. If one's goal is to help others, then it is merely efficient to help those one can help the most.

Individual benefit has advantages over social worth that make it more acceptable to reasonable persons. First, analyses of individual benefit are less complex than those of social worth. To determine individual benefit, one need consider the effects on only one person, whereas to determine social worth one must consider effects on the whole of society. Second, the value of effects on a given individual is much less likely to be controversial than those on society as a whole. Frequently, that individual can simply say whether an effect is good or bad. This point is partially recognized by the informed desire condition for membership in the potential recipient pool. Of course, opportunities for paternalism can arise. But if resources are scarce, the doubt about benefit raised by a potential recipient's rejection is surely sufficient to justify allocating resources among those who do want them. Third, because the decisionmaker is not a person whose benefit is in question, there is less room for conflicts of interest. Individual benefit thus offers less opportunity and motivation for abuse than social worth and is more likely to be workable. However, there are problems of this sort that require further discussion.

Elements.   Individual benefit from a resource is a function of three factors: the probability of success, the length of life achieved, and the value of life at a moment to the person whose life it is. The last two factors can be called life expectancy and momentary value. The value of life for some period is the integral of its momentary values from starting to end point. An allocation of a scarce medical resource can affect either or both the length of life and its momentary values. A heart transplant will clearly affect length of life, but it can also affect the momentary value of life—permitting a more active one with less pain.

The basic conception of the individual benefit (IB) expectable from allocating a resource to a given patient is represented by the following formula:[5]

$$(1)\ IB = p \times (V_w - V_o)$$

where p is the probability of success, V_w the value of life with the resource, and V_o the value of life without the resource. Thus $(V_w - V_o)$ is the net benefit to the individual if the treatment from allocating the resource is successful. Although this formula gives a correct account of individual benefit, because of difficulties discussed below it is not workable and permits partiality.

The probability of success and life expectancy with and without the resource are matters of medical judgment. Though often difficult to determine, physicians constantly make rough and sometimes even statistically fine judgments about them. For example, rates of one and five year life expectancy with various treatments are common. Life expectancy with complete success can simply be taken from life expectancy tables for persons of that age. Considerations of general health, other ailments, and so forth, can sometimes be factored in for particular individuals. Of course, people can still disagree in specific cases.

The difficult variable in the formula is the value of life. The concept is that of the value of the life to the individual whose life it is. (Hereafter "valuable life" is used in this sense.) The formula does not specify what makes life valuable for a person, and it probably differs from person to person. Both theoretical problems of interpersonal comparison and the test for impartiality among conceptions of a good life call for leaving this matter open for individual differences. Thus, more objective determinants of individual benefit are needed.

One cannot distribute valuable life, only resources that provide opportunities for it. In medicine, the resources distributed vary, so one must look to their effects on opportunities for valuable life. Decisions whether or not to treat seriously ill newborns are often made on the basis of the child's best interest, that is, individual benefit. Three factors are usually taken into account in decisions to treat infants: pain, physical handicap, and mental handicap. The greater the pain or physical or mental handicap, the less the opportunity for valuable life. In short, these are factors that affect one's opportu-

nities for valuable life whatever one's conception of a valuable life.

Thus, instead of determining individual benefit directly by the value of life, a more operational conception determines it by opportunity for valuable life as indicated by pain and mental and physical handicap. If we let OV_w measure the opportunity for value with the resource, and OV_o the opportunity without the resource, then this conception of individual benefit can be represented in the following formula:

$$(2)\ IB = p \times (OV_w - OV_o)$$

This conception should be further [developed].

Objections and Replies.   Three central objections indicate further modifications needed for an acceptable operational conception of individual benefit. The first objection is that the factors in the opportunity for valuable life will be the same for everyone considered. Because the resource allocated is the same, for example, an organ, the pain or physical handicap one might remove is the same. The only factor then is length of life. When that is not affected, individual benefit interpreted as opportunity for valuable life cannot provide a basis for priority so the criterion is inadequate.

The objection is not correct. Potential recipients of, say, a hip replacement, can have different degrees of pain and handicap and thus different benefits from receiving one. More interestingly, with older children and mature adults, one can sometimes distinguish the significance of the opportunities provided by removing handicaps. Unlike newborn infants, adults have life plans which should be distinguished from life styles; they are primary activities such as occupation, housekeeping, major leisure activities, and so on. Some capacities are more important than others for these plans. For example, a kidney transplant would provide more significant opportunity to a person whose job requires frequent travel away from town than for a person whose employment does not require such travel and can more readily be available for dialysis. Such a consideration can outweigh some difference in tissue matching that would affect probability of success.

The general question is the significance or importance of a handicap for a person's life plans. Answering it does not normally involve a valuation of those life plans and thus preserves substantive impartiality. Loss of a dominant hand is more significant for a painter's than a teacher's opportunity for valuable life, regardless of the respective social values of the two occupations. Thus, if a hand surgery center is confronted with a painter and teacher with damaged dominant hands who are otherwise comparable and does not have time to save both, the individual benefit criterion supports operating on the painter. Social value should enter only if the person's life plans have been officially judged antisocial, that is, criminal. Thus, if a hand surgery center is faced with a choice between a teacher and a pickpocket, it should prefer the teacher even though the use of the hand might be more central to the pickpocket's life plans.

One cannot individualize such considerations too finely. Doing so would be a mere pretense and provide an opportunity for abuse. To avoid this, opportunities should be presumed the same unless shown by clear and convincing evidence to differ importantly or significantly for persons' life plans. Consequently, differences in benefit due to differences in life plans will not often be found. The primary opportunity differences will be due to differences in pain and handicap.

A second objection is that the individual benefit criterion discriminates against handicapped persons, at least when the extension is involved. By the factors used, the opportunities for a handicapped person will be less than those of a nonhandicapped person. Consequently, if the lives of a handicapped and a nonhandicapped person would be lengthened the same amount, the nonhandicapped person would benefit more.[6]

A bias against handicapped persons can be eliminated by considering the proportional benefit for an individual rather than the mere quantum of increased benefit. This revised conception of individual benefit can be represented in the following formula:

$$(3)\ IB = p \times [(OV_w - OV_o)/OV_o]$$

By this conception, benefit is determined by the proportional gain for an individual. Thus, a nonhandicapped person does not have an advantage simply due to not having a handicap.

However, this formula has an implication to which some people might object. If the same quantity of benefit can be provided a handicapped or a nonhandicapped person, the handicapped person will have a proportionally greater benefit. Consequently, there will be a preference for allocating resources to handicapped persons.

This preference is acceptable. Suppose a hand surgery center is faced with a choice between a dominant hand for a paraplegic and a nonhandicapped person. Not knowing which one would be, one could accept preference for the paraplegic; the loss of a hand if one has already lost the use of one's legs seems a greater loss than if one can still use one's legs. The benefit is probably more central to the paraplegic's life plans, and the proportional benefit merely captures this element. Moreover, the proportional benefit conception does not imply that a neonatal ICU should expend all its resources on very seriously handicapped infants, because the probability of success and expectation of length of life strongly favor allocating them to more infants who are less seriously ill and thus producing greater individual benefit.

The third objection is that proportional benefit violates impartiality by discriminating against the elderly. Suppose a resource merely extends life. Further suppose two candidates are thirty and sixty years old and that the resource would provide each with five more years. By the proportional opportunity for value formula, five years for the younger person is a gain of one-sixth, while for the older person it is merely a gain of one-twelfth.

The appropriate conception is proportional benefit from the time benefit is realized. Usually benefit is added at the time of intervention, which has been implicit in the previous discussion, but when only life extension is in question, benefit is added at the end of life. From that point, there is no opportunity for valuable life without the resource. Hence, proportionality does not make sense (it involves division by zero). Consequently, the only consideration is length of life added and the following formula should be used:

$$(3a)\ IB = p \times LG$$

where LG is length of life gained from the resource. This formula is merely an emendation of (3) for cases in which opportunity for value is not affected.

Nevertheless, one might object that the operational criteria—(3) and (3a)—still inherently discriminate on the basis of age. Given the prominence of life expectancy in the determination of individual benefit even on (3), the young will normally receive priority over the elderly. Usually, a life-saving resource will provide greater life expectancy to a younger than an older person. Consequently, both criteria should be rejected as discriminatory.

Although age is often important in applying the criteria, it is neither the decisive nor sole factor. An older person can have a greater life expectancy than a younger one with other potentially fatal conditions. Moreover, an older person in generally good health might have a significantly greater probability of success than a younger person in poor health.

Any remaining preference for younger persons would be acceptable to a reasonable person. As that preference is strongest in (3a), if it is acceptable there it is acceptable in (3). First, expectable life is implicitly weighted in considering prospect of success in allocating life-saving resources. Other factors equal, the lower the probability of success, the less the expectable life gained. Thus, one cannot entirely eliminate a preference for the young or expectable life without dropping probability for success as a factor. However, with randomization and a very minimal requirement of success to be in a potential recipient pool, expectable life is a negligible consideration.

Second, the issue is less whether expectable life is acceptable than the weight to be accorded it. Holding constant opportunity for life found valuable, if one's goal is to maximize one's expectable life, (3a) will do so and be acceptable. If one drops the assumption of self-interest and instead assumes limited benevolence, the argument for (3a) is more complex. Consider the benevolent concern parents have for their children. If it is equal to that for themselves, then they would prefer the criterion. If their concern for their children is less than for themselves, then they might put less weight on life expectancy. However, most actual parents would prefer more years of life for their children to fewer for themselves. One could put the choice as between prolonging one's mother's life three years or one's child's life four years. Preferring the young in such a case is acceptable. Randomization with a weak criterion of medical success would decide all such cases either by drawing lots or by first come. Its ignoring of such differences in individual benefit would not be acceptable to reasonable persons.

Thus, the individual benefit criterion is capable of meeting the impartiality test. Any effect due to age is acceptable. The chief factors in determining individual benefit are relatively objective medical criteria—probability of success, length of life, pain, and physical or mental handicap. Of course, these factors do not admit of precise measurement. Moreover, anyone using the criterion might be subconsciously biased and, say, prefer physicians to

manual laborers. The greatest possibility of such abuse arises in using the effect on life plans, but that is largely contained by requiring a significant difference established by clear and convincing evidence. The possibility of abuse can be further limited by having policies made, or even the operation of a system overseen, by a committee or group composed of persons from various walks of life. Reasonable persons could accept the still somewhat greater risk of abuse than with a randomization criterion because of the greater chance of valuable life.

Application

Various acceptable criteria and subcriteria have been identified. To satisfy the test of workability, a scheme is needed to indicate how they can be used together. Such a scheme indicates their relative importance. Unfortunately, the arguments above are not sufficiently powerful to provide a clear priority in all cases. Consequently, plausible variations are mentioned.

General Principles. First, a pool of potential recipients is determined. There are two main criteria for admission to the pool other than jurisdiction. Only people who voluntarily make an informed choice for the resources, or whose representatives do so, are to be in the pool. Moreover, some probability of success should be required for entry. What the probability will be depends on the success rates that can be achieved with a medical treatment and the ratio of resources to persons. One can set the requirement to pick out two or three times as many persons as there are resources to serve. Occasionally, depending on the resource, a social worth criterion might be used to exclude people, for example, convicted rapists from AIDS treatment.

Second, if there are clear indices of personal responsibility for the condition requiring the resource, the pool is divided into two groups—those responsible and those not responsible for their condition. Although this is a supplemental principle, it is organizationally easier (at least for purposes of exposition) to apply it first. For many if not most resources, such a division is not possible.

Third, one sorts each group into subgroups based on individual benefit. How many subgroups there should be and how large they will be depends on how precise one can make judgments of probability of success, life expectancy, and opportunity for value of life. It is unlikely that in practice one can get more than three or four groups.[7]

At this point, there are one or two groups (responsible, R, and not responsible, NR) divided into three or four subgroups—R1, R2, R3 and NR1, NR2, and NR3. If one has not distinguished between those responsible and not responsible for their condition, then one simply allocates resources down the list of subgroups, providing for all those in 1 before 2. One can use a lottery to choose among members of a subgroup when there are not enough for all members.

If one has divided into two groups, R and NR, then the process is more complex. Resources permitting, one can provide them to everyone in the top group of persons not responsible for their condition, NR1. The remaining resources can then be allocated by lottery among a group consisting of NR2 and RI. If all of them can be provided treatment, then one takes the remaining resources and randomly allocates among a group consisting of R2 and NR3. One could place less emphasis on responsibility by selecting some proportion of R1 persons by lottery and putting them with NR1, the remaining RI persons being grouped with NR2 and a proportion of R2. The many possible mathematical variations are of no practical interest.

In practice, such precision is usually not workable. Instead, on the basis of individual benefit one will pick out a few persons to be assured of receiving the resource, and then a much larger group among whom decisions are made by a random procedure, and another group that will not be considered unless more resources become available. With organ transplants, one might simply have a recipient group two or three times the number likely to receive organs.[8]

The procedure thus differs significantly from other major proposals. Throughout, the emphasis is on individual benefit for membership in a group both for those who are assured the resources and for determining who is in the group from whom persons are chosen by lottery. The procedure thus differs significantly from Childress's proposal.[9] He uses only a weak medical criterion for a patient pool and then first come selection, whereas here individual benefit is used to divide the pool into subgroups and lottery randomization rather than first come is used to select among members. It also importantly differs from Rescher's proposal.[10] Although Rescher uses constituency, likelihood of success, and life expec-

tancy, he strongly weights social worth considerations and ignores opportunity for valuable life except as affected by life expectancy. In contrast, here individual benefit is dominant and social worth considered only for special exclusions from the patient pool or exceptions. Moreover, both Childress and Rescher ignore the responsibility criterion.

An Example.   Patient selection for *in vitro* fertilization can illustrate the principles. Although it does not involve life expectancy, it makes clear how opportunity for a valuable life and responsibility enter. First, entry into the potential recipient pool requires some probability of success. Severe adhesions of the ovaries preventing retrieval of ova would be a ground for exclusion, assuming donated ova or embryos are not available. A social value criterion can also be used to exclude patients if they or their partners were previously convicted of child abuse or neglect; this is based on past desert as well as possible future effects on the child. However, given that life plans are to be considered equally valuable, the marital status of the woman would not be considered. Second, patients can be divided into two groups depending on whether their infertility results from previous voluntary sterilization, provided such a condition for access was known at the time of sterilization. Each of these groups could be divided into two depending on whether they already have a living child. Presumably, the proportional benefit of a child to a person who does not have any children is greater than for a person who already has a living child. The probability of success might divide into two groups—those with normal chance of success and those who have a lower chance of success.

The resulting groups are presented in the appended table.

		PROBABILITY OF SUCCESS	
		HIGH	LOW
NOT RESPONSIBLE	no child	1	3
	child	2	4
RESPONSIBLE	no child	2	4
	child	3	5

The numbers in the table indicate the order of preference in which groups are to be chosen. Those with the same number are to be considered together. For simplicity, responsibility for infertility is taken to lower ranking one unit. If one does not believe responsibility for infertility significant, one would not make that division. Probability of success is given a strong ranking, that is, taken to outweigh parity. One could, of course, reverse this weighting. The decision depends on how much one thinks already having a child decreases the proportional opportunity for value. However one weights the factors the resultant allocation will differ greatly from a random allocation or one based on social worth. This example thus shows that the various principles can be combined into one workable scheme that is both adequate and reasonably workable.

Notes

1. See, for example, Nicholas Rescher, "The Allocation of Exotic Medical Lifesaving Therapy"; James F. Childress, "Who Shall Live When Not All Can Live?"; and George J. Annas, "The Prostitute, the Playboy, and the Poet: Rationing Schemes for Organ Transplantation"; all collected in *Intervention and Reflection,* ed. Ronald Munson, 3rd ed. (Belmont, Calif.: Wadsworth Publishing Co., 1988), pp. 492–515.

2. See further my *Principles of Law* (Dordrecht: Reidel Publishing Co., 1987), pp. 4–7; Richard B. Brandt, *A Theory of the Good and the Right* (Oxford: Clarendon Press, 1979), pp. 10–16.

3. See, for example, Dan E. Beauchamp, "Public Health and Individual Liberty"; Daniel Wikler, "Persuasion and Coercion for Health: Ethical Issues in Government Efforts to Change Lifestyles"; and Robert M. Veatch, "Voluntary Risks to Health: The Ethical Issues"; all collected in *Contemporary Issues in Bioethics,* ed. Tom L. Beauchamp and LeRoy Walters, 2d ed. (Belmont, Calif.: Wadsworth Publishing Co., 1982), pp. 442–63.

4. See Annas, "The Prostitute, the Playboy, and the Poet," p. 514. Such a procedure may be used under the United Network for Organ Sharing.

5. With a resource, one could have different probabilities of life with various values. A person might have a lower probability of life with a greater value than with a lower one. Although this could theoretically be factored in by averaging or some other method, the subject does not admit of mathematically precise calculations.

6. Brandt has argued that the utility of income to handicapped and nonhandicapped persons is basically the same, except that handicapped persons need more to reach the same point on a utility curve (*Theory of the Good and the Right,* pp. 316–19). Even if correct, this point is not relevant to the present concern with allocating medical resources. People's opportunities for valuable life are not independent of pain and handicaps.

7. Theoretically, one could use a point system, assigning rough numbers for each factor. For example, probability of success might be classified as below average, average, and above average. Length of life might be done by groups, such as less than one year, one to five years, five to ten years, and more than ten. One could rank average opportunity for valuable life on a scale of one to three.

8. If tissue typing is crucial to success, the group might be much larger to allow for the variability of tissue. In effect, such tissue typing leaves the judgment of probability of success until an organ is found. Still, significantly greater proportional value should outweigh a somewhat smaller chance of success.

9. "Who Shall Live When Not All Can Live?" pp. 503–11.

10. "The Allocation of Exotic Medical Lifesaving Therapy," pp. 492–503.

Take My Kidney, Please

Michael Kinsley

Michael Kinsley examines the issue of whether we should permit the sale of transplant organs. How far, he asks, are we willing to pursue the logic of capitalism? Kinsley shows that, in the final analysis, when we react with horror to the spectacle of a man forced to sell a kidney to pay for his daughter's operation, we are actually reacting to the injustices of life.

Even Margaret Thatcher's devotion to the free market has some limits, it seems. Reacting to newspaper reports that poor Turkish peasants are being paid to go to London and give up a kidney for transplant, the British Prime Minister said that "the sale of kidneys or any organs of the body is utterly repugnant." Emergency legislation is now being prepared for swift approval by Parliament to make sure that capitalism does not perform its celebrated magic in the market for human organs.

Commercial trade in human kidneys does seem grotesque. But it's a bit hard to say why. After all, the moral logic of capitalism does not stop at the epidermis. That logic holds, in a nutshell, that if an exchange is voluntary, it leaves both parties better off. In one case, a Turk sold a kidney for £2,500 ($4,400) because he needed money for an operation for his daughter. Capitalism in action: one person had $4,400 and wanted a kidney, another person had a spare kidney and wanted $4,400, so they did a deal. What's more, it seems like an advantageous deal all around. The buyer avoided a lifetime of dialysis. The seller provided crucial help to his child, at minimum risk to himself. (According to the *Economist*, the chance of a kidney donor's dying as a result of the loss is 1 in 5,000.)

Nevertheless, the conclusion that such trade is abhorrent is not even controversial. Almost everyone agrees. Is almost everyone right? This question of how far we are willing to push the logic of capitalism will be thrust in our faces increasingly in coming years. Medical advances are making it possible to buy things that were previously unobtainable at any price. (The Baby M. "womb renting" case is another example.) Meanwhile, the communications and transportation revolutions are breaking down international borders, making new commercial relations possible between the comfortably rich and the desperately poor. On what basis do we say to a would-be kidney seller, "Sorry, this is one deal you just can't make?"

One widely accepted category of forbidden deals involves health and safety regulations: automobile standards, bans on food additives, etc. Although we quarrel about particular instances, only libertarian cranks reject in principle the idea that government sometimes should protect people from themselves. But it is no more dangerous to sell one of your kidneys than it is to give one away to a close relative—a transaction we not only allow but admire. On health grounds alone, you can't ban the sale without banning the gift as well. Furthermore, the sale of a kidney is not necessarily a foolish decision that society ought to protect you from. To pay for a daughter's operation, it seems the opposite.

But maybe there are some things money just shouldn't be allowed to buy, sensibly or otherwise. Socialist philosopher Michael Walzer added flesh to this ancient skeleton of sentiment in his 1983 book, *Spheres of Justice*. Walzer argued that a just society is not necessarily one with complete financial equality—a hopeless and even destructive goal—but one in which the influence of money is not allowed to dominate all aspects of life. By outlawing organ sales, you are indeed keeping the insidious influence of money from leaching into a new sphere and are thereby reducing the power of the rich. Trouble is, you are also reducing opportunity for the poor.

The grim trade in living people's kidneys would not be necessary if more people would voluntarily offer their kidneys (and other organs) when they die. Another socialist philosopher, Richard Titmuss, wrote a famous book two decades ago called *The Gift Relationship*, extolling the virtues of donated blood over purchased blood and, by extension, the superiority of sharing over commerce. Whatever you may think of Titmuss's larger point, the appeal of the blood-donor system as a small testament to our shared humanity is undeniable. Perhaps we should do more to encourage organ donation at death for the same reason. On the other hand, however cozy and egalitarian it might seem, a system that supplied all the kidneys we need through voluntary donation would be no special favor to our Turkish friend, who would be left with no sale and no $4,400. Why not at least let his heirs sell his kidneys when he dies? A commercial market in cadaver organs would wipe out the sale of live people's parts a lot more expeditiously than trying to encourage donations.

The logic of capitalism assumes knowledgeable, reasonably intelligent people on both sides of the transaction. Is this where the kidney trade falls short? At $4,400, the poor Turk was probably underpaid for his kidney. But in an open, legal market with protections against exploitation, he might have got more. At some price, the deal would make sense for almost anyone. I have no sentimental attachment to my kidneys. Out of prudence, I'd like to hang on to one of them, but the other is available. My price is $2 million.

Of course, I make this offer safe in the knowledge that there will always be some poor Turk ready to undercut me. So maybe, because of who the sellers inevitably will be, the sale of kidneys is by its very nature exploitation. A father shouldn't have to sacrifice a kidney to get a necessary operation for his daughter. Unfortunately, banning the kidney sale won't solve the problem of paying for the operation.

Nor can the world yet afford expensive operations for everyone who needs one. And leaving aside the melodrama of the daughter's operation, we don't stop people from doing things to support their families—working in coal mines, for example—that reduce their life expectancies more than would the loss of a kidney. In fact, there are places in the Third World where even $4,400 can do more for a person's own life expectancy than a spare kidney.

The horror of kidney sales, in short, is a sentimental reaction to the injustice of life—injustice that the transaction highlights but does not increase. This is not a complaint. In fact, it may even be the best reason for a ban on such transactions. That kind of sentiment ought to be encouraged.

Rights, Symbolism, and Public Policy in Fetal Tissue Transplants

John A. Robertson

John Robertson examines some moral objections raised by opponents of fetal tissue transplants. To those who charge that fetal tissue transplants encourage or abet abortion, he argues that the decision to end an unwanted pregnancy is a separate issue; the use of fetal tissue from such cases does not entail approval of abortion any more than the use of an organ from a homicide victim entails approval of homicide.

Also, in Robertson's view, whether it is legitimate to abort (or conceive and abort) a fetus to obtain material for transplant is more morally complex than usually recognized and in some circumstances "may be more justified than previously thought."

As to recruiting unrelated donors of fetal tissue, Robertson sees the possibility of becoming a donor as within the range of a woman's autonomy. The fear that women will become "tissue farms" is wholly unfounded.

Fetal tissue transplants hold great hope for many patients. Extensive work with animal models has shown that human fetal brain cells transplanted into the substantia nigra of monkeys with oxogenously produced Parkinson's disease have restored their function. Physicians expect similar results in humans, to the benefit of thousands of patients.[1] Experimental evidence is also strong that fetal islet cell transplants will restore normal insulin function in diabetics.[2] And fetal thymus and liver transplants may have utility for blood and immune system disorders.

Reprinted by permission of the author and the publisher from Hastings Center Report, *December 1988, pp. 5–9. Copyright © The Hastings Center. (Excerpt from whole article, pp. 5–12.) Footnotes have been renumbered.*

Clarifying the Issues

As with many issues in bioethics, careful analysis will help elucidate the normative conflict, showing both areas of agreement and irreducible conflict. An essential distinction in the fetal tissue controversy is between procuring tissue from family planning abortions and procuring tissue from abortions performed expressly to provide tissue for transplant. Although opponents of fetal tissue transplants have often conflated the two, tissue from family planning abortions may be used without implying approval of abortions to produce tissue. Indeed, with ample tissue available from family planning abortions, the latter scenario may never occur.

A second important distinction is that between retrieving tissue for transplant from dead and from live fetuses. Only the use of tissue from dead fetuses is at issue. Researchers are not proposing to maintain nonviable fetuses ex utero to procure tissue, or to take tissue from them before they are dead, practices that current regulations and law prohibit.[3] . . .

Tissue from Family Planning Abortions

Fetal tissue transplant research for Parkinson's disease, diabetes, and other disorders will use tissue retrieved from the one and a half million abortions performed annually in the United States to end unwanted pregnancies. Nearly 80 percent of induced abortions are performed between the sixth and eleventh weeks of gestation, at which time neural and other tissue is sufficiently developed to be retrieved and transplanted.[4] Abortions performed at fourteen to sixteen weeks provide pancreatic tissue used in diabetes research, but it may prove possible to use pancreases retrieved earlier.[5]

No need now or in the foreseeable future exists to have a family member conceive and abort to produce fetal tissue. The neural tissue to be transplanted in Parkinson's disease lacks antigenicity, thus obviating the need for a close match between donor and recipient. Fetal pancreas is more antigenic, but processing can reduce this, also making family connection less important.

The key question is whether women who abort to end unwanted pregnancies may donate the aborted fetuses for use in medical research or therapy by persons who have no connection with or influence on the decision to terminate the pregnancy. One's views on abortion need not determine one's answer to this question, because the abortion and subsequent transplant use are clearly separated. But some opposed to abortion object that transplanting fetal tissue involves complicity in an immoral act and will legitimate and even encourage abortion. Analysis of these concerns will show that they are insufficient to justify a public policy that bans or refuses to fund research or therapy with fetal tissue from induced abortion.

Complicity in Abortion

Even proponents of the complicity argument recognize that not all situations of subsequent benefit make one morally complicitous in a prior evil act. For example, James Burtchaell claims that complicity occurs not merely from partaking of benefit but only when one enters into a "supportive alliance" with the underlying evil that makes the benefit possible. He distinguishes "a neutral or even an opponent and an ally" of the underlying evil by "the way in which one does or does not hold oneself apart from the enterprise and its purposes."[6]

On this analysis, a researcher using fetal tissue from an elective abortion is not necessarily an accomplice with the abortionist and woman choosing abortion. The researcher and recipient have no role in the abortion process. They will not have requested it, and may have no knowledge of who performed the abortion or where it occurred since a third-party intermediary will procure the tissue. They may be morally opposed to abortion, and surely are not compromised because they choose to salvage some good from an abortion that will occur regardless of their research or therapeutic goals.

A useful analogy is transplant of organs and tissue from homicide victims. Families of murder victims are often asked to donate organs and bodies for research, therapy, and education. If they consent, organ procurement agencies retrieve the organs and distribute them to recipients. No one would seriously argue that the surgeon who transplants the victim's kidneys, heart, liver, or corneas, or the recipient of the organs, becomes an accomplice in the homicide that made the organs available, even if aware of the source. Nor is the medical student who uses the cadaver of a murder victim to study anatomy.

If organs from murder victims may be used without complicity in the murder that makes the organs available, then fetal remains could also be used without complicity in the abortion. Burtchaell's approach to the problem of complicity assumes that researchers necessarily applaud the underlying act of abortion. But one may benefit from another's evil act without applauding or approving of that evil. X may disapprove of Y's murder of Z, even though X gains an inheritance or a promotion as a result. Indeed, one might even question Burtchaell's assumption that X becomes an accomplice in Y's prior act if he subsequently applauds it. Applauding Y's murder of Z might be insensitive or callous. But that alone would not make one morally responsible for, complicitous in, the murder that has already occurred. In any event, the willingness to derive benefit from another's wrongful death does not create complicity in that death because the beneficiary played no role in causing it.

The complicity argument against use of aborted fetuses often draws an analogy to a perceived reluctance to use the results of unethical medical research carried out by the Nazis. Burtchaell and others have claimed that it would make us retroactively accomplices in the Nazi horrors to use the results of their unethical and lethal research.[7] This ignores, however, the clear separation between the perpetrator and beneficiary of the immoral act that breaks the chain of moral complicity for that act.

Thus one could rely on Nazi-generated data while decrying the horrendous acts of Nazi doctors that produced the data. Nor would it necessarily dishonor those unfortunate victims. Indeed, it could reasonably be viewed as retrospectively honoring them by saving others. The Jewish doctors who made systematic studies of starvation in the Warsaw ghetto to reap some good from the evil being done to their brethren were not accomplices in that evil, nor are doctors and patients who now benefit from their studies.[8]

If the complicity claim is doubtful when the underlying immorality of the act is clear, as with Nazi-produced data or transplants from murder victims, it is considerably weakened when the act making the benefit possible is legal and its immorality vigorously debated, as is the case with abortion. Even persons opposed to abortion might agree that

perceptions of complicity should not determine public policy on fetal tissue transplants.

Legitimizing, Entrenching, and Encouraging Abortion

A second objection is that salvaging tissue for transplant from aborted fetuses will make abortion more morally offensive and more easily tolerated both by individual pregnant women and by society, and perhaps transform it into a morally positive act. This will encourage abortions that would not otherwise occur, and dilute support for reversing the legal acceptability of abortion, in effect creating complicity in future abortions.[9]

But the feared impact on abortion practices and attitudes is highly speculative, particularly at a time when few fetal transplants have occurred. The main motivation for abortion is the desire to avoid the burdens of an unwanted pregnancy. The fact that fetal remains may be donated for transplant will continue to be of little significance in the total array of factors that lead a woman to abort a pregnancy.

Having decided to abort, a woman may feel better if she then donates the fetal remains. But this does not show that tissue donation will lead to a termination decision that would not otherwise have occurred, particularly if the decision to abort is made before the opportunity to donate the remains is offered. Perhaps a few more abortions will occur because of the general knowledge that tissue can be donated for transplant, but it is highly unlikely that donation—as opposed to contraceptive practices and sex education—will contribute significantly to the rate of abortion.[10]

Nor does the use of fetal remains for transplant mean that a public otherwise ready to outlaw abortion would refrain from doing so. Legal acceptance of abortion flows from the wide disagreement that exists over early fetal status. If a majority agreed that fetuses should be respected as persons despite the burdens placed on pregnant women, such possible secondary benefits of induced abortion as fetal tissue transplants would not prevent a change in the legality of abortion.

Indeed, one could make the same argument against organ transplants from homicide, suicide, and accident victims. The willingness to use their organs might be seen to encourage or legitimate such deaths, or at least make it harder to enact lower speed limits, seatbelt, gun control, and drunk driving laws to prevent them. After all, the need to prevent murder, suicide, and fatal accidents becomes less pressing if some good to others might come from use of victims' organs for transplant. In either case, the connection is too tenuous and speculative to ban organ or fetal tissue transplants.

In sum, fetal tissue transplants are practically and morally separate from decisions to end unwanted pregnancy. Given that abortion is legal and occurring on a large scale, the willingness to use resulting tissue for transplant neither creates complicity in past abortions nor appears significantly to encourage more future abortions. Such ethical concerns and speculations are not sufficient, given the possible good to others, to justify banning use of fetal tissue for research or therapy.

Aborting to Obtain Tissue for Transplant

Central to the argument for transplanting fetal tissue from family planning abortions has been the assumption that the abortion occurs independently of the need for tissue, and that permitting such transplants does not also entail pregnancy and abortion to produce fetal tissue.

But successful tissue transplants may create the need to abort to produce fetal tissue in two future situations. One situation would arise if histocompatability between the fetus and recipient were necessary for effective fetal transplants. Female relatives, spouses, or even unrelated persons might then seek to conceive to provide properly matched fetal tissue for transplant.

The second situation would arise if fetal transplants were so successful that demand far outstripped supply, such as might occur if the treatment were advantageous to most patients with Parkinson's disease and diabetes, or if the number of surgical family planning abortions decreased. Pressure on supply might also occur if tissue from several aborted fetuses were needed to produce one viable transplant.

The hypothetical possibility of such situations is not a sufficient reason to ban all tissue transplants from family planning abortions. But should such abortions be banned if the imagined situations occurred? Most commentators assume that conception and abortion for tissue procurement is so clearly unethical that the prospect hardly merits discus-

sion.[11] Accordingly, they would ban all tissue transplants from related persons and deny the donor the right to designate the recipient of a fetal tissue transplant.

Analysis will show, however, that the question is more ethically complicated than generally assumed, and should not be the driving force in setting policy for tissue transplants from family planning abortions.

A Hypothetical Situation

Consider first the situation where a woman pregnant with her husband's child learns that tissue from her fetus could cure severe neurologic disease in herself or a close relative, such as her husband, child, parent, father or mother-in-law, sibling, or brother or sister-in-law. May she ethically abort the pregnancy to obtain tissue for transplant to the relative? Or may a woman not yet pregnant conceive a fetus that she will then abort to provide tissue for transplant to herself or to her relative?

To focus analysis on fetal welfare, assume in each case that no other viable tissue source exists, and that the advanced state of neurologic disease has become a major tragedy for the patient and family. The woman has broached the question of abortion to obtain tissue without any direct pressure or inducements from the family or others. Her husband accepts an abortion for transplant purposes if she is willing, but exerts no pressure on her to abort.

The woman is already pregnant. If the woman is already pregnant, the question is whether a first trimester fetus that would otherwise have been carried to term may be sacrificed to procure tissue for transplant to the woman herself or to a sick family member. The answer depends on the value placed on early fetuses and on the acceptable reasons for abortion. One may distinguish between fetuses that have developed the neurologic and cognitive capacity for sentience and interests in themselves, and those so neurologically immature that they cannot experience harm.[12] While aborting fetuses at that earlier stage prevents them from achieving their potential, it does not harm or wrong them, since they are insufficiently developed to experience harm.[13]

Although aborting the fetus at that early stage does not wrong the fetus, it may impose symbolic costs measurable in terms of the reduced respect for human life generally that a willingness to abort early fetuses connotes. Still the abortion may be ethically acceptable if the good sought sufficiently outweighs the symbolic devaluation of life that occurs when fetuses that cannot be harmed in their own right are aborted. Many persons find that the burdens of unwanted pregnancy outweigh the symbolic devaluation of human life. Others would require a more compelling reason for abortion, such as protecting the mother's life or health, avoiding the birth of a handicapped child, or avoiding the burdens of a pregnancy due to rape or incest.

By comparison, abortion to obtain tissue to save one's own life or the life of a close relative seems equally, if not more compelling. If abortion in the case of an unwanted pregnancy is deemed permissible, surely abortion to obtain tissue to save another person's life is. Indeed, aborting to obtain tissue would seem as compelling as the most stringent reasons for permitting abortion. In fact, many would find this motive more compelling than the desire to end an unwanted pregnancy.

Of course, aborting a wanted pregnancy to prevent severe neurologic disease in oneself or a close relative will hardly be done joyfully, and will place the mother in an excruciating dilemma. A fetus that could be carried to term will have to be sacrificed to save a parent, spouse, sibling, or child who already exists. Such a tragic choice will induce fear and trembling, and engender loss or grief whatever the decision. Yet one cannot say that the choice to abort is ethically impermissible. There is no sound ethical basis for prohibiting *this* sacrifice of the fetus when its sacrifice to end an unwanted pregnancy or pursue other goals is permitted.

Public attitudes toward a woman aborting an otherwise wanted pregnancy to benefit a family member would most likely reflect attitudes toward abortion generally. Those who are against abortion in all circumstances will object to abortions done to treat severe neurologic disease in the mother or in a family member. Similarly, persons who accept family planning abortions should have no objection to abortion to procure tissue for transplant, since fetal status is no more compelling and the interest of the woman in controlling her body and reproductive capacity is similar.

Since neither group forms a majority, however, persons who object to family planning abortions but accept abortions necessary to protect the mother's health, in cases of rape or incest, or to prevent the birth of a handicapped child will determine whether a majority of people approve.[14] It is conceivable that many persons in this swing group would find abortion to produce tissue for transplant to a family member to be acceptable. The benefit of alleviating severe neurologic disease is arguably as great as the benefits in the cases they accept as justifiable abortion, and more compelling than abortions done for family planning purposes.

Conceiving and aborting for transplant purposes. What is the objection, then, when a woman not yet pregnant seeks to conceive in order to abort and provide tissue for transplant?

In terms of fetal welfare, no greater harm occurs to the fetus conceived expressly to be aborted, as long as the abortion occurs at a stage at which the fetus is insufficiently developed to experience harm, such as during the first trimester. Of course, such deliberate creation may have greater symbolic significance, because it denotes a willingness to use fetuses as a means or object to serve other ends. However, aborting when already pregnant to procure tissue for transplant (or aborting for the more customary reasons) also denotes a willingness to use the fetus as a means to other ends.

As long as abortion of an existing pregnancy for transplant purposes is ethically accepted, conceiving in order to abort and procure tissue for transplant should also be ethically acceptable when necessary to alleviate great suffering in others.[15] People could reasonably find that the additional symbolic devaluation is negligible, or in any case, insufficient to outweigh the substantial gain to transplant recipients that deliberate creation provides.

Many people, no doubt, will resist this conclusion, even if they accept abortion to procure tissue when the woman is already pregnant. Whether rational or not, they assign moral or symbolic significance to deliberate creation, and are less ready to sanction such a practice. Others who accept abortion for tissue procurement when the woman is already pregnant will find an insufficient difference in deliberate creation to outweigh the resulting good. Public acceptability of such a practice thus depends on how the swing group that views abortion as acceptable only for very stringent reasons views the fact of deliberate creation for the purpose of abortion. If it would accept abortion to produce tissue when the pregnancy is unplanned, it might accept conception to produce fetal tissue as well.

In sum, deliberate creation of fetuses to be aborted for tissue procurement is more ethically complex, and more defensible, than its current widespread dismissal would suggest. Such a practice is, of course, not in itself desirable, but in a specific situation of strong personal or familial need may be more justified than previously thought. In any case, the fear that fetal tissue transplants will lead to abortions performed solely to obtain tissue for transplant should not prevent use of tissue from abortions not performed for that purpose.

Recruiting Unrelated Fetal Tissue Donors

The strongest case for conception and abortion to produce fetal tissue—if the need arose—is to save oneself or a close relative from death or serious harm. But many patients in need would lack a female relative willing to donate. May unrelated women be recruited for this purpose?

If the hypothetical need arose, a strong case for unrelated fetal tissue donors can be made. If a relative may provide tissue, why not a stranger who chooses to do so altruistically? At this point concerns about fetal status become less important, and the focus shifts toward the welfare of the donor. But the physical effects of pregnancy and abortion to produce fetal tissue are roughly comparable to the effects of kidney or bone marrow donation, though somewhat less since general anesthesia will not be involved. While few unrelated persons now act as kidney donors, there is a national registry for unrelated bone marrow donors. Even if fetal tissue donation were psychologically more complicated, the risks to the woman would appear to be within the boundaries of autonomous choice.

Some persons might object that this will turn women into "fetal tissue farms," thus denigrating their inherent worth as persons. This charge could also be made against any living donor, whether of kidney, bone marrow, blood, sperm, or egg. Insofar as persons donate body parts, they may be viewed as mere tissue or organ producers. Indeed, women who bear children are always in danger of being viewed as "breeders." But such views oversimplify the complex emotional reality of organ and tissue donation and of human reproduction. The risk of misperception does not justify barring women from freely choosing to be fetal tissue donors.

Special attention should be given to consent procedures that will protect the woman from being coerced or unduly pressured by prospective recipients and their families, just as occurs with living related kidney and marrow donors. Waiting periods, consent advisors and monitors, and other devices to guarantee free, informed consent are clearly justified.[16]

References

The author gratefully acknowledges the helpful comments of Richard Markovits, Douglas Laycock, Michael Sharlot, Alan Fine, Albert R. Jonsen, George J. Annas, Arthur L. Caplan, Pat Cain, and Jean Love on a much longer version of this article.

1. Alan Fine, "The Ethics of Fetal Tissue Transplants," *Hastings Center Report* 18:3 (June 1988), 5–8.

2. Kevin Lafferty, statement to the Fetal Tissue Transplantation Research Panel, National Institutes of Health, September 15, 1988.

3. 45 CFR 46.209; John A. Robertson, "Relaxing the Death Standard for Pediatric Organ Donations," in *Organ Substitution Technology:* Ethical, Legal, and Public Policy Issues (Boulder, CO: Westview Press, 1988), 69–77.

4. Stanley K. Henshaw *et al.* "A Portrait of American Women Who Obtain Abortions," *Family Planning Perspectives* 17:2 (1985), 90–96.

5. Lafferty, "Statement."

6. James Burtchaell, "Case Study: University Policy on Experimental Use of Aborted Fetal Tissue," *IRB: A Review of Human Subjects Research* 10:4 (July/August 1988), 7–11.

7. Burtchaell, "Case Study," 10: Phillip Shabecott. "Head of E.P.A. Bars Nazi Data in Study on Gas," *New York Times*, March 23, 1988, 1.

8. Leonard Tushnet, *The Uses of Adversity: Studies of Starvation in the Warsaw Ghetto* (New York: Thomas Yoseloff, 1966); "Minnesota Scientist Plans to Publish a Nazi Study," *New York Times*, May 12, 1988, 9.

9. Tamar Lewin, "Medical Use of Fetal Tissue Spurs New Abortion Debate." *New York Times*, Aug. 16, 1987, A1.

10. John A. Robertson, "Fetal Tissue Transplants," *Washington University Law Quarterly* 66:3 (November 1988) (forthcoming).

11. Mary B. Mahowald, Jerry Silver, and Robert A. Ratcheson, "The Ethical Options in Transplanting Fetal Tissue," *Hastings Center Report* 17:2 (February 1987), 9–15; Mark Danis, "Fetal Tissue Transplants:

Restricting Recipient Designation," *Hastings Law Journal* 39:5 (July 1988), 1079–1107.

12. Clifford Grobstein, *Science and the Unborn* (New York: Basic Books, 1988).

13. John A. Robertson, "Gestational Burdens and Fetal Status: A Defense of *Roe v. Wade.*" *American Journal of Law and Medicine* 13:2/3 (1988), 189–212; John Bigelow and Robert Pargetter, "Morality, Potential Persons, and Abortion," *American Philosophical Quarterly* 25 (1988), 173–81.

14. See, for example, "America's Abortion Dilemma," *Newsweek*, January 14, 1985, 22–26.

15. John A. Robertson, "Embryos, Families, and Procreative Liberty: The Legal Structure of the New Reproduction," *Southern California Law Review* 59 (1986), 939–1041.

16. John A. Robertson, "Taking Consent Seriously: IRB Interventions in the Consent Process," *IRB: A Review of Human Subjects Research* 4:5 (May 1982), 1–5.

Decision Scenario 1 ·

"What do you mean, you don't know who he is?" asked Dr. Bridewell, the head of the Oakbrook Hospital Renal Unit.

"He was unconscious when the police brought him to the ER. We started the IV, stopped his bleeding, and patched him up. But he still hasn't recovered consciousness. The police think it was a hit-and-run driver." Dr. Kathy McDowell spoke in a precise, matter-of-fact voice. Dr. Bridewell always frightened her, but she was determined not to show it.

"He didn't have any identification?"

"That's right. They think that either the driver robbed him or somebody else who came along did. Anyway, he was wearing jeans and a sweatshirt, nothing that gives any clue as to his background. There is one thing we do know definitely."

"What's that?" asked Dr. Bridewell.

"Both of his kidneys were hopelessly damaged, but his general physical condition is good. We think he's a good candidate for a transplant."

"Then you know we've got a guy whose brain waves we're waiting to flatten out?"

"Dr. Liebsbaum told me."

"He ought to keep his mouth shut," Dr. Bridewell said. "Oh, don't take that seriously. I'm just upset because this faces us with a big problem. We're only going to have one kidney to transplant. The other one's shot."

"That's all we want," said McDowell.

Bridewell ignored her. "You did a tissue check?" he asked.

"It's close enough."

"Too bad. What I mean is that I've got another candidate. Now we have to decide which of the two gets the kidney."

"Who's the other candidate?"

"A Mrs. Benson. She's a woman in her early sixties who's active in local affairs. She was on the school board. Her husband's a rich lawyer, and both of them move in high social circles. She does a lot of work now with a foundation that's supposed to help minority children in school. She also happens to be a pretty good candidate physically for a transplant."

"So you'll choose her over my patient?" McDowell felt herself getting angry.

"I didn't say that. How old is this guy?"

"I would estimate that he's in his early or middle thirties. He seems to be in good physical condition."

"But we don't know anything about him," said Dr. Bridewell. "He might just be a drifter passing through town. He's probably not a member of the community that this hospital is supposed to serve, the one that pays bills and makes donations."

"Not that we know of," Dr. McDowell admitted. "But he might be. He might be a person of great value. Maybe he's even a physician."

"But we don't know for sure, do we?" said Dr. Bridewell.

1. *Suppose you are Dr. Bridewell and have to decide between the unknown man and Mrs. Benson. On what grounds might you make your decision?*

2. *In the absence of any information about "social worth" and "family role," is it possible to apply Rescher's criteria in this case?*

3. *Does Annas's position suggest that the best way to solve the problem is just by tossing a coin?*

4. *Suppose the unknown patient regains consciousness and reveals that he is a state senator, the father of a*

two-year-old child, and a writer of detective novels. Might this information alter the way in which the decision would be made according to Annas? Might *it alter the outcome of a decision based on the use of Rescher's criteria?*

Decision Scenario 2 . . . .

Colin Benton, a British citizen, died in the summer of 1988 of renal disease after a kidney transplant failed. Benton's widow later revealed that the donor kidney has been obtained from a Turkish citizen who traveled to London for the surgery. The kidney donor was paid the equivalent of around $4,400. When asked why he had sold the organ, the man explained that he needed the money to pay for medical treatment for his daughter. It was this case that led the British Parliament to outlaw organ sales.

1. *If we can be considered to own our own bodies, then on what grounds could selling one of our kidneys be said to be wrong?*

2. *What view of selling an organ might be taken by a natural law theorist? For such a theorist, is there a moral distinction between donating a kidney out of benevolence and selling one for financial gain?*

3. *If a father has no other way to raise money for surgery necessary to preserve the life of his child, would it be morally permissible for him to sell a kidney? Should we hold him morally blameworthy if, given the opportunity, he refused to do so?*

4. *Is selling one's kidney different in any morally relevant way from selling one's labor under potentially hazardous conditions (e.g., mining coal)?*

Decision Scenario 3 . . . .

Valdez Regional Hospital is the primary medical facility for the residents of Valdez County, Arizona. Its intensive-care unit is the only one available in the entire county, and the closest comparable unit is eighty-five miles away in Somora County.

The Valdez ICU is a twelve-bed facility and, from the statistical point of view, it is generally adequate to serve the needs of its patient population. That is, the cost of adding extra equipment and staff to increase the size of the facility is much greater than its actual use would justify.

Valdez's ICU policy, which is similar to policies of hospitals everywhere, requires that the staff make the effort to keep at least one of the twelve beds free for use in a genuine emergency.

On a bright, clear afternoon one day after Christmas, sixty-eight-year-old Harry Aveni was brought to the emergency room of Valdez after he had collapsed on the patio of his house. Mr. Aveni had been brought to the emergency room twice before. Both were episodes of congestive heart failure, and this third occasion was no different. Mr. Aveni had broken his diet during the holidays and consumed an unaccustomed amount of salt.

Mr. Aveni responded well to emergency treatment. The fluid surrounding his heart was with-drawn, a glycoside medication was administered, and his condition seemed to stabilize. Then, that evening, there was a sudden onset of fibrillation—his heart started beating erratically. Again, Mr. Aveni responded well to treatment, and after emergency defibrillation his condition again stabilized.

"He needs to be put into the ICU," Dr. Ellen Gracian said. "We can't care for him sufficiently on the wards, because he's got to have constant monitoring."

"I don't think Dr. Franklin is going to want to admit him," the nurse said. "There's only one bed left."

Dr. Gracian immediately left the floor and went to the ICU director's office. She explained what she wanted and waited while he seemed to be thinking it over.

"I don't think I can admit him," Dr. Franklin said. "Here we have an elderly gentleman who has now gone through three episodes of congestive failure and also seems to have something wrong to cause the fibrillation. He didn't stick to his diet, and in general his days are likely to be in the rather small numbers."

"But if he doesn't have intensive care, the numbers may be even smaller," Dr. Gracian said.

"That's no doubt true. But as things are, we've got eleven people who need to stay right where they are for God knows how long, and we've got just one bed at our disposal."

"But that's all I need, just one bed."

"I understand that," said Dr. Franklin. "But let's suppose we install your patient in the ICU and fifteen minutes after we put him there an eighteen-year-old accident victim is brought in. She's going to have to have emergency treatment, then close and constant monitoring, or she's likely to die."

"But you don't know that somebody like that is going to come in," Dr. Gracian said. "And Mr. Aveni is here right now and is in need right now."

"I'm sorry," said Dr. Franklin. "But the chances are very good that somebody is going to need that bed, somebody we can do more for than we can do for your patient. Somebody who's got a better chance to live a longer and more normal life."

"I see," Dr. Gracian said. "But I thought we were in the business of saving lives."

"We are. But we can't save them all, and that's where the problems come in."

1. *What argument can be made from the point of view of an act utilitarian to support Dr. Franklin's decision?*

2. *Would a selection procedure of the sort favored by Bayles secure a bed in the ICU for Mr. Aveni?*

3. *Is the fact that Mr. Aveni broke his diet and so is, in some sense, responsible for being in immediate need relevant to deciding whether he should be admitted to the ICU?*

4. *Would any of the criteria presented by Rescher lead to the selection of Mr. Aveni over an eighteen- year-old accident victim?*

5. *Would Annas's recognition of immediate need as a justification for selection in transplants also justify granting intensive care to Mr. Aveni?*

Decision Scenario 4 . . . .

The microsurgical team at Benton Public Hospital consisted of twenty-three people. Five were surgeons, three were anesthesiologists, three were internists, two were radiologists, and the remaining members were various sorts of nurses and technicians.

Early Tuesday afternoon on a date late in March, the members of the team that had to be sterile were scrubbing while the others were preparing to start operating on Mr. Hammond Cox. Mr. Cox was a fifty-nine-year-old unmarried African American who worked as a janitor in a large apartment building. While performing his duties, Mr. Cox had caught his hand in the mechanism of a commercial trash compactor. The bones of his wrist had been crushed and the blood vessels severed.

The head of the team, Dr. Herbert Lagorio, believed that it was possible to restore at least partial functioning to Mr. Cox's hand. Otherwise, the hand would have to be amputated.

Mr. Cox had been drunk when the accident happened. When the police ambulance brought him to the emergency room, he was still so drunk that a decision was made to delay surgery for almost an hour to give him a chance to burn up some of the alcohol he had consumed. As it was, administering anesthesia to Mr. Cox would incur a greater-than-average risk. Furthermore, blood tests had shown that Mr. Cox already suffered from some degree of liver damage. In both short- and long-range terms, Mr. Cox was not a terribly good surgical risk.

Dr. Lagorio was already scrubbed when Dr. Carol Levine, a resident in emergency medicine, had him paged.

"This had better be important," he told her. "I've got a guy prepped and waiting."

"I know you do," Dr. Levine said. "But there's something you ought to know about before you start."

"Tell me quickly."

"They just brought in a thirty-five-year-old white female with a totally severed right hand. She's a biology professor at Columbia and was working late in her lab when some maniac looking for drugs came in and attacked her with a cleaver."

"What shape is the hand in?"

"Excellent. The campus cops were there within minutes, and there was ice in the lab. One of the cops had the good sense to put the hand in a plastic bag and bring it with her."

"Is she in good general health?"

"It seems excellent," Dr. Levine said.

"This is a real problem."

"You can't do two cases at once?"

"No way. We need everybody we've got to do one."

"How about sending her someplace else?"

"No place else is set up to do what has to be done," Dr. Lagorio said.

"So what are you going to do?"

"That's what I've got to decide," Dr. Lagorio said.

1. *Does a "first-come, first-served" criterion like that defended by Annas require that Mr. Cox receive the surgery?*

2. *Does a "social-value" criterion require that the biology professor receive the surgery?*

3. *Can the chance of a successful outcome in each case be used as a criterion without violating the notion that all people are of equal inherent worth?*

4. *Does Bayles's criterion of "individual patient benefits" point to an answer?*

5. *In your view, who should have the potential benefits of the surgery? Give reasons to support your view.*

Decision Scenario 5 ·

"Your baby's pituitary gland is not fully developed," Dr. Robert Amatin said.

Clarissa Austin nodded to show that she understood that at least something was wrong with her child. She had already made up her mind to do whatever she had to do to see to it that her baby was all right.

"That means he's not getting enough of a hormone—a chemical—produced there," Dr. Amatin went on. "He won't undergo the normal course of development without that chemical."

"Can you give it to him?"

Dr. Amatin avoided answering the question directly. "A transplant is the best hope," he said. "If we can surgically remove the malformed pituitary and attach a new one, then the baby has a very good chance of being normal."

"I'll be happy to give my permission, if that's what you're waiting for," Clarissa said.

"It's not that simple," Dr. Amatin said. He looked uncomfortable. "It really comes down to a matter of money."

"I don't have much money," Clarissa said. "You know my bills are being paid by Medicaid."

"I know that, and the government won't pay for transplant organs."

"How much does it cost?"

"I've got a family right now that says it wants $5,000 for the pituitary of their baby. She just died this morning."

"I can't get money like that," Clarissa said.

"I can ask them to come up and talk to you. Maybe they would take less, or maybe you could work out some kind of deferred payment with them."

"What if I can't?"

Dr. Amatin shook his head. "I can't arrange for a transplant without an organ, and I suspect they will just try to find somebody else to sell it to."

"That don't seem fair," Clarissa said. "Just because I haven't got the money, my little baby is going to have to be some kind of cripple and maybe die."

1. *Does the possibility of such situations demonstrate that the present policy of relying on donated organs is a superior one?*

2. *If organs are sold on the open market, are such situations inevitable?*

3. *What other organ procurement policy, besides voluntary donation and organ sales, might be worth considering as a means to increase the number of transplant organs available?*

4. *Is Ms. Austin correct in saying that it would be unfair for her child not to have the organ because she cannot afford to pay the asking price? After all, surely it is not unfair for her child not to have, say, a silver drinking cup because she cannot afford to pay the asking price.*

5. *On what grounds does Annas object to the market approach? What position might Kinsley take?*

Decision Scenario 6 •

Jean-Pierre Bosze, twelve years old, had leukemia. The disease was under control for a while, but then Jean-Pierre had a relapse. His father was told that his son's only hope was to have a bone marrow transplant, but neither the boy's father nor his mother was a suitable match. Bosze's twenty-two-year-old son from a previous marriage also failed to be a match, and his thirteen-month-old daughter by another woman was too young to be a donor.

In desperation, Tamas Bosze turned to his other children, Jimmy and Allison Curran, three-year-old twins by yet another woman. The chance of a tissue match between them and their half-brother would be much greater than the 1-in-20,000 chance offered by an unrelated individual.

However, the mother of the twins, Nancy Curran, from whom Tamas Bosze was estranged, refused to permit the children to be tested. Curran explained that she did not want the twins to suffer the pain of having the marrow extracted or to be subjected to the risk involved. General anesthesia carries a risk of death in 1 in 10,000 cases and of complications in about 1 in 300 cases.

Bosze's paternity had been established in a suit by Curran seeking child support. The blood tests showed that the twins matched Jean-Pierre in two of the six factors considered basic for compatibility.

"Strangers are calling up to offer bone marrow and blood, and she won't help," Bosze said. He decided to file suit to force Curran to allow the twins to be tested.

"I don't feel that I'm killing this boy," Curran said. "I could be killing my own children if I let this happen."

On September 28, 1990, the Illinois Supreme Court ruled that the mother of the twins could not be compelled to permit them to be tested as potential bone marrow donors for Jean-Pierre. Jean-Pierre Bosze died early in 1991.

1. The court offered no reasons for its decision. What grounds might be offered?

2. Might a utilitarian argue that the twins should be tested, because the slight risk it poses to them is offset by the potentially great advantage to Jean-Pierre?

3. Would putting the twins at any risk to provide benefit to someone else violate the Kantian notion that it is wrong to treat persons as a means only?

4. What reasons might be presented in favor of a national policy of testing that would make virtually every citizen a potential organ donor? What might be said in criticism of such a policy?

Decision Scenario 7 •

"My client asked me not to tell you his name, but he did want me to be perfectly explicit about everything else," Consuelo Cortez said. "He's married and has two children, but he also suffers from Parkinson's disease. His doctors think that a transplant of fetal cells has a good chance of stopping or at least slowing the progress of his disease."

"He wants me to get pregnant," Alice Williams said, cutting into the other woman's explanation.

"Well, yes," Cortez said. "He wants you to get pregnant and then have an abortion at a time the doctors think best. My client will then become owner of the fetal tissue, and it will be used to treat him."

"Who does he want me to become pregnant with?"

"That's entirely up to you. I think you should work this out with your husband. If he doesn't want to make you pregnant, then artificial insemination is always a possibility."

"Twenty thousand and expenses?" Williams asked.

"Five thousand when you get pregnant, and the rest of the money when my client receives the tissue."

"But would I be doing something wrong?" Williams asked.

1. Apart from the issue of abortion, is there anything inherently wrong in selling fetal tissue?

2. If the tissue were going to be donated to someone in

need, would this change the moral character of the act?

3. Suppose that abortion was not involved and the tissue in question was from miscarriages. Would it be wrong to sell this tissue?

4. Why does Robertson think that the issue of conception with the aim of having an abortion to obtain fetal tissue is more morally complicated than is usually recognized?

5. If Williams is already pregnant and planning to have an abortion, would it necessarily be wrong, according to Robertson, to employ the fetal tissue in a medical treatment? How does he answer the charge that to do so would be to encourage abortion and contribute to its entrenchment as a social practice?

CHAPTER 10

THE CLAIM TO HEALTH CARE

CASE PRESENTATION
Drawing the Line in Oregon: Rationing Health Care

A new law took effect in Oregon in June 1988: No longer would the state pay for heart, liver, pancreas, or bone marrow transplants for the poor.

States typically pay 25–40% of the $100,000 to $200,000 cost of a transplant under the Medicaid program for the poor, and the federal government pays the rest. However, no one is eligible for federal funds until the state has agreed to pay its share. Oregon decided to use the $1.1 million it annually spent on organ transplants to increase the funding for prenatal care, a program it believed would provide more health benefits.

A consequence of this decision was immediately obvious. Oregon residents began seeing posters with photographs of children needing organ transplants. The children's parents, unable to get support from the state and unable to pay the bills themselves, were desperately trying to keep their children alive by raising enough money from donations to meet the enormous costs of transplants.

Coby Howard, a seven-year-old boy, was the first to appear on a poster. He needed $100,000 for a bone marrow transplant, but before the last $30,000 could be raised he died.

Donna Arnason and her fourteen-year-old son were luckier. Through their "Save a Mom" campaign, they were able to raise all of the $100,000 needed for a liver transplant.

At least five states have followed Oregon's lead in eliminating or restricting payments for transplants. So individuals who are poor and live in the wrong state cannot get organ transplants for themselves or their children. However, even in states that pay a share of transplant costs, people who lack the proper kind of insurance, do not qualify for Medicaid, or are unable to afford the cost may also not be able to secure most organ transplants.

Oregon is in the process of taking the lead in another and even more far-reaching respect. The transplant issue convinced some in the Oregon legislature that it made little sense to consider the relative value of the money spent on transplants without going on to consider the relative value of other medical services. As a result, Oregon has thus become the first state to develop a plan for rationing health care for the poor.

Oregon's problems in financing and distributing health care are not significantly different from those in other states. The legislature's decision to address the rationing question was influenced to a considerable extent by the public discussion of health-care issues promoted by a group called Oregon Health Decisions. The organization was founded in 1981 by psychiatrist Ralph Crawshaw to provide a forum for addressing the moral and economic issues in health care. The group's 1984 report, "Society Must Decide," played a major role in shaping the views of both citizens and legislators on matters of fairness in health care. The legislature's efforts to address issues of fairness in allotting state-funded medical services led to a program of establishing relative values to govern their distribution.

According to the Oregon plan, the legislature must decide who is eligible for Medicaid assistance and how much money it is going to allocate as the state contribution to the program. The money will then be spent in accordance with a list of priorities drawn up by the Oregon Medicaid Priority Executive Group. The group developed a formula to rank each procedure covered by Medicaid based on three factors: the cost of the procedure, the number of people who would be helped by it, and the length of time a patient would be healthy after treatment.

In effect, the group asked "How much health are we buying per dollar spent?" Medical procedures that provided a poor return on money invested were ranked lowest on the list.

The ranking system the group devised makes 10 the highest priority and 1 the lowest. A number of medical services may be ranked at the same level. When it comes to spending allotted money, this means that the demands for services at a given rank must be met before services at the next lowest rank are provided. In effect, then, a line will be drawn below which no services can be provided. This means that, although procedures like liver transplants were still on the list, since they were ranked 3, the chances were good that no money would be available to fund them.

Here is a selection from the original list. It is divided into the four main headings of Medicaid funding.

1. Reproductive Services

    Rank 10. Family Planning Services: Preconception counseling based on risk; Pregnancy testing; Reversible and irreversible methods of contraception; Genetic counseling and services; Termination of pregnancy; Prenatal Care; Prenatal visits; Counseling and education; Case management, including home visits, child care, regular exams, and outreach programs to achieve equitable access to care; Lab studies; Ultrasound, stress testing, biophysical profile, genetic counseling, amniocentesis, and, as appropriate, fetal maturity studies; Labor and Delivery Services in Certified Birth Settings; Uncomplicated vaginal and Caesarean-section births; Ectopic pregnancy; Electronic fetal monitoring; Fetal scalp sampling; Postpartum care; Pap test and pelvic exam; High-Risk Pregnancy Services; Home care services.

    Rank 3. Infertility Counseling and Workup Services

2. Health Promotion and Disease Prevention

    Rank 10. Immunizations; Nutritional Supplements; Providing food to hungry people whose poor nutrition makes them a significant health risk, meant as an addition to federal Women, Infant and Children program and food stamps. The age priority is: children and the elderly, adults. Screenings for Children from Birth to 2.

Rank 9. Periodic Focused Screening Based on Risk.

Rank 7. Periodic Screening for Other People, e.g., Pap smears, mammograms; Prevention and education programs in the following order: sexually transmitted diseases and teen parents; quitting smoking and alcohol and drug abuse; safety, suicide prevention, and physical and sexual abuse; and eating disorders.

3. Chronic Disease Management

    Rank 10. Procedures, Therapies, or Interventions That Can Restore Patients with Chronic Diseases to Near-Full or Manageable Levels of Function and Independence: Including cataract surgery, lens implants, or corneal transplants.

    Rank 9. Procedures, Therapies, or Interventions That Would Maintain Patients in the Least Restrictive and Most Appropriate Environment: Including therapy and clinical case management; education and training for primary care givers; provision of appropriate support services, for example, respite care, homemaker services, transport, child care, and delivery of medicine.

4. Acute Illnesses and Episodic Treatment

    Rank 10. Diagnosis and Treatment of Acute Illnesses, Conditions, and Episodes: In-hospital care, including intensive-care units; Emergency and trauma care; Anesthesia and surgery; Diagnostic and therapeutic radiology and nuclear medicine; Diagnostics, lab and pathology studies; Medications; Appropriate transport and transfer; Inpatient Admissions for Psychiatric Emergencies and Crises: Including incapacitating depression, attempted suicide, or suicidal tendencies or acute psychoses.

    Rank 9. Preventive Dentistry for Children; Restorative Dental Care for Adults Where Necessary for Nutrition; Occupational Therapy and Speech Therapy with Predictable Return of Functions; Eye Exams and Eyeglasses for Children and Elderly Every Two Years; Hearing Exams and Aids for Children and Elderly Every Three Years.

    Rank 8. Orthopedic Procedures for Replacement of Total Hip for Intractable Pain or Because of Absence of Mobility; Restorative Dentistry for Children's Permanent Teeth;

Routine Dental Care for the Elderly; Necessary Reconstructive Surgery.

Rank 7. Rehabilitation for Improvement of Function.

Rank 6. Therapy for Alcohol and Drug Abuse; Foot Care for Elderly.

Rank 5. Eye Exams and Glasses for Others Every Two Years; Hearing Exams and Aids for Others Every Three Years.

Rank 4. Routine Dental Care for Adults.

Rank 3. Organ Transplantation.

The list developed in accordance with the group's criteria gave priority to prenatal care, disease prevention, and the treatment of acute and chronic diseases. It gave low priority to dental procedures, plastic surgery, and infertility treatments. Age alone was not considered a reason to restrict access to a service, although the treatment of diseases and conditions affecting mostly the elderly was ranked much lower than that for younger people or women of childbearing age.

In February 1991 the Oregon Health Services Commission, responding to intense criticism, significantly revised its original rationing plan and produced a new ranked list. Conditions now receiving the highest benefit are infectious diseases (e.g., various types of pneumonia, tuberculosis) and acute disorders (e.g., peritonitis, appendicitis, ectopic pregnancy). Those given the lowest ranking are superficial wounds, benign conditions (e.g., kidney cysts), and untreatable disorders (e.g., chronic pancreatitis, terminal HIV disease, anencephaly). Organ transplants were moved from near the bottom of the list to around the middle.

The new list uses the same cost–benefit formula, but the final version was also based on polls, interviews with state citizens, and item-by-item votes by the eleven members of the Commission. "We realized that the initial formula did not take into account what people were telling us in public hearings and polls," one member said. Although the same principles were followed, common-sense judgment was used to modify the results of the formula, and many consider the new list to come much closer to capturing popular sentiment than did the original one.

John Kitzhaber, a physician and the president of the Oregon Senate, was a sponsor of the 1988 law that eliminated Medicaid payments for most transplants. He has also been one of the strongest proponents of the rationing plan. "Although we prefer not to recognize it, we do ration health care in this country," he says. "But that rationing is enormously inequitable and not based on any consistent social policy or sound clinical criteria."

Officials in Oregon say their concern is not only to find a rational and just way of distributing medical resources to the poor, but also to develop a model for health-care rationing that could be adopted by the federal government and insurance companies as ways of bringing health-care costs under control. Under Oregon's present Medicaid system, almost all medical services are available, but access is limited to only the poorest segment of the population. Under the proposed rationing scheme, officials estimate that the number of people eligible for Medicaid can be almost doubled.

Rationing systems have had several other advocates in recent years. Notably, Daniel Callahan in his book *Setting Limits* has argued for an age-based rationing of health-care costs. As our population ages, Callahan points out, it will produce an increasing demand for very expensive medical services, such as coronary-artery bypass surgery and organ transplants. The $80 billion spent for the care of older people in 1981 may rise to $200 billion by the end of the century.

Furthermore, when long-term care is needed in nursing homes or similar facilities, the money spent to care for the elderly reduces the amount available to Medicaid for other purposes. This reduction leads to a tightening of the eligibility requirements. Hence, large numbers of people who are young and poor are denied the medical care they need. Rationing care to the elderly, although providing different forms of care, would make available funds that could be used to care for younger people in need.

According to Callahan, the strain on the health-care system is also the result of our commitment to the development and use of high-technology devices and surgical procedures. He advocates that we more carefully review the social and economic consequences of medical technology before we attempt to develop it or make it available.

Not everyone sees rationing health care and placing limits on the development of medical technology as responses that are either necessary or desirable. A number of economists, in opposition to Callahan, say that a reduction in costs should be enough to postpone, if not eliminate, the need for rationing. For example, Alain Enthoven points to large numbers of inappropriate medical procedures (as many as one-third of coronary-artery bypass procedures) and unnecessary hospitalizations (as many as one-fourth) as evidence that health-care costs could be reduced by as much as a third.

Others claim that discouraging the development of high-technology care will, in the long run, work to the detriment of all. The use of medical imaging devices like the CT- and PET-scanners has eliminated the need for much of the expensive exploratory surgery of the past, made diagnoses more reliable, and so in general led to more appropriate and effective treatments. Those who initially opposed buying imaging devices for hospitals can now be shown to have been advocating a false economy. The technology of the future may turn out to be an even better bargain.

Finally, with respect to rationing plans like the one in Oregon, critics point out that the plans are inherently unfair. The rationing is not to everyone in the society but just to the poor—to those who must depend on Medicaid for their medical care.

Alameda County, California, which includes Oakland, felt itself so threatened by medical costs connected with AIDS and the problems of the urban poor that, when it learned of the Oregon rationing plan, it began to develop one of its own. "Decision making by default masks the reality of the choices that have to be made," the head of the county health department said.

After almost a year of meetings and discussions, a commission set up to devise a list of priorities similar to Oregon's turned in a report that declared the entire procedure "immoral." According to the report, the health-care needs of the poor people in Alameda County are so severe that no list could be established. All forms of care were essential.

Americans have mixed feelings about providing access to medical care. They want every sick or suffering person to have access to every treatment that will help, but they don't want to pay for it. This ambivalent attitude is borne out by statistical surveys. According to a 1987 Harris poll, 91% of Americans agreed with the statement that "everybody should have the right to get the best possible health care—as good as the treatment a millionaire gets."

Similarly, in a survey by the Public Agenda Foundation, a strong majority said they would support a federal plan to provide catastrophic health coverage for everyone, even if it costs $10 billion a year. However, when people were asked if they would be willing to pay $125 a year more in taxes tỏ support this universal coverage, 90% said they would not.

Oregon's list of priorities was supposed to have been submitted to the legislature in June of 1990. However, claims that many of the rankings were based on inadequate or incorrect information resulted in a postponement of its legislative consideration until a revision could be made. The Oregon Health Services Commission now plans to reconsider the details of more than 1,600 procedures to decide where they should be placed on the list. If rationing goes into effect at all, no one expects it to happen before 1992.

Discussions of rationing health care are just now beginning in earnest. In the years ahead, the issues are likely to provoke public and political debates as serious and acrimonious as those surrounding abortion. Should the poor quietly accept a state of affairs in which their children go without liver transplants while the children of the rich and the middle class have their lives prolonged?

Susan McGee, Coby Howard's aunt, remembers his final days with anger and regret. "In his last few weeks, the family spent every minute trying to raise funds," she said. "We are bitter that we had to market Coby Howard so that the public would want to save his life."

Can we continue to tolerate circumstances that make such responses necessary? Do we want our society to be one in which poor children must beg to raise money to pay for the only surgery that may save their lives? If not, are we willing to make the changes and sacrifices necessary to keep this from happening?

SOCIAL CONTEXT: THE CONTINUING CRISIS IN HEALTH CARE

A crisis exists in a social institution when there are factors present that tend to destroy the institution or render it ineffective in achieving its goals. Two major factors have led observers to say that the American health-care system is in a state of crisis: the increasing cost to the society of health care and the failure to deliver health care to those who need it. We will examine each factor briefly and then consider some solutions that have been offered.

COST OF HEALTH CARE

After defense, health care is the most expensive item in the federal budget, and policy analysts have repeatedly issued strong warnings about the need to take measures to curb its rising cost.

In 1960 health expenditures in the United States amounted to some $27 billion; in 1970 they were up to $75 billion, and in 1983 they increased to $356 billion. By 1989, the last year for which complete figures are available, spending had climbed to an incredible $600 billion. This represents an expenditure of $1,926 per capita, compared to the 1960 figure of $145. As a percentage of the gross national product (GNP), the cost of health care has more than doubled, from 5.3% to 11.5%.

Unless changes are made, future increases are expected to resemble past ones. Costs in 1990 are projected to be $690 billion, and those in the year 2000 are estimated to be $1.9 trillion. This amounts to an increase of expenditure to about $6,000 per capita.

Analysts see the spiraling costs of health care as threatening the economic welfare of the country. The almost $2,000 per person the United States spends on health costs is not matched by other industrialized nations. Japan spends less than half this amount and Great Britain about one-third. Because the United States spends such a large percentage of its GNP on health care, the costs of U.S. goods will be comparatively higher than those of other exporting nations. (Health-care expenditures contribute about 10% to the cost of a car.) Consequently, the United States will not be as effective a competitor in world trade and will be faced with an ever more serious balance-of-payments problem and with the loss of even more domestic industries.

Other serious problems are connected with increasing health-care costs. The Medicare system, which was established in 1965 to provide medical care for the elderly and the handicapped, turned out to cost much more than predicted, and some economists have predicted that, unless more effective ways are found to limit health costs, either the system will become bankrupt or far fewer people will be provided assistance.

Various explanations have been given for the spiraling costs of health care. Stanley Hwang suggests that one factor is the lack of financial accountability from those responsible for operating the health-care system. Most Americans are covered by employee group insurance that pays physicians and hospitals on a fee-for-service basis. The system serves to hide the cost of medical care from the consumer. Because the consumer gets a relatively unlimited number of medical services for a fixed premium, and because the premium itself is hidden in the form of payroll deductions, the consumer has no incentive to avoid unnecessary or expensive medical services. Physicians and hospitals have no incentive to trim costs because the consumer is not concerned, and insurers respond to rising costs by passing them on in the form of increased premiums. In such a situation, no one is forced to be concerned about costs.

This situation is changing, however. Employers, faced with 20–25% increases in group premiums, are passing along the costs to employees in noticeable ways. Higher deductibles and required co-payments now mean that a family of four can pay as much as $2,000 a year for ordinary care, about ten times the amount they would have paid ten years ago.

Apart from whatever flaws there may be in the way the health-care system operates, other factors having to do with a changing population and the state of medicine itself are no doubt responsible to some extent for increasing costs. Here are three of them:

- As children born during the baby boom of the 1940s have reached adulthood, the median age of the population has increased. An aging population requires more medical care and more expensive medical care than a population with a lower median age.

- Improvements in medical technology now make it possible to provide a greater number of services to hospitalized patients. This also means that more people are likely to be hospitalized in order to receive the services.

- Improvements in medicine now make it possible to provide therapies for illnesses that once would not have been treated. The very availability of such treatments means increases in the hospital population, and the very success of such treatments means that more people will be alive who can benefit from additional care.

Such considerations as these have persuaded nearly everyone concerned with the formulation and implementation of health-care policies that the current state of affairs needs to be changed. A general belief is that, if matters are not altered, the health-care system will become so economically unrealistic that it will collapse.

HEALTH-CARE DELIVERY

Despite the great economic investment in health care, the U.S. medical system has a great many shortcomings. Some studies show that more than 10% of the population receives no care at all and that more than 4 million people in need of care do not get it. Furthermore, the life expectancy in the United States is 75 years, which puts it about in the middle of the range for industrialized countries, all of which spend less money for medical care. Similarly, the infant mortality rate in the United States is much higher than for other industri-

alized countries: 11 deaths per 1,000, compared to 7 in Canada and 9 in Great Britain.

Although efforts over the past two decades have improved access to health care for low-income and minority groups, a significant portion of the population is still not receiving needed care. The situation seems to be growing worse. The tightening of federal and state regulations determining eligibility for Medicaid and Medicare has led to a sharp decline in the percentage of poor people receiving benefits.

Furthermore, according to a Census Bureau survey, the number of people without medical insurance has reached 31.1 million, up from 29 million in 1979. (Some consider the real figure closer to 37 million.) Half of those without insurance are children or families with children. Thus, millions of Americans are unable to pay the expenses that accompany serious illness or injury. This result is partly due to the loss of jobs in industries that provided insurance coverage for their workers and to the rise in part-time jobs in companies that offer no health insurance. The "working poor" often find that they make too much money to be eligible for the increasingly stringent requirements of Medicaid, yet they make too little money to buy health insurance after they have paid for rent and housing. The increased number of people with AIDS or with chronic diseases who are rejected by insurance companies has also contributed to the number of uninsured. Furthermore, insurance companies have been accused of blacklisting groups of workers and denying them coverage. Bartenders, dentists, AIDS workers, gas-station attendants, and oil drillers are a few of the more than forty occupational groups declared uninsurable.

The loss of the ability to pay for medical care by low-income people has put great stress on university and public hospitals that have traditionally provided care for the indigent. Historically, these hospitals have recouped the cost of caring for the poor by cost shifting— that is, by charging higher rates to those who can afford to pay or who have an insurer that will pay. However, increasing costs have made the federal government, health maintenance organizations, business groups with insurance programs, and private insurance companies balk at paying inflated rates for their patients. The private organizations are concerned with increasing their profits, and they reject the idea that they should, directly or indirectly, subsidize medical care for the poor.

Recent studies show that, when uninsured people are admitted to hospitals, they are discharged earlier and receive fewer diagnostic and therapeutic procedures than those who have insurance. Some see results of this kind as evidence that the United States has already moved to a two-tier medical system in which the poor are provided with second-class care, while those able to pay receive the best care available.

The failure of the current medical system to supply an adequate level of health care (a "decent minimum," as it is often phrased) to everyone in the society in need of it is a major force behind recent efforts to establish some version of a national health plan. We need such a plan, advocates say, because we now live with a system offering two kinds of medicine—one for the rich and one for the poor. And it too often happens that the medicine for the poor is none at all.

POSSIBLE SOLUTIONS AND ACTUAL PROBLEMS

Recent analyses of public-opinion polls reveal that Americans hold inconsistent attitudes about health-care costs. In particular:

- Increasing costs are regarded by both the public and elected officials as the major problem in health care. Yet the problem does not appear in rankings of the top ten problems facing the country. People report that they are deeply disturbed by the rising cost of health care, yet they are not disturbed by the proportion of the economy devoted to it. Most respondents believe we spend too little on health care, rather than too much.

- Most people are unwilling to give up their own physicians, but they favor requiring low-income people to use HMOs (see below) or clinics.

- Most people say they believe that present health-care arrangements are not satisfactory, yet they are not prepared to endorse basic changes in the health-care system.

- An overwhelming majority (91%) of people favor a national plan to provide care for everyone in need, yet almost the same majority does not favor even a rather modest tax increase to make it possible.

Policy analysts point out that public opinion is only one of the many factors that influence health-care policy. However, as they also note, there are practical and political limits on the changes that will be accepted by the society. Mostly, people are unwilling to see any changes that would produce a major alteration in the way they currently arrange for their own medical care. However, people are willing to approve of a variety of cost-containment programs that would make a cumulative difference in slowing or halting the increase in costs.

In fact, recent changes in the ways in which health care is paid for have not been ones requiring a major restructuring of social arrangements, and they have mostly been accepted without complaint by the public.

Medicare and Diagnosis Related Groups (DRGs)

In 1983 about $60 billion was spent under the Medicare program to provide medical services for the elderly. In 1970 its cost was $7.5 billion. To attempt to gain control over escalating costs, in 1983 Congress mandated that the Department of Health and Human Services put into operation a plan for paying hospitals a predetermined price for each Medicare patient. At the heart of this "prospective payment plan" are the Diagnosis Related Groups (DRGs) that determine the price Medicare will pay for a service.

The DRGs consist of 468 categories, and associated with each is an index number representing the relative number of medical resources required to treat a patient with that diagnosis. The patient's diagnosis at the time of discharge from the hospital (the patient's DRG) determines the payment the hospital will receive. The actual payment is calculated by multiplying the index number by the average dollar cost per patient at hospitals within the geographical region.

If the actual cost of treating a patient exceeds the DRG-determined price by more than 150%, Medicare will consider the patient a statistical "outlier" and pay 60% of the costs above the 150%. In such a case, the hospital must take a loss amounting to the difference between 100% and 150% plus 40% of the amount above 150%.

Under the traditional "retrospective payment" plan, hospitals were simply reimbursed for the actual cost of treating a Medicare patient. Neither the patient nor the hospital had an incentive to control costs, and the DRG plan was intended to introduce a motive for cost containment. If hospital costs are higher than the DRG amount, the hospital will lose money. However, if the costs are lower, the hospital still will receive the allowable amount.

In the long run, however, hospitals cannot gain from reducing their costs. If they lower their overall costs to make up the difference in those cases in which the actual costs of treating Medicare patients are not fully paid for by the DRG amounts, they will lower the average cost per patient in their region. An annual review of regional rates will reflect this, and the next year's DRG payments will be smaller. Hospitals are thus forced to cut costs, but they are not rewarded for it.

When the prospective payment plan was introduced, critics argued that the elderly, who are the great majority of Medicare recipients, might not be provided with the highest quality care. Hospitals would be tempted to spend no more in caring for a Medicare patient than they could expect to be reimbursed for. Thus, relevant laboratory tests and treatments might not be offered. Given an option, hospitals might choose the least expensive methods, supplies, and devices. (Hip-replacement joints might come in deluxe and Medicare models.) Thus, critics said, people who can afford to pay for the best of care will get it, while those wholly dependent on Medicare may not.

From the perspective of several years' experience with DRGs, analysts now have a sense of whether they have produced the results intended while avoiding the problems feared. The outcome has been viewed generally as positive. A recent study of 14,000 Medicare patients in 297 hospitals in 30 geographical regions indicates that, overall, the prospective payment system has been successful in controlling the costs of medical care and also meeting the health needs of the Medicare population.

Hospital stays are the most expensive item in the medical-care budget, and DRGs cut the length of stays in short-term hospitals from 10 days in 1963 to 8.5 days in 1989. The study showed a 1.1% drop in death rates from the five most serious diseases covered by the program in the 30 days after admission, the period when most deaths occur. Overall, hospital stays declined from 14.4 days to 11 days, a difference of 24%, and some decline took place for each of the diseases.

The quality of care was also considered. An examination of patient records suggested that physicians and other health-care workers seemed to be providing better physical examinations, diagnostic testing, and treatment. The percentage of patients receiving care that was described as "poor or very poor" declined from 25% to 12%. Despite this decline, 30% of the patients were judged to have received very poor care, and their death rate during the 30 days after admission was 17% higher than for patients who received "very good" care.

On the negative side, the study showed that the DRG system makes it more likely that a patient will be discharged from the hospital in a medically unstable condition. The percentage rose from 10.3% to 17%. Early discharge can have grave consequences, and those discharged "quicker and sicker" were 50% more likely to die within 90 days than those who were medically stable. This slowed the trend toward improved survival rates as a result of care given during hospitalization, but it did not reverse it.

Many private insurers and group health organizations have followed the lead of Medicare and adopted prospective payment plans. Thus it is reasonable to expect that in the future virtually all health care in the United States will be under the control of DRGs.

This prospect makes it especially important to keep in mind that, although early experience with DRGs is somewhat encouraging, not all aspects of the program have been studied, nor are all aspects studied satisfactory. The program should be subjected to a constant and critical review to find ways to eliminate or reduce its actual shortcomings and potential hazards. If we do not monitor the program and correct its failures, there is a risk that the entire medical system will decline in both the quantity and quality of service it can provide.

Physicians' Fee Schedule

In 1989 Congress directed the Department of Health and Human Services to establish a national fee schedule for physicians providing services to Medicare patients. The schedule is supposed to be based an a "relative value scale" that considers a physician's time, overhead, and insurance costs in setting fees. The final version of the plan is supposed to be in operation by January 1, 1992. The schedule will cover about 1,400 commonly performed medical procedures, and it is intended to control physicians' fees the way DRG schedules have controlled hospital costs.

The fee system involves "value units" based on time, overhead, and insurance costs. These units are then multiplied by a conversion factor to determine a dollar amount. For example, a comprehensive examination is worth 61.8 points: 35.9 (physician's time) + 22.9 (overhead) + 3 (malpractice insurance). In comparison, a CT-scan of the abdomen is worth 220.9 points: 57.6 (time) + 146.9 (overhead/equipment) + 16.4 (insurance).

The 1,400 procedures with already assigned values represent about two-thirds of the money spent yearly by Medicare. The number of procedures to be added to the list is expected to bring the total to around 7,000.

Medicare began by paying considered "current and prevailing" fees, but this practice had two objectionable consequences. First, it perpetuated the fee disparities existing among medical specialties and geographical regions. Second, the system was inherently inflationary: when fees were raised by increasing the customary rates, Medicare payments had to be raised to match them.

Physicians' fees were frozen by Medicare in 1984, and, as inflation continued, physicians treating Medicare patients began to get only 25–30% of amounts billed. Physicians could accept that amount or ask patients for the rest. Patients with "medi-gap" insurance could pay, but others had to find physicians willing to accept the Medicare amount as full payment. Consequently, to avoid a situation that worked a hardship on both patients and physicians, many physicians are pleased to see Medicare alter the way they are reimbursed for their services.

Also, physicians in some specialties will benefit by the adoption of the fee schedules. Studies show that surgeons, in particular, are overpaid in comparison with those in other medical specialties. Fee schedules are likely to raise the rates for those in internal medicine, pediatrics, and family practice.

As of January 1991, physicians who do not accept Medicare payments as full compensation for services are not allowed to charge more than an additional 25%. In 1992, the amount will be limited to 20%; in 1993 the limit will be 15%. Some states, such as New York, have already placed restrictions on the amounts allowable above Medicare figures.

This is seen as a significant step in controlling medical costs, but medical groups have not welcomed this new policy. Some have claimed that it is a form of price fixing that is unfairly applied to physicians. Others claim that it may lead to a decline in medical care for those receiving Medicare. Physicians may avoid accepting Medicare patients or will tend to build their practices in areas in which there are few such patients. The elderly, particularly the elderly poor, will be underserved. Although no physician's organization says so, it is also possible to imagine Medicare patients receiving less attention from their physicians than full-paying patients.

Mandated fee schedules give rise to some of the same fears of compromised quality of care as DRG-based hospital payments. It may be possible to control costs through fee schedules, but whether doing so will compromise the strengths of the present medical system to an unacceptable degree remains open.

Health-Care Organizations

In the last fifteen years, the United States has moved away from group health insurance and toward establishing health maintenance organizations (HMOs). An HMO is a medical plan in which an individual pays a fixed annual fee to an organized group of physicians. The group then undertakes to supply the individual with most kinds of needed medical services, at no additional charge.

HMOs hold out the possibility of lowered medical costs. They avoid unnecessary tests and procedures because the profit of the group is determined by the money remaining after the expenses of patients have been paid. Better patient care may result, because the HMO encourages patients to consult a physician at the beginning of an illness rather than waiting until it grows serious.

In a variation on the HMO concept, some businesses and unions have established contracts with physicians to provide medical services for their employees or members. These Preferred Provider Organizations (PPOs) have the advantage of allowing individuals to choose their physicians from a list of those who have entered into the arrangement. In this way a major complaint against HMOs—that the individual is required to receive care from a group and has no physician of his or her own—is avoided.

HMOs and PPOs have made a contribution to reducing health-care costs. To some extent, however, this result has been achieved by providing less than a full range of services. As businesses and other contracting groups begin to demand more services for their members, the cost of providing them will rise. Organizations that have attracted clients by setting their prices too low have been forced out of business by the increasing costs of medical equipment, supplies, and personnel.

Critics have also pointed out that health-care organizations have inherent weaknesses. The possibility that managers will encourage physicians to provide inferior care in order to maximize profits is very real. Furthermore, patients may be dissatisfied with the care they receive, for physicians are empowered to turn down their requests for medical services if the physician believes they are unnecessary.

It is still too early to tell how successful health-care organizations will be in providing high-quality care at a reasonable price. However, experiences in California suggest that such organizations can work very well. The Kaiser plan, which was started in 1945, owns 23 hospitals and 158 clinics and has 20% of the residents of the San Francisco area as members. Over 6 million people in California are members of either the Kaiser plan or the Ross-Loos plan. In the view of some analysts, health-care organizations offer the best approach to providing national health insurance that attempts to meet the medical needs of all citizens.

Alternative Solutions

Some have argued that more radical solutions to the health-care problems of the United States are required than would be provided by health-care organizations, employee-option insurance, or particular cost-containment policies. Some claim that the entire medical-delivery system of the country needs to be totally altered. Only then, they say, can costs be controlled, medical needs met, and justice done. The following are among the many recommendations that have been made:

- Issue health stamps to those whose income shows them to be in need. Health-stamp recipients could then shop around for medical services. This would introduce an element of competition among health-care providers and lead to a reduction in costs.

- Place all pharmaceutical and medical equipment manufacturers under public ownership. By eliminating excessive profits, the costs of drugs and equipment would come closer to reflecting their true development and production costs.

- Eliminate all fee-for-service transactions between physicians and patients, and remove the profit motive from health care.

- Introduce rationing of health care, and apply the restrictions to everyone. Make considerations of age and possible benefit relevant criteria. Also, rank medical procedures by their cost and expected benefit, and fund only those with the best ratios. This would emphasize prevention and primary care and eliminate expensive operations (like most organ transplants) that cost a lot and benefit few.

(See the Case Presentation for a discussion of Oregon's plan.)

- Require that everyone pay premiums for a national health insurance program, but allow claims beyond a certain limit only by those who cannot afford to pay. (See the next Social Context for a discussion of comprehensive health plans.)

Not all of these proposals are equally sound, of course. Some are politically and socially unrealistic at the present time. They are suggestive, however, and they do provide alternative views about how a system that is almost universally regarded as dangerously unworkable might be modified. That such proposals should now be at the focus of national debate is itself evidence that the health-care system is indeed in crisis.

SOCIAL CONTEXT: A COMPREHENSIVE HEALTH-CARE PROGRAM FOR THE UNITED STATES ON THE CANADIAN MODEL?

"Socialized medicine" was the phrase once used to condemn plans to provide comprehensive medical coverage for all U.S. citizens, regardless of their ability to pay. The label suggested something like political heresy. How could a capitalist society adopt a plan exempting medical care from the rules of the market economy? Medical care, like house painting, was a service one could purchase from a provider for an agreed-upon fee. The physician-provider, like the painter-provider, was an independent economic agent, and to suggest otherwise would be to recommend the practice of socialism.

Of course, those unable to pay a physician's fee would have to do without the service. A charitable organization or benevolent physician might provide treatment for some individuals truly in need. This wasn't something to be counted on, and in neither case was need a basis for demanding the service. Clearly, just as you couldn't expect a painter to paint your house without payment, you couldn't expect a physician to provide you with medical care for nothing. Nor did anyone expect the government to pick up the bill. The role of the government in a market economy is not to provide some citizens with free goods or services, whether they be painting their houses or providing them with medical care.

For decades this view dominated public discussions about national health programs. Critics of a proposed program hardly had to do more than apply the label "socialized medicine" to bring discussion to a close. Then attitudes began to change for a complex of reasons, including the spiraling cost of health care, the increasing power of medical intervention, and the growing number of citizens needing care but lacking insurance.

The introduction of the Medicare program in 1965 provided care to millions of elderly people, many of whom would have received no medical assistance at all. Medicaid played a similar role in the lives of those whose low income qualified them for help. These two programs, along with private insurance, group health plans, and health maintenance organizations, now provide medical help to the great majority of people in the society.

Still, the very success of this combination of programs casts into sharp relief the plight of those lacking insurance and unable to pay for even basic medical care. The number of people in this predicament is estimated at 31 to 37 million, and this group grows at a rate of a million per year. An awareness of so many people in need may have been a factor prompting 60% of the respondents in a 1988 survey to say that "fundamental changes are needed to make the American health-care system work better." In another survey, 75% said they were in favor of the government's establishing a national health system.

The general public is not alone in its belief that a change is needed. Executives in the au-

tomobile industry, in particular, faced with paying out $5 billion in employee medical costs, have suggested that efforts to control costs in the private fee-for-service medical system have not been successful enough, and some are calling for a program of national health insurance.

THE BIPARTISAN COMMISSION ON COMPREHENSIVE HEALTH CARE

In response to the demands of various groups, in 1988 Congress established the Bipartisan Commission on Comprehensive Health Care. In March 1990, the Commission recommended that Congress pass legislation establishing a program to provide health insurance and long-term nursing care to any American needing them.

The insurance program would be a public/private partnership that would include some government insurance, but it would also require businesses to provide coverage for their employees. Thus, there would continue to be a role for private health-insurance industry. The program combining public with private insurance would be designed so that every person, employed or not, would have some form of medical coverage. The Commission also recommended that the insurance industry be prohibited from blacklisting groups and refusing to sell policies to people with health problems.

Nursing-home coverage would also be expanded in the Commission's plan. Anyone of any age who is "severely disabled" and individuals with assets of less than $30,000 (or, if married, with joint assets twice this amount) would receive three months of free care. At present, only the elderly qualify for nursing-home care, and they must pay for a percentage of it. If they need more than 100 days of care, they must divest themselves of their assets to pay for it. When they have less than $2,000, they then qualify for Medicaid. The Commission's plan would help with, though not eliminate, the present difficulty faced by spouses who must impoverish themselves to provide care for husbands or wives.

The proposals would cost $86.2 billion to implement, and the Commission made no suggestions about how the money might be raised. Since the proposals would leave the fee-for-service system intact, they were praised by the American Medical Association as making "the American people the real winners." But, because of the restrictions that would be placed on the insurance industry, the Health Insurance Association of America called them "an economic disaster." Other critics thought the plan offered an improvement over the present system, even though the changes it would introduce were not sufficiently far-reaching.

The Commission had considered introducing a health-care plan resembling the system currently in effect in Canada. That they did not was primarily due (according to a staff member), to the opposition they knew could be expected from the health providers, "physicians in particular." However, many in the United States still consider the Canadian system a model for what the American system should become.

THE CANADIAN HEALTH-CARE SYSTEM

Canada established universal health insurance coverage in 1971. It did not nationalize hospitals or make physicians government employees, as did Great Britain. Rather, it eliminated most forms of private medical insurance and enrolled citizens in a government plan administered by the ten provinces.

Every Canadian citizen is guaranteed access to a physician, and he may see any primary-care physician he chooses. If hospitalization, testing, or surgery is necessary, then the government insurance plan will pay for it without any direct cost to the patient. The medical program has become highly popular with Canadian citizens. In one survey, 7 out of 10 said they receive good or excellent care, and 9 out of 10 said the health-care system "is one of the things that makes Canada the best country in the world in which to live." Various objective measures of health care show that the system is successful. The infant mortality rate of 9.6 per 1,000 live births is superior to the U.S. rate of 12.6, and the Canadian life-expectancy rate is higher than that of the United States.

Cost control also has been successful under the plan. Before 1971, the United States and Canada spent about the same percentage of their GNP on health care; since the introduction of the new system, Canada spends 9%, while the United States spends almost 12%. This aspect of the system has appealed strongly to legislators, manufacturing executives, and union leaders.

Canadian physicians were initially bitterly opposed to the universal health-care system. Many now approve of it, though, for it has turned out to have aspects they like. Although they cannot charge as much as physicians in the United States, they need not contend with the paperwork burden. Nor do they have to argue with insurance representatives who challenge their judgment about a needed medical service.

Physicians' fees in the United States are 2.4 times Canadian fees. However, Canadian physicians have incomes equal to two-thirds those of U.S. physicians. The reason the incomes are not lower is that Canadian physicians see more patients.

The system has negative aspects, however. One of the ways in which costs are kept down is by restricting investment in high-cost medical technology. The United States has 1,500 cardiac catheterization labs (166 people per unit), while Canada has 31 (816 people per unit). Canada has 12 magnetic resonance imagers (2,108 people per unit), while the United States has 1,375 (182 people per unit). Similarly, Canada has increased the number of general practitioners and pediatricians, but it has cut back the number of people in medical specialties. Canada has only 11 heart-surgery units, while the United States has 793.

The strength of the Canadian system is its emphasis on basic care and prevention. Its weakness is the restricted access it permits to specialized care, equipment, and procedures. Patients may have to wait from three to six months for heart surgery, a hip replacement, or a bed in a cancer unit. Care is not explicitly rationed, but it is organized so that those with a greater need are given higher priorities.

Would the centralized Canadian system work in the United States? Many observers who know both systems well express doubts. According to economist Victor Fuchs:

> There is reason to doubt that the quality of our civil services is up to the quality of the Canadian civil services. There is also reason to question whether the organization and degree of discipline in the [medical] profession is as strong as in Canada. We are very much individualists, and that includes physicians.

Similar doubts have been expressed by David Woods, who sees the different systems of health care as expressions of "national character." "Canada's system is a centralized public enterprise, cautious and based upon ingrained notions (or delusions) of egalitarianism. America's system is decentralized, market-driven, entrepreneurial, and with 37 million citizens uninsured by it, certainly unequal in terms of access." Further, the fact that access to specialized care and technology is highly restricted in the Canadian system is something that Americans would find particularly galling. Moreover, Canada has indicated a greater willingness to pay much higher taxes, both explicit and hidden, to guarantee universal access than has the United States.

Finally, John Iglehart, in a study of the Canadian system published in the *New En-gland Journal of Medicine,* suggests that all is not as well with the system as may seem from the outside:

> Canada's Health Insurance Program resembles a pressure cooker that is building up steam on a hot stove. The federal government is reducing its financial commitment, the supply of physicians is increasing, and the physical plants of many Canadian hospitals— particularly the teaching institutions—are nearing obsolescence.

Does this mean that the present health-care system in the United States is the way it should be? No one believes this. What remains unclear to all is how the virtues of the system can be preserved, the cost controlled, and access to medical care expanded to include all who need it.

INTRODUCTION

It has been estimated that it was not until the middle 1930s that the intervention of a physician in the treatment of an illness was likely to affect the outcome in a substantial way. The change was brought about by the discovery and development of antibiotic agents such as penicillin and sulfa drugs. They made it possible, for the first time, both to control infection and to provide specific remedies for a variety of diseases. Additional advances in treatment modalities, procedures, and technology have helped establish contemporary medicine as an effective enterprise.

Before these dramatic changes occurred, there was little reason for anyone to be particularly concerned with the question of the distribution of medical care within society. The situation in the United States has altered significantly, and a number of writers have recently argued that everyone ought to be guaranteed at least some form of medical care.

In part this is a reflection of the increased effectiveness of contemporary medicine, but it is also no doubt due to a growing awareness of the serious difficulties faced by disadvantaged groups within society.

In the last chapter we discussed one aspect of the problem of the distribution of medical resources—that of allocating limited resources among competing individuals in a particular situation. Here we need to call attention to some of the broader social issues. These are ones that transcend moral decisions about particular people and raise questions about the basic aims and obligations of society.

A great number of observers believe that the United States is currently faced with a health-care crisis. Some of the reasons supporting this belief, as well as some proposed solutions, are outlined in the Social Context parts of this chapter, and we need not repeat them here. But one element of the crisis is often said to be the lack of any program to provide health care for everyone in the society. That there should be people forced to do without needed health care for primarily financial reasons has seemed to some a morally intolerable state of affairs.

This point of view has frequently been based on the claim that everyone has a *right* to health care. Thus, it has been argued, society has a duty to provide that care; if it does not, then it is sanctioning a situation that is inherently wrong. To remedy the situation requires redesigning the health-care system and present practices to see to it that all who need and want health care have access to it.

The language of "rights" is very slippery. To understand and evaluate arguments that involve claiming (or denying) rights to health care, it is important to understand the nature of the claim. The word "rights" is used in several distinct ways, and a failure to be clear about the use in any given case leads only to unproductive confusion.

The following distinctions may help capture some of the more important sorts of things that people have in mind when they talk about rights.

CLAIM-RIGHTS, LEGAL RIGHTS, AND STATUTORY RIGHTS

Suppose I own a copy of the book *Anne of Green Gables*. If so, then I may be said to have a right to do with the book whatever I choose. Other people may be said to have a duty to recognize my right in appropriate ways. Thus, if I want to read the book, burn it, or sell it, others have a duty not to interfere with me. If I lend the book to someone, then he or she has a duty to return it.

It is generally agreed in the philosophy of law that a claim-right to something serves as a ground for other people's duties. A *claim-right*, then, always entails a duty or duties on the part of someone else. Right and duty thus go together like parent and child—one is not possible without the other.

Generally speaking, *legal rights* are claim-rights. Someone has a legal right when someone else has a definable duty, and legal remedies are available when the duty is not performed. Either the person can be forced to perform the duty, or damages of some sort can be collected for failure to perform. If I pay someone to put a new roof on my house by a certain date, she has contracted a duty to perform the work we have agreed to. If the task is not performed, then I can turn to the legal system for enforcement or damages.

Statutory rights are claim-rights that are explicitly recognized in legal statutes or laws. They impose duties on certain classes of people under specified conditions. A hospital contractor, for example, has a duty to meet certain building codes. If he fails to meet them, he is liable to legal penalties. But not all legal rights are necessarily statutory rights. Such considerations as "customary and established practices" may sometimes implicitly involve a legally enforceable claim-right.

MORAL RIGHTS

Generally speaking, a *moral right* is one that is stated in or derived from the principles of a moral theory. More specifically, to say that someone has a moral right to certain goods or manner of treatment is to say that others have a moral duty to see to it that she receives what she has a right to. A moral right is a certain kind of claim-right. Here, though, the source of justification for the right and for the corresponding duty lies in moral principles and not in the laws or practices of a society.

According to Ross, for example, people have a right to expect benevolent treatment from others—we have a duty to treat other people benevolently. This is a right that is not recognized by our legal system. We may, if we wish, treat others in a harsh and unsympathetic manner and in doing so violate no law.

Of course, many rights and duties that are based upon the principles of moral theories are also embodied in our laws. Thus, to take Ross again as an example, we have a prima facie duty not to injure or kill anyone. This duty, along with its correlative right to be free from injury or death at the hands of another, is reflected in the body of statutory law and common law that deals with bodily harm done to others and with killing.

The relationship between ethical theories and the laws of a society is complicated and controversial. The fundamental question is always the extent to which laws should reflect or be based upon an ethical theory. In a society such as ours, it does not seem proper that an ethical theory accepted by only a part of the people should determine the laws that govern us all. It is for this reason that some object to laws regulating sexual activity, pornography, and abortion. These are considered best regarded as a part of personal morality.

At the same time, however, it seems that we must rely upon ethical theories as a basis for evaluating laws. Unless we are prepared to say that what is legal is, in itself, what is right, we must recognize the possibility of laws that are bad or unjust. But what makes a law bad? A possible answer is that a law is bad when it violates a right derived from the principles of an ethical theory. Similarly, both laws and social practices may be criticized for failing to recognize a moral right. A moral theory, then, can serve as the basis for a demand for the reform of laws and practices.

Clearly there is no sharp line separating the moral and the legal. Indeed, virtually all of the moral theories we discussed in the introductory chapter have been used by philosophers and other thinkers as the basis for principles applying to society as a whole. Within such frameworks as utilitarianism, natural law theory, and Rawls's theory of a just society, legal and social institutions are assigned roles and functions in accordance with more general moral principles.

POLITICAL RIGHTS

Not everyone attempts to justify claims to rights by referring such claims directly to a moral theory. Efforts are frequently made to provide justification by relying upon principles or commitments that are generally acknowledged as basic to our society. (Of course, to answer how these are justified may force us to invoke moral principles.) Our society, for example, is committed to individual autonomy and equality, among other values. It is by reference to commitments of this sort that we evaluate proposals and criticize practices.

From this point of view, to recognize health care as a right is to acknowledge it as a *political* right. This means showing that it is required by our political commitments or principles. Of course, this may also mean resolving any conflicts that may arise from other rights that also seem to be demanded by our principles. But this is a familiar state of affairs. We are all aware that the constitutional guarantee of freedom of speech, for example, is not absolute and unconditional. It can conflict with other rights or basic commitments, and we look to the courts to provide us with guidelines to resolve the conflicts.

With the distinctions that we have discussed in mind, let us return now to the question of a general right to health care. What can those who make such a claim be asserting?

Obviously everyone in our society is free to seek health care and, when the proper arrangements are made, to receive it. That is, health care is a service available in society, and people may avail themselves of it. At the same time, however, no physician or hospital has a duty to provide health care that is sought. The freedom to seek does not imply that others have a duty to provide what we seek.

There is not in our society a legally recognized claim-right to health care. Even if I am sick, no one has a legal duty to see to it that I receive treatment for my illness. (A few states, such as New York, do impose legal duties on physicians and hospitals to treat people faced with life-threatening emergencies. Even this is not generally the case, however.) I may request care, or I may attempt to persuade a physician that it is his or her moral duty to provide me with care. But I have no legal right to health care, and, if someone refuses to provide it, I cannot seek a legal remedy.

Of course, I may contract with a physician, clinic, or hospital for care, either in general or for a certain ailment. If I do this, then the other party acquires a legally enforceable duty to provide me the kind of care that we agreed upon. In this respect, contracting for health care is not relevantly different from contracting for a new roof on my house.

Those who assert that health care is a right cannot be regarded as merely making the obviously false claim that there is a legal right to care. Their claim, rather, must be interpreted as one of a moral or political sort. They might be taken as asserting something like "Everyone in the society *ought* to be entitled to health care, regardless of his or her financial condition."

Anyone making such a claim must be prepared to justify it by offering reasons and evidence in support of it. The ultimate source of the justification is most likely to be the principles of a moral theory. For example, Kant's principle that every person is of inherent and equal worth might be used to support the claim that every person has an equal right to medical care, simply by virtue of being a person.

Justification might also be offered in terms of principles that express the aims and commitments of the society. A society that endorses justice and equality, it might be argued, must be prepared to offer health care to all if it offers it to anyone.

However justification is offered, it is clear that to claim that health care is a right is to go beyond merely expressing an attitude. It is to say more than something like "Everyone would like to have health care" or "Everyone needs health care." It is true that the language of "rights" is frequently used in a rhetorical way to encourage us to recognize the wants and needs of people—or even other organisms, such as animals and trees. This is a perfectly legitimate way of talking. But, at bottom, to urge that something be considered a right is to make a claim requiring justification in terms of some set of legal, social, or moral principles.

Why not recognize health care for all as a right? Certainly virtually everyone would admit that in the abstract it would be a good thing. If this is so, then why should anyone wish to oppose it? Briefly stated, arguments against a right to health care are most frequently of two kinds.

First, those who subscribe to a position sometimes called "medical individualism" argue that to recognize a right to health care would have the consequence of violating the rights of physicians and other medical practitioners. Physicians, they claim, would be required to employ their intelligence, knowledge, and skills in a way dictated by society. Thus, physicians would be deprived of their autonomy and, in a very real sense, made slaves of the state.

Second, some writers have pointed out that, while it is possible to admit health care to the status of a right, we must also recognize that health care is just one social good among others. Education, transportation, housing, legal assistance, and so on are other goods that are also sought and needed by members of our society. It is impossible to admit all of these (and perhaps others) to the status of rights, for the society simply cannot afford to pay for them.

The first line of argument, medical individualism, fails to recognize that the health-care situation is perhaps best regarded as one in which there is a *conflict* of rights (between patients and providers) and not just one in which the rights of physicians are being restricted.

The second line of argument does not necessarily lead to the conclusion that we should not recognize a right to health care. It does serve to warn us that we must be very careful to specify just what sort of right—if any—we want to support. Do we want to claim, for example, that everyone has a right to a certain *minimum* of health care? Or do we want to claim that everyone has a right to *equal* health care (whatever anyone can get, everyone can demand)?

Furthermore, this line of argument warns us that we have to make decisions about what we, as a society, are willing to pay for. Would we, for example, be willing to give up all public support for education in order to use the money for health care? Probably not. But we might be willing to reduce the level of support for education in order to increase that for health care. Whatever we decide, we have to face up to the problem of distributing our limited resources. This is an issue that is obviously closely connected with what sort of right to health care (or, really, the right to what sort of health care) we are prepared to endorse.

None of the selections in this chapter attempt to provide detailed answers to the multitude of questions that swarm around the issues of a public health-care policy. Yet each of them calls attention to some of the fundamental issues of rights, values, and social goals that must be resolved before any practical policy can be accepted as legitimate. If we are to recognize a right to health care, then we must be clear about exactly what is involved in recognizing such a right. Are we prepared to offer only a "decent minimum"? Does justice require that we make available to all whatever is available to any? Are we prepared to restrict the wants of some people in order to satisfy the basic needs of all people?

The issues discussed in this chapter are of more than academic interest, and they concern more than just a handful of patients and physicians. How they are resolved will affect us all, both directly and indirectly, through the character of our society.

Social Justice and Equal Access to Health Care ⸺⸺⸺

Gene Outka

Gene Outka argues that concepts of justice that grant access to health care on the basis of personal merit, societal contribution, or market considerations all rely on factors that are not sufficiently relevant to the special nature of health care. Justice demands that we treat people differently only when there are relevant differences between them, and factors such as personal accomplishments, social merit, and income level are not relevant to health care.

Need, Outka claims, is the sole standard for determining who shall receive care. People who need health care are people who are ill, and being ill is the only relevant factor in determining access to care. However, because medical resources are finite, access may have to be restricted. Thus, the formal principle of justice as treating similar cases in a similar way becomes relevant. (See the discussion of this principle in the general introduction.)

Outka suggests that restrictions might be imposed by refusing to treat some categories of illness, by employing a procedure to select patients randomly, or by excluding some components of a comprehensive medical-care system. In any case, whatever services are available to some who need them would be available to all who need them. Thus, even with restrictions, the social goal of equal access would retain its authority.

I want to consider the following question. Is it possible to understand and to justify morally a societal goal that increasing numbers of people, including Americans, accept as normative? The goal is: the assurance of comprehensive health services for every person irrespective of income or geographic location. Indeed, the goal now has almost the status of a platitude. Currently in the United States politicians in various camps give it at least verbal endorsement.[1] I do not propose to examine the possible sociological determinants in this emergent consensus. I hope to show that whatever these determinants are, one may offer a plausible case in defense of the goal on reasonable grounds. To demonstrate why appeals to the goal get so successfully under our skins, I shall have recourse to a set of conceptions of social justice. Some of the standard conceptions, found in a number of writings on justice, will do.[2] By reflecting on them it seems to me a prima facie case can be established, namely, that every person in the entire resident population should have equal access to health care delivery.

The case is prima facie only. I wish to set aside as far as possible a related question which comes readily enough to mind. In the world of "suboptimal alternatives," with the constraints, for example, that impinge on the government as it makes decisions about resource allocation, what is one to say? What criteria should be employed? Paul Ramsey in *The Patient as Person* thinks that the large question of how to choose between medical and other societal priorities is "almost, if not altogether, incorrigible to

moral reasoning."[3] Whether it is or not is a matter that must be ignored for the present. One may simply observe in passing that choices are unavoidable nonetheless, as Ramsey acknowledges, even where the government allows them to be made by default, so that in some instances they are determined largely by which private pressure groups prove to be dominant. In any event, there is virtue in taking up one complicated question at a time, and we need to get the thrust of the case for equal access before us. It is enough to observe now that Americans attach an obviously high priority to organized health care. National health expenditures for the fiscal year 1972 were $83.4 billion.[4] Even if such an enormous sum is not entirely adequate, we may still ask: How are we to justify spending whatever we do in accordance as far as possible with the goal of equal access? The answer I propose involves distinguishing various conceptions of social justice and trying to show which of these apply or fail to apply to health care considerations. . . .

Which then among the standard conceptions of social justice appear to be particularly relevant or irrelevant? Let us consider the following five:

1. To each according to his merit or desert.
2. To each according to his societal contribution.
3. To each according to his contribution in satisfying whatever is freely desired by others in the open marketplace of supply and demand.
4. To each according to his needs.
5. Similar treatment for similar cases.

From the Journal of Religious Ethics, Vol. 2, no. 1 (Spring 1974), pp. 11–32. Reprinted by permission.

In general I shall argue that the first three of these are less relevant because of certain distinctive features that health crises possess. I shall focus on crises here not because I think preventive care is unimportant (the opposite is true), but because the crisis situation shows most clearly the special significance we attach to medical treatment as an institutionalized activity or social practice, and the basic purpose we suppose it to have.

To Each According to His Merit or Desert

Meritarian conceptions, above all perhaps, are grading ones: advantages are allocated in accordance with amounts of energy expended or kinds of results achieved. What is judged is particular conduct that distinguishes persons from one another and not only the fact that all the parties are human beings. Sometimes a competitive aspect looms large.

In certain contexts it is illuminating to distinguish between efforts and achievements. In the case of efforts one characteristically focuses on the individual: rewards are based on the pains one takes. Some have supposed, for example, that entry into the kingdom of heaven is linked more directly to energy displayed and fidelity shown than to successful results attained.

To assess achievements is to weigh actual performance and productive contributions. The academic prize is awarded to the student with the highest grade-point average, regardless of the amount of midnight oil he or she burned in preparing for the examinations. Sometimes we may exclaim, "It's just not fair," when person X writes a brilliant paper with little effort while we are forced to devote more time with less impressive results. But then our complaint may be directed against differences in innate ability and talent which no expenditure of effort altogether removes.

After the difference between effort and achievement, and related distinctions, have been acknowledged, what should be stressed is the general importance of meritarian or desert criteria in the thinking of most people about justice. These criteria may serve to illuminate a number of disputes about the justice of various practices and institutional arrangements in our society. It may help to explain, for instance, the resentment among the working class against the welfare system. However wrong-headed or self-deceptive the resentment often is, particularly when directed toward those who want to work but for various reasons beyond their control cannot, at its better moments it involves in effect an appeal to desert considerations. "Something for nothing" is repudiated as unjust; benefits should be proportional (or at least related) to costs; those who can make an effort should do so, whatever the degree of their training or significance of their contribution to society; and so on. So, too, persons deserve to have what they have labored for; unless they infringe on the works of others their efforts and achievements are justly theirs. . . .

. . . I would simply hold now (1) that the idea of justice is not exhaustively characterized by the notion of desert, even if one agrees that the latter plays an important role; and (2) that the notion of desert is especially ill suited to play an important role in the determination of policies that should govern a system of health care.

Why is it so ill suited? Here we encounter some of the distinctive features that health crises possess. Health crises seem nonmeritarian because they occur so often for reasons beyond our control or power to predict. They frequently fall without discrimination on the (according-to-merit) just and unjust, i.e., the virtuous and the wicked, the industrious and the slothful alike.

While we may believe that virtues and vices cannot depend upon natural contingencies, we are bound to admit, it seems, that many health crises do. It makes sense therefore to say that we are equal in being randomly susceptible to these crises. Even those who ascribe a prominent role to desert acknowledge that justice has also properly to do with pleas of "But I could not help it."[5] One seeks to distinguish such cases from those acknowledged to be praiseworthy or blameworthy. Then it seems unfair as well as unkind to discriminate among those who suffer health crises on the basis of their personal deserts. For it would be odd to maintain that a newborn child deserves his hemophilia or the tumor afflicting her spine.

These considerations help to explain why the following rough distinction is often made. Bernard Williams, for example, in his discussion of "equality in unequal circumstances," identifies two different sorts of inequality, inequality of merit and inequality of need, and two corresponding goods, those earned by effort and those demanded by need.[6] Medical treatment in the event of illness is located under the umbrella of need. He concludes: "Leaving aside preventive medicine, the proper ground of distribution of medical care is ill health: this is a necessary truth."[7] An irrational state of affairs is held to obtain if those whose needs are the same are treated unequally, when needs are the ground of the treatment. One might put the point this way. When people are equal in the relevant respects—in this case when their needs are the same and occur in a context of random, undeserved susceptibility—that by itself is a good reason for treating them equally.[8]

In many societies, however, a second necessary condition for the receipt of medical treatment exists de facto: the possession of money. This is not the place to consider the general question of when inequalities in health may be regarded as just. It is enough to note that one can plausibly appeal to all of the conceptions of justice we are embarked in sorting out. A person may be thought to be entitled to a higher income when he works more, contributes more, risks more, and not simply when he needs more. We may think it fair that the industrious should have more money than the slothful and the surgeon more than the tobacconist. The difficulty comes in the misfit between the reasons for differential incomes and the reasons for receiving medical treatment. The former may include a pluralistic set of claims in which different notions of justice must be meshed. The latter are more monistically focused on needs, and the other notions not accorded a similar relevance. Yet money may nonetheless remain as a causally necessary condition for receiving medical treatment. It may be the power to secure what one needs. The senses in which health crises are distinctive may then be insufficiently determinative for the policies which govern the actual availability of treatment. The nearly automatic links between income, prestige, and the receipt of comparatively higher quality medical treatment should then be subjected to critical scrutiny. For unequal treatment of the rich ill and the poor ill is unjust if, again, needs rather than differential income constitute the ground of such treatment.

Suppose one agrees that it is important to recognize the misfit between the reasons for differential incomes and the reasons for receiving medical treatment, and that therefore income as such should not govern the actual availability of treatment. One may still ask whether the case so far relies excessively on "pure" instances where desert considerations are admittedly out of place. That there are such pure instances, tumors afflicting the spine, hemophilia, and so on, is not denied. Yet it is an exaggeration if we go on and regard all health crises as utterly unconnected with desert. Note for example that Williams leaves aside preventive medicine. And if in a cool hour we examine the statistics, we find that a vast number of deaths occur each year due to causes not always beyond our control, e.g., automobile accidents, drugs, alcohol, tobacco, obesity, and so on. In some final reckoning it seems that many persons (though crucially, not all) have an effect on, and arguably a responsibility for, their own medical needs. Consider the following bidders for emergency care: (1) a person with a heart attack who is seriously overweight; (2) a football hero who has suffered a concussion; (3) a man with lung cancer who has smoked cigarettes for forty years; (4) a sixty-year-old man who has always taken excellent care of himself and is suddenly stricken with leukemia; (5) a three-year-old girl who has swallowed poison left out carelessly by her parents; (6) a fourteen-year-old boy who has been beaten without provocation by a gang and suffers brain damage and recurrent attacks of uncontrollable terror; (7) a college student who has slashed his wrists (and not for the first time) from a psychological need for attention; (8) a woman raised in the ghetto who is found unconscious due to an overdose of heroin.

These cases help to show why the whole subject of medical treatment is so crucial and so perplexing. They attest to some melancholy elements in human experience. People suffer in varying ratios the effects of their natural and undeserved vulnerabilities, the irresponsibility and brutality of others, and their own desires and weaknesses. In some final reckoning, then, desert considerations seem not irrelevant to many health crises. The practical applicability of this admission, however, in the instance of health care delivery, appears limited. We may agree that it underscores the importance of preventive health care by stressing the influence we sometimes have over our medical needs. But if we try to foster such care by increasing the penalties for neglect, we normally confine ourselves to calculations about incentives. At the risk of being denounced in some quarters as censorious and puritannical, perhaps we should for example levy far higher taxes on alcohol and tobacco and pump the dollars directly into health care programs rather than (say) into highway building. Yet these steps would by no means lead necessarily to a demand that we correlate in some strict way a demonstrated effort to be temperate with the receipt of privileged medical treatment as a reward. Would it be feasible to allocate the additional tax monies to the man with leukemia before the overweight man suffering a heart attack on the ground of a difference in desert? At the point of emergency care at least, it seems impracticable for the doctor to discriminate between these cases, to make meritarian judgments at the point of catastrophe. And the number of persons who are in need of medical treatment for reasons utterly beyond their control remains a datum with tenacious relevance. There are those who suffer the ravages of a tornado, are handicapped by a genetic defect, beaten without provocation, etc. A commitment to the basic purpose of medical care and to the institutions for achieving it involves the recognition of this persistent state of affairs.

To Each According to His Societal Contribution

This conception gives moral primacy to notions such as the public interest, the common good, the welfare of the community, or the greatest good of the greatest number. Here one judges the social consequences of particular conduct. The formula can be construed in at least two ways.[9] It may refer to the interest of the social group considered collectively, where the group has some independent life all its own. The group's welfare is the decisive criterion for determining what constitutes any member's proper share. Or the common good may refer only to an aggregation of distinct individuals and considered distributively.

Either version accords such a primacy to what is socially advantageous as to be unacceptable not only to defenders of need, but also, it would seem, of desert. For the criteria of effort and achievement are often conceived along rather individualistic lines. The pains an agent takes or the results he brings about deserve recompense, whether or not the public interest is directly served. No automatic harmony then is necessarily assumed between his just share as individually earned and his proper share from the vantage point of the common good. Moreover, the test of social advantage *simpliciter* obviously threatens the agapeic concern with some minimal consideration due each person which is never to be disregarded for the sake of long-range

social benefits. No one should be considered as *merely* a means or instrument.

The relevance of the canon of social productiveness to health crises may accordingly also be challenged. Indeed, such crises may cut against it in that they occur more frequently to those whose comparative contribution to the general welfare is less, e.g., the aged, the disabled, children.

Consider for example Paul Ramsey's persuasive critique of social and economic criteria for the allocation of a single scarce medical resource. He begins by recounting the imponderables that faced the widely discussed "public committee" at the Swedish Hospital in Seattle when it deliberated in the early 1960s. The sparse resource in this case was the kidney machine. The committee was charged with the responsibility of selecting among patients suffering chronic renal failure those who were to receive dialysis. Its criteria were broadly social and economic. Considerations weighed included age, sex, marital status, number of dependents, income, net worth, educational background, occupation, past performance, and future potential. The application of such criteria proved to be exceedingly problematic. Should someone with six children always have priority over an artist or composer? Were those who arranged matters so that their families would not burden society to be penalized in effect for being provident? And so on. Two critics of the committee found "a disturbing picture of the bourgeoisie sparing the bourgeoisie," and observed that "the Pacific Northwest is no place for a Henry David Thoreau with bad kidneys."[10]

The mistake, Ramsey believes, is to introduce criteria of social worthiness in the first place. In those situations of choice where not all can be saved and yet all need not die, "the equal right of every human being to live, and not relative personal or social worth, should be the ruling principle."[11] The principle leads to a criterion of "random choice among equals" expressed by a lottery scheme or a practice of "first come, first served." Several reasons stand behind Ramsey's defense of the criterion of random choice. First, a religious belief in the equality of persons before God leads intelligibly to a refusal to choose between those who are dying in any way other than random patient selection. Otherwise their equal value as human beings is threatened. Second, a moral primacy is ascribed to survival over other (perhaps superior) interests persons may have, in that it is the condition of everything else. "Life is a value incommensurate with all others, and so not negotiable by bartering one man's worth against another's."[12] Third, the entire enterprise of estimating a person's social worth is viewed with final skepticism. "We have no way of knowing how really and truly to estimate a man's societal worth or his worth to others or to himself in unfocused social situations in the ordinary lives of men in their communities."[13] This statement, incidentally, appears to allow something other than randomness in *focused* social situations; when, say, a president or prime minister and the owner of the local bar rush for the last place in the bomb shelter, and the knowledge of the former can save many lives. In any event, I have been concerned with a restricted point to which Ramsey's discussion brings illustrative support. The canon of social productiveness is notoriously difficult to apply as a workable criterion for distributing medical services to those who need them.

One can go further. A system of health care delivery that treats people on the basis of the medical care required may often go against (at least narrowly conceived) calculations of societal advantage. For example, the health care needs of people tend to rise during that period of their lives, signaled by retirement, when their incomes and social productivity are declining. More generally:

> Some 40 to 50 per cent of the American people—
> the aged, children, the dependent poor, and
> those with some significant chronic disability
> are in categories requiring relatively large
> amounts of medical care but with inadequate
> resources to purchase such care.[14]

If one agrees, for whatever reasons, with the agapeic judgment that each person should be regarded as irreducibly valuable, then one cannot succumb to a social productiveness criterion of human worth. Interests are to be equally considered even when people have ceased to be, or are not yet, or perhaps never will be, public assets.

To Each According to His Contribution in Satisfying Whatever Is Freely Desired by Others in the Open Marketplace of Supply and Demand

Here we have a test which, though similar to the preceding one, concentrates on what is desired de facto by certain segments of the community rather than the community as a whole, and on the relative scarcity of the service rendered. It is tantamount to the canon of supply and demand as espoused by various laissez-faire theoreticians.[15] Rewards should be given to those who by virtue of special skill, prescience, risk-taking, and the like discern what is desired and are able to take the requisite steps to bring satisfaction. A surgeon, it may be argued, contributes more than a nurse because of the greater training and skill required, burdens borne, and effective care provided, and should be compensated accordingly. So too, perhaps, a star quarterback on a pro football team should be remunerated even more highly because of the rare athletic prowess needed, hazards involved, and widespread demand to watch him play.

This formula does not then call for the weighing of the value of various contributions, and tends to conflate needs and wants under a notion of desires. It also assumes that a prominent part is assigned to consumer free choice. The consumer should be at liberty to express his preferences, and to select from a variety of competing goods and services. Those who resist many changes currently proposed in the organization and financing of health care delivery in the U.S.A.—such as national health insurance— often do so by appealing to some variant of this formula.

Yet it seems health crises are often of overriding importance when they occur. They appear therefore not satisfactorily accommodated to the context of a free marketplace where consumers may freely choose among alternative goods and services.

To clarify what is at stake in the above contention, let us examine an opposing case. Robert M. Sade, M.D., published an article in *The New England Journal of Medicine* entitled "Medical Care as a Right: A Refutation." He attacks programs of national health insurance in the name of a person's right to select one's own values, determine how they may be realized, and dispose of them if one chooses without coercion from other men. The values in question are construed as economic ones in the context of supply and demand. So we read:

> In a free society, man exercises his right to sustain his own life by producing economic values in the form of goods and services that he is, or should be, free to exchange with other men who are similarly free to trade with him or not. The economic values produced, however, are

not given as gifts by nature, but exist only by virtue of the thought and effort of individual men. Goods and services are thus owned as a consequence of the right to sustain life by one's own physical and mental effort.[16]

Sade compares the situation of the physician to that of the baker. The one who produces a loaf of bread should as owner have the power to dispose of his own product. It is immoral simply to expropriate the bread without the baker's permission. Similarly, "medical care is neither a right nor a privilege: it is a service that is provided by doctors and others to people who wish to purchase it."[17] Any coercive regulation of professional practices by the society at large is held to be analogous to taking the bread from the baker without his consent. Such regulation violates the freedom of the physician over his own services and will lead inevitably to provider apathy.

The analogy surely misleads. To assume that doctors autonomously produce goods and services in a fashion closely akin to a baker is grossly oversimplified. The baker may himself rely on the agricultural produce of others, yet there is a crucial difference in the degree of dependence. Modern physicians depend on the achievements of medical technology and the entire scientific base underlying it, all of which is made possible by a host of persons whose salaries are often notably less. Moreover, the amount of taxpayer support for medical research and education is too enormous to make any such unqualified case for provider autonomy plausible.

However conceptually clouded Sade's article may be, its stress on a free exchange of goods and services reflects one historically influential rationale for much American medical practice. And he applies it not only to physicians but also to patients or "consumers."

> The question is whether the decision of how to allocate the consumer's dollar should belong to the consumer or to the state. It has already been shown that the choice of how a doctor's services should be rendered belongs only to the doctor: in the same way the choice of whether to buy a doctor's service rather than some other commodity or service belongs to the consumer as a logical consequence of the right to his own life.[18]

This account is misguided, I think, because it ignores the overriding importance that is so often attached to health crises. When lumps appear on someone's neck, it usually makes little sense to talk

of choosing whether to buy a doctor's service rather than a color television set. References to just tradeoffs suddenly seem out of place. No compensation suffices, since the penalties may differ so much.

There is even a further restriction on consumer choice. One's knowledge in these circumstances is comparatively so limited. The physician makes most of the decisions: about diagnosis, treatment, hospitalization, number of return visits, and so on. In brief:

> The consumer knows very little about the medical services he is buying—probably less than about any other service he purchases. . . . While [he] can still play a role in policing the market, that role is much more limited in the field of health care than in almost any other area of private economic activity.[19]

For much of the way, then, an appeal to supply and demand and consumer choice is not quite fitting. It neglects the issue of the value of various contributions. And it fails to allow for the recognition that medical treatments may be overridingly desired. In contexts of catastrophe, at any rate, when life itself is threatened, most persons (other than those who are apathetic or seek to escape from the terrifying prospects) cannot take medical care to be merely one option among others.

To Each According to His Needs

The concept of needs is sometimes taken to apply to an entire range of interests that concern a person's "psychophysical existence."[20] On this wide usage, to attribute a need to someone is to say that the person lacks what is thought to conduce to his or her "welfare"—understood in both a physiological sense (e.g., for food, drink, shelter, and health) and a psychological one (e.g., for continuous human affection and support).

Yet even in the case of such a wide usage, what the person lacks is typically assumed to be basic. Attention is restricted to recurrent considerations rather than to every possible individual whim or frivolous pursuit. So one is not surprised to meet with the contention that a preferable rendering of this formula would be: "to each according to his essential needs."[21] This contention seems to me well taken. It implies, for one thing, that basic needs are distinguishable from felt needs or wants. For the latter may encompass expressions of personal preference unrelated to considerations of survival or subsistence, and sometimes artificially generated by circumstances of rising affluence in the society at large.

Essential needs are also typically assumed to be given rather than acquired. They are not constituted by any action for which the person is responsible by virtue of his or her distinctively greater effort. It is almost as if the designation "innocent" may be linked illuminatingly to need, as retribution, punishment, and so on, are to desert, and in complex ways, to freedom. Thus essential needs are likewise distinguishable from deserts. Where needs are unequal, one thinks of them as fortuitously distributed; as part, perhaps, of a kind of "natural lottery."[22] So very often the advantages of health and the burdens of illness, for example, strike one as arbitrary effects of the lottery. It seems wrong to say that a newborn child deserves as a reward all of his faculties when he has done nothing in particular that distinguishes him from another newborn who comes into the world deprived of one or more of them. Similarly, though crudely, many religious believers do not look on natural events as personal deserts. They are not inclined to pronounce sentences such as, "That evil person with incurable cancer got what he deserved." They are disposed instead to search for some distinction between what they may call the conditions of finitude on the one hand and sin and moral evil on the other. If the distinction is "ultimately" invalid, in this life it seems inscrutably so. Here and now it may be usefully drawn. Inequalities in the need for medical treatment are taken, it appears, to reflect the conditions of finitude more than anything else.

One can even go on to argue that among our basic or essential needs, the case of medical treatment is conspicuous in the following sense. While food and shelter are not matters about which we are at liberty to please ourselves, they are at least predictable. We can plan, for instance, to store up food and fuel for the winter. It may be held that responsibility increases along with the power to predict. If so, then many health crises seem peculiarly random and uncontrollable. Cancer, given the present state of knowledge at any rate, is a contingent disaster, whereas hunger is a steady threat. Who will need serious medical care, and when, is then perhaps a classic example of uncertainty . . . .

. . .[J]ustice has properly to do with pleas of "But I could not help it." It seeks to distinguish such cases from those acknowledged to be praiseworthy or blameworthy. The formula "to each according to his needs" is one cogent way of identifying the moral relevance of these pleas. To ignore them may be thought to be unfair as well as unkind when they arise from the deprivation of some essential need. The move to confine the notion of justice wholly to desert considerations is thereby resisted as well. Hence we may say that sometimes "questions of social justice arise just because people are unequal in ways they can do very little to change and . . . only by attending to these inequalities can one be said to be giving their interests equal consideration."[23]

Similar Treatment for Similar Cases

This conception is perhaps the most familiar of all. Certainly it is the most formal and inclusive one. It is frequently taken as an elementary appeal to consistency and linked to the universalizability test. One should not make an arbitrary exception on one's own behalf, but rather should apply impartially whatever standards one accepts. The conception can be fruitfully applied to health care questions and I shall assume its relevance. Yet as literally interpreted, it is necessary but not sufficient. For rightly or not, it is often held to be as compatible with no positive treatment whatever as with active promotion of other peoples' interests, as long as all are equally and impartially included. Its exponents sometimes assume such active promotion without demonstrating clearly how this is built into the conception itself. Moreover, it may obscure a distinction that we have seen agapists and other[s] make: between equal consideration and identical treatment. Needs may differ and so treatments must, if benefits are to be equalized.

I have placed this conception at the end of the list partly because it moves us, despite its formality, toward practice. Let me suggest briefly how it does so. Suppose first of all one agrees with the case so far offered. Suppose, that is, it has been shown convincingly that a need conception of justice applies with greater relevance than the earlier three when one reflects about the basic purpose of medical care. To treat one class of people differently from another because of income or geographic location should therefore be ruled out, because such reasons are irrelevant. (The irrelevance is conceptual, rather than always, unfortunately, causal.) In short, all persons should have equal access, "as needed, without financial, geographic, or other barriers, to the whole spectrum of health services."[24]

Suppose however, second, that the goal of equal access collides on some occasions with the realities of finite medical resources and needs that prove to be insatiable. That such collisions occur in fact it would be idle to deny. And it is here that the practical bearing of the formula of similar treatment for similar cases should be noticed. Let us recall Williams's conclusion: "the proper ground of distribution of medical care is ill health: this is a necessary truth." While I agree with the essentials of his argument—for all the reasons above—I would prefer, for practical purposes, a slightly more modest formulation. Illness is the proper ground for the *receipt* of medical care. However, the *distribution* of medical care in less-than-optimal circumstances requires us to face the collisions. I would argue that in such circumstances the formula of similar treatment for similar cases may be construed so as to guide actual choices in the way most compatible with the goal of equal access. The formula's allowance of no positive treatment whatever may justify exclusion of entire classes of cases from a priority list. Yet it forbids doing so for irrelevant or arbitrary reasons. So (1) if we accept the case for equal access, but (2) if we simply cannot, physically cannot, treat all who are in need, it seems more just to discriminate by virtue of categories of illness than, for example, between the rich ill and poor ill. All persons with a certain rare, noncommunicable disease would not receive priority, let us say, where the costs were inordinate, the prospects for rehabilitation remote, and for the sake of equalized benefits to many more. Or with Ramsey we may urge a policy of random patient selection when one must decide between claimants for a medical treatment unavailable to all. Or we may acknowledge that any notion of "comprehensive benefits" to which persons should have equal access is subject to practical restrictions that will vary from society to society depending on resources at a given time. Even in a country as affluent as the United States there will surely always be items excluded, e.g., perhaps over-the-counter drugs, some teenage orthodontia, cosmetic surgery, and the like.[25] Here, too, the formula of similar treatment for similar cases may serve to modify the application of a need conception of justice in order to address the insatiability problem and limit frivolous use. In all of the foregoing instances of restriction, however, the relevant feature remains the illness, discomfort, etc., itself. The goal of equal access then retains its prima facie authoritativeness. It is imperfectly realized rather than disregarded.

Notes

1. Edward M. Kennedy, *In Critical Condition: The Crisis in America's Health Care* (New York: Simon and Schuster, 1972), pp. 234–52; Richard M. Nixon, "President's Message on Health Care System," Document No. 92-261 (March 2, 1972), House of Representatives, Washington, D.C., 1.

2. Hugo A. Bedau, "Radical Egalitarianism," pp. 168–80, in *Justice and Equality*, ed. by Hugo A. Bedau (Englewood Cliffs, N.J.: Prentice-Hall, 1971); John Haspers, *Human Conduct* (New York: Harcourt, Brace, 1961), 416–68; J. R. Lucas, "Justice," *Philosophy* 47, No. 181 (July 1972), 229–48; Ch. Perelman, *The Idea of Justice and the Problem of Argument*, trans. by John Petrie (London: Routledge and Kegan Paul, 1963); Nicholas Rescher, *Distributive Justice* (Indianapolis: Bobbs-Merrill, 1966), Gregory Vlastos, "Justice and Equality," pp. 31–72 in *Social Justice*, ed. by Richard B. Brandt (Englewood Cliffs, N.J.: Prentice-Hall, 1962).

3. Paul Ramsey, *The Patient as Person: Explorations in Medical Ethics* (New Haven: Yale University Press, 1970), p. 240.

4. Nancy Hicks, "Nation's Doctors Move to Police Medical Care," *New York Times* (Sunday, October 28, 1973), 52.

5. Lucas, 321.

6. Bernard A. O. Williams, "The Idea of Equality," pp. 116–37 in *Justice and Equality*, ed. by Hugo A. Bedau (Englewood Cliffs, N.J.: Prentice-Hall, 1971), pp. 126–37.

7. Ibid., 127.

8. See also Thomas Nagel, "Equal Treatment and Compensatory Discrimination," *Philosophy and Public Affairs* 2, No. 4, 348–63 (Summer 1973), 354.

9. Rescher, pp. 79–80.

10. Quoted in Ramsey, p. 248.

11. Ramsey, p. 256.

12. Ibid.

13. Ibid.

14. Anne R. Somers, *Health Care in Transition: Directions for the Future* (Chicago: Hospital Research and Educational Trust, 1971), p. 20.

15. Cf. Rescher, pp. 80–81.

16. Robert M. Sade, "Medical Care as a Right: a Refutation," *The New England Journal of Medicine* 285, 1288–92 (December 1971), 1289.

17. Ibid.

18. Ibid., p. 1291.

19. Charles L. Schultze, Edward R. Fried, Alice M. Rivlin, and Nancy H. Teeters, *Setting National Priorities: The 1973 Budget* (Washington, D.C.: The Brookings Institution, 1972), pp. 214–15.

20. Gene Outka, *Agape: An Ethical Analysis* (New Haven: Yale University Press, 1972), pp. 264–65.

21. Perelman, p. 22.

22. See John Rawls, *A Theory of Justice* (Cambridge: Harvard University Press, 1971), e.g., 104.

23. Benn, Stanley, I., "Egalitarianism and the Equal Consideration of Interests," pp. 152–67 in *Justice and Equality*, ed. by Hugo A. Bedau (Englewood Cliffs, N.J.: Prentice-Hall, 1971), p. 164.

24. Anne R. Somers and Herman M. Somers, "The Organization and Financing of Health Care: Issues and Directions for the Future," *American Journal of Orthopsychiatry* 42, 119–36 (January 1972), 122.

25. Anne R. Somers and Herman M. Somers, "Major Issues in National Health Insurance," *Milbank Memorial Fund Quarterly* 50, No. 2, Part 1, 177–210 (April 1972), 182.

Equality and Rights in Medical Care

Charles Fried

Charles Fried maintains that we cannot afford to accept the view that everyone has a right to equal health care. If everyone were given equal access to the *best* health care, Fried argues, this would absorb an intolerable portion of our gross national income. Fried is willing to grant a right to a "decent minimum" of health care to all. But, as he points out, this means that we have to face the problem of determining this minimum.

Furthermore, Fried recommends that we consider how to change the present "medical guild" so that highly paid and trained physicians might be replaced by people with less training who can provide a number of services more cheaply. Fried also suggests that we allow patients more choice in the "medical marketplace" by giving each person a certain amount of money to buy the medical services that he or she chooses. This might encourage the development of a variety of medical delivery systems suited to consumers' needs. Also, those who want fancier or more individualized medical care could get it by paying additional money out of their own pocket.

In this article I present arguments intended to support the following conclusions:

1. To say there is a right to health care does not imply a right to equal access, a right that whatever is available to any shall be available to all.

2. The slogan of equal access to the best health care available is just that, a dangerous slogan which could be translated into reality only if we submitted either to intolerable government controls of medical practice or to a thoroughly unreasonable burden of expense.

3. There is sense to the notion of a right to a decent standard of care for all, dynamically defined, but still not dogmatically equated with the best available.

4. We are far from affording such a standard to many of our citizens and that is profoundly wrong.

5. One of the major sources of the exaggerated demands for equality are the pretensions, inflated claims, inefficiencies, and guild-like, monopolistic practices of the health professions.

I. Background

The notion of some kind of a right to health care is not likely to be found in any but the most recent writings, not to mention legislation. After all, even the much more well-established institution of free, universal public education has not achieved the status of a federal constitutional right, is not a constitutional right by the law of many states, and stands as a right more as an inference from the practices and legislation of states, counties, and municipalities. The federal constitutional litigation regarding rights in that area has been restricted to the provision *equally* of whatever public education is in fact provided. So it should not be surprising that the notion of a right to health care is something of a novelty. Moreover, it is only fairly recently that health care could deliver a product which was as unambiguously beneficial as elementary schooling. Nevertheless, if one looks to the laws, practices, and understandings of states, counties, and municipalities, one sees growing up through the last century, and certainly in the twentieth century, an understanding which might be thought of as the inchoate recognition of a right to health care. Indeed, there are those who might say that such an inchoate recognition might be discerned as far back as Elizabethan England.

As one considers this progress, one should not misrepresent history, for in that history lies an important lesson. For the progress may represent not simply a progress in our ideas of social justice, but a progress in what medicine could do. The fact is that the increasingly general provision of medical care may be correlated as well with what medical care could accomplish as with any changing social doctrines. What could medicine accomplish a hundred or even fifty years ago? It is well known that the improvements in health that were wrought in those days were largely the result of improved sanitation, working conditions, diet, and the like. Beyond that, specifically medical ministrations could do very little. They could provide ease, amenities, relief, but rarely a cure. So society may be forgiven if it did not provide elaborate medical care to the poor until recently, since provision of medical care in essence would have meant simply the provision of amenities and placebos. And since society appeared little concerned to assure the amenities to its poor generally, it is no great surprise that it had scant inclination to provide these amenities to the sick poor.

The detailed history of the extension of medical care to the poor, and indeed to those who were not poor but lived in out-of-the-way places, has yet to be written. The emergence of a notion of a right to health care and the embodiment of such a notion in legislation and court decisions must also await difficult historical research. Nevertheless, it is worth noting that, at least in American public discourse, the idea of a right to medical care developed into something which had the appearance of inevitability only recently, in what might be called the intermediate, perhaps golden, age of modern medicine. This was a period when advances in treating acute illness, advances such as the antibiotics, could really make a large difference in prolonging life or restoring health; but the most elaborate technologies which may make only marginal improvements in situations previously thought to be hopeless had not yet been generally developed. In this recent "Golden Age" we could unambiguously afford a notion of a general right to medical care because there were a number of clear successes available to medicine, and these successes were not unduly costly. Having conquered the infectious diseases, medical science has undertaken the degenerative diseases, the malignant neoplasms, and the diseases of unknown etiology; and one must say that the ratio between expense and benefit has become exponentially more unfavorable. So it is really only now that the notion of a right to health care poses acute analytical and social problems. It is for that reason that neither history nor legal analysis will much illuminate our future course. What we do now will be a matter of our choosing, and for this reason careful analysis of the notion of a right to health care is crucial.

II. Equality and Rights: Analytical Distinctions

First, something should be said by way of at least informal definition of this term "right." A right is more than just an interest that an individual might have, a state of affairs or a state of being which an individual might prefer. A claim of right invokes entitlements; and when we speak of entitlements, we mean not those things which it would be nice for people to have, or which they would prefer to have, but which they must have, and which if they do not have they may demand, whether we like it or not. Although I would not want to say that a right is something we must recognize "no matter what," nevertheless a right is something we must accord unless _____ and what we put in to fill in the unless clause should be tightly confined and specific.

This notion of rights has interesting and not altogether obvious relations to the concept of equality, and confusions about those relations are very likely to lead to confused arguments about the very area before us—rights to health care and equality in respect to health care.

First, it should be noted that equality itself may be considered a right. Thus, a person can argue that he is not necessarily entitled to any particular thing—whether it be income, or housing, or education, or health care—but that he is entitled to equality in respect to that thing, so that whatever anyone gets he should get, too. And this is a nice example of my previous proposition about the notion of rights generally. For to recognize a right to equality may very well be—I suppose it often is—contrary to many other policies that we may have, and particularly contrary to attempts to attain some kind of efficiency. Yet, by the very notion of rights, if there is a right to equality, then granting equality cannot depend on whether or not it is efficient to do so.

Second, there is the relation between rights and equality which runs the other way, too: to say that a class of persons, or all persons, have a certain right implies that they all have that right equally. If it is said that all persons within the jurisdiction of the United States have a constitutionally protected right to freedom of speech, whatever that may mean, one thing seems clear: that this right should not depend on what it is one wants to say, who one is, and the like. Indeed, if the government against whom this right is protected were to make such distinctions, for instance, subjecting to constraints the speech of "irresponsible persons," that would be the exact concept of denial of freedom of speech to those persons.

These relations between the notion of right and of equality suggest the great importance of being very clear and precise about how a particular right is conceived: confusions in this regard are rampant in respect to health, and are the source of much pointless controversy. But because the point is quite

general, let me first take an example from another area. If we were sloppy in our thinking about what the right of freedom of speech is—and many people are as sloppy about that as they are about their definition of the rights in the area which is our immediate concern—if we were sloppy about that definition, we might, for instance, consider that there has been a denial of right because some people have access to radio or television in getting their ideas across, while others have only the street-corner soapbox to broadcast their views. Indeed, there are those who might find it unjust that even on the soapbox the timid or inarticulate are much less effective than the bold or eloquent. All of these disparities, of course, may or may not be regrettable but they have nothing to do with freedom of speech as a right, given the premise that there is a right to free speech and that this right must be an equal right. It seems clear to me that it is very different from the right to be heard, believed, admired, and applauded. The right to speak freely is just that: a right to be free of constraints and impositions on whatever speaking one might wish to do, should you be able to find someone to listen.

Now this analogy is offered as more than a distant irrelevance. Is it not very similar to many things that are said in the area of health? For analogous to the claim that the right to freedom of speech really implies a right to be heard by the multitude, is the notion that whatever rights might exist in respect to health care are rights to health, rather than to health *care*. And of course the claim is equally absurd in both instances. We may sensibly guarantee that all will be equally free of constraints on the speaking they wish to do, but we should not guarantee that all will be equally effective in getting their views across. Similarly, we may or may not choose to guarantee all equality of access to health care, but we cannot possibly guarantee to all equality of health.

Consider how these clarifications operate upon the historical development I alluded to at the beginning of this analysis. The right whose recognition might be said to have been implicit in social practices throughout the past hundred years was a right not to health care as such, nor yet a right to health, but rather a right to a certain standard of health care, which was defined in terms of what medicine could reasonably do for people. It is this notion which has become so difficult in our present situation, where the apparatus of medicine has become so much more elaborate, pretentious, and costly than it was in earlier times.

Bringing together the historical and the analytical sides, we might conclude that our present dilemma comes from the fact that there are very many expensive things that medicine can do which might possibly help. And if we commit ourselves to the notion that there is a right to whatever health care might be available, we do indeed get ourselves into a difficult situation where overall national expenditure on health must reach absurd proportions—absurd in the sense that far more is devoted to health at the expense of other important social goals than the population in general wants. Indeed, more is devoted to health than the population wants relative not only to important social goals—for example, education or housing—but relative to all the other things which people would like to have money left over to pay for. And if we recognize that it would be absurd to commit our society to devote more than a certain proportion of our national income to health, while at the same time recognizing a "right to health care," we might then be caught on the other horn of the dilemma. For we might then be required to say that because a right to health care implies a right to equality of health care, then we must limit, we must lower the quality of the health care that might be purchased by some lest our commitment to equality require us to provide such care to all and thus carry us over a reasonable budget limit.

Consider the case of the artificial heart. It seems to me not too fanciful an assumption that such a device is technically feasible within a reasonable time, and likely to be hugely expensive both in terms of its actual implantation and in terms of the subsequent care required by those benefiting from the device. Now if the right to health care is taken to mean the right to whatever health care is available to anybody, and if this entails that it is a right to an equal enjoyment of whatever care anyone else enjoys, then what are we to do with respect to the artificial heart? Might we decide not to develop such a device? Though the development and experimental use of it involves an entirely tolerable burden, the general provision of the artificial heart would be an intolerable burden, and since if we provide it to any we must provide it to all, therefore perhaps we should provide it to none.

This solution seems to me to be both uncomfortable and unstable. For surely there is something odd, if not perverse, about foregoing research on such devices, not because the research might fail, but because it might succeed. Might not this research then go on under some kinds of private auspices if such a governmental decision were made? Would we then go further and forbid even private research, rather than simply refusing to fund it? I can well imagine the next step, where artificial heart research and implantation would become like abortion or sex change operations in the old days: something one went to Sweden or Denmark for. Nor is a lottery device for distributing a limited number of artificial hearts likely to be more stable or satisfactory. For there, too, would we forbid people to go outside the lottery? Would it be a crime to cross national boundaries with the intent of obtaining an artificial heart? The example makes a general point about instituting an all-inclusive "right to health care," with the necessary concomitant of an equal right to whatever health care is available. For if we really instituted such a right and limited the provision of health care to a reasonable level, we would have to institute as well a degree of stringent state control, which it is both unlikely we can achieve and undesirable for us even to try to achieve. There is something that goes very deeply against the grain about any scheme which prohibits scientists from making discoveries which no one claims are harmful as such, but which will cause trouble because we can't give them to everybody. There is something which goes against the grain in a system which might forbid individual doctors to render a service, not because it is harmful, but because its benefits are not available to all.

Or take a much less dramatic case—dental care. It is said that ordinary basic prophylactic care is so lacking for tens of millions of our citizens that quite unnecessarily they do not have their own teeth while still in their prime. I take it that to provide the kind of elaborate dental care deployed on affluent suburban families to rural populations, and to all even poorer urban dwellers, would be a prodigiously expensive undertaking, one that would cost each of us quite heavily. But if we followed the slogan, "The best available made available to all," that is what is meant. My guess is the American people would not want to bear this burden and that as a form of transfer payment the poor would prefer just to have the money to spend on other things. But this shows the dangerousness of slogans, for perhaps the greatest part of the dental damage could be remedied at far less cost by fluoridation and by relatively routine care provided by a type of modestly trained person who is only now beginning to exist. Care of this sort can be afforded and should be provided. But this would mean abandoning the concept of equality and accepting the fact that the poor would be getting less elaborate care than those who are not poor.

Now it might be said that I am exaggerating. The case put forward is the British National Health Service, which is alleged to provide a model of high level care at reasonable costs with equality for all. But I would caution planners and enthusiasts from drawing too much from this example. The situation in Great Britain is very different in many ways. The country is smaller and more homogeneous. Moreover, even in Great Britain there are disparities between the care available between urban and rural areas; there are long waits for so-called "elective procedures"; and there is a small but significant and distinguished private sector outside of National Health which is the focus of great controversy and rancor. Finally, Great Britain is a country where a substantial portion of the citizenry is committed to the socialist ideal of equalizing incomes and nationalizing the provisions of all vital services. Surely this is a very different situation from that in the United States. Indeed, it may be that the cry for equality of access to health care bears to a general yearning for social equality much the same relation that the opposition to fetal research bears to the opposition to abortion. In each case it is a very large ideological tail wagging a relatively small and confused dog.

My point is analytical. My point is that apart from a rather general commitment to equality and, indeed, to state control of the allocation and distribution of resources, to insist on the right to health care, where that right means a right to equal access, is an anomaly. For as long as our society considers that inequalities of wealth and income are morally acceptable—acceptable in the sense that the system that produces these inequalities is in itself not morally suspect—it is anomalous to carve out a sector like health care and say that *there* equality must reign.

III. Towards a Better Definition of the Rights Involved

After all, is health care so special? Is it different from education, housing, food, legal assistance? In respect to all of these things, we recognize in our society a right, whose enjoyment may not be made wholly dependent upon the ability to pay. But just as surely in respect to all these things, we do not believe that this right entails equality of enjoyment, so that whatever diet one person or class of persons enjoys must be enjoyed by all. The argument, put forward for instance by some members of the Labor Party in Great Britain, that the independent schools in that country should be abolished because they offer a level of education better than that available in state schools, is an argument which would be found strange and repellent in the United States. Rather, in all of these areas—education, housing, food, legal assistance—there obtains a notion of a decent, fair standard, such that when this standard is satisfied all that exists in the way of *rights* has been accorded. And it is necessarily so; were we to insist on equality all the way up, that is, past this minimum, we would have committed ourselves to a political philosophy which I take it is not the dominant one in our society.

Is health care different? Everything that can be said about health care is true of food and is at least by analogy true of education, housing, and legal assistance. The real task before us is not, therefore, I think, to explain why there must be complete equality in medicine, but the more subtle and perilous task of determining the decent minimum in respect to health which accords with sound ethical judgments, while maintaining the virtues of freedom, variety, and flexibility which are thought to flow from a mixed system such as ours. The decent minimum should reflect some conception of what constitutes tolerable life prospects in general. It should speak quite strongly to things like maternal health and child health, which set the terms under which individuals will compete and develop. On the other hand, techniques which will offer some remote relief from conditions that rarely strike in the prime of life, and which strike late in life because something must, might be thought of as too esoteric to be part of the concept of minimum decent care.

On the other hand, the notion of a decent minimum should include humane and, I would say, worthy surroundings of care for those whom we know we are not going to be able to treat. Here, it seems to me, the emphasis on technology and the attention of highly trained specialists is seriously mistaken. Not only is it unrealistic to imagine that such fancy services can be provided for everyone "as a right," but there is serious doubt whether these kinds of services are what most people really want or can benefit from.

In the end, I will concede very readily that the notion of minimum health care, which it does make sense for our society to recognize as a right, is itself an unstable and changing notion. As my initial historical remarks must have suggested, the concept of a decent minimum is always relative to what is available over all, and what the best which is available might be. I suppose (to revert to my parable of the artificial heart) that if we allowed an artificial heart to be developed under private auspices and to be available only to those who could pay for it, or who could obtain it from specialized eleemosynary institutions, then the time might well come when it would have been so perfected that it would be a reasonable component of what one would consider minimum decent care. And the process of arriving at this new situation would be a process imbued with struggle and political controversy. But since I do not believe in utopias or final solutions, a resolution of the problem of the right to health care having these kinds of tensions within it neither worries me nor leads me to suspect that I am on the wrong track. To my mind, the right track consists in identifying what it is that health care can and cannot provide, in identifying also the cost of health care, and then in deciding how much of this health care, what level of health care, we are ready to underwrite as a floor for our citizenry.

IV. Practical Proposals

Although the process of defining the decent minimum is inherently a political process, there is a great deal which analysis and research can do to make the process rational and satisfactory. Much of this is a negative service, clearing away misconceptions and fallacies. For instance, as I have already argued, to state that our objective is to provide the best medical care for all, regardless of the ability to pay, must be shown up for the misleading slogan that it is. But there are more subtle misconceptions as well. The most pervasive of these deal with the situation of the medical profession.

Many observers look at the medical profession, its history of resistance to social change, and the fact that doctors as a profession enjoy the highest incomes of any group in the nation—somewhere around $50,000 a year on the average—and they draw their own conclusions. They draw the conclu-

sion that therefore what is needed is necessarily more regulation. They look at the oversupply of surgeons in this country. They note the obvious fact of over-recourse to surgery which seems to result, and they conclude that what is needed is more government regulation. For instance, the problems of supply would be met by a kind of doctors' draft, requiring service in underserved rural areas. Now I would, for a moment, suggest that we consider some alternative explanations and alternative reforms. Perhaps, after all, the irrationalities in the supply of medical personnel, together with the high incomes earned, are the result not of market forces run wild, but the result of a guild system as tight and self-protective as any we know. It is, perhaps, an irony that the medical profession, having persuaded the public of the necessity of strictly limiting entry into the profession, having persuaded the public of the indispensability of highly trained specialists, is now faced with the threat of a kind of doctors' draft to make these rare specialists available to all. Perhaps clearer thinking might indicate that many of the things which highly paid and highly trained doctors do might be done by an army of less pretentious persons.

It is well known, of course, that doctors' fees as such represent the smaller portion of the total health care budget, so it might be thought that I am taking aim at an obvious, vulnerable, and somewhat irrelevant target. Yet this is not so. Though the fees of doctors represent the smaller portion of the medical budget, doctors themselves control almost all of the decisions—from the decision about hospitalization, to the decision whether to prescribe drugs by brand or generic name—which do influence the total cost of medical care. And it is in this respect that doctors have resisted most attempts to make their behavior rational and cost-effective. In general, it is said that this is because no doctor would sacrifice the individual interests of his patient, and this may be a sincere claim. But a certain skepticism is in order. What choice do the patients have to choose more economical systems of delivery? What doctor, for that matter, even gives his patient the choice between a brand and a generic prescription drug?

But it is in the choice of delivery systems themselves that the consumer is most restricted. Most consumers do not have the choice between a variety of delivery systems from prepaid group plans to the present individual fee-for-service system, with each plan costing what it really costs. If the consumer did have this choice, we might soon find out whether the alleged advantages of the fee-for-service system were something the consumer was willing to pay for. But of course we will never find this out if we are committed to underwrite, out of general revenues, the cost of this most expensive possible delivery system. "The best available to all." That is what we tend to do today for those groups whose medical care we do underwrite. The result is that we are trying to drive down the cost of this most expensive delivery system not by changing its organization but by bureaucratic control. What if, instead, each person were assured a certain amount of money to purchase medical services as he chose? If the restrictive practices of the profession itself could be avoided, would this not help a vast variety of delivery systems to grow up, all competing for the consumer's federally assured dollar? And then those who would want what might be considered as fancier or more individualized services could get them, provided only that they were willing to pay more for them.

Finally, there is a feature of our modern situation which is responsible for the present crisis in health care, and for the impossible dilemma posed by the promise of a right to health care. This is a feature of the society and the culture as a whole. I refer to our culture's inability to face and cope with the persistent facts of illness, old age, and death. Because we are little able to come to terms with the hazards which illness proposes, because the old are a burden and an embarrassment, because we pretend that death does not exist, we employ elaborate ruses to put these things out of the ambit of our ordinary lives. The reason why we hospitalize so much more than is rationally required surely goes beyond the vagaries of the health insurance system. Is it not also the result of the fact that the ill are an embarrassment to us, and that we seek to put them away, so we do not have to care for them, while assuaging our consciences that those "best qualified" to care for them are doing so? And in order that the ruse will work, we greatly overstate what it is that these "qualified" people can do for the ill. Needless to say, they are our willing accomplices in this piece of deception. So it is with the mentally retarded, the aged, and the dying. All of these persons are defined as having an abnormal condition not only justifying but requiring their isolation from us and their care in the hands of "specialists." Perhaps it is time that we recognize that this is part of the neurosis of our age. And of course, those whom we hire to perform our proper human role toward the sick, the old, and the dying can get away with charging a very high price for relieving us of our ordinary human obligations. But is this medical care?

Finally, to avoid misunderstanding, a general theoretic point must be made. My argument must sound harsh and callous—unfeelingly, if not unerringly economic. I have elsewhere argued that it is of the essence of the physician's role and of the patient's expectations that the doctor faced with the patient's need will do everything in his power to alleviate that need.[1] I believe that. I believe that for the individual physician to do less than his best because of some economic calculation of equity or efficiency is a breach of trust. The doctor in his dealings with his patient must not act like a bureaucrat, policy maker, or legislator. But policy makers, voters, and legislators must think in different terms. It is monstrous if an individual doctor thinks like a budget officer when he cares for his patient in need; but it is chaotic and incoherent if budget officers and voters making general policy think like doctors at the bedside.

Note

1. In my book, *Medical Experimentations: Personal Integrity and Social Policy* (Amsterdam and New York: Associated Scientific Publishers/Elsevier, 1974).

Cost Containment, Justice, and Provider Autonomy ——————

Norman Daniels

Norman Daniels points out that rationing health care is inescapable. No principle of justice entitles a patient (or class or patients) to every useful treatment, for others may have a better claim on the resources. If health care is considered an ordinary commodity, fairness of distribution is based on the ability to pay. For Daniels, though, health care is a "good of special moral importance," because it is necessary to preserve the normal range of opportunities available in society. Granted that we have a duty to provide equal opportunity, we also have a duty to provide nondiscriminatory access to services that "adequately protect and restore normal functioning."

Rationing in the British system operates under two constraints: (1) universal access, even though beneficial care may sometimes be denied; (2) a centralized budgeting system within which decisions to deny care are made. Under a rationing constraint, the physician still can do the best for a patient, knowing that the denial of a resource will bring benefit to others in the system. Under the U.S. system, when physicians decide to restrict care, it may be to make money for a hospital, reduce costs for an HMO, or (in some cases) increase their own profits. Patients have no guarantee that their physician is their advocate, and the physician has no guarantee that restricting a patient's care will provide health benefits to others in the system.

Daniels concludes by pointing out that current cost-containment incentives "are not a substitute for social decisions about health care priorities and the just design of health care institutions."

If cost-containment measures, such as the use of Medicare's diagnosis-related groups (DRGs), involved trimming only unnecessary health care services from public budgets, they would pose no moral problems. Instead, such measures lead physicians and hospitals to deny some possibly beneficial care, such as longer hospitalization or more diagnostic tests, to their own patients—that is, at the "micro" level.[1] Similarly, if the "macro" decision not to disseminate a new medical procedure, such as liver transplantation, resulted only in the avoidance of waste, then it would pose no moral problem. When is it morally justifiable to say no to beneficial care or useful procedures? And why is it especially difficult to justify saying no in the United States?

Justice and Rationing

Because of scarcity and the inevitable limitation of resources even in a wealthy society, justice—however we elucidate it—will require some no-saying at both the macro and micro levels of allocation.

No plausible principles of justice will entitle an individual patient to every potentially beneficial treatment. Providing such treatment might consume resources to which another patient has a greater claim. Similarly, no class of patients is entitled to whatever new procedure offers them some benefit. New procedures have opportunity costs, consuming resources that could be used to produce other benefits, and other classes of patients may have a superior claim that would require resources to be invested in alternative ways.

How rationing works depends on which principles of justice apply to health care. For example, some people believe that health care is a commodity or service no more important than any other and that it should be distributed according to the ability to pay for it. For them, saying no to patients who cannot afford certain services (quite apart from whether income distribution is itself just or fair) is morally permissible. Indeed, providing such services to all might seem unfair to the patients who are required to pay.

Reprinted by permission from The New England Journal of Medicine, *Vol. 314, No. 21, May 22, 1986.*
Supported by grants from the Retirement Research Foundation and the National Endowment of the Humanities.

In contrast, other theories of justice view health care as a social good of special moral importance. In one recent discussion,[2] health care was seen to derive its moral importance from its effect on the normal range of opportunities available in society. This range is reduced when disease or disability impairs normal functioning. Since we have social obligations to protect equal opportunity, we also have obligations to provide access, without financial or discriminatory barriers, to services that adequately protect and restore normal functioning. We must also weigh new technological advances against alternatives, to judge the overall effect of their introduction on equal opportunity. This gives a slightly new sense to the term "opportunity cost." As a result, people are entitled only to services that are part of a system that on the whole protects equal opportunity. Thus, even an egalitarian theory that holds health care as of special moral importance justifies sometimes saying no at both the macro and micro levels.

Saying No in the British National Health Service

Aaron and Schwartz have documented how beneficial services and procedures have had to be rationed within the British National Health Service, since its austerity budget allows only half the level of expenditures of the United States.[3] The British, for example, use less x-ray film, provide little treatment for metastatic solid tumors, and generally do not offer renal dialysis to the elderly. Saying no takes place at both macro and micro levels.

Rationing in Great Britain takes place under two constraints that do not operate at all in the United States. First, although the British say no to some beneficial care, they nevertheless provide universal access to high-quality health care. In contrast, over 10 percent of the population in the United States lacks insurance, and racial differences in access and health status persist.[4,5] Second, saying no takes place within a regionally centralized budget. Decisions about introducing new procedures involve weighing the net benefits of alternatives within a closed system. When a procedure is rationed, it is clear which resources are available for alternative uses. When a procedure is widely used, it is clear which resources are unavailable for other uses. No such closed system constrains American

decisions about the dissemination of technological advances except, on a small scale and in a derivative way, within some health maintenance organizations (HMOs).

These two constraints are crucial to justifying British rationing. The British practitioner who follows standard practice within the system does not order the more elaborate x-ray diagnosis that might be typical in the United States, possibly even despite the knowledge that additional information would be useful. Denying care can be justified as follows: Though the patient might benefit from the extra service, ordering it would be unfair to other patients in the system. The system provides equitable access to a full array of services that are fairly allocated according to professional judgments about which needs are most important. The salve of this rationale may not be what the practitioner uses to ease his or her qualms about denying beneficial treatment, but it is available.

A similar rationale is available at the macro level. If British planners believe alternative uses of resources will produce a better set of health outcomes than introducing coronary bypass surgery on a large scale, they will say no to a beneficial procedure. But they have available the following rationale: Though they would help one group of patients by introducing this procedure, its opportunity cost would be too high. They would have to deny other patients services that are more necessary. Saying yes instead of no would be unjust.

These justifications for saying no at both levels have a bearing on physician autonomy and on moral obligations to patients. Within the standards of practice determined by budget ceilings in the system, British practitioners remain autonomous in their clinical decision making. They are obliged to provide the best possible care for their patients within those limits. Their clinical judgments are not made "impure" by institutional profit incentives to deny care.

The claim made here is not that the British National Health Service is just, but that considerations of justice are explicit in its design and in decisions about the allocation of resources. Because justice has this role, British rationing can be defended on grounds of fairness. Of course, some no-saying, such as the denial of renal dialysis to elderly patients, may raise difficult questions of justice.[2] The issue here, however, is not the merits of each British decision, but the framework within which they are made.

Saying No in the United States

Cost-containment measures in the United States reward institutions, and in some cases practitioners, for delivering treatment at a lower cost. Hospitals that deliver treatment for less than the DRG rate pocket the difference. Hospital administrators therefore scrutinize the decisions of physicians to use resources, pressuring some to deny beneficial care. Many cannot always act in their patients' best interests, and they fear worse effects if DRGs are extended to physicians' charges.[6] In some HMOs and preferred-provider organizations, there are financial incentives for the group to shave the costs of treatment—if necessary, by denying some beneficial care. In large HMOs, in which risks are widely shared, there may be no more denial of beneficial care than under fee-for-service reimbursement.[7] But in some capitation schemes, individual practitioners are financially penalized for ordering "extra" diagnostic tests, even if they think their patient needs them. More ominously, some hospital chains are offering physicians a share of the profits made in their hospitals from the early discharge of Medicare patients.

When economic incentives to physicians lead them to deny beneficial care, there is a direct threat to what may be called the ethic of agency. In general, granting physicians considerable autonomy in clinical decision making is necessary if they are to be effective as agents pursuing their patients' interests. The ethic of agency constrains this autonomy in ways that protect the patient, requiring that clinical decisions be competent, respectful of the patient's autonomy, respectful of the other rights of the patient (e.g., confidentiality), free from consideration of the physician's interests, and uninfluenced by judgments about the patient's worth. Incentives that reward physicians for denying beneficial care clearly risk violating the fourth-mentioned constraint, which, like the fifth, is intended to keep clinical decisions pure—that is, aimed at the patient's best interest.

Rationing need not violate the constraint that decisions must be free from consideration of the physician's interest. British practitioners are not rewarded financially for saying no to their patients. Because our cost-containment schemes give incentives to violate this constraint, however, they threaten the ethic of agency. Patients would be foolish to think the physician who benefits from saying no is any longer their agent. (Of course, patients in the United States traditionally have had to guard against unnecessary treatments, since reimbursement schemes provided incentives to overtreat.)

American physicians face a problem even when the only incentive for denying beneficial care is the hospital's, not theirs personally. For example, how can they justify sending a Medicare patient home earlier than advisable? Can they, like their British peers, claim that justice requires them to say no and that therefore they do no wrong to their patients?

American physicians cannot make this appeal to the justice of saying no. They have no assurance that the resources they save will be put to better use elsewhere in the health care system. Reducing a Medicare expenditure may mean only that there is less pressure on public budgets in general, and thus more opportunity to invest the savings in weapons. Even if the savings will be freed for use by other Medicare patients, American physicians have no assurance that the resources will be used to meet the greater needs of other patients. The American health care system, unlike the British one, establishes no explicit priorities for the use of resources. In fact, the savings from saying no may be used to invest in a procedure that may never provide care of comparable importance to that the physician is denying the patient. In a for-profit hospital, the profit made by denying beneficial treatment may be returned to investors. In many cases, the physician can be quite sure that saying no to beneficial care will lead to greater harm than providing the care.

Saying no at the macro level in the United States involves similar difficulties. A hospital deciding whether or not to introduce a transplantation program competes with other medical centers. To remain competitive, its directors will want to introduce the new service. Moreover, they can point to the dramatic benefit the service offers. How can opponents of transplantation respond? They may (correctly) argue that it will divert resources from other projects—projects that are perhaps less glamorous, visible, and profitable but that nevertheless offer comparable medical benefits to an even larger class of patients. They insist that the opportunity costs of the new procedure are too great.

This argument about opportunity costs, so powerful in the British National Health Service, loses its force in the United States. The alternatives to the transplantation program may not constitute real options, at least in the climate of incentives that exists in America. Imagine someone advising the Humana Hospital Corporation, "Do not invest in artificial hearts, because you could do far more good if you established a prenatal maternal care program in the catchment area of your chain." Even if correct, this appeal to opportunity costs is unlikely to be persuasive, because Humana responds to the incentives society offers. Artificial hearts, not prenatal maternal-care programs, will keep its hospitals on the leading technological edge, and if they become popular, will bring far more lucrative reimbursements than the prevention of low-birth-weight morbidity and mortality. The for-profit Humana, like many nonprofit organizations, merely responded to existing incentives when it introduced a transplantation program during the early 1980s, at the same time prenatal care programs lost their federal funding. Similarly, cost-containment measures in some states led to the cutting of social and psychological services but left high-technology services untouched.[8] Unlike their British colleagues, American planners cannot say, "Justice requires that we forgo this procedure because the resources it requires will be better spent elsewhere in the system. It is fair to say no to this procedure because we can thereby provide more important treatments to other patients."

The failure of this justification at both the micro and macro levels in the United States has the same root cause. In our system, saying no to beneficial treatments or procedures carries no assurance that we are saying yes to even more beneficial ones. Our system is not closed; the opportunity costs of a treatment or procedure are not kept internal to it. Just as important, the system as a whole is not governed by a principle of distributive justice, appeal to which is made in decisions about disseminating technological advances. It is not closed under constraints of justice.

Some Consequences

Saying no to beneficial treatments or procedures in the United States is morally hard, because providers cannot appeal to the justice of their denial. In ideally just arrangements, and even in the British system, rationing beneficial care is nevertheless fair to all patients in general. Cost-containment measures in our system carry with them no such justification.

The absence of this rationale has important effects. It supports the feeling of many physicians that current measures interfere with their duty to act in their patients' best interests. Of course, physicians should not think that duty requires them to reject any resource limitations on patient care. But it is legitimate for physicians to hope they may act as their patients' advocate within the limits allowed by the just distribution of resources. Our cost-containment measures thus frustrate a legitimate expectation about what duty requires. Eroding this sense of duty will have a long-term destabilizing effect.

The absence of a rationale based on justice also affects patients. Resource constraints mean that each patient can legitimately expect only the treatments due him or her under a just or fair distribution of health care services. But if beneficial treatment is denied even when justice does not require or condone it, then the patient has reason to feel aggrieved. Patients will not trust providers who put their own economic gain above patient needs. They will be especially distrustful of schemes that allow doctors to profit by denying care. Conflicts between the interests of patients and those of physicians or hospitals are not a necessary feature of a just system of rationing care. The fact that such conflicts are central in our system will make patients suspect that there is no one to be trusted as their agent. In the absence of a concern for just distribution, our cost-containment measures may make patients seek the quite different justice afforded by tort litigation, further destabilizing the system.

Finally, these effects point to a deeper issue. Economic incentives such as those embedded in current cost-containment measures are not a substitute for social decisions about health care priorities and the just design of health care institutions. These incentives to providers, even if they do eliminate some unnecessary medical services, will not ensure that we will meet the needs of our aging population over the next several decades in a morally acceptable fashion or that we will make effective—and just—use of new procedures. These hard choices must be faced publicly and explicitly.

References

1. Diagnosis-related groups (DRGs) and the Medicare program: implications for medical technology.

Washington D.C.: U.S. Congress, 1983. (Office of Technology Assessment OTA-TM-H-17.)

2. Daniels N. Just health care. New York: Cambridge University Press, 1985.

3. Aaron HJ, Schwartz, WB. The painful prescription: rationing hospital care. Washington D.C.: The Brookings Institution, 1984.

4. President's Commission for the Study of Ethical Problems in Medicine and Biomedical and Behavioral Research. Securing access to health care: ethical implications of differences in the accessibility of health services. Vol. 1. Washington D.C.: Government Printing Office, 1983.

5. Iglehart JK. Medical care of the poor—a growing problem. N Engl J Med 1985; 313:59–63.

6. Jencks SF, Dobson A. Strategies for reforming Medicare's physician payments: physician diagnosis-related groups and other approaches. N Engl J Med 1985; 312:1492–9.

7. Yelin EH, Hencke CJ, Kramer JS, Nevitt MC, Shearn M, Epstein, WV. A comparison of the treatment of rheumatoid arthritis in health maintenance organizations and fee-for-service practices. N Engl J Med 1985; 312:962–7.

8. Cromwell J, Kanak J. The effects of prospective reimbursement on hospital adoption and service sharing. Health Care Financ Rev 1982; 4:67.

A National Health Program for the United States: A Physicians' Proposal

David U. Himmelstein, Steffie Woolhandler, and the Writing Committee of the Working Group on Program Design

This proposal for a comprehensive health-care plan was developed by a group of over 400 physicians. Its main features include: (1) a single public insurance plan covering everyone; (2) a single annual payment to hospitals and nursing homes for expenses; (3) pay for physicians' services by fee, by capitation, or by assignment; and (4) funding from current sources initially, though centrally administered, with cost containment achieved by centralizing administration and improving planning. Among expected benefits are the extension of medical care and the improvement of health. Cost savings in acute care might be offset by increased costs of long-term care.

This proposal was drafted by a 30-member Writing Committee, then reviewed and endorsed by 412 other physicians representing virtually every state and medical specialty. A full list of the endorsers is available on request. The members of the Writing Committee were as follows: David U. Himmelstein, M.D., Cambridge, Mass. (cochair); Steffie Woolhandler, M.D., M.P.H., Cambridge, Mass. (cochair); Thomas S. Bodenheimer, M.D., San Francisco; David H. Bor, M.D., Cambridge, Mass.; Christine K. Cassel, M.D., Chicago; Mardge Cohen, M.D., Chicago; David A. Danielson, M.P.H., Newton, Mass.; Alan Drabkin, M.D., Cambridge, Mass.; Paul Epstein, M.D., Brookline, Mass.; Kenneth Frisof, M.D., Cleveland; Howard Frumkin, M.D., M.P.H., Philadelphia; Martha S. Gerrity, M.D., Chapel Hill, N.C.; Jerome D. Gorman, M.D., Richmond, Va.; Michelle D. Holmes, M.D., Cambridge, Mass.; Henry S. Kahn, M.D., Atlanta; Robert S. Lawrence, M.D., Cambridge, Mass.; Joanne Lukomnik, M.D.,

Bronx, N.Y.; Arthur Mazer, M.P.H., Cambridge, Mass.; Alan Meyers, M.D., Boston; Patrick Murray, M.D., Cleveland; Vicente Navarro, M.D., Dr.P.H., Baltimore; Peter Orris, M.D., Chicago; David C. Parish, M.D., M.P.H., Macon, Ga.; Richard J. Pels, M.D., Boston; Leonard S. Rodberg, Ph.D., New York City; Jeffrey Scavron, M.D., Springfield, Mass.; Gordon Schiff, M.D., Chicago; Isaac M. Taylor, M.D., Boston; Howard Waitzkin, M.D., Ph.D., Anaheim, Calif.; Paul H. Wise, M.D., M.P.H., Boston; and William Zinn, M.D., Cambridge, Mass.

Our health care system is failing. It denies access to many in need and is expensive, inefficient, and increasingly bureaucratic. The pressures of cost control, competition, and profit threaten the traditional tenets of medical practice. For patients, the

Reprinted by permission from The New England Journal of Medicine, *Vol. 320, No. 2, Jan. 12, 1989.*

misfortune of illness is often amplified by the fear of financial ruin. For physicians, the gratifications of healing often give way to anger and alienation. Patchwork reforms succeed only in exchanging old problems for new ones. It is time to change fundamentally the trajectory of American medicine—to develop a comprehensive national health program for the United States.

We are physicians active in the full range of medical endeavors. We are primary care doctors and surgeons, psychiatrists, and public health specialists, pathologists and administrators. We work in hospitals, clinics, private practices, health maintenance organizations (HMOs), universities, corporations, and public agencies. Some of us are young, still in training; others are greatly experienced, and some have held senior positions in American medicine.

As physicians, we constantly confront the irrationality of the present health care system. In private practice, we waste countless hours on billing and bureaucracy. For uninsured patients, we avoid procedures, consultations, and costly medications. Diagnosis-related groups (DRGs) have placed us between administrators demanding early discharge and elderly patients with no one to help at home—all the while glancing over our shoulders at the peer-review organization. In HMOs we walk a tightrope between thrift and penuriousness, too often under the pressure of surveillance by bureaucrats more concerned with the bottom line than with other measures of achievement. In public health work we are frustrated in the face of plenty; the world's richest health care system is unable to ensure such basic services as prenatal care and immunizations.

Despite our disparate perspectives, we are united by dismay at the current state of medicine and by the conviction that an alternative must be developed. We hope to spark debate, to transform disaffection with what exists into a vision of what might be. To this end, we submit for public review, comment, and revision a working plan for a rational and humane health care system—a national health program.

We envisage a program that would be federally mandated and ultimately funded by the federal government but administered largely at the state and local level. The proposed system would eliminate financial barriers to care; minimize economic incentives for both excessive and insufficient care, discourage administrative interference and expense, improve the distribution of health facilities, and control costs by curtailing bureaucracy and fostering health planning. Our plan borrows many features from the Canadian national health program and adapts them to the unique circumstances of the United States. We suggest that, as in Canada's provinces, the national health program be tested initially in statewide demonstration projects. Thus, our proposal addresses both the structure of the national health program and the transition process necessary to implement the program in a single state. In each section below, we present a key feature of the proposal, followed by the rationale for our approach. Areas such as long-term care; public, occupational, environmental, and mental health; and medical education need much more development and will be addressed in detail in future proposals.

Coverage

Everyone would be included in a single public plan covering all medically necessary services, including acute, rehabilitative, long-term, and home care; mental health services; dental services; occupational health care; prescription drugs and medical supplies; and preventive and public health measures. Boards of experts and community representatives would determine which services were unnecessary or ineffective, and these would be excluded from coverage. As in Canada, alternative insurance coverage for services included under the national health program would be eliminated, as would patient copayments and deductibles.

Universal coverage would solve the gravest problem in health care by eliminating financial barriers to care. A single comprehensive program is necessary both to ensure equal access to care and to minimize the complexity and expense of billing and administration. The public administration of insurance funds would save tens of billions of dollars each year. The more than 1500 private health insurers in the United States now consume about 8 percent of revenues for overhead, whereas both the Medicare program and the Canadian national health program have overhead costs of only 2 to 3 percent. The complexity of our current insurance system, with its multiplicity of payers, forces U.S. hospitals to spend more than twice as much as Canadian hospitals on billing and administration and requires U.S. physicians to spend about 10 percent of their gross incomes on excess billing costs.[1] Eliminating insurance programs that duplicated the national health program coverage, though politically thorny, would clearly be within the prerogative of the Congress.[2] Failure to do so would require the continuation of the costly bureaucracy necessary to administer and deal with such programs.

Copayments and deductibles endanger the health of poor people who are sick,[3] decrease the use of vital inpatient medical services as much as they discourage the use of unnecessary ones,[4] discourage preventive care,[5] and are unwieldy and expensive to administer. Canada has few such charges, yet health costs are lower than in the United States and have risen slowly.[6,7] In the United States, in contrast, increasing copayments and deductibles have failed to slow the escalation of costs.

Instead of the confused and often unjust dictates of insurance companies, a greatly expanded program of technology assessment and cost-effectiveness evaluation would guide decisions about covered services, as well as about the allocation of funds for capital spending, drug formularies, and other issues.

Payment for Hospital Services

Each hospital would receive an annual lump-sum payment to cover all operating expenses—a "global" budget. The amount of this payment would be negotiated with the state national health program payment board and would be based on past expenditures, previous financial and clinical performance, projected changes in levels of services, wages and other costs, and proposed new and innovative programs. Hospitals would not bill for services covered by the national health program. No part of the operating budget could be used for hospital expansion, profit, marketing, or major capital purchases or leases. These expenditures would also come from the national health program fund, but monies for them would be appropriated separately.

Global prospective budgeting would simplify hospital administration and virtually eliminate billing, thus freeing up substantial resources for increased clinical care. Before the nationwide implementation of the national health program, hospitals in the states with demonstration programs could bill out-of-state patients on a simple per diem basis. Prohibiting the use of operating funds for capital purchases or profit would eliminate the main financial incentive for both excessive intervention (under fee-for-service payment) and skimping on care (under DRG-type prospective-payment systems), since neither inflating revenues nor limiting care could result in gain for the institution. The separate appropriation of funds explicitly designated for capital expenditures would facilitate rational health planning. In Canada, this method of hospital payment has been successful in containing costs, minimizing bureaucracy, improving the distribution of health resources, and maintaining the quality of care.[6-9] It shifts the focus of hospital administration away from the bottom line and toward the provision of optimal clinical services.

Payment for Physicians' Services, Ambulatory Care, and Medical Home Care

To minimize the disruption of existing patterns of care, the national health program would include three payment options for physicians and other practitioners: fee-for-service payment, salaried positions in institutions receiving global budgets, and salaried positions within group practices or HMOs receiving per capita (capitation) payments.

Fee-for-Service Payment

The state national health program payment board and a representative of the fee-for-service practitioners (perhaps the state medical society) would negotiate a simplified, binding fee schedule. Physicians would submit bills to the national health program on a simple form or by computer and would receive extra payment for any bill not paid within 30 days. Payments to physicians would cover only the services provided by physicians and their support staff and would exclude reimbursement for costly capital purchases of equipment for the office, such as CT scanners. Physicians who accepted payment from the national health program could bill patients directly only for uncovered services (as is done for cosmetic surgery in Canada).

Global Budgets

Institutions such as hospitals, health centers, group practices, clinics serving migrant workers, and medical home care agencies could elect to receive a global budget for the delivery of outpatient, home care, and physicians' services, as well as for preventive health care and patient-education programs. The negotiation process and the regulations covering capital expenditures and profits would be similar to those for inpatient hospital services. Physicians employed in such institutions would be salaried.

Capitation

HMOs, group practices, and other institutions could elect to be paid fees on a per capita basis to cover all outpatient care, physicians' services, and medical home care. The regulations covering the use of such payments for capital expenditures and for profits would be similar to those that would apply to hospitals. The capitation fee would not cover inpatient services (except care provided by a physician), which would be included in hospitals' global budgets. Selective enrollment policies would be prohibited, and patients would be permitted to leave an HMO or other health plan with appropriate notice. Physicians working in HMOs would be salaried, and financial incentives to physicians based on the HMO's financial performance would be prohibited.

The diversity of existing practice arrangements each with strong proponents, necessitates a pluralistic approach. Under all three proposed options, capital purchases and profits would be uncoupled from payments to physicians and other operating costs—a feature that is essential for minimizing entrepreneurial incentives, containing costs, and facilitating health planning.

Under the fee-for-service option, physicians' office overhead would be reduced by the simplification of billing.[1] The improved coverage would encourage preventive care.[10] In Canada, fee-for-service practice with negotiated fee schedules and mandatory assignment (acceptance of the assigned fee as total payment) has proved to be compatible with cost containment, adequate incomes for physicians, and a high level of access to and satisfaction with care on the part of patients.[6,7] The Canadian provinces have responded to the inflationary potential of fee-for-service payment in various ways: by limiting the number of physicians, by monitoring physicians for outlandish practice patterns, by setting overall limits on a province's spending for physicians' services (thus relying on the profession to police itself), and even by capping the total reimbursement of individual physicians. These regulatory options have been made possible (and have not required an extensive bureaucracy) because all payment comes from a single source. Similar measures might be needed in the United States, although our penchant for bureaucratic hypertrophy might require a concomitant cap on spending for the regulatory apparatus. For example, spending for program administration and reimbursement bureaucracy might be restricted to 3 percent of total costs.

Global budgets for institutional providers would eliminate billing, while providing a predictable and stable source of income. Such funding could also encourage the development of preventive health programs in the community, such as education programs on the acquired immunodeficiency syndrome (AIDS), whose costs are difficult to attribute and bill to individual patients.

Continuity of care would no longer be disrupted when patients' insurance coverage changed as a result of retirement or a job change. Incentives for providers receiving capitation payments to skimp on care would be minimized, since unused operating funds could not be devoted to expansion or profit.

Payment for Long-Term Care

A separate proposal for long-term care is under development, guided by three principles. First, access to care should be based on need rather than on age or ability to pay. Second, social and community-based services should be expanded and integrated with institutional care. Third, bureaucracy and entrepreneurial incentives should be minimized through global budgeting with separate funding for capital expenses.

Allocation of Capital Funds, Health Planning, and Return on Equity

Funds for the construction or renovation of health facilities and for purchases of major equipment would be appropriated from the national health program budget. The funds would be distributed by state and regional health-planning boards composed of both experts and community representatives. Capital projects funded by private donations would require approval by the health-planning board if they entailed an increase in future operating expenses.

The national health program would pay owners of for-profit hospitals, nursing homes, and clinics a reasonable fixed rate of return on existing equity. Since virtually all new capital investment would be funded by the national health program, it would not be included in calculating the return on equity.

Current capital spending greatly affects future operating costs, as well as the distribution of resources. Effective health planning requires that funds go to high-quality, efficient programs in the areas of greatest need. Under the existing reimbursement system, which combines operating and capital payments, prosperous hospitals can expand and modernize, whereas impoverished ones cannot, regardless of the health needs of the population they serve or the quality of services they provide. The national health program would replace this implicit mechanism for distributing capital with an explicit one, which would facilitate (though not guarantee) allocation on the basis of need and quality. Insulating these crucial decisions from distortion by narrow interests would require the rigorous evaluation of the technology and assessment of needs, as well as the active involvement of providers and patients.

For-profit providers would be compensated for existing investments. Since new for-profit investment would be barred, the proprietary sector would gradually shrink.

Public, Environmental, and Occupational Health Services

Existing arrangements for public, occupational, and environmental health services would be retained in the short term. Funding for preventive health care would be expanded. Additional proposals dealing with these issues are planned.

Prescription Drugs and Supplies

An expert panel would establish and regularly update a list of all necessary and useful drugs and outpatient equipment. Suppliers would bill the national health program directly for the wholesale cost, plus a reasonable dispensing fee, of any item in the list that was prescribed by a licensed practitioner. The substitution of generic for proprietary drugs would be encouraged.

Funding

The national health program would disburse virtually all payments for health services. The total expenditure would be set at the same proportion of the gross national product as health costs represented in the year preceding the establishment of the national health program. Funds for the national health program could be raised through a variety of mechanisms. In the long run, funding based on an income tax or other progressive tax might be the fairest and most efficient solution, since tax-based funding is the least cumbersome and least expensive mechanism for collecting money. During the transition period in states with demonstration programs, the following structure would mimic existing funding patterns and minimize economic disruption.

Medicare and Medicaid

All current federal funds allocated to Medicare and Medicaid would be paid to the national health program. The contribution of each program would be based on the previous year's expenditures, adjusted for inflation. Using Medicare and Medicaid funds in this manner would require a federal waiver.

State and Local Funds

All current state and local funds for health care expenditures, adjusted for inflation, would be paid to the national health program.

Employer Contributions

A tax earmarked for the national health program would be levied on all employers. The tax rate would be set so that total collections equaled the previous year's statewide total of employers' expenditures for health benefits, adjusted for inflation. Employers obligated by preexisting contracts to provide health benefits could credit the cost of those benefits toward their national health program tax liability.

Private Insurance Revenues

Private health insurance plans duplicating the coverage of the national health program would be phased out over three years. During this transition period, all revenues from such plans would be turned over to the national health program, after the deduction of a reasonable fee to cover the costs of collecting premiums.

General Tax Revenues

Additional taxes, equivalent to the amount now spent by individual citizens for insurance premiums and out-of-pocket health costs, would be levied.

It would be critical for all funds for health care to flow through the national health program. Such single-source payment (monopsony) has been the cornerstone of cost containment and health planning in Canada. The mechanism of raising funds for the national health program would be a matter of tax policy, largely separate from the organization of the health care system itself. As in Canada, federal funding could attenuate inequalities among the states in financial and medical resources.

The transitional proposal for demonstration programs in selected states illustrates how monopsony payment could be established with limited disruption of existing patterns of health care funding. The employers' contribution would represent a decrease in costs for most firms that now provide health insurance and an increase for those that do not currently pay for benefits. Some provision might be needed to cushion the impact of the change on financially strapped small businesses. Decreased individual spending for health care would offset the additional tax burden on individual citizens. Private health insurance, with its attendant inefficiency and waste, would be largely eliminated. A program of job placement and retraining for insurance and hospital-billing employees would be an important component of the program during the transition period.

Discussion

The Patient's View

The national health program would establish a right to comprehensive health care. As in Canada, each person would receive a national health program card entitling him or her to all necessary medical care without copayments or deductibles. The card could be used with any fee-for-service practitioner and at any institution receiving a global budget. HMO members could receive nonemergency care only through their HMO, although they could readily transfer to the non-HMO option.

Thus, patients would have a free choice of providers, and the financial threat of illness would be eliminated. Taxes would increase by an amount equivalent to the current total of medical expenditures by individuals. Conversely, individuals' aggregate payments for medical care would decrease by the same amount.

The Practitioner's View

Physicians would have a free choice of practice settings. Treatment would no longer be constrained by the patient's insurance status or by bureaucratic dicta. On the basis of the Canadian experience, we anticipate that the average physician's income would change little, although differences among specialties might be attenuated.

Fee-for-service practitioners would be paid for the care of anyone not enrolled in an HMO. The entrepreneurial aspects of medicine—with the attendant problems as well as the possibilities—would be limited. Physicians could concentrate on medicine; every patient would be fully insured, but physicians could increase their incomes only by providing more care. Billing would involve imprinting the patient's national health program card on a charge slip, checking a box to indicate the complexity of the procedure or service, and sending the slip (or a computer record) to the physician-payment board. This simplification of billing would save thousands of dollars per practitioner in annual office expenses.[1]

Bureaucratic interference in clinical decision making would sharply diminish. Costs would be contained by controlling overall spending and by limiting entrepreneurial incentives, thus obviating the need for the kind of detailed administrative oversight that is characteristic of the DRG program and similar schemes. Indeed, there is much less administrative intrusion in day-to-day clinical practice in Canada (and most other countries with national health programs) than in the United States.[11,12]

Salaried practitioners would be insulated from the financial consequences of clinical decisions. Because savings on patient care could no longer be used for institutional expansion or profits, the pressure to skimp on care would be minimized.

The Effect on Other Health Workers

Nurses and other health care personnel would enjoy a more humane and efficient clinical milieu. The burdens of paperwork associated with billing would be lightened. The jobs of many administrative and insurance employees would be eliminated, necessitating a major effort at job placement and retraining. We advocate that many of these displaced workers be deployed in expanded programs of public health, health promotion and education, and home care and as support personnel to free nurses for clinical tasks.

The Effect on Hospitals

Hospitals' revenues would become stable and predictable. More than half the current hospital bureaucracy would be eliminated,[1] and the remaining administrators could focus on facilitating clinical care and planning for future health needs.

The capital budget requests of hospitals would be weighed against other priorities for health care investment. Hospitals would neither grow because they were profitable nor fail because of unpaid bills—although regional health planning would undoubtedly mandate that some expand and others close or be put to other uses. Responsiveness to community needs, the quality of care, efficiency, and innovation would replace financial performance as the bottom line. The elimination of new for-profit investment would lead to a gradual conversion of proprietary hospitals to not-for-profit status.

The Effect on the Insurance Industry

The insurance industry would feel the greatest impact of this proposal. Private insurance firms would have no role in health care financing, since the public administration of insurance is more efficient[1,13] and single-source payment is the key to both equal access and cost control. Indeed, most of the extra funds needed to finance the expansion of care would come from eliminating the overhead and profits of insurance companies and abolishing the billing apparatus necessary to apportion costs among the various plans.

The Effect on Corporate America

Firms that now provide generous employee health benefits would realize savings, because their contribution to the national health program would be less than their current health insurance costs. For example, health care expenditures by Chrysler, currently $5,300 annually per employee,[14] would fall to about $1,600, a figure calculated by dividing the total current U.S. spending on health by private employers by the total number of full-time-equivalent, nongovernment employees. Since most firms

that compete in international markets would save money, the competitiveness of U.S. products would be enhanced. However, costs would increase for companies that do not now provide health benefits. The average health care costs for employers would be unchanged in the short run. In the long run, overall health costs would rise less steeply because of improved health planning and greater efficiency. The funding mechanism ultimately adopted would determine the corporate share of those costs.

Health Benefits and Financial Costs

There is ample evidence that removing financial barriers to health care encourages timely care and improves health. After Canada instituted a national health program, visits to physicians increased among patients with serious symptoms.[15] Mortality rates, which were higher than U.S. rates through the 1950s and early 1960s, fell below those in the United States.[16] In the Rand Health Insurance Experiment, free care reduced the annual risk of dying by 10 percent among the 25 percent of U.S. adults at highest risk.[3] Conversely, cuts in California's Medicaid Program led to worsening health.[17] Strong circumstantial evidence links the poor U.S. record on infant mortality with inadequate access to prenatal care.[18]

We expect that the national health program would cause little change in the total costs of ambulatory and hospital care; savings on administration and billing (about 10 percent of current health spending[1]) would approximately offset the costs of expanded services.[19,20] Indeed, current low hospital-occupancy rates suggest that the additional care could be provided at low cost. Similarly, many physicians with empty appointment slots could take on more patients without added office, secretarial, or other overhead costs. However, the expansion of long-term care (under any system) would increase costs. The experience in Canada suggests that the increased demand for acute care would be modest after an initial surge[21,22] and that improvements in health planning[8] and cost containment made possible by single-source payment[9] would slow the escalation of health care costs. Vigilance would be needed to stem the regrowth of costly and intrusive bureaucracy.

Unsolved Problems

Our brief proposal leaves many vexing problems unsolved. Much detailed planning would be needed to ease dislocations during the implementation of the program. Neither the encouragement of preventive health care and healthful life styles nor improvements in occupational and environmental health would automatically follow from the institution of a national health program. Similarly, racial, linguistic, geographic, and other nonfinancial barriers to access would persist. The need for quality assurance and continuing medical education would be no less pressing. High medical school tuitions that skew specialty choices and discourage low-income applicants, the underrepresentation of minorities, the role of foreign medical graduates, and other issues in medical education would remain. Some patients would still seek inappropriate emergency care, and some physicians might still succumb to the temptation to increase their incomes by encouraging unneeded services. The malpractice crisis would be only partially ameliorated. The 25 percent of judgments now awarded for future medical costs would be eliminated, but our society would remain litigious, and legal and insurance fees would still consume about two-thirds of all malpractice premiums.[23] Establishing research priorities and directing funds to high-quality investigations would be no easier. Much further work in the area of long-term care would be required. Regional health planning and capital allocation would make possible, but not ensure, the fair and efficient allocation of resources. Finally, although insurance coverage for patients with AIDS would be ensured, the need for expanded prevention and research and for new models of care would continue. Although all these problems would not be solved, a national health program would establish a framework for addressing them.

Political Prospects

Our proposal will undoubtedly encounter powerful opponents in the health insurance industry, firms that do not now provide health benefits to employees, and medical entrepreneurs. However, we also have allies. Most physicians (56 percent) support some form of national health program, although 74 percent are convinced that most other doctors oppose it.[24] Many of the largest corporations would enjoy substantial savings if our proposal were adopted. Most significant, the great majority of Americans support a universal, comprehensive, publicly administered national health program, as shown by virtually every opinion poll in the past 30 years.[25,26] Indeed, a 1986 referendum question in Massachusetts calling for a national health program was approved two to one, carrying all 39 cities and 307 of the 312 towns in the commonwealth.[27] If mobilized, such public conviction could override even the most strenuous private opposition.

References

1. Himmelstein DU, Woolhandler S. Cost without benefit: administrative waste in U.S. health care. N Engl J Med 1986; 314:441–5.

2. Advisory opinion regarding House of Representatives Bill 85-H-7748 (No. 86-269-MP, R.I. Sup. Ct. Jan 5, 1987).

3. Brook RH, Ware JE Jr, Rogers WH, et al. Does free care improve adults' health? Results from a randomized controlled trial. N Eng J Med 1983; 309:1426–34.

4. Siu AL, Sonnenberg FA, Manning WG, et al. Inappropriate use of hospitals in a randomized trial of health insurance plans. N Engl J Med 1986; 315:1259–66.

5. Brian EW, Gibbens SF. California's Medi-Cal copayment experiment. Med Care 1974; 12:Suppl 12:1–303.

6. Iglehart JK. Canada's health care system. N Engl J Med 1986; 315:202–8, 778–84.

7. *Idem.* Canada's health care system: addressing the problem of physician supply. N Engl J Med 1986; 315:1623–8.

8. Detsky AS, Stacey SR, Bombardier C. The effectiveness of a regulatory strategy in containing hospital costs: the Ontario experience, 1967–1981. N Engl J Med 1983; 309:151–9.

9. Evans RG. Health care in Canada: patterns of funding and regulation. In: McLachlan G, Maynard A, eds. The public/private mix for health: the relevance and effects of change. London: Nuffield Provincial Hospitals Trust, 1982: 369–424.

10. Woolhandler S, Himmelstein DU. Reverse targeting of preventive care due to lack of health insurance. JAMA 1988; 259:2872–4.

11. Reinhardt UE. Resource allocation in health care: the allocation of lifestyles to providers. Milbank Q 1987; 65:153–76.

12. Hoffenberg R. Clinical freedom. London: Nuffield Provincial Hospitals Trust, 1987.

13. Horne JM, Beck RG. Further evidence on public versus private administration of health insurance. J Public Health Policy 1981; 2:274–90.

14. Cronin C. Next Congress to grapple with U.S. health policy, competitiveness abroad. Bus Health 1986; 4(2):55.

15. Enterline PE, Salter V, McDonald AD, McDonald JC. The distribution of medical services before and after "free" medical care—the Quebec experience. N Engl J Med 1973; 289:1174–8.

16. Roemer R, Roemer MI. Health manpower policy under national health insurance: the Canadian experience. Hyattsville, Md.: Health Resources Administration, 1977. (DHEW publication no. (HRA) 77-37.)

17. Lurie N, Ward NB, Shapiro MF, et al. Termination of Medi-Cal benefits: a follow-up study one year later. N Engl J Med 1986; 314:1266–8.

18. Institute of Medicine. Preventing low birthweight. Washington, D.C.: National Academy Press, 1985.

19. Newhouse JP, Manning WG, Morris CN, et al. Some interim results from a controlled trial of cost sharing in health insurance. N Engl J Med 1981; 305:1501–7.

20. Himmelstein DU, Woolhandler S. Free care: a quantitative analysis of the health and cost effects of a national health program. Int J Health Serv 1988; 18:393–9.

21. LeClair M. The Canadian health care system. In: Andreopoulos S, ed. National health insurance: can we learn from Canada? New York: John Wiley, 1975: 11–92.

22. Evans RG. Beyond the medical marketplace: expenditure, utilization and pricing of insured health care in Canada. In: Andreopoulos S, ed. National health insurance: can we learn from Canada? New York: John Wiley, 1975: 129–78.

23. Danzon PM. Medical malpractice: theory, evidence, and public policy. Cambridge, Mass.: Harvard University Press, 1985.

24. Colombotas J, Kirchner C. Physicians and social change. New York: Oxford University Press, 1986.

25. Navarro V. Where is the popular mandate? N Engl J Med 1982; 307:1516–8.

26. Pokorny G. Report card on health care. Health Manage Q 1988: 10(1):3–7.

27. Danielson DA, Mazer A. Results of the Massachusetts Referendum on a national health program. J Public Health Policy 1987; 8:28–35.

Decision Scenario 1 . . . .

The Cashier's Office of Archway Memorial Hospital is, even for the wealthy and best educated, a place of frustration. Bills are presented in the form of long computer printouts, covered with unfamiliar names referring to supplies, medical treatment, and diagnostic tests. Associated with each item is a price that seems absurdly high.

For someone without any form of medical insurance, being faced with such a bill can be more than confusing—it can be frightening. And that is just the situation that Marvin Baldesi found himself in.

"Your age makes you ineligible for Medicare," said Ms. Kearney, the Archway billing officer. "And you say you aren't covered by Blue Cross or a private insurance plan."

"That's right," said Mr. Baldesi. "I own my own business. My wife and me, we run a small upholstery shop. We decided we couldn't afford to keep up our insurance."

"Normally we wouldn't have admitted you," said Ms. Kearney. "It's only because you came in as an acute emergency that you were allowed to run up such a bill."

Mr. Baldesi looked down to keep from meeting Ms. Kearney's eyes. He felt embarrassed. He had always paid his bills, and now this woman didn't bother to disguise the fact that she saw him as a deadbeat.

"I don't guess you have any money in savings?" Ms. Kearney asked.

"About fifty dollars. Just enough to keep the account open."

"Then it looks to me like you've only got two choices," Ms. Kearney said. "You've got to borrow the money or you've got to declare yourself bankrupt. If you do that, then you'll be eligible for Medicaid payments, and the hospital may be able to collect from the government. I'm not sure of the legal process."

"But the bill is almost fifty thousand dollars," Mr. Baldesi said. "I can't borrow money like that. My family and friends don't have it, and no bank would loan it to me without collateral."

"Then you'll just have to get a lawyer and get yourself declared bankrupt."

"But if I do that, I'll lose my business. My credit will be ruined, and I won't be able to get the materials I need from suppliers. Isn't there any other way?"

"I don't know of any," said Ms. Kearney. "But that's not really my problem. All I know is that Archway has to be paid. You received our services, and we have to have the money for them."

1. Is Mr. Baldesi's predicament possible in the U.S. today? If the "Physicians' Proposal" were implemented, would it eliminate such cases? How would Archway Hospital get paid?

2. How might the health-care proposal outlined by Fried apply to such a case?

3. Archway (through Ms. Kearney) is asserting its claim as an agent in a market economy. Why does Outka regard market considerations as irrelevant in determining the distribution of health care? Is Daniels's notion that a commitment to equal opportunity requires a commitment to some form of universal health care compatible with Outka's position?

4. Suppose Mr. Baldesi's illness is connected with his failure to give up smoking and drinking, even though advised to do so by his physician. Would this lead you to view his situation any differently?

Decision Scenario 2 . . . .

"There's more than one way to get to Rome," Dr. Kenton said. "And we've got a couple of options to offer you."

"I'll take anything that will make the pain stay away," Mr. Czahz said.

"We can do a surgical procedure that we call a coronary-artery bypass. In your case, there are two arteries involved so it would be a double bypass."

"This is not something experimental, is it?"

"No, it's a well-established procedure with a pretty good safety record. Now something like 80% of the people who have the bypass get rid of their angina pains."

"I don't much like the idea of being cut, but I'd do most anything to stop those chest pains."

"Let me tell you the other option. We can treat you medically instead of surgically. That is, we can try you on some drugs and see how you do, put you on a diet, and keep a close watch on you. Now people we treat this way do a little bit better in terms of living longer than those treated surgically do. That's a little misleading, though, because those who have surgery usually have worse cases of the disease."

"What about the angina pains?" Mr. Czahz asked.

"There's the problem. Medical treatment can do something about the pains, but it's really not as effective as surgery."

"So I'll take the surgery."

"Aren't you on health stamps?" Dr. Kenton asked.

"That's right."

"We've got a problem then. You see, health stamps won't cover the cost of bypass surgery. It's an optional procedure under the HHS guidelines, and they won't kick in the extra money to pay for it."

"So I have to make up the difference myself?"

"That's right," Dr. Kenton said. "You're going to have to come up with about two thousand in cash."

"Dr. Kenton, there's no way I can do that."

"Okay, then. I just wanted you to know what the possibilities were. We can put you on a treatment program, and I'm sure you'll do just fine."

"But what about the angina pain?"

"We'll do what we can," Dr. Kenton said.

1. A health-stamp program might operate by granting a fixed amount of money to each person below a certain income level. This would permit someone to shop around for the best health-care bargain she or he could afford. What might be the advantages and disadvantages of such a program?

2. Would such a program be likely to provide the sort of equal access of health care argued for by Outka?

3. According to Fried's position, should Mr. Czahz be entitled to anything more than basic medical treatment for his heart condition?

4. Is such a double-level health care system compatible with the position on justice and equal opportunity taken by Daniels?

Decision Scenario 3 •

When the pain began, Alan Warfard was certain he was having a heart attack. The pain lasted more than an hour, and when it was finally over he was weak and exhausted. He knew there was something seriously wrong with him, and as soon as he was able he called his next-door neighbor and asked her to drive him to Southwest Hospital.

"You have no insurance coverage, except for Medicare?" the man at the admitting desk asked Mr. Warfard. "No private insurance at all?"

"Just Medicare," Mr. Warfard said.

"Can you show us any financial records, such as savings-account passbooks, to establish that you are able to pay your charges here?"

"I live on my Social Security check, and I don't have a savings account."

"Do you have any relatives who would be willing to sign a statement assuming financial responsibility for your treatment here?"

"I'm afraid not," Mr. Warfard said. "But I don't see what the problem is. I told you—I'm covered by Medicare. Isn't that enough?"

The admitting clerk shook his head. "I'm afraid it's not. We don't know what your treatment is likely to cost, and we don't know whether Medicare would pay for all of it. You know, they pay only a certain amount, and you might run up bills above that. This is a private hospital, and I'm afraid that,

without your being able to guarantee that you can pay us, I can't admit you for treatment."

"But I'm sick," Mr. Warfard said. "What am I supposed to do, just go home and die?"

"That's not really our concern," the clerk said. "But I suggest you see if you can get yourself admitted to a public hospital. Taking care of people like you is their responsibility."

The phrase "people like you" stung Mr. Warfard's pride. After all those years of paying his taxes and being a good citizen, how could he be dismissed so easily?

1. *How does Mr. Warfard's case illustrate some of the drawbacks of the current prospective payment plan (DRGs) employed by Medicare? What are some of the other drawbacks of the plan?*

2. *Do private, for-profit hospitals pose particular difficulties for public hospitals and the public financing of health care?*

3. *How might it be argued that health care is such a special commodity that it should not be bought and sold on the open market the way that other goods are?*

4. *When cost control is at issue, why does Daniels think British physicians are in a better position to act for the sake of patients, even under constraints, than their American counterparts?*

Decision Scenario 4 •

"Let me see if I understand you correctly," Mrs. Burgone said. "I need a liver transplant, but I'm not allowed to have such an operation?"

"That's correct," Dr. Popp said. "The National Health policy stipulates that transplant surgery cannot be performed on patients over the age of seventy."

Mrs. Burgone shook her head. "But I don't expect National Health to pay for it. I'm able to pay for it myself."

"That doesn't matter. It's a matter of social policy, not medicine. The idea is that we can't afford, as a society, to do everything for every patient. You might be able to pay for such an operation, but not everybody can. Then society would have to pay for those who can't afford it, and society can't afford

to do that. Consequently, to be fair, the operation is denied to everyone above the age of seventy."

"That doesn't seem fair to me," Mrs. Burgone said. "How can it be fair to condemn someone to pain and a greater risk of death when a way of changing this is available?"

"I didn't make the policy," Dr. Popp said.

1. *According to Outka, the standard for determining who shall receive medical care is need alone. However, since resources are finite, he admits that access may have to be restricted and suggests that the principle of treating similar cases similarly might be used to limit access. Would the policy described above be a legitimate restriction on access? Is the age require-*

ment relevant to determining whether the restriction is legitimate?

2. *Is the policy compatible with the position taken by Fried? On Fried's view, is the policy one that might legitimately be followed by Medicare and Medicaid?*

3. *Is the "opportunity cost" view of health care taken by Daniels compatible with such a social policy?*

Decision Scenario 5 ·

"Let me explain it to you, Mr. Faust," Charles Young said. "Although your wife is covered by Medicare, we cannot pay for the care she is receiving in the nursing home. As an Alzheimer's patient, she is receiving what we consider to be 'custodial' care, and that is explicitly excluded from Medicare coverage. Do you have any private insurance?"

"Yes, I do. But you're telling me exactly the same thing I heard from my insurance company. My policy doesn't cover long-term, chronic, or custodial care."

"I'm sorry to hear that," Charles Young said. "That means that you will have to pay the total cost of the care yourself."

"Where can I get that kind of money?" Mr. Faust said. "A nursing home will cost me thirty or forty thousand dollars a year. If I sell our house and use all our savings, I could pay for maybe a year, but then I wouldn't have anything to live on myself. Where could I live? How could I eat?"

"I understand. But the only alternative is to divest yourself of your assets so that you cannot be held legally responsible for paying for your wife's care. Then you and she can both get assistance under the Medicaid program."

"Then I have to literally bankrupt myself and become a pauper before I can get any help?"

"I'm sorry to say that's true."

1. *Should a national health-care program pay for the custodial care that is required by patients with Alzheimer's and similar diseases?*

2. *Should family members (adult children or grandchildren) be required by law to help pay the health-care expenses of other family members?*

3. *Since people with such severe diseases are not able to take advantage of the "normal range of opportunity," and since access to treatment is not likely to "restore normal functioning," would it be legitimate, given Daniels's principle of justice, to withhold health care from such people?*

4. *Should people with incomes adequate to cover the cost of their health care or to buy private insurance be ineligible to participate in a national health-insurance plan?*

5. *We expect people to pay for the goods and services that they receive. Since Mrs. Faust is receiving goods and services in getting custodial care, why is it unfair to expect her husband to pay for them?*

Decision Scenario 6 ·

"I've decided to do something that may cause me a lot of trouble," Dr. Miles Toliver said.

Alan Burford took a sip of his drink and sat back in his chair. He had known Miles for a long time and knew he could be counted on to see most things in a novel way. Sometimes Miles could be annoying, but he always made you think.

"I'm not going to accept women as patients anymore," Toliver said. "I don't like dealing with them, and there's nothing that says I have to. From now on, I'm restricting my practice to men only."

"I don't think you can do that," Burford said. "I suspect that involves civil rights violations of some sort. You know, discriminating on the basis of race or sex or something like that."

"Then I'll get a lawyer and show that the government can't force me to treat women without violating my own rights."

"I don't follow you."

"Look at it this way," Toliver said. "My medical knowledge and skills belong to me. I acquired them through the exercise of my own mind, and I have a constitutional right to privacy and freedom of expression. Therefore, I have a right to exercise my knowledge and skills in the way I see fit. Therefore, if I don't want to treat women, then I don't have to."

"That's an argument I've never heard," Burford said.

"The government can't force me to do what I don't want to do without violating my rights and being despotic."

"I suspect you'll have to prove that in court."

"I'm prepared to," Toliver said.

1. *State explicitly (and more fully if it seems necessary) the argument presented by Dr. Toliver.*

2. *Toliver's argument might be construed as one supporting what is sometimes called "medical individualism." Do the objections to medical individualism made by Outka also apply to Toliver's argument?*

NOTES AND REFERENCES FOR INTRODUCTIONS, CASES, AND SCENARIOS

Moral Principles, Ethical Theories, and Medical Decisions: An Introduction

I learned much about medical ethics and about presenting it to a general audience from those who have gone before me. I have benefited from the example (among others) of Samuel Gorovitz et al., eds., *Moral Problems in Medicine* (Englewood Cliffs, N.J.: Prentice-Hall, 1976), Robert Hunt and John Arras, eds., *Ethical Issues in Modern Medicine* (Palo Alto, Calif.: Mayfield, 1977), and Richard W. Wertz, ed., *Readings on Ethical and Social Issues in Biomedicine* (Englewood Cliffs, N.J.: Prentice-Hall, 1973). All three have informative introductions, but the one by Hunt and Arras I found most helpful and most philosophically interesting.

My discussion of ethical theories is generally indebted to Richard B. Brandt, *Ethical Theory* (Englewood Cliffs, N.J.: Prentice-Hall, 1959) and William K. Frankena, *Ethics*, 2d ed. (Englewood Cliffs, N.J.: Prentice-Hall, 1973). My treatment of utilitarianism owes much to the excellent introductory essay by Paul Taylor in his *Problems of Moral Philosophy* (Belmont, Calif.: Dickenson, 1971), pp. 137–151. Mill's statement of the principle of utility is from *Utilitarianism* (Indianapolis: Bobbs-Merrill, 1971), p. 18; the second quotation is from p. 24. In the discussion of act and rule utilitarianism and their attendant difficulties, I am indebted to Michael D. Bayles and Kenneth Henley's introduction in their *Right Conduct* (New York: Random House, 1983), pp. 86–94, and to Carl Wellman, *Morals and Ethics* (New York: Scott, Foresman, 1975), pp. 39–42, 47–50. The quotation from Wellman is on p. 49.

The statements of Kant's categorical imperative are more paraphrases than literal translations. They are from his *Groundwork of the Metaphysics of Morals*, translated by H. J. Paton (New York: Harper & Row, 1964). Other translations and editions are easily available. Some of the criticisms of Kant are based on those of Brandt (*Ethical Theory*, pp. 27–35) and Frankena (*Ethics*, pp. 30–33).

The quotation from Ross is from his *The Right and the Good* (New York: Oxford University Press, 1930), p. 24. The prima facie duties are found on pp. 21–22 and the "rules" for resolving conflict on pp. 41–42. My exposition is indebted, in part, to G. J. Warnock, *Contemporary Moral Philosophy* (New York: St. Martin's Press, 1967) and to Fred Feldman, *Introductory Ethics* (Englewood Cliffs, N.J.: Prentice-Hall, 1978), pp. 149–160.

Rawls's theory is presented in *A Theory of Justice* (Cambridge, Mass.: Harvard University Press, 1971). The principles are quoted from p. 203; "natural duties" are discussed on pp. 340–350. My statement of the theory is indebted to Norman Daniels's introduction to his anthology *Reading Rawls* (New York: Basic Books, 1976). The first criticism is one made by Thomas Nagel, "Rawls on Justice" (Daniels, pp. 1–16) and Ronald Dworkin, "The Original Position" (Daniels, pp. 16–53). The second criticism is urged by R. M. Hare, "Rawls's Theory of Justice" (Daniels, pp. 81–108) and David Lyons, "Nature and Soundness of the Contract and Coherence Arguments" (Daniels, pp. 141–169). A relatively easy entrance into Rawls's theory is provided by the general reviews of the book that are listed in the Bibliography.

For Aquinas's view on "man," see his *Summa Theologica*, Part II (First Part), vol. 6, translated by Fathers of the English Dominican Province (London: Burns Oates and Washbourne, 1914). For his views on natural law and law in general, see vol. 8, "Treatise on Law." For an interpretation of Aquinas, see Frederick Copleston, *A History of Philosophy*, vol. 2, part 2 (New York: Doubleday, 1962), pp. 126–131, to which my account is indebted. For the presentation of the current Catholic natural law view I am indebted to Charles J. McFadden, *Medical Ethics*, 6th ed. (Philadelphia: F. A. Davis, 1967). The doctrine of double effect is treated on pp. 121–155; euthanasia, extraordinary means, and medical experimentation, pp. 239–270. The quotations from

627

the Directives are from the appendix in McFadden: abortion, p. 441, euthanasia, p. 442.

My discussion of moral principles is indebted to Tom. L. Beauchamp and James F. Childress, *Principles of Biomedical Ethics* (New York: Oxford University Press, 1979), pp. 56–201, and to Beauchamp's and LeRoy Walters's introduction in *Contemporary Issues in Bioethics*, 2d ed. (Belmont, Calif.: Wadsworth, 1982), pp. 26–32. The discussion of liberty-limiting principles is based on Joel Feinberg, *Social Philosophy* (Englewood Cliffs, N.J.: Prentice-Hall, 1973), pp. 20–33, as is the discussion of principles of justice, pp. 98–119.

Chapter 1: Abortion

The Case Presentation has been fictionalized, but it is based on the case of an unnamed minor in the United Press International story "Court Orders Abortion for a Rape Victim, 12" (Oklahoma City, 29 September 1981).

The Social Context draws information from *Newsweek*, 1 May 1989; 17 July 1989—the Guttmacher statistical data are from these sources— and *Time*, 1 May 1989. Response to the *Webster* decision is based on Linda Greenhouse, "Supreme Court Upholds Sharp State Limits on Abortion," *New York Times*, 4 July 1980 and E. Dionne, "On Both Sides, Advocates Predict a 50-State Battle" in the same issue; the Minnesota and Akron cases are based on material from Linda Greenhouse, "States May Require a Girl to Notify Her Parents Before Having an Abortion," *New York Times*, 26 June 1990.

The Social Context on RU 486 is based on *New York Times* stories: 27 July 1990; 22 June 1990; 23 September 1989; 26, 27, 29, 30 October 1988; 22 February 1988. It also draws from *Time*, 7 November 1988, and Steven Greenhouse, "A Fierce Battle," *New York Times Magazine*, 12 February 1989. More background material can be found in *New York Times*: 6 April 1990; 15 June 1988; 9 March 1990; 14 February 1990; 6 April 1990; 11 May 1990; 30 June 1990.

Information on fetal development is found in Arthur J. Vender, J. H. Sherman, and D. S. Luciano, *Human Physiology*, chapter 15 (New York: McGraw-Hill, 1970).

The Finkbine Case Retrospective is based on Allen F. Guttmacher, *The Case for Legalized Abortion* (Berkeley, Calif.: Diablo Press, 1977), pp. 15–17. The Bishop Scenario is based on a case reported in the *New York Times*, 11 April 1982. The procedure de-

scribed was developed at Mount Sinai Medical Center by Drs. Thomas Kerenyi and Usha Chitkara.

Chapter 2: Treating or Terminating: The Problem of Impaired Infants

"Social Context: The Baby Doe Cases" is based on information from the following sources: George J. Annas, "Disconnecting the Baby Doe Hotline," *Hastings Center Report* 13 (June 1983): 14–16, and "Baby Doe Redux," *Hastings Center Report* 13 (October 1983): 26–27; Bonnie Steinbock, "Baby Jane Doe in the Courts," *Hastings Center Report* 14 (February 1984): 13–19; Thomas H. Murray, "The Final Anticlimactic Rule on Baby Doe," *Hastings Center Report* 15 (June 1985): 5–9; *Time*, 14 November 1983, p. 107. Also the following articles from the *New York Times*: Marcia Chambers, "U.S. Suing for L.I. Records of Baby in Surgery Dispute," 3 November 1983, and "Letting Panels Decide the Fate of Defective Infants," 15 January 1984; Harold M. Schmeck, Jr., "Life, Death and the Rights of Handicapped Babies," 18 June 1985; Stuart Taylor, Jr., "High Court Upsets U.S. Intervention on Infants' Lives," 10 June 1986; Andrew H. Malcolm, "Ruling on Baby Doe: Impact Limited," 11 June 1986.

The Case Presentation is based on an actual case presented in James M. Gustafson, "Mongolism, Parental Desires, and the Right to Life," *Perspectives in Biology and Medicine* 16 (1973): 529–557, and in Milton D. Heifetz and Charles Mangel, *The Right to Die* (New York: G. P. Putnam's, 1975), pp. 59–60.

For a discussion of the medical and biological aspects of birth defects, see E. P. Volpe, *Human Heredity and Birth Defects* (New York: Pegasus, 1971). On prenatal diagnosis, see Theodore Friedman, "Prenatal Diagnosis of Genetic Disease," *Scientific American* 225 (November 1971): 34–42.

The R. S. Duff and A. G. M. Campbell article referred to is "Moral and Ethical Dilemmas in the Special-Care Nursery," *New England Journal of Medicine* 289 (1973): 75–78.

The "Juli" Decision Scenario is based on a case reported in B. D. Colen, *Karen Ann Quinlan: Dying in the Age of Eternal Life* (New York: Nash, 1976), pp. 130–137. The "Susan Roth" scenario is based on a case reported in Richard Trubo, *An Act of Mercy* (Los Angeles: Nash, 1973), pp. 149–150. The "Irene Towers" scenario is based on a Chicago case reported by the Associated Press, 18 May 1981.

The "Dr. Daniel McKay" Decision Scenario is based on information from E. R. Shipp, "Mistrial in Killing of Malformed Baby Leaves Town Uncertain about Law," *New York Times*, 18 February 1985.

The AMA policy decision is reported in Andrew H. Malcolm, "Reassessing Care of the Dying," *New York Times*, 16 March 1986.

The information about the Bartling case is drawn from the *New York Times*, 28 December 1984, and George J. Annas, "Prisoner in the ICU: The Tragedy of William Bartling," *Hastings Center Report* 14 (December 1984): 28–29.

The "Virginia Crawford" Decision Scenario is based on a Baltimore case reported by United Press International on 25 February 1979.

The facts in the Shick case are from a United Press International story of 8 February 1983; the Dohr-Engel case was reported in the *New York Times*, 20 March 1985; the Montigny case was reported by the Associated Press on 8 August 1985; the Gilbert case was reported by the *New York Times* on 9 August 1985 and the Associated Press on 26 August 1985. The policy endorsed by the Netherlands Supreme Court was outlined by a *New York Times* story, 27 November 1984.

Chapter 3: Euthanasia

The Social Context on the Cruzan case draws from: *Time* (11 December 1989; 19 March 1990; 9 July 1990); *Newsweek*, Marcia Angell, "The Right to Die in Dignity" (23 July 1990); *New York Times* (17 November 1988; 29 July 1988; 25 July 1989; 19 January 1990; 26, 27 June 1990; 23 July 1990).

The discussion of euthanasia in the Netherlands is based on F. X. Klines, "Dutch Quietly in Lead in Euthanasia Requests," *New York Times*, 31 October 1986. The California proposal is discussed in *New York Times*, 18 May 1988.

For a discussion of covert and unilateral decisions made about euthanasia by physicians, see Milton D. Heifetz and Charles Mangel, *The Right to Die* (New York: G. P. Putnam's, 1975). The information about and the criticisms of the California Natural Death Act are from Karen Lebacqz, "On 'Natural Death,' " *Hastings Center Report* 7 (1977): 14. An excellent discussion of the history and practice of euthanasia and of euthanasia legislation is O. Ruth Russell, *Freedom to Die: Moral and Legal Aspects of Euthanasia* (New York: Dell, 1976).

By far the most detailed account of the Karen Quinlan case is Joseph and Julia Quinlan with Phyllis Battelle, *Karen Ann Quinlan* (New York: Doubleday, 1977). The facts in the Case Presentation are mostly from Phyllis Battelle, "The Story of Karen Quinlan," *Ladies' Home Journal* 93 (September 1976): 69–76, 172–180. Direct quotations are from Battelle. I have also drawn from B. D. Colen, *Karen Ann Quinlan: Dying in the Age of Eternal Life* (New York: Nash, 1976), and *In the Matter of Karen Quinlan: The Complete Legal Briefs, Court Proceedings, and Decisions* (Arlington, Va.: University Publications of America, 1975).

The "Elizabeth Bouvia" Case Presentation draws heavily upon George J. Annas, "When Suicide Prevention Becomes Brutality," *Hastings Center Report* 14 (April 1984): 20–21, 46. Additional information is from the United Press International article of 2 November 1983, the Associated Press article of 23 May 1985, and Robert Lindsy, "Ruling Is Upheld in Suicide Appeal," *New York Times*, 20 January 1983. More recent events are reported in the following *New York Times* articles: Marcia Chambers, "Woman Who Fought to Die Is Back in Court," 9 February 1986; "Winner of Right to Starve Faces New Fight at Hospital," 20 April 1986; "Quadriplegic Obtains Court Help on Morphine," 24 April 1986.

No philosophical or legal analysis has so far been made of the J. K. Collums case. The facts and quotations in the Case Presentation are from the account by William K. Stevens, *New York Times*, 9 December 1981. The facts and quotations about the punishment hearing are from a United Press International news story of 5 February 1982. Information about the sentencing is from a United Press International story of 5 March 1982.

Chapter 4: AIDS and Its Issues

The Compound Q Social Context is based on information from Gina Kolata's reports in the *New York Times*: "Group Conducts Secret AIDS Drug Tests," 28 June 1989; "Critics Fault Secret Effort to Test AIDS Drug," 21 September 1989; and "Unorthodox Trials of AIDS Drug Are Allowed by FDA to Go On," 9 March 1990. For the panel recommendation, see Robert Pear, "Faster Approval of AIDS Drugs Is Urged," *New York Times*, 15 April 1990. The DDI information is reported in Gina Kolata, "Odd Surge in Deaths of Those Taking AIDS Drug," *New York Times*, 12 March 1990.

The Tod Thompson case is wholly fictional, but it is based on first-person accounts of a number of people with AIDS. The issue of AIDS and suicide is reported by Seth Mydans, "AIDS Patients' Silent Companion Is Often Suicide," *New York Times*, 25 February 1990. The basic account of the AIDS struggle from the point of view of the homosexual community is from Randy Shilts, *And the Band Played On* (New York: Viking Penguin, 1987).

The best general biomedical account of AIDS is Eve K. Nichols, *Mobilizing Against AIDS*, rev. ed. (Cambridge, Mass.: Harvard University Press, 1989). Nichols is a clear and helpful writer. Also useful is "What Science Knows About AIDS," *Scientific American*, October 1988; the entire issue is devoted to the topic. A helpful collection is I. B. Corless and M. Pitman-Lindeman, eds., *AIDS: Principles, Practices, and Politics* (New York: Hemisphere, 1988). The statistics and quotation are from Dick Thompson, "A Losing Battle with AIDS," *Time*, 2 June 1990. Data about Africa are from Erik Eckholm, "AIDS in Africa," *New York Times*, 16 September 1990. The study showing that DDI delays onset is reported in P. J. Hilts, "Drug Found to Delay AIDS Onset 15 Months," *New York Times*, 30 August 1990. The new blood test is described in *New York Times*, 11 July 1989. Early treatment results are reported in Lawrence K. Altman, "Advances in Treatment Change Face of AIDS," *New York Times*, 12 June 1990. Information about anonymous testing is found in *New York Times*, 9 July 1989. The Behringer case is discussed in J. F. Sullivan, "Should a Hospital Inform Patients If One of Its Surgeons Has AIDS?" *New York Times*, 12 December 1989. The autopsy data and the problem of confidentiality are reported in Bruce Lambert, "Autopsies in N.Y. Find 1 in 7 People Infected with AIDS," *New York Times*, 29 August 1990. The study of how many would warn partners is reported in an Associated Press story, Chicago, 8 January 1988. The studies of testing without consent are reported in *New York Times*, 8 January 1988; 16 February 1990. The AMA proposal is reported in *New York Times*, 31 June 1988, and the movement toward more aggressive testing and notification in Bruce Lamber, "AIDS: Keeping Track of the Infected," 13 May 1990. The issues surrounding privacy and testing are thoroughly laid out in Martin Gunderson, D. J. Mayo, and F. S. Rhame, *AIDS: Testing and Privacy* (Salt Lake City: University of Utah Press, 1989). The insurance problems are discussed in W. C. Gifford III, "An Insidious Test for AIDS," *New York Times*, 14 December 1989, and Bob Hunter and Jay Angoff, "Insurers Are Right on

AIDS Testing," 18 September 1987. Policies concerning testing in the military and in immigration are reported in *New York Times*, 9 June 1987; 13 December 1988; 18 June 1988; 28 February 1990. Dick Thompson's discussion of whether AIDS is claiming too many resources is from "The AIDS Political Machine," *Time*, 22 January 1990.

In the decision scenarios, the solicitation of volunteers was reported by the Associated Press, 12 March 1990, the "Johnson" case in *New York Times*, 4 March 1988, and the Owens case in P. S. Gutis, "AIDS Cited in Killing of Sex Partner," *New York Times*, 4 March 1987.

Chapter 5: Physicians, Patients, and Others

The Social Context on pregnancy and prosecution is based on: Martha Field, "Controlling the Woman to Protect the Fetus," *Law Medicine and Health Care* 2 (1989): 114–129, for the Monson and similar cases; *New York Times*, 15 January 1986 and 30 August 1988, for effects of alcohol and other drugs; 4 May 1989 and 9 May 1989 for the Illinois cases; 2 February 1990 for the Wyoming case; 30 May 1990 for New York court ruling; 19 July 1990 for racial bias; *Time*, 19 September 1988 for statistics about crack babies and hospital experiences in California and South Carolina. The factual account of the Carter case is based on the Field article mentioned above, pp. 117–118.

The Twitchell Case Presentation draws substantially from David Margolic, "Death and Faith, Law and Christian Science," *New York Times*, 6 August 1990; other sources were *New York Times*, 3 and 6 July 1990, and "Convicted of Relying on Prayer," *Time*, 16 July 1990.

The quotations and facts in the "Gonzalez" Case Presentation are from Daniel Goleman, "Emergency Room Struggle: Deciding Who Is Dangerous," *New York Times*, 13 July 1986, and Frank Trippett, "The Madman on the Ferry," *Time*, 21 July 1986, p. 28.

For an account of the physician-patient relationship and the development of licensing procedures for physicians in the United States, see John Duffy, *The Healers: The Rise of the Medical Establishment* (New York: McGraw-Hill, 1977). Duffy also deals with American medical quackery, but the classic works in this area are James Harvey Young, *The Toadstool Millionaires: A Social History of Patent Medicines in America before Federal Regulation* (Princeton, N.J.: Princeton University Press, 1961), and *The*

Medical Messiahs (Princeton, N.J.: Princeton University Press, 1971). An influential sociological account of the nature of the doctor-patient relationship as a social role is Talcott Parsons, "Illness and the Role of the Physician: A Sociological Perspective," in Clyde Kluckhohn and H. A. Murray, eds., *Personality in Nature, Society, and Culture* (New York: Knopf, 1961).

The multiple sclerosis study is reported in *Hastings Center Report* 13 (June 1983): 2–3. The "Korin" Decision Scenario is based on information in Dudley Clendinen, "Therapist's Notes Issue in Fraud Case," *New York Times*, 17 March 1985. For an account of the VD inspection program mentioned, see Clyde Haberman, "New York Testing Prostitutes for V.D.," *New York Times*, 5 March 1982.

Chapter 6: Medical Experimentation and Informed Consent

"The Artificial Heart" Case Presentation draws from the following sources: for a discussion of the Cooley controversy, see Thomas Thompson, *Hearts* (New York: Fawcett, 1971), pp. 227–235; for current criticisms, see Philip M. Boffey, "Artificial Heart: Should It Be Scaled Back?" *New York Times*, 3 December 1985; for questions about terminating the experiment and DeVries's responses, see L. K. Altman, "The Ongoing Ordeal of a 'Human Experiment,' " New York Times, 14 May 1985.

The quotations from Lenfant and DeVries are from Malcolm Browne, "U.S. Halts Funds to Develop Artificial Hearts for Humans," *New York Times*, 13 May 1988. For a negative response, see P. M. Boffey, "Panel Appeals for Funds in Artificial Heart Work," *New York Times*, 19 May 1988.

For information about foreign testing, see Elisabeth Rosenthal, "For More Drugs, First Test Is Abroad," *New York Times*, 7 August 1990.

The "Baby Fae" Case Presentation is based on information from the following *New York Times* stories: L. K. Altman, "Learning from Baby Fae," 18 November 1984; Philip M. Boffey, "Medicine Under Scrutiny," 20 November 1984; Sandra Blakeslee, "Baboon Implant in Baby Fae Assailed," 20 December 1985; and Erik Eckholm, "Baby Death Laid to Wrong Blood," 17 October 1985. The NIH report is summarized in the Associated Press story "Baby Fae's Survival Chances Overstated, U.S. Report Says," 14 March 1985, and in "NIH Approves the Consent for Baby Fae, or Does It?" *Hastings Center Report* 15 (April 1985): 2.

The "Kaimowitz" Case Presentation is based on the opinion of the Wayne County Circuit Court (references cited in the selection). (The quotation from the consent form is from the notes of the opinion.) But it is most indebted to the excellent account by Ronald S. Gass, "*Kaimowitz* v. *Department of Mental Health*," W. M. Gaylin and J. S. Meister, eds., *Operating on the Mind* (New York: Basic Books, 1975), pp. 73–87. Anyone seriously concerned with the Detroit case should read Gass's article. The full opinion is reprinted as an appendix to the book.

The details of the experiments in the "Willowbrook" Case Presentation are taken from Saul Krugman and Joan P. Giles, "Viral Hepatitis: New Light on an Old Disease," *Journal of the American Medical Association* 212 (1970): 1019–21.

The description of Nazi medical experiments is from the indictment in *United States* v. *Karl Brandt*, a selection from which is reprinted in *Hastings Center Report*, "Special Supplement: Biomedical Ethics and the Shadow of Nazism," 6 (August 1976): 5.

The description of drug testing is based on the account by Ross J. Baldessarini, *Chemotherapy in Psychiatry* (Cambridge, Mass.: Harvard University Press, 1977), pp. 4–11.

For a discussion of some of the problems of providing information, testing understanding, and getting consent, I am indebted to William Shebar's unpublished paper "Understanding and Informed Consent in Psychiatric Research." The paternalistic view that physicians must decide because patients can never understand is expressed in Eugene G. Laforet, "The Fiction of Informed Consent," *Journal of the American Medical Association* 235 (12 April 1976): 1579–85. Problems with placebos are discussed in Sissela Bok, "The Ethics of Giving Placebos," *Scientific American* 231 (November 1974): 17–23. The discussion of research and children is indebted to Jean D. Lockhart, "Pediatric Drug Testing," *Hastings Center Report* 7 (June 1977): 8–10. Prisoners and research is discussed at length in Jessica Mitford, *Kind and Usual Punishment* (New York: Knopf, 1973). The historical cases of research on the poor are from M. H. Pappworth, *Human Guinea Pigs* (Boston: Beacon Press, 1961), pp. 61–62. The details of the Tuskegee case are from the "Final Report of the Tuskegee Syphilis Study Ad Hoc Advisory Panel," U.S. Public Health Service (Washington, D.C., 1973), part of which is reprinted in S. J. Reiser et al., *Ethics in Medicine* (Cambridge, Mass.: MIT

Press, 1977), pp. 316–321. I am indebted to the letter by Jay Katz, in particular. In the discussion of fetal experimentation, I am indebted to "Individual Risks vs. Societal Benefits: The Fetus," a forum appearing in *Experiments and Research with Humans: Values in Conflict* (Washington, D.C.: National Academy of Sciences, 1975), pp. 59–90.

HHS regulations on using children as research subjects were published in the Federal Register, 8 March 1983. They are summarized in "Finally, Final Rules on Children Who Become Research Subjects," *Hastings Center Report* 13 (August 1983): 2–3.

The "Phoenix heart" Decision Scenario draws information and quotations from the following articles in the *New York Times*: Lawrence K. Altman, "Anguish, Hope, a Moment of Fame," 19 March 1985; Irvin Molotsky, "F.D.A. Ponders Action on Unsanctioned Implant," 8 March 1985. The questions raised reflect the doubts expressed by George J. Annas in "The Phoenix Heart: What We Have to Lose," *Hastings Center Report* 15 (June 1985): 15–16.

The "Boyd Rush" Decision Scenario is drawn from information cited in George J. Annas, "Baby Fae: The 'Anything Goes' School of Human Experimentation," *Hastings Center Report* 15 (February 1985): 15–17. The original source is Jurgen Thorwald, *The Patients* (New York: Harcourt Brace Jovanovich, 1972).

The case of Ms. Mink presented in the Decision Scenario is based on a report in *Time*, 9 May 1977, p. 44, and on Marlene Cimons's article in the *Los Angeles Times*, 16 May 1977. The quotations are from these sources.

A report on the charges of "guinea-pig" surgery involving mental patients in Chicago is to be found in the *New York Times*, 19 April 1979. Additional information is from *Time*, 23 April 1979.

Chapter 7: Genetics: Intervention, Control, and Research

The "Huntington's disease" Case Presentation relies heavily on information from Gina Kolata, "Closing in on a Killer Gene," *Discover* (March 1984): 83–87. See also Lawrence K. Altman, "Researchers Report Genetic Test Detects Huntington's Disease," *New York Times*, 9 November 1983, and Albert Rosenfeld, "At Risk for Huntington's Disease," *Hastings Center Report* 14 (June 1984): 5–8.

The plan to initiate ADA gene therapy is described in Natalie Angier, "Gene Implant Therapy," *New York Times*, 8 March 1990, and her account of

the first case is in "Girl, 4, Becomes First Human to Receive Engineered Genes," 15 September 1990. The best account of the topic is Eve K. Nicholas, *Human Gene Therapy* (Cambridge, Mass.: Harvard University Press, 1988).

The "gene therapy" Case Presentation is based on information from the following *New York Times* articles: 8 September 1981; Harold M. Schmeck, "Activity of Genes Reported Altered in Treating Man," 9 December 1982; Walter Sullivan, "Transplanting Cells into Brain Offers Promise as Therapy," 11 September 1984; Harold M. Schmeck, "Hereditary Disease: Therapies Are Closer," 28 January 1986. I am also indebted to the Fletcher article reprinted here and to Clifford Grobstein and Michael Flower, "Gene Therapy: Proceed with Caution," *Hastings Center Report* 14 (April 1984): 13–17.

Other information relevant to the topic is drawn from these *New York Times* articles: Walter Sullivan, "Transplanting Cells into Brain Offers Promise as Therapy," 11 September 1984; Harold M. Schmeck, Jr., "U.S. Sets Guidelines on Using Gene Transplants in Humans," 23 September 1985.

The discovery of the cystic fibrosis gene is from Sandra Blakeslee, "Discovery May Help Cystic Fibrosis Victims," *New York Times*, 24 August 1989. For new drugs developed by recombinant techniques, see Harold M. Schmeck, Jr., "An Era Opens as Scientists Reproduce Drugs Made in the Body," *New York Times*, 16 June 1987, and Sandra Blakeslee, "Human Genes Turn Plants into Factories for Medicines," 16 January 1990. The Argentina case is reported in Warren E. Leary, "Altered Virus Said to Cause Infection," *New York Times*, 22 January 1988. The account of the human genome project is indebted to Leon Jaroff's excellent "The Gene Hunt," *Time*, 20 March 1989, pp. 22–67. For a discussion of genetic discrimination, see *Science News* (21 January 1989): 40–42.

For an account of diseases currently screened for and their relation to legal and social issues, see George Annas and B. Coyne, "Fitness for Birth and Reproduction: Legal Implications of Genetic Screening," *Family Law Quarterly* 9 (Fall 1975): 463–490, and Marc Lappé, "The Predictive Powers of the New Genetics," *Hastings Center Report* 14 (October 1984): 18–21. A review of recent diagnostic possibilities is offered by Harold M. Schmeck, Jr., "Fetal Tests Can Now Find Many More Genetic Flaws," *New York Times*, 11 March 1986. A critical look at Tay-Sachs screening is offered in Madeleine J. Goodman and

Lenn E. Goodman, "The Overselling of Genetic Anxiety," *Hastings Center Report* 12 (October 1982): 20–27.

A general survey of the types of screening that are current and the ethical problems they pose is presented by Tabitha M. Powledge, "Genetic Screening," in Warren T. Reich, ed., *Encyclopedia of Bioethics*, vol. 2 (New York: Free Press, 1978), pp. 567–573. The account of the experiences and problems (social and scientific) in PKU screening is found in National Academy of Sciences, *Genetic Screening: Programs, Principles, and Research* (Washington, D.C.: National Academy of Sciences, 1975). For an account of alpha-fetoprotein screening, see Barbara Gastel et al., eds., *Maternal Serum Alpha-Fetoprotein: Issues in the Prenatal Screening and Diagnosis of Neural Tube Defects* (U.S. Department of Health and Human Services Publication HE 20.2: M41, 1981). For a discussion of social problems caused by PKU laws and sickle-cell screening, see Philip Reilly, "There's Another Side to Genetic Screening," *Prism* (January 1976): 55–57.

Genetic screening and the problems it poses for rights is considered by Susan West, "Genetic Testing on the Job," *Science 82* (September 1982): 16. See also Phillip M. Boffey, "Rapid Advances Point to the Mapping of All Human Genes," *New York Times*, 15 July 1986, and Morton Hunt, "The Total Gene Screen," *New York Times Magazine*, 19 January 1986.

For the controversy over genetic-engineering guidelines, testing genetically altered substances, and the potential hazards of altered organisms, see the following *New York Times* articles (when no name is given, the author is Keith Schneider): "Field-Testing Permit for Genetic Concern Lifted for False Data," 26 March 1986; "U.S. Quietly Approved the Sale of Genetically Altered Vaccine," 4 April 1986; "Biology's Unknown Risks," 4 April 1986; "Release of a Gene-Altered Virus Is Halted by U.S. After Challenge," 8 April 1986; "Genetic Field Test Faces a Challenge," 7 April 1986; "U.S. Ends Curb on a Vaccine Using Altered Virus," 23 April 1986; " '84 Test of Altered Virus Stirs Concern," 29 April 1986; "Field Tests Backed for Gene-Altered Pesticide," 25 April 1986; "Another Inquiry Set for Gene-Altered Virus," 1 May 1986; William Dicke, "Gene Splicing Suit Dismissed," 8 May 1986; "President Weighs Easing of Controls for Gene-Splicing," 22 May 1986; "Tests Set for a Pesticide Made by Biotechnologists," 13 June 1986; "U.S. Unveils Rules on Biotechnology," 20 June 1986. See also

Time, 21 April 1986, pp. 52–54. Jeremy Rifkin's views are stated in his book, written in collaboration with Nicanor Perlas, *Algeny* (New York: Viking Press, 1983). For both scientific and social issues, see G. V. Nossal, *Reshaping Life: Key Issues in Genetic Engineering* (New York: Cambridge University Press, 1985). Quite important and useful also is the report of the President's Commission for the Study of Ethical Problems in Medicine and Biomedical and Behavioral Research, *Splicing Life: The Social and Ethical Issues of Genetic Screening with Human Beings* (Washington, D.C.: President's Commission, 1982).

Chapter 8: Reproductive Control: In Vitro Fertilization, Artificial Insemination, and Surrogate Pregnancy

The basic information for the "Louise Brown" Case Presentation is from *Newsweek*, 7 August 1978; *Time*, 7 August 1978; and *U.S. News & World Report*, 7 August 1978. For a discussion of the techniques and issues of in vitro fertilization, in addition to the popular accounts cited above, see R. G. Edwards, "Fertilization of Human Eggs In Vitro: Morals, Ethics, and the Law," *Quarterly Review of Biology* 49 (March 1974): 3–26. I am also indebted for information to George H. Kieffer, "Reproductive Technology: The State of the Art," in Thomas A. Mappes and Jane S. Zembaty, eds., *Biomedical Ethics* (New York: McGraw-Hill, 1981), pp. 485–490.

The "Unclaimed Infant" Case Presentation employs facts and quotations from the Associated Press story "Surrogate Infant Left Unclaimed," 22 January 1983, and from Iver Peterson, "Legal Snarl Developing Around Case of a Baby Born to Surrogate Mother," *New York Times*, 7 February 1983.

Information about sterility, the Norfolk clinic, and the moratorium on in vitro research in the U.S. is found in Michael Gold, "The Baby Makers," *Science 85* (April 1985): 26–38. The history of the moratorium and survey results about public attitudes are based on Susan Abramowitz, "A Stalemate on Test-Tube Baby Research," *Hastings Center Report* 14 (February 1984): 5–9. Abramowitz's analysis of present concerns and problems is highly recommended. For a general survey of all the issues in reproductive technology from a feminist perspective, see Gena Corea, *The Mother Machine* (New York: Harper & Row, 1985).

The historical background on artificial insemination is presented in R. Snowden and G. D. Mitchell, *The Artificial Family* (London: Allen and Unwin, 1981). The technical aspects of the process and the statistics mentioned are discussed in Ronald P. Goldstein, "Artificial Insemination by Donor—Status and Problems," in Aubrey Milunsky and George J. Annas, eds., *Genetics and the Law* (New York: Plenum Press, 1976), pp. 197–202. I am also indebted for information to Donald A. Goss, "Current Status of Artificial Insemination with Donor Semen," *American Journal of Obstetrics and Gynecology* 122 (May 1975): 246–249. For general objections to artificial insemination and other forms of reproductive technology, see Paul Ramsey, *Fabricated Man* (New Haven, Conn.: Yale University Press, 1970), particularly chapter 3.

Statistics and issues surrounding surrogate mothers are presented in Nadine Brozan, "Surrogate Mothers: Problems and Goals," *New York Times*, 27 February 1984. The nonsurgical technique of ova recovery is discussed in Walter Sullivan, "Clinic Offers Aid for Fertilization," *New York Times*, 30 January 1986. The "Rios" Case Presentation is based on information from the Associated Press story "Australians Reject an Effort to Destroy Frozen Embryos," 23 October 1984. For a general review of most of the issues in the current social context, see "Making Babies: The New Science of Conception," *Time*, 10 September 1984, pp. 46–56. The legal issues in reproductive technology are well reviewed by George Annas, "Surrogate Embryo Transfer" and "Redefining Parenthood and Protecting Embryos," *Hastings Center Report* 14 (June 1984): 25–26 and 14 (October 1984): 50–52. The Kim Cotton case is reported in the Associated Press story "Surrogate Mother's Child in English Court Custody," 9 January 1985.

Information on the Davis case is from United Press International stories of 21 September 1989; *New York Times*, 22 April 1989 and 8 August 1989; and Associated Press stories of 26 May 1990 and 13 September 1990.

Recent information about the Rios case is from James Lieber, "The Case of the Frozen Embryos," *The Saturday Evening Post*, October 1989, pp. 50–53.

Recent information about the Stiver case is from "In Brief," *Hastings Center Report* 16 (April 1986): 2.

The new approach to IVF is described in Claude Ranoux et al., "A New In Vitro Fertilization Technique," *Fertility and Sterility* 49 (1988): 654 ff.

The Calvert case is based on materials from Carol Lawson, "Couple's Own Embryos Used in Birth Surrogacy," *New York Times* 12 August 1990; Seth Mydans, "Surrogate Loses Custody Bid in Case Defining Motherhood," *New York Times*, 22 October 1990; and *Time*, 22 August 1990.

Information about the Baby M case is drawn from the *New York Times* articles of 4, 5, 6, 10, 26, 27 January 1987; 2, 3, 9, 10, 11, 17 February 1987; 5, 9, 10, 31 March 1987; 2 April 1987. Information about the Vatican "Instruction" and reaction to it is from *New York Times*, 10, 11 March 1987.

Chapter 9: Acquiring and Allocating Scarce Medical Resources

The developing story of fetal cell implants and the public debate told in the Social Context section is drawn, in part, from the following *New York Times* articles: Walter Sullivan, "Transplanting Cells into Brain Offers Promise as Therapy," 11 September 1984; Tamar Lewin, "Medical Uses of Fetal Tissues Spurs New Abortion Debate, 16 August 1987; Warren Leary, "Panel Supports Research Uses of Fetal Tissues," 17 September 1988, and "Panel Says Use of Fetal Tissue 'Is Acceptable Public Policy,' " 21 October 1988; Tamar Lewin, "Reagan Signs Bill to Bar Sale of Fetal Organs and Tissues," 6 November 1988; William Regelson, "A Wise Fetal Tissue Policy," 14 November 1988; Gina Kolata, "Fetal Tissue Implant Said to Be Aiding a Parkinson Patient," 2 February 1990. See also Howard Wolinsky, "Transplants from the Unborn," *American Health* (April 1988): 47–49.

The facts and opinions in the Ayala case are presented in the Associated Press story "Mom, 43, Having Baby to Save Daughter's Life," 17 February 1990, and Irene Chang, "Bone Marrow Baby Is Born to the Ayalas," *Los Angeles Times*, 6 April 1990.

For the current status of transplants, see D. R. Zimmerman, "Organ Transplantation: From the Experiment to the Routine," in *Next: The Coming Era in Medicine*," ed. H. B. Noble (Boston: Little, Brown, 1987), pp. 61–78.

For the Bosze case, see Isabel Wilkerson, "Search for Marrow Donor Questions Nature of Altruism and Child Rights," *New York Times*, 30 July 1990, and "Setback for Boy Needing Marrow," Associated Press, 28 September 1990. For the Benton case, see Terry Trucco, "Sales of Kidneys Prompt New Laws and Debate," *New York Times*, 1 August 1990.

The "Policy Decision" Case Presentation is based on a real incident. See the St. Louis *Post-Dis-*

patch, 5 July 1981, for an account of the policy at Tampa General Hospital.

There is no Brattle County, Texas, and the Case Presentation is wholly fictional. It does represent, however, the problem that was faced by some dialysis centers when programs were just starting. For a fine account of the workings of a real committee (the one at Swedish Hospital, Seattle, Washington, in 1961), see Shana Alexander, "They Decide Who Lives, Who Dies." The piece first appeared in *Life* magazine in 1962, but it is usefully reprinted in Robert Hunt and John Arras, eds., *Ethical Issues in Modern Medicine* (Palo Alto, Calif.: Mayfield, 1977), pp. 409–424.

Information in the Social Context section about organ transplants and the problems of allocation can be found in Susan Jacoby, "Lifesavers: The Drive for More Organ Donations," *New York Magazine*, 18 July 1983, pp. 39–43; Donald Sullivan, "New York to Require That Hospitals Seek Donation of Organs," *New York Times*, 14 August 1985; H. Tristram Engelhardt, Jr., "Allocating Scarce Medical Resources and the Availability of Organ Transplantation," *New England Journal of Medicine* 311 (5 July 1984): 66–71. The debate about means of increasing the supply is rehearsed in the following *Hastings Center Report* articles: Arthur L. Caplan, "Organ Transplants: The Costs of Success," 13 (December 1983): 23–32; George J. Annas, "Life, Liberty, and the Pursuit of Organ Sales," 14 (February 1984): 22–23; Alfred M. Sadler, Jr., and B. L. Sadler, "A Community of Givers, Not Takers," 14 (October 1984): 6–9; Arthur L. Caplan, "Organ Procurement: It's Not in the Cards," 14 (October 1984): 9–12; "In Minn. and Mass., No Transplants for the Sickest?" 15 (April 1985): 2–3.

The story of cyclosporine and its successful use in organ transplants is presented in Carol Bolotin, "Drug as Hero," *Science 85* (June 1985): 68–71. For the debate over the cost of the Medicare kidney program and relevant statistics, see Robert Reinhold, "Economics of Life and Death Arises in Debate over Kidney Therapy," *New York Times*, 28 May 1982.

For an account of how dialysis takes place and of what it is like from a personal point of view, see Lee Foster, "Man and Machine: Life without Kidneys," *Hastings Center Report* 6 (June 1976): 5–8. I have drawn heavily from Foster's account. The lifeboat analogy is discussed by Paul Ramsey in *The Patient as Person* (New Haven, Conn.: Yale University Press, 1970).

An important sociological study on dialysis and transplants is Reneé C. Fox, "A Sociological Perspective on Organ Transplantation and Hemodialysis," *New Dimensions in Legal and Ethical Concepts for Human Research, Annals of the New York Academy of Sciences* 169 (1970): 406–428. A volume that concentrates on the transplant issue is G. W. Wostenholme and M. O'Connor, eds., *Ethics in Medical Progress: With Special Reference to Transplantation* (Boston: Little, Brown, 1966). See also the relevant chapters in Paul Ramsey, *The Patient as Person* (New Haven, Conn.: Yale University Press, 1970). The ethical issues involved in transplants go beyond the question of distribution, of course.

Chapter 10: The Claim to Health Care

Information about Oregon's rationing efforts is drawn from Ira Mothner, "Drawing the Line," *American Health* (July/August 1989); John Elson, "Rationing Medical Care," *Time*, 27 March 1989; Mary Cantwell, "The Death Dilemma," *New York Times*, 14 February 1990; Jane Gross, "What Medical Care the Poor Can Have: Lists Are Drawn Up," *New York Times*, 27 March 1990; Timothy Egan, "Controversial Oregon Health Plan Delayed," *San Francisco Chronicle*, 31 July 1990; L. A. Chung, "Alameda County Admits Health Rationing Failed," *San Francisco Chronicle*, 2 August 1989; L. A. Chung, "Rationing Health Care—Oregon Lists Priorities," *San Francisco Chronicle*, 4 April 1989. The list of ratings is from the last source.

The Comprehensive Health Care plan is reported in Martin Tochin, "Panel Says Broad Health Care Would Cost $86 Billion a Year," *New York Times*, 2 March 1990. The Canadian system is discussed in the following *New York Times* pieces: Milt Freudenhen, "Debating Canadian Health Model," 29 June 1989; David Woods, "Health Care Canadian Style: Americans Beware," 4 July 1989; H. M. Lerner, "Don't Look to Canada's Health System," 3 February 1990; letters by Mark Warren and Janey Joy; Shanke K. Cobb; I. S. Tummon under the title "Canada's Health Care Succeeds Where Ours Doesn't," 26 February 1990.

The Social Context section on crisis is indebted to Stanley Hwang, "Dissecting the Health Care Beast," *Harvard Political Review* 6 (Fall 1977): 12–15, and Bernard Winter, "The Problem of Profits," *The Progressive* 41 (October 1977): 16–19. Statistics are from U.S. Health Care Financing Administration, *Health Care Financing Review* (Winter 1984). Information on DRGs and their difficulties is from Danielle A. Dolenc and Charles J. Dougherty, "DRGs: The Counterrevolution in Financing Health Care," *Hastings Center Report* 15 (June 1985): 20–29, and John K. Inglehart, "Medicare Begins Prospective Payment of Hospitals," *New England Journal of Medicine* 308 (9 June 1983): 1428–1432. Information about using DRGs to establish fee schedules for physicians can be found in Robert Pear, "Rx for Fees," *New York Times*, 24 August 1985. Problems caused public and teaching hospitals by DRGs and the increasing number of uninsured poor are discussed in Dudley Clendinen, "Meeting on Poor and Health Care," *New York Times*, 9 October 1985, and in Robert Pear, "White House Acting to End Rules Requiring Hospitals to Help Poor," *New York Times*, 4 November 1985. Problems associated with for-profit hospitals are discussed in Arnold S. Relman, "Investor-Owned Hospitals and Health-Care Costs," *New England Journal of Medicine* 309 (11 August 1983): 370–372, and Donald O. Nutter, "Access to Care and the Evolution of Corporate, For-Profit Medicine," *New England Journal of Medicine* 311 (4 October 1984): 917–919. The survey of public attitudes is found in Robert J. Blendon and Drew Altman, "Public Attitudes about Health-Care Costs," *New England Journal of Medicine* 311 (30 August 1984): 613–616.

The discussion of rights in the introduction is indebted to Joel Feinberg, "The Nature and Value of Rights," *Journal of Value Inquiry* 4 (1970): 243–257. For a discussion of the legal status of claims to health care, see Edward V. Sparer, "The Legal Right to Health Care: Public Policy and Equal Access," *Hastings Center Report* 6 (1976): 39–47.

For a discussion of the idea of health stamps or vouchers, see John Arras, "Health Care Vouchers and the Rhetoric of Equity," *Hastings Center Report* 11 (August 1981). A potential health-stamp plan is discussed by Gordon K. MacLeod, "Health Stamps, Maybe?" *New York Times*, 8 April 1980.

BIBLIOGRAPHY

The number of books and articles dealing with medical ethics is staggering, and it is growing larger at a rapid rate. The materials listed here are no more than a sample of those currently available. Thus, this bibliography is best thought of as a guide to further reading. The general and special bibliographies listed below—some book-length works—will provide guides for those who are looking for comprehensiveness.

I have tried to select works with substantial philosophical content. Thus, with a few exceptions, I have not listed publications that are primarily medical, biological, sociological, or otherwise scientific. Furthermore, I have not attempted to duplicate the references given in the selections or in the chapter introductions, and for the most part I have restricted this bibliography to works that have appeared in the last five to ten years.

General Works and Anthologies

American Medical Association. *Current Opinions of the Judicial Council.* Chicago: American Medical Association, 1991.

Arras, John and Nancy Rhoden. *Ethical Issues in Modern Medicine,* 3rd ed. Palo Alto, Calif.: Mayfield, 1989.

Augenstein, Leroy. *Come, Let Us Play God.* New York: Harper & Row, 1969.

Bandman, Elsie and Bertram Bandman, eds. *Bioethics and Human Rights: A Reader for Health Professionals.* Boston: Little, Brown, 1978.

Beauchamp, Tom L. and LeRoy Walters, eds. *Contemporary Issues in Bioethics.* 3d ed. Belmont Calif.: Wadsworth, 1989.

Benjamin, Martin and Joy Curtis. *Ethics in Nursing.* New York: Oxford University Press, 1981.

British Medical Association. *Handbook of Medical Ethics.* London: British Medical Association, 1981.

Brody, Howard. *Ethical Decisions in Medicine.* Boston: Little, Brown, 1976.

Chapman, Carleton, B. "The Importance of Being Ethical." *Perspectives in Biology and Medicine* 24 (Spring 1981): 422–439.

Clouser, K. Danner. "Medical Ethics: Some Uses, Abuses, and Limitations." *Arizona Medicine* 33 (January 1976): 44–49.

Copp, David and David Zimmerman, eds. *Morality, Reason and Truth: New Essays on the Foundations of Ethics.* Totowa, N.J.: Rowman and Allanheld, 1984.

Curran, William J. "The Proper and Improper Concerns of Medical Law and Ethics." *New England Journal of Medicine* 259 (4 November 1976): 1057–58.

Curtin, Leah and M. Josephine Flaherty. *Nursing Ethics: Theories and Pragmatics.* Bowie, Md.: Robert J. Brady, 1982.

Cutler, Donald R., ed. *Updating Life and Death.* Boston: Beacon Press, 1969.

Duncan, A. S. et al., eds. *Dictionary of Medical Ethics.* London: Darton, Longman, and Todd, 1975.

Engelhardt, H. Tristram. *The Foundations of Bioethics.* New York: Oxford University Press, 1986.

Engelhardt, H. Tristram, Jr., and Daniel Callahan, eds. *Science, Ethics and Medicine.* Hastings-on-Hudson, N.Y.: Institute of Society, Ethics and the Life Sciences, 1976.

Fletcher, Joseph. *Morals and Medicine.* Boston: Beacon Press, 1954. A classic book stating the "situation ethics" view of euthanasia, truth telling, contraception, etc.

Francoeur, Robert T. *Biomedical Ethics: A Guide to Decision Making.* New York: Wiley, 1983.

Giles, James E. *Medical Ethics: A Patient-Centered Approach.* Cambridge: Schenkman, 1983.

Glover, Jonathan. *Causing Death and Saving Lives.* New York: Penguin Books, 1977.

Gorovitz, Samuel et al., eds. *Moral Problems in Medicine.* 2nd ed. Englewood Cliffs, N.J.: Prentice-Hall, 1983.

Gribetz, Donald and Moshe D. Tendler, guest eds. "Medical Ethics: The Jewish Point of View." *The Mount Sinai Journal of Medicine.* Special Issue 51 (January/February 1984).

Harris, John. *The Value of Life: An Introduction to Medical Ethics.* London: Routledge & Kegan Paul, 1985.

Harrison, Beverly Wildung. *Making the Connections: Essays in Feminist Social Ethics.* Boston: Beacon Press, 1985.

Humber, James M. and Robert F. Almeder, eds. *Biomedical Ethics Reviews—1983.* Clifton, N.J.: Humana Press, 1983.

_____ . *Biomedical Ethics and the Law.* New York: Plenum, 1976.

Jonsen, Albert R., Mark Siegler, and William J. Winslade. *Clinical Ethics.* New York: Macmillan, 1982.

Labby, Daniel H., ed. *Life or Death: Ethics and Options.* Seattle: University of Washington Press, 1968.

Levine, Carol, ed. *Taking Sides: Clashing Views on Controversial Bio-Ethical Issues.* Guilford, Conn.: Dushkin, 1984.

Lockwood, Michael, ed. *Moral Dilemmas in Modern Medicine.* Oxford: Oxford University Press, 1985.

Mappes, Thomas A. and Jane S. Zembaty, eds. *Biomedical Ethics.* 2d ed. New York: McGraw-Hill, 1986.

Martin, Rex. *Rawls and Rights.* Lawrence: University of Kansas Press, 1985.

McIntyre, Neil and Karl Popper. "The Critical Attitude in Medicine: The Need for a New Ethics." *British Medical Journal* 287 (24–31) (December 1983): 1919–23.

Ostheimer, Nancy and John Ostheimer, eds. *Life or Death—Who Controls?* New York: Springer, 1976.

Peters, Karl E., ed. "Is Ethics a Science?" *Zygon* 15 (March 1980). Articles by Abraham Edel, R. B. Brandt, and Marcus Singer.

President's Commission for the Study of Ethical Problems in Medicine and Biomedical and Behavioral Research. *Summing Up.* Washington, D.C.: President's Commission, 1983.

Rachels, James. "Can Ethics Provide Answers?" *Hastings Center Report* 10 (1980): 32–40.

_____ . *The Elements of Moral Philosophy.* Philadelphia: Temple University Press, 1986.

Ramsey, Paul. *Ethics at the Edges of Life: Medical and Legal Intersections.* New Haven, Conn.: Yale University Press, 1978.

_____ . *The Patient as Person.* New Haven, Conn.: Yale University Press, 1970. A classic work by a Christian theologian that presents influential views on experimentation, transplantation, allocation of resources, etc.

Reich, W. T., ed. *Encyclopedia of Bioethics.* New York: Macmillan, 1978. A wide-ranging collection of articles by many scholars. Good for a quick survey of major issues.

Reidy, Maurice. *Foundations for a Medical Ethic.* New York: Paulist Press, 1979.

Reiser, S. J., A. J. Dyck, and W. J. Curran, eds. *Ethics in Medicine: Historical Perspectives and Contemporary Concerns.* Cambridge, Mass.: MIT Press, 1977. A large book, strong on historical writings and documents but not on philosophy.

Rivlin, Alice M. and P. Michael Timpane, eds. *Ethical and Legal Issues of Social Experimentation.* Washington, D.C.: The Brookings Institution, 1975. See in particular "Ethical Principles in Medical Experimentation," by Robert M. Veatch.

Shannon, Thomas. *Twelve Problems in Health Care Ethics.* Lewiston, N.Y.: Edwin Mellen Press, 1985.

Shannon, Thomas A. and Jo Ann Manfra, eds. *Law and Bioethics.* Ramsey, N.J.: Paulist Press, 1982.

_____ . *Bioethics.* New York: Paulist Press, 1981.

Shelp, Earl E., ed. *Virtue and Medicine: Explorations in the Character of Medicine.* Boston: D. Reidel, 1985.

Skegg, P. D. G. *Law, Ethics, and Medicine.* Oxford: Clarendon Press, 1984.

Spicker, Stuart F. and H. Tristram Engelhardt, Jr., eds. *Philosophical Medical Ethics: Its Nature and Significance.* Boston: D. Reidel, 1977.

Thompson, Ian E., Kath M. Melia, and Kenneth M. Boyd. *Nursing Ethics.* New York: Churchill Livingstone, 1983.

Trial 16 (December 1980). An issue devoted to bioethical and biolegal issues.

Varga, Andrew C., S. J. *The Main Issues in Bioethics.* New York: Paulist Press, 1980.

Vaux, Kenneth. *Biomedical Ethics: Morality for the New Medicine.* New York: Harper & Row, 1974.

Veatch, Robert M. *Case Studies in Medical Ethics.* Cambridge, Mass.: Harvard University Press, 1977.

_____ . *Death, Dying, and the Biological Revolution.* New Haven, Conn.: Yale University Press, 1976. Deals with dying patients, euthanasia, birth defects, defining death, and transplant organs. Contains much information.

_____ . *A Theory of Medical Ethics.* New York: Basic Books, 1981.

Wall, Thomas F. *Medical Ethics: Basic Moral Issues.* Lanham, Md.: University Press of America, 1980.

Williams, Bernard. *Ethics and the Limits of Philosophy.* Cambridge, Mass.: Harvard University Press, 1985.

Williams, Granville. *The Sanctity of Life and the Criminal Law.* New York: Knopf, 1957.

Williams, Preston, ed. *Ethical Issues in Biology and Medicine.* Cambridge, Mass.: Schenkman, 1973. Original papers, several with a theological orientation.

Williams, Robert H., ed. *To Live and to Die: When, Why, and How.* New York: Springer-Verlag, 1973.

Wojcik, Jan. *Muted Consent: A Case Book of Modern Medical Ethics.* West Lafayette, Ind.: Purdue University Press, 1978.

Yezzi, Ronald. *Medical Ethics: Thinking About Unavoidable Questions.* New York: Holt, Rinehart and Winston, 1980.

Bibliographies

American Nurses' Association. *Ethics References for Nurses.* Kansas City, Mo.: American Nurses' Association, 1982.

American Nurses' Association, Committee on Ethics. *Ethics in Nursing: References and Resources.* Kansas City, Mo.: American Nurses' Association, 1979.

"Bioethics and the Law: A Bibliography, 1974–1976." *American Journal of Law and Medicine* 2 (Winter 1976–1977): 263–281.

Calhoun, Cheryl. *Annotated Bibliography of Medical Oaths, Codes, and Prayers.* Washington, D.C.: Kennedy Institute of Ethics, 1975.

Carmody, James. *Ethical Issues in Health Services: A Report and Annotated Bibliography.* Washington, D.C.: U.S. Department of Health, Education and Welfare, 1974.

Clouser, K. Danner and Arthur Zucker. *Abortion and Euthanasia: An Annotated Bibliography.* Philadelphia: Society for Health and Human Values, 1974.

A Comprehensive Set of Bibliographies on Voluntary Sterilization. New York: The International Project of the Association for Voluntary Sterilization, January 1976.

Euthanasia: An Annotated Bibliography. New York: Euthanasia Educational Fund, 1970.

Goldstein, Doris M. *Bioethics: A Guide to Information Sources.* Detroit: Gale Research, 1982.

Kalish, Richard A. "Death and Dying: A Briefly Annotated Bibliography." In *The Dying Patient.* Edited by Orville G. Brim, Jr., et al. New York: Russell Sage Foundation, 1970, pp. 323–380.

Kutscher, A. *Bibliography of Books on Death, Bereavement, Loss, and Grief: 1955–1968.* New York: Health Sciences, 1969.

Lineback, Richard H., ed. *Philosopher's Index.* Vols. 1–. Bowling Green, Ohio: Philosophy Documentation Center, Bowling Green State University. Issued quarterly.

Nevins, Madeline M., ed. *Annotated Bibliography of Bioethics: Selected 1976 Titles.* Rockville, Md.: Information Planning Associations, 1977.

Pence, Terry. *Ethics in Nursing: An Annotated Bibliography.* New York: National League for Nursing, 1983.

Sollitto, Sharmon and Robert M. Veatch. Revised by Ira D. Singer. *Bibliography of Society, Ethics and the Life Sciences: 1979–1980.* Hastings-on-Hudson, N.Y.: Institute of Society, Ethics and the Life Sciences, 1978. This is the best general bibliography and also the best guide to philosophical articles on medical ethics. It is partially annotated and brought up to date periodically.

Sorenson, James R. *Social and Psychological Aspects of Applied Human Genetics: A Bibliography.* Washington, D.C.: Department of Health, Education and Welfare, 1973.

Vernick, Joel J. *Selected Bibliography on Death and Dying.* Washington, D.C.: U.S. Department of Health, Education and Welfare, National Institutes of Health, n.d.

Walters, LeRoy and Tamar Joy Kahn, eds. *Bibliography of Bioethics.* Vols. 1–13. Washington, D.C.: Kennedy Institute of Ethics, Georgetown University. Published annually.

Computer Databases

AIDSLINE, National Library of Medicine, indexes over 3,000 journals in the clinical, research, epidemiology, and social policy literature of the disease.

BIOETHICSLINE, National Library of Medicine, covers relevant literature in medicine, law, religion, philosophy, and the social sciences.

FACTS ON FILE contains the full text of the weekly printed reference publication of the same name. Topics include news concerning abortion (specifically) and medicine in general.

MEDLINE, National Library of Medicine, contains summaries of articles in clinical and research medicine and related areas. Includes articles on ethics, economics, and society as related to medicine, and over 250,000 records are added each year.

PHILOSOPHER'S INDEX provides indexes and abstracts from journals and books in philosophy and related fields. The journals are indexed from 1940, and the file contains more than 140,000 items.

Moral Principles, Ethical Theories, and Medical Decisions: An Introduction

A. General Works on Ethics

Beauchamp, Tom L. and Terry Pinkard, eds. *Ethics and Public Policy: An Introduction to Ethics.* Englewood Cliffs, N.J.: Prentice-Hall, 1983.

Brandt, Richard B. *Ethical Theory.* Englewood Cliffs, N.J.: Prentice-Hall, 1959.

Ewing, A. C. *Ethics.* New York: Free Press, 1965.

Feinberg, Joel. *Doing and Deserving: Essays in the Theory of Responsibility.* Princeton, N.J.: Princeton University Press, 1970.

——— . *Social Philosophy.* Englewood Cliffs, N.J.: Prentice-Hall, 1973.

——— . *Rights, Justice, and the Bounds of Liberty.* Princeton, N.J.: Princeton University Press, 1980.

Frankena, William K. *Ethics.* 2d ed. Englewood Cliffs, N.J.: Prentice-Hall, 1973.

Gert, Bernard. *The Moral Rules.* New York: Harper & Row, 1970.

Ladd, John. *Ethical Relativism.* Belmont, Calif.: Wadsworth, 1973.

MacIntyre, Alasdair. *After Virtue.* Notre Dame, Ind.: University of Notre Dame Press, 1981.

Rachels, James. *Understanding Moral Philosophy.* Encino, Calif.: Dickenson, 1976. A short, readable introduction.

Taylor, Paul W., ed. *The Moral Judgment: Readings in Contemporary Meta-Ethics.* Englewood Cliffs, N.J.: Prentice-Hall, 1963.

——— , ed. *Problems of Moral Philosophy.* Belmont, Calif.: Dickenson, 1971. Clear and sophisticated introduction.

Warnock, Geoffrey James. *Contemporary Moral Philosophy.* New York: St. Martin's Press, 1967.

Wellman, Carl. *Morals and Ethics.* New York: Scott, Foresman, 1975.

White, Alan R. *Rights.* Oxford: Clarendon Press, 1984.

Williams, Bernard. *Morality: An Introduction to Ethics.* New York: Harper & Row, 1972.

B. Utilitarianism

Bayles, Michael D., ed. *Contemporary Utilitarianism.* New York: Doubleday, 1968.

Bentham, Jeremy. *A Fragment on Government and An Introduction to the Principles of Morals and Legislation.* Edited by Wilfried Harrison. Oxford: Blackwell, 1967.

Hodgson, D. H. *Consequences of Utilitarianism: A Study in Normative Ethics and Legal Theory.* Oxford: Clarendon Press, 1967.

Lyons, David. *Forms and Limits of Utilitarianism.* New York: Oxford University Press, 1965.

_____ . *In the Interest of the Governed: A Study in Bentham's Philosophy of Utility and Law.* Oxford: Oxford University Press, 1973.

Mill, John Stuart. *Utilitarianism: With Critical Essays.* Edited by Samuel Gorovitz. Indianapolis: Bobbs-Merrill, 1971.

Quinton, A. M. *Utilitarian Ethics.* New York: St. Martin's Press, 1973.

Regan, Donald H. *Utilitarianism and Co-operation.* New York: Oxford University Press, 1980.

Sen, Amartya and Bernard Williams, eds. *Utilitarianism and Beyond.* New York: Cambridge University Press, 1982.

Smart, J. J. C. and Bernard Williams. *Utilitarianism: For and Against.* New York: Cambridge University Press, 1973.

C. Kant

Beck, L. W. *Studies in the Philosophy of Kant.* Indianapolis: Bobbs-Merrill, 1965.

Kant, Immanuel. *Foundations of the Metaphysics of Morals: Text and Critical Essays.* Edited by Robert P. Wolff. New York: Bobbs-Merrill, 1969.

_____ . *Lectures on Ethics.* New York: Harper & Row, 1963.

Paton, H. J. *The Categorical Imperative: A Study of Kant's Moral Philosophy.* New York: Harper & Row, 1967.

Singer, Marcus G. *Generalization in Ethics: An Essay in the Logic of Ethics with the Rudiments of a System of Moral Philosophy.* New York: Atheneum, 1971.

Wolff, R. P., ed. *Kant: A Collection of Critical Essays.* Garden City, N.Y.: Doubleday, 1967.

D. Ross

Ross, W. D. *Foundations of Ethics.* Oxford: Oxford University Press, 1963. A reissue of the 1939 edition.

_____ . *The Right and the Good.* Oxford: Clarendon Press, 1930. (For evaluations of Ross, see relevant sections of Frankena, Brandt, Ewing, Rachels, and Taylor listed above.)

E. Rawls

Barry, Brian. *The Liberal Theory of Justice.* New York: Oxford University Press, 1974. An exposition and criticism of Rawls.

Chen, Marshall. "The Social Contract Explained and Defended." *New York Book Review,* 16 July 1972, p. 1.

Daniels, Norman, ed. *Reading Rawls.* New York: Basic Books, 1976. This volume has a helpful introduction and contains some of the more important critical articles.

F. Aquinas and Natural Law

Copleston, F. C. *Aquinas.* Baltimore: Penguin Books, 1965.

Gilson, Etienne. *The Philosophy of St. Thomas Aquinas.* 3d ed. Translated by Edward Bullough. St. Louis: Herder, 1937.

Kelly, Gerald. *Medico-Moral Problems.* St. Louis: Catholic Hospital Association, 1958.

McFadden, Charles J. *Medical Ethics.* 6th ed. Philadelphia: F. A. Davis, 1967.

O'Connor, D. J. *Aquinas and Natural Law.* New York: St. Martin's Press, 1969.

Pegis, Anton, ed. *Basic Writings of St. Thomas Aquinas.* New York: Random House, 1945.

Tuck, Richard. *Natural Rights Theories: Their Origin and Development.* New York: Cambridge University Press, 1980.

Part I: Termination

Chapter 1: Abortion

Altman, Andrew. "Abortion and the Indigent." *Journal of Social Philosophy* 11 (1980): 5–9. Favors the Supreme Court decision that states need not fund abortions.

Annis, David. "Self-Consciousness and the Right to Life." *Southwestern Journal of Philosophy* 6 (1975): 123–128.

Bagley, C. "On the Sociology and Social Ethics of Abortion." *Ethics in Science and Medicine* 3 (1976): 21–32.

Becker, Laurence C. "Human Being: The Boundaries of the Concept." *Philosophy and Public Affairs* 4 (1975): 334–359. Attempts to develop a biological concept relevant to abortion and euthanasia.

Bok, Sissela. "Ethical Problems of Abortion." *Hastings Center Report* 2 (1974): 33–52.

_____ . "Who Shall Count as a Human Being? A Treacherous Question in the Abortion

Discussion." In **Robert L. Perkins, ed.** *Abortion: Pro and Con.* Cambridge, Mass.: Schenkman, 1974, pp. 91–105.

Bondeson, William B., H. Tristram Engelhardt, Jr., Stuart F. Spicker, and Daniel H. Winship, eds. *Abortion and the Status of the Fetus.* Boston: D. Reidel, 1983.

Brandt, R. B. "The Morality of Abortion." *Monist* 56 (1972): 503–526.

Brody, Baruch. *Abortion and the Sanctity of Human Life.* Cambridge, Mass.: MIT Press, 1975. Brody's several papers are embodied here.

_____ . "Thomson on Abortion." *Philosophy and Public Affairs* 1 (1972): 335–340.

Callahan, Daniel. *Abortion: Law, Choice and Morality.* New York: Macmillan, 1970.

Callahan, Sidney. "Abortion and the Sexual Agenda." *Commonweal* 113(8) (25 April 1986): 232–238.

Callahan, Sidney and Daniel Callahan, eds. *Abortion: Understanding Differences.* New York: Plenum Press, 1984.

Camenisch, Paul F. "Abortion: For the Fetus's Own Sake?" *Hastings Center Report* 6 (1976): 38–41.

_____ . "Abortion Analogies and the Emergence of Value." *Journal of Religious Ethics* 4 (1976): 131–158.

Chervenak, Frank A. et al. "When Is Termination of Pregnancy During the Third Trimester Morally Justifiable?" *New England Journal of Medicine* 310 (23 February 1984): 501–504.

Cohen, Marshall et al., eds. *The Rights and Wrongs of Abortion.* Princeton, N.J.: Princeton University Press, 1974.

Connery, John R. *Abortion: The Development of the Roman Catholic Perspective.* Chicago: Loyola University Press, 1977.

Daniels, Charles B. "Abortion and Potential." *Dialogue* 18 (June 1979): 220–223.

Davis, Michael. "Fetuses, Famous Violinists, and the Right to Continued Aid." *Philosophical Quarterly* 33 (July 1983): 259–278.

Davis, Nancy. "Abortion and Self-Defense." *Philosophy and Public Affairs* 13(3) (Summer 1984): 175–207.

Engelhardt, H. Tristram. "The Ontology of Abortion." *Ethics* 84 (April 1974): 217–234.

English, Jane. "Abortion and the Concept of a Person." *Canadian Journal of Philosophy* 5 (October 1975): 233–243.

Feinberg, Joel. "Abortion." In **Tom Regan, ed.** *Matters of Life and Death.* New York: Random House, 1980, pp. 183–217.

_____ . "Is There a Right to Be Born?" In **James Rachels, ed.** *Understanding Moral Philosophy.* Belmont, Calif.: Dickenson, 1976.

_____ , ed. *The Problem of Abortion.* 2d ed. Belmont, Calif.: Wadsworth, 1984.

Finnis, John, Judith Thomson, Michael Tooley, and Roger Wertheimer. *The Rights and Wrongs of Abortion.* Princeton, N.J.: Princeton University Press, 1974. A collection of influential articles.

Fleming, Lorette. "The Moral Status of the Fetus: A Reappraisal." *Bioethics* 1 (January 1987): 15–34.

Fletcher, Joseph. "Four Indicators of Humanhood—The Enquiry Matures." *Hastings Center Report* 4 (December 1974): 4–7.

Foot, Phillippa. "The Problem of Abortion and the Doctrine of Double Effect." *Oxford Review* 5 (1967): 5–15.

Frohock, Fred M. *Abortion: A Case Study in Law and Morals.* Westport, Conn.: Greenwood Press, 1983.

Garfield, Jay L. and Patricia Hennessey, eds. *Abortion: Moral and Legal Perspectives.* Amherst: University of Massachusetts Press, 1984.

Gerber, D. "Abortion: The Uptake Argument." *Ethics* 83 (1972): 80–83.

Gerber, R. J. "Abortion: Parameters for Decision." *Ethics* 82 (1972).

Gertler, Gary B. "Brain Birth: A Proposal for Defining When a Fetus Is Entitled to Human Life Status." *Southern California Law Review,* 59(5) (July 1986): 1061–78.

Gillespie, Norman C. "Abortion and Human Rights." *Ethics* 87 (April 1977): 237–243.

Goldenring, John. "The Brain-Life Theory: Towards a Consistent Biological Definition of Humaneness." *Journal of Medical Ethics* 11 (December 1985): 194–204.

Goldman, Alan H. "Abortion and the Right to Life." *Personalist* 60 (October 1979): 402–406.

Goodrich, T. "The Morality of Killing." *Philosophy* 44 (1969): 127–139.

Gordon, Robert M. "The Abortion Issue." In **Eugene Freeman, ed.** *The Abdication of Philosophy: Essays in Honor of Paul A. Schilpp.* Chicago: Open Court, 1974, pp. 267–277.

Granfield, David. *The Abortion Decision.* New York: Doubleday, 1971. A Catholic point of view.

Grobstein, Clifford. "The Early Development of Human Embryos." *Journal of Medicine and Philosophy* 10 (August 1985): 213–236.

Hall, Robert E., ed. *Abortion in a Changing World.* New York: Columbia University Press, 1970.

Hare, R. M. "Abortion and the Golden Rule." *Philosophy and Public Affairs* 4 (1975): 201–222.

Harrison, Beverly Wildung. *Our Right to Choose: Toward a New Ethic of Abortion.* Boston: Beacon Press, 1983.

Harrison, S. M. "The Unwilling Dead." *Proceedings of the Catholic Philosophical Association* 46 (1972): 199–208. Argues that the concept of a person is central to the abortion issue and offers one based on C. S. Peirce.

Herbewick, Raymond M. "Remarks on Abortion, Abandonment and Adoption Opportunities." *Philosophy and Public Affairs* 5 (Fall 1975): 98–104.

Humber, James M. "The Case against Abortion." *The Thomist* 39 (1975): 65–84. A criticism of major arguments.

Jaffee, Frederick, Barbara Lindheim, and Philip Lee. *Abortion Politics: Private Morality and Public Policy.* New York: McGraw-Hill, 1981.

Kohl, Marvin. "Abortion and the Argument from Innocence." *Inquiry* 14 (1971): 147–151.

―――― , ed. *Infanticide and the Value of Life.* Buffalo, N.Y.: Prometheus Books, 1978.

Kushner, Thomasine. "Having a Life versus Being Alive." *Journal of Medical Ethics* 10 (March 1984): 5–8.

Langham, Paul. "Between Abortion and Infanticide." *Southern Journal of Philosophy* 17 (1979): 465–471.

Levy, Steven R. "Abortion and Dissenting Parents: A Dialogue." *Ethics* 90 (1980): 162–163.

Manier, Edward, William Liu, and David Solomon. *Abortion: New Directions for Policy Studies.* Notre Dame, Ind.: University of Notre Dame Press, 1977.

Margolis, Joseph. "Abortion." *Ethics* 84 (1973): 51–61.

Moore, E. C. et al. "Abortion: The New Ruling." *Hastings Center Report* 3 (1973): 4–7.

Moore, Harold F. "Abortion and the Logic of Moral Justification." *Journal of Value Inquiry* 9 (1975): 140–151.

Noonan, John T. *A Private Choice: Abortion in America in the Seventies.* New York: Free Press, 1979.

Parness, Jeffrey. "Crimes Against the Unborn: Protecting and Respecting the Potentiality of Human Life." *Harvard Journal on Legislation* 22(1) (Winter 1985): 97–172.

Petchesky, Rosalind Pollack. *Abortion and Woman's Choice: The State, Sexuality, and Reproductive Freedom.* New York: Longman, 1984.

Pole, Nelson. "To Respect Human Life." *Philosophical Context* 2 (1973): 16–22. Argues that a right to abortion promotes human dignity.

Quinn, Warren. "Abortion: Identity and Loss." *Philosophy and Public Affairs* 13 (Winter 1984): 24–54.

Regan, Tom. *Matters of Life and Death.* New York: Random House, 1980.

Rorty, Amelie O. "Persons, Policies, and Bodies." *International Philosophical Quarterly* 13 (March 1973): 63–80.

Schneider, Carl E. and Maris A. Vinouskis, eds. *The Law and Politics of Abortion.* Lexington, Mass.: D.C. Heath, 1980.

Shea, M. C. "Embryonic Life and Human Life." *Journal of Medical Ethics* 11 (June 1984): 79–81.

Sher, George. "Hare, Abortion and the Golden Rule." *Philosophy and Public Affairs* 6 (Winter 1977): 185–190.

Sumner, L. W. *Abortion and Moral Theory.* Princeton, N.J.: Princeton University Press, 1981.

Talmage, R. S. "Utilitarianism and the Morality of Killing." *Philosophy* 47 (1972): 55–63.

Tauer, Carol. "Personhood and Human Embryos and Fetuses." *Journal of Medicine and Philosophy* 10 (August 1985): 253–266.

Thomson, Judith Jarvis. "Rights and Deaths." *Philosophy and Public Affairs* 2 (1973): 146–159.

Tietze, Christopher. *Induced Abortion: A World Review, 1981.* New York: Population Council, 1981.

Tooley, Michael. *Abortion and Infanticide.* New York: Oxford University Press, 1983.

Vandever, Donald. "Justifying Wholesale Slaughter." *Canadian Journal of Philosophy* 5 (1975): 245–258.

Wade, Francis C. "Potentiality in the Abortion Discussion." *Review of Metaphysics* 29 (December 1975): 239–255.

Warren, Mary Anne. "Do Potential People Have Moral Rights?" *Canadian Journal of Philosophy* 7 (June 1977): 275–289.

Wasserstrom, Richard. "The Status of the Fetus." *Hastings Center Report* 5 (June 1975): 18–22.

Weiss, Roslyn. "The Perils of Personhood." *Ethics* 89 (October 1978): 66–75.

Werner, Richard. "Abortion: The Moral Status of the Unborn." *Social Theory and Practice* 3 (Fall 1974): 201–222.

———. "Abortion: The Ontological and Moral Status of the Unborn." In **Richard A. Wasserstrom, ed.** *Today's Moral Problems.* 2d ed. New York: Macmillan, 1979, pp. 51–74.

Wertheimer, Roger. "Understanding the Abortion Argument." *Philosophy and Public Affairs* 1 (1971): 67–95. A clear statement of issues.

Wicclair, Mark R. "The Abortion Controversy and the Claim That This Body is Mine." *Social Theory* 7 (Fall 1981): 337–346.

Zaitchik, Alan. "Viability and the Morality of Abortion." *Philosophy and Public Affairs* 10 (Winter 1981): 18–26.

Chapter 2: Treating or Terminating: The Problem of Impaired Infants

Abrams, Natalie. "Defective Newborns: A Framework for a Case Analysis." *Westminister Institute Review* 2 (Winter 1983): 3–7.

American Academy of Pediatrics, ed. "Selected Readings on Infant Care Review Committees and Bioethical Issues in the Care of Seriously Ill and Disabled Newborns." May 1984.

Augenstein, Leroy. "Birth Defects, The Ethical Problem." *Humanist* 28 (1968): 18–20.

Coburn, Robert C. "Morality and the Defective Newborn." *Journal of Medicine and Philosophy* 5 (December 1980): 340–357.

Corr, Charles A. and Donna M. Corr, eds. *Hospice Approaches to Pediatric Care.* New York: Springer, 1985.

Darling, Rosalyn Benjamin. "Parents, Physicians, and Spina Bifida." *Hastings Center Report* 7 (August 1977): 10–13.

Drane, James F. "The Defective Child: Ethical Guidelines for Painful Dilemmas." *Journal of Obstetric Gynecologic and Neo-Natal Nursing* 13 (January/February 1984): 42–48.

Duff, R. S. and A. G. M. Campbell. "Moral and Ethical Dilemmas in the Special Care Nursery." *New England Journal of Medicine* 289 (1973): 890–894.

Engelhardt, H. T. "Euthanasia and Children: The Inquiry of Continued Existence." *Journal of Pediatrics* 83 (1973): 170–171.

Fletcher, John C. "Abortion, Euthanasia, and Care of Defective Newborns." *New England Journal of Medicine* 292 (1975): 75–78.

———. "Attitudes toward Defective Newborns." *Hastings Center Studies* 2 (1974): 21–32.

———. "Choices for Life or Death in the Case of Defective Newborns." *Social Responsibility: Journalism, Law, Medicine.* Program on Society and the Professions: Studies in Applied Ethics. Lexington, Va.: Washington and Lee University, 1975, pp. 62–78.

Freeman, J. M. "To Treat or Not to Treat: Ethical Dilemmas of Treating the Infant with a Myelomeningocele." *Clinical Neurosurgery* 20 (1973): 134–146.

Gostin, Larry. "A Moment in Human Development: Legal Protection, Ethical Standards and Social Policy on the Selective Non-Treatment of Handicapped Neonates." *American Journal of Law & Medicine* 11(1) (1985): 31–78.

Gustafson, James M. "Mongolism, Parental Desires, and the Right to Life." *Perspectives in Biology and Medicine* 16 (1973): 529–557.

Gustaitis, Rasa and Ernle W. D. Young. *A Time to Be Born, A Time to Die: Conflicts and Ethics in an Intensive Care Nursery.* Reading, Mass.: Addison-Wesley, 1986.

Hemphill, M. et al. "Ethical Aspects of Care of the Newborn with Serious Neurological Disease." *Clinical Perinatology* 4 (March 1977): 201–209.

Hetmann, Philip B. and Sara Holtz. "The Severely Defective Newborn: The Dilemma and the Decision Process." *Public Policy* 23 (Fall 1975): 381–418.

Horan, Dennis, J. and Melinda Delaboyde, eds. *Infanticide and the Handicapped Newborn.* Provo, Utah: Brigham Young University Press, 1982.

Johnson, Paul R. "Selective Nontreatment and Spina Bifida: A Case Study in Ethical Theory and Application." *Bioethics Quarterly* 3 (Summer 1981): 91–111.

Jonsen, A. R. et al. "Critical Issues in Newborn Intensive Care: A Conference Report and Policy Proposal." *Pediatrics* 55 (1975): 756–768.

_____ and Michael J. Garland, eds. *Ethics of Newborn Intensive Care.* Berkeley: University of California, Institute of Governmental Studies, 1976.

Kelly, S. et al., eds. *Birth Defects.* New York: Academic Press, 1976.

Kelsey, Beverly. "Which Infants Shall Live?" *Hastings Center Report* 5 (April 1975): 5–7.

Kohl, Marvin, ed. *Infanticide and the Value of Life.* Buffalo, N.Y.: Prometheus Books, 1978. See in particular papers by Richard Brandt and R. S. Duff.

Lorber, John. "Selective Treatment of Myelomeningocele." *Pediatrics* 53 (1974): 307–308.

Lund, Nelson. "Infanticide, Physicians, and the Law: The 'Baby Doe' Amendments to the Child Abuse Prevention and Treatment Act." *American Journal of Law and Medicine* 11(1) (1985): 1–30.

Lyon, Jeff. *Playing God in the Nursery.* New York: W. W. Norton, 1985.

Magnet, Joseph E. and Eike-Henner W. Kluge. *Withholding Treatment from Defective Newborn Children.* Cowansville, Quebec: Brown Legal Publications, 1985.

McCormick, Richard A. "To Save or Let Die: The Dilemma of Modern Medicine." *Journal of the American Medical Association* 229 (1974): 172–176.

Paris, John J. and Anne B. Fletcher. "Infant Doe Regulations and the Absolute Requirement to Use Nourishment and Fluids for the Dying Infant." *Law, Medicine and Health Care* 11 (October 1983): 210–213.

Rhoden, Nancy K. "The New Neonatal Dilemma: Live Births from Late Abortions." *Georgetown Law Journal* 72 (June 1984): 1451–1509.

_____. "Treatment Dilemmas for Imperiled Newborns: Why Quality of Life Counts." *Southern California Law Review* 58(6) (September 1985): 1283–1347.

_____ and John D. Arras. "Withholding Treatment from Baby Doe: From Discrimination to Child Abuse." *Milbank Memorial Fund Quarterly/Health and Society* 63(1) (1985).

Shapiro, Robyn. "Medical Treatment of Defective Newborns: An Answer to the 'Baby Doe' Dilemma." *Harvard Journal on Legislation* 20 (1983): 137–152.

Shatten, Deborah A. and Robert S. Chabon. "Decision-Making and the Right to Refuse Lifesaving Treatment for Defective Newborns." *Journal of Legal Medicine* 3 (March 1982): 57–79.

Shelp, Earl E. *Born to Die? Deciding the Fate of Critically Ill Newborns.* New York: Free Press, 1986.

Sherlock, Richard. "Selective Non-Treatment of Defective Newborns: A Critique." *Ethics in Science and Medicine* 7 (1980): 111–117.

Singer, Peter et al. "The Treatment of Newborn Infants with Major Handicaps: A Survey of Obstetricians and Paediatricians in Victoria." *The Medical Journal of Australia* (17 September 1983): 274–278.

Smith, David H. "On Letting Some Babies Die." *Hastings Center Studies* 2 (1974): 37–46.

Smith, G. and E. D. Smith. "Selection for Treatment in Spina Bifida Cystica." *British Medical Journal* 27 (October 1973): 189–204.

Swinyard, Chester A., ed. *Decision Making and the Defective Newborn.* Springfield, Ill.: Charles C Thomas, 1978.

Veatch, Robert M. "The Technical Criteria Fallacy." *Hastings Center Report* 7 (August 1977): 15–16.

Waldman, A. M. "Medical Ethics and the Hopelessly Ill Child." *Journal of Pediatrics* 88 (1976): 890–892.

Weir, Robert. *Selective Nontreatment of Handicapped Newborns.* New York: Oxford University Press, 1984.

Chapter 3: Euthanasia

Annas, George J. "In re Quinlan: Legal Comfort for Doctors." *Hastings Center Report* 6 (1976): 29–31. A criticism of the grounds of the New Jersey Supreme Court decision.

Arras, John. "The Right to Die on the Slippery Slope." *Social Theory and Practice* 8 (Fall 1982): 285–328.

Battin, M. Pabst. *Ethical Issues in Suicide.* Englewood Cliffs, N.J.: Prentice-Hall, 1982.

Bayles, Michael D. "The Value of Life—By What Standard?" *American Journal of Nursing* 80 (December 1980): 2226–30.

Baylor Law Review 27 (Winter 1975). Entire issue on euthanasia.

Beauchamp, Tom L. "The Moral Justification for Withholding Heroic Procedures." In **Nora K. Bell, ed.** *Who Decides? Conflicts of Rights in Health Care.* Clifton, N.J.: Humana Press, 1982.

——— . "A Reply to Rachels on Active and Passive Euthanasia." In **Wade L. Robinson and Michael S. Pritchard, eds.** *Medical Responsibility.* Clifton, N.J.: Humana Press, 1979, pp. 182–195. See also Rachels below.

——— and S. Perlin, eds. *Ethical Issues in Death and Dying.* Englewood Cliffs, N.J.: Prentice-Hall, 1978.

Behnke, John A. and Sissela Bok. *The Dilemmas of Euthanasia.* New York: Doubleday Anchor, 1975.

Benjamin, Martin. "Moral Agency and Negative Acts in Medicine." In **Wade L. Robinson and Michael S. Pritchard, eds.** *Medical Responsibility.* Clifton, N.J.: Humana Press, 1979, pp. 170–181.

Black, Peter M. "Focusing on Some Ethical Problems Associated with Death and Dying." *Geriatrics* 31 (1976): 138–141.

——— . "Three Definitions of Death." *Monist* 60 (January 1977): 136–146.

Bok, Sissela. "Personal Directions for Care at the End of Life." *New England Journal of Medicine* 295 (12 August 1976): 367–369.

Cahill, L. S. "A 'Natural Law' Reconsideration of Euthanasia." *Linacre Quarterly* 44 (February 1977): 47–63.

Callahan, Daniel. "Feeding the Dying Elderly." *Generations: In-Depth Views of Issues in Aging* (Winter 1985): 15–17.

Cantor, Norman L. "A Patient's Decision to Decline Lifesaving Medical Treatment." *Rutgers Law Review* 26 (1973): 228.

Carmi, A., ed. *Euthanasia.* New York: Springer-Verlag, 1984.

Cassem, Ned. "When Illness Is Judged Irreversible: Imperative and Elective Treatments." *Man and Medicine* 5 (1980): 154–166.

Childress, James F. "To Live or Let Die." In his *Priorities in Biomedical Ethics.* Philadelphia: Westminster Press, 1981, pp. 34–50.

Cohen, Cynthia B. "Interdisciplinary Consultation on the Care of the Critically Ill and Dying: The Role of One Hospital Ethics Committee." *Critical Care Medicine* 10 (November 1982): 776–784.

Committee on Policy for DNR Decisions, Yale New Haven Hospital. "Report on Do Not Resuscitate Decisions." *Connecticut Medicine* 47 (August 1983): 477–483.

Devine, Philip E. *The Ethics of Homicide.* Ithaca, N.Y.: Cornell University Press, 1978.

Dimler, G. Richard, ed. *Thought* 47 (December 1982). Whole issue on "Issues of Life and Death."

Downing, A. B., ed. *Euthanasia and the Right to Die: The Case for Voluntary Euthanasia.* London: Peter Owen, 1969. See in particular the article by Anthony Flew.

Dyck, Arthur J. "Ethical Aspects of Care for the Dying Incompetent." *Journal of the American Geriatrics Society* 32 (September 1984): 661–664.

Eisendrath, Stuart J. and Albert R. Jonsen. "The Living Will: Help or Hindrance?" *Journal of the American Medical Association* 249 (15 April 1983): 2054–58.

Engelhardt, H. Tristram, Jr., and Michelle Malloy. "Suicide and Assisting Suicide: A Critique of Legal Sanctions." *Southwestern Law Journal* 36 (November 1982): 1003–37.

Evans, Andrew L. and Baruch A. Brody. "The Do-Not-Resuscitate Order in Teaching Hospitals." *Journal of the American Medical Association* 253 (19 April 1985): 2236–39.

Feinberg, Joel. "Voluntary Euthanasia and the Inalienable Right to Life." *Philosophy and Public Affairs* 7 (Winter 1978): 93–123.

Fitzgerald, P. J. "Acting and Refraining." *Analysis* 27 (1974): 133–139.

Fletcher, Joseph. "Elective Death." In E. F. Torrey, ed. *Ethical Issues in Medicine*. Boston: Little, Brown, 1968.

____. "Ethics and Euthanasia." In Robert H. Williams, ed. *To Live and to Die: When, Why, and How*. New York: Springer-Verlag, 1973, pp. 113–122.

____. "The 'Right' to Live and the 'Right' to Die." *The Humanist* 34 (1974): 12–15.

Fried, Charles. "Terminating Life Support: Out of the Closet." *New England Journal of Medicine* 295 (12 August 1976): 390–391.

Gillick, Muriel. "The Ethics of Cardiopulmonary Resuscitation: Another Look." *Ethics in Science and Medicine* 7 (1980): 161–169.

Gillon, Raanan. "Acts and Omissions, Killing and Letting Die." *British Medical Journal* 292 (January 1986): 126–127.

Goodrich, T. "The Morality of Killing." *Philosophy* 44 (1969): 127–129. Euthanasia and abortion.

Green, Michael B. and Daniel Wikler. "Brain Death and Personal Identity." *Philosophy and Public Affairs* 9 (Winter 1980): 105–133.

Grisez, Germain and Joseph M. Boyle, Jr. *Life and Death with Liberty and Justice: A Contribution to the Euthanasia Debate*. Notre Dame, Ind.: University of Notre Dame Press, 1979.

Hare, R. M. "Euthanasia: A Christian View." *Proceedings of the Center for Philosophic Exchange* 2 (1975): 43–52.

Hausman, David B. "On Abandoning Life Support: An Alternative Proposal." *Man and Medicine* 2 (Spring 1977): 169–177. Also see 178–188 for commentaries.

Horan, Dennis J. and Edward R. Grant. "The Legal Aspects of Withdrawing Nourishment." *Journal of Legal Medicine* 5(4) (1984): 595–632.

____ and David Mall, eds. *Death, Dying, and Euthanasia*. Washington, D.C.: University Publications of America, 1977.

Human Life Review 2 (Spring 1976): 27–70. Three articles on euthanasia.

Institute of Society, Ethics and the Life Sciences, Task Force on Death and Dying. "Refinements in Criteria for the Determination of Death." *Journal of the American Medical Association* 221 (3 July 1972): 48–53.

Jonsen, Albert R. "Dying Right in California: The Natural Death Act." *Clinical Research* 26 (February 1978): 55–60.

Kamisar, Yale. "Some Non-Religious Views against Proposed 'Mercy-Killing' Legislation." *Minnesota Law Review* 42 (1958): 969–1042.

Kelly, Gerald. "The Duty of Using Artificial Means of Preserving Life." *Theological Studies* 11 (1950): 203–220.

Kohl, Marvin, ed. *Beneficent Euthanasia*. Buffalo, N.Y.: Prometheus Books, 1975. Contains several interesting philosophical articles.

____. "Beneficent Euthanasia." *The Humanist* 34 (1974): 9–11.

____. "Understanding the Case for Beneficent Euthanasia." *Science, Medicine and Man* 1 (1973): 111–121.

____. "The Word 'Mercy' and the Problem of Euthanasia." *The American Rationalist* 9 (1965): 5–7.

Kuhse, Helga. "A Modern Myth. That Letting Die Is Not the Intentional Causation of Death: Some Reflections on the Trial and Acquittal of Dr. Leonard Arthur." *Journal of Applied Philosophy* 1 (1984): 21–38.

Ladd, John, ed. *Ethical Issues Relating to Life and Death*. New York: Oxford University Press, 1979.

Levin, Donald L. and Nancy R. Levin. "DNR: An Objectionable Form of Euthanasia." *University of Cincinnati Law Review* 49 (1980): 567–579.

Lombardi, Joseph L. "Killing and Letting Die: What Is the Moral Difference?" *New Scholasticism* 54 (1980): 200–212.

Long, P. H. "On the Quantity and Quality of Life: Fruitless Longevity." *Physician* 6 (1960): 69–70.

Maguire, Daniel C. "A Catholic View of Mercy Killing." *The Humanist* 34 (1974): 16–18.

——— . *Death by Choice.* New York: Doubleday, 1974.

Margolis, Joseph. "On Being Allowed to Die." *The Humanist* 36 (1976): 17–19.

McIntyre, R. V. "Voluntary Euthanasia: The Ultimate Perversion." *Medical Counterpoint* 2 (1970): 26–29.

Meilaender, Gilbert. "The Distinction between Killing and Allowing to Die." *Theological Studies* 37 (September 1976): 467–470.

Menzel, Paul T. "Are Killing and Letting Die Morally Different in Medical Contexts?" *Journal of Medicine and Philosophy* 4 (September 1979): 269–293.

Middleton, Carl L., Jr. "Principles of Life-Death Decision Making." *Linacre Quarterly* 42 (1975): 268–278.

Monagle, John F. "Living Will Does Not Resolve Medical-Ethical-Legal Dilemma." *Hospital Progress* 57 (1976): 76–79.

Moore, F. D. "Medical Responsibility for the Prolongation of Life." *Journal of the American Medical Association* 206 (1968): 384–386.

Morrison, Robert and Leon Kass. "Death—Process or Event?" *Science* 173 (20 August 1971): 694–702.

Neu, Steven and Carl M. Kjellstrand. "Stopping Long-Term Dialysis: An Empirical Study of Withdrawal of Life-Supporting Treatment." *New England Journal of Medicine* 314(1) (2 January 1986): 14–20.

Potter, Ralph B. "The Paradoxical Preservation of a Principle." *Villanova Law Review* 13 (1968): 874–892.

President's Commission for the Study of Ethical Problems in Medicine and Biomedical and Behavioral Research. *Deciding to Forego Life Sustaining Treatment.* Washington, D.C.: President's Commission, 1983.

Rachels, James. "Euthanasia." In **Tom Regan, ed.** *Matters of Life and Death.* New York: Random House, 1980, pp. 28–66.

——— . "Euthanasia, Killing, and Letting Die," in **Wade L. Robinson and Michael S. Pritchard, eds.** *Medical Responsibility.* Clifton, N.J.: Humana Press, 1979, pp. 153–169. See also Beauchamp.

——— . "Killing and Starving to Death." *Philosophy* 54 (1979): 159–171.

——— . *The End of Life: Euthanasia and Morality.* New York: Oxford University Press, 1986.

Ramsey, Paul. "The Two-Step Fantastic: The Continuing Case of Brother Fox." *Theological Studies* 42 (March 1981): 122–134.

Reichenbach, Bruce R. "Euthanasia and the Active-Passive Distinction." *Bioethics* 1 (January 1987): 51–73.

Rhodes, Jonathan E. "The Right to Die and the Chance to Live." *Journal of Medical Ethics* 6 (1980): 53–54.

Robertson, John A. and Norman Fost. "Passive Euthanasia of Defective Newborn Infants: Legal Considerations." *Journal of Pediatrics* 88 (May 1976): 883–889.

Russell, O. Ruth. *Freedom to Die: Moral and Legal Aspects of Euthanasia.* New York: Human Sciences Press, 1975 (also New York: Dell, 1976). Contains a clear review of objections.

Saunders, Cicely and Mary Baines. *Living with Dying: The Management of Terminal Disease.* New York: Oxford University Press, 1983.

Showalter, J. Stuart and Brian L. Andrew. *To Treat or Not to Treat: A Working Document for Making Critical Life Decisions.* St. Louis: Catholic Health Association, 1984.

Strong, Carson. "Euthanasia: Is the Concept Really Nonevaluative?" *Journal of Medicine and Philosophy* 5 (December 1980): 313–325.

Suber, Daniel G. and William J. Tabor. "Withholding of Life-Sustaining Treatment from the Terminally Ill, Incompetent Patient: Who Decides?" Parts I and II. *Journal of the American Medical Association* 248 (12 and 19 November 1982): 2250–51, 2431–32.

Suckiel, Ellen K. "Death and Benefit in the Permanently Unconscious Patient: A Justification of Euthanasia." *Journal of Medicine and Philosophy* 3 (March 1978): 38–52.

Sullivan, Thomas D. "Active and Passive Euthanasia: An Impertinent Distinction?" *Human Life Review* 3 (Summer 1977): 40–47.

Trammell, Richard L. "The Presumption Against Taking Life." *Journal of Medicine and Philosophy* 3 (March 1978): 53–67.

Vanderpool, H. Y. "The Ethics of Terminal Care." *Journal of the American Medical Association* 239 (27 February 1978): 850–852.

Veatch, Robert M. "An Ethical Framework for Terminal Care Decisions: A New Classification of Patients." *Journal of the American Geriatrics Society* 32 (September 1984): 665–669.

Walton, Douglas N. *Ethics of Withdrawing Life-Support Systems: Case Studies on Decision Making in Intensive Care.* Westport, Conn.: Greenwood Press, 1983.

_____ . "Omissions and Other Negative Actions." *Metamedicine* 1 (1980): 305–324.

_____ . *On Defining Death: An Analytic Study of the Concept of Death in Philosophy and Medical Ethics.* Montreal: McGill-Queen, 1979.

Weir, Robert F., ed. *Ethical Issues in Death and Dying.* New York: Columbia University Press, 1977.

Williams, Glanville. "Mercy-Killing Legislation—A Rejoinder." *Minnesota Law Review* 43 (1958): 1–12.

Williams, Peter C. "Rights and the Alleged Rights of Innocents to Be Killed." *Ethics* 87 (July 1977): 383–394.

Winslade, William J. and Judith Wilson Ross. *Choosing Life or Death: A Guide for Patients, Families, and Professionals.* New York: Free Press, 1986.

Wolstenholme, Gordon et al. "Euthanasia." *Proceedings of the Royal Society of Medicine* 63 (1970): 659–670.

Young, Robert. "Voluntary and Involuntary Euthanasia." *Monist* 59 (April 1976): 264–283.

Part II: Rights

Chapter 4: AIDS and Its Issues

AIDS: From the Beginning. Chicago: American Medical Association, 1986.

AIDS: Public Health and Civil Liberties. *The Hastings Center Report* 16 (December 1986): 1–36. Special supplement.

Altman, Dennis. *AIDS in the Mind of America.* Garden City, N.Y.: Doubleday, 1986.

American Council of Life Insurance. "White Paper: The Acquired Immunodeficiency Syndrome and HTLV-III Testing." *AIDS & Public Policy Journal* 2 (1987): 32–41.

Bayer, Ronald, C. Levine, and S. M. Wolf. "HIV Antibody Screening: An Ethical Framework for Evaluating Proposed Programs." In **P. O'Malley, ed.** *The AIDS Epidemic.* Boston: Beacon Press, 1989.

Black, David. *The Plague Years: A Chronicle of AIDS, the Epidemic of Our Times.* New York: Simon & Schuster, 1986.

Blaine, Jack H. "AIDS: Regulatory Issues for Life and Health Insurers." *AIDS & Public Policy Journal* 2 (1987): 2–10.

Cahill, Kevin M., ed. *The AIDS Epidemic.* New York: St. Martin's Press, 1983.

Childress, James F. "An Ethical Framework for Assessing Policies to Screen for Antibodies to HIV." *AIDS & Public Policy Journal* 2 (1987): 28–31.

Cooper, Ellen R. "AIDS in Children: An Overview of the Medical, Epidemiological, and Public Health Problems." In **P. O'Malley, ed.** *The AIDS Epidemic.* Boston: Beacon Press, 1989.

Dixon, John. *Catastrophic Rights: Experimental Drugs & AIDS.* Vancouver: New Star Books, 1990.

Fox, Daniel M. "The Cost of AIDS from Conjecture to Research." *AIDS & Public Policy Journal* 2 (1987): 25–27.

Gallagher, Thomas A., ed. "Twenty-third Annual Symposium: AIDS: At the Limits of the Law." *Villanova Law Review* 34(5) (September 1989).

Gostin, Lawrence O. "The AIDS Litigation Project: A National Review of Court and Human Rights Commission Decisions." *Journal of the American Medical Association* 263(14,15), Part 1 (11 April 1990): 1961–74; Part 2 (18 April 1990): 2086–93.

_____ , **ed.** *AIDS and the Health Care System.* New Haven, Conn.: Yale University Press, 1990.

_____ , **William J. Curran, and Mary E. Clark.** "The Case Against Compulsory Casefinding in Controlling AIDS—Testing, Screening, and Reporting." *American Journal of Law and Medicine* 12 (1987): 17–53.

Gray, Alec. "The AIDS Epidemic: A Prism Distorting Social and Legal Principles." In **P. O'Malley, ed.** *The AIDS Epidemic.* Boston: Beacon Press, 1989.

Grodin, Michael A., P. V. Kaminow, and R. Sassower. "Ethical Issues in AIDS Research." In **P. O'Malley, ed.** *The AIDS Epidemic.* Boston: Beacon Press, 1989.

Holder, Angela R. "Is This a Job for the IRB? The Case of the ELISA Assay." *IRB: A Review of Human Subjects Research* 7 (November/December 1985): 7–8.

Hummel, Robert F. "AIDS, Public Policy, and Insurance." *AIDS & Public Policy Journal* 2 (1987): 1.

——— **et al., eds.** *AIDS: Impact on Public Policy.* New York: Plenum Press, 1986.

Institute of Medicine of the National Academy of Science. *Mobilizing Against AIDS.* Cambridge, Mass.: Harvard University Press, 1986.

Iuculano, Russel P. "D.C. Act 6–170: The Five-Year Ban on Risk-Based Pricing for AIDS." *AIDS & Public Policy Journal* 2 (1987): 15–18.

Kulstad, Ruth, ed. *AIDS: Papers from* Science *1982–1985.* Washington, D.C.: American Association for the Advancement of Science, 1986.

Landesman, Sheldon H., Harold M. Ginzberg, and Stanley H. Weiss. "Special Report: The AIDS Epidemic." *New England Journal of Medicine* 312(8) (21 February 1985): 521–525.

Law, Medicine, and Health Care 15 (Summer 1987). Special issue on "AIDS: Law and Policy."

Levine, Carol and Ronald Bayer. "The Ethics of Screening for Early Intervention in HIV Disease." *American Journal of Public Health* 79(12) (December 1989): 1661–67.

Miller, David et al. "HTLV-III: Should Testing Ever Be Routine?" *British Medical Journal* 292 (5 April 1986): 941–943.

Mohr, Richard D. "AIDS: What to Do—And What Not to Do." *Report from the Center for Philosophy and Public Policy* 5 (1985): 6–9.

Nichols, Chris D. "AIDS—A New Reason to Regulate Homosexuality?" *Journal of Contemporary Law* 11 (1984): 315–343.

Oppenheimer, Gerald M. and Robert A. Padgug. "AIDS and Health Insurance: Social and Ethical Issues." *AIDS & Public Policy Journal* 2 (1987): 11–14.

——— . "AIDS: The Risk to Insurers, the Threat to Equity." *Hastings Center Report* 16 (October 1986): 18–22.

Pascal, Anthony et al. "State Policies and the Financing of Acquired Immunodeficiency Syndrome." *Health Care Financing Review* 11(1) (Fall 1989): 91–104.

Pierce, Christine and Donald VanDeVeer, eds. *AIDS: Ethics and Public Policy.* Belmont, Calif.: Wadsworth, 1988.

Scherzer, Mark. "AIDS and Insurance: The Case Against HIV Antibody Testing." *AIDS & Public Policy Journal* 2 (1987): 19–24.

Sieghart, Paul. *AIDS & Human Rights: A UK Perspective.* London: British Medical Association Foundation for AIDS, 1989.

"Special Section: AIDS—Responding to the Crisis." *Health Progress* (May 1986): 29–56.

Walters, LeRoy. "Ethical Issues in the Prevention and Treatment of HIV Infection and AIDS." *Science* 239 (5 February 1988): 597–603.

Winston, Morton and Sheldon H. Landesman. "AIDS and a Duty to Protect." *Hastings Center Report* 17 (February 1987): 22–23.

Chapter 5: Physicians, Patients, and Others

Annas, George J. "Confidentiality and the Duty to Warn." *Hastings Center Report* 6 (December 1976): 6–8.

——— **and Joan E. Densberger.** "Competence to Refuse Medical Treatment: Autonomy vs. Paternalism." *The University of Toledo Law Review* 15 (Winter 1984): 561–596.

Appelbaum, Paul S. et al. "Confidentiality: An Empirical Test of the Utilitarian Perspective." *Bulletin of the American Academy of Psychiatry Law* 12(2) (1984): 109–116.

——— . "Researchers' Access to Patient Records: An Analysis of the Ethical Problems." *Clinical Research* 32 (October 1984): 399–403.

Barber, Barry et al. "Some Problems of Confidentiality in Medical Computing." *Journal of Medical Ethics* 2 (June 1976): 71–73.

Bassford, H. A. "The Justification of Medical Paternalism." *Social Science and Medicine* 16(6) (1982): 731–739.

Basson, Marc, ed. *Rights and Responsibilities in Modern Medicine.* New York: Alan R. Liss, 1981.

Beauchamp, Tom L. and Lawrence B. McCullough. *Medical Ethics: The Moral Responsibilities of Physicians.* Englewood Cliffs, N.J.: Prentice-Hall, 1984.

Beigler, Jerome (American Psychiatric Association Committee on Confidentiality). "Statement of the American Psychiatric Association Before the Subcommittee on Government Information and Individual Rights." *New York State Journal of Medicine* 79 (December 1979): 2088–92.

Bell, Nora K., ed. *Who Decides? Conflicts of Rights in Health Care.* Clifton, N.J.: Humana Press, 1982.

British Medical Association. "New Horizons in Medical Ethics: Confidentiality." *British Medical Journal* (23 June 1973): 700–705.

Brody, Howard. "The Physician-Patient Contract: Legal and Ethical Aspects." *Journal of Legal Medicine* 4 (1976): 25–29.

Byrn, Robert M. "Compulsory Life-Saving Treatment for the Competent Adult." *Fordham Law Review* 44 (1975): 1–36.

Cantor, Norman L. "A Patient's Decision to Decline Life-Saving Medical Treatment: Bodily Integrity vs. the Preservation of Life." *Rutgers Law Review* 26 (1972): 228–264.

Childress, James F. *Who Should Decide? Paternalism in Health Care.* New York: Oxford University Press, 1982.

Coleman, Lee. *The Reign of Error.* Boston: Beacon Press, 1984.

"Compulsory Medical Treatment: The State's Interest Re-evaluated." *Minnesota Law Review* 51 (1966): 293–305.

"The Confidentiality of Health Records." *Psychiatric Opinion* 12 (January 1975). Entire issue on confidentiality and society.

Cousins, Norman. "A Layman Looks at Truth-Telling in Medicine." *Journal of the American Medical Association* 244 (24 October 1980): 1929–30.

Cranford, Ronald E. et al. "Institutional Ethics Committees: Issues of Confidentiality and Immunity." *Law, Medicine, and Health Care* 13 (April 1985): 52–60.

Curran, William J. "Ethical and Legal Problems in Medical Participation in Criminal Investigations." *New England Journal of Medicine* 249 (1976): 764–765.

_____ . "Protecting Confidentiality in Epidemiologic Investigations by the Centers for Disease Control." *New England Journal of Medicine* 314 (17 April 1986): 1027–28.

_____ et al. "Protection of Privacy and Confidentiality." *Science* 182 (1973): 797–802.

Davies, Edmund. "The Patient's Right to Know the Truth." *Proceedings of the Royal Society of Medicine* 66 (1973): 533–536.

Dougherty, Charles J. "The Right to Begin Life with Sound Body and Mind: Fetal Patients and Conflicts with Their Mothers." *University of Detroit Law Review* 63 (1 and 2) (Fall 1985): 89–117.

Eck, Marcel. *Lies and Truth.* New York: Macmillan, 1970.

Ellin, Joseph S. "Lying and Deception: The Solution to a Dilemma in Medical Ethics." *Westminster Institute Review* 1(2) (May 1981): 3–6.

Everstine, Louis et al. "Privacy and Confidentiality in Psychotherapy." *American Psychologist* 35 (September 1980): 828–840.

Ford, John C. "Refusal of Blood Transfusions by Jehovah's Witnesses." *Catholic Law* 10 (1964): 212–226.

Freedman, Alfred. "Threats to Confidentiality." *Journal of the American Academy of Psychoanalysis* 7 (January 1979): 1–5.

Fry, John. *A New Approach to Medicine: Principles and Priorities in Health Care.* Baltimore: University Park Press, 1978.

Gaylin, Willard and Daniel Callahan. "The Psychiatrist as Double Agent." *Hastings Center Report* 4 (February 1974): 11–14.

Gazza, B. A. "Compulsory Medical Treatment and Constitutional Guarantees: A Conflict?" *University of Pittsburgh Law Review* 33 (1972): 628–637.

Gewirth, Alan. "Human Rights and the Prevention of Cancer." *American Philosophical Quarterly* 17 (April 1980): 117–125.

Gibbs, R. F. "Money and Medical Ethics." *Journal of Legal Medicine* 4 (1976): 3–4.

Gilbert, Richard M. "Ethical Considerations in the Prevention of Smoking in Adults and Children." *Medicolegal News* 8 (June 1980): 4–7.

Gillon, Raanan. "Telling the Truth and Medical Ethics." *British Medical Journal* 291 (30 November 1985): 1556–57.

Gordis, Leon and Ellen Gold. "Privacy, Confidentiality, and the Use of Medical Records in Research." *Science* 207 (11 January 1980).

Grossman, M. "Confidentiality in Medical Practice." *Annual Review of Medicine* 28 (1977): 43–55.

Gurevitz, Howard. "Tarasoff: Protective Privilege Versus Public Peril." *American Journal of Psychiatry* 134 (March 1977): 289–292.

Havard, John. "Medical Confidence." *Journal of Medical Ethics* 11 (March 1985): 8–11.

Horn, Sheila E. "What's in a Name?" *Journal of Medical Humanities and Bioethics* 6 (Fall/Winter 1985): 99–108.

Journal of Medical Ethics 2 (1976): 28–33. "Limits of Confidentiality."

Kelman, Steven. "Regulation and Paternalism," *Public Policy* 29(2) (Spring 1981): 219–254.

Kelsey, Jennifer L. "Privacy and Confidentiality in Epidemiological Research Involving Patients." *IRB: A Review of Human Subjects Research* 3 (February 1981): 1–4.

Kleinig, John. *Paternalism.* Totowa, N.J.: Rowman and Allanheld, 1984.

Lasagna, Louis. "The Boston State Hospital Case (Rogers v. Okin): A Legal, Ethical and Medical Morass." *Perspectives in Biology and Medicine* 25 (Spring 1982): 382–403.

Litin, E. M. "Should the Cancer Patient Be Told?" *Postgraduate Medicine* 28 (November 1960): 470–475.

Lomasky, Loren E. and Michael Detlefsen. "Medical Paternalism Reconsidered." *Pacific Philosophical Quarterly* 62 (1981): 95–98.

Mahowald, Mary B. "Against Paternalism: A Developmental View." *Philosophy Research Archives* 6, no. 1386 (1980).

Marsh, Frank. "The 'Deeper Meaning' of Confidentiality within the Physician-Patient Relationship." *Ethics in Science and Medicine* 6 (1979): 131–136.

Merton, Vanessa. "Confidentiality and the 'Dangerous' Patient: Implications of Tarasoff for Psychiatrists and Lawyers." *Emory Law Journal* 31(2) (Spring 1982): 263–343.

Meyer, B. C. "Truth and the Physician." *Bulletin of the New York Academy of Medicine* 45 (January 1969): 59–71.

Nesbitt, Nancy A. "Tarasoff v. Regents of the University of California: Psychotherapist's Obligation of Confidentiality Versus the Duty to Warn." *Tulsa Law Journal* 12 (1977): 747–757.

Noll, John O. and Mark J. Hanlon. "Patient Privacy and Confidentiality at Mental Health Centers." *American Journal of Psychiatry* 133 (November 1976): 1286–89.

Oken, Donald. "What to Tell Cancer Patients." *Journal of the American Medical Association* 175 (1961): 1120–28.

Parness, Jeffrey A. "The Duty to Prevent Handicaps: Laws Promoting the Prevention of Handicaps to Newborns." *Western New England Law Review* 5(3) (Winter 1983): 431–464.

Pemberton, L. B. "Diagnosis: Can/Should We Tell the Truth?" *Bulletin of the American College of Surgeons* (May 1971): 7–13.

Perr, I. N. "Confidentiality and Consent in the Psychiatric Treatment of Minors." *Journal of Legal Medicine* 4 (1976): 9–13.

Phillips, William R. "Patients, Pills, and Professionals: The Ethics of Placebo Therapy." *The Pharos* 44 (Winter 1981): 21–25.

Public Responsibility in Medicine and Research. *Privacy and Confidentiality: Can They Be Protected?* Boston: PRIM & R, 1982.

Roth, L. H. et al. "Dangerousness, Confidentiality, and the Duty to Warn." *American Journal of Psychiatry* 134 (March 1977): 508–511.

Samuels, Alec. "The Duty of the Doctor to Respect the Confidence of the Patient." *Medicine, Science, and the Law* 20 (January 1980): 58–66.

Schöne-Seifert, Bettina and James F. Childress. "How Much Should the Patient Know and

Decide?" *CA-A Cancer Journal for Clinicians* 36 (March–April 1986): 85–94.

Sheldon, Mark. "Truth Telling Medicine." *Journal of the American Medical Association* 247 (5 February 1982): 651–654.

Sissons, P. L. "The Place of Medicine in the American Prison: Ethical Issues in the Treatment of Offenders." *Journal of Medical Ethics* 2 (1976): 173–179.

Standard, Samuel and Helmuth Nathan, eds. *Should the Patient Know the Truth?* New York: Springer, 1955.

Stein, Eugene J. "Doctors and Patients: Partners or Adversaries?" *Bioethics Quarterly* 2 (Summer 1980): 118–122.

Thomson, Judith J. "The Right to Privacy." *Philosophy and Public Affairs* 4 (1975): 295–314.

Van de Veer, Donald. "Autonomy Respecting Paternalism." *Social Theory Practice* 6 (Summer 1980): 187–208.

_____ . "The Contractual Argument for Withholding Medical Information." *Philosophy and Public Affairs* 9 (Winter 1980): 198–205.

_____ . "Paternalism and Subsequent Consent." *Canadian Journal of Philosophy* 9 (1979): 631–642.

_____ . *Paternalistic Intervention: The Moral Bounds of Benevolence.* Princeton, N.J.: Princeton University Press, 1986.

Wangenstein, O. H. "Should Patients Be Told They Have Cancer?" *Surgery* 27 (1950): 944–947.

Weir, Robert. "Truthtelling in Medicine." *Perspectives in Biology and Medicine* 24 (Autumn 1980): 95–112.

Wexler, David B. "Patients, Therapists, and Third Parties: The Victimological Virtues of Tarasoff." *International Journal of Law and Psychiatry* 2 (1979): 1–28.

Whyman, Fran Lochan. "Laissez Faire in the Medical Marketplace—Recognition of a Constitutional Right to Un-Conventional Medical Treatment: Andrews v. Ballard." *New England Law Review* 18(1) (1982–83): 149–181.

Zimmerman, David R. "An Ethical Dilemma: Patient Privacy vs. His Insurability." *Modern Medicine* 42 (1974): 18–24.

Chapter 6: Medical Experimentation and Informed Consent

AAP Task Force on Pediatric Research, Informed Consent and Medical Ethics. "AAP Code of Ethics for the Use of Fetuses and Fetal Material for Research." *Pediatrics* 56 (August 1975): 304–305.

Abrams, Natalie. "Justice in Fetal Experimentation." *Journal of Value Inquiry* 13 (1979): 103–113.

Annas, George J. *Informed Consent to Human Experimentation: The Subject's Dilemma.* Cambridge, Mass.: Ballinger, 1977.

_____ . "Report on the National Commission: Good as Gold." *Bioethics Quarterly* 2 (Summer 1980): 84–93. On the protection of human subjects.

_____ . *The Rights of Hospital Patients.* New York: Avon Books, 1975.

Barber, Bernard. "The Ethics of Experimentation with Human Subjects." *Scientific American* 234 (1976): 25–31.

_____ et al. *Research on Human Subjects: Problems of Social Control in Medical Experimentation.* New York: Russell Sage Foundation, 1973 (reprinted New Brunswick, N.J.: Transaction Books, 1979).

Bartholome, William G. "Parents, Children, and the Moral Benefits of Research." *Hastings Center Report* 6 (December 1976): 44–45.

Beauchamp, Tom L. and Ruth R. Faden. "Decision-Making and Informed Consent: A Study of the Impact of Disclosed Information." *Social Indicators Research* 7 (1980): 313–336. An empirical and normative study.

Beecher, H. K. "Ethics and Clinical Research." *New England Journal of Medicine* 274 (1966): 1354–60.

_____ . "Experimentation in Man." *Journal of the American Medical Association* 169 (1959): 461–478.

_____ . *Research and the Individual: Human Studies.* Boston: Little, Brown, 1970.

Bloomberg, Seth Allan and Leslie Wickins. "Ethics of Research Involving Human Subjects in Criminal Justice." *Crime and Delinquency* (October 1977): 435–444.

Bogomolny, Robert L., ed. *Human Experimentation.* Dallas: Southern Methodist University Press, 1976.

British Medical Association. "New Horizons in Medical Ethics: Research Investigation and the Fetus." *British Medical Journal* (26 May 1973): 464–468.

Capron, Alexander. "Informed Consent in Catastrophic Disease Research." *University of Pennsylvania Law Review* 123 (1974): 340–438.

Cooke, Robert E. "An Ethical and Procedural Basis for Research on Children." *Journal of Pediatrics* 90 (April 1977): 681–682.

Cowles, Jane. *Informed Consent.* New York: Coward, McCann and Geoghegan, 1976.

Curran, W. J. "The Tuskegee Syphilis Study." *New England Journal of Medicine* 289 (4 October 1973): 730–731.

Drane, James F. "Competence to Give Informed Consent: A Model for Making Clinical Assessments." *Journal of the American Medical Association* 252(7) (17 August 1984): 925–927.

Eisenberg, Leon. "The Social Imperatives of Medical Research." *Science* 198 (December 1977): 1105–10.

Experiments and Research with Humans: Values in Conflict. Washington, D.C.: National Academy of Sciences, 1975.

Faden, Ruth R., Carol Lewis, Catherine Becker, Alan I. Faden, and John Freeman. "Disclosure Standards and Informed Consent." *Journal of Health Politics, Policy and Law* 6 (Summer 1981): 255–284.

Federal Proceedings 36 (September 1977): 2344–64. Special section on drugs and human research.

Fletcher, John. "Human Experimentation: Ethics in the Consent Situation." *Law and Contemporary Problems* 32 (1967): 620–649. A good general review.

Forssman, Werner. *Experiments on Myself. Memoirs of a Surgeon in Germany.* New York: St. Martin's Press, 1974. An experimenter who used himself as a research subject for cardiac catheterization.

Freund, Paul A. "Ethical Problems in Human Experimentation." *New England Journal of Medicine* 273 (1965): 687–692.

——, ed. *Experimentation with Human Subjects.* New York: George Braziller, 1970. An influential collection of twenty articles.

Fried, Charles. *Medical Experimentation: Personal Integrity and Social Policy.* New York: American Elsevier, 1974.

—— **and Marc Lappé.** "Fetal Policies: The Debate on Experimenting with the Unborn." *Atlantic Monthly* 235 (May 1975): 66–71.

Furrow, Barry R. "Informed Consent: A Thorn in Medicine's Side? An Arrow in Law's Quiver?" *Law, Medicine & Health Care* 12(6) (December 1984): 268–273, 278.

Gardner, E. Clifton. "Ethical Issues in the Testing of New Drugs in Man." *Journal of Drug Issues* 7 (Summer 1977): 275–286.

Gaylin, Willard and Ruth Macklin, eds. *Who Speaks for the Child: The Problems of Proxy Consent.* New York: Plenum Press, 1982.

Goldiamond, Israel. "Protection of Human Subjects and Patients: A Social Contingency Analysis of Distinctions between Research and Practice and Its Implications." *Behaviorism* 4 (1976): 1–41.

Gorovitz, Samuel. "The Artificial Heart: Questions to Ask and Not to Ask." *Hastings Center Report* 14 (October 1984): 15–17.

Graham, John B. "Ethical and Social Issues Posed by Genetic Studies of Cardiovascular Disease." *Perspectives in Biology and Medicine* 20 (Winter 1977): 260–270.

Guttentag, O. E. "Ethical Problems in Human Experimentation." In **E. F. Torrey, ed.** *Ethical Issues in Medicine.* Boston: Little, Brown, 1968.

Halper, Thomas. "Ethics and Medical Experimentation: Some Unconfronted Problems." *Connecticut Medicine* 40 (1976): 267–268.

Hastings Center Report 5 (June 1975): 13–46. Special issue on fetal research.

Hatfield, Frank. "Prison Research: The View from Inside." *Hastings Center Report* 7 (February 1977): 11–12.

Heller, P. "Informed Consent and the Old-Fashioned Conscience of the Physician-Investigator." *Perspectives in Biology and Medicine* 20 (Spring 1977): 434–438.

Hilton, Bruce and Daniel Callahan, eds. *Ethical Issues in Human Genetics: Genetic Counseling and the Use of Genetic Knowledge.* New York: Plenum Press, 1976.

Hubbard, Ruth. " 'Fetal Rights' and the New Eugenics." *Science for the People* 16(2) (March/April 1984): 7–9, 27–29.

The Human Life Review 1 (Fall 1975). "A Symposium: Fetal Research."

Jones, James H. *Bad Blood: The Tuskegee Syphilis Experiment.* New York: Free Press, 1981.

Katz, Jay. *Experimentation with Human Beings.* New York: Russell Sage Foundation, 1972.

Kidd, Alexander M. "Limits of the Right of a Person to Consent to Experimentation on Himself." *Science* 117 (1953): 211–212.

Kushner, Thomasine Kimbrough and Raymond Belliotti. "Baby Fae: A Beastly Business." *Journal of Medical Ethics* 11 (December 1985): 178–183.

Ladimer, Irving, ed. "New Dimensions in Legal and Ethical Concepts for Human Research." *Annals of the New York Academy of Sciences* 169 (1970): 293–593.

____ **and R. W. Newman, eds.** *Clinical Investigation in Medicine: Legal, Ethical and Moral Aspects.* Boston: Boston University Press, 1963.

Laforet, Eugene G. "The Fiction of Informed Consent." *Journal of the American Medical Association* 235 (12 April 1976): 1579–85.

Langer, E. "Human Experimentation: New York Verdict Affirms Patients' Rights." *Science* 151 (1966): 663–666. On the Sloan-Kettering case.

Lebacqz, Karen and Robert Levine. "Respect for Persons and Informed Consent to Participate in Research." *Clinical Research* 25 (April 1977): 101–107.

Levine, Robert J. *Ethics and Regulation of Human Research.* 2d ed. Baltimore: Urban & Schwarzenberg, 1986.

Lewis, Melvin. "Comments on Some Ethical, Legal, and Clinical Issues Affecting Consent in Treatment, Organ Transplants, and Research in Children." *Journal of the American Academy of Child Psychiatry* 20 (1981): 581–596.

Lipsett, Mortimer B. "On the Nature and Ethics of Phase I Clinical Trials of Cancer Chemotherapies." *Journal of the American Medical Association* 248 (27 August 1982): 941–942.

Lower, Charles U. et al. "Nontherapeutic Research on Children: An Ethical Dilemma." *Journal of Pediatrics* 84 (April 1974): 468–473.

Ludlum, James E. *Informed Consent.* Chicago: American Hospital Association, 1978.

Luker, Kristin. *Abortion and the Politics of Motherhood.* Berkeley: University of California Press, 1984.

Macklin, Ruth. "Some Problems in Gaining Informed Consent from Psychiatric Patients." *Emory Law Journal* 31(2) (Spring 1982): 345–374.

____ . "Consent, Coercion, and Conflicts of Rights." *Perspectives in Biology and Medicine* 20 (Spring 1977): 360–371.

____ **and Susan Sherwin.** "Experimenting on Human Subjects: Philosophical Perspectives." *Case-Western Reserve Law Review* 25 (1975): 434–471. A good review of issues with respect to Mill, Kant, and Rawls. Part of a symposium on human experimentation.

Margolis, Joseph. "Conceptual Aspects of a Patient's Bill of Rights." *Journal of Value Inquiry* 11 (Summer 1977): 126–135.

Martin, Michael M. "Ethical Standards for Fetal Experimentation." *Fordham Law Review* 43 (1975): 548–570.

McCormick, Richard A. "Proxy Consent in the Experimentation Situation." *Perspectives in Biology and Medicine* 18 (Autumn 1974): 2–20.

____ . "A Reply to Paul Ramsey—Experimentation in Children: Sharing in Sociality." *Hastings Center Report* 6 (December 1976): 41–46.

McKinley, Sonja M., ed. "Experimental Evidence and Social Policy." *Milbank Memorial Fund Quarterly/Health and Society* (Summer 1981). Special issue.

Meisel, Alan. "Informed Consent—The Rebuttal." **And Mills, Don Harper.** "Informed Consent—The Rejoinder." *Journal of the American Medical Association* 234 (1975): 615–616.

____ **and Lisa Kabnick.** "Informed Consent to Medical Treatment: An Analysis of Recent Legislation." *University of Pittsburgh Law Review* 41 (Spring 1980): 407–564.

____ **and Loren H. Roth.** "Toward an Informed Discussion of Informed Consent: A Review and

Critique of the Empirical Studies." *Arizona Law Review* 25(2) 1983.

—— **and Loren H. Roth.** "What We Do and Do Not Know About Informed Consent." *Journal of the American Medical Association* 246 (27 November 1981): 2473–77.

Meyers, David W. *The Human Body and the Law.* Chicago: Aldine, 1970.

Miller, Leslie J. "Informed Consent: I, II, III, IV." *Journal of the American Medical Association* 244 (7 November 1980–12 December 1980): 2100–03, 2347–50, 2556–58, 2661–62.

Mills, D. H. "Whither Informed Consent?" *Journal of the American Medical Association* 229 (1974): 305–310.

Mistichelli, Judith. "Baby Fae: Ethical Issues Surrounding Cross-Species Organ Transplantation." *Scope Note #5.* Washington, D.C.: Kennedy Institute of Ethics, 1985.

Montange, C. H. "Informed Consent and the Dying Patient." *Yale Law Journal* 83 (1974): 1632–64.

Morrissey, James M., Adele D. Hofmann, and Jeffrey C. Thrope. *Consent and Confidentiality in the Health Care of Children and Adolescents: A Legal Guide.* New York: Free Press, 1986.

Murphy, Jeffrie G. "Therapy and the Problem of Autonomous Consent." *International Journal of Law and Psychiatry* 2 (1979): 415–430.

——. "Total Institution and the Possibility of Consent to Organic Therapies." *Human Rights* 5 (Fall 1975): 25–45.

Nicholson, Richard H., ed. *Medical Research with Children: Ethics, Law, and Practice.* Oxford: Oxford University Press, 1986.

Norton, Martin L. "When Does an Experimental/Innovative Procedure Become an Accepted Procedure?" *Pharos* 38 (October 1975): 161–165.

President's Commission for the Study of Ethical Problems in Medicine and Biomedical and Behavioral Research. *Implementing Human Research Regulations.* Washington, D.C.: President's Commission, 1983.

——. *Making Health Care Decisions: Empirical Studies of Informed Consent.* Volume Two: Appendices. Washington, D.C.: President's Commission, 1982.

——. *Making Health Care Decisions: The Ethical and Legal Implications of Informed Consent in the Patient-Practitioner Relationship.* Washington, D.C.: President's Commission, 1982.

——. *Protecting Human Subjects: First Biennial Report on the Adequacy and Uniformity of Federal Rules and Policies, and Their Implementation, for the Protection of Human Subjects in Biomedical and Behavioral Research.* Washington, D.C.: President's Commission, 1981.

Ramsey, Paul. "Children as Research Subjects—A Reply." *Hastings Center Report* 7 (April 1977): 40–41.

——. "A Reply to Richard McCormick—The Enforcement of Morals: Nontherapeutic Research on Children." *Hastings Center Report* 6 (August 1976): 21–30.

——. "The Enforcement of Morals: Nontherapeutic Research on Children." *Hastings Center Report* 6 (1975): 21–30.

——. "The Ethics of a Cottage Industry in an Age of Community and Research Medicine." *New England Journal of Medicine* 284 (1971): 700–706.

——. *The Ethics of Fetal Research.* New Haven, Conn.: Yale University Press, 1975.

Robinson, Wade L. and Michael S. Pritchard, eds. *Medical Responsibility: Paternalism, Informed Consent, and Euthanasia.* Clifton, N.J.: Humana Press, 1979. See in particular articles by Abrams, Browne, and Toulmin.

Schreiner, G. E. "The Ethics of Human Experimentation." *Pharos* 29 (1966): 78–83.

Schultz, Marjorie Maguire. "From Informed Consent to Patient Choice: A New Protected Interest." *Yale Law Journal* 95(2) (December 1985): 219–299.

Science **198** (18 November 1977): 677–705. "Medical Research: Statistics and Ethics."

Shaw, Margery W., ed. *After Barney Clark: Reflections on the Utah Artificial Heart Program.* Austin: University of Texas Press, 1984.

Smith, Richard. "Prison Doctors: Ethics, Invisibility, and Quality." *British Medical Journal* 288 (10 March 1984): 781–783.

Swazey, Judith P., Judith C. Watkins, and Renee Fox. "Assessing the Artificial Heart: The Clinical Moratorium Revisited." *International*

Journal of Technology Assessment in Health Care 2 (July 1986): 387–410.

Varley, A. B. "Protection of Human Research Subjects: Are Ethics Necessary?" *Journal of Legal Medicine* 4 (1976): 23–26.

Veatch, Robert M. "Human Experimentation: The Crucial Choices Ahead." *Prism* 2 (1974): 58 ff.

_____ . " 'Experimental' Pregnancy." *Hastings Center Report* 1 (1971): 2–3. About the Goldzieher experiment, in which placebos were used instead of contraceptive pills.

Visscher, Maurice B. *Ethical Constraints and Imperatives in Medical Research.* Springfield, Ill.: Charles C Thomas, 1975.

Walters, LeRoy. "Ethical Issues in Experimentation on the Human Fetus." *Journal of Religious Ethics* 2 (1974): 33–54.

_____ . "Some Ethical Issues in Research Involving Human Subjects." *Perspectives in Biology and Medicine* 20 (Winter 1977): 193–211.

Wecht, C. H. "Medical, Legal and Moral Considerations in Human Experiments Involving Minors and Incompetent Adults." *Journal of Legal Medicine* 4 (1976): 27–30.

Weisbard, Alan J. "Informed Consent: The Law's Uneasy Compromise with Ethical Theory." *Nebraska Law Review* 65(4) (1986): 749–767.

Welt, L. G. "Reflections on the Problems of Human Experimentation." *Connecticut Medicine* 25 (1961): 75–78.

White, L. P. "Biomedical Experimentation on Prisoners." *Western Journal of Medicine* 124 (1976): 514–516.

Willis, David P., ed. "The Problem of Personhood: Biomedical, Social, Legal, and Policy Views." *Milbank Memorial Fund Quarterly* 61(1) (Winter 1983).

Wolfenberger, W. "Ethical Issues in Research with Human Subjects." *Science* 155 (1967): 47–51.

Animal Experimentation

Bateson, Patrick. "When to Experiment on Animals." *New Scientist* 109 (February 1986): 30–32.

Cohen, Carl. "The Case for the Use of Animals in Research." *New England Journal of Medicine* 315 (1986): 865–870.

Fox, Michael Allen. *The Case for Animal Experimentation: An Evolutionary and Ethical Perspective.* Berkeley: University of California Press, 1986.

Frey, R. G. "Animal Parts, Human Wholes: On the Use of Animals as a Source of Organs for Human Transplants." In **James M. Humber and Robert F. Almeder, eds.** *Biomedical Ethics Reviews: 1987.* Clifton, N.J.: Humana Press, 1987, pp. 89–107.

Gallup, Gordon and Susan D. Suarez. "Alternatives to the Use of Animals in Psychological Research." *American Psychologist* 40 (October 1985): 1104–11.

Great Britain. *The Animals (Scientific Procedures) Act,* 1986.

Jamieson, Dale and Tom Regan. "On the Ethics of the Use of Animals in Science." In **Tom Regan and Donald VanDeVeer, eds.** *And Justice for All.* Totowa, N.J.: Rowman and Allanheld, 1982, pp. 169–196.

Kuhse, Helga. "Interests." *Journal of Medical Ethics* 11 (September 1985): 146–149.

Leader, Robert W. and Dennis Stark. "The Importance of Animals in Biomedical Research." *Perspectives in Biology and Medicine* 30(4) (Summer 1987): 470–485.

Paton, William. *Man & Mouse: Animals in Medical Research.* New York: Oxford University Press, 1984.

Rowan, Andrew N. *Of Mice, Models, and Men: A Critical Evaluation of Animal Research.* Albany, N.Y.: State University of New York Press, 1984.

Ryder, Richard. *Victims of Science: The Use of Animals in Research.* Rev. ed. London: Anti-Vivisection Society, 1983.

Singer, Peter. *Animal Liberation.* 2d ed. New York: New York Review (Random House), 1990.

_____ , ed. *In Defense of Animals.* New York: Blackwell, 1985.

Tannenbaum, Jerry and Andrew N. Rowan. "Rethinking the Morality of Animal Research." *Hastings Center Report* 15 (October 1985): 32–43.

Part III: Controls

Chapter 7: Genetics: Intervention, Control, and Research

The Ann Arbor Science for the People Editorial Collective. *Biology as a Social Weapon.* Minneapolis: Burgess, 1977.

Annas, George J. and Brian Cogne. "Fitness for the Birth and Reproduction: Legal Implications of Genetic Screening." *Family Law Quarterly* 9 (Fall 1975): 463–489.

Applebaum, Eleanor Gordon and Stephen K. Firestein. *A Genetic Counseling Casebook.* New York: Free Press, 1983.

Ausubel, F., J. Beckwith, and K. Janssen. "The Politics of Genetic Engineering: Who Decides Who's Defective." *Psychology Today* 7 (June 1974): 30–43. The authors are members of Science for the People.

Baker, Robert. "Protecting the Unconceived." In **John W. Davis, Barry Hoffmaster, and Sarah Shorten, eds.** *Contemporary Issues in Biomedical Ethics.* Clifton, N.J.: Humana Press, 1978, pp. 89–100.

Bass, I. Scott. "Governmental Control of Research in Positive Eugenics." *Journal of Law Reform* 8 (Spring 1974): 615–630.

Bayles, Michael D. *Reproductive Ethics.* Englewood Cliffs, N.J.: Prentice-Hall, 1984.

———. "Harm to the Unconceived." *Philosophy and Public Affairs* 5 (Spring 1976): 292–304.

Beckwith, Jon and Jonathan King. "The XYY Syndrome: A Dangerous Myth." *New Scientist* 14 (November 1974): 474–476.

Beers, Roland F., Jr., and Edward G. Bassett, eds. *Recombinant Molecules: Impact on Science and Society.* New York: Raven Press, 1977.

Berg, Paul et al. "Asilomar Conference on Recombinant DNA Molecules." *Science* 188 (1975): 991–994.

Breyer, Stephan and Richard Zeckhauser. "The Regulation of Genetic Engineering." *Man and Medicine* 1 (Winter 1976): 1–9.

Buckley, John J., Jr., ed. *Genetics Now: Ethical Issues in Genetic Research.* Washington, D.C.: University Press of America, 1978.

Capron, Alexander. *Genetic Counseling: Facts, Values and Norms.* New York: Alan R. Liss, 1979.

———. "Reflections on Issues Posed by Recombinant DNA Molecule Technology." *Annals of the American Academy of Sciences* 265 (1976): 71–81. Entire issue is devoted to genetic issues.

Carmen, Ira H. *Cloning and the Constitution: An Inquiry into Governmental Policymaking and Genetic Experimentation.* Madison: University of Wisconsin Press, 1986.

Culliton, Barbara. "Gene Therapy: Research in Public." *Science* 227 (February 1985): 493–496.

Curran, William J. "The Questionable Virtues of Genetic Screening Laws." *American Journal of Public Health* 64 (1974): 1003–04.

Daedalus **90** (1961). "Evolution and Man's Progress." See in particular the articles by Muller and Crow.

Danielli, James F. "Industry, Society, and Genetic Engineering." *Hastings Center Report* 2 (December 1972): 5–7.

Davidson, Michael D. "First Amendment Protection for Biomedical Research." *Arizona Law Review* 19 (1977): 893–918.

Davis, Bernard D. "Prospects for Genetic Intervention in Man." *Science* 170 (1970): 1279–83.

———. *Storm over Biology: Essays on Science, Sentiment, and Public Policy.* Buffalo, N.Y.: Prometheus Books, 1986.

Edwards, Robert G. "Fertilization of Human Eggs In Vitro: Morals, Ethics, and the Law." *Quarterly Review of Biology* 49 (March 1974): 3–26.

Ellison, Craig W., ed. *Modifying Man.* Washington, D.C.: University Press of America, 1978. A "Christian evangelical" view.

Esbjorson, Robert, ed. *The Manipulation of Life.* San Francisco: Harper & Row, 1984.

Etzioni, Amitai. "Amniocentesis: A Case Study of the Management of 'Genetic Engineering.' " *Ethics in Science and Medicine* 2 (May 1975): 13–24.

———. *Genetic Fix: The Next Technological Revolution.* New York: Harper & Row, 1975.

———. "Sex Control, Science and Society." *Science* 161 (1968): 1107–12.

Ferguson, James R. "Scientific Inquiry and the First Amendment." *Cornell Law Review* 64 (April 1979): 639–665.

Fletcher, John C. "Ethical Issues in and Beyond Prospective Clinical Trials of Human Gene Therapy." *Journal of Medicine and Philosophy* 10 (August 1985): 293–309.

____ . "Ethics and Trends in Applied Human Genetics." *Birth Defects* 19(5) (1983): 143–158.

____ . "Moral Problems and Ethical Issues in Prospective Human Gene Therapy." *Virginia Law Review* 69(3) (April 1983): 515–546.

____ . "Ethical Issues in Genetic Screening and Antenatal Diagnosis." *Clinical Obstetrics and Gynecology* 24 (December 1981): 1151–68.

____ . "Ethics and Amniocentesis for Fetal Sex Identification." *Hastings Center Report* 10 (1980): 15–17.

____ . "Moral and Ethical Problems of PreNatal Diagnosis." *Clinical Genetics* 8 (1975): 251–257.

Fletcher, Joseph. "Ethical Aspects of Genetic Controls." *New England Journal of Medicine* 285 (1971): 776–783.

Frankel, Charles. "The Specter of Eugenics." *Commentary* 57 (1974): 25–33.

Frankel, Mark S. "The Application of Genetic Technology: Ethics and Pitfalls." *Impact of Science on Society* 25 (1975): 85–90.

Friedman, Theodore. "The Future of Gene Therapy: A Reevaluation." *Annals of the American Academy of Sciences* 265 (1976): 141–152.

Fudenberg, H. Hugh and Vijaya Melnick, eds. *Biomedical Scientists and Public Policy.* New York: Plenum Press, 1978.

Gastel, Barbara. *Maternal Serum Alpha-Fetoprotein: Issues in the Prenatal Screening and Diagnosis of Neural Tube Defects.* Washington, D.C.: Government Printing Office, 1981.

Gaylin, Willard. "Genetic Screening: The Ethics of Knowing." *New England Journal of Medicine* 286 (22 June 1972): 1361–62.

Georgia Law Review II (Summer 1977): 785–878. "Recombinant DNA and Technology Assessment." Special issue.

Golding, Martin. "Obligations to Future Generations." *The Monist* 56 (January 1972); 85–99.

Goodfield, June. *Playing God: Genetic Engineering and the Manipulation of Life.* New York: Random House, 1977.

Green, Harold P. "The Boundaries of Scientific Freedom." *Newsletter on Science, Technology, and Human Values* 20 (June 1977): 17–21.

Grobstein, Clifford. *A Double Image of the Double Helix: The Recombinant-DNA Debate.* San Francisco: W. H. Freeman, 1979.

Harris, Maureen, ed. *Early Diagnosis of Human Genetic Defects: Scientific and Ethical Considerations.* Fogarty International Center Proceedings, no. 6, 1972.

Harzanyi, Zsolt and Richard Hutton. *Genetic Prophecy: Beyond the Double Helix.* New York: Rawson, Wade, 1981.

Hilton, Bruce et al., eds. *Ethical Issues in Human Genetics: Genetic Counseling and the Use of Genetic Knowledge.* New York: Plenum Press, 1973.

Hoffman, John C. *Ethical Confrontation in Counseling.* Chicago: University of Chicago Press, 1979.

Holton, Gerald, ed. "Limits of Scientific Inquiry." *Daedalus* 107 (Spring 1978): 1–234. Special issue.

Hull, R. T. "Philosophical Considerations in the Growing Potential for Human Genetic Control." *Annals of the American Academy of Sciences* 265 (1976): 118–126.

Humber, James M. and Robert F. Almeder, eds. *Biomedical Ethics and the Law.* New York: Plenum Press, 1976.

Ingle, D. J. "Ethics of Genetic Intervention." *Medical Opinion Review* 3 (1967): 54–61.

Institute of Society, Ethics and the Life Sciences: Research Group on Ethical, Social and Legal Issues in Genetic Counseling and Genetic Engineering. "Ethical and Social Issues in Screening for Genetic Disease." *New England Journal of Medicine* 286 (25 May 1972): 1129–32.

Jackson, David A. and Stephen P. Stich, eds. *The Recombinant DNA Debate.* Englewood Cliffs, N.J.: Prentice-Hall, 1979.

Kass, Leon. "Implications of Prenatal Diagnosis for the Human Right to Life." In **Bruce Hilton, et al., eds.** *Ethical Issues in Human Genetics.* New York: Plenum Press, 1973.

____ . "Making Babies: The New Biology and the 'Old' Morality." *Public Interest* 26 (1972): 18–56.

____ . "New Beginning in Life." In **Michael Hamilton, ed.** *The New Genetics and the Future*

Man. Grand Rapids, Mich.: Eerdmans, 1972, pp. 15–63. On in vitro fertilization.

Kelly, Patricia T. *Dealing with Dilemma: A Manual for Genetic Counselors*. New York: Springer-Verlag, 1977.

Kevles, Daniel J. *In the Name of Eugenics: Genetics and the Uses of Human Heredity*. New York: Knopf, 1985.

Klein, David. "Genetic Manipulations." *Impact of Science on Society* 23 (1973): 21–27.

Kolata, Gina B. "Prenatal Diagnosis of Neural Tube Defects." *Science* 209 (12 September 1980): 1216–18.

Kopelman, Loretta. "Genetic Screening in Newborns: Voluntary or Compulsory?" *Perspectives in Biology and Medicine* 22 (Autumn 1978): 83–89.

Lakoff, Sanford A. "Moral Responsibility and the 'Galilean Imperative.' " *Ethics* 91 (October 1980): 100–116.

Lappé, Marc. *Broken Code: The Exploitation of DNA*. San Francisco: Sierra Club Books, 1984.

——— et al. "Ethical and Social Issues in Screening for Genetic Disease." *New England Journal of Medicine* 286 (1972): 1129–32. Problems and guidelines in social programs.

——— . *Genetics Politics: The Limits of Biological Control*. New York: Simon & Schuster, 1979.

——— . "Moral Obligations and the Fallacies of Genetic Control." *Theological Studies* 33 (1972): 411–427.

——— and Robert S. Morrison, eds. "Ethical and Scientific Issues Posed by Human Uses of Molecular Genetics." *Annals of the New York Academy of Sciences* 265 (1976): 1–208.

——— and Peter Steinfels. "Choosing the Sex of Our Children." *Hastings Center Report* 4 (1974): 1–4.

Lederberg, Joshua. "DNA Splicing: Will Fear Rob Us of Its Benefits?" *Prism* 2 (November 1975): 33–37.

——— . "Experimental Genetics and Human Evolution." *American Naturalist* 100 (1966): 519–531.

——— . "Orthobiosis: The Perfection of Man." In **Nicholas Rescher, ed.** *The Place of Value in a World of Facts*. New York: Wiley, 1970.

Leiser, Burton M. "The New Genetics and Lives Not Worth Living." In **John J. Buckley, Jr., ed.** *Genetics Now: Ethical Issues in Genetic Research*. Washington, D.C.: University Press of America, 1982, pp. 41–58.

Lenzer, Gertrud. "Gender Ethics." *Hastings Center Report* 10 (1980): 18–19.

Leonard, C. O. et al. "Genetic Counseling: A Consumer's View." *New England Journal of Medicine* 287 (1972): 433–449. An empirical survey of consumer attitudes and information.

Lipkin, Mack, Jr., and P. T. Rowley, eds. *Genetic Responsibility: On Choosing Our Children's Genes*. New York: Plenum Press, 1974.

Ludmerer, Kenneth M. *Genetics and American Society*. Baltimore: Johns Hopkins University Press, 1972. A history of the eugenics movement.

Man and Medicine 2 (Winter 1977): 78–132. Special issue on recombinant DNA.

McCormick, Richard. "Genetic Medicine: Notes on the Moral Literature." *Theological Studies* 33 (September 1972): 531–532.

——— . "Genetic Technology and our Common Future." *America* 152(16) (27 April 1985): 337–342.

Mercola, Karen and Martin Cline. "The Potentials of Inserting New Genetic Information." *New England Journal of Medicine* 303 (27 November 1980): 1297–1300.

Milunsky, A. and G. J. Annas, eds. *Genetics and the Law*. New York: Plenum Press, 1976.

Muller, H. J. "The Guidance of Human Evolution." *Perspectives in Biology and Medicine* 3 (1959): 1–43.

——— . "What Genetic Course Will Man Steer?" In **J. F. Crow and J. V. Neel, eds.** *Proceedings of the Third International Congress of Human Genetics*. Baltimore: Johns Hopkins University Press, 1967.

National Academy of Sciences. *Genetic Screening: Programs, Principles, and Research*. Washington, D.C.: National Academy of Sciences, 1975.

——— . *Research with Recombinant DNA: An Academy Forum, 7–9 March 1977*. Washington, D.C.: National Academy of Sciences, 1977.

National Research Council, Committee for the Study of Inborn Errors of Metabolism. *Genetic*

Screening: Programs, Principles, and Research. Washington, D.C.: National Academy of Sciences, 1975.

Neville, Robert. "Gene Therapy and the Ethics of Genetic Therapeutics." *Annals of the New York Academy of Sciences* 265 (1976): 153–161.

Nichols, Eve K. *Human Gene Therapy.* Cambridge, Mass.: Harvard University Press, 1988.

Omenn, Gilbert. "Genetics and Epidemiology: Medical Interventions and Public Policy." *Social Biology* 26 (Summer 1979): 117–125.

Osborn, Frederick. "The Emergence of a Valid Eugenics." *American Scientist* 61 (1973): 425–429.

Panel on Bioethical Concerns, National Council of Churches of Christ/U.S.A. *Genetic Engineering: Social and Ethical Consequences.* New York: Pilgrim Press, 1984.

Powledge, Tabitha. "The New Ghetto Hustle." *Saturday Review of the Sciences* (February 1973): 38–47.

____ . "There's Another Side to Genetic Screening." *Prism* 3 (1976): 55–57.

____ and John Fletcher. "Guidelines for the Ethical, Social, and Legal Issues in Prenatal Diagnosis." *New England Journal of Medicine* 300 (January 1979): 168–172.

President's Commission for the Study of Ethical Problems in Medicine and Biomedical and Behavioral Research. *Screening and Counseling for Genetic Conditions: The Ethical, Social, and Legal Implications of Genetic Screening, Counseling, and Education Programs.* Washington, D.C.: President's Commission, 1983.

____ . *Splicing Life: The Social and Ethical Issues of Genetic Engineering with Human Beings.* Washington, D.C.: President's Commission, 1982.

Ramsey, Paul. *Fabricated Man: The Ethics of Genetic Control.* New Haven, Conn.: Yale University Press, 1970.

____ . "Genetic Engineering." *Bulletin of the Atomic Scientists* 29 (December 1972): 14–17.

Reed, Sheldon. *Counseling in Medical Genetics.* New York: Alan R. Liss, 1980.

Reilly, Philip. *Genetics, Law and Social Policy.* Cambridge, Mass.: Harvard University Press, 1977.

Richards, John, ed. *Recombinant DNA: Science, Ethics and Politics.* New York: Academic Press, 1978.

Robertson, John A. "Procreative Liberty and the Control of Conception, Pregnancy, and Childbirth." *Virginia Law Review* 69(3) (April 1983): 405–464.

____ . "The Right to Procreate and in Utero Fetal Therapy." *Journal of Legal Medicine* 3 (September 1982): 333–366.

Robitscher, Jonas. *Eugenic Sterilization.* Springfield, Ill.: Charles C Thomas, 1973.

Rogers, Michael. *Biohazard.* New York: Knopf, 1977.

Ruse, Michael. "Genetics and the Quality of Life." *Social Indicators Research* 7 (January 1980): 419–441.

Sinsheimer, Robert. "An Evolutionary Perspective for Genetic Engineering." *New Scientist* 73 (20 January 1977): 150–152.

____ . "Troubled Dawn for Genetic Engineering." *New Scientist* 68 (1975): 148–151. An excellent review of problems.

Sorenson, James R., Judith P. Swazey, and Norman A. Scotch. *Reproductive Pasts, Reproductive Futures: Genetic Counseling and Its Effectiveness.* New York: Alan R. Liss, 1982.

Southern California Law Review 51 (September 1978): 969–1573. "Biotechnology and the Law: Recombinant DNA and the Control of Scientific Research." Special issue.

Stetten, DeWitt. "Freedom of Enquiry." *Genetics* 81 (November 1975): 415–425.

Sylvester, Edward J. and Lynn C. Klotz. *The Gene Age: Genetic Engineering and the Next Industrial Revolution.* New York: Scribner's, 1983.

Thomas, Lewis. "The Hazards of Science." *New England Journal of Medicine* 296 (10 February 1977): 324–328.

Tormey, Judith F. "Ethical Considerations of Prenatal Genetic Diagnosis." *Clinical Obstetrics and Gynecology* 19 (1976): 957–963.

Tsuang, Ming T. and Randall VanderMey. *Genes and the Mind: Inheritance of Mental Illness.* New York: Oxford University Press, 1980.

Twiss, S. B., Jr. "Ethical Issues in Priority Setting for the Utilization of Genetic Technologies."

Annals of the New York Academy of Sciences 265 (1976): 22–45.

Ulrich, Lawrence P. "Reproductive Rights and Genetic Disease." In **James M. Humber, ed.** *Biomedical Ethics and the Law*. New York: Plenum Press, 1976, pp. 351–360.

Veatch, Robert M. "Ethical Issues in Genetics." In **Arthur G. Steinberg and Alexander G. Bearn, eds.** *Progress in Medical Genetics*, vol. X. New York: Grune and Stratton, 1974.

Wade, Nicholas. "Genetics: Conference Sets Strict Controls to Replace Moratorium." *Science* 187 (1975): 931–935.

_____ . *The Ultimate Experiment*. New York: Walker, 1977.

Walters, LeRoy. "Genetics, Reproductive Biology, and Bioethics." In **Marguerite Neumann, ed.** *The Tricentennial People: Human Applications of the New Genetics*. Ames: Iowa State University Press, 1978, pp. 66–80.

Watson, James D. "Moving toward Clonal Man: Is That What We Want?" *Atlantic Monthly* 227 (1971): 50–53.

Wautz, Jon R. and Carol R. Thigpen. "Genetic Screening and Counseling: The Legal and Ethical Issues." *Northwestern University Law Review* 68 (September–October 1973): 696–767.

Westoff, Charles F. and R. R. Rindfuss. "Sex Preselection in the U.S.: Some Implications." *Science* 184 (1974): 633–636.

Williamson, Bob. "Gene Therapy." *Nature* 298 (July 1982): 416–418.

Yoxen, Edward. *The Gene Business: Who Should Control Biotechnology?* New York: Oxford University Press, 1983.

Zimmerman, Burke K. *Biofuture Confronting the Genetic Era*. New York: Plenum Press, 1984.

Chapter 8: Reproductive Control: In Vitro Fertilization, Artificial Insemination and Surrogate Pregnancy

Amicus, 2 (February 1977): 33–47. "Society's Right to Sterilize: What Are the Limits?" A special issue.

Annas, George J. "The Baby Broker Boom." *Hastings Center Report* 16 (June 1986): 30–31.

_____ and Sherman Elias. "In Vitro Fertilization and Embryo Transfer: Medicolegal Aspects of a New Technique to Create a Family." *Family Law Quarterly* 17(2) (Summer 1983): 199–223.

Beck, William W., Jr. "A Critical Look at the Legal, Ethical, and Technical Aspects of Artificial Insemination." *Fertility and Sterility* 27 (January 1976): 1–8.

Bellotis, Raymond A. "Morality and In Vitro Fertilization." *Bioethics Quarterly* 2 (1980): 6–19.

Brahams, Diana. "Surrogacy, Adoption and Custody." *Lancet* 1 (4 April 1987): 817.

Burgdorf, Robert and Marcia Burgdorf. "The Wicked Witch Is Almost Dead: Buck vs. Bell and the Sterilization of Handicapped Persons." *Temple Law Quarterly* 50 (1977): 995–1034.

Burt, Robert and Monroe E. Price. "Sterilization, State Action and the Concept of Consent." *Law and Psychology Review* (Spring 1975): 57–78.

Callahan, Daniel et al. "In Vitro Fertilization: Four Commentaries." *Hastings Center Report* 8 (October 1978): 7–14.

Cohen, Barbara. "Surrogate Mothers: Whose Baby Is It?" *American Journal of Law & Medicine* 10(3) (Fall 1984): 243–285.

Cushan, Anna Marie, ed. *Adoption and A.I.D.: Access to Information?* Melbourne: Monash Centre for Human Bioethics, 1984.

Davis, Morris E. "Involuntary Sterilization: A History of Social Control." *Journal of Black Health* 1 (August–September 1974).

Deroulin, Judy. "In re Guardianship of Eberhardy: The Sterilization of the Mentally Retarded." *Wisconsin Law Review* 6 (1982): 1199–1227.

Donovan, Patricia. "Sterilization and the Poor: Two Views on the Need for Protection from Abuse." *Family Planning/Population Reporter* 5 (April 1976): 28–30.

Eaton, Thomas A. "Comparative Responses to Surrogate Motherhood." *Nebraska Law Review* 65(4) (1986): 686–727.

Edwards, Robert G. "Fertilization of Human Eggs in Vitro: Morals, Ethics, and the Law." *Quarterly Review of Biology* 49 (March 1974): 3–26.

_____ and D. J. Sharpe. "Social Values and Research in Human Embryology." *Nature* 231 (14 May 1971): 87–91.

Flynn, Eileen P. *Human Fertilization In Vitro: A Catholic Moral Perspective*. Lanham, Md.: University Press of America, 1984.

Frankel, Mark S. "Human Semen Banking: Social and Public Policy Issues." *Man and Medicine* 1 (Summer 1976): 289–309.

Hellegers, Andre and Richard A. McCormick. "Unanswered Questions on Test-Tube Life." *America* 139 (August 1978): 74–78.

Holder, A. R. "Voluntary Sterilization." *Journal of the American Medical Association* 225 (24 September 1973): 1743–44.

Horne, Herbert, Jr. "Artificial Insemination Donor: An Issue of Ethical and Moral Values." *New England Journal of Medicine* 293 (23 October 1975): 873–874.

Kass, Leon R. "Babies by Means of In Vitro Fertilization: Unethical Experiments on the Unborn?" *New England Journal of Medicine* 285 (18 November 1971): 1174–79.

_____ . "Making Babies: The New Biology and the Old Morality." *Public Interest* 26 (Winter 1972): 18–56.

Keane, Noel P. with Dennis L. Breo. *The Surrogate Mother*. New York: Everest House, 1981.

Law and Ethics of A.I.D. and Embryo Transfer. CIBA Foundation Symposium 17. New York: Associated Scientific Publishers, 1973.

Macklin, Ruth and William Gaylin, eds. *Mental Retardation and Sterilization: A Problem of Competency and Paternalism*. New York: Plenum Press, 1981.

Marsh, Frank H. and Donnie L. Self. "In Vitro Fertilization: Moving from Theory to Therapy." *Hastings Center Report* (10 January 1980): 5–6.

Marx, Jean L. "Embryology: Out of the Womb—Into the Test Tube" and "In Vitro Fertilization of Human Eggs: Bioethical and Legal Considerations." *Science* 182 (23 November 1973): 811–814.

McGarrah, Robert E., Jr., and Susan L. Peck. "Voluntary Female Sterilization." *Hastings Center Report* 4 (June 1974): 5–10.

Meyers, David. *The Human Body and the Law*. Chicago: Aldine, 1970.

Parker, Philip J. "Surrogate Motherhood, Psychiatric Screening and Informed Consent, Baby Selling, and Public Policy." *Bulletin of the American Academy of Psychiatry and the Law* 12(1) (1984): 21–39.

Peckins, David M. "Artificial Insemination and the Law." *Journal of Legal Medicine* (July–August 1976): 17–22.

Perrin, J. C. et al. "A Considered Approach to Sterilization of Mentally Retarded Youths." *American Journal of Diseases of Children* 130 (March 1976): 288–290.

Ramsey, Paul. "Shall We Reproduce?" *Journal of the American Medical Association* 220 (5 June 1972): 1346–50.

Reilly, Philip. "The Surgical Solution: The Writings of Activist Physicians in the Early Days of Eugenical Sterilization." *Perspectives in Biology and Medicine* 26 (Summer 1983): 637–653.

Robertson, John A. "Embryos, Families, and Procreative Liberty: The Legal Structure of the New Reproduction." *Southern California Law Review* 59 (July 1986): 939–1041.

Robitscher, Jonas, ed. *Eugenic Sterilization*. Springfield, Ill.: Charles C Thomas, 1973.

Rosoff, Jennie. "Sterilization: The Montgomery Case." *Hastings Center Report* 3 (September 1973): 6.

Rothman, Barbara Katz. *The Tentative Pregnancy: Prenatal Diagnosis and the Future of Motherhood*. New York: Viking Penguin, 1986.

Schima, Marilyn and Ira Lumbell, eds. *Advances in Voluntary Sterilization*. New York: Elsevier, 1974.

Shannon, Thomas A. *Surrogate Motherhood: The Ethics of Using Human Beings*. New York: Crossroad, 1989.

Singer, Peter and Deane Wells. *Making Babies: The New Science and Ethics of Conception*. New York: Scribner's, 1985.

Smith, George P., II. "Through a Test Tube Darkly: Artificial Insemination and the Law." *Michigan Law Review* 67 (1968): 127–150.

Snowden, R., G. D. Mitchell, and E. M. Snowden. *Artificial Reproduction: A Social Investigation*. Winchester, Mass.: Allen and Unwin, 1983.

Uniacke, Suzanne. "In Vitro Fertilization and the Right to Reproduce." *Bioethics* 1 (July 1987): 241–254.

U.S. Congress, Office of Technology Assessment. *Infertility: Medical and Social Choices.* Washington, D.C.: OTA [OTA-BA-358], May 1988.

Veatch, Robert M. "Sterilization: Its Socio-Cultural and Ethical Determinants." In **Marilyn E. Schima and Ira Lumbell, eds.** *Advances in Voluntary Sterilization.* New York: Elsevier, 1974, pp. 138–150.

Wadlington, Walter. "Artificial Insemination: The Dangers of a Poorly Kept Secret." *Northwestern University Law Review* 64 (January–February): 777–807.

Walters, LeRoy. "Human In Vitro Fertilization." *Hastings Center Report* 9 (August 1979): 23–43.

_____ , issue ed. "Genetics and Reproductive Engineering." *Journal of Medicine and Philosophy* 10 (August 1985).

Walters, William and Peter Singer, eds. *Test-Tube Babies.* New York: Oxford University Press, 1982.

Warnock, Mary. *A Question of Life: The Warnock Report on Human Fertility and Embryology.* New York: Blackwell, 1985.

Working Party Council for Science and Society. *Human Procreation: Ethical Aspects of the New Techniques.* Oxford: Oxford University Press, 1984.

Zaner, Richard M. "A Criticism of Moral Conservatism's View of In Vitro Fertilization and Embryo Transfer." *Perspectives in Biology and Medicine* 27(2) (Winter 1984): 201–212.

Part IV: Resources

Chapter 9: Acquiring and Allocating Scarce Medical Resources

Aaron, Henry J. and William B. Schwartz. *The Painful Prescription: Rationing Hospital Care.* Washington, D.C.: The Brookings Institution, 1984.

American Medical Association Judicial Council. "Ethical Guidelines for Organ Transplantation." *Journal of the American Medical Association* 25 (1968): 341–342.

Anscombe, G. E. M. "Who Is Wronged?" *Oxford Review* 5 (1967): 16–17. A general argument relating to distribution.

Beecher, Henry K. "Scarce Resources and Medical Advancement." In **Paul Freund, ed.** *Experimentation with Human Subjects.* New York: George Braziller, 1970.

Bermant, Gordon, Peter Brown, and Gerald Dworkin. "Of Morals, Markets, and Medicine." *Hastings Center Report* 5 (1975): 14–16.

Caplan, Arthur L. "Kidneys, Ethics, and Politics: Lessons of the ESRD Program." *Journal of Health Politics, Policy and Law* 6(3) (Fall 1981): 488–503.

Coward, Howard and Donald E. Larsen, eds. *Ethical Issues in the Allocation of Health Care Resources.* Calgary: University of Calgary, 1982.

Daniels, Norman. "Am I My Parents' Keeper?" *Midwest Studies in Philosophy* VII (1982): 517–540.

_____ . "Cost-Effectiveness and Patient Welfare." In **Marc Basson, ed.** *Rights and Responsibilities in Medicine.* New York: Alan R. Liss, 1981, pp. 159–170.

Dougherty, Charles J. "A Proposal for Ethical Organ Donation." *Health Affairs* 5(3) (Fall 1986): 105–110.

_____ . "The Right to Health Care: First Aid in the Emergency Room." *Public Law Forum* 4(1) (1984) 101–128.

Dukeminier, J., Jr., and D. Sanders. "Organ Transplantation: A Proposal for Routine Salvaging of Cadaver Organs." *New England Journal of Medicine* 279 (22 August 1968): 413–419.

Engelhardt, H. Tristram, Jr., "Shattuck Lecture: Allocating Scarce Medical Resources and the Availability of Organ Transplantation: Some Moral Presuppositions." *New England Journal of Medicine* 331(1) (5 July 1984): 66–71.

Evans, Roger W. "Health Care Technology and the Inevitability of Resource Allocation and Rationing Decisions." Parts I and II. *Journal of the American Medical Association* 249 (15 and 16) (15 and 22/29 April 1983): 2047–53, 2208–19.

Ezorsky, Gertrude. "How Many Lives Shall We Save?" *Metaphilosophy* 3 (1972): 156–162. Includes a criticism of Anscombe's "Who Is Wronged?"

Fellner, Carl H. "Altruism in Disrepute." *New England Journal of Medicine* 284 (1973): 589–592.

_____ . "Kidney Donors—The Myth of Informed Consent." *American Journal of Psychiatry* 126 (1970): 9.

_____ . "Organ Donation: For Whose Sake?" *Annals of Internal Medicine* (October 1973): 589–592.

Fox, R. C. and J. P. Swazey. *The Courage to Fail: A Social View of Organ Transplants and Dialysis.* Chicago: University of Chicago Press, 1974.

Gorovitz, Samuel. "Ethics and the Allocation of Medical Resources." *Medical Research Engineering* 5 (1966): 5–7.

Hanink, J. G. "On the Survival Lottery." *Philosophy* 51 (1976): 223–225. Criticism of John Harris's "The Survival Lottery."

Harris, John. "The Survival Lottery." *Philosophy* 50 (1975): 81–87. Argues that perfection of transplants would make it right to sacrifice a healthy person chosen by lottery to save lives of several people needing organs.

Harrison, Michael R. "Organ Procurement for Children: The Anencephalic Fetus as Donor." *Lancet* 2 (December 1986): 1383–86.

_____ and Gilbert Meilander. "The Anencephalic Newborn as Organ Donor." *Hastings Center Report* 16 (April 1986): 21–23.

Havighurst, Clark C. "The Ethics of Cost Control in Medical Care." *Soundings* 60 (Spring 1977): 22–39.

Hiatt, H. "On the Distribution of Resources." *New England Journal of Medicine* 293 (1975).

Kaplan, M. B. "The Case of the Artificial Heart Panel." *Hastings Center Report* 5 (1975): 41–48.

Katz, Jay and Alexander Morgan Capron. *Catastrophic Diseases: Who Decides What? A Psychological and Legal Analysis of the Problems Posed by Hemodialysis and Organ Transplantation.* New York: Russell Sage Foundation, 1975.

Kemna, Donald J. "Confidentiality of Organ Donor Registry Records Versus the Interest in Preserving Human Life: A Proposal." *Journal of Legal Medicine* 5(1) (1984): 117–145.

Kilner, John F. "A Moral Allocation of Scarce Lifesaving Medical Resources." *Journal of Religious Ethics* 9 (Fall 1981): 245–285.

Knutson, A. L. "Body Transplants and Ethical Values." *Social Science and Medicine* 2 (1968–1969): 393–414.

Leake, C. D. "Technical Triumph and Moral Muddle." In T. E. Sturzl, ed. *Experience in Renal Transplantation.* Philadelphia: Saunders, 1964.

Leenen, H. J. J. "The Selection of Patients in the Event of a Scarcity of Medical Facilities—An Unavoidable Dilemma." *International Journal of Medicine and Law* (1980): 161–180.

Levy, Norman B. "Renal Transplantation and the New Medical Era." *Advances in Psychosomatic Medicine* 15 (1986): 167–179.

Lyons, Catherine. *Organ Transplants: The Moral Issues.* Philadelphia: Westminister Press, 1970.

Mack, Eric. "Bad Samaritanism and the Causation of Harm." *Philosophy and Public Affairs* 9 (Spring 1980): 230–259.

Mechanic, David. *Future Issues in Health Care: Social Policy and the Rationing of Medical Sources.* New York: Free Press, 1979.

Miller, George W. *Moral and Ethical Implications of Human Organ Transplants.* Springfield, Ill.: Charles C Thomas, 1971.

Mooney, Gavin. "Cost-Benefit Analysis and Medical Ethics." *Journal of Medical Ethics* 6 (December 1980): 177–179.

Peters, David A. "Protecting Autonomy in Organ Procurement Procedures: Some Overlooked Issues." *Milbank Memorial Fund Quarterly* 64(2) (1986): 241–270.

Plant, Raymond. "Gifts, Exchanges and the Political Economy of Health Care." Part 1: "Should Blood Be Bought and Sold?" *Journal of Medical Ethics* 3 (December 1977): 166–173; and Part 2: "How Should Health Care Be Distributed?" (March 1978): 5–11.

Ramsey, Paul. "Choosing How to Choose: Patients and Sparse Medical Resources." In *The Patient as Person.* New Haven, Conn.: Yale University Press, 1980, chapter 7.

Rhoads, Steven E. "How Much Should We Spend to Save a Life?" *Public Interest* 51 (Spring 1978): 74–92.

"The Sale of Human Body Parts." *Michigan Law Review* 72 (1974): 1182–1264.

"Scarce Medical Resources." *Columbia Law Review* 69 (1969): 620–692.

Robertson, John A. "Extracorporeal Embryos and the Abortion Debate." *Journal of Contemporary Health Law and Policy* 2 (Spring 1986): 53–70.

_____ . "Supply and Distribution of Hearts for Transplantation: Legal, Ethical, and Policy Issues." *Circulation* 75 (January 1987): 77–87.

Schiffer, R. M. and Benjamin Freedman. "Case Studies in Bioethics: The Last Bed in the ICU." *Hastings Center Report* 7 (December 1977): 21–22.

Shapiro, M. H. "Who Merits Merit? Problems in Distributive Justice and Utility Posed by the New Biology." *California Law Review* 48 (1974): 318–370.

Simmons, Roberta G. et al. *Gift of Life: The Social and Psychological Impact of Organ Transplantation.* New York: Wiley, 1977.

Smith, Harmon L. "Distributive Justice and American Health Care." In **W. M. Finnin, Jr., ed.** *The Morality of Scarcity.* Baton Rouge: Louisiana State University Press, 1977, pp. 67–80.

Taurek, John M. "Should the Numbers Count?" *Philosophy and Public Affairs* 6 (Summer 1977): 293–316.

U.S. Department of Health and Human Services, Task Force on Organ Transplantation. *Report of the Task Force on Organ Transplantation: Issues and Recommendations.* Washington, D.C.: DHHS, 1986.

Westervelt, B., Jr. "The Selection Process Viewed from Within: A Reply to Childress." *Soundings* 53 (1970): 154–158.

Winslow, Gerald R. *Triage and Justice: The Ethics of Rationing Life-Saving Medical Resources.* Berkeley: University of California Press, 1982.

Youngner, Stuart J. et al. "Psychosocial and Ethical Implications of Organ Retrieval." *New England Journal of Medicine* 313(5) (1 August 1985): 321–324.

Chapter 10: The Claim to Health Care

Alford, Robert R. *Health Care Politics: Ideological Interest Group Barriers to Reform.* Chicago: University of Chicago Press, 1975.

Anderson, Gerald and Earl Steinberg. "To Buy or Not to Buy: Technology Acquisition Under Prospective Payment." *New England Journal of Medicine* 311(3) (19 July 1984): 182–185.

Angell, Marcia. "Special Communications: Cost-Containment and the Physician." *Journal of the American Medical Association* 254(9) (6 September 1985): 1203–07.

Arrow, Kenneth J. et al. "Government Decision Making and the Preciousness of Life." In **Lawrence R. Ranoredi, ed.** *Ethics of Health Care.* Washington D.C.: National Academy of Sciences, 1974, pp. 33–64.

Battin, Margaret P. "Age Rationing and the Just Distribution of Health Care: Is There a Duty to Die?" *Ethics* 97 (January 1987): 317–340.

Bayer, Ronald, Arthur Caplan, and Norman Daniels, eds. *In Search of Equity: Health Needs and the Health Care System.* New York: Plenum Press, 1983.

Bayles, Michael D. "National Health Insurance and Non-Covered Services." *Journal of Health Politics, Policy and Law* 2 (Fall 1977): 335–348.

Birnbaum, Morton. "The Right to Treatment." *American Bar Association Journal* 46 (1960): 499–505.

Black, M. M. and C. Riley. "Moral Issues and Priorities in Biomedical Engineering." *Science, Medicine and Man* 1 (1973): 67–74.

Blackstone, William T. "On Health Care as a Legal Right: Philosophical Justifications, Political Activity, and Adequate Health Care." *Georgia Law Review* 10 (Winter 1976): 391–418.

Blank, Robert. *Rationing Medicine.* New York: Columbia University Press, 1988.

Brown, Lawrence D. "The Scope and Limits of Equality as a Normative Guide to Federal Health Care Policy." *Public Policy* 26 (Fall 1978): 481–532.

Buxton, M. J. and R. R. West. "Cost-Benefit Analysis of Long-Term Hemodialysis for Chronic Renal Failure." *British Medical Journal* 17 (May 1975): 376–379. A caution about instituting similar programs for other diseases.

Cairl, R. E. et al. "National Health Insurance Policy in the United States: A Case of Non-Decision-Making." *International Journal of Health Services* 7 (1977): 167–178.

Califano, Joseph A., Jr. *America's Health Care Revolution: Who Lives? Who Dies? Who Pays?* New York: Random House, 1986.

Callahan, Daniel. "Adequate Health Care and an Aging Society: Are They Morally Compatible?" *Daedalus* (Winter 1986): 247–267.

_____ . *Setting Limits: Medical Goals in an Aging Society.* New York: Simon & Schuster, 1987.

_____ . "How Much Is Enough? A National Perspective." *Alabama Journal of Medical Sciences* 17 (January 1980): 76–80.

_____ and Bruce Jennings, eds. *Ethics, the Social Sciences, and Policy Analysis.* New York: Plenum Press, 1983.

Childress, James F. *Priorities in Biomedical Ethics.* Philadelphia: Westminster Press, 1981.

Churchill, Larry M. *Rationing Health Care in America: Perceptions and Principles of Justice.* Notre Dame, Ind.: University of Notre Dame Press, 1987.

Cleverly, W. "Cost Containment in the Health Care Industry." *Topics in Health Care Financing* 3 (Spring 1977): 1–17.

Crawshaw, Ralph et al. "Oregon Health Decisions: An Experiment with Informed Community Consent." *Journal of the American Medical Association* 254(22) (13 December 1985): 3213–16.

Curran, William J. "The Right to Health in National and International Law." *New England Journal of Medicine* 284 (1971): 1258.

Daniels, Norman. "A Reply to Some Stern Criticisms and a Remark on Health Care Rights." *Journal of Medicine and Philosophy* 8 (November 1983): 363–371.

_____ . "Equity of Access to Health Care: Some Conceptual and Ethical Issues." *Milbank Memorial Fund Quarterly: Health and Society* 60(1) (1982): 51–81.

_____ . *Just Health Care.* New York: Cambridge University Press, 1985.

de Kervasdoué, Jean, John R. Kimberly, and Victor G. Rodwin, eds. *The End of an Illusion: The Future of Health Policy in Western Industrialized Nations.* Berkeley: University of California Press, 1984.

Devries, Andre. "Health Care Responsibility." *Metamedicine* 1 (Fall 1980): 95–106.

Dougherty, Charles J. "The Right to Health Care: First Aid in the Emergency Room." *Public Law Forum* 4(1) (1984): 101–128.

"Due Process in the Allocation of Scarce Lifesaving Medical Resources." *Yale Law Journal* 84 (1975): 1734–49.

Edwards, Marvin Henry. *Hazardous to Your Health: A New Look at the "Health Care Crisis" in America.* New York: Arlington House, 1972.

Ehrenreich, Barbara and John Ehrenreich. *The American Health Empire: Power, Profits and Politics.* New York: Random House, 1970.

Falk, I. S. "Proposals for National Health Insurance in the USA: Origins and Evolution, and Some Perceptions for the Future." *Milbank Memorial Fund Quarterly: Health and Society* (Spring 1977): 161–191.

Fein, Rashi. "On Achieving Access and Equity in Health Care." *Milbank Memorial Fund Quarterly* 50 (1972): 157–190.

Feldstein, Paul J. "National Health Insurance: An Approach to the Redistribution of Medical Care." In *Health Care Economics.* New York: Wiley, 1979, chapter 19.

Freedman, Benjamin. "The Case for Medical Care: Inefficient or Not." *Hastings Center Report* 7 (April 1977): 31–39.

Fried, Charles. "Rights and Health Care—Beyond Equity and Efficiency." *New England Journal of Medicine* 293 (31 July 1975): 241–245.

Fromer, Margot Joan. *Ethical Issues in Health Care.* St. Louis: Mosby, 1981.

Fuchs, Victor. *Who Shall Live?* New York: Basic Books, 1974.

Garfield, Sidney. "The Delivery of Medical Care." *Scientific American* 222 (1970): 15–23.

Ginzberg, Eli. *The Limits of Health Reform: The Search for Realism.* New York: Basic Books, 1977.

_____ and Miriam Ostow. *Men, Money and Medicine.* New York: Columbia University Press, 1969.

Greenberg, Selig. *The Quality of Mercy.* New York: Atheneum, 1971.

Gutmann, Amy and Dennis Thompson, eds. *Ethics and Politics: Cases and Comments.* Chicago: Nelson-Hall, 1984.

Halberstam, Michael. "Liberal Thought, Radical Theory and Medical Practice." *New England Journal of Medicine* 284 (1971): 1180–85.

Hiatt, Howard H. *America's Health in the Balance: Choice or Chance?* New York: Harper and Row, 1987.

_____ . "Protecting the Medical Commons: Who Is Responsible?" *New England Journal of Medicine* 293 (31 July 1975): 235–241.

Hodgson, Godfrey. "The Politics of American Health Care." *Atlantic* (October 1973): 45–61.

Iglehart, John K., ed. "Special Issue: HMOs." *Health Affairs* 5(1) (Spring 1986).

Illich, Ivan. *Medical Nemesis.* New York: Pantheon, 1976.

Jennings, Bruce, Daniel Callahan, and Arthur Caplan. "Ethical Challenges of Chronic Illness." *Hastings Center Report* 18 (March 1988). Special supplement, 1–16.

Journal of Medicine and Philosophy 4 (1979). Special issue on the right to health care.

Journal of Medicine and Philosophy 13 (1988). Special issue on "Justice Between Generations and Health Care for the Elderly."

Kass, Leon R. "Reading the End of Medicine and the Pursuit of Health." *The Public Interest* 40 (1975): 11–42.

Kelman, Steven. "Cost-Benefit Analysis: An Ethical Critique." *Regulation* 5 (January/February 1981): 33–40.

Knowles, John H., ed. *Doing Better and Feeling Worse: Health Care in the United States.* New York: W. W. Norton, 1977.

Krizay, John and Andrew Wilson. *The Patient as Consumer: Health Care Financing in the United States.* Lexington, Mass.: D. C. Heath, 1974.

Lesser, Paul B. "A Right to Health?" *Forum on Medicine* 3 (October 1980): 667–669.

Lewis, Charles E. et al. *A Right to Health—The Problem of Access to Medical Care.* New York: Wiley, 1976.

Lomasky, Loren E. "Medical Progress and National Health Care." *Philosophy and Public Affairs* 10 (Winter 1981): 65–88.

MacLeon, Gordon and Jeffrey A. Prussin. "Continuing Evolution and Health Maintenance Organizations." *New England Journal of Medicine* 288 (1973): 439–443.

McCreadie, Claudine. "Rawlsian Justice and Financing of the National Health Service." *Journal of Social Policy* 5 (April 1976): 113–130.

Mechanic, David. "Approaches to Controlling the Costs of Medical Care: Short-Range Alternatives." *New England Journal of Medicine* 298 (2 February 1978): 249–254.

————. *From Advocacy to Allocation: The Evolving American Health Care System.* New York: Free Press, 1986.

————. *The Growth of Bureaucratic Medicine: An Inquiry into the Dynamics of Patient Behavior and the Organization of Medical Care.* New York: Wiley, 1976.

————. "Rationing Health Care: Public Policy and the Medical Marketplace." *Hastings Center Report* 6 (1976): 34–37.

Mistichelli, Judith. "Diagnosis Related Groups (DRGs) and the Prospective Payment System: Forecasting Social Implications." *Scope Note* 4 (June 1984).

Morison, Robert S. "Rights and Responsibilities: Redressing the Uneasy Balance." *Hastings Center Report* 4 (1974): 1–4.

Moskop, John C. "Rawlsian Justice and a Human Right to Health Care." *Journal of Medicine and Philosophy* 8 (November 1983): 329–338.

Navarro, Vicente. "Justice, Social Policy, and the Public's Health." *Medical Care* 15 (May 1977): 363–370.

New England Journal of Medicine 293 (31 July 1975). A large part of this issue is devoted to health-care delivery. See, in particular, the articles by Hiatt and Fried.

Northwestern University Law Review 70 (1975). "Current Problems in Health Care: A Symposium."

Omenn, Gilbert S. and Douglas A. Conrad. "Implications of DRGs for Clinicians." *New England Journal of Medicine* 311 (15 November 1984): 1314–17.

Outka, Gene. "Social Justice and Equal Access to Health Care." *Journal of Religious Ethics* 2 (1974): 11–32.

Pellegrino, Edmund D. "Rationing Health Care: The Ethics of Medical Gatekeeping." *Journal of Contemporary Health Law and Policy* 2 (Spring 1986): 23–45.

Pilpel, Harriet F. "Minors' Rights to Medical Care." *Albany Law Review* 36 (1972): 462–487.

President's Commission for the Study of Ethical Problems in Medicine and Biomedical and Behavioral Research. *Securing Access to Health Care: The Differences in the Availability of Health Services.* Washington, D.C.: President's Commission, 1982.

Raffel, Marshall W., ed. *Comparative Health Systems: Descriptive Analyses of Fourteen National Health Systems.* University Park: Pennsylvania State University Press, 1984.

Review of Radical Political Economics 9 (Spring 1977). A special issue entitled "The Political Economy of Health."

Sade, R. "Concepts of Rights: Philosophy and Application to Health Care." *Linacre Quarterly* 46 (November 1979): 330–344.

Schlesinger, Mark. "On the Limits of Expanding Health Care Reform: Chronic Care in Prepaid Settings." *Milbank Memorial Fund Quarterly* 64(2) (1986): 189–215.

Schwartz, William B. "Policy Analysis, Politics and the Problems of Health Care." *New England Journal of Medicine* 286 (1972): 1057–58.

Seham, Max. *Blacks and American Medical Care.* Minneapolis: University of Minnesota Press, 1973.

Sheldon, Mark. "Ethical Issues in the Cost-Containment of Modern Medicine." *Urban Health* 13(8) (September 1984): 25, 48.

Shelp, Earl, ed. *Justice and Health Care.* Boston: D. Reidel, 1981.

Slaby, Andrew E. and Laurance R. Tancredi. "The Economics of Moral Values: Policy Implications." *Journal of Health Politics, Policy, and Law* 2 (Spring 1977): 20–31.

Soble, Alan. "On Health Care as a Right: More on the Right to Health Care." *Georgia Law Review* 10 (Winter 1976): 525–544.

Sparer, Edward V. "The Legal Right to Health Care: Public Policy and Equal Access." *Hastings Center Report* 6 (October 1976): 39–47.

Steiner, Hillel. "The Just Provision of Health Care: A Reply to Elizabeth Telfer." *Journal of Medical Ethics* 2 (December 1976): 185–189.

Stevens, Rosemary. *American Medicine and the Public Interest.* New Haven, Conn.: Yale University Press, 1971.

Tancredi, Laurence, ed. *Ethics of Health Care.* Washington, D.C.: National Academy of Sciences, 1975.

Taylor, Vincent. "How Much Is Good Health Worth?" *Policy Sciences* 1 (1970): 49–72.

Telfer, Elizabeth. "Justice, Welfare and Health Care." *Journal of Medical Ethics* 2 (September 1976): 107–111.

Veatch, R. M. and Roy Branson, eds. *Ethics and Health Policy.* Cambridge, Mass.: Ballinger, 1976.

Weaver, Jerry L. *National Health Policy and the Underserved: Ethnic Minorities, Women, and the Elderly.* St. Louis: Mosby, 1976.

Yaggy, Duncan and William G. Anlyan, eds. *Financing Health Care: Competition Versus Regulation.* Cambridge, Mass.: Ballinger, 1982.

Ziegenfuss, James T., Jr. *Law, Medicine and Health Care: A Bibliography.* New York: Facts on File, 1984.